BLUEPRINTS
OBSTETRICS & GYNECOLOGY

Sixth Edition

BLUEPRINTS
OBSTETRICS & GYNECOLOGY

Sixth Edition

Tamara Callahan, MD, MPP
Assistant Professor
Department of Obstetrics and Gynecology
Division of Gynecologic Specialties
Vanderbilt University Medical Center
Nashville, Tennessee

Aaron B. Caughey, MD, MPP, MPH, PhD
Professor and Chair
Department of Obstetrics and Gynecology
Oregon Health and Science University
Portland, Oregon

Wolters Kluwer | Lippincott Williams & Wilkins
Health
Philadelphia • Baltimore • New York • London
Buenos Aires • Hong Kong • Sydney • Tokyo

Acquisitions Editor: Susan Rhyner
Product Manager: Jennifer Verbiar
Marketing Manager: Joy Fisher-Williams
Vendor Manager: Bridgett Dougherty
Manufacturing Coordinator: Margie Orzech
Design Coordinator: Terry Mallon
Production Services: S4Carlisle Publishing Services

351 West Camden Street
Baltimore, MD 21201

Two Commerce Square
2001 Market Street
Philadelphia, PA 19103

Printed in China

Library of Congress Cataloging-in-Publication Data

Callahan, Tamara L.
Blueprints obstetrics & gynecology / Tamara L. Callahan, Aaron B. Caughey. — 6th ed.
p. ; cm.
Obstetrics & gynecology
Blueprints obstetrics and gynecology
Includes bibliographical references and index.
ISBN 978-1-4511-1702-8 (alk. paper)
I. Caughey, Aaron B. II. Title. III. Title: Obstetrics & gynecology. IV. Title: Blueprints obstetrics and gynecology.
[DNLM: 1. Pregnancy Complications--Examination Questions. 2. Genital Diseases, Female--Examination Questions. WQ 18.2]

618.0076--dc23

2012028782

To purchase additional copies of this book, call our customer service department at (800) 638-3030 or fax orders to (301) 223-2320. International customers should call (301) 223-2300.

Visit Lippincott Williams & Wilkins on the Internet: http://www.lww.com. Lippincott Williams & Wilkins customer service representatives are available from 8:30 am to 6:00 pm, EST.

RRS1211

Contents

Contributors

Jeff Andrews, MD, FRCSC
Associate Professor
Department of Obstetrics and Gynecology
Division of General Obstetrics and Gynecology
Vanderbilt University School of Medicine
Nashville, Tennessee

Suzanne Barakat
Medical student
University of North Carolina
Chapel Hill, North Carolina

Alison Barlow, WHNP
Assistant Professor
Department of Obstetrics and Gynecology
Division of Midwifery and Advanced Practice Nursing
Vanderbilt University School of Medicine
Nashville, Tennessee

Lisa Bayer, MD
Fellow, Family Planning
Oregon Health & Science University
Portland, Oregon

Daniel H. Biller, MD
Assistant Professor
Department of Obstetrics and Gynecology
Division of Female Pelvic Medicine and Reconstructive Surgery
Vanderbilt University School of Medicine
Nashville, Tennessee

Yvonne W. Cheng, MD, PhD
Assistant Professor
University of California, San Francisco
San Francisco, California

Howard Curlin, MD
Department of Obstetrics and Gynecology
Madigan Army Medical Center
Tacoma, Washington

Amy Doss, MD
Fellow, Maternal-Fetal Medicine
Oregon Health & Science University
Portland, Oregon

Sharon Engel, MD
Resident, Obstetrics and Gynecology
Oregon Health & Science University
Portland, Oregon

Abby Furukawa, MD
Resident, Obstetrics and Gynecology
Oregon Health & Science University
Portland, Oregon

Karen Gold, MD, MSCI
Assistant Professor
Director of Resident Education
Department of Obstetrics and Gynecology
Division of Female Pelvic Medicine and Reconstructive Surgery
University of Oklahoma - Tulsa
Tulsa, Oklahoma

Meghana Gowda, MD
Clinical Instructor
Department of Obstetrics and Gynecology
Division of Female Pelvic Medicine and Reconstructive Surgery
Vanderbilt University School of Medicine
Nashville, Tennessee

William J. Kellett, DO
Assistant Professor
Department of Obstetrics and Gynecology
Division of General Obstetrics and Gynecology
Vanderbilt University School of Medicine
Nashville, Tennessee

Tamara Keown, MSN, WHNP-BC
Assistant Professor
Department of Obstetrics and Gynecology
Division of Midwifery and Advanced Practice Nursing
Vanderbilt University School of Medicine
Nashville, Tennessee

Dineo Khabele, MD, FACOG, FACS
Assistant Professor
Department of Obstetrics and Gynecology
Division of Gynecologic Oncology
Vanderbilt University School of Medicine
Nashville, Tennessee

John Lucas, MD
Assistant Professor
Department of Obstetrics and Gynecology
Division of Reproductive Endocrinology and Infertility
Vanderbilt University School of Medicine
Nashville, Tennessee

Lucy Koroma, MSN, WHNP-BC
Department of Obstetrics and Gynecology
Divisions of Reproductive Endocrinology and Gynecology
Vanderbilt University School of Medicine
Nashville, Tennessee

Erica Marsh, MD
Assistant Professor
Department of Obstetrics and Gynecology
Divisions of Reproductive Endocrinology and Infertility and Reproductive Biology Research
Feinberg School of Medicine - Northwestern University
Evanston, Illinois

John Mission, MD
Resident
Obstetrics and Gynecology
Oregon Health and Science University
Portland, Oregon

Melinda New, MD
Assistant Professor
Director of Resident Education
Department of Obstetrics and Gynecology
Division of Gynecology
Vanderbilt University School of Medicine
Nashville, Tennessee

Brian Nguyen, MD
Resident, Obstetrics and Gynecology
Oregon Health & Science University
Portland, Oregon

Rachel Pilliod, MD
Resident, Obstetrics and Gynecology
Brigham & Women's Hospital
Boston, Massachusetts

Stacey Scheib, MD
Assistant Professor
Department of Gynecology and Obstetrics
Division of Minimally Invasive Gynecology
Johns Hopkins Hospital
Baltimore, Maryland

Brian L. Shaffer, MD
Director, Fetal Diagnosis & Treatment Center
Oregon Health & Science University
Portland, Oregon

Jonas Swartz, MD
Resident, Obstetrics and Gynecology
Oregon Health & Science University
Portland, Oregon

May Thomassee, MD
Clinical Instructor
Department of Obstetrics and Gynecology
Division of Minimally Invasive Gynecology
Vanderbilt University School of Medicine
Nashville, Tennessee

Susan H. Tran, MD
Assistant Professor, Maternal-Fetal Medicine
Oregon Health & Science University
Portland, Oregon

Ashlie Tronnes, MD
Fellow, Maternal-Fetal Medicine
University of Washington
Seattle, Washington

Gina Westhoff, MD
Fellow, Gynecologic Oncology
University of California, San Francisco

Keenan Yanit, MD
Resident, Obstetrics and Gynecology
Oregon Health & Science University
Portland, Oregon

Jessica L. Young, MD
Assistant Professor
Department of Obstetrics and Gynecology
Division of General Obstetrics and Gynecology
Vanderbilt University School of Medicine
Nashville, Tennessee

Amanda Yunker, DO
Assistant Professor
Department of Obstetrics and Gynecology
Division of Minimally Invasive Gynecology
Vanderbilt University School of Medicine
Nashville, Tennessee

Contributors to Previous Editions

Stephanie Beall, MD
Section Implantation & Oocyte Physiology
National Institutes of Health
Bethesda, Maryland

Nicole S. Carroll, MD
Department of Obstetrics and Gynecology
Wilmington Health
Wilmington, North Carolina

Annette Chen, MD
Department of Obstetrics and Gynecology
Division of Gynecologic Oncology
Kaiser Permanente
Oakland, California

Bruce B. Feinberg, MD
Department of Obstetrics and Gynecology
Division of Maternal-Fetal Medicine
Brigham and Women's Hospital
Boston, Massachusetts

Linda J. Heffner, MD, PhD
Professor and Chair
Department of Obstetrics and Gynecology
Boston University Medical School
Boston, Massachusetts

Celeste O. Hemingway, MD
Assistant Professor
Department of Obstetrics and Gynecology
Division of General Obstetrics and Gynecology
Vanderbilt University School of Medicine
Nashville, Tennessee

Sarah E. Little, MD
Fellow
Maternal-Fetal Medicine
Brigham and Women's Hospital
Boston, Massachusetts

Sara Newmann, MD, MPH
Assistant Clinical Professor
Department of Obstetrics and Gynecology
San Francisco General Hospital
San Francisco, California

Susan H. Tran, MD
Assistant Professor, Maternal-Fetal Medicine
Oregon Health & Science University
Portland, Oregon

Jing Wang Chiang, MD
Department of Obstetrics and Gynecology
Division of Gynecologic Oncology
Stanford Women's Cancer Center
Palo Alto, California

Preface

In 1997, the first five books in the Blueprints series were published as board review for medical students, interns, and residents who wanted high-yield, accurate clinical content for USMLE Steps 2 and 3. Fifteen years later, we are proud to report that the original books and the entire Blueprints brand of review materials have far exceeded our expectations.

The feedback we've received from our readers has been tremendously helpful and pivotal in deciding what direction the sixth edition of the core books would take. To ensure that the sixth edition of the series continues to provide the content and approach that made the original Blueprints a success, we have expanded the text to include the most up-to-date topics and evidence-based research and therapies. Information is provided on the latest changes in the management of cervical dysplasia and cervical cancer screening, abnormal uterine bleeding, hypertension in pregnancy, cervical insufficiency, and preterm labor. The newest and future techniques in contraception and sterilization and hormone replacement therapies are covered, as are contemporary treatment options for uterine fibroids and invasive breast cancer.

The succinct and telegraphic use of tables and figures was highly acclaimed by our readers, so we have redoubled our efforts to expand their usefulness by adding updated and improved artwork, including the section of color plates. In each case, we have tried to include only the most helpful and clear tables and figures to maximize the reader's ability to understand and remember the material.

We have likewise updated our bibliography to include evidence-based articles as well as references to classic articles and textbooks in both obstetrics and gynecology. These references are now provided in electronic format. It was also suggested that the review questions should reflect the current format of the boards. We are particularly proud to include new and revised board-format questions in this edition with full explanations of both correct and incorrect options provided in the answers. In particular, we have added a section of case-based clinical vignettes questions at the end of each chapter to facilitate review of the topics and practice for the boards.

That said, we have also learned from our readers that Blueprints is more than just board review for USMLE Steps 2 and 3. Students use the books during their clerkship rotations, subinternships, and as a quick refresher while rotating on various services in early residency. Residents studying for USMLE Step 3 often use the books for reviewing areas outside their specialty. Students in physician assistant, nurse practitioner, and osteopath programs use Blueprints as a companion to review materials in their own areas of expertise.

When we first wrote the book, we had just completed medical school and started residency training. Thus, we hope this new edition brings both that original viewpoint as well as our clinical experience garnered over the past 15 years. However you choose to use Blueprints, we hope that you find the books in the series informative and valuable to your own continuing education.

Tamara L. Callahan, MD, MPP
Aaron B. Caughey, MD, MPP, MPH, PhD

Acknowledgments

I would like to express my sincere and deep appreciation to my coauthor, Dr. Caughey, and to the OB/Gyn residents and faculties at Harvard and Vanderbilt who gave liberally of their time and expertise to make this book something of which we can all be proud. Without the extraordinary talent and commitment of these physicians and providers, this project would not have been possible. This accomplishment is also credited in no small part to an incredible core of family and friends who lovingly and selflessly allow me to follow my passion for education and women's health. And to my children, Connor and Jaela, being your mother has been an indescribable honor and an immeasurable joy—a blessing which I try to earn each and every day. I would also like to acknowledge my mentors, Dr. William F. Crowley, Jr., Dr. Janet Hall, Dr. Linda J. Heffner, Dr. Nancy Chescheir, Dr. Robert Barbieri, and Dr. Nancy E. Oriol, whose strength, insight, leadership, and drive are exemplary of what it means to be an active contributor to academic medicine and women's health. Lastly, I'd like to thank the many medical students and residents who have shared their input and enthusiasm with us along this exciting journey. Their support has been paramount to the success of this project and to our quest to make this book the very best it can be. It has truly been a privilege to be a small part of their never-ending learning experience.

Tamara L. Callahan, MD, MPP

I would like to acknowledge and extend my thanks to everyone involved in the sixth edition of our book, most importantly my coauthor, Dr. Callahan, as well as all of those who contributed to the first five editions, particularly Drs. Chen, Feinberg, and Heffner, and the staff at both Blackwell and LWW. I would also like to thank my colleagues and mentors for the supportive environment in which I work, in particular, the residents and faculty in the department of Obstetrics and Gynecology at OHSU as well as my mentors, Drs. Washington, Norton, Kuppermann, Ames, Repke, Blatman, Robinson, and Norwitz. I would also like to acknowledge the suggestions and critiques from medical students around the country and particularly those at Harvard, UCSF, and OHSU who keep pushing us to produce better editions of this work. I would also like to thank my parents, Bill and Carol, for their support for all these years. To my children, Aidan, Ashby, Amelie, and our little man, Atticus—and of course, to my wife, Susan— thank you for all your patience and support during all my projects. I love you all so very much.

Aaron B. Caughey, MD, MPP, MPH, PhD

Abbreviations

3β-HSD	3β-hydroxysteroid dehydrogenase
5-FU	5-fluorouracil
17α-OHP	17α-hydroxyprogesterone
ACTH	adrenocorticotropic hormone
AD	autosomal dominant
ADH	antidiuretic hormone
AED	antiepileptic drug
AFE	amniotic fluid embolus
AFI	amniotic fluid index
AFLP	acute fatty liver of pregnancy
AFP	α-fetoprotein
AGC	atypical glandular cells
AIDS	acquired immunodeficiency syndrome
ALT	alanine transaminase
AMA	advanced maternal age
AMH	Antimullerian Hormone
APA	antiphospholipid antibody
AR	autosomal recessive
ARDS	adult respiratory distress syndrome
AROM	artificial rupture of membranes
ART	assisted reproductive technology
ASC	atypical squamous cells
ASC-H	atypical squamous cells cannot exclude high-grade squamous intraepithelial lesion
ASC-US	atypical squamous cells of undetermined significance
AST	aspartate transaminase
AV	arteriovenous
AZT	analogs—zidovudine
β-hCG	beta human chorionic gonadotropin
BID	twice a day
BP	blood pressure
BPP	biophysical profile
BUN	blood urea nitrogen
BV	bacterial vaginosis
CAH	congenital adrenal hyperplasia
CBC	complete blood count
CCCT	clomiphene citrate challenge test
CF	cystic fibrosis
CHF	congestive heart failure
CIN	cervical intraepithelial neoplasia
CKC	cold-knife conization (biopsy)
CMV	cytomegalovirus
CNS	central nervous system
CPD	cephalopelvic disproportion
CRS	congenital rubella syndrome
CSF	cerebrospinal fluid
CT	computed tomography (CAT scan)
CVA	cerebrovascular accident
CVAT	costovertebral angle tenderness
CVD	collagen vascular disorders
CVS	chorionic villus sampling
CXR	chest x-ray
DA	developmental age
D&C	dilation and curettage
D&E	dilation and evacuation
DCIS	ductal carcinoma in situ
DES	diethylstilbestrol
DEXA	dual-energy x-ray absorptiometry
DHEA	dehydroepiandrosterone
DHEAS	dehydroepiandrosterone sulfate
DHT	dihydrotestosterone
DIC	disseminated intravascular coagulation
DMPA	depot medroxyprogesterone acetate (Depo-Provera)
DTRs	deep tendon reflexes
DUB	dysfunctional uterine bleeding
DVT	deep venous thrombosis
ECG	electrocardiogram
EDC	estimated date of confinement
EDD	estimated date of delivery
EFW	estimated fetal weight
EIF	echogenic intracardiac focus
ELISA	enzyme-linked immunosorbent assay
EMB	endometrial biopsy
ERT	estrogen replacement therapy
ESR	erythrocyte sedimentation rate
FAS	fetal alcohol syndrome
FH	fetal heart
FHR	fetal heart rate
FIGO	International Federation of Gynecology and Obstetrics
FIRS	fetal immune response syndrome
FISH	fluorescent in situ hybridization
FNA	fine-needle aspiration
FSE	fetal scalp electrode
FSH	follicle-stimulating hormone
FTA-ABS	fluorescent treponemal antibody absorption
FTP	failure to progress
G	gravidity
GA	gestational age
GBS	group B *streptococcus*

GDM	gestational diabetes mellitus
GFR	glomerular filtration rate
GH	gestational hypertension
GI	Gastrointestinal
GLT	glucose loading test
GnRH	gonadotropin-releasing hormone
GTD	gestational trophoblastic disease
GTT	glucose tolerance test
GU	genitourinary
HAART	highly active antiretroviral therapy
Hb	hemoglobin
HbH	hemoglobin H disease
hCG	human chorionic gonadotropin
hCS	human chorionic somatomammotropin
Hct	hematocrit
HDL	high-density lipoprotein
HELLP	hemolysis, elevated liver enzymes, low platelets
HIV	human immunodeficiency virus
hMG	human menopausal gonadotropin
HPL	human placental lactogen
HPV	human papillomavirus
HR	heart rate
HRT	hormone replacement therapy
HSG	hysterosalpingogram
HSIL	high-grade squamous intraepithelial lesion
HSV	herpes simplex virus
I&D	incision and drainage
ICSI	intracytoplasmic sperm injection
Ig	Immunoglobulin
IM	Intramuscular
INR	International Normalized Ratio
ITP	idiopathic thrombocytopenic purpura
IUD	intrauterine device
IUFD	intrauterine fetal demise or death
IUGR	intrauterine growth restricted
IUI	intrauterine insemination
IUP	intrauterine pregnancy
IUPC	intrauterine pressure catheter
IUT	intrauterine transfusion
IVC	inferior vena cava
IVF	in vitro fertilization
IVP	intravenous pyelogram
KB	Kleihauer-Betke test
KOH	potassium hydroxide
KUB	kidneys/ureter/bladder (x-ray)
LBW	low birth weight
LCHAD	long-chain hydroxyacyl-CoA dehydrogenase
LCIS	lobular carcinoma in situ
LDH	lactate dehydrogenase
LDL	low-density lipoprotein
LEEP	loop electrosurgical excision procedure
LFT	liver function test
LGA	large for gestational age
LGV	lymphogranuloma venereum
LH	luteinizing hormone
LIQ	lower inner quadrant
Lletz	large loop excision of the transformation zone
LMP	last menstrual period
LOQ	lower outer quadrant
LOT	left occiput transverse
LSIL	low-grade squamous intraepithelial lesion
LTL	laparoscopic tubal ligation
MAO	monoamine oxidase
MESA	microsurgical epididymal sperm aspiration
MHATP	microhemagglutination assay for antibodies to *T. pallidum*
MI	myocardial infarction
MIF	müllerian inhibiting factor
MLK	myosin light-chain kinase
MRI	magnetic resonance imaging
MRKH	Mayer-Rokitansky-Küster-Hauser (syndrome)
MSAFP	maternal serum α-fetoprotein
MTHFR	methyl tetrahydrofolate reductase
NPO	nil per os (nothing by mouth)
NPV	negative predictive value
NRFT	nonreassuring fetal testing
NSAID	nonsteroidal anti-inflammatory drug
NST	nonstress test
NSVD	normal spontaneous vaginal delivery
NT	nuchal translucency
NTD	neural tube defect
OA	occiput anterior
OCP	oral contraceptive pill
OCT	oxytocin challenge test
OI	ovulation induction
OP	occiput posterior
OT	occiput transverse
OTC	over-the-counter
P	parity
PCOS	polycystic ovarian syndrome
PCR	polymerase chain reaction
PDA	patent ductus arteriosus
PE	pulmonary embolus
PFTs	pulmonary function tests
PID	pelvic inflammatory disease
PIH	pregnancy-induced hypertension
PMDD	premenstrual dysphoric disorder
PMN	polymorphonuclear leukocyte
PMOF	premature ovarian failure
PMS	premenstrual syndrome
PO	per os (by mouth)
POCs	products of conception
POP	progesterone-only contraceptive pills
POP-Q	pelvic organ prolapse quantification system
PPCM	peripartum cardiomyopathy
PPD	purified protein derivative
PPROM	preterm premature rupture of membranes
PPS	postpartum sterilization
PPV	positive predictive value
PROM	premature rupture of membranes
PSTT	placental site trophoblastic tumor
PT	prothrombin time

PTL	preterm labor
PTT	partial thromboplastin time
PTU	propylthiouracil
PUBS	percutaneous umbilical blood sampling
QD	each day
QID	four times a day
RBC	red blood cell
RDS	respiratory distress syndrome
ROM	rupture of membranes
ROT	right occiput transverse
RPR	rapid plasma reagin
RR	respiratory rate
SAB	spontaneous abortion
SCC	squamous cell carcinoma
SERM	selective estrogen receptor modulator
SGA	small for gestational age
SHBG	sex hormone binding globulin
SIDS	sudden infant death syndrome
SLE	systemic lupus erythematosus
SNRIs	serotonin and norepinephrine reuptake inhibitors
SPT	septic pelvic thrombophlebitis
SROM	spontaneous rupture of membranes
SSRIs	selective serotonin reuptake inhibitors
STD	sexually transmitted disease
STI	sexually transmitted infection
SVT	superficial vein thrombophlebitis
TAB	therapeutic abortion
TAC	transabdominal cerclage
TAHBSO	total abdominal hysterectomy and bilateral salpingo-oophorectomy
TBG	thyroid binding globulin
TENS	transcutaneous electrical nerve stimulation
TFTs	thyroid function tests
TLC	total lung capacity
TNM	tumor/node/metastasis
TOA	tubo-ovarian abscess
TOLAC	trial of labor after cesarean
TOV	transposition of the vessels
TPAL	term, preterm, aborted, living
TRH	thyrotropin-releasing hormone
TSE	testicular sperm extraction
TSH	thyroid-stimulating hormone
TSI	thyroid-stimulating immunoglobulins
TSS	toxic shock syndrome
TSST	toxic shock syndrome toxin
TTTS	twin-to-twin transfusion syndrome
UA	urinalysis
UAE	uterine artery embolization
UG	urogenital
UIQ	upper inner quadrant
UOQ	upper outer quadrant
UPI	uteroplacental insufficiency
US	ultrasound
UTI	urinary tract infection
V/Q	ventilation/perfusion ratio
VAIN	vaginal intraepithelial neoplasia
VBAC	vaginal birth after cesarean
V_D	volume of distribution
VDRL	Venereal Disease Research Laboratory
VIN	vulvar intraepithelial neoplasia
VSD	ventricular septal defect
VZIG	varicella zoster immune globulin
VZV	varicella zoster virus
WBC	white blood cell
XR	x-ray

Part I Obstetrics

Chapter 1 Pregnancy and Prenatal Care

PREGNANCY

Pregnancy is the state of having products of conception implanted normally or abnormally in the uterus or occasionally elsewhere. It is terminated by spontaneous or elective abortion or by delivery. A myriad of physiologic changes occur in a pregnant woman, which affect every organ system.

DIAGNOSIS

In a patient who has regular menstrual cycles and is sexually active, a period delayed by more than a few days to a week is suggestive of pregnancy. Even at this early stage, patients may exhibit signs and symptoms of pregnancy. On physical examination, a variety of findings indicate pregnancy (Table 1-1).

Many over-the-counter (OTC) urine pregnancy tests have a high sensitivity and will be positive around the time of the missed menstrual cycle. These urine tests and the hospital laboratory serum assays test for the beta subunit of human chorionic gonadotropin (β-hCG). This hormone produced by the placenta will rise to a peak of 100,000 mIU/mL by 10 weeks of gestation, decrease throughout the second trimester, and then level off at approximately 20,000 to 30,000 mIU/mL in the third trimester.

A viable pregnancy can be confirmed by ultrasound, which may show the gestational sac as early as 5 weeks on a transvaginal ultrasound or at a β-hCG of 1,500 to 2,000 mIU/mL. Fetal heart motion may be seen on transvaginal ultrasound as soon as 6 weeks or at a β-hCG of 5,000 to 6,000 mIU/mL.

TERMS AND DEFINITIONS

From the time of fertilization until the pregnancy is 8 weeks along (10 weeks' gestational age [GA]), the conceptus is called an **embryo**. After 8 weeks until the time of birth, it is designated a **fetus**. The term **infant** is used for the period between delivery and 1 year of age. Pregnancy is divided into trimesters. The **first trimester** lasts until 12 weeks but is also defined as up to 14 weeks' GA, the **second trimester** lasts from 12 to 14 until 24 to 28 weeks' GA, and the **third trimester** lasts from 24 to 28 weeks until delivery. An infant delivered prior to 24 weeks is considered to be **previable**, delivered between 24 and 37 weeks is considered **preterm**, and between 37 and 42 weeks is considered **term**. A pregnancy carried beyond 42 weeks is considered **postterm**.

Gravidity (G) refers to the number of times a woman has been pregnant, and **parity** (P) refers to the number of pregnancies that led to a birth at or beyond 20 weeks' GA or of an infant weighing more than 500 g. For example, a woman who has given birth to one set of twins would be a G1 P1, as a multiple gestation is considered as just one pregnancy. A more specific designation of pregnancy outcomes divides parity into **term** and **preterm** deliveries and also adds the number of **abortuses** and the number of **living** children. This is known as the TPAL designation. Abortuses include all pregnancy losses prior to 20 weeks, both therapeutic and spontaneous, as well as ectopic pregnancies. For example, a woman who has given birth to one set of preterm twins, one term infant, and had two miscarriages would be a G4 P1-1-2-3.

The prefixes nulli-, primi-, and multi- are used with respect to gravidity and parity to refer to having 0, 1, or more than 1, respectively. For example, a woman who has been pregnant twice, one ectopic pregnancy and one full-term birth, would be multigravid and primiparous. Unfortunately, this terminology often gets misused with individuals referring to women with a first pregnancy as primiparous, rather than nulliparous. Obstetricians also use the term **grand multip**, which refers to a woman whose parity is greater than or equal to 5.

Dating of Pregnancy

The GA of a fetus is the age in weeks and days measured from the last menstrual period (LMP). **Developmental age** (DA) or conceptional age or embryonic age is the number of weeks and days since fertilization. Because fertilization usually occurs about 14 days after the first day of the prior menstrual period, the GA is usually 2 weeks more than the DA.

Classically, the **Nagele rule** for calculating the **estimated date of confinement** (EDC), or estimated date of delivery (EDD), is to subtract 3 months from the LMP and add 7 days. Thus, a pregnancy with an LMP of January 16, 2012 would have an EDC of 10/23/12. Exact dating uses an EDC calculated as 280 days after a certain LMP. If the date of ovulation is known, as in assisted reproductive technology (ART), the EDC can be calculated by adding 266 days. Pregnancy dating can be confirmed and should be consistent with the examination of the uterine size at the first prenatal appointment.

TABLE 1-1 Signs and Symptoms of Pregnancy

Signs
Bluish discoloration of vagina and cervix (Chadwick sign)
Softening and cyanosis of the cervix at or after 4 wk (Goodell sign)
Softening of the uterus after 6 wk (Ladin sign)
Breast swelling and tenderness
Development of the linea nigra from umbilicus to pubis
Telangiectasias
Palmar erythema
Symptoms
Amenorrhea
Nausea and vomiting
Breast pain
Quickening—fetal movement

With an uncertain LMP, ultrasound is often used to determine the EDC. Ultrasound has a level of uncertainty that increases during the pregnancy, but it is rarely off by more than 7% to 8% at any GA. A safe rule of thumb is that the ultrasound should not differ from LMP dating by more than 1 week in the first trimester, 2 weeks in the second trimester, and 3 weeks in the third trimester. The dating done with crown–rump length in the first half of the first trimester is probably even more accurate, to within 3 to 5 days.

Other measures used to estimate GA include pregnancy landmarks such as auscultation of the fetal heart (FH) at 20 weeks by nonelectronic fetoscopy or at 10 weeks by Doppler ultrasound, as well as maternal awareness of fetal movement or "quickening," which occurs between 16 and 20 weeks.

Because ultrasound dating of pregnancy decreases in accuracy as the pregnancy progresses, determining and confirming pregnancy dating at the first interaction between a pregnant woman and the health care system is imperative. A woman who presents to the emergency department may not return for prenatal care, so dating should be confirmed at that visit. Pregnancy dating is particularly important because a number of decisions regarding care are based on accurate dating. One such decision is whether to resuscitate a newborn at the threshold of viability, which may be at 23 or 24 weeks of gestation depending on the institution. Another is the induction of labor at 41 weeks of gestation. Approximately 5% to 15% of women may be oligo-ovulatory, meaning they ovulate beyond the usual 14th day of the cycle. Thus, their LMP dating may overdiagnose a prolonged (≥41 weeks' gestation) or postterm pregnancy (≥42 weeks' gestation). Thus, early verification or correction of dating can correct such misdating.

PHYSIOLOGY OF PREGNANCY

Cardiovascular

During pregnancy, **cardiac output** increases by 30% to 50%. Most increases occur during the first trimester, with the maximum being reached between 20 and 24 weeks' gestation and maintained until delivery. The increase in cardiac output is first due to an increase in stroke volume and is then maintained by an increase in heart rate as the stroke volume decreases to near prepregnancy levels by the end of the third trimester. **Systemic vascular resistance** decreases during pregnancy, resulting in a fall in arterial blood pressure. This decrease is most likely due to elevated progesterone, leading to smooth muscle relaxation. There is a decrease in systolic blood pressure of 5 to 10 mm Hg and in diastolic blood pressure of 10 to 15 mm Hg that nadirs at week 24. Between 24 weeks' gestation and term, the blood pressure slowly returns to prepregnancy levels but should never exceed them.

Pulmonary

There is an increase of 30% to 40% in tidal volume (V_T) during pregnancy (Fig. 1-1) despite the fact that the total lung capacity (TLC) is decreased by 5% due to the elevation of the diaphragm. This increase in V_T decreases the expiratory reserve volume by about 20%. The increase in V_T with a constant respiratory rate leads to an increase in minute ventilation of 30% to 40%, which in turn leads to an increase in alveolar (PAO_2) and arterial (PaO_2) PO_2 levels and a decrease in $PACO_2$ and $PaCO_2$ levels.

$PaCO_2$ decreases to approximately 30 mm Hg by 20 weeks' gestation from 40 mm Hg during prepregnancy. This change leads to an increased CO_2 gradient between mother and fetus and is likely caused by elevated progesterone levels that either increase the respiratory system's responsiveness to CO_2 or act as a primary stimulant. This gradient facilitates oxygen delivery to the fetus and carbon dioxide removal from the fetus. Dyspnea of pregnancy occurs in 60% to 70% of patients. This is possibly secondary to decreased $PaCO_2$ levels, increased V_T, or decreased TLC.

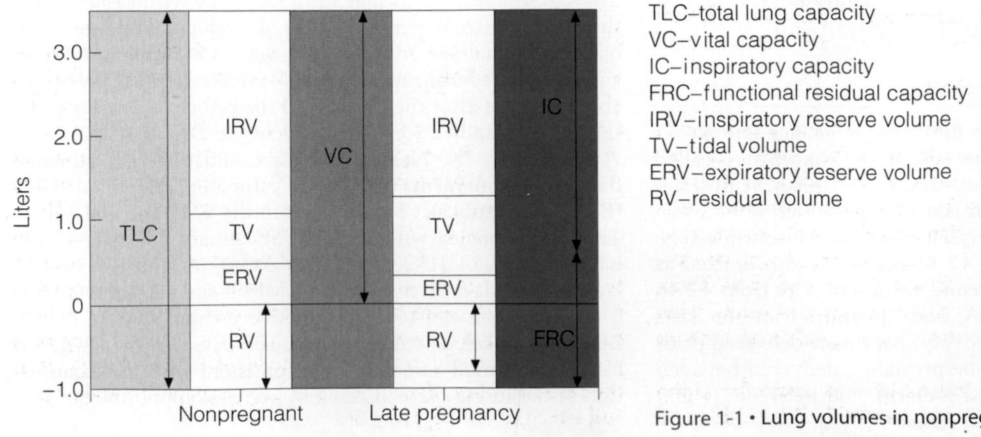

Figure 1-1 • Lung volumes in nonpregnant and pregnant women.

Gastrointestinal

Nausea and vomiting occur in more than 70% of pregnancies. This has been termed **morning sickness** even though it can occur anytime throughout the day. These symptoms have been attributed to the elevation in estrogen, progesterone, and hCG. They may also be due to hypoglycemia and can be treated with frequent snacking. The nausea and vomiting typically resolve by 14 to 16 weeks' gestation. **Hyperemesis gravidarum** refers to a severe form of morning sickness associated with weight loss ($\geq$5% of prepregnancy weight) and ketosis.

During pregnancy, the stomach has prolonged gastric emptying times and the gastroesophageal sphincter has decreased tone. Together, these changes lead to reflux and possibly combine with decreased esophageal tone to cause ptyalism, or spitting, during pregnancy. The large bowel also has decreased motility, which leads to increased water absorption and constipation.

Renal

The kidneys increase in size and the ureters dilate during pregnancy, which may lead to increased rates of pyelonephritis. The glomerular filtration rate (GFR) increases by 50% early in pregnancy and is maintained until delivery. As a result of increased GFR, blood urea nitrogen and creatinine decrease by about 25%. An increase in the renin–angiotensin system leads to increased levels of aldosterone, which results in increased sodium resorption. However, plasma levels of sodium do not increase because of the simultaneous increase in GFR.

Hematology

Although the plasma volume increases by 50% in pregnancy, the RBC volume increases by only 20% to 30%, which leads to a decrease in the hematocrit, or dilutional anemia. The WBC count increases during pregnancy to a mean of 10.5 million/mL with a range of 6 to 16 million. During labor, stress may cause the WBC count to rise to over 20 million/mL. There is a slight decrease in the concentration of platelets, probably secondary to increased plasma volume and an increase in peripheral destruction. Although in 7% to 8% of patients the platelet count may be between 100 and 150 million/mL, a drop in the platelet count below 100 million/mL over a short time is not normal and should be investigated promptly.

Pregnancy is considered to be a hypercoagulable state with an increase in the number of thromboembolic events. There are elevations in the levels of fibrinogen and factors VII–X. However, the actual clotting and bleeding times do not change. The increased rate of thromboembolic events in pregnancy may also be secondary to the other elements of Virchow triad, that is an increase in venous stasis and vessel endothelial damage.

Endocrine

Pregnancy is a hyperestrogenic state. The increased estrogen is produced primarily by the placenta, with the ovaries contributing to a lesser degree. Unlike estrogen production in the ovaries, where estrogen precursors are produced in ovarian theca cells and transferred to the ovarian granulosa cells, estrogen in the placenta is derived from circulating plasma-borne precursors produced by the maternal adrenal glands. Fetal well-being has been correlated with maternal serum estrogen levels, with low estrogen levels being associated with conditions such as fetal death and anencephaly.

The hormone hCG is composed of two dissimilar alpha and beta subunits. The alpha subunit of hCG is identical to the alpha subunits of luteinizing hormone (LH), follicle-stimulating hormone (FSH), and thyroid-stimulating hormone (TSH), whereas the beta subunits differ. Levels of hCG double approximately every 48 hours during early pregnancy, reaching a peak at approximately 10 to 12 weeks, and thereafter declining to reach a steady state after week 15.

The placenta produces hCG, which acts to maintain the corpus luteum in early pregnancy. The corpus luteum produces progesterone, which maintains the endometrium. Eventually, the placenta takes over progesterone production and the corpus luteum degrades into the corpus albicans. Progesterone levels increase over the course of pregnancy. Progesterone causes relaxation of smooth muscle, which has multiple effects on the gastrointestinal, cardiovascular, and genitourinary systems. **Human placental lactogen** (hPL) is produced in the placenta and is important for ensuring a constant nutrient supply to the fetus. hPL, also known as human chorionic somatomammotropin (hCS), induces lipolysis with a concomitant increase in circulating free fatty acids. hPL also acts as an insulin antagonist, along with various other placental hormones, thereby having a diabetogenic effect. This leads to increased levels of insulin and protein synthesis. Levels of **prolactin** are markedly increased during pregnancy. These levels decrease after delivery but later increase in response to suckling.

There are two major changes in thyroid hormones during pregnancy. First, estrogen stimulates thyroid binding globulin (TBG), leading to an elevation in total T3 and T4, but free T3 and T4 remain relatively constant. Second, hCG has a weak stimulating effect on the thyroid, likely because its alpha subgroup is similar to TSH. This leads to a slight increase in T3 and T4 and a slight decrease in TSH early in pregnancy. Overall, however, pregnancy is considered a euthyroid state.

Musculoskeletal and Dermatologic

The obvious change in the center of gravity during pregnancy can lead to a shift in posture and lower back strain, which worsens throughout pregnancy, particularly during the third trimester. Numerous changes occur in the skin, including spider angiomata and palmar erythema secondary to increased estrogen levels and hyperpigmentation of the nipples, umbilicus, abdominal midline (the **linea nigra**), perineum, and face (**melasma** or **chloasma**) secondary to increased levels of the melanocyte-stimulating hormones and the steroid hormones. Pregnancy is also associated with carpal tunnel syndrome, which results from compression of the median nerve. The incidence in pregnancy varies greatly and symptoms are usually self-limited.

Nutrition

Nutritional requirements increase during pregnancy and breastfeeding. An average woman requires 2,000 to 2,500 kcal/day. The caloric requirement is increased by 300 kcal/day during pregnancy and by 500 kcal/day when breastfeeding. Thus, pregnancy is not the caloric equivalent of eating for two; more accurately, it is approximately eating for 1.15. Most patients should gain between 20 and 30 lb during pregnancy. Overweight women are advised to gain less, between 15 and 25 lb; underweight women are advised to gain more, 28 to 40 lb. Unfortunately, a large proportion of women gain more than the recommended amount, which contributes to a number of complications in pregnancy plus postpartum weight retention and downstream obesity. It is the responsibility of each prenatal care provider to review diet and exercise during pregnancy.

In addition to the increased caloric requirements, there are increased nutritional requirements for protein, iron, folate, calcium, and other vitamins and minerals. The protein requirement increases from 60 to 70 or 75 g/day. Recommended calcium intake is 1.5 g/day. Many patients develop iron deficiency anemia because of the increased demand on hematopoiesis both by the mother and the fetus. Folate requirements increase from 0.4 to 0.8 mg/day and are important in preventing neural tube defects.

All patients are advised to take prenatal vitamins during pregnancy. These are designed to compensate for the increased nutritional demands of pregnancy. Furthermore, any patient whose hematocrit falls during pregnancy is advised to increase iron intake with oral supplementation (Table 1-2).

PRENATAL CARE

Prenatal visits are designed to screen for various complications of pregnancy and to educate the patient. They include a series of outpatient office visits that involve routine physical examinations and various screening tests that occur at different points in the prenatal care. Important issues of prenatal care include initial patient evaluation, routine patient evaluation, nutrition, disease states during the pregnancy, and preparing for the delivery.

INITIAL VISIT

This is often the longest of the prenatal visits because it involves obtaining a complete history and performing a physical examination as well as a battery of initial laboratory tests. It should occur early in the first trimester, between 6 and 10 weeks, although occasionally patients will not present for their initial prenatal visit until later in their pregnancy. At this visit, diet, exercise, and weight gain goals should also be discussed.

History

The patient's history includes the present pregnancy, the LMP, and symptoms during the pregnancy. After this, an obstetric history of prior pregnancies, including date, outcome (e.g., SAB [spontaneous abortion], TAB [therapeutic abortion], ectopic pregnancy, term delivery), mode of delivery, length of time in labor and second stage, birth weight, and any complications, should be obtained. Finally, a complete medical, surgical, family, and social history should be obtained.

Physical Examination

A complete physical examination is performed, paying particular attention to the patient's prior medical and surgical history. The pelvic examination includes a Pap smear, unless one has been done in the past 6 months, and cultures for gonorrhea and

TABLE 1-2 Recommended Daily Dietary Allowances for Nonpregnant, Pregnant, and Lactating Women

	Nonpregnant Women by Age					Pregnant Women	Lactating Women
	11–14 y	15–18 y	19–22 y	23–50 y	51+ y		
Energy (kcal)	2,400	2,100	2,100	2,000	1,800	+300	+500
Protein (g)	44	48	46	46	46	+30	+20
Fat-soluble vitamins	800	800	800	800	800	1,000	1,200
Vitamin A activity (RE) (IU)	4,000	4,000	4,000	4,000	4,000	5,000	6,000
Vitamin D (IU)	400	400	400	—	—	400	400
Vitamin E activity (IU)	12	12	12	12	12	15	15
Water-soluble vitamins							
Ascorbic acid (mg)	45	45	45	45	45	60	80
Folacin (mg)	400	400	400	400	400	800	600
Niacin (mg)	16	14	14	13	12	+2	+4
Riboflavin (mg)	1.3	1.4	1.4	1.2	1.1	+0.3	+0.5
Thiamin (mg)	1.2	1.1	1.1	1	1	+0.3	+0.3
Vitamin B_6 (mg)	1.6	2	2	2	2	2.5	2.5
Vitamin B_{12} (mg)	3	3	3	3	3	4	4
Minerals							
Calcium (mg)	1,200	1,200	800	800	800	1,200	1,200
Iodine (mg)	115	115	100	100	80	125	150
Iron (mg)	18	18	18	18	10	+18	18
Magnesium (mg)	300	300	300	300	300	450	450
Phosphorus (mg)	1,200	1,200	800	800	800	1,200	1,200
Zinc (mg)	15	15	15	15	15	20	25

IU, International Unit. From Gabbe SG, Niebyl JR, Simpsen JL. *Obstetrics: Normal and Problem Pregnancies*, 4th ed. New York, NY: Churchill Livingstone; 2002:196.

chlamydia. On bimanual examination, the size of the uterus should be consistent with the GA from the LMP. If a woman is unsure of her LMP or if size and dates are not consistent, one should obtain an ultrasound for dating. Accurate dating is crucial for all subsequent obstetrical evaluations and interventions.

Diagnostic Evaluation

The panel of tests in the first trimester includes a complete blood count, primarily for hematocrit, blood type, antibody screen, rapid plasma reagin (RPR) or VDRL screening for syphilis, rubella antibody screen, hepatitis B surface antigen, urinalysis, and urine culture. If a patient has no history of chickenpox, a titer for varicella zoster virus (VZV) antibodies is sent. A purified protein derivative (PPD) is usually placed during the first or second trimester to screen for tuberculosis in high-risk patients. A urine pregnancy test should be sent if the patient is not entirely certain she is pregnant. If there has been any bleeding or cramping, a serum β-hCG level should be obtained. While there is some debate over the use of routine toxoplasma titers, they are often ordered as well. All patients are counseled about HIV, and testing should be offered routinely (Table 1-3). In addition, first-trimester screening tests for aneuploidy with nuchal translucency (NT) by ultrasound and serum markers are increasingly being obtained in most women via referral to a prenatal diagnosis unit. In addition to this battery of tests, there are a variety of other screens offered to high-risk patients (Table 1-4).

ROUTINE PRENATAL VISITS

Blood pressure, weight, urine dipstick, measurement of the uterus, and auscultation of the FH are performed and assessed on each follow-up prenatal care visit. Maternal blood pressure decreases during the first and second trimesters and slowly returns to baseline during the third trimester; elevation may be a sign of preeclampsia. Maternal weight is followed serially throughout the pregnancy as a proxy for adequate nutrition. Also, large weight gains toward the end of pregnancy can be a sign of fluid retention and preeclampsia. Measurement of the uterine fundal height in centimeters corresponds roughly to the weeks of gestation. If the fundal height is progressively decreasing or is 3 cm less than GA, an ultrasound is done to more accurately assess fetal growth. After 10 to 14 weeks, Doppler ultrasound is used to auscultate the fetal heart rate (FHR). Urine is routinely dipped for protein, glucose, blood, and leukocyte esterase. The presence of protein may be indicative of preeclampsia, glucose of diabetes, and leukocyte esterase of urinary tract infection (UTI). Pregnant women are at an increased risk for complicated UTIs such as pyelonephritis, given increased urinary stasis from mechanical compression of the ureters and progesterone-mediated smooth muscle relaxation.

At each visit, the patient is asked about symptoms that indicate complications of pregnancy. These symptoms include vaginal bleeding, vaginal discharge or leaking of fluid, and urinary symptoms. In addition, after 20 weeks, patients are asked about contractions and fetal movement. Vaginal bleeding is a sign of possible miscarriage or ectopic pregnancy in the first trimester and of placental abruption or previa as the pregnancy advances. Vaginal discharge may be a sign of infection or cervical change, whereas leaking fluid can indicate ruptured fetal membranes. While irregular (Braxton Hicks) contractions are common throughout the third trimester, regular contractions more frequent than five or six per hour may be a sign of preterm labor and should be assessed. Changes in or absence of fetal movement should be evaluated by auscultation of the FH in the previable fetus and with further testing such as a nonstress test or biophysical profile in the viable fetus.

First-Trimester Visits

During the first trimester, patients—particularly nulliparous women—need to be familiarized with pregnancy. The symptoms of pregnancy and what will occur at each prenatal visit should be reviewed. At the second prenatal visit, all of the initial laboratory test results should be reviewed with the patient. Those with poor weight gain or decreased caloric

TABLE 1-3 Routine Tests in Prenatal Care

Initial Visit and First Trimester	Second Trimester	Third Trimester
Hematocrit	MSAFP/triple or quad screen	Hematocrit
Blood type and screen	Obstetric ultrasound	RPR/VDRL
RPR/VDRL	Amniocentesis for women interested in prenatal diagnosis	GLT
Rubella antibody screen		Group B streptococcal culture
Hepatitis B surface antigen		
Gonorrhea culture		
Chlamydia culture		
PPD		
Pap smear		
Urinalysis and culture		
VZV titer in patients with no history of exposure		
HIV offered		
Early screening for aneuploidy (NT plus serum markers)		

TABLE 1-4 Initial Screens in Specific High-Risk Groups

High-Risk Group	Specific Test
African American, Southeast Asian, MCV <70	Sickle cell prep for African Americans; Hgb electrophoresis
Family history of genetic disorder (e.g., hemophilia, sickle cell disease, fragile X syndrome), maternal age 35 or older at time of EDC	Prenatal genetics referral
Prior gestational diabetes, family history of diabetes, Hispanic, Native American, Southeast Asian	Early GLT
Pregestational diabetes, unsure dates, recurrent miscarriages	Dating sonogram at first visit
Hypertension, renal disease, pregestational diabetic, prior preeclampsia, renal transplant, SLE	BUN, Cr, uric acid, and 24 h urine collection for protein and creatinine clearance (to establish a baseline)
Pregestational diabetes, prior cardiac disease, hypertension	ECG
Pregestational diabetes	Hgb A1C, ophthalmology for eye examination
Graves disease	Thyroid-stimulating immunoglobulins (can cause fetal disease)
All thyroid disease	TSH, possibly free T4
PPD+	Chest X-ray after 16 weeks' gestation
SLE	AntiRho, antiLa antibodies (can cause fetal complete heart block)

intake secondary to nausea and vomiting may be referred to a nutritionist. Patients treated for infections noted at the initial prenatal visit should be cultured for test of cure. Additionally, early screening for aneuploidy, with an ultrasound for NT and correlation with serum levels of pregnancy-associated plasma protein A (PAPP-A) and free β-hCG, is offered between 11 and 13 weeks of gestation to all women.

Second-Trimester Visits

During the second trimester, much of the screening for genetic and congenital abnormalities is done. This allows a patient to obtain an elective termination if there are abnormalities. Screening for **maternal serum alpha fetoprotein** (MSAFP) is usually performed between 15 and 18 weeks. An elevation in MSAFP is correlated with an increased risk of neural tube defects, and a decrease is seen in some aneuploidies, including Down syndrome. The sensitivity of aneuploidy screening is augmented using β-hCG and estriol along with MSAFP called the **triple screen**. The addition of inhibin A to this screening test further enhances the ability to detect abnormalities and is known as the **quad screen**. Between 18 and 20 weeks' gestation, most patients are offered a screening ultrasound. This provides the opportunity to screen for common fetal abnormalities. Also noted are the amniotic fluid volume, placental location, and GA.

The FH is usually first heard during the second trimester, as is the first fetal movement, or "quickening," felt usually between 16 and 20 weeks' GA. Most patients have resolution of their nausea and vomiting by the second trimester, although some continue with these symptoms throughout their pregnancy. Because the risk of spontaneous abortions decreases after 12 weeks of gestation, childbirth classes and tours of the labor floor are usually offered in the second and third trimesters.

Third-Trimester Visits

During the third trimester, the fetus is viable. Patients will begin to have occasional Braxton Hicks contractions and, if these contractions become regular, the cervix is examined to rule out preterm labor. Prenatal visits increase to every 2 to 3 weeks from 28 to 36 weeks and then to every week after 36 weeks. In addition, patients who are Rh negative should receive RhoGAM at 28 weeks. Beyond 32 to 34 weeks, Leopold maneuvers (see Fig. 3-1) are performed to determine fetal presentation. Either as a routine or if there is any question, an office ultrasound may be used at 35 to 36 weeks to confirm fetal presentation. In the setting of breech presentation, women are offered external cephalic version of the fetus at 37 to 38 weeks of gestation.

Beyond 37 weeks, which is considered term, the cervix is usually examined at each visit. Because a vigorous examination of the cervix, known as "sweeping" or "stripping" the membranes, has been demonstrated to decrease the probability of progressing postterm or requiring an induction of labor, this is commonly offered at all term pregnancy prenatal visits.

Third-Trimester Laboratory Test Results

At 27 to 29 weeks, the third-trimester laboratory test results are ordered. These consist of the hematocrit, RPR/VDRL, and **glucose loading test** (GLT). At this time, the hematocrit is getting close to its nadir. Patients with a hematocrit below 32% to 33% (hemoglobin <11 mg/dL) are usually started on iron supplementation. Because this will cause further constipation, stool softeners are given in conjunction. The GLT is a screening test for gestational diabetes. It consists of giving a 50-g oral glucose loading dose and checking serum glucose 1 hour later. If this value is greater than or equal to 140 mg/dL, a **glucose tolerance test** (GTT) is administered, though some institutions use a lower threshold of 130 or 135 mg/dL.

The GTT is the diagnostic test for gestational diabetes. It consists of a fasting serum glucose measurement and then administration of a 100-g oral glucose loading dose. The serum glucose is then measured at 1, 2, and 3 hours after the oral dose is given. This test is indicative of gestational diabetes if there is an elevation in two or more of the following threshold values: the fasting glucose, 95 mg/dL; 1 hour, 180 mg/dL; 2 hour, 155 mg/dL; or 3 hour, 140 mg/dL.

In high-risk populations, vaginal cultures for gonorrhea and chlamydia are repeated late in the third trimester. These infections are transmitted vertically during birth and should be treated if cultures or DNA tests return positive. In women with latent herpes simplex virus (HSV), antiviral prophylaxis can be initiated at 36 weeks. Active HSV would be an indication for cesarean delivery. At 36 weeks, screening for group B streptococcal infection is also performed. Patients who have a positive culture should be treated with intravenous penicillin when they present in labor to prevent potential neonatal group B streptococcal infection.

ROUTINE PROBLEMS OF PREGNANCY

BACK PAIN

During pregnancy, low back pain is quite common, particularly in the third trimester when the patient's center of gravity has shifted and there is an increased strain on the lower back. Mild exercise—particularly stretching—may release endorphins and reduce the amount of back pain. Gentle massage, heating pads, and Tylenol can be used for mild pain. For patients with severe back pain, muscle relaxants or, occasionally, narcotics can be used. Physical therapy can also be helpful in these patients.

CONSTIPATION

The decreased bowel motility secondary to elevated progesterone levels leads to increased transit time in the large bowel. In turn, there is greater absorption of water from the gastrointestinal tract. This can result in constipation. Increased oral (PO) fluids, particularly water, should be recommended. In addition, stool softeners or bulking agents may help. Laxatives can be used, but are usually avoided in the third trimester because of the theoretical risk of preterm labor.

CONTRACTIONS

Occasional irregular contractions that do not lead to cervical change are considered Braxton Hicks contractions and will occur several times per day up to several times per hour. Patients should be warned about these and assured that they are normal. Dehydration may cause increased contractions, and patients should be advised to drink many (10 to 14) glasses of water per day. Regular contractions, as often as every 10 minutes, should be considered a sign of preterm labor and should be assessed by cervical examination. If a patient has had several days of contractions and no documented cervical change, this is reassuring to both the obstetrician and the patient that delivery is not imminent.

DEHYDRATION

Because of the expanded intravascular space and increased third spacing of fluid, patients have a difficult time maintaining their intravascular volume status. Dietary recommendations should include increased fluids. As mentioned above, dehydration may lead to uterine contractions, possibly secondary to cross-reaction of vasopressin with oxytocin receptors.

EDEMA

Compression of the inferior vena cava (IVC) and pelvic veins by the uterus can lead to increased hydrostatic pressure in the lower extremities and eventually to edema in the feet and ankles. Elevation of the lower extremities above the heart can ease this. Also, patients should be advised to sleep on their sides to decrease compression. Severe edema of the face and hands may be indicative of preeclampsia and merits further evaluation.

GASTROESOPHAGEAL REFLUX DISEASE

Relaxation of the lower esophageal sphincter and increased transit time in the stomach can lead to reflux and nausea. Patients with reflux should be started on antacids, advised to eat multiple small meals per day, and should avoid lying down within an hour of eating. For patients with continued symptoms, H_2 blockers or proton pump inhibitors can be given.

HEMORRHOIDS

Patients will have increased venous stasis and IVC compression, leading to congestion in the venous system. Congestion of the pelvic vessels combined with increased abdominal pressure with bowel movements secondary to constipation can lead to hemorrhoids. Hemorrhoids are treated symptomatically with topical anesthetics and steroids for pain and swelling. Prevention of constipation with increased fluids, increased fiber in the diet, and stool softeners may prevent or decrease the exacerbation of hemorrhoids.

PICA

Rarely, a patient will have cravings for inedible items such as dirt or clay. As long as these substances are nontoxic, the patient is advised to maintain adequate nutrition and encouraged to stop ingesting the inedible items. However, if the patient has been consuming toxic substances, immediate cessation along with a toxicology consult is advised.

ROUND LIGAMENT PAIN

Usually late in the second trimester or early in the third trimester, there may be some pain in the adnexa or lower abdomen. This pain is likely secondary to the rapid expansion of the uterus and stretching of the ligamentous attachments, such as the round ligaments. This is often self-limited but may be relieved with warm compresses or acetaminophen.

URINARY FREQUENCY

Increased intravascular volumes and elevated GFR can lead to increased urine production during pregnancy. However, the most likely cause of urinary frequency during pregnancy is increasing compression of the bladder by the growing uterus. A UTI may also be present with isolated urinary frequency but is often accompanied by dysuria. A urinalysis and culture should therefore be ordered to rule out infection. If no infection is present, patients can be assured that the increased voiding is normal. Patients should be advised to keep up PO hydration despite urinary frequency.

VARICOSE VEINS

The lower extremities or the vulva may develop varicosities during pregnancy. The relaxation of the venous smooth muscle and increased intravascular pressure, probably both, contribute to the pathogenesis. Elevation of the lower extremities or the use of pressure stockings may help reduce existing varicosities and prevent more from developing. If the problem does not resolve by 6 months' postpartum, patients may be referred for surgical therapy.

PRENATAL ASSESSMENT OF THE FETUS

Throughout pregnancy, the fetus is screened and diagnosed by a variety of modalities. Parents can be screened for common diseases such as cystic fibrosis, Tay-Sachs disease, sickle cell disease, and thalassemia. If both parents are carriers of recessive genetic diseases, the fetus can then be diagnosed. Fetal karyotype and genetic screens can be obtained via amniocentesis or chorionic villus sampling (CVS). The fetus can be imaged and many of the congenital anomalies diagnosed via second-trimester ultrasound. First- and second-trimester genetic screening and prenatal diagnosis is discussed further in Chapter 3. Other fetal testing includes fetal blood sampling, fetal lung maturity testing, and assessment of fetal well-being.

ULTRASOUND

Ultrasound can be used to date a pregnancy with an unknown or uncertain LMP and is most accurate in the first trimester. To detect fetal malformations, most patients undergo a routine screening ultrasound at 18 to 20 weeks. Routinely, an attempt is made to identify placental location, amniotic fluid volume, GA, and any obvious malformations. Of note, most patients will think of this ultrasound as the time to find out the fetal sex. While determination of fetal sex is medically indicated in some settings (e.g., history of fragile X syndrome or other X-linked disorders), it is not necessarily a part of the routine level I obstetric ultrasound. It is useful to clarify this point with patients to establish proper expectations for the ultrasound.

In high-risk patients, careful attention is paid to commonly associated anomalies such as cardiac anomalies in pregestational diabetics. Fetal echocardiography and, rarely, MRI are used to augment assessment of the FH and brain, respectively.

In the third trimester, ultrasound can be used to monitor high-risk pregnancies by obtaining **biophysical profiles** (BPP), fetal growth, and fetal Doppler studies. The BPP looks at five categories and gives a score of either 0 or 2 for each: amniotic fluid volume, fetal tone, fetal activity, fetal breathing movements, and the **nonstress test** (NST), which is a test of the FHR. A BPP of 8 to 10 or better is reassuring. Ultrasound with Doppler flow studies can also be used to assess the blood flow in the umbilical cord. A decrease, absence, or reversal of diastolic flow in the umbilical artery is progressively more worrisome for placental insufficiency and resultant fetal compromise.

ANTENATAL TESTING OF FETAL WELL-BEING

Formal antenatal testing includes the NST, the oxytocin challenge test (OCT), and the BPP. The NST is considered formally reactive (a reassuring sign) if there are two accelerations of the FHR in 20 minutes that are at least 15 beats above the baseline heart rate and last for at least 15 seconds. An OCT or contraction stress test (CST) is obtained by getting at least three contractions in 10 minutes and analyzing the FHR tracing during that time. The reactivity criteria are the same as for the NST. In addition, late decelerations with at least half of the contractions constitute a positive test and are worrisome. Commonly, most antenatal testing units use the NST beginning at 32 to 34 weeks of gestation in high-risk pregnancies and at 40 to 41 weeks for undelivered patients. If the NST is nonreactive, the fetus is assessed via ultrasound. If the FH tracing has any worrisome decelerations or the BPP is not reassuring, an OCT is usually performed or, in more severe cases, consideration is given to delivery.

FETAL BLOOD SAMPLING

Percutaneous umbilical blood sampling (PUBS) is performed by placing a needle transabdominally into the uterus and phlebotomizing the umbilical cord. This procedure may be used when the fetal hematocrit needs to be obtained, particularly in the setting of Rh isoimmunization, other causes of fetal anemia, and hydrops. PUBS is also used for fetal transfusion, karyotype analysis, and assessment of fetal platelet count in alloimmune thrombocytopenia.

FETAL LUNG MATURITY

To test for fetal lung maturity, an amniotic fluid sample obtained through amniocentesis is analyzed. Classically, the lecithin to sphingomyelin (L/S) ratio has been used as a predictor of fetal lung maturity. Type II pneumocytes secrete a surfactant that uses phospholipids in its synthesis. Commonly, lecithin increases as the lungs mature, whereas sphingomyelin decreases beyond about 32 weeks. The L/S ratio should therefore increase as the pregnancy progresses. Repetitive studies have shown that an L/S ratio of greater than 2 is associated with only rare cases of **respiratory distress syndrome** (RDS). Examples of other fetal lung maturity tests include measuring the levels of phosphatidylglycerol (PG), saturated phosphatidyl choline (SPC), the presence of lamellar body count, and surfactant to albumin ratio (S/A).

KEY POINTS

- A urine pregnancy test will often be positive at the time of the missed menstrual cycle.
- Physiologic changes during pregnancy, mediated by the placental hormones, affect every organ system.
- Cardiovascular changes include a decrease in systemic vascular resistance and blood pressure and an increase in cardiac output.
- The initial prenatal visit is designed to screen for many of the problems that can occur in pregnancy and to verify dating of the pregnancy.
- Much of the screening for genetic and congenital abnormalities is performed in the second trimester.
- Blood pressure, weight gain, fundal height, FHR, and symptoms including contractions, vaginal bleeding or discharge, and perceived fetal movement are assessed at each prenatal visit.
- Many of the routine problems of pregnancy are related to hormonal effects of the placenta.
- It is important to discuss the side effects of pregnancy in order to best prepare the patient.
- Although pregnancy is often the cause of many somatic complaints, other causes should still be ruled out as in a nonpregnant patient.
- Common screening tests for fetal abnormalities include MSAFP and the triple screen.
- The fetus may be diagnosed for abnormalities, using amniocentesis, CVS, and ultrasound.
- Fetal status can be assessed antepartum with ultrasound, NST, BPP, and OCT.

C Clinical Vignettes

Vignette 1

A 27-year-old woman comes to your practice desiring pregnancy. She has a history of regular, 28-day cycles and has been using oral birth control pills for contraception. She has had two pregnancies in the past, one ending in miscarriage at 9 weeks and one vaginal delivery at 39 weeks. Her last Pap smear was 10 months ago and she has never had an irregular Pap. She is not taking any medications and has no known medical allergies.

1. On the basis of this woman's obstetrical history, find out what is her TPAL designation?
   a. G3P1011
   b. G3P2001
   c. G2P1011
   d. G2P1101
   e. G1P1001

2. Nutritional supplements she should begin before she gets pregnant include which of the following:
   a. Folate to reduce neural tube defects
   b. Vitamin B_{12} to increase RBC production prior to pregnancy
   c. Vitamin B_1 to reduce beriberi
   d. Vitamin C to reduce scurvy
   e. No supplementation is necessary until pregnancy is confirmed

3. Before leaving your office, she asks how reliable over-the-counter (OTC) pregnancy tests are and how quickly after conceiving she should expect to test positive. You inform her that:
   a. urine pregnancy tests are notoriously unreliable and that she should come in for blood tests if she thinks she is pregnant
   b. OTC tests have high sensitivity for human placental lactogen (hPL) and will be positive around the time of the missed menstrual cycle
   c. OTC tests have high sensitivity for β-hCG and will be positive around the time of the missed period
   d. OTC tests have high specificity, but low sensitivity, so she should repeat the test twice at home to confirm the results
   e. OTC tests are typically positive the day after conception

4. She returns to your office 2 months later pregnant. Her initial prenatal visit should include:
   a. quad screen
   b. abdominal ultrasound
   c. pelvic examination
   d. titer for herpes simplex virus (HSV)
   e. Leopold maneuvers

Vignette 2

A 33-year-old G0P0 woman comes to your office for her initial prenatal visit. She tested positive with two home pregnancy tests and has been experiencing breast tenderness and mild nausea for a few weeks. She has a history of regular menstrual periods occurring every 28 to 30 days. This was a planned pregnancy and is the first child for her and for her partner.

1. Your patient was actively tracking her menstrual cycle and is certain that the first day of her last menstrual period (LMP) was 12/2/11. Using Nägele rule, estimate her date of delivery.
   a. 7/5/12
   b. 9/2/12
   c. 9/16/12
   d. 9/9/12
   e. 8/26/12

2. As her pregnancy continues, you would expect her cardiac output to increase by which of the following mechanisms:
   a. First an increase in stroke volume, then an increase in heart rate
   b. A decrease in systemic vascular resistance
   c. Cardiac output would not change significantly until the third trimester
   d. An increase in systemic vascular resistance facilitated by elevated progesterone levels
   e. Increased heart rate alone

3. Which of the following is true regarding the physiologic changes she might expect during her pregnancy?
   a. Gastric emptying and large bowel motility are increased in pregnancy
   b. BUN and creatinine will decrease by 25% as a result of an increase in glomerular filtration rate (GFR), which will be maintained until delivery
   c. An overall decrease in the number of WBC and platelets
   d. Nausea and vomiting that should be treated aggressively with antiemetics and intravenous hydration
   e. An increase in the tidal volume along with an increase in total lung capacity (TLC)

4. Which of the following is true regarding hCG in your patient?
   a. The corpus luteum produces hCG throughout pregnancy
   b. It is composed of two dissimilar alpha and beta units
   c. Levels double every 3 to 4 days in early pregnancy

d. Levels peak after 24 weeks of pregnancy
e. The alpha subunits are identical to subunits of prolactin and human growth hormone

5. The major function of human placental lactogen is:
a. To cause a diuretic effect
b. To cause relaxation of smooth muscle
c. To maintain the corpus luteum in early pregnancy
d. To act as an insulin agonist
e. To induce lipolysis and protein synthesis leading to a constant nutrient supply to the fetus

Vignette 3

A 36-year-old G1P0 is 31 weeks and 5 days by LMP and is sure of her dates. Her pregnancy has been complicated by persistent nausea and vomiting, back pain, and lower extremity swelling. She comes to you for a routine prenatal visit. She had a quad screen at 16 weeks that was normal. She is having a girl.

1. On this visit her urine is assessed for the presence of protein, glucose, blood, and leukocyte esterase. Which of the following results would be most concerning?
a. Absent leukocyte esterase
b. Negative glucose
c. Trace blood
d. 4+ protein
e. Leukocyte esterase positive

2. Her low back pain is no longer relieved with a heating pad and she finds that she needs pain relief to make it through each work day. Which of the following options would be safest for her?
a. Ibuprofen
b. Aspirin
c. Oxycodone
d. Flexeril
e. Tylenol

3. Her nausea and vomiting has extended past the first trimester when most women stop experiencing these symptoms. What would suggest that she has hyperemesis gravidarum?
a. Less than 5% loss of prepregnancy weight
b. Jaundice
c. Syncopal episodes
d. Ketonuria
e. Metabolic acidosis

4. She has started experiencing lower abdominal pain and tightening that occurs infrequently (1 to 2 times per hour) and irregularly. This is most likely:
a. a preterm labor
b. round ligament pain
c. Braxton Hicks contractions
d. an indication of fetal distress
e. related to constipation

Vignette 4

A G3P2002 woman at 35 weeks is seen in your office for her prenatal visit. She is concerned because she has not felt her baby moving as much as she used to. Her pregnancy has been uncomplicated and her past two pregnancies ended in full term, normal spontaneous vaginal deliveries.

1. A biophysical profile (BPP) is done to assess which of the following?
a. Diastolic flow in the umbilical artery
b. Lung maturity
c. Blood flow in the middle cerebral artery
d. Fetal well-being
e. Genetic abnormalities

2. An indication for early delivery is identified, but first a test for fetal lung maturity is done. Which of the following is true?
a. Type I pneumocytes secrete surfactant
b. A lecithin to sphingomyelin (L/S) ratio greater than 2 is ideal if an early delivery is indicated
c. A low L/S ratio is associated with fewer cases of respiratory distress syndrome (RDS)
d. Typically, lecithin decreases as the lung matures
e. Sphingomyelin decreases beyond 24 weeks

3. When formal antenatal testing is done, which of the following is most reassuring?
a. Late decelerations on fetal monitoring
b. A contraction stress test (CST) with variable fetal heart rate (FHR) decelerations with contractions, but moderate variability
c. A nonstress test (NST) with two accelerations of the FHR in 20 minutes that are at least 15 beats above baseline and last for at least 15 seconds
d. An increase in the systolic to diastolic ratio in the umbilical artery blood flow
e. A score of 6 on a BPP

A Answers

Vignette 1 Question 1
Answer C: TPAL designation is written in the following order to reflect the total number of pregnancies: term deliveries, preterm deliveries, abortions including all pregnancy losses prior to 20 weeks, and living children. She has been pregnant twice (G2) and had one term delivery leading to one living child and one spontaneous miscarriage prior to 20 weeks. Although she desires pregnancy, she is not yet pregnant, and so G3 is not correct.

Vignette 1 Question 2
Answer: A Women can reduce the risk of neural tube defects by taking 400 μg folic acid supplements the month before conception and during the first trimester. The other supplements would not harm, but are not routinely recommended in the time before conception.

Vignette 1 Question 3
Answer C Many OTC pregnancy tests have improved in recent decades. These are highly sensitive for urine β-hCG and are typically positive around the time of the missed menstrual cycle.

Vignette 1 Question 4
Answer C: A pelvic examination should be conducted, feeling for the size of the uterus, and should include a Pap smear if one has not been done in the past 6 months. Quad screen is done in the second trimester and Leopold maneuvers are done beyond 32 to 34 weeks to determine fetal presentation. HSV treatment or prophylaxis is initiated on the basis of clinical examination or patient history and not laboratory data. Transvaginal ultrasound is typically used to date the pregnancy in initial, first-trimester visits.

Vignette 2 Question 1
Answer D: Nägele rule gives an estimated date of delivery by subtracting 3 months and adding 7 days from the LMP.

Vignette 2 Question 2
Answer A: Cardiac output increases by 30% to 50% during pregnancy as a result of, first, an increase in stroke volume and is then maintained by an increase in heart rate. Progesterone levels lead to a decrease in systemic vascular resistance, resulting in a fall in arterial blood pressure.

Vignette 2 Question 3
Answer B: BUN and creatinine will decrease because of a 50% increase in the GFR, which occurs early in pregnancy. Gastric emptying and large bowel motility are decreased as a result of progesterone, leading to reflux and constipation, respectively. WBCs increase in pregnancy, but an increase in plasma volume results in a decrease in the concentration of both platelets and WBCs. Nausea and vomiting is common in early pregnancy and is most often mild. These symptoms should be treated with frequent snacking and oral hydration, though some patients will require more aggressive treatment. Tidal volume increases, but TLC decreases in pregnancy.

Vignette 2 Question 4
Answer B: The placenta produces hCG. Levels double approximately every 48 hours in early pregnancy and peak at 10 to 12 weeks. The alpha subunits are identical to luteinizing hormone, follicular-stimulating hormone, and thyroid-stimulating hormone.

Vignette 2 Question 5
Answer e: Human placental lactogen (also known as human chorionic somatomammotropin) is an insulin antagonist, and its major function is not a diuretic effect. In its role as an insulin antagonist progesterone causes relaxation of smooth muscle and hCG maintains the corpus luteum in early pregnancy. It contributes to the development of gestational diabetes as well.

Vignette 3 Question 1
Answer D: Leukocyte esterase and trace blood may be indicative of urinary tract infection, which could be complicated by pyelonephritis, but is treatable. Large amounts of blood could be nephrolithiasis, bladder injury, nephritic syndrome, or even cancer. Absent glucose is normal, whereas the presence of glucose may indicate diabetes. Large amounts of protein is concerning for preeclampsia, which demands a broader assessment. While trace or 1+ protein has only a modest positive predictive value, 3+ or 4+ protein has a very high positive predictive value for significant proteinuria and deserves immediate attention.

Vignette 3 Question 2
Answer E: Ibuprofen and aspirin are contraindicated in pregnancy. While NSAIDs are occasionally prescribed in the midtrimester for acute pain, in the latter part of the third trimester, they are absolutely contraindicated as they are associated with premature closure of the ductus arteriosus. Narcotics and muscle relaxants are options for patients with severe back pain, but it would be safest to start with Tylenol and gentle massage.

Vignette 3 Question 3
Answer D: Hyperemesis gravidarum is a severe form of morning sickness in which women lose more than 5% of their prepregnancy weight and go into ketosis. With severe vomiting, a metabolic alkalosis would be expected. Syncopal episodes may occur secondary to dehydration but are not a part of the diagnosis. Jaundice is not associated with hyperemesis gravidarum.

Vignette 3 Question 4

Answer C: Occasional irregular contractions that do not lead to cervical change are considered Braxton Hicks contractions and will occur several times per day up to several times per hour. Patients should be warned about these and reassured that they are normal. However, if contractions are more frequent or painful, the patient should be assessed for preterm labor.

Vignette 4 Question 1

Answer D: A BPP is particularly helpful in monitoring high-risk pregnancies. The BPP assesses fetal well-being using amniotic fluid volume, fetal tone, activity, breathing movements, and a nonstress test receiving either 0 or 2 points for each of the five categories. A score of 8 to 10 is reassuring. A BPP is often done in conjunction with fetal Doppler studies, which assess flow in the umbilical artery. Genetic abnormalities are screened for in the second trimester, using the triple or quad screen. Blood flow in the middle cerebral artery is used when evaluating for fetal anemia in the setting of Rh isoimmunization. Lung maturity is assessed through amniocentesis.

Vignette 4 Question 2

Answer B: An L/S ratio greater than 2 is associated with only rare cases of RDS. Type II pneumocytes secrete surfactant. Lecithin increases as the lung matures and sphingomyelin decreases beyond 32 weeks.

Vignette 4 Question 3

Answer C: This answer describes a formally reactive NST, which is a reassuring sign. On fetal monitoring, late FHR decelerations are concerning for uteroplacental insufficiency. Similarly, on a CST, FHR decelerations with contractions are considered nonreassuring. The fact that the decelerations are variable is a bit less worrisome, but certainly not reassuring. Decreased diastolic flow in the umbilical artery, which leads to an increased systolic to diastolic ratio, is concerning for increased placental resistance. While a 6/10 on a BPP is not particularly worrisome, it is not formally reassuring and demands a plan for further follow up.

Chapter 2 Early Pregnancy Complications

ECTOPIC PREGNANCY

An **ectopic pregnancy** is one that implants outside the uterine cavity. Implantation occurs in the fallopian tube in 95% to 99% of patients (Fig. 2-1). The most common site of implantation in a tubal pregnancy is the ampulla (70%), followed by the isthmus (12%) and fimbriae (11%). Implantation may also occur on the ovary, the cervix, the outside of the fallopian tube, the abdominal wall, or the bowel. The incidence of ectopic pregnancies has been increasing over the past 10 years. Currently, more than 1:100 of all pregnancies are ectopic. This is thought to be secondary to the increase in assisted fertility, sexually transmitted infections (STIs), and pelvic inflammatory disease (PID). Patients who present with vaginal bleeding and/or abdominal pain should always be evaluated for ectopic pregnancy because a ruptured ectopic pregnancy is a true emergency. It can result in rapid hemorrhage, leading to shock and eventually death. While early diagnosis and treatment of this condition has dramatically decreased the mortality risk, ruptured ectopic pregnancies are still responsible for 6% of all maternal deaths in the US. (*NEJM*. 2009;361:379–387.)

RISK FACTORS

Several risk factors predispose patients to extrauterine implantation (Table 2-1). Many of the risk factors commonly affect the fallopian tubes causing either tubal scarring or decreased peristalsis of the tube which may lead to abnormal implantation of a pregnancy. One of the strongest risk factors is prior ectopic pregnancy. The risk of a subsequent ectopic pregnancy is 10% after one prior ectopic pregnancy and increases to 25% after more than one prior ectopic pregnancy. (*NEJM*. 2009;361:379–387.) It has been noted that there is an increased risk (up to 1.8%) of ectopic implantation in pregnancies produced by assisted reproductive technology (ART). Whether this is due primarily to the techniques utilized or the underlying tubal disease and pelvic adhesions in such patients is unclear. While use of an intrauterine device (IUD) for birth control decreases the overall rate of pregnancy, in case the contraceptive fails, there is an increased rate of ectopic pregnancy in those women who become pregnant because the IUD prevents normal intrauterine implantation. This risk may be as high as 25% to 50%. (*NEJM*. 2009;361:379–387.)

DIAGNOSIS

The diagnosis of ectopic pregnancy is made by history, physical examination, laboratory tests, and ultrasound. On history, patients often complain of unilateral pelvic or lower abdominal pain and vaginal bleeding. Physical examination, including speculum and bimanual examination, may reveal an adnexal mass that is often tender, a uterus that is small for gestational age, and bleeding from the cervix. Patients with ruptured ectopic pregnancies may be hypotensive, tachycardic, unresponsive, or show signs of peritoneal irritation secondary to hemoperitoneum. Importantly, however, because many women with ectopic pregnancies are young and otherwise healthy, such signs of intra-abdominal hemorrhage may not occur until the patient has lost a large amount of blood.

On laboratory studies, the classic finding is a beta human chorionic gonadotropin (β-hCG) level that is low for gestational age and does not increase at the expected rate. In patients with a normal **intrauterine pregnancy** (IUP), the trophoblastic tissue secretes β-hCG in a predictable manner that should lead to doubling (or at least an increase of two-third or more) approximately every 48 hours. An ectopic pregnancy has a poorly implanted placenta with less blood supply than in the endometrium, thus levels of β-hCG do not double every 48 hours. The hematocrit may be low or may drop in patients with ruptured ectopic pregnancies.

Ultrasound may reveal an adnexal mass or an extrauterine pregnancy (Fig. 2-2). A gestational sac with a yolk sac seen in the uterus on ultrasound indicates an IUP. However, there is always a small risk of **heterotopic pregnancy**, a multiple gestation with at least one IUP and at least one ectopic pregnancy. This is of particular concern in the setting of IVF pregnancies when more than one embryo is transferred. At early gestations, neither an IUP nor an adnexal mass can be seen on ultrasound. A hemorrhaging, ruptured ectopic pregnancy may reveal intra-abdominal fluid throughout the pelvis and abdomen.

Patients who cannot be definitively diagnosed with an ectopic versus an IUP are labeled rule-out ectopic. If such patients are stable on examination, they may be followed with serial β-hCG levels every 48 hours. β-hCG levels that do not double (or increase by at least two-third) every 48 hours might indicate ectopic pregnancy. As a guideline, an IUP should be seen on transvaginal ultrasonography with β-hCG levels between 1,500 and 2,000 mIU/mL. A fetal heartbeat should be seen with β-hCG level greater than 5,000 mIU/mL.

TREATMENT

If a patient presents with a ruptured ectopic pregnancy and is unstable, the first priority is to stabilize with intravenous fluids, blood products, and vasopressor medications if necessary. The patient should then be taken to the operating room where exploratory laparotomy can be performed to stop the bleeding and remove the ectopic pregnancy. If the patient is stable with a likely ruptured ectopic pregnancy, the procedure of choice at many institutions is an exploratory laparoscopy, which can be performed to evacuate the hemoperitoneum, coagulate any ongoing bleeding, and resect the ectopic pregnancy. Resection can be either through a salpingostomy where the ectopic

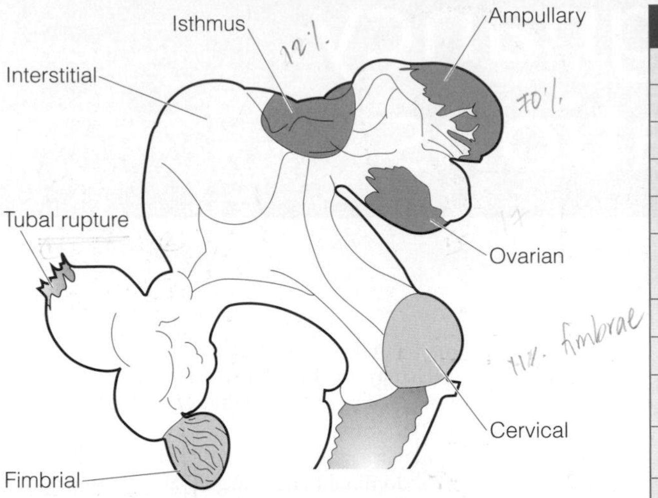

Figure 2-1 • Sites of ectopic pregnancies.

TABLE 2-1 Risk Factors for Ectopic Pregnancy
History of STIs or PID
Prior ectopic pregnancy
Previous tubal surgery
Prior pelvic or abdominal surgery resulting in adhesions
Endometriosis
Current use of exogenous hormones including progesterone or estrogen
IVF and other assisted reproduction
DES-exposed patients with congenital abnormalities
Congenital abnormalities of the fallopian tubes
Use of an IUD for birth control
Smoking

pregnancy is removed leaving the fallopian tube in place or a salpingectomy where the entire ectopic pregnancy is removed. In the rare case of a cornual (or interstitial) ectopic pregnancy, a cornual resection can be performed.

Patients who present with an unruptured ectopic pregnancy can be treated either surgically (as described above) or medically. At most institutions, clinicians prescribe **methotrexate** in order to treat uncomplicated, nonthreatening, ectopic pregnancies. It is appropriate to use methotrexate for patients who have small ectopic pregnancies (as a general rule, <4 cm, serum β-hCG level <5,000, and without a fetal heartbeat) and for those patients who will be reliable with follow-up. Of note, ectopic pregnancies outside of these parameters have also been treated with methotrexate, but the failure risks are higher, and such patients deserve careful attention and follow-up.

Care of such women involves assessment of baseline transaminases and creatinine, intramuscular methotrexate, and serially following the β-hCG levels. Both single- and multidose methotrexate regimens are available. A single-dose regimen most commonly uses a 50 mg/m^2 dose of intramuscular methotrexate and requires fewer clinic or emergency department visits. However, the success rate is slightly lower with a single- versus a multidose regimen (93% vs. 88% respectively). Commonly, the β-hCG level will rise the first few days after methotrexate therapy, but should fall by 10% to 15% between days 4 and 7 of the treatment. If β-hCG does not fall to these levels, the patient requires a second dosage of methotrexate. Additionally, these women should be monitored for signs and symptoms of rupture—increased abdominal pain, bleeding, or signs of shock—and advised to come to the emergency department immediately in case of such symptoms.

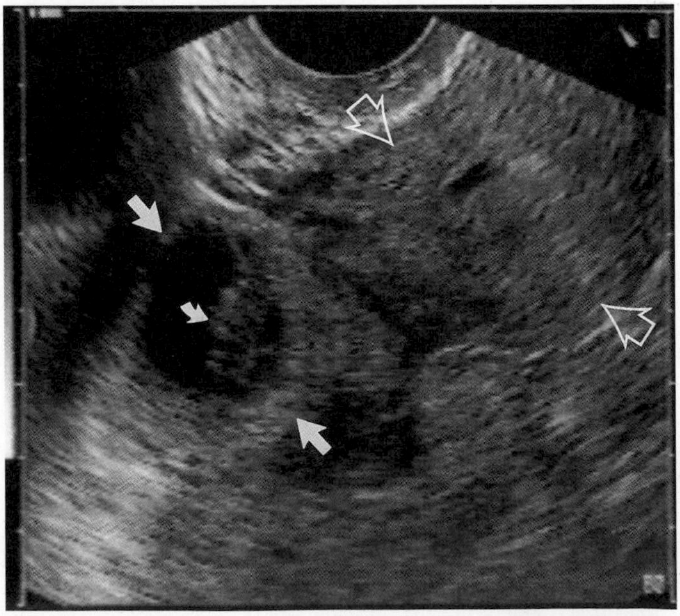

Figure 2-2 • Endovaginal view of a right adnexal ectopic pregnancy with a gestational sac (*large arrows*) and fetal pole (*small arrow*). The uterus is seen to the right of the image, with a small amount of endometrial fluid (*hollow arrows*).

SPONTANEOUS ABORTION

A **spontaneous abortion (SAB)**, or miscarriage, is a pregnancy that ends before 20 weeks' gestation. SABs are estimated to occur in 15% to 25% of all pregnancies. This number may be even higher because losses that occur at 4 to 6 weeks' gestational age are often confused with late menses. The type of SAB is defined by whether any or all of the **products of conception** (POC) have passed and whether or not the cervix is dilated. Definitions are as follows:

- **Abortus**—fetus lost before 20 weeks' gestation or less than 500 g
- **Complete abortion**—complete expulsion of all POC before 20 weeks' gestation (Fig. 2-3).
- **Incomplete abortion**—partial expulsion of some but not all POC before 20 weeks' gestation.
- **Inevitable abortion**—no expulsion of products, but vaginal bleeding and dilation of the cervix such that a viable pregnancy is unlikely.
- **Threatened abortion**—any vaginal bleeding before 20 weeks, without dilation of the cervix or expulsion of any POC (i.e., a normal pregnancy with bleeding).
- **Missed abortion**—death of the embryo or fetus before 20 weeks with complete retention of all POC.

FIRST-TRIMESTER ABORTIONS

It is estimated that 60% to 80% of all SABs in the first trimester are associated with abnormal chromosomes, of which 95% are due to errors in maternal gametogenesis. In these 95%, autosomal trisomy is the most common chromosomal abnormality. Other factors associated with SABs include infections, maternal anatomic defects, immunologic factors, environmental exposures, and endocrine factors. A large number of first-trimester abortions have no obvious cause.

DIAGNOSIS

Most patients present with bleeding from the vagina (Table 2-2). Other findings include cramping, abdominal pain, and decreased symptoms of pregnancy. The physical examination should include vital signs to rule out shock and febrile illness. A pelvic examination can be performed to look for sources of bleeding other than uterine and for changes in the cervix suggestive of an inevitable abortion. The laboratory tests to be ordered include a quantitative level of β-hCG, complete blood cell count (CBC), blood type, and antibody screen. An ultrasound can assess fetal viability and placentation. As ectopic pregnancies can also present with vaginal bleeding, this must also be considered in the differential diagnosis.

TREATMENT

The treatment plan is based on specific diagnosis and on the decisions made by the patient and her caregivers. Initially, all pregnant and bleeding patients need to be stabilized if hypotensive. A complete abortion can be followed for recurrent bleeding and signs of infection such as elevated temperature. Any tissue that the patient may have passed at home and at the hospital may be sent to pathology, both to assess that POC have passed and for chromosome analysis if applicable.

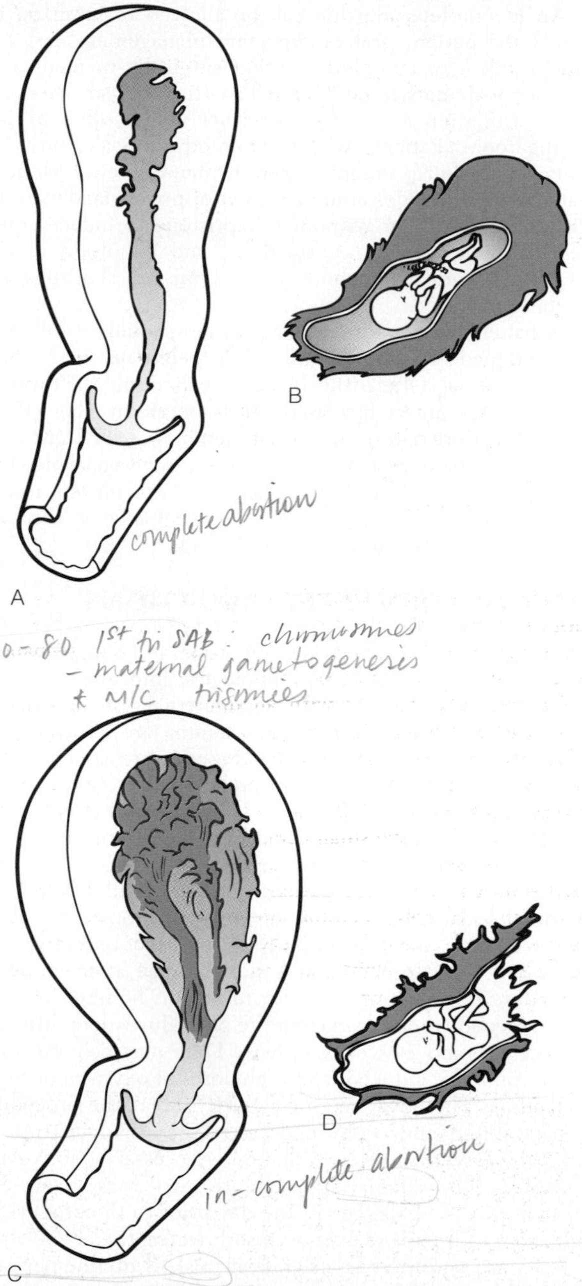

Figure 2-3 • **(A)** Complete abortion. **(B)** Product of complete abortion. **(C)** Incomplete abortion. **(D)** Product of incomplete abortion.

TABLE 2-2 Differential Diagnosis of First-Trimester Bleeding
SAB
Postcoital bleeding
Ectopic pregnancy
Vaginal or cervical lesions or lacerations
Extrusion of molar pregnancy
Nonpregnancy causes of bleeding

An incomplete abortion can be allowed to finish on its own if the patient prefers expectant management, but can also be taken to completion either surgically or medically. The surgical management of a first-trimester abortion requires a dilation and curettage either in the office or operating room. Patients who are hemodynamically unstable generally require urgent surgical management. Medical management includes administration of prostaglandins (e.g., misoprostol) with or without mifepristone to induce cervical dilatation, uterine contractions, and expulsion of the pregnancy. Inevitable abortions and missed abortions are similarly managed.

A patient with a threatened abortion should be followed for continued bleeding and placed on pelvic rest with nothing per vagina. Often, the bleeding will resolve. However, these patients are at increased risk for preterm labor (PTL) and preterm premature rupture of membranes (PPROM). All Rh-negative pregnant women who experience vaginal bleeding during pregnancy should receive RhoGAM to prevent isoimmunization. Finally, all patients who experience an abortion should be offered contraception if desired.

SECOND-TRIMESTER ABORTIONS

Second-trimester abortions (i.e., abortion at 12 to 20 weeks' gestational age) have multiple etiologies. Infection, maternal uterine or cervical anatomic defects, maternal systemic disease, exposure to fetotoxic agents, and trauma are all associated with late abortions. Abnormal chromosomes are not a frequent cause of late abortions. Late second-trimester abortions and periviable deliveries are also seen with PTL and incompetent cervix. As in first-trimester abortions, the treatment plan is based on the specific clinical scenario.

Incomplete and missed abortions can be allowed to finish on their own, but are often taken to completion with a D&E (dilation and evacuation). The distinction between a D&C and D&E depends on gestational age at the time of procedure (i.e., first or second trimester). The fetus is larger in the second trimester making the procedure more difficult. Between 16 and 24 weeks, either a D&E may be performed or labor may be induced with high doses of oxytocin or prostaglandins. The advantage of a D&E is that the procedure is self-limited and performed faster than an induction of labor. However, aggressive dilation is necessary prior to the procedure with laminaria (which are small rods of seaweed that are placed in the cervix the day prior to the procedure, and these rods expand as they absorb water, thereby dilating the cervix), and there is a significant risk of uterine perforation and cervical lacerations. An induction of labor can take longer, but allows completion of the abortion without the inherent risks of instrumentation. An induction of labor also allows for the possibility of an external genetics examination or autopsy of the POC. Patient preference as well as the capabilities of the facility should be considered when choosing medical or surgical options. With either method, great care should be taken to ensure the complete evacuation of all POC.

In the second trimester, the diagnoses of PTL and incompetent cervix need to be ruled out. Particularly in the setting of inevitable abortions or threatened abortions, the etiology is likely to be related to the inability of the uterus to maintain the pregnancy. PTL begins with contractions leading to cervical change, whereas an incompetent cervix is characterized by painless dilation of the cervix. In the case of an incompetent cervix, an emergent cerclage may be offered. PTL can potentially be managed with tocolysis.

INCOMPETENT CERVIX

Patients with an **incompetent cervix** or cervical insufficiency present with painless dilation and effacement of the cervix, often in the second trimester of pregnancy. As the cervix dilates, the fetal membranes are exposed to vaginal flora and risk of increased trauma. Thus, infection, vaginal discharge, and rupture of the membranes are common findings in the setting of incompetent cervix. Patients may also present with short-term cramping or contracting, leading to advancing cervical dilation or pressure in the vagina with the chorionic and amniotic sacs bulging through the cervix. Cervical incompetence is estimated to cause approximately 15% of all second-trimester losses.

RISK FACTORS

Surgery or other cervical trauma is the most common cause of cervical incompetence (Table 2-3). Causes of cervical trauma might include dilation and curettage, loop electrocautery excisional procedure (LEEP), or cervical conization. The other possible cause is a congenital abnormality of the cervix that can sometimes be attributed to diethylstilbestrol (DES) exposure in utero. However, many patients who present with cervical incompetence have no known risk factors.

DIAGNOSIS

Patients with incompetent cervix often present with a dilated cervix noted on routine examination, ultrasound, or in the setting of bleeding, vaginal discharge, or rupture of membranes. Occasionally, patients experience mild cramping or pressure in the lower abdomen or vagina. On examination, the cervix is dilated more than expected with the level of contractions experienced. It is often difficult to differentiate between incompetent cervix and PTL. However, patients who present with mild cramping and have advancing cervical dilation on serial examinations and/or an amniotic sac bulging through the cervix (Fig. 2-4) are more likely to have an incompetent cervix, with the cramping being instigated by the dilated cervix and exposed membranes rather than the contractions/cramping leading to cervical change as in the case of PTL.

TREATMENT

Individual obstetric issues should be treated accordingly. If the fetus is previable (i.e., <24 weeks' gestational age), expectant

TABLE 2-3 Risk Factors for Cervical Incompetence

History of cervical surgery, such as a cone biopsy or dilation of the cervix
History of cervical lacerations with vaginal delivery
Uterine anomalies
History of DES exposure

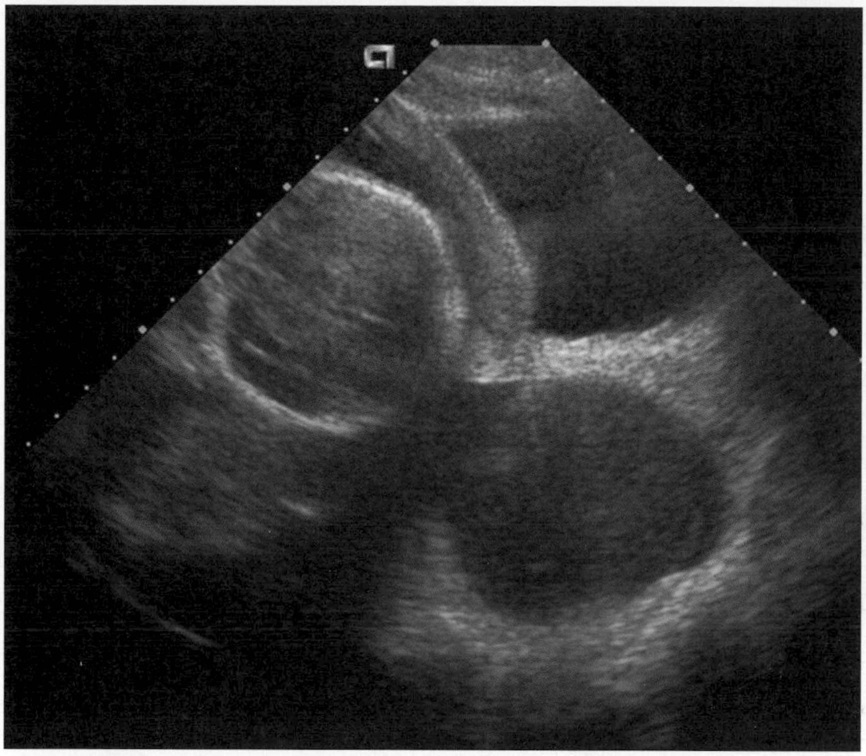

Figure 2-4 • Hourglass membranes.

management and elective termination are options. Patients with viable pregnancies are treated with betamethasone to decrease the risk of prematurity and are managed expectantly with strict bed rest. If there is a component of preterm contractions or PTL, tocolysis may be used with viable pregnancies.

One alternative course of management for incompetent cervix in a previable pregnancy is the placement of an emergent **cerclage**. The cerclage is a suture placed vaginally around the cervix either at the cervical–vaginal junction (McDonald cerclage) or at the internal os (Shirodkar cerclage). The intent of a cerclage is to close the cervix. Complications include rupture of membranes, PTL, and infection.

If incompetent cervix was the suspected diagnosis in a previous pregnancy, the patient is usually offered an elective cerclage with subsequent pregnancies (Fig. 2-5). Placement of the elective cerclage is similar to that of the emergent cerclage (with either the McDonald or Shirodkar methods being used), usually at 12 to 14 weeks' gestation. The cerclage is maintained until 36 to 38 weeks of gestation if possible. At that point it is removed and the patient is followed expectantly until labor ensues. Both types of prophylactic cerclage are associated with 85% to 90% successful pregnancy rate. In patients for whom one or both of the vaginal cerclages have failed, a transabdominal cerclage (TAC) is often the next management offered. This is placed around the cervix at the level of the internal os during a laparotomy. This can be placed electively either prior to the pregnancy or at 12 to 14 weeks. Patients with a TAC need to be delivered via cesarean section.

RECURRENT PREGNANCY LOSS

A recurrent or habitual aborter is a woman who has had three or more consecutive SABs. Less than 1% of the population is diagnosed with **recurrent pregnancy loss**. The risk of an SAB after one prior SAB is 20% to 25%; after two consecutive SABs, 25% to 30%; and after three consecutive SABs, 30% to 35%.

PATHOGENESIS

The etiologies of recurrent pregnancy loss are generally similar to those of SABs. These include chromosomal abnormalities, maternal systemic disease, maternal anatomic defects, and infection. Fifteen percent of patients with recurrent pregnancy loss have **antiphospholipid antibody** (APA) **syndrome**. Another group of patients are thought to have a **luteal phase defect** and lack an adequate level of progesterone to maintain the pregnancy.

DIAGNOSIS

Patients who are habitual aborters should be evaluated for the etiology. Patients with only two consecutive SABs are occasionally assessed as well, particularly those with advancing maternal age or for whom continued fertility may be an issue. Patients are often screened in the following manner. First, a karyotype of both parents is obtained, as well as the karyotypes of the POC from each of the SABs if possible. Of note, often obtaining a karyotype from the aborted tissue is impossible; new technology, particularly array complete

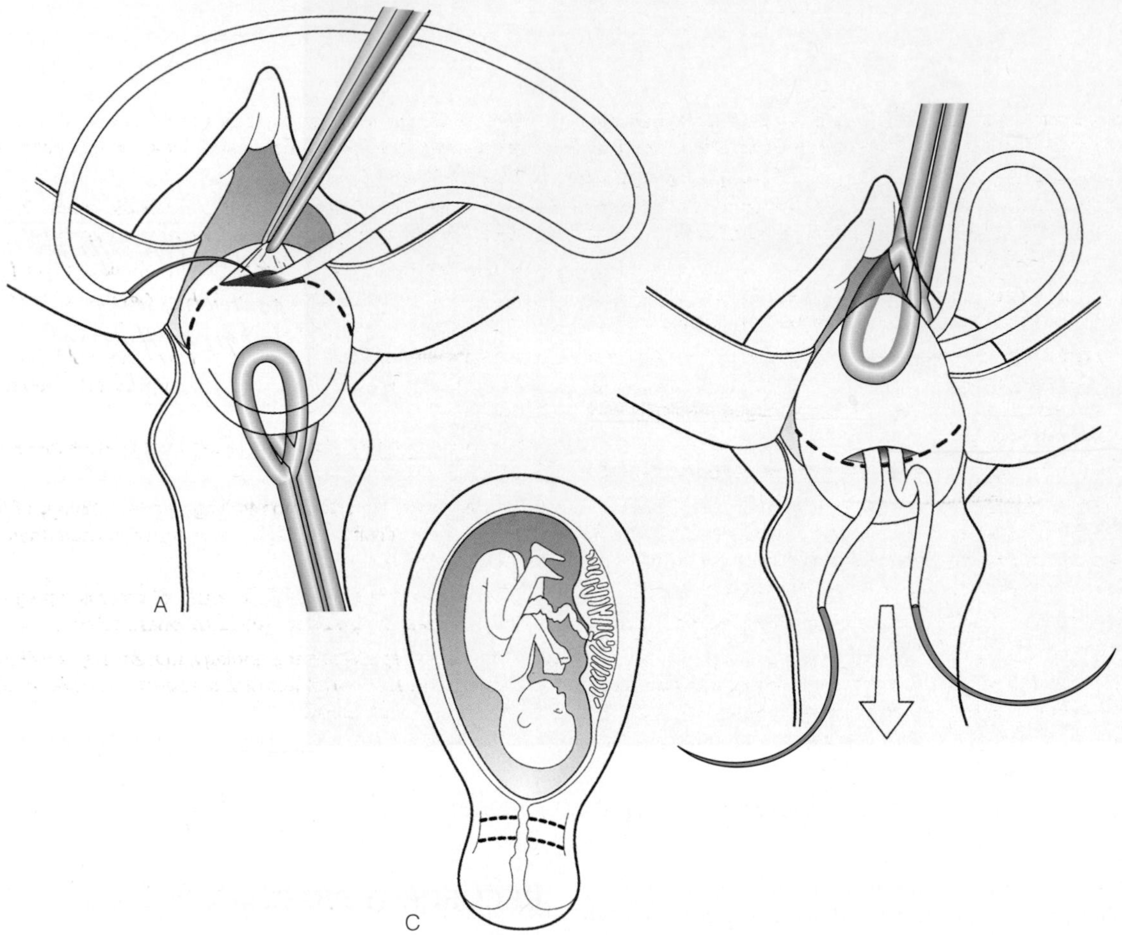

Figure 2-5 • Cervical cerclage (Shirodkar) for incompetent cervix in pregnant patient. **(A)** Placement of the suture. **(B)** Cinching the suture down to tie the knot posteriorly. **(C)** The tightened cerclage almost at the internal os.

genome hybridization (CGH) can be used to identify chromosomal abnormalities as well with much more success. Second, maternal anatomy should be examined, initially with a hysterosalpingogram (HSG). If the HSG is abnormal or nondiagnostic, a hysteroscopic or laparoscopic exploration may be performed. Third, screening tests for hypothyroidism, diabetes mellitus, APA syndrome, hypercoagulability, and systemic lupus erythematosus (SLE) should be performed. These tests should include lupus anticoagulant, factor V Leiden deficiency, prothrombin G20210A mutation, ANA, anticardiolipin antibody, Russell viper venom, antithrombin III, protein S, and protein C. Fourth, a level of serum progesterone should be obtained in the luteal phase of the menstrual cycle. Finally, cultures of the cervix, vagina, and endometrium can be taken to rule out infection. An endometrial biopsy can be done during the luteal phase as well to look for proliferative endometrium.

TREATMENT

Treatment of patients with recurrent pregnancy loss depends on the etiology of the SABs. For many (approximately 30% to 50%), no etiology is ever found. For others, the etiology itself needs to be diagnosed (as described above) and can often be treated on an individual basis. For patients with chromosomal abnormalities such as balanced translocations, IVF can be performed using donor sperm or ova. More recently, such patients may undergo preimplantation diagnosis (PGD) in order to maximize fertilization with their own normal chromosomes. This is where one cell of an embryo harvested through IVF is removed and karyotyped so that abnormal embryos are not implanted. Anatomic abnormalities may or may not be correctable. If incompetent cervix is suspected, a cerclage may be placed. If a luteal phase defect is suspected, progesterone may be given. Patients with APA syndrome are treated with low-dose aspirin. In the presence of a thrombophilia, SQ heparin (either low molecular weight or unfractionated) may be used. Maternal diseases should be treated with the appropriate therapy (e.g., hypothyroidism with thyroid hormone, infection with antibiotics). However, with some systemic diseases, treatment may not decrease the risk of SAB. Because even patients with three prior consecutive SABs will have a subsequent normal pregnancy two-thirds of the time, it is difficult to estimate whether certain treatments of recurrent abortions are effective.

KEY POINTS

- Approximately 1% of pregnancies are ectopic; that is, implantation of the pregnancy has occurred outside the uterine cavity.
- Initially, when a pregnant woman presents with vaginal bleeding and abdominal pain, an ectopic pregnancy must be ruled out or diagnosed with physical examination, laboratory assessment, and pelvic ultrasound.
- β-hCG levels double approximately every 48 hours in normal intrauterine pregnancies but not in ectopic pregnancies.
- Treatment of ectopic pregnancies is often surgical and includes stabilizing the patient and removing the pregnancy. Stable, unruptured ectopic pregnancies can be managed medically with methotrexate therapy.
- The most common cause of first-trimester abortions is fetal chromosomal abnormality.
- Incomplete, inevitable, and missed abortions are usually completed with a D&C or medical management with prostaglandins, although expectant management can also used.
- RhoGAM should be given to all Rh-negative pregnant patients who experience vaginal bleeding.
- Most second-trimester abortions are secondary to uterine or cervical abnormalities, trauma, systemic disease, or infection.
- D&E, prostaglandins, or oxytocic agents can be used for the management of SABs in the second trimester that needs assistance to completion.
- Incompetent cervix is a painless dilation of the cervix. This dilation may lead to infection, rupture of membranes, or PTL.
- If the fetus is previable, incompetent cervix is treated with expectant management, elective termination, or emergent cerclage.
- Patients with a history of incompetent cervix should be offered an elective, prophylactic cerclage at 12 to 14 weeks' gestational age.
- Recurrent pregnancy loss is defined as three or more consecutive SABs.
- Despite extensive evaluation to diagnose the etiology of SABs, the cause of recurrent SABs is undiagnosed in more than one-third of all cases.
- The most common diagnosed causes of recurrent pregnancy loss include APA syndrome and luteal phase defects.
- Treatment is specific to the etiology, but efficacy is difficult to measure because two-thirds of subsequent pregnancies will be normal without therapy.

magnesium is mainstay of [illegible] during labor + for 24 hours postpartum to [illegible] seizure [illegible]

Therapeutic mag = 4-7 mEq/L
Loss of patellar reflex at 7-10; > [illegible] resp. depression, cardiac arrest

- [illegible] to control [illegible] in [illegible]

Contraindications to expectant management of severe preeclampsia: thrombocytopenia < 100,000, inability to control BP w/ 2 meds [illegible], [illegible] symptoms [illegible]; LFT elevated 2x more than normal, persistent CNS symptoms, oliguria.

delivery is not based on degree of proteinuria

C Clinical Vignettes

Vignette 1

A 28-year-old P0010 woman presents to the emergency department with abdominal pain since the past day. She reports a 1-week history of nausea with occasional vomiting. She has noticed some breast tenderness as well. She denies dysuria, vaginal bleeding, or any bowel symptoms. She reports that her last period was 4 weeks ago, but was lighter than normal. She has been using condoms for contraception. On arrival, her vital signs include a temperature of 37°C, BP of 117/68, pulse rate of 78 beats per minute, and respiratory rate of 16 breaths per minute. Cardiovascular and respiratory examinations are normal. She notes some suprapubic abdominal discomfort with palpation, but she does not have rebound tenderness or guarding. A speculum examination reveals a closed cervix without bleeding. A pelvic examination is mildly uncomfortable and reveals a normally sized, anteverted uterus, and palpably normal adnexa. A urine pregnancy test is positive.

1. What is the test you should order first?
   a. Type and cross
   b. CBC
   c. Quantitative level of β-hCG
   d. Pelvic ultrasound
   e. Urine gonorrhea and chlamydia testing

2. The quantitative β-hCG level is 1,300 mIU/mL. The patient reveals that this was an unplanned, but desired pregnancy. What follow-up recommendations do you give this patient?
   a. Make an appointment with her primary OB/GYN for an initial prenatal visit
   b. This is likely an ectopic pregnancy and she should proceed with methotrexate therapy
   c. She should undergo urgent laparoscopy for evacuation of an ectopic pregnancy
   d. She should return in 48 hours for a repeat β-hCG
   e. She has likely had a SAB and does not need further follow-up

3. The patient returns 48 hours later per your recommendations. She reports that her abdominal pain is worse and is left-sided. Yesterday, she also had a small amount of vaginal bleeding that has since subsided. She has not been lightheaded, short of breath, or had palpations and she has been able to tolerate food and drink without difficulty. Her vital signs remain stable. You repeat a β-hCG and the level is now 1,700 mIU/mL. A pelvic ultrasound reveals a left adnexal mass and nothing in the uterine cavity. What is the most common site of an ectopic pregnancy?
   a. Ampulla
   b. Ovary
   c. Fimbriae
   d. Isthmus
   e. Cervix

4. You explain to the patient that she most likely has an ectopic pregnancy that requires treatment. She would like to avoid surgery. You draw a type and screen, CBC, and complete metabolic panel. Her blood type is O positive, antibody negative. Her hemoglobin is normal as are her liver enzymes. What is your next recommendation?
   a. Her vaginal bleeding suggests an inevitable abortion and she does not need further treatment at this time
   b. Her abdominal pain is concerning and she must undergo urgent laparoscopy for evacuation of the ectopic pregnancy
   c. This is a desired pregnancy, she should return in 48 hours to continue to follow the β-hCG level
   d. She should proceed with methotrexate therapy
   e. She should proceed with mifepristone and misoprostol therapy

5. What additional recommendation would you make at this time?
   a. The patient should receive RhoGAM
   b. She should return in 48 hours for a follow-up test of β-hCG level
   c. She should return in 96 hours for a follow-up test of β-hCG level
   d. She should return in 1 week for a follow-up test of β-hCG level
   e. She should return in 48 hours for a follow-up ultrasound

Vignette 2

A 35-year-old G3P0020 woman presents to the hospital with vaginal bleeding and abdominal pain. She appears pale and states that she feels lightheaded when sitting up or standing. She reports that she is currently 9 weeks' pregnant. On arrival, her temperature is 37°C, BP is 86/50, pulse rate is 110 beats per minute, and respiratory rate is 18 breaths per minute. Abdominal examination reveals a rigid abdomen with rebound tenderness to palpation. Pelvic examination reveals a small amount of vaginal bleeding, a 6-week-size uterus, and fullness at the right adnexa. A urine β-hCG confirms that she is pregnant. The nurse works to obtain IV access and draw blood for laboratory tests.

1. What is your first step?
   a. Proceed immediately to the operating room for emergency laparotomy

b. Perform an emergency dilation and suction curettage in the emergency department
c. Obtain a pelvic ultrasound
d. Give the patient IM methotrexate
e. Give the patient oral misoprostol

2. A pelvic ultrasound reveals a right-sided ectopic pregnancy as well as large amounts of fluid, thought to be blood in the abdomen. She now has IV access and a bolus of IV fluids is being given. Her BP is now 78/45 and her pulse rate is 112 beats per minute. Her hematocrit returns as 27.2%. How will you proceed?
   a. Administer IM methotrexate
   b. Transfuse the patient with two units of packed RBCs and transfer her to the ICU
   c. Proceed with a laparoscopic salpingectomy
   d. Proceed with emergent laparotomy
   e. Start vasopressors and transfer the patient to the ICU

3. The patient undergoes emergency laparotomy with evacuation of the hematoperitoneum as well as right salpingectomy for removal of the ectopic pregnancy. On postoperative day 1, she explains that this pregnancy was conceived via IVF and was highly desired. What is her risk of having a future ectopic pregnancy?
   a. 1% to 2%
   b. 5%
   c. 10%
   d. 15%
   e. 25%

Vignette 3

A 22-year-old P0 woman presents to the clinic for an annual examination. She reports that her last normal menstrual period was 5 weeks prior. Her menstrual cycles are irregular and she reports that she frequently skips a month between periods. She reports that she is sexually active and uses condoms sporadically for birth control. Pelvic examination reveals a mildly enlarged, anteverted, nontender uterus with palpably normal adnexa bilaterally. The patient consents to a urine pregnancy test that returns as positive. The patient expresses that she is uncertain if this is a desired pregnancy. You perform an in-office transvaginal ultrasound; however, neither an ectopic or IUP are visualized.

1. What step do you take next?
   a. Obtain a serum quantitative β-hCG level
   b. Explain that the patient likely has a chemical pregnancy that will not develop into a viable pregnancy
   c. Explain to the patient that she likely had a miscarriage
   d. Offer the patient IM methotrexate for a presumed ectopic pregnancy
   e. Send the patient for an official ultrasound with a high-resolution machine

2. The patient consents to a blood draw before leaving the clinic. Later that day, the patient's β-hCG level returns at 1,300 mIU/mL. You call the patient with the results and she informs you that she would like to continue the pregnancy. What do you recommend next?
   a. You inform her that ultrasound should have detected a pregnancy and she has likely had a miscarriage
   b. She should return in 48 hours for a follow-up β-hCG
   c. She should return in 1 week for a follow-up β-hCG
   d. She should return in 48 hours for a follow-up ultrasound
   e. She should return in 1 week for a follow-up ultrasound

3. Forty-eight hours later, the patient has a repeat β-hCG level that returns at 2,700 mIU/mL. An office ultrasound reveals an intrauterine gestational sac with yolk sac consistent with a 5-week pregnancy. You prescribe a prenatal vitamin and ask the patient to return in 4 weeks for an official prenatal visit. At 8 weeks' gestation, she returns to the clinic with vaginal spotting. A pelvic examination reveals minimal old blood in the vagina and closed cervix. What test or procedure do you perform first?
   a. CBC
   b. Quantitative β-hCG level
   c. Dilation and curettage
   d. Pelvic ultrasound
   e. Gonorrhea and chlamydia testing

4. Fetal heart tones are confirmed with an office ultrasound. What test should you obtain next?
   a. CBC
   b. Gonorrhea and chlamydia
   c. Saline wet mount
   d. Blood type
   e. Quantitative β-hCG level

Vignette 4

A 34-year-old G3P0020 woman presents to the office at 8 weeks' gestation for her first prenatal visit. This is a planned and desired pregnancy. Her obstetric history is significant for one prior elective termination and one SAB. It took her and her partner just over 1 year to conceive this pregnancy. She is afebrile, normotensive with a normal pulse. Pelvic examination reveals a 7- to 8-week-sized uterus with normal adnexa. Her cervix is closed and there is no vaginal bleeding. An office ultrasound is performed and an IUP is seen with a crown–rump length consistent with 7 weeks and 2 days gestation. Unfortunately, no fetal heart beat is seen.

1. What is your diagnosis?
   a. Incomplete abortion
   b. Threatened abortion
   c. Ectopic pregnancy
   d. Missed abortion
   e. Inevitable abortion

2. You offer the patient either medical or surgical management. She opts for medical management and takes mifepristone in the office with the plan to take misoprostol the next day. The following evening, you receive a call that the patient has presented to the emergency department with heavy vaginal bleeding. Her vital signs are as follows: temperature, 37°C; BP, 90/52; pulse rate, 100 beats per minute; respirations, 16 breaths per minute; and 100% oxygen saturation on room air. Pelvic examination reveals active bleeding from an open cervical os. Pelvic ultrasound reveals partial retention of fetal products. What is your new diagnosis?
   a. Incomplete abortion
   b. Threatened abortion
   c. Ectopic pregnancy
   d. Missed abortion
   e. Inevitable abortion

3. The emergency department team obtains IV access and draws blood for a CBC, type and screen and quantitative β-hCG level. An IV fluid bolus is given. Her hematocrit is 30.6%, she is RH positive, and the β-hCG is pending. What is your next step in the management of this patient?
   a. Reassure that patient and send her home
   b. Proceed with dilation and curettage

c. Administer RhoGAM
d. Administer vasopressors
e. Transfer the patient to the ICU

4. The patient stabilizes and is discharged. She follows up in your office 1 week later and wants to know why she had a miscarriage as well as her risk of future miscarriages. Which of the following is not true?

a. As much as 80% of first-trimester SABs are due to abnormal chromosomes
b. The most common chromosomal abnormality is autosomal trisomy
c. Ninety-five percent of the chromosomal abnormalities are due to errors in paternal gametogenesis
d. Her risk of a third miscarriage is 25% to 30%
e. Because of her advancing age, she should consider evaluation for recurrent pregnancy loss, starting with parental karyotyping

A Answers

Vignette 1 Question 1
Answer C: The next best test is to obtain a quantitative β-hCG level. This will help determine an approximate gestational age for the pregnancy as well as whether you would expect to see anything on ultrasound. Recall that in most institutions, ultrasound should be able to detect an IUP at β-hCG levels between 1,500 and 2,000 mIU/mL. While a CBC may be ordered to ensure hemodynamic stability, her vital signs are stable and she is not having vaginal bleeding. Similarly, a type and cross is not immediately necessary, as there is no evidence of hemodynamic instability. Given the unremarkable pelvic examination, a pelvic ultrasound may be deferred until you are certain that the β-hCG levels are above the discriminatory zone. Gonorrhea and chlamydia testing is part of routine prenatal care, but is not the best first step.

Vignette 1 Question 2
Answer D: The patient's β-hCG level is below the discriminatory zone and you would not expect to see anything on ultrasound. The patient should return for a repeat β-hCG level in 48 hours so that you can trend the values. With only one β-hCG level, you cannot definitively determine whether this is an intrauterine or ectopic pregnancy. Her abdominal pain is concerning, but not diagnostic for an ectopic pregnancy and it would be premature to recommend methotrexate therapy given that the pregnancy is desired. She is hemodynamically stable and does not need surgery at this point. She has not had any vaginal bleeding to suggest that she has had a SAB. Because you do not know yet if this is an IUP, it would be premature to send the patient for routine prenatal care (a).

Vignette 1 Question 3
Answer A: The most common site of implantation in a tubal pregnancy is the ampulla (70%), followed by the isthmus (12%) and fimbriae (11%). While an ectopic pregnancy may implant in the cervix or ovary, this is rare.

Vignette 1 Question 4
Answer D: The patient's β-hCG level did not rise by more than two-third in 48 hours, which is suggestive of an abnormal pregnancy. This in conjunction with the adnexal mass on ultrasound is highly suggestive of an ectopic pregnancy. She should proceed with treatment. Her β-hCG level is well below the cut-off of 5,000 mIU/mL, that is, at an appropriate level for methotrexate therapy and this would be the recommended first-line therapy. Vaginal bleeding is a common presenting symptom in an ectopic pregnancy. However, unlike in an IUP, vaginal bleeding does not signify that the pregnancy will pass on its own. Again, the patient's vital signs and CBCs are stable. She has proven that she is reliable as she returned for her follow-up visit as recommended. She may be offered surgery at this time, but it is not mandatory. Once the diagnosis of ectopic pregnancy is made, the patient should no longer be managed expectantly. Mifepristone and misoprostol therapy is reserved for the treatment of intrauterine pregnancies.

Vignette 1 Question 5
Answer C: The β-hCG level commonly rises in the first few days after methotrexate therapy with a fall of 10% to 15% between days 4 and 7 after administration. Checking β-hCG levels at 48 hours may raise a false concern that the patient needs additional treatment. However, the patient should be seen sooner than 1 week so that additional methotrexate may be administered if necessary. The patient's blood type is Rh positive and RhoGAM is not indicated. Ultrasound is not commonly used to follow the resolution of an ectopic pregnancy.

Vignette 2 Question 1
Answer: C The patient is hemodynamically stable. The first steps should be to obtain IV access with a large-bore IV catheter, bolus the patient with IV fluids, and draw blood for a CBC and a type and screen and/or cross for units of blood. While the nurse helps with these important steps, it would be prudent to perform an urgent ultrasound to determine if this is an intrauterine versus an ectopic pregnancy, as this will dictate your next steps. The patient will likely need to undergo an urgent procedure, but the type of pregnancy will determine whether a D&C versus abdominal surgery is most appropriate. As the patient is not hemodynamically stable, she is not a candidate for medical therapy at this time.

Vignette 2 Question 2
Answer D: The patient is hemodynamically unstable and has evidence of a rupture ectopic pregnancy on ultrasound as well as acute blood loss anemia and possible hematoperitoneum. She should be taken for emergent exploratory laparotomy to control the bleeding and remove the ectopic pregnancy. While a more stable patient may be offered laparoscopy, it is not the best choice in an unstable patient. The patient may require a blood transfusion, vasopressor support, and ICU care, but not without concurrent surgery to control the bleeding. She is not a candidate for methotrexate because of her hemodynamic instability.

Vignette 2 Question 3
Answer C: The risk of an ectopic pregnancy after IVF has been estimated to be between 1% and 2% and this was likely the patient's baseline risk of ectopic pregnancy. However, after one prior ectopic pregnancy, the risk of a subsequent ectopic pregnancy increases

to 10% that is likely the patient's new risk. The risk of a subsequent ectopic pregnancy after more than one prior ectopic pregnancy increases to 25%.

Vignette 3 Question 1
Answer A: An IUP should be seen on ultrasound with β-hCG levels between 1,500 and 2,000 mIU/mL. Without knowing the patient's β-hCG level, you cannot give any additional advice about the status of the pregnancy.

Vignette 3 Question 2
Answer B: In an IUP, the β-hCG level can be expected to increase by 60% or more every 48 hours. An ectopic pregnancy would be expected to have a slower rate of increase in β-hCG level because of decreased blood supply due to abnormal placentation. Therefore, the next best step would be to ask the patient to return in 48 hours for a repeat β-hCG level. A β-hCG level of 1,300 mIU/mL is not above the discriminatory zone for detection of pregnancy and cannot rule out pregnancy. Repeating an ultrasound in 48 hours may not be necessary if the patient has a normal rise in β-hCG level and is not symptomatic. Returning in 1 week for laboratory tests and/or ultrasound would not be advised prior to determining whether the pregnancy is intrauterine or ectopic.

Vignette 3 Question 3
Answer D: The current diagnosis based on your clinical assessment is a threatened abortion. It is important to confirm the presence or absence of fetal heart tones with ultrasound to appropriately counsel the patient regarding the next steps. She does not have heavy vaginal bleeding and does not need an urgent CBC. At this gestational age, a quantitative β-hCG level will not offer additional information. It would be premature to proceed with dilation and curettage for a desired pregnancy. Cervicitis may cause vaginal spotting, but this is not the initial test of choice.

Vignette 3 Question 4
Answer D: With any bleeding in pregnancy, the patient's Rh status should be obtained. All patients with Rh-negative status should receive RhoGAM to prevent maternal isoimmunization. Again, the patient is not bleeding heavily so obtaining a CBC would not be the first step. While gonorrhea, chlamydia, or other vaginal infections may cause spotting, these tests are less urgent than obtaining the patient's blood type. A quantitative β-hCG level does not offer any additional information at this point.

Vignette 4 Question 1
Answer D: Missed abortion is the death of an embryo with complete retention of all POCs. An incomplete abortion is partial expulsion of POCs prior to 20 weeks. This patient has not had any tissue expelled. A threatened abortion does present with vaginal bleeding, but in this type of abortion the patient does not have cervical dilation. This patient has an IUP as confirmed by an intrauterine gestational sac and yolk sac. An inevitable abortion is a pregnancy complicated by vaginal bleeding with a dilated cervix such that the pregnancy is unlikely to be viable.

Vignette 4 Question 2
Answer A: Missed abortion is the death of an embryo with complete retention of all POCs. An incomplete abortion is partial expulsion of POC prior to 20 weeks. This patient has not had any tissue expelled. A threatened abortion does present with vaginal bleeding, but in this type of abortion the patient does not have cervical dilation. This patient has an IUP as confirmed by an intrauterine gestational sac and yolk sac. An inevitable abortion is a pregnancy complicated by vaginal bleeding with a dilated cervix such that the pregnancy is unlikely to be viable.

Vignette 4 Question 3
Answer B: The patient is actively bleeding and controlling this is the first step after stabilizing the patient. Performing a dilation and curettage to remove the remaining fetal tissues will allow the uterus to contract and will likely stop the bleeding. The patient should not be sent home with heavy vaginal bleeding and unstable vital signs. She is Rh positive and does not require RhoGAM. She has not yet become so unstable as to require vasopressors or be transferred to the ICU.

Vignette 4 Question 1
Answer C: Ninety-five percent of the chromosomal abnormalities are due to errors in maternal gametogenesis. All of the other statements are true.

Chapter

3 Prenatal Screening, Diagnosis, and Treatment

Prenatal screening, diagnosis, and treatment is a relatively new field within obstetrics. It has been particularly tied to the advent and advancement of real-time ultrasound imaging over the past two decades as well as the new kinds of genetic testing that are being rapidly introduced today. Prenatal genetic diagnoses are and will be increasingly available as the association between specific genes, large chromosomal aberrations, and submicroscopic chromosomal losses and gains and their phenotypes are discovered. Imperative to understanding prenatal diagnosis is the distinction between screening and diagnostic tests. **Screening** allows high-risk individuals to be selected out of a low-risk population at risk for a given diagnosis or complication. The sensitivity and specificity and resulting false-negative and false-positive rates of screening tests are highly important both because of the number of patients missed by a screen as well as the number of patients who are falsely concerned. The so called noninvasive prenatal diagnosis is a recently developed screening tool that may maximize sensitivity and minimize false positives, but is not currently a diagnostic test. **Prenatal diagnosis** is nearly always diagnostic and usually far more specific than screening, but diagnostic procedures such as amniocentesis and chorionic villus sampling (CVS) bear a greater risk of complications, in particular, pregnancy loss.

SCREENING PATIENTS FOR GENETIC DISEASES

Many diseases are passed genetically from parents to their offspring. This is best understood using the principles of Mendelian genetics. **Autosomal dominant** (**AD**) diseases are usually inherited from one parent with the disease via a single gene defect. Risk of disease and recurrence (if the partners choose to have another child) is usually 50%. **Autosomal recessive** (**AR**) diseases require two affected alleles. Thus, assuming both parents are carriers, the risk to the child is 25%. **X-linked disorders** (e.g., hemophilia, fragile X) are usually carried by the mother who is unaffected (in X-linked recessive) or mildly affected (X-linked dominant) and passed only to her sons. The sons are affected 50% of the time and the daughters are unaffected or mildly affected carriers 50% of the time. **X-linked dominant** disorders can be passed from mothers to their sons and daughters and theoretically from fathers to their daughters. In some X-linked dominant disorders, the disorder is lethal in males, as in Aicardi syndrome. One important tenet of X-lined inheritance is that there is no male-to-male transmission, which is a key component of the family history. Phenotypes can vary, especially in females, because of X-chromosome lyonization. The first step in determining fetal risk is to screen the mother for the disease, which is usually done in higher risk groups (e.g., by ethnicity or family history). In this section, we review several of the common genetic diseases that have prenatal screening and diagnosis.

CYSTIC FIBROSIS

Cystic fibrosis (**CF**) is an AR disease resulting from an abnormality in the cystic fibrosis transmembrane conductance regulator (CFTR), which is the gene responsible for chloride channels. Almost all CF patients have chronic lung disease because of recurrent infections, leading eventually to irreversible lung damage and strain on the right ventricle (cor pulmonale). Eighty-five percent of CF patients have pancreatic insufficiency manifested by chronic malabsorption and failure to thrive. Chronic lung disease and its sequelae are the life-limiting factors for most CF patients. Median survival is close to 40 years for CF patients born today in the United States with high phenotypic variability.

In CF two mutant copies (gene changes) of the CFTR gene are required (homozygosity) for disease, though, for the majority of AR disorders, affected individuals have two different allelic mutations at the same locus (compound heterozygote). For example, ΔF508/G542X are two of the most common mutations in CF. These two specific mutations can be screened for in asymptomatic carrier patients. If the mother has a positive screen, her partner can be screened as well and if he is also positive, then the risk of the fetus being affected is 25%. If desired, amniocentesis or CVS can then be performed to diagnose the fetus. The CF mutations are more common in Caucasians (approximately 1:25 to 29 is a carrier). One challenge in screening for CF is that more than 1,300 disease-causing mutations have been identified in the CFTR gene. Therefore, even with a negative screen of the most common disease causing mutations, there remains a small probability that a child could be affected. While the risk of carrier status is less common in other races/ethnicities (e.g., Asian, Hispanic), the relative proportion of disease common mutations is fewer as well, making the screening test less sensitive in these women. One way to improve the sensitivity of screening is to screen for additional mutations, and a number of commercial laboratories offer screening for up to 97 mutations.

SICKLE CELL ANEMIA

Sickle cell anemia is an AR disease caused by a single point mutation in the gene for the beta chain in hemoglobin. The resulting hemoglobin (Hb S) forms polymers that when deoxygenated cause the cells to lose their biconcave shape and become "sickled" in appearance. As a result, patients have a hemolytic anemia, shortened life expectancy, and frequent pain crises secondary to vaso-occlusion of small vessels by the dysmorphic erythrocytes. Because this disease is more common among African Americans, all persons of African descent should be screened during pregnancy. Individuals with one abnormal sickle cell allele are known as having sickle cell trait. It is likely that the increased carrier status in those of African ancestry was selected because of **heterozygote advantage**. This is observed because resistance to malaria in individuals heterozygous for sickle cell anemia was greater than those without the gene defect. In these individuals, RBCs function in normal conditions but are inhospitable to *Plasmodium vivax*, the parasitic protozoan responsible for malaria. Interestingly, a recent study demonstrated a lower rate of preterm birth among women with sickle cell trait.

The maternal screen is usually accomplished with a hemoglobin electrophoresis. This test distinguishes Hb S from normal Hb A. If the patient is positive, then her partner can also be screened. If he is also positive, then the fetus carries a 25% chance of being affected, and the couple can choose to undergo invasive fetal diagnosis.

TAY-SACHS DISEASE

Tay-Sachs is an AR disease that is most commonly observed in Eastern European Jews and French Canadians. Approximately 1 in 27 to 31 Ashkenazi Jews is a carrier for an abnormal Tay-Sachs allele, which means that the incidence of Tay-Sachs in this population is approximately 100 times greater than in other populations. It is thought that this is due to a **founder effect**, in which the high frequency of a mutant gene in a population is founded by a small ancestral group when one or more individuals are a carrier for the mutation.

Infants with Tay-Sachs disease develop symptoms approximately 3 to 10 months after birth. These symptoms include a loss of alertness and an excessive reaction to noise (hyperacusis). There is a progressive developmental delay and neurologic degeneration in intellectual and neurologic function. Myoclonic and akinetic seizures can present 1 to 3 months later. One physical examination finding is a cherry-red spot seen on funduscopic eye examination where the prominent red macular fovea centralis is contrasted by the pale retina. These children eventually suffer from paralysis, blindness, and dementia, and typically die by age 4 years.

Tay-Sachs disease occurs due to the deficiency of hexosaminidase A (hex A), the enzyme responsible for the degradation of GM2 gangliosides. Hex A is a multimeric protein composed of three parts: alpha and beta subunits, which comprise the enzyme, and an activator protein. The activator protein must associate with both the enzyme and the substrate before the enzyme can cleave the ganglioside between the *N*-acetyl-α-galactosamine and galactose residues. Gangliosides are continually degraded in lysosomes, where multiple degradative enzymes function to sequentially remove terminal sugars from the gangliosides. The impact of Tay-Sachs disease is primarily in the brain, which has the highest concentrations of gangliosides, particularly in the gray matter. The deficiency of hex A results in the accumulation of gangliosides in the lysosomes, which in turn results in enlarged neurons containing lipid-filled lysosomes, cellular dysfunction, and ultimately neuronal death.

Similar to other AR syndromes, Tay-Sachs is screened for particularly among high-risk patients (e.g., Ashkenazi Jews), and their partners if they are positive. Fetal diagnosis can then be performed if both partners are carriers.

THALASSEMIA

The **thalassemias** are a set of hereditary hemolytic anemias that are caused by mutations that result in the reduction in the synthesis of either the α or β chains that make up the hemoglobin molecule. The reduction of a particular chain leads to the imbalance of globin chain synthesis and subsequently a distortion in the α:β ratio. As a result, unpaired globin chains produce insoluble tetramers that precipitate in the cell and cause damage to membranes. The RBCs are susceptible to premature red cell destruction by the reticuloendothelial system in the bone marrow, liver, and spleen.

Beta-Thalassemia

In **β-thalassemia**, there is an impairment of β-chain production that leads to an excess of alpha chains. These disorders are typically diagnosed several months after birth because the presence of β-chain is important only postnatally when it would normally replace the γ-chain as the major non-α chain. There are multiple mutations that can lead to β-thalassemia. Almost any point mutation that causes a decrease in the synthesis of mRNA and the subsequent protein can cause this disease. β-Thalassemia is essentially an AR disorder seen more commonly among patients of Mediterranean descent as well as Asians and Africans. Because the heterozygotes will have a mild hemolytic anemia and low MCV (<80 fL), they can be screened by getting a CBC. Confirmation can then be made by hemoglobin electrophoresis, which will show an increase in α:β ratio (Hgb A_2).

Alpha-Thalassemia

The alpha chain is encoded by four alleles on two chromosomes. Additionally, two out of four mutations can occur *cis* or *trans*, with *cis* being on the same chromosome and *trans* being on two different chromosomes. *cis* mutations are seen more commonly among women of Southeast Asian descent, whereas *trans* mutations are seen more commonly among women of African descent. With α-thalassemia, deletions or alterations of two, three, or four genes cause an increasingly severe phenotype; however, deletion of one allele has no clinical significance. The most severe form of α-thalassemia causes fetal hydrops and is incompatible with life. The infants are delivered premature and are pale, hydropic, severely anemic, and have splenomegaly. A fetal hemoglobin electrophoresis would reveal no HbF, no HbA, and approximately 90% to 100% Hbα4 also referred to as **Hb Bart**. **Hemoglobin H disease** (HbH) is due to the deletion of three alpha globin genes, resulting in the accumulation of excess beta chains in the red cell. Beta tetramers form, which are unstable and undergo oxidation. Membrane damage results, and these RBCs are susceptible to early clearance and destruction. These infants develop moderate hemolytic anemia, and the initial hemoglobin electrophoresis shows some Hb Bart and some HbH. Within the following few months, Hb Bart disappears and the hemoglobins detected are HbH and HbA. **α-Thalassemia**

trait (two deletions) carries a milder phenotype with mainly a microcytic anemia and a normal hemoglobin electrophoresis. Patients with only one gene deletion are silent carriers and usually have an MCV of less than 85 fL. In such a case, diagnosis is confirmed by targeted mutation analysis.

Like β-thalassemia, α-thalassemia is also screened for with a CBC in high-risk groups. Patients can then undergo hemoglobin electrophoresis if they have a microcytic anemia, which is typically normal. Molecular testing is needed to determine the number of genes lost. Sorting out whether patients are *cis* or *trans* is particularly important. When both partners have a *cis* mutation, their child has a 25% chance of getting the most severe variant that usually results in fetal death. If they both have the *trans* mutation, the child will end up with the *trans* mutation, as well, and primarily remain an asymptomatic carrier.

CHROMOSOMAL ABNORMALITIES

In addition to genetic disorders caused by single gene mutations, another family of genetic disorders in the fetus is caused by chromosomal abnormalities. Aneuploidy, that is, extra or missing chromosome(s), is generally the cause of these syndromes. These chromosomal abnormalities are usually accompanied by obvious phenotypic differences and congenital anomalies. However, these may not always be appreciated on prenatal ultrasound. Thus, fetal karyotype remains the only way to achieve a definitive diagnosis of aneuploidy. Screening tests exist for some types of aneuploidy—specifically trisomies 21 and 18. Women may choose to undergo first-trimester screening at 11 to 14 weeks, second-trimester screening, or a combination of the two called sequential screening. The components of first-trimester screening include a nuchal translucency, which is combined with pregnancy-associated plasma protein A (PAPP-A) and β-hCG. The second-trimester portion is called the quadruple (quad) screen and includes MSAFP, estriol, β-hCG, and inhibin. Recent advancements have allowed researchers to examine cell-free fetal DNA in maternal serum to make a "noninvasive prenatal diagnosis." Preliminary results suggest that these tests are highly sensitive and specific in women at high risk for having a fetus with aneuploidy, but have a number of limitations (e.g., not applicable in twins, chromosomal mosaicism, etc.) and do not currently assess all chromosomes as one can do with a karyotype. While trisomy and monosomy of any of the chromosomes theoretically exist, most result in early miscarriage. In addition, triploidy (i.e., three sets of chromosomes) may also occur and usually results in miscarriage or gestational trophoblastic disease. Despite the high rate of miscarriage, an infant is occasionally born with triploidy and survival for up to 1 year has been described.

DOWN SYNDROME

Trisomy 21, or an extra chromosome 21, is the most common cause of **Down syndrome**. This chromosomal aneuploidy results in higher rates of both miscarriage and stillbirth. However, several thousand infants with Down syndrome are born each year. Because chromosomal abnormalities increase with maternal age, the overall average risk per patient is increasing in the United States as more women delay childbearing. The typical phenotype of Down syndrome is that of a short stature, classic facies, developmental delay, and mental retardation with IQs ranging from 40 to as high as 90. Associated anomalies include cardiac defects, duodenal atresia or stenosis, and short limbs. Some of these anomalies can be seen by ultrasound, but up to 40% to 50% of fetuses with Down syndrome will not have diagnosable anomalies by ultrasound, making this a poor screening tool.

Currently, women undergo screening for Down syndrome using the first-trimester screen (nuchal translucency with PAPP-A and hCG) and/or the quad screen (MSAFP, hCG, estriol, and inhibin A) between 15 and 20 weeks' gestation. The sensitivity of the first-trimester screen is 82% to 87% for Down syndrome and for the quad screen alone has just more than 80% sensitivity. The combination of these two tests results in a sensitivity of 95% with a screen positive rate of 5%, while the sensitivity of the nuchal translucency alone is 64% to 70%. When the serum analytes are used alone, free β-hCG and PAPP-A, can achieve a 60% sensitivity. First-trimester screening has been studied in several large trials and affords women to have information earlier in gestation to allow decisions on prenatal diagnostic testing as early as 12 weeks. The newer, noninvasive prenatal diagnostic tests have been focused on identifying trisomy 21, and early reports suggest sensitivity and specificity both in the 98% to 99% range or better.

TRISOMY 18

Trisomy 18 (Edward syndrome) is another common trisomy that can also be screened for using the first- and second-trimester screening with a sensitivity approaching 90% in women who choose sequential screening. Noninvasive prenatal diagnosis has been shown in recent studies to be greater than 97% sensitive at a much lower screen positive rate (0.3%) in high-risk populations. Trisomy 18 is a lethal aneuploidy and nearly all neonates die in the first 2 years of life. This syndrome is associated with multiple congenital anomalies, which are typically seen on ultrasound (in approximately 95% of cases), making this modality a reasonable screening tool. Edward syndrome is classically associated with clenched fists, overlapping digits, and rocker bottom feet. Cardiac defects including ventricular septal defect (VSD) and tetralogy of Fallot, omphalocele, congenital diaphragmatic hernia, neural tube defects, and choroid plexus cysts have also been associated with trisomy 18 (Fig. 3-1). While the newer, noninvasive prenatal diagnostic tests have been focused on

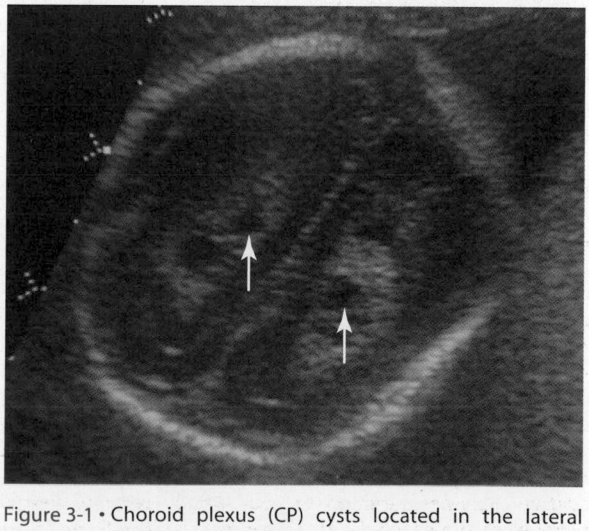

Figure 3-1 • Choroid plexus (CP) cysts located in the lateral ventricles of the brain.
(Image provided by Departments of Radiology and Obstetrics & Gynecology, University of California, San Francisco, CA.)

identifying trisomy 21, most are being augmented to identify trisomy 18 as well. Although trisomy 18 is rarely missed on ultrasound, the advantage of early diagnosis with a screening test is an earlier, safer, termination of pregnancy.

TRISOMY 13

Trisomy 13 (Patau syndrome) has many findings similar to trisomy 18. Eighty-five percent of these newborns will not live past the first year of life. Commonly associated anomalies include holoprosencephaly, cleft lip and palate, cystic hygroma, single nostril or absent nose, omphalocele, cardiac anomalies including hypoplastic left heart, and limb anomalies including clubfoot and clubhand, polydactyly, and overlapping fingers. Unfortunately, the serum analytes of the first trimester and quad screen are variable in these pregnancies, making this a poor screening test, and thus it is typically not reported. Early studies of noninvasive prenatal diagnosis suggest that detection of trisomy may also be possible. It is very rare that trisomy 13 fetuses would not have anomalies visible on ultrasound, and thus will be commonly diagnosed by routine ultrasound examination. Similar to trisomy 18, the newer, noninvasive prenatal diagnostic are being augmented to identify trisomy 13 too. While trisomy 13 is likely missed even less than trisomy 18 on ultrasound, the advantage of early diagnosis with a screening test is an earlier, safer, termination of pregnancy.

SEX CHROMOSOMAL ABNORMALITIES

45,X (**Turner syndrome**, or monosomy X) and 47,XXY (**Klinefelter syndrome**) are the most common sex chromosome aneuploidies. This may be because 47,XXX and 47,XYY karyotypes exhibit little variation from standard phenotypes and are not identified as often. Individuals affected by Turner syndrome are phenotypically female and of short stature. They experience primary amenorrhea, sexual infantilism, webbed neck, low-set ears, low posterior hairline, epicanthal folds, wide carrying angle of the arms, shield-like chest, wide-set nipples, short fourth metacarpal, renal anomalies, lymphedema of the extremities at birth, and cardiovascular anomalies, especially coarctation of the aorta. The only anomaly in Turner syndrome commonly seen on ultrasound is cystic hygroma. Unfortunately, no screening test for Turner syndrome is currently available; however, detection of Turner syndrome and the other sex chromosome aneuploidies may be possible with noninvasive prenatal diagnostic techniques.

There is currently no screening test for Klinefelter syndrome also; however, both this and other sex chromosome abnormalities are diagnosed by karyotype when patients undergo amniocentesis or CVS. Testicular development is initially normal in these individuals. However, the presence of at least two X chromosomes causes the germ cells to die when they enter meiosis, eventually resulting in small, firm testes and hyalinization of the seminiferous tubules. Other classic findings in Klinefelter syndrome include infertility, gynecomastia, mental retardation, and elevated gonadotropin levels due to the decreased levels of circulating androgens.

FETAL CONGENITAL ANOMALIES

Congenital anomalies can occur in any organ system and may be due to an intrinsic abnormality such as a gene change, aneuploidy, or related to a teratogenic agent. The affected organ system often depends on which time during gestation a teratogenic insult is received by the fetus. These teratogens can include medications ingested by the mother or infections, most commonly a viral infection that the mother contracts and transmits transplacentally, and rarely chemotherapy. Radiation doses resulting in a congenital malformation are considerably higher than any diagnostic radiologic study (>20 rads). In order to better understand how these anomalies occur, a review of organogenesis is useful.

EARLY EMBRYOGENESIS AND ORGANOGENESIS

After fertilization of the ovum by the sperm, the resulting zygote undergoes a series of cell divisions, reaching the 16-cell morula stage by day 4 (Fig. 3-2). After the morula enters the uterine cavity, an influx of fluid separates the morula into the inner and outer cell masses, which forms the blastocyst. This gives rise to the embryo and the trophoblast, respectively. The blastocyst implants into the endometrium by the end of week 1. By the start of week 2, the trophoblast begins to differentiate into the inner cytotrophoblast and the outer syncytiotrophoblast, and together they eventually give rise to the placenta. Meanwhile, the inner cell mass divides into the bilaminar germ disc composed of the epiblast and the hypoblast.

During week 3 of development, the embryo is primarily preoccupied with the process of gastrulation. This is characterized by the formation of the primitive streak on the epiblast, followed by the invagination of epiblast cells to form the three germ layers of the embryo: the inner endoderm, the middle mesoderm, and

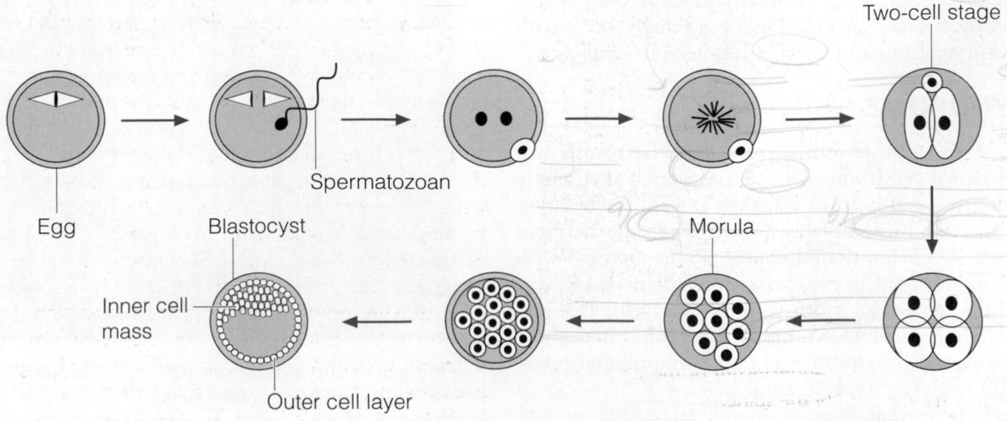

Figure 3-2 • Progression of the ova through fertilization to the blastula phase.

ectoderm: nervous sensory organs skin

+ large ventricles
+ clubfeet

the outer ectoderm. The endodermal layer eventually gives rise to the gastrointestinal and respiratory systems. The mesoderm forms the cardiovascular, musculoskeletal, and genitourinary systems. The ectoderm layer will differentiate into the nervous system, skin, and many sensory organs (e.g., hair, eyes, nose, and ears). The period of organogenesis primarily lasts from weeks 3 to 8 after conception (i.e., weeks 5 to 10 gestational age) and is the time when most of the major organ systems are formed.

NEURAL TUBE DEFECTS

day 22–23 = wk 4

The formation of the neural tube begins on days 22 to 23 after conception (week 4) in the region of the fourth and sixth somites. Fusion of the neural folds occurs in cranial and caudal directions. The anterior neuropore (future brain) closes by day 25 and the posterior pore (future spinal cord) closes by day 27. Closure of the neural tube coincides with establishment of its vascular supply. The majority of **neural tube defects (NTDs)** develop as a result of defective closure by week 4 of development (6 weeks' gestational age by LMP dating).

day 25 cranial
caudal day 27
vascular supply

NTDs, including spina bifida and anencephaly, are classic examples of multifactorial inheritance, emphasizing the interactions between environmental and genetic factors. Geographic and ethnic variations may reflect environmental and genetic influences on the incidence of NTDs. Decreased levels of maternal folic acid are associated with the development of NTDs. Supplementation with periconceptional folic acid effectively reduces the incidence as well as recurrence of NTDs. The risk of NTDs is doubled in cases of homozygosity for a common mutation in the gene for methyl tetrahydrofolate reductase (MTHFR), the C677T allelic variant that encodes an enzyme with reduced activity. However, even if the association were causal, this MTHFR variant would account for only a small fraction of NTDs prevented by folic acid. The risk of NTDs seen with certain genotypes may vary depending on maternal factors, such as the blood levels of vitamin B_{12} or folate.

NTDs multi factorial geo ethnic

MTHFR mutation

Fetuses with **spina bifida** can be identified on ultrasound, which is accomplished not by visualization of the opening of the spinal canal (Fig. 3-3), but by the associated findings. Spina

u/s associated findings

concave frontal bones.

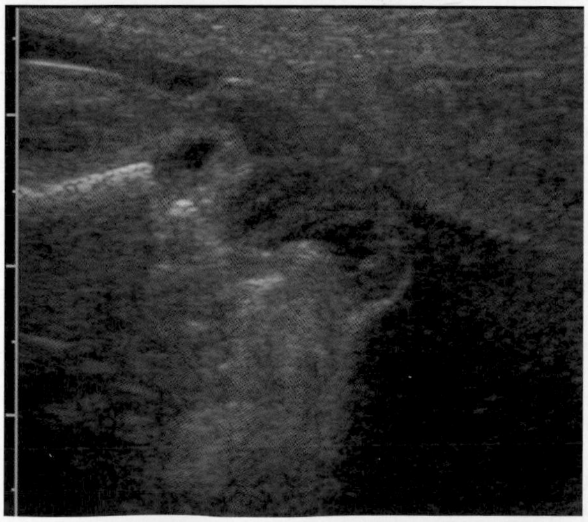

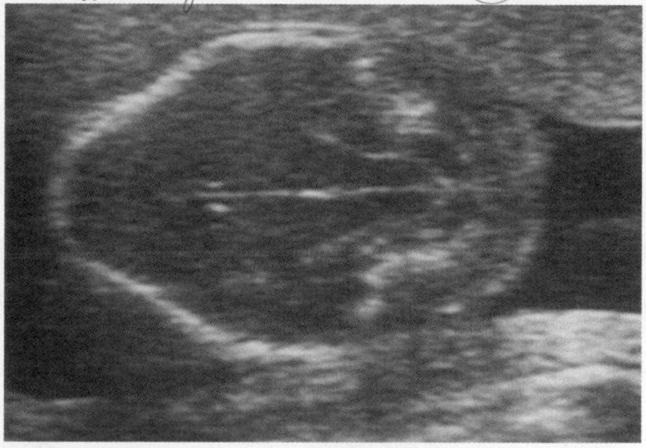

Figure 3-4 • Cerebral findings of the "lemon" and "banana" signs in spina bifida.
(Image provided by Departments of Radiology and Obstetrics & Gynecology, University of California, San Francisco, CA.)

↑ AFP leak from NT to maternal

bifida leads to classic ultrasound findings of the "lemon" sign (concave frontal bones), and the "banana" sign (a cerebellum that is pulled caudally and flattened) (Fig. 3-4). Ventriculomegaly and clubfeet are also seen. Prior to the existence of real-time ultrasound, one of the first prenatal screening programs was created using MSAFP to screen for NTDs. An open neural tube leads to elevated amniotic fluid α-fetoprotein (AFP) that crosses into the maternal serum.

Function of the infant and child with spina bifida is entirely dependent on the level of the spinal lesion. If the lesion is quite low in the sacral area, bowel and bladder function may be normal, and ambulation can be achieved with assistance. However, in higher lesions, there may be complete inability to use the lower extremities as well as lack of bowel or bladder control. Currently, there is a trial under way to see if in utero surgical repair can help those who are severely affected.

CARDIAC DEFECTS

23–28 d: cardiac loop

While the heart is merely a four-chamber pump, there are a number of ways to change the structure that can lead to some interesting pathophysiology. Cardiac development begins during week 3 after conception, when an angiogenic cell cluster forms at the anterior central portion of the embryo. As the embryo folds cephalocaudally, the cardiogenic area also folds into a heart tube. Even at this early stage, the embryonic heart tube is already receiving venous flow from its caudal end and pumping blood through the first aortic arch and into the dorsal aorta. Simultaneously, mesoderm around the endocardial tube forms the three layers of the heart wall composed of an outer epicardium, a muscular wall of myocardium, and the endocardium that is the internal endothelial lining. Between days 23 and 28, the heart tube elongates and bends to create the cardiac loop with a common atrium and a narrow atrioventricular junction connecting it to the primitive ventricle. The bulbus cordis is the caudal section of the heart tube and will eventually form three structures: the proximal third will form the trabeculated part of the right ventricle, the midportion (conus cordis) will form the outflow tracts of the ventricles, and the distal segment (truncus arteriosus) will eventually give rise to the proximal portions of the aorta and pulmonary artery (Fig. 3-5).

Between days 27 and 37, the heart continues to develop through the formation of the major septa. Septum formation

Figure 3-3 • Meningomyelocele—nonclosure of the neural tube at the lower aspect of the spine.
(Image provided by Departments of Radiology and Obstetrics & Gynecology, University of California, San Francisco, CA.)

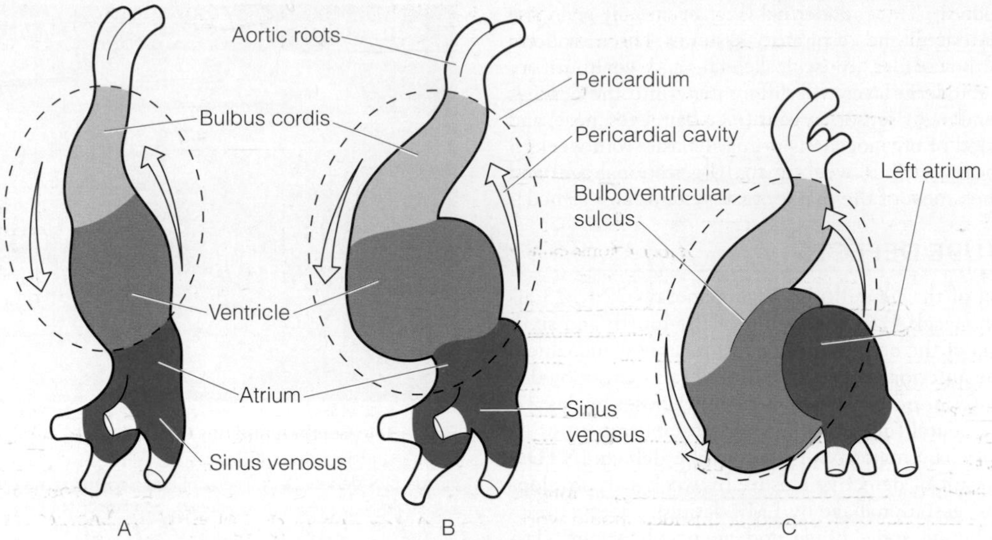

Figure 3-5 • (A–C) Folding of the heart tube into the four-chamber heart.

is achieved via the formation of tissue, called endocardial cushions, which subdivide the lumen into two cavities. The right and left atria are created by the formation of the septum primum and septum secundum that subdivides the primitive atrium while allowing for an interatrial opening (foramen ovale) to continue the right-to-left shunting of blood. At the end of week 4, endocardial cushions also appear in the atrioventricular canal to form the right and left canals as well as the mitral and tricuspid valves. During this time, the medial walls of the ventricles gradually fuse together to form the muscular interventricular septum. The conus cordis comprises the middle third of the bulbus cordis, and during week 5 of development, cushions subdivide the conus to form the outflow tract of the right and left ventricle as well as the membranous portion of the interventricular septum. Cushions also appear in the truncus arteriosus (distal third of bulbus cordis) and grow in a spiral pattern to form the aorticopulmonary septum and divide the truncus into the aortic and pulmonary tracts.

Any of these points of development can go awry, leading to disastrous complications. For example, if the ventricular walls fail to fuse, there is a VSD, which, if not repaired, can lead to Eisenmenger physiology, that is, right ventricular hypertrophy, pulmonary hypertension, and a right-to-left shunt. A commonly seen constellation of cardiac findings is tetralogy of Fallot. This is a VSD with an overriding aorta, pulmonary stenosis (or atresia), and right ventricular hypertrophy. Just as the chambers and valves can be anomalous, so can the great vessels as seen in transposition of the vessels (TOV), where the pulmonary artery and the aorta are connected to the wrong ventricles. Other common anomalies of vessels are coarctation of the aorta, an atretic portion prior to the insertion of the ductus arteriosus; and a patent ductus arteriosus (PDA), which can also lead to Eisenmenger physiology.

Diagnosis of these anomalies varies widely and depends on the lesion and the quality of the sonologist or sonographer imaging the fetal heart. Some of the more common lesions will be identified by the standard four-chamber view of the heart, but many—including coarctation of the aorta, small VSDs, and ASD—often will not. Outcomes of these congenital anomalies are quite variable. Most of these may be surgically repaired, although hypoplastic left heart, in particular, can have high mortality at a young age.

POTTER SYNDROME

Potter syndrome results from renal failure leading to anhydramnios, which in turn causes pulmonary hypoplasia and contractures or deformations of the limbs in the fetus. Potter disease is a bilateral renal agenesis. However, a fetus can also develop renal failure if there is distal obstruction of the urinary system as with posterior urethral valves. To better understand the etiology of this system, we should consider its embryology.

The kidneys are formed from intermediate mesoderm. Kidney development begins in week 4 with the formation of the first of three kidney scaffolds that arise and regress sequentially before the permanent kidney develops. This first scaffold is the pronephros, which is nonfunctional. In week 5, the *meso*nephros develops and functions briefly, creating the *meso*nephric duct (Wolffian duct). The ureteric bud is an offshoot of the mesonephric duct that dilates and subdivides to form the urinary collecting system (collecting tubules, calyces, renal pelvis, and ureter) in both males and females. In the presence of testosterone, the mesonephric duct in males also forms the vas deferens, epididymis, ejaculatory duct, and seminal vesicles. In females, it degenerates entirely except for the vestigial Gartner's duct that can form a benign cyst along the broad ligament. The third scaffold—the *meta*nephros—also appears in week 5 of gestation and becomes the functioning kidney by week 9 of gestation. The ureteric bud from the *meso*nephric duct contacts the *meta*nephros and induces it to form nephrons. If this contact does not occur, renal agenesis results. The adjacent dorsal aorta also sends out collaterals into the *meta*nephros that ultimately develop into glomerular tufts.

Before week 7, the cloaca (the proximal portion of the allantois distally connected to the yolk sac) is divided into the urogenital (UG) sinus and the anorectal canal. During this process, the caudal-most portion of the mesonephric duct is absorbed. Thus, the ureteric bud no longer buds off of the mesonephric duct but enters the UG sinus directly. As such, the UG sinus forms the bladder and the ureteric buds form the ureters. The UG sinus forms the bladder and is continuous with the urethra caudally and the allantois cranially. The urachus is the fibrotic cord that remains when the allantois is obliterated and becomes the median umbilical ligament in the adult.

There are many renal anomalies (e.g., horseshoe kidney, ectopic kidney, double ureter) that go undiagnosed and are without much consequence. Renal agenesis, however, is not one of these. Without kidneys, the fetus can still excrete waste via placental exchange; however, in the setting of renal agenesis resulting in anhydramnios leads to other potentially lethal issues. Without amniotic fluid, the fetal lungs do not have constant pressure on them, causing them to expand and grow. This leads to pulmonary hypoplasia. Without amniotic fluid, the fetus cannot move much and so develops dramatic deformations called contractures of the limbs. There have been attempts to put amniotic fluid into the amniotic cavity via amniocentesis. However, this has been unsuccessful because the fluid is resorbed rapidly. An indwelling catheter has also been considered, but the infectious risks are quite high. At this point in time, there is minimal treatment available for Potter disease. However, in Potter syndrome secondary to bladder outlet obstruction, there have been attempts to place catheters into the bladder or to perform in utero laser ablation of the obstruction. In theory, as long as the fetal kidneys have not been damaged, this idea should work. However, the recent trials indicate that pulmonary function may be improved but renal injury is much more difficult to prevent.

PRENATAL SCREENING

Screening for fetal chromosomal and congenital anomalies is dependent on developing screens that are both sensitive and specific for the condition being screened. Before we move on to discuss these modalities, we should quickly review the terms used with screening tests.

EPIDEMIOLOGY

The classic two-by-two table in epidemiology is divided into cases and controls versus exposed and unexposed. In screening tests, the two dimensions are affected/not affected versus screen positive/screen negative (Table 3-1).

TABLE 3-1 Epidemiology

	Screen Positive (Pos)	Screen Negative (Neg)
Affected	a	b
Not affected	c	d

Sensitivity (sens) = a/(a + b); specificity (spec) = d/(c + d); false negative = b/(a + b); false positive = c/(c + d); positive predictive value (PPV) = a/(a + c); negative predictive value (NPV) = d/(b + d); positive likelihood ratio (LR+) = sens/(1 − spec) = [a/(a + b)]/[c/(c + d)]; negative likelihood ratio (LR−) = (1 − sens)/spec = [b/(a + b)]/[d/(c + d)].

As can be seen in Table 3-1, the sensitivity is the proportion of individuals who are affected and test positive. On the other hand, the specificity is that proportion of individuals who are unaffected and test negative. Sometimes we are more interested in what it means to have a particular test result. In this setting, the positive predictive value (PPV) reports what percentage of patients with a positive screen is affected. The negative predictive value (NPV) is the percentage of people with a negative screen who indeed are not affected. Another set of useful test characteristics are likelihood ratios. The positive likelihood ratio (LR+) tells how much to multiply the prior odds to get the posterior odds; that is, if one knows the odds of some event occurring is 1:100, and runs a test with an LR of 5, then the odds after getting a positive result is 5:100. Similarly, the negative likelihood ratio (LR–) does the same for a negative result.

FIRST-TRIMESTER SCREENING

First trimester was traditionally the time for the first prenatal visit and to get laboratory tests done. However, first-trimester screening has become a routine part of prenatal care and this has two theoretical benefits. One is to find screening tests that are more sensitive than the current second-trimester tests. The other is that by making the diagnosis sooner, the option of termination is safer. **Nuchal translucency (NT)** appears to be an excellent way to screen for aneuploidy and Down syndrome in particular. NT involves a measurement of the posterior fetal neck taken in profile view (Fig. 3-6). Its sensitivity for Down syndrome has been reported to be between 60% and 90% and is generally assumed to be about 70% or greater.

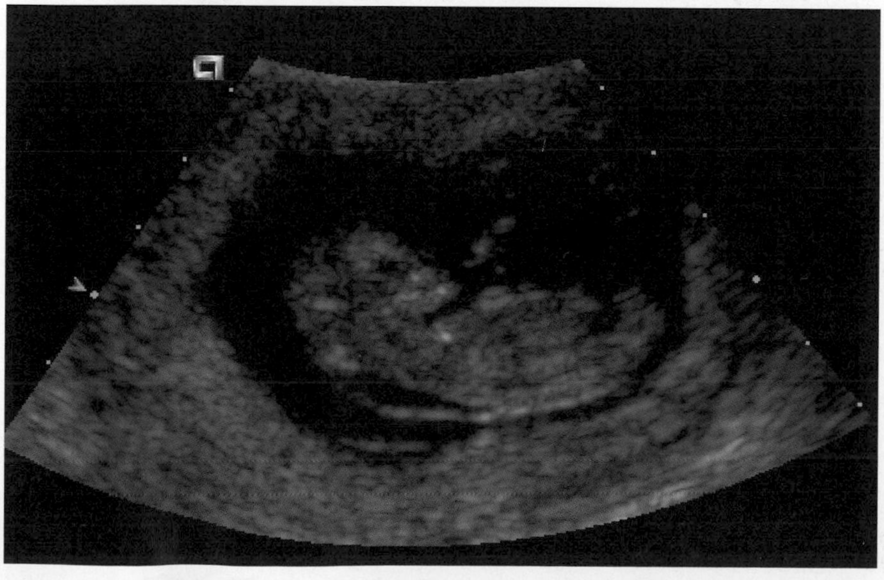

Figure 3-6 • Posterior fetal neck, posterior view.

Several maternal serum analytes have been studied to generate a first-trimester serum screen. Currently, a combination of free or total β-hCG and PAPP-A is being studied alone and in combination with NT. Using a 5% false-positive rate, they appear to have a sensitivity of approximately 60% when used alone, and when combined, the two appear to give an approximate sensitivity of 80%. Commonly, thresholds for these tests are established at a 5% false-positive rate, or where the posterior probability of disease is somewhere between 1:190 and 1:300.

SECOND-TRIMESTER SCREENING

The initial second-trimester serum screen was the MSAFP. This was designed to screen for fetuses with NTDs. When the data from studies was being analyzed, it was noted that the cases of Down syndrome had low MSAFP. This has been combined with low serum estriol and high β-hCG and inhibin as the quadruple screen (Table 3-2). Overall, the quadruple screen has only a 75% to 80% sensitivity for Down syndrome with a 5% false-positive rate. Maternal age is essentially another screening tool because it has been found that the risk of aneuploidy increases exponentially beyond age 35 (Fig. 3-7). At age 35, the overall risk is about 1:190 of aneuploidy. The quad screen is combined with maternal age to generate an overall risk profile of both Down syndrome and trisomy 18. Among women older than age 35, the quadruple (quad) screen has a sensitivity of more than 80%, whereas in women younger than age 35, the sensitivity drops to about 60%. One advantage of the quad screen over the first-trimester screens is that specially trained ultrasound technologists and sonologists are not necessary for performing the test so it is more widely available. Also, because a proportion of the pregnant population does not present for care in the first trimester, the quad screen is the only test available for them.

TABLE 3-2 Quadruple Screen Table

	Trisomy 21	Trisomy 18	Trisomy 13
MSAFP	Decreased	Decreased	Depends on defects
Estriol	Decreased	Decreased	Depends on defects
β-hCG	Elevated	Decreased	Depends on defects
Inhibin	Elevated	Decreased	Depends on defects

Another finding from studies of MSAFP has been in patients whose MSAFP was elevated, but did not have an open NTD. Common reasons for this include inaccurate dating (MSAFP increases with gestation), abdominal wall defects, multiple gestations, placental abnormalities, and fetal demise. Patients whose MSAFP is elevated without an elevated amniotic fluid AFP or these other etiologies have been found to be at greater risk of pregnancy complications associated with the placenta: placental abruption, preeclampsia, IUGR, and possibly IUFD. These problems have been associated with elevated β-hCG as well.

Real-time ultrasound is used to document a singleton, viable gestation and a rudimentary anatomy scan in more than 90% of pregnancies in the United States. The level I or screening obstetric ultrasound scan is a fair screening tool, but its sensitivity varies between providers. One study showed that there was a two- to threefold difference in the number of anomalies identified between primary and tertiary medical centers. The level I ultrasound is not designed to be all encompassing and does not look at fetal limbs, identify sex, show the face, or provide extensive views of the heart. These are generally all done in a level II, detailed or targeted ultrasound. A level II

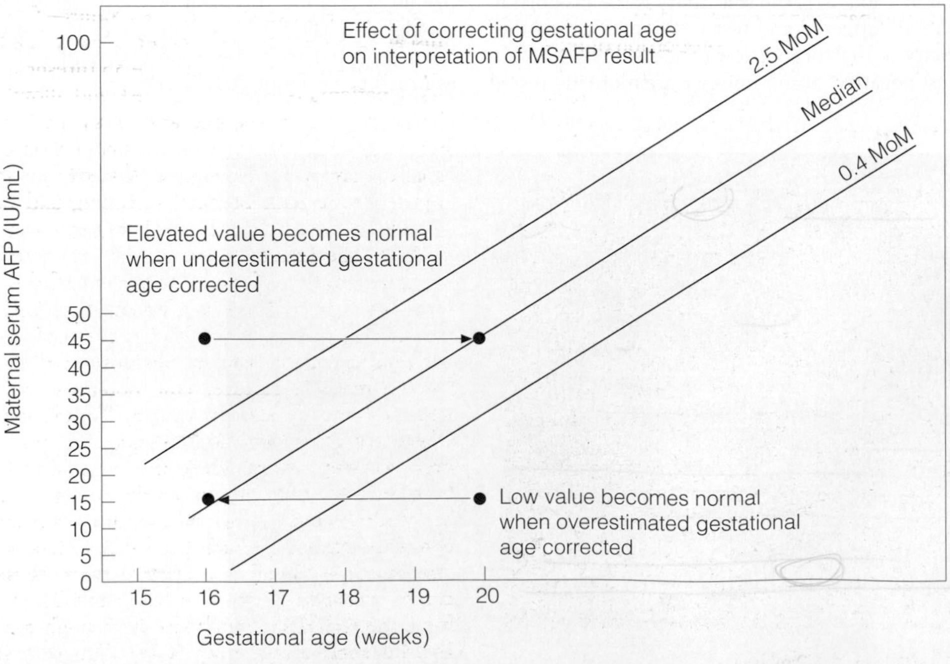

Figure 3-7 • Median maternal serum α-fetoprotein levels throughout gestation. Increasing values with increasing gestational age require accurate dating to interpret low or high MSAFP.

ultrasound is used in patients who are at risk for congenital anomalies or who have had an abnormal level I scan. These tests are generally performed by specially trained perinatologists or radiologists.

There are a number of "soft" findings on obstetric ultrasound that have been associated with aneuploidies. Trisomy 18 has been associated with the finding of a choroid plexus cyst, and Down syndrome has been associated with many ultrasound findings, most notably the **echogenic intracardiac focus (EIF)**. Pathologically, the EIF (Fig. 3-8) is a calcification of the papillary muscle without any particular pathophysiology. It is seen in 5% of pregnancies and is more common in the fetuses of Asian women. Unfortunately, the LR for this test is 1.5 to 2.0, so it at most doubles the pretest odds. For example, a young, 25-year-old woman whose Down syndrome risk is 1:1,000 prior to finding the EIF will therefore have an "increased" risk of 1:500 after finding the EIF. Thus, these tests end up needlessly worrying many patients only to identify a few abnormal fetuses.

NONINVASIVE PRENATAL DIAGNOSIS

Noninvasive prenatal diagnosis has been thought about and discussed for more than 20 years. It is known that both fetal cells and fetal DNA end up in the maternal circulation. Thus, it would be much less invasive to extract this genetic information from a blood draw from the mother than from either the amniotic fluid around the baby (amniocentesis) or a placental biopsy (CVS). Currently, there are several noninvasive prenatal diagnostic tests on the market. These tests are relatively new and therefore should still be considered very good screening tests as opposed to perfectly diagnostic. The currently available tests all rely on the fact that there are free fetal DNA fragments circulating in the maternal plasma. From a maternal blood draw, a technique call massive parallel sequencing is performed in which millions of small fragments of DNA are sequenced and counted. The relative ratio of fetal chromosome 21 is compared to the maternal 21 (and any other chromosome of interest) based on the proportion of fetal DNA in the maternal circulation. Potential advantages of this test include the high sensitivity (>98%), low false-positive rates (approximately 0.2%), and the ability to obtain samples early in pregnancy (10 weeks). Disadvantages of this test are that this has not been assessed in a low-risk population, is not useful in twins or cases of mosaicism, and is costly and available only in a few laboratories in the United States.

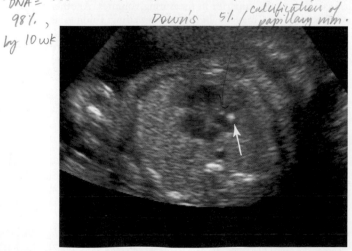

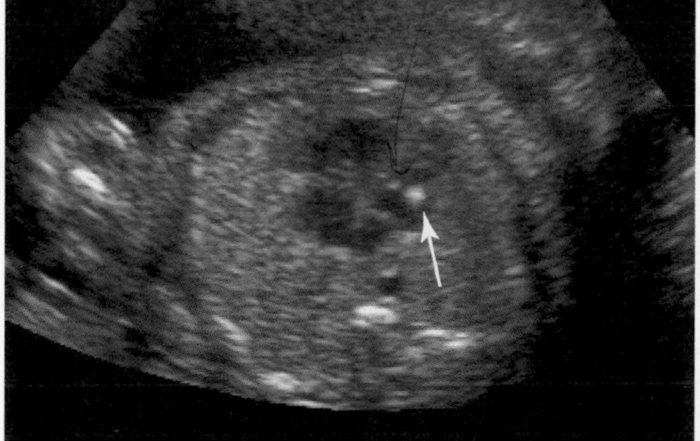

Figure 3-8 • Echogenic intracardiac focus.
(Image provided by Departments of Radiology and Obstetrics & Gynecology, University of California, San Francisco, CA.)

Patients who are known carriers of a genetic disease, at high risk for aneuploidy based on age, or who have a positive screening test may choose to undergo a prenatal diagnostic test. This involves obtaining fetal cells in order to perform a karyotype and possibly DNA tests. There are currently three ways that fetal cells are obtained: amniocentesis, CVS, and percutaneous umbilical blood sampling (PUBS).

AMNIOCENTESIS

An amniocentesis is generally performed beyond 15 weeks to obtain a fetal karyotype, once the chorion and amnion have fused. Early amniocentesis prior to that has been studied and appears to be associated with higher pregnancy loss rates. **Amniocentesis** involves placing a needle transabdominally through the uterus, into the amniotic sac, and withdrawing some of the fluid. The fluid contains sloughed fetal cells that can be cultured. These cultured cells can then be karyotyped and also used in DNA tests.

The cultures take about 5 to 7 days to grow, and additional techniques—**fluorescent in-situ hybridization** (FISH)—can be used to identify aneuploidy and gives results in 24 to 48 hours. Additionally, chromosomal abnormalities (e.g., deletions) that are below the detection threshold of the traditional karyotype may be detected by FISH or microarray comparative genomic hybridization (CGH). Generally, the risk of complications secondary to amniocentesis is considered to be about 1:200, but more recent studies indicate a lower risk, perhaps 1 in approximately 350 or even less. The common risks are rupture of membranes, preterm labor, and, rarely, fetal injury. This risk of 1:200 is one of the reasons why the threshold risk for offering patients fetal diagnosis is about 1:200, which is roughly equivalent to age 35. While it is true that the numbers are approximately the same, the outcomes—Down syndrome and miscarriage—are quite different. Thus, there has been a recent push to discard the maternal age 35 threshold in favor of counseling patients regarding their risk and allowing them to make their own decision incorporating risks and benefits of screening and diagnosis. The most recent bulletin on prenatal diagnosis from the American College of Obstetricians and Gynecologists suggests that both prenatal screening and prenatal diagnosis should be made available to all pregnant women.

With the improvement in maternal serum screening tests for aneuploidy, and now the advent of the noninvasive free fetal DNA tests, there is a de-emphasis on invasive prenatal diagnostic testing. While this is a personal, individual decision for each pregnant woman, obviously, patients can be swayed by the medical culture. One potential issue with screening tests is that they look for trisomy 21, 18, and occasionally 13. There are other common aneuploidies, for example, the sex chromosomal aneuploidies, that some couples would choose to terminate. But, they often do not even know about these anomalies. Another relatively common chromosomal problem is a microdeletion, which is a break or loss of a small piece of chromosome. Small is a relative term, these microdeletions can be missing thousands of base pairs. The best way to screen for a microdeletion syndrome is through a complete genome hybridization array (array cGH). This test will identify these microdeletions and research studies are being done to determine the clinical utility for these tests. If a couple wants such a test, currently fetal DNA from an invasive prenatal diagnostic test would be necessary.

Thus, while there are improvements in sensitivity and specificity, in the end, one cannot replace the certainty of a diagnostic test. It is important for patients to understand the difference between a screening and diagnostic test when they are being seen for prenatal care. If the primary clinician is not comfortable explaining the tests, referral to a genetic counselor or other expert in prenatal diagnosis is merited.

CHORIONIC VILLUS SAMPLING

Chorionic villus sampling (CVS) can be used to obtain a fetal karyotype sooner than amniocentesis because it can be performed between 9 and 12 weeks. CVS involves placing a catheter into the intrauterine cavity, either transabdominally or transvaginally, and aspirating a small quantity of chorionic villi from the placenta. The risk of complications from CVS is likely higher than the amniocentesis rate of 1:200. Because a greater amount of cells are obtained, CVS results are often faster than those of amniocentesis. However, the cells are from the placenta; therefore, in rare cases of confined placental mosaicism, the cells may be misleading. Complications include preterm labor, premature rupture of membranes, previable delivery, and fetal injury. When performed earlier than 9 weeks of gestation, CVS has been associated with fetal limb anomalies, which is assumed to be secondary to vascular interruption.

FETAL BLOOD SAMPLING

Percutaneous umbilical blood sampling (PUBS) is performed by placing a needle transabdominally into the uterus and phlebotomizing the umbilical cord. This procedure may be used when a fetal hematocrit or platelet count needs to be obtained, particularly in the setting of Rh alloimmunization and other causes of fetal anemia. PUBS may also used for rapid karyotype analysis. The PUBS needle can also be used to transfuse the fetus in cases of fetal anemia. Intrauterine transfusion (IUT) was performed before the advent of real-time ultrasound by placing needles into the fetal peritoneal cavity and performing intraperitoneal transfusions, but transumbilical transfusions are more effective.

FETAL IMAGING

Currently, ultrasound is used most commonly to image a fetus prenatally. As described above, a level I or level II ultrasound is commonly performed between 18 and 22 weeks. The fetal anatomy can be difficult to visualize well prior to 18 weeks of gestation, giving the lower threshold for detection of anomalies. For the upper threshold, if an anomaly is seen, the further workup can take more than a week, giving the patient just a few days prior to 24 weeks of gestation to decide about termination of the pregnancy in the setting of congenital anomalies. A targeted, level II ultrasound can identify cleft lip, polydactyly, clubfoot (Fig. 3-9), fetal sex, NTDs, abdominal wall defects, and renal anomalies. It can usually identify some cardiac and brain anomalies as well, but may not be able to make a specific diagnosis. It is poor at identifying esophageal atresia and tracheoesophageal fistula, in which sometimes the only sign may be a small or nonvisualized stomach in the setting of polyhydramnios.

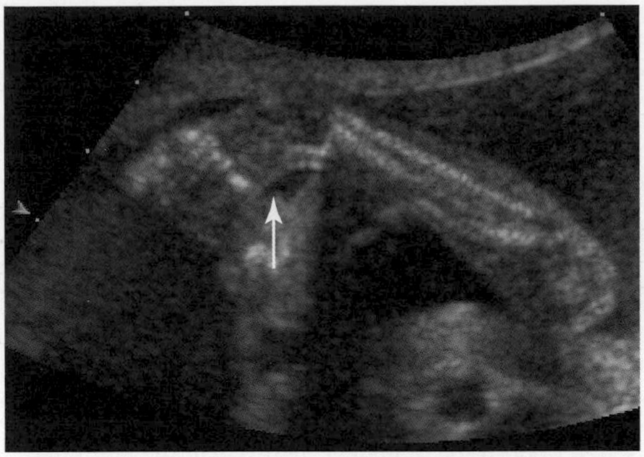

Figure 3-9 • Clubfoot—The fibula and tibia can be seen with the foot at almost a right angle to them.
(Image provided by Departments of Radiology and Obstetrics & Gynecology, University of California, San Francisco, CA.)

Fetal echocardiogram is usually used to make specific diagnoses of fetal cardiac anomalies detected on ultrasound. Doppler ultrasound can characterize the blood flow through the chambers of the heart as well as the vessels entering and leaving the heart. Fetal echo is used in some institutions as the first-line diagnostic modality in patients at high risk for cardiac anomalies, in particular, pregestational diabetic patients.

Fetal MRI is one of the newest modalities to image a fetus. It is particularly useful in examining the fetal brain and may recognize changes associated with hypoxic damage sooner than ultrasound. It is also superior in measuring volumes. Another new modality that may be better in measuring volumes is three-dimensional (3-D) ultrasound. While the image provided certainly looks more like an actual fetus than the more common 2-D images, it is unclear whether 3-D ultrasound offers increased diagnostic capabilities.

KEY POINTS

- Mothers can be asymptomatic carriers of AR diseases and can often be screened for carrier status. Geographic ancestry is used to provide pretest counseling and inform testing.
- If a mother is a carrier, the father of the baby can be screened as well to determine his carrier status. If the father is negative, there is no risk to the baby; if he is positive, there is a 25% chance of the disease in the fetus.
- The two common ways that AR disorders are introduced and maintained in a population are the founder effect (Tay-Sachs) and heterozygote advantage (sickle cell disease).
- Having an abnormal number of chromosomes usually leads to miscarriage. However, several aneuploidies exist that commonly survive until birth and beyond.
- Of all the autosomal trisomies, Down syndrome is the hardiest. While they have foreshortened life expectancies, these individuals commonly survive into their 50s.
- The most common aneuploidies are those of the sex chromosomes. These individuals are less severely affected than the autosomal aneuploidies.

- Fetal congenital anomalies primarily arise during embryogenesis. However, they can progress (as seen in Potter syndrome) as development continues.
- NTDs are associated with folate deficiency and can be screened for by noting an elevated MSAFP.
- Cardiac anomalies that are surgically repaired can often result in minimal impairment, although this is highly lesion dependent.
- Organ systems are often interconnected during development, as in the case of the lungs and kidneys in Potter syndrome.
- The sensitivity of a screening test is that percentage of patients who would be identified by the test.
- Common screening tests for fetal abnormalities include first-trimester screening, the quad screen and level I ultrasound.
- Noninvasive prenatal diagnosis appears to have great sensitivity and specificity for trisomy 21 but has limitations.
- Karyotype and DNA tests require fetal or trophoblastic cells for analysis.
- Fetal diagnosis in the first trimester is by CVS, which obtains trophoblastic cells.
- In the second trimester, amniocentesis is used to obtain fetal cells in the amniotic fluid.
- Prenatal diagnosis can also be made by imaging studies, most commonly 2-D ultrasound. Fetal echocardiogram, MRI, and 3-D ultrasound are also used.

C Clinical Vignettes

Vignette 1

A 40-year-old G_2P_0 woman at 7 weeks GA by LMP presents for her first prenatal visit. She spontaneously conceived after 18 months of trying. She is excited about the pregnancy, but at the same time is concerned about potential risks for herself as well as the baby because of her age. Her husband is 52 years old, healthy, and has fathered two children from a prior marriage. The week prior to the visit, she experienced spotting that lasted 3 days and then resolved. Currently, she has no complaints. She has no past medical or surgical history except for a miscarriage 3 years ago. She has regular periods every 30 days.

1. You offer her which of the following prenatal screening/diagnostic tests?
   a. CVS
   b. Amniocentesis
   c. First-trimester screening
   d. Quad screening
   e. All of the above
2. She undergoes both first- and second-trimester screening. All of the screening tests are relatively reassuring as her risk of Down syndrome is reduced below the screen positive threshold at 1 in 967. She also has a normal screening ultrasound. You explain that these are screening tests and that she still has some risk for aneuploidy. Which of the following aneuploidies would be most common in the setting of otherwise normal screening?
   a. Trisomy 21
   b. Trisomy 18
   c. Trisomy 13
   d. Sex chromosomal aneuploidy
   e. None of the above
3. Because of the lack of certainty, she is considering an amniocentesis. The risks of amniocentesis include which of the following?
   a. Alloimmunization of an Rh-negative woman carrying an Rh-positive fetus
   b. Preeclampsia
   c. Premature rupture of membranes
   d. a, b, and c
   e. a and c only
4. In the end, she decides not to undergo amniocentesis. She goes on to deliver a normal-appearing baby boy at 39 weeks' gestation without complications. The counseling you gave to facilitate her decision making specifically emphasized which of the following?
   a. Beneficence
   b. Justice
   c. Autonomy
   d. Paternalism
   e. None of the above

Vignette 2

You are providing prenatal care to a 22-year-old G_1P_0 woman at 16 weeks GA by LMP. She has had a relatively smooth pregnancy without complications thus far. At 5′5″ and 215 lb she has an obese BMI, otherwise without medical or surgical history. She presented to prenatal care at 14½ weeks, and so missed first-trimester screening. She undergoes the quad screen and has an elevated level of maternal serum alpha-fetoprotein (MSAFP).

1. Given the elevation in MSAFP, her pregnancy is at increased risk for which of the following?
   a. Gestational diabetes
   b. Gastroschisis
   c. Down syndrome
   d. Klinefelter syndrome
   e. All of the above
2. You discuss the potential meaning of the elevated MSAFP. After a long conversation, the patient decides to undergo her second-trimester ultrasound. Which of the following findings seen on ultrasound would NOT be an explanation for the elevated MSAFP?
   a. Double bubble-duodenal atresia
   b. A membrane-covered mass protruding through the abdominal wall
   c. Fetal bowel floating around in the amniotic fluid
   d. Lack of a fetal skull
   e. A small membrane-covered outpouching in the lower back/spine
3. The ultrasound reveals a myelomeningocele. Which of the following is true and may be used in counseling?
   a. This is generally a lethal anomaly
   b. Delivery must be by cesarean to protect the baby
   c. Fetal surgery includes laser therapy
   d. Fetal surgery has been shown to improve some outcomes
   e. Fetal surgery is experimental and has no known benefits
4. The increased incidence of this finding is associated with which of the following medications when used in pregnancy?
   a. Valproic acid
   b. Lithium

c. Fluoxetine
d. Prednisone
e. Acetaminophen

5. In a subsequent pregnancy, prevention of recurrence would include:
   a. low-dose aspirin
   b. low molecular weight heparin
   c. prenatal vitamins taken twice per day
   d. 4 mg folic acid
   e. increased dietary calcium

Vignette 3

A 25-year-old G2P1 woman presents at 9 weeks' gestation for routine prenatal care. She has a history of a prior term birth 2 years earlier in which she developed preeclampsia and required induction of labor at 38 weeks' gestation, leading to a vaginal delivery of a viable baby girl. She is interested in first-trimester screening.

1. Which of the following is true about first-trimester screening?
   a. First-trimester serum screening has an 80% sensitivity for Down syndrome
   b. NT screening alone has a 70% sensitivity for Down syndrome
   c. Combined first-trimester screening has a 90% sensitivity for Down syndrome
   d. Increased NT in the setting of normal karyotype is associated with limb anomalies
   e. First-trimester screening has a sensitivity for Down syndrome that is greater than the sequential screen

2. Her tests come back with a risk for Down syndrome of 1 in 420 at 11 weeks' gestation. What do you report to the patient?
   a. The test is negative
   b. The test is positive
   c. The risk for Down syndrome is 1 in 420
   d. She will need an amniocentesis
   e. She will not need an amniocentesis

3. The patient chooses to delay prenatal diagnosis at this time and plans on obtaining second-trimester screening and an obstetric ultrasound. Which of the following is true about obstetric ultrasound and Down syndrome
   a. Ultrasound has a higher sensitivity for Down syndrome than the first-trimester screening
   b. Ultrasound has higher sensitivity for Down syndrome than the quad screening
   c. A finding of caudal regression syndrome on ultrasound is pathognomonic for Down syndrome
   d. Down syndrome fetuses with normal ultrasound findings have lower IQs than those with major anomalies
   e. Classic findings of Down syndrome on obstetric ultrasound are an AV canal and pyloric stenosis

Vignette 4

A 24-year-old G1P0 woman presents for prenatal care at 8 weeks by LMP. She has regular menses every 28 to 30 days and you confirm her gestational age with an ultrasound today in the office. She has no past medical or surgical history. She and her husband of 6 months planned the pregnancy and they have both been reading about pregnancy and prenatal care. You discuss the prenatal tests for the first visit as well as the plan throughout the rest of the pregnancy.

1. As part of this discussion, you offer her which of the following prenatal screening/diagnostic tests?
   a. CVS
   b. Amniocentesis
   c. First-trimester screening
   d. Quad screening
   e. All of the above

2. The patient opts to undergo first-trimester screening, which returns with a risk for Down syndrome of 1 in 1,214 and risk of trisomy 18 of 1 in 987. At 18 weeks, she gets a quad screen, and her estriol, β-hCG, and α-fetoprotein (AFP) were all low. She has an ultrasound, which shows a fetus consistent with 16 weeks' size, increased amniotic fluid, clubfoot, omphalocele, choroid plexus cyst, and possible heart defect. On the basis of the patient's history and data provided, what is the most likely diagnosis?
   a. Trisomy 21
   b. Trisomy 18
   c. Trisomy 13
   d. Turner syndrome
   e. Klinefelter syndrome

3. The patient and her husband wish to have a definitive diagnosis. Which of the following tests do you offer her?
   a. Amniocentesis
   b. CVS
   c. Array CGH
   d. Quad screen
   e. Noninvasive prenatal diagnosis

4. Because of their anxiety about the diagnosis, the patient and her husband wonder if there is a faster test one could do to obtain a diagnosis more quickly. Which of the following do you offer them?
   a. Array CGH
   b. Fetal MRI
   c. FISH
   d. MCA Doppler
   e. Quad screen

CLINICAL VIGNETTES

A Answers

Vignette 1 Question 1
Answer E: Decision making about prenatal screening and diagnosis are going to be different for each woman/couple, instead of as with much of medical care where clinicians make strong recommendations. In prenatal diagnosis, the key is to not make specific recommendations, but to educate regarding the options. Because there are some young women who would prefer not to have a child with aneuploidy and are willing to bear the risk of invasive prenatal diagnosis, all pregnant women should be offered invasive prenatal diagnosis alongside options of screening. Conversely, older women who historically were recommended to undergo invasive prenatal diagnosis may wish to have a screening test and will live with the uncertainty of a screening test to avoid the risk of a pregnancy loss from invasive prenatal diagnosis.

Vignette 1 Question 2
Answer D: The sex chromosomal abnormalities include 45 X,O—Turner's syndrome, 47 XXY—Klinefelter's syndrome, as well as the less commonly diagnosed 47 XXX and 47 XYY. Unfortunately, the serum screens in the first and second trimester do not screen for the sex chromosomal abnormalities, so having a normal screen does not reduce the risk. Turner's syndrome will commonly be found on first trimester NT screen because these patients may have a cystic hygroma. However, this still does not reduce the risk of sex chromosomal abnormality below a screening threshold. Trisomy 21 thresholds are generally 1 in 200 to 1 in 300 varying by states and countries. Trisomy 18 and 13 will also commonly manifest multiple congenital anomalies, so their risk is quite low after a normal ultrasound. The four most common sex chromosomal abnormalities range in risk from approximately 1 in 500 to 1 in 1,000 live births, and the most common, Turner syndrome and Klinefelter syndrome appear to be due to paternal nondysjunction rather than maternal, thus maternal age itself does not appear to be a risk factor.

Vignette 1 Question 3
Answer E: There are risks of amniocentesis that include pregnancy loss, infection (chorioamnionitis), preterm premature rupture of the membranes (PPROM), risk of fetal injury with the needle, risk of puncturing the umbilical cord leading to loss of fetal blood, exposure to the fetus of maternal infection (e.g., HIV), and exposure to the mother of the fetal cells (e.g., alloimmunization of mother). There is no evidence that the risk of preeclampsia is any higher in the setting of amniocentesis.

Vignette 1 Question 4
Answer C: In many aspects of medical decision making, it is important to emphasize patient autonomy in the decision-making process. This is because while the patient may not have as much information about the medical issues, she will have the most information about her preferences toward the outcomes. Thus, shared medical decision making is at its best when the clinician provides information, pros and cons, and the patient incorporates her values and preferences to make the ultimate decision.

Vignette 2 Question 1
Answer B: Elevated MSAFP can be seen in a variety of pregnancy complications. It is primarily used to screen for NTDs such as spina bifida, meningomyelocele, or anencephaly. It is also elevated in pregnancies that are not dated as far along as they should be, have abdominal wall defects such as omphalocele or gastroschisis, and have placental abnormalities like previa or accreta. MSAFP is decreased in Down syndrome and has no relationship with Klinefelter syndrome.

Vignette 2 Question 2
Answer A: Double bubble is seen in the setting of duodenal atresia, which is seen more commonly in Down syndrome and is not associated with an elevated MSAFP. The membrane-covered mass through the abdominal wall is an omphalocele. Along with the bowel floating in the amniotic fluid, gastroschisis, these abdominal wall defects are associated with an increased MSAFP. NTDs such as anencephaly, no skull or cerebral cortex, or spina bifida, a lack of closure of the neural tube at various levels of the spine lead to an increased MSAFP.

Vignette 2 Question 3
Answer D: Myelomeningocele, a common form of spina bifida, is not usually lethal, but leads to long-term morbidity in a large majority of affected children. In order to reduce the morbidity, a recent prospective trial of closure of the defect while the fetus was still in utero was conducted. The study demonstrated improvement in several outcomes including ambulation at 30 months of age. Laser is used for in utero ablation of connecting vessels in the setting of twin-to-twin transfusion syndrome, not in myelomeningocele repair. Some providers recommend cesarean delivery for fetuses with NTDs. This is not a uniform recommendation and is not accompanied with much evidence in favor of its practice.

Vignette 2 Question 4
Answer A: NTDs are increased in the setting of diabetes and women with seizure disorders. The latter is thought to be associated with the use of several antiepileptic drugs (AEDs), including carbamazepine and valproic acid. Lithium is associated with Ebstein's anomaly, a displacement of the tricuspid valve. Fluoxetine and several

other SSRIs have been associated with an increase in fetal cardiac anomalies. Prednisone does not cross the placenta. However, it can lead to hyperglycemia, which may, in turn, cause fetal effects. It is important to have women on prednisone in pregnancy check blood glucose values. Acetaminophen has not been associated with any fetal anomalies.

Vignette 2 Question 5

Answer D: Folic acid supplementation has been shown to decrease the risk of NTDs. Folic acid has been added to grains in the United States, which has led to lower rates of NTDs. There is 0.4 mg of folic acid in standard prenatal vitamins. However, in high-risk patients, the recommendation is currently to take 10 times that dose, or 4 mg/day. Further work delineating the dose response and threshold effect still needs to be done. Low-dose aspirin has been shown to slightly reduce the risk of preeclampsia and both low-dose aspirin and LMWH have been used in women with known thrombophilias. Low dietary calcium intake has been shown to be associated with preeclampsia, but intervention trials are equivocal on the potential benefits.

Vignette 3 Question 1

Answer B: First-trimester screening for Down syndrome has become the standard of care, though not all women can get access to the testing because of the lack of availability of trained sonologists to provide NT ultrasound and variability in the insurance coverage for first-trimester testing. The serum screen is composed of PAPP-A and free β-hCG and has a 60% sensitivity for Down syndrome alone. NT alone has a 70% sensitivity and when added to the serum screen, the two together have an 80% sensitivity. If the NT is increased and there is no aneuploidy, the fetus is at increased risk, in particular, for cardiac anomalies. The sequential screen is a test that combines the first-trimester and second-trimester tests. This combination gets to a 90% to 95% sensitivity, so it has a greater sensitivity than first-trimester screening alone.

Vignette 3 Question 2

Answer C: The question is not meant as a trick question, but to make the point that across most clinical settings, clinicians think of the Down syndrome screening tests as positive or negative. However, in the setting of Down syndrome screening because patient preferences are so important, the best way to counsel women is to present them with the absolute risks instead of calling a test positive or negative. Now, it is true that most Down syndrome screening thresholds range from 1 in 150 to 1 in 350, so this 1 in 420 would be considered a "negative" test from that standpoint. However, given that this risk is approximately twice her age-related risk should also be mentioned.

Vignette 3 Question 3

Answer E: Down syndrome fetuses will have findings on ultrasound about 60% of the time. This makes obstetric ultrasound a poor screening test for Down syndrome, worse than both first-trimester combined screening and quad screening. There are no good studies that suggest that the function of individuals with Down syndrome varies by ultrasound findings. However, mortality and some morbidity will be greater in those with serious cardiac anomalies. The classic cardiac anomaly in Down syndrome is the AV canal defect. Pyloric stenosis is also common and should raise concern for Down syndrome. Caudal regression is seen in diabetic pregnancies.

Vignette 4 Question 1

Answer E: As explained in Case 1, all prenatal screening and diagnostic options should be offered to all women. Case 1 discussed a 40-year-old woman and this one is about a 24-year-old woman; however, all options should be made available to both women. This is contrary to historic practice and teaching as recently as 5 to 10 years ago when clinicians would recommend invasive prenatal diagnosis to higher risk women and recommend against in lower risk women. Many clinicians today, because they were trained in this prior era, still practice this way. Thus, in contrast to much of medical care wherein clinicians make strong recommendations, nondirective counseling by clinicians will make decision making about prenatal screening and diagnosis different for each woman/couple. In prenatal diagnosis, the key is to not make specific recommendations, but to educate regarding the options. Because there are some young women who would prefer not to have a child with aneuploidy and are willing to bear the risk of invasive prenatal diagnosis, all pregnant women should be offered invasive prenatal diagnosis alongside options of screening. Conversely, older women who historically were recommended to undergo invasive prenatal diagnosis may wish to have a screening test and will live with the uncertainty of a screening test to avoid the risk of a pregnancy loss from invasive prenatal diagnosis.

Vignette 4 Question 2

Answer B: The quad screen with low estriol, β-hCG, and MSAFP is consistent with trisomy 18. So is the finding of the multiple anomalies on ultrasound, including the growth restriction. Trisomy 13 may also have multiple anomalies on ultrasound, though these findings are more consistent with trisomy 18. Trisomy 21, Turner syndrome, and Klinefelter syndrome will all often have a normal ultrasound, though trisomy 21 will have soft findings or anomalies on ultrasound about 60% of the time. One part of the case that may have been confusing was her first-trimester test results, which revealed a risk of approximately 1 per 1,000 of both trisomy 21 and 18. Of note, while a 1 per 1,000 risk of trisomy 21 is roughly the background baseline, the risk of trisomy 18 of 1 per 1,000 is an increase over the background risk, which is 1 per 5,000 to 1 per 10,000. Further, this reminds us that these are simply screening tests, not diagnostic tests.

Vignette 4 Question 3

Answer B: In order to achieve a definitive diagnosis, one must obtain fetal DNA, this is usually done via CVS or amniocentesis. At 18 weeks' gestation, the preferred route is amniocentesis. Array CGH can be performed on the cells from the amniocentesis to look for microdeletions. This is relatively new technology and is not universally covered by insurance, so one would obtain a karyotype first and then order CGH if karyotype was negative. The quad screen was already performed on the patient and is just a screening test. Noninvasive prenatal diagnostic testing using free fetal DNA in the maternal circulation is available for trisomies 21, 18, and 13. However, this is still thought of as a high-order screening test, not a diagnostic test.

Vignette 4 Question 4

Answer C: A karyotype usually takes 5 to 10 business days to return a result. FISH (fluorescent in situ hybridization) can be used to get quick results in 2 to 3 days for commonly known problems such as trisomies 21, 18, 13, and aneuploidies of X or Y. FISH can also be used to screen for particular aberrations in components of the genome such as the 22q deletion seen in DiGeorge syndrome. Array CGH could also give the results potentially sooner than amniocentesis. However, currently turnaround times are not as fast as FISH and there are still relatively few laboratories performing this test. Fetal MRI can allow better visualization of anomalies, but would not give a genetic diagnosis. MCA Doppler is used to screen for fetal anemia by measuring the peak systolic velocity in the middle cerebral artery. As mentioned previously the quad screen is a screening test that she has already had. She obtains the FISH testing, which is consistent with trisomy 18 as is the follow-up karyotype.

Chapter

4 Normal Labor and Delivery

LABOR AND DELIVERY

When a patient first presents to the labor floor, a quick initial assessment is made using the history of present pregnancy, obstetric history, and the standard medical and social history. Routinely, patients are queried regarding contractions, vaginal bleeding, leakage of fluid, and fetal movement. Beyond the standard physical examination, the obstetric examination includes maternal abdominal examination for contractions and the fetus (**Leopold maneuvers**), cervical examination, fetal heart tones, and a sterile speculum examination if rupture of membranes is suspected. Increasingly, this obstetric examination is augmented with obstetric ultrasound evaluation of the cervical length and fetal presentation.

OBSTETRIC EXAMINATION

The physical examination includes determination of fetal lie and presentation and a cervical examination. **Fetal lie**, that is, whether the infant is longitudinal or transverse within the uterus, is relatively easy to determine with Leopold maneuvers (Fig. 4-1). The maneuvers involve palpating first at the fundus of the uterus in the maternal upper abdominal quadrants, then on either side of the uterus (maternal left and right), and finally, palpation of the presenting part just above the pubic symphysis. Determination of **fetal presentation**, either breech or vertex (cephalic), can be more difficult, and even the most experienced examiner may require ultrasound to confirm presentation, particularly in the obese patient.

RUPTURE OF MEMBRANES

In 10% of pregnancies, the membranes surrounding the fetus rupture prior to the onset of labor; this is called premature rupture of membranes (PROM). When PROM occurs more than 18 hours before labor, it is considered prolonged PROM and puts both mother and fetus at increased risk for infection. PROM is often confused with PPROM, which is preterm, premature rupture of membranes, with preterm being before 37 weeks of gestation.

Diagnosis

Diagnosis of rupture of membranes (ROM) is suspected with a history of a gush or leaking of fluid from the vagina, although sometimes it is difficult to differentiate between stress incontinence and small leaks of amniotic fluid. Diagnosis can be confirmed by the **pool**, **nitrazine**, and **fern** tests.

Using a sterile speculum to examine the vaginal vault, the pool test is positive if there is a collection of fluid in the vagina. This can be augmented by asking the patient to cough or bear down, potentially allowing one to observe fluid escaping from the cervix. Vaginal secretions are normally acidic, whereas amniotic fluid is alkaline. Thus, when amniotic fluid is placed on nitrazine paper, the paper should immediately turn blue. The estrogens in the amniotic fluid cause crystallization of the salts in the amniotic fluid when it dries. Under low microscopic power, the crystals resemble the blades of a fern, giving the test its name (Fig. 4-2). Caution should be exercised to sample fluid that is not directly from the cervix because cervical mucus also ferns and may result in a false-positive reading. If these tests are equivocal, an ultrasound examination can determine the quantity of fluid around the fetus. If the fluid volume was previously normal and there is no other reason to suspect low fluid, **oligohydramnios** is indicative of ROM. In situations when an accurate diagnosis is necessary (e.g., PPROM where antibiotic prophylaxis would be indicated), amniocentesis may be used to inject dilute indigo carmine dye into the amniotic sac to look for leakage of fluid from the cervix onto a tampon (the amnio dye test or tampon test). More recently, a rapid test called Amnisure has been described. This test uses rapid molecular testing to identify placental alpha-microglobulin-1 via immunoassay, which appears to have a higher sensitivity and specificity than conventional tests for PROM. The clinical utility and cost-effectiveness of using this test requires further research.

CERVICAL EXAMINATION

The cervical examination allows the obstetrician to determine whether a patient is in labor, the phase of labor, and how labor is progressing. The five components of the cervical examination are dilation, effacement, fetal station, cervical position, and consistency of the cervix. These five aspects of the examination make up the **Bishop score** (Table 4-1). A Bishop score greater than 8 is consistent with a cervix favorable for both spontaneous labor and, as it is more commonly used, induced labor.

Dilation is assessed by using either one or two fingers of the examining hand to determine how open the cervix is at the level of the **internal os**. The measurements are in centimeters and range from closed, or 0 cm, to fully dilated, or 10 cm. On average, a 10-cm dilation is necessary to accommodate the term infant's biparietal diameter.

Effacement is also a subjective measurement made by the examiner. It determines how much length is left of the cervix and how effaced (i.e., thinned out) it is (Fig. 4-3). Effacement can commonly be reported by percent or by cervical length. The typical cervix is 3 to 5 cm in length; thus, if the cervix feels like it is about 2 cm from external to internal os, it is 50%

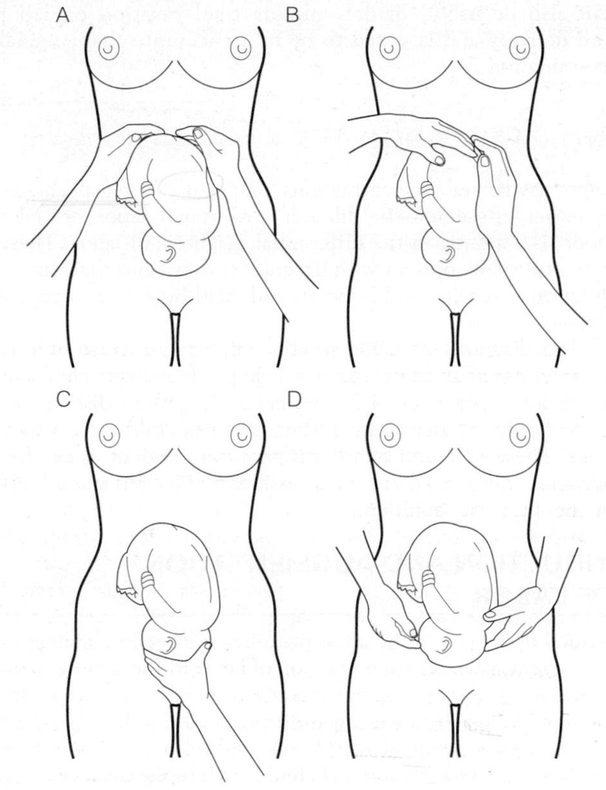

Figure 4-1 • (A–D) Leopold maneuvers used to determine fetal presentation, position, and engagement.

(N) 3–5 cm from internal to external OS

effaced. Complete or 100% effacement occurs when the cervix is as thin as the adjoining lower uterine segment.

The relation of the fetal head to the ischial spines of the female pelvis is known as **station** (Fig. 4-4). When the most *station* descended aspect of the presenting part is at the level of the ischial spines, it is designated 0 station. Station is negative when the presenting part is above the ischial spines and positive when it is below. There are two systems of measuring the distance of the presenting part in relation to the ischial spines. One divides the distance to the pelvic inlet into thirds and thus station is −3 to 0 and then 0 to +3, which is at the level of the introitus. The other system uses centimeters, which gives

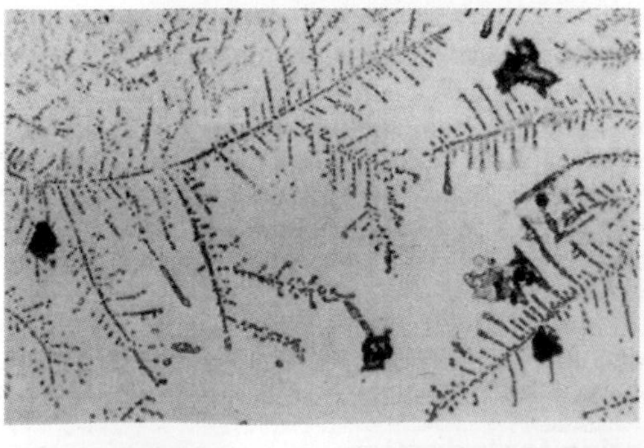

Figure 4-2 • Fern test.
(From Beckmann CRB, Ling LW, Laube DW, et al. *Obstetrics and Gynecology*, 4th ed. Baltimore, MD: Lippincott Williams & Wilkins; 2002.)

■ **TABLE 4-1** The Bishop Score				
Score	**0**	**1**	**2**	**3**
Cervical (cm)	Closed	1–2	3–4	<5 dilation
Cervical (%)	0–30	40–50	60–70	<80 effacement
Station	−3	−2	−1, 0	<+1
Cervical consistency	Firm	Medium	Soft	
Cervical position	Posterior	Mid	Anterior	

stations of −5 to +5. Either system is effective and both are widely used among different institutions; however, the American College of Obstetricians and Gynecologists (ACOG) recommends the usage of the 5 system in its clinical guidelines. *ACOG: 5 system*

Cervical **consistency** is self-explanatory. Whether the cervix feels firm, soft, or somewhere in between should be noted. Cervical **position** ranges from posterior to mid to anterior. A posterior cervix is high in the pelvis, located behind the fetal head and often quite difficult to reach, let alone examine. The anterior cervix can usually be felt easily on examination and is often lower down in the vagina. During early labor, the cervix often changes its consistency to soft and advances its position from posterior to mid to anterior.

While cervical evaluation through a physical examination has been the standard throughout modern obstetrics, cervical evaluation through ultrasound has become increasingly common. There are clinical studies that find greater interobserver reliability with ultrasound measures of cervical length as opposed to a digital physical examination of the cervix. So, particularly in the evaluation of preterm patients with concern for preterm labor, many clinicians will use ultrasound to measure the cervical length. *use U/S in preterm*

FETAL PRESENTATION AND POSITION

The fetal presentation can be **vertex** (head down), **breech** (buttocks down), or **transverse** (neither down). Although presentation may already be known from the Leopold maneuvers, it can be confirmed by examination of the presenting part during cervical examination. Assuming that the cervix is somewhat dilated, the fetal presenting part may be palpated as well during this examination. In the early stages of labor when the cervix is not very dilated, digital examination of the presenting part can be difficult, leading to inaccurate determination of presentation. However, palpation of hair or sutures on the fetal vertex or the gluteal cleft or anus on the breech usually leaves little doubt. A fetus presenting head-first should actually be designated cephalic rather than vertex, unless the head is flexed and the vertex is truly presenting. If the fetus is cephalic with an extended head, it may be presenting with either the face or brow. If the fetal vertex is presenting along with a fetal extremity such as an arm, this is deemed a compound presentation.

With face presentations, the chin or mentum is the fetal reference point, while with breech presentations the reference is the fetal sacrum (Fig. 4-5). If fetal presentation cannot be determined by physical examination, ultrasound can confirm presentation. Ultrasound is also useful in determining whether

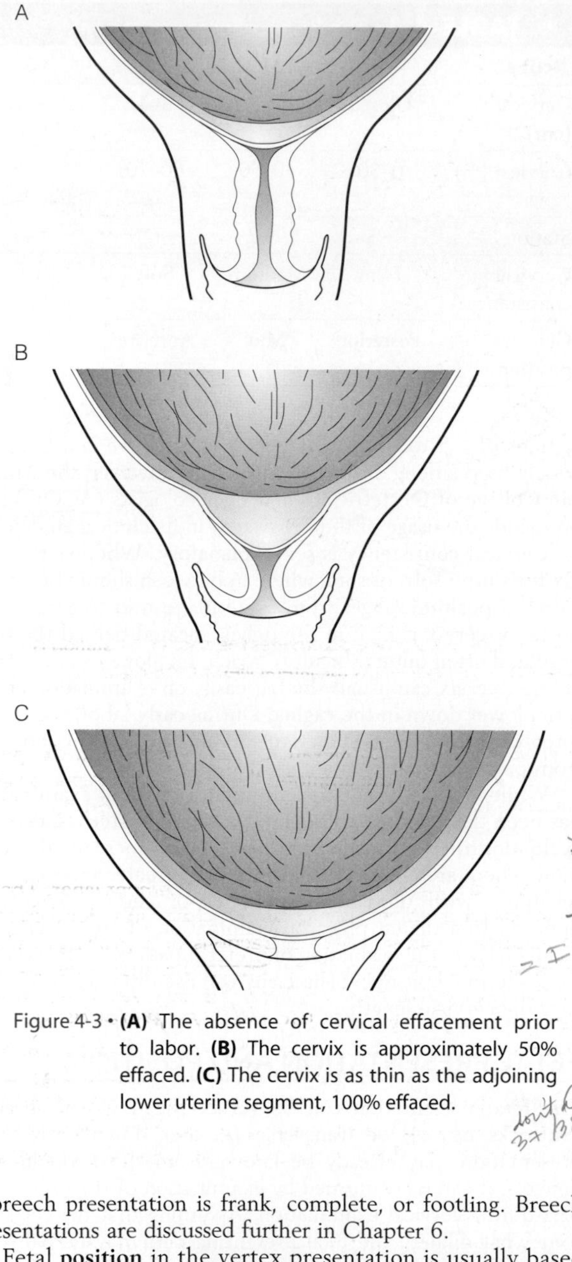

Figure 4-3 • **(A)** The absence of cervical effacement prior to labor. **(B)** The cervix is approximately 50% effaced. **(C)** The cervix is as thin as the adjoining lower uterine segment, 100% effaced.

a breech presentation is frank, complete, or footling. Breech presentations are discussed further in Chapter 6.

Fetal **position** in the vertex presentation is usually based on the relationship of the fetal occiput to the maternal pelvis. An abnormal fetal position such as occiput transverse (OT) or occiput posterior (OP) can lead to prolonged labor and a higher rate of cesarean delivery. Thus, OT or OP position may be suspected with an abnormally long labor. Position is determined by palpation of the sutures and fontanelles. The vault, or roof, of the fetal skull is composed of five bones: two frontal, two parietal, and one occipital. The **anterior fontanelle** is the junction between the two frontal bones and two parietal bones and is larger and diamond-shaped. The **posterior fontanelle** is the junction between the two parietal bones and the occipital bone and is smaller and more triangular-shaped. In the setting of extensive molding of the fetal skull or asynclitism, where the sagittal suture is not midline within the maternal pelvis, palpation of the fetal ear can be used to determine position. Ultrasound can also be useful in determining fetal position on labor and delivery and is noted to be more accurate than vaginal examination.

NORMAL LABOR

Labor is defined as contractions that cause cervical change in either effacement or dilation. **Prodromal labor** or "false labor" is common in the differential diagnosis of labor. These patients usually present with irregular contractions that vary in duration, intensity, and intervals and yield little or no cervical change.

The diagnosis of labor strictly defined is regular uterine contractions that cause cervical change. However, clinicians use many other signs of labor, including patient discomfort, bloody show, nausea and vomiting, and palpability of contractions. These signs and symptoms vary from patient to patient; although they can add to the assessment, clinicians should rely on an objective definition.

INDUCTION AND AUGMENTATION OF LABOR

Induction of labor is the attempt to begin labor in a nonlaboring patient, whereas **augmentation of labor** is intervening to increase the already present contractions. Labor is induced with **prostaglandins**, **oxytocic agents**, mechanical dilation of the cervix, and/or **artificial ROM**. The indications for induction are based on either maternal, fetal, or fetoplacental reasons. Common indications for induction of labor include postterm pregnancy, preeclampsia, diabetes mellitus, nonreassuring fetal testing, and intrauterine growth restriction. The patient's desire to end the pregnancy is *not* an indication for induction of labor, and is characterized as an elective induction of labor.

Induction of labor has become increasingly common in the United States with as many as one in five pregnancies ending up with an induction of labor. It has been conjectured that the rise in inductions of labor, particularly those at 35 and 36 weeks of gestation, has contributed to the overall rise in the rate of preterm birth. Elective inductions at 37 and 38 weeks of gestation, while technically at term, have been shown to lead to higher rates of neonatal morbidity and should be avoided. While elective induction of labor at 39 and 40 weeks of gestation has been demonized as contributing to the overall rise in cesarean delivery, it is unclear whether elective induction is truly associated with an increase in cesareans. The majority of studies compare elective induction to spontaneous labor, but the actual clinical decision is between induction and expectant management. Expectant management can lead to spontaneous labor, but it also leads to a larger fetus, an older placenta, and a proportion of these patients will go on to develop preeclampsia or a postterm pregnancy requiring induction of labor as well. In studies of elective induction of labor at 41 weeks of gestation, there appears to be a decrease in the overall rate of cesarean. In three very small, non-US studies of elective induction of labor prior to 41 weeks of gestation, there appears to be a decrease in the overall rate of cesarean as well. Future studies, particularly ones that will reflect practice in a variety of settings, will be necessary to demonstrate such a potential benefit.

Preparing for Induction

When proper indications for induction exist, the situation should be discussed with the patient and a plan for induction

IUPC : intrauterine pressure catheter

strength of CTX

BPD : widest part

Symphysis pubis

Biparietal diameter

Above the pelvic inlet

Ischial spine

Sacral promontory

Vertex above ischial spines

-2
-1
0
+1
+2
+3

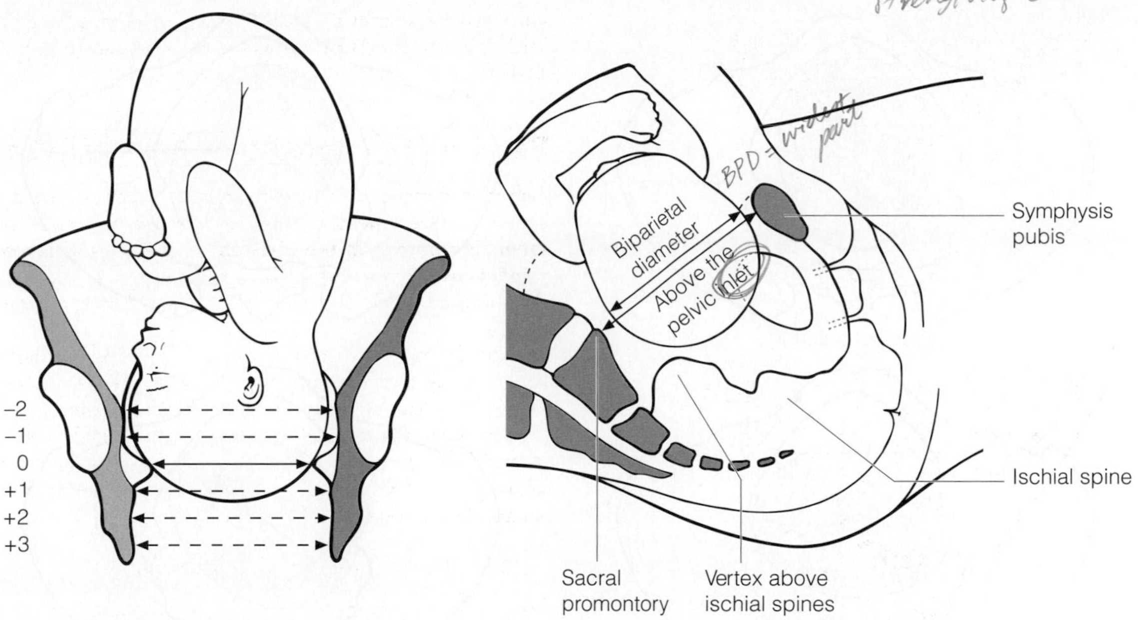

Figure 4-4 • The relationship of the leading edge of the presenting part of the ischial spine determines the station. +1 station is depicted in the frontal view on the left; approximately −2 station is depicted in the lateral view on the right.

10L reduce c/s

formed. When the indication is more pressing, induction should be started without significant delay. The success of an induction (defined as achieving vaginal delivery) is higher with favorable cervical status as defined by the Bishop score. A Bishop score of 5 or less may lead to a failed induction as often as 50% of the time. In these patients, prostaglandin E_2 (PGE$_2$) gel, PGE$_2$ pessary (Cervidil), or PGE$_1$M (misoprostol) is often used to "ripen" the cervix. The use of cervical ripening agents with prostaglandins or a mechanical means to dilate the cervix can reduce the risk of cesarean delivery.

There are both maternal and obstetric contraindications for the use of prostaglandins. Maternal reasons include asthma and glaucoma. Obstetric reasons include having had a prior cesarean delivery and nonreassuring fetal testing. Because PGE$_2$ gel cannot be turned off with the ease of oxytocin, there is a risk of uterine hyperstimulation and tetanic contractions. In this setting, a mechanical dilator such as a 30 cc or 60 cc Foley bulb can be used. The Foley is placed inside the cervix adjacent to the amniotic sac, inflated, and placed on gentle traction. It usually dilates the cervix to 2 to 3 cm within 4 to 6 hours.

contraind. for PG's
- glaucoma
- asthma
- prev. c/s
- NST ↑
(?)

Induction

Labor may begin with the ripening and dilation of the cervix performed with prostaglandins or mechanical means. However, labor induction is usually formally begun pharmacologically with oxytocin (Pitocin). This is a synthesized, but identical, version of the octapeptide oxytocin normally released from the posterior pituitary that causes uterine contractions. Pitocin is given continuously via IV drip because it is rapidly metabolized.

Labor may also be induced by amniotomy. Amniotomy is performed with an amnio hook that is used to puncture the amniotic sac around the fetus and release some of the amniotic fluid. After the amniotomy is performed, a careful examination should be performed to ensure that prolapse of the umbilical cord has not occurred. When performing amniotomy,

it is important not to elevate the fetal head from the pelvis to release more of the amniotic fluid because this may lead to prolapse of the umbilical cord beyond the fetal head.

Augmentation

Pitocin and amniotomy are also used to augment labor. The indications for augmentation of labor include those for induction in addition to inadequate contractions or a prolonged phase of labor. The adequacy of contractions is indirectly assessed by the progress of cervical change. It may also be measured directly using an **intrauterine pressure catheter** (IUPC) that determines the absolute change in pressure during a contraction and thus estimates the strength of contractions. Aggressive augmentation, deemed active management of labor, involves both oxytocin and amniotomy and has been demonstrated to lead to shorter labor courses but no difference in cesarean delivery rates.

MONITORING OF THE FETUS IN LABOR

It is easy to monitor the mother in labor with vital signs and laboratory studies. Monitoring the infant is indirect and thus more difficult than maternal assessment. Determination of the baseline rate and assessment of fetal heart rate variations with contractions can be done by auscultation. The normal range for the fetal heart rate is between 110 and 160 beats per minute. With baselines above 160, fetal distress secondary to infection, hypoxia, or anemia is of concern. Any prolonged fetal heart rate deceleration of greater than 2 minutes' duration with a heart rate less than 90 beats per minute is of concern and requires immediate action.

External Electronic Monitors

Since the advent of electronic fetal monitoring, auscultation is rarely used. Continuous fetal heart monitors are standard in most hospitals in the United States because they afford several

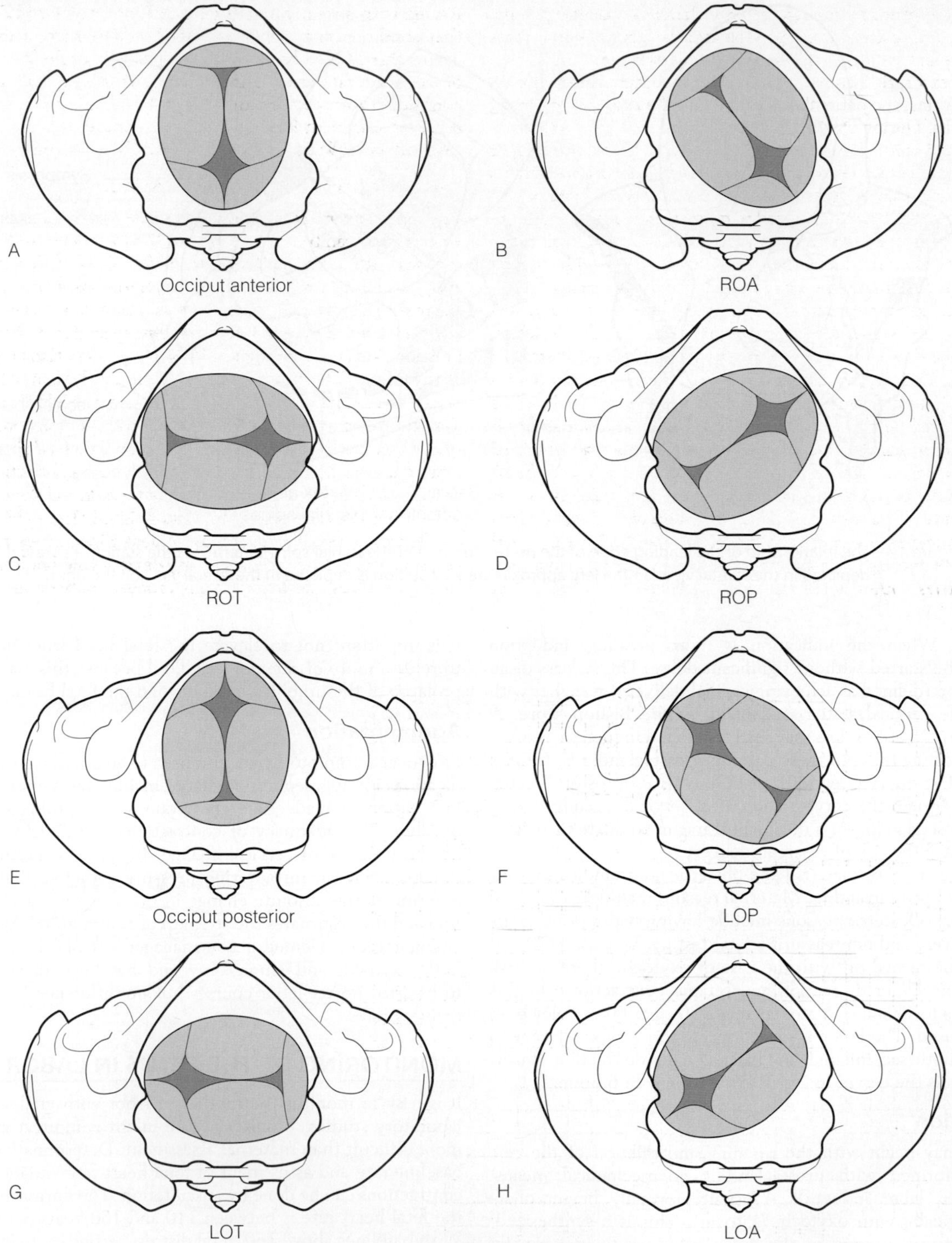

Figure 4-5 • (A–H) Various possible positions of the fetal head in the maternal pelvis.

advantages over auscultation. The information gathered is more subtle and includes variations in heart rate. Arguably, the greatest advantage is that the information is easier to gather and record. This allows more time for analyzing the data and has economic advantages as one nurse can readily monitor multiple patients. In one of the largest studies conducted in Dublin at the National Maternity Hospital and published in 1985, the rate of cesarean was a little bit greater in the continuous fetal monitoring group (2.4% vs. 2.2%) and the rate of operative vaginal delivery was higher (8.2% vs. 6.3%). However, there were more fetuses identified with abnormal umbilical cord pH values. There are few other studies that directly compare continuous fetal heart rate monitoring to intermittent auscultation and none recently. The decision making surrounding the use of such monitoring varies in different labor and delivery units. Intermittent auscultation is predominantly driven by midwives and pregnant women who desire less intervention.

The external tocometer has a pressure transducer that is placed against the patient's abdomen, usually near the fundus of the uterus. During uterine contractions, the abdomen becomes firmer, and this pressure is transmitted through the transducer to a tocometer that records the contraction. The relative heights of the tracings on different patients or at different locations on the same patient cannot be used to compare strength of contractions. External tocometers are most useful for measuring the frequency of contractions and comparing to the fetal heart rate tracing to determine the type of decelerations occurring.

A fetal heart rate tracing is examined for several characteristics that are considered reassuring. First, the baseline is determined and should be in the normal range (110 to 160 beats per minute). Then the variations from the baseline should be examined. The moment-to-moment variation from the baseline is called fetal heart rate variability. Fetal heart rate variability is defined as absent (<3 beats per minute of variation), minimal (3 to 5 beats per minute of variation), moderate (5 to 25 beats per minute of variation), and marked (more than 25 beats per minute of variation). The tracing should be jagged from the beat-to-beat variability of the heart rate. Although a fetal heart rate tracing with minimal variability is not reassuring, this may also occur while the fetus is asleep or inactive. A flat tracing with absent variability is more worrisome and demands that another test to determine fetal well-being be conducted. There should also be at least three to five cycles per minute of the heart rate around the baseline. Finally, a tracing can be considered formally reactive (Fig. 4-6) if there are at least two accelerations of at least 15 beats per minute over the baseline that last for at least 15 seconds within 20 minutes.

Decelerations of the Fetal Heart Rate

The fetal heart rate tracing should also be used to examine decelerations and can be used along with the tocometer to determine the type and severity. There are three types of decelerations: early, variable, and late. **Early decelerations** begin and end approximately at the same time as contractions (Fig. 4-7A). They are a result of increased vagal tone secondary to head compression during a contraction. **Variable decelerations** can occur at any time and tend to drop more precipitously than either early or late decelerations (Fig. 4-7C). They are a result of umbilical cord compression. Repetitive variables with contractions can be seen when the cord is entrapped either under a fetal shoulder or around the neck and is compressed with each contraction. **Late decelerations** begin at the peak of a contraction and slowly return to baseline after the contraction has finished (Fig. 4-7B). These decelerations are a result of uteroplacental insufficiency and are the most worrisome type. They may degrade into bradycardias as labor progresses, particularly with stronger contractions.

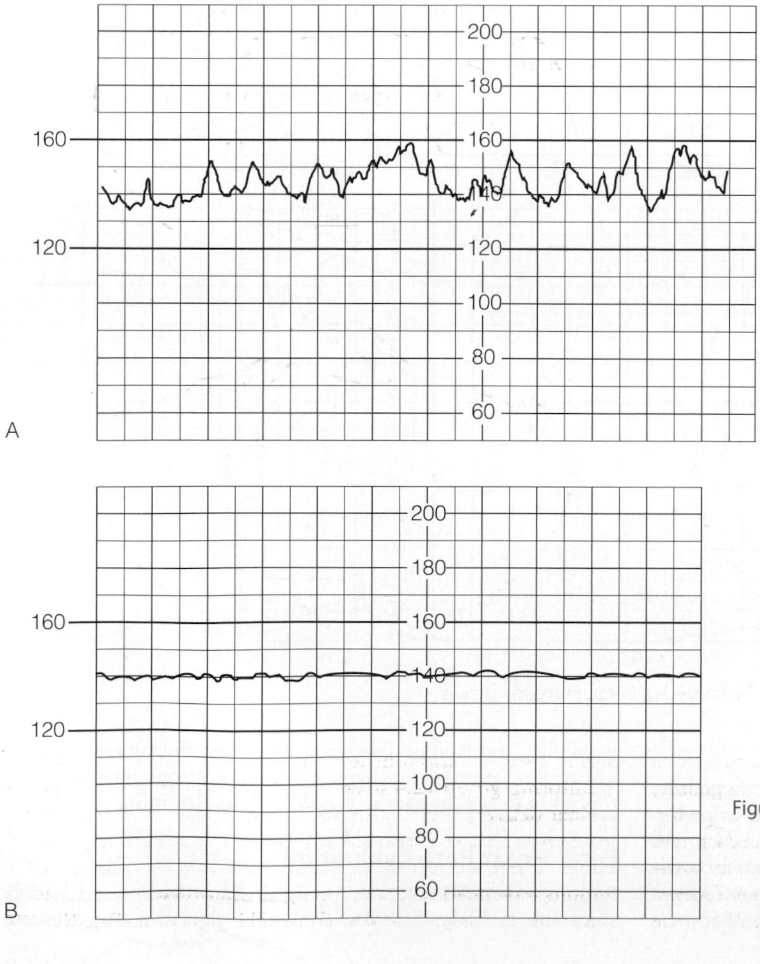

Figure 4-6 • **(A)** Normal short- and long-term beat-to-beat variability. **(B)** Reduced variability. This may occur during fetal sleep, following maternal intake of drugs, or with reduced fetal CNS function, as in asphyxia.

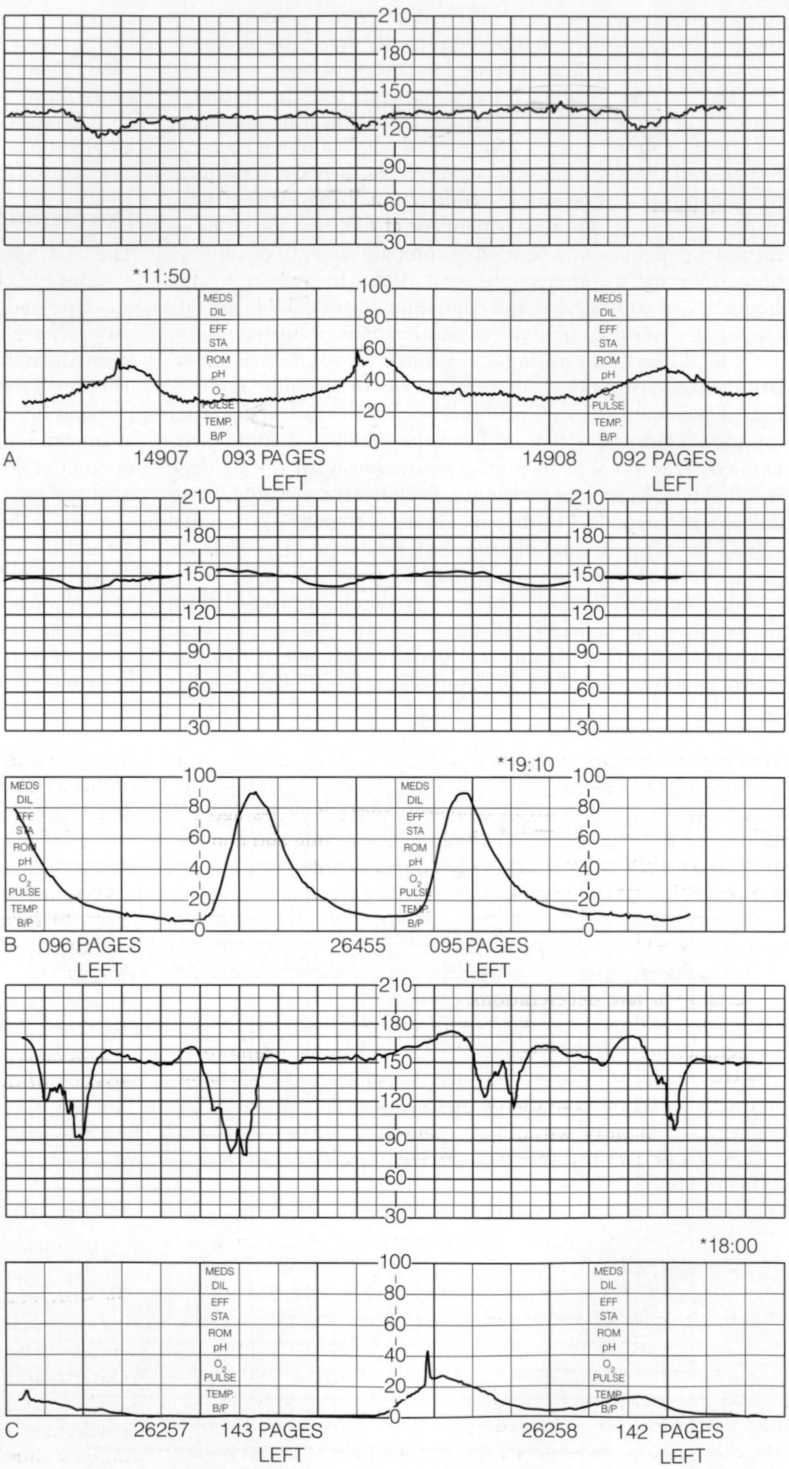

Figure 4-7 • **(A)** An early deceleration pattern is depicted in this FHR tracing. Note that each deceleration returns to baseline before the completion of the contraction. The remainder of the FHR tracing is reassuring. **(B)** Repetitive late decelerations in conjunction with decreased variability. **(C)** Variable decelerations are the most common periodic change of the FHR during labor. Repetitive mild to moderate variable decelerations are present. The baseline is normal.

Fetal Scalp Electrode

In the case of repetitive decelerations or in fetuses who are difficult to trace externally with Doppler, a **fetal scalp electrode** (FSE) is often used. A small electrode is attached to the fetal scalp that senses the potential differences created by the depolarization of the fetal heart. The information obtained from the scalp electrode is more sensitive in terms of the beat-to-beat variability and is in no danger of being lost during contractions as the fetal position changes. Contraindications include a history of maternal hepatitis or HIV or fetal thrombocytopenia.

Fetal Heart Rate Evaluation

Although fetal heart rate monitoring has been used widely since the 1970s and 1980s, consistent algorithms to evaluate

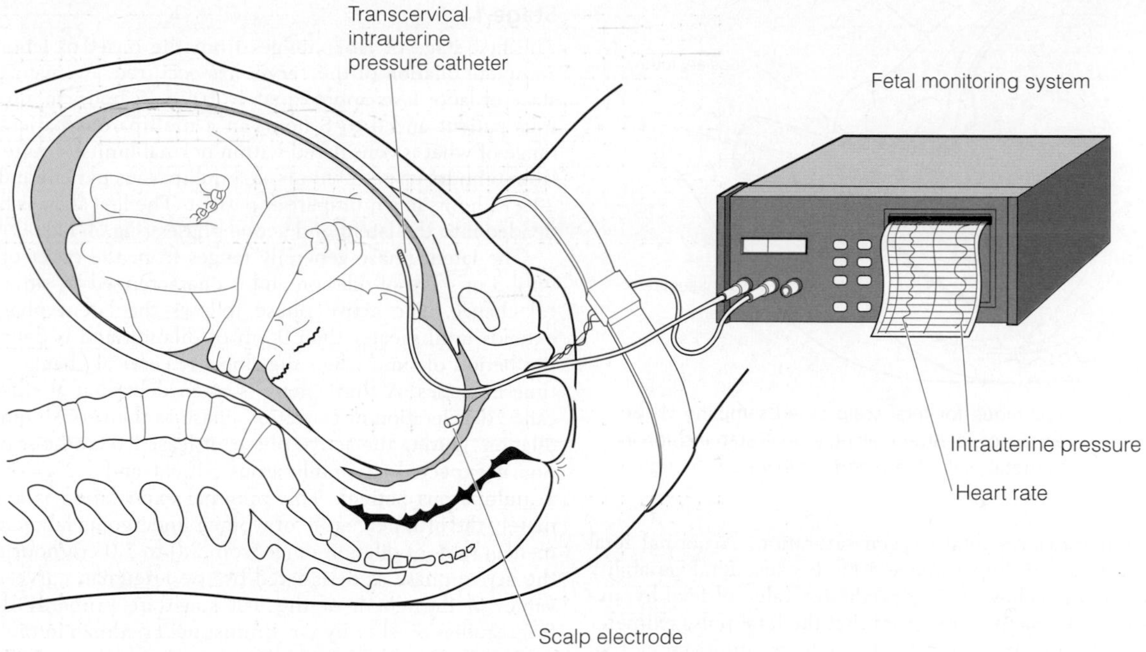

Figure 4-8 • Technique for continuous electronic monitoring of FHR and uterine contractions.

the tracing have not been developed and adopted. Thus, the fetal heart rate abnormalities that were thought to contribute to the rapid rise in cesarean deliveries three decades ago are still poorly understood. This lack of understanding and consensus led to an NIH conference in 2008. This conference arrived at a three-tier categorization of the fetal heart rate:

Category I—This is a normal fetal heart rate tracing characterized by a normal baseline, moderate variability, and no variable or late decelerations.

Category II—This is an indeterminate fetal heart tracing and includes many variety of fetal heart tracings including those with variable and late decelerations, bradycardia and tachycardia, minimal variability, marked variability, and even absent variability without decelerations. The best way to remember Tier II is that it is not Tier I and not Tier III, but every other fetal heart tracing.

Category III—This is an abnormal fetal heart rate tracing. Category III tracings consist of those with absent fetal heart variability and recurrent late or variable decelerations or bradycardia. The other fetal heart rate tracing that also is Category III is the sinusoidal pattern consistent with fetal anemia.

While these categories are a step in the right direction to provide a consistent approach to fetal heart rate monitoring, they should not be perceived as the final word on fetal heart rate monitoring. In particular, there has been criticism of the three-tiered system as not being granular enough and having too broad of a range of tracings in Category II. Ongoing work will hopefully shed light on this incredibly important topic to allow us to better identify those fetuses at risk for injury and also maintaining or even decreasing the cesarean delivery rate.

Intrauterine Pressure Catheter

The external tocometer records the onset and end of contractions. The absolute values of the readings mean little and are entirely position dependent. Further, on some patients—particularly those who are obese—the tocometer does not show much in the way of fluctuation from the baseline. If it is particularly important to determine the timing or strength of contractions, an IUPC may be used (Fig. 4-8). This catheter is threaded past the fetal presenting part into the uterine cavity to measure the pressure changes during contractions. The baseline intrauterine pressure is usually between 10 and 15 mm Hg. Contractions during labor will increase by 20 to 30 mm Hg in early labor and by 40 to 60 mm Hg as labor progresses. The most commonly used measurement of uterine contractions is the **Montevideo unit**, which is an average of the variation of the intrauterine pressure from the baseline multiplied by the number of contractions in a 10-minute period. Some institutions use the Alexandria unit, which multiplies the Montevideo units by the length of each contraction as well.

Fetal Scalp pH and Pulse Oximetry

If a fetal heart rate tracing is nonreassuring, the fetal scalp pH may be obtained to directly assess fetal hypoxia and acidemia (Fig. 4-9). Fetal blood is obtained by making a small nick in the fetal scalp and drawing up a small amount of fetal blood into capillary tubes. The results are reassuring when the scalp pH is greater than 7.25, indeterminant when it is between 7.20 and 7.25, and nonreassuring when it is less than 7.20. Care must be taken to avoid contamination of the blood sample with amniotic fluid, which is basic and will elevate the results falsely. Although this tool is used less frequently now that technology has improved fetal monitoring, it can still provide additional information on fetal well-being. Interestingly, it is almost never used in the United States any longer, but still used in 5% or more of fetuses in the United Kingdom.

Another modality for assessing fetal status that is still experimental at this point is fetal pulse oximetry. Using technology similar to the monitors placed on ears, fingers, and toes, the fetal pulse oximeter is placed intrauterine along the fetal

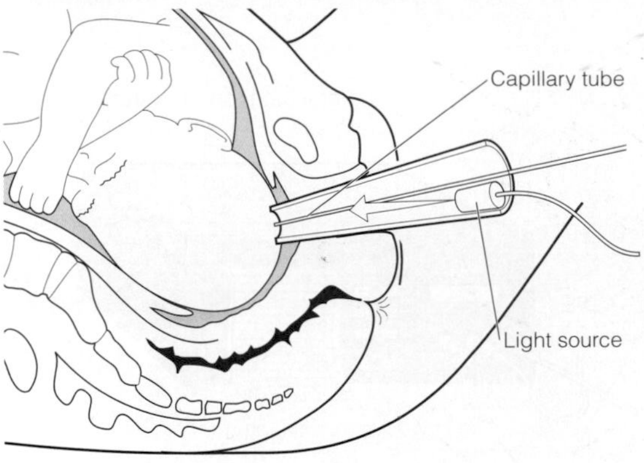

Figure 4-9 • Technique for fetal scalp blood sampling via an amnioscope. After making a small stab incision in the fetal scalp, the blood is drawn off through a capillary tube.

cheek and measures fetal oxygen saturation. A normal fetal pulse oximeter reading is above 30%. Because fetal variability and decelerations have a poor predictive value of fetal hypoxemia and acidemia, it is theorized that the fetal pulse oximeter would be useful in such patients. A large, multicenter trial demonstrated that many of these fetuses with nonreassuring tracings do have normal pulse oximeter readings. However, the use of the pulse oximeter did not have an effect on either the cesarean delivery rate or fetal outcomes. Thus, the FDA did not approve fetal pulse-oximetry and it is unclear whether this technology has the potential for future use.

THE PROGRESSION OF LABOR

Labor is assessed by the progress of cervical effacement, cervical dilation, and descent of the fetal presenting part. To assess the progress of labor, it is important to understand the cardinal movements or mechanisms of labor.

Cardinal Movements of Labor

The cardinal movements are engagement, descent, flexion, internal rotation, extension, and external rotation (also called restitution or resolution) (Fig. 4-10). When the fetal presenting part enters the pelvis, it is said to have undergone **engagement**. The head will then undergo **descent** into the pelvis, followed by **flexion**, which allows the smallest diameter to present to the pelvis. With descent into the midpelvis, the fetal vertex undergoes **internal rotation** from an OT position so that the sagittal suture is parallel to the anteroposterior diameter of the pelvis, commonly to the occiput anterior (OA) position. Disruption of the internal rotation or improper rotation can lead to a fetus maintained in OT position or malrotated to the OP position. As the vertex passes beneath and beyond the pubic symphysis, it will **extend** to deliver. Once the head delivers, **external rotation** occurs and the shoulders may be delivered.

Stages of Labor

Labor and delivery are divided into three stages. Each stage involves different concerns and considerations. Stage 1 begins with the onset of labor and lasts until dilation and effacement of the cervix are completed. Stage 2 is from the time of full dilation until delivery of the infant. Stage 3 begins after delivery of the infant and ends with delivery of the placenta.

Stage 1

The first stage of labor ranges from the onset of labor until complete dilation of the cervix has occurred. An average first stage of labor lasts approximately 10 to 12 hours in a nulliparous patient and 6 to 8 hours in a multiparous patient. The range of what is considered within normal limits is quite wide, from 6 hours up to 20 hours in a nulliparous patient and from 2 to 12 hours in a multiparous patient. The first stage is further divided into the latent and active phases (Fig. 4-11).

The **latent phase** generally ranges from the onset of labor until 3 or 4 cm of dilation and is characterized by slow cervical change. The **active phase** follows the latent phase and extends until greater than 9 cm of dilation and is defined by the period of time when the slope of cervical change against time increases. A third phase is often delegated at this point called deceleration or transition phase as the cervix completes dilation. During the active phase, at least 1.0 cm/hour of dilation is expected in a nulliparous patient and 1.2 cm/hour in a multiparous patient. This minimal expectation is approximately the fifth percentile of women undergoing labor and the median rates of dilation range from 2.0 to 3.0 cm/hour during the active phase as designated by the Friedman curve. These values of the length of the first stage are primarily derived from studies of labor by Dr. Emmanuel Friedman in the 1950s and 1960s. Studies over the last decade reveal longer first and second stages of labor and variation by maternal race/ethnicity, age, and body habitus.

The three "Ps"—powers, passenger, and pelvis—can all affect the transit time during the active phase of labor. The "powers" are determined by the strength and frequency of uterine contractions. The size and position of the infant affect the duration of the active phase, as do the size and shape of the maternal pelvis. If the "passenger" is too large for the "pelvis," **cephalopelvic disproportion** (CPD) results. If the rate of change of cervical dilation falls below the fifth percentile (1.0 cm/hour), these three Ps should be assessed to determine whether a vaginal delivery can be expected. Strength of uterine contractions can be measured with an IUPC and is considered adequate with greater than 200 Montevideo units. Signs of CPD include development of fetal caput and extensive molding of the fetal skull with palpable overlapping sutures.

If there is no change in either cervical dilation or station for 2 hours in the setting of adequate Montevideo units during the active phase of labor, this is deemed active phase arrest and is an extremely common indication for cesarean. However, in the past decade, several studies have indicated that if clinicians exhibited more patience in this setting by waiting up to 4 or more hours to make this diagnosis, then more than half of these women will go on to deliver vaginally. While the issue deserves more research, in a setting with continuous fetal monitoring and no worrisome signs from either the mother or fetus, it appears reasonable to manage such pregnancies expectantly to allow for the possibility of vaginal birth.

Stage 2

When the cervix has completely dilated, stage 2 has begun. Stage 2 is completed with delivery of the infant. Stage 2 is considered prolonged if its duration is longer than 2 hours in a nulliparous patient, although 3 hours are allowed in patients who have epidurals. In multiparous women, stage 2 is prolonged if its duration is longer than 1 hour without an epidural and 2 hours with an epidural. In multiparous women without an epidural, it is rare for stage 2 to last longer than 30 minutes unless there is fetal macrosomia, persistent occiput posterior

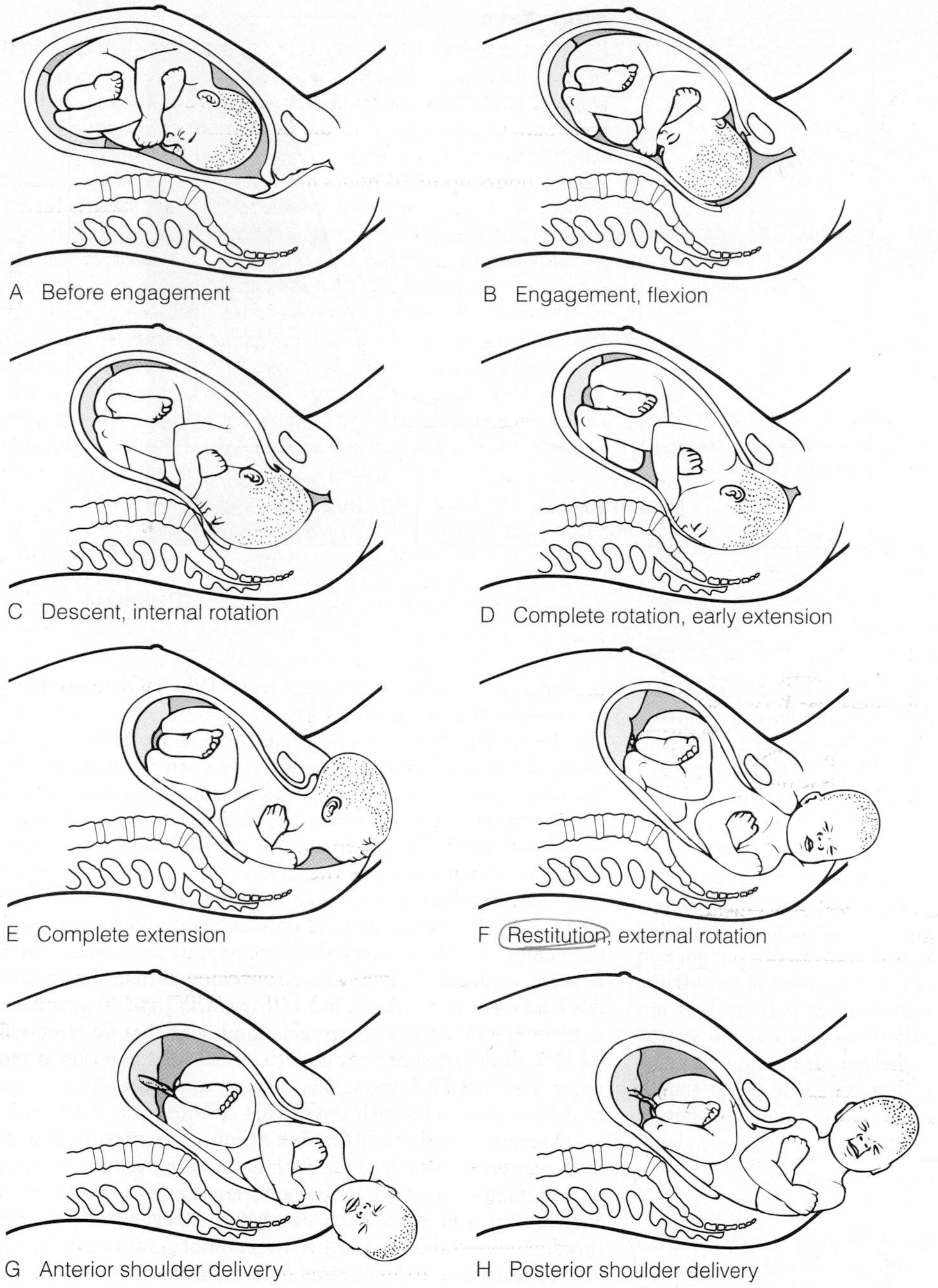

Figure 4-10 • (A–H) Cardinal movements of labor.

or transverse position, compound presentation, or asynclitism. However, epidurals can have a profound effect on the length of the second stage in both nulliparous and multiparous women.

One reason for the effect on second stage is that often women will have little urge to push, little sensation, and even a strong motor block and so have less ability to push. Often, such patients are given an hour or two without pushing at the beginning of second stage; this is called "laboring down" or "passive descent." Prospective randomized trials of laboring down do not demonstrate universal benefit, and all find that women will have a longer second stage with laboring down. Traditionally, it was perceived that a prolonged second stage of labor may lead to worse neonatal outcomes. However, recent studies of the length of the second stage of labor have not actually demonstrated a difference in neonatal outcomes with prolonged second stage of labor in the setting of fetal heart rate monitoring. There also remains a concern that prolonged second stage of labor will lead to higher rates of maternal urinary incontinence and pelvic relaxation, but to date, no large, prospective studies have been performed. Thus, management of the second stage of labor remains somewhat controversial.

Monitoring

Repetitive early and variable decelerations are common during the second stage. The clinician can be reassured if these decelerations resolve quickly after each contraction and there is no

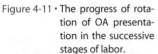

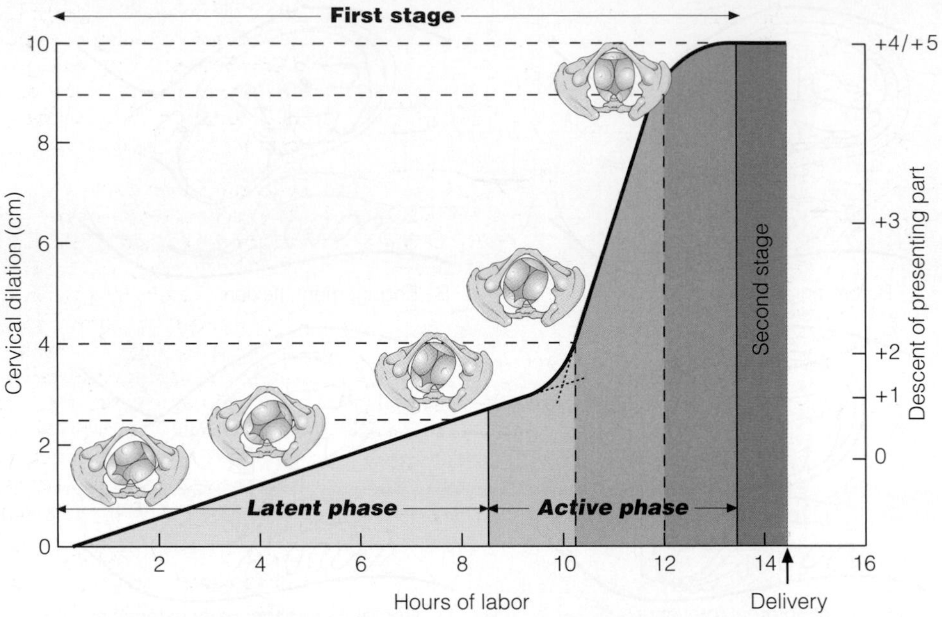

Figure 4-11 • The progress of rotation of OA presentation in the successive stages of labor.

loss of variability in the tracing. Repetitive late decelerations, bradycardias, and loss of variability are all signs of nonreassuring fetal status. With these tracings, the patient should be placed on face mask O_2, turned onto her left side to decrease inferior vena cava (IVC) compression and increase uterine perfusion; if it is being used, the oxytocin should be immediately discontinued until the tracing resumes a reassuring pattern. If a prolonged deceleration is felt to be the result of uterine **hypertonus** (a single contraction lasting 2 minutes or longer) or **tachysystole** (greater than five contractions in a 10-minute period), which can be diagnosed by palpation or examination of the tocometer, the patient can be given a dose of terbutaline to help relax the uterus. If a nonreassuring pattern does not resolve with these interventions, the fetal position and station should be assessed to determine whether an operative vaginal delivery can be performed. If fetal station is above 0 station (though many clinicians will require the fetus to be +2 station or lower) or the position cannot be determined, cesarean delivery is the mode of choice.

Vaginal Delivery

As the fetus begins crowning, the delivering clinician should be dressed with eye protection, sterile gown, and sterile gloves (for self-protection as much as for prevention of maternal/fetal infection) and have two clamps, scissors, and suction bulb. When meconium is suspected or confirmed many units will use a DeLee suction trap to aspirate meconium from the neonatal airway after the head is delivered and prior to delivery of the rest of body before breaths can be taken. However, after a large, prospective, randomized trial was conducted and demonstrated no benefit from such suctioning, the use of the DeLee has declined.

Various approaches can be taken to vaginal delivery, but most clinicians would agree that a smooth, controlled delivery leads to less perineal trauma. Thus, one hand is commonly used to support or massage the perineum while the other hand is used to flex the head to keep it from extending too quickly and causing periurethral or labial lacerations. The fingers on the hand controlling the fetal head can also be used to massage the labia over the head during delivery. When a delivery needs to be expedited, a modified Ritgen maneuver (Fig. 4-12) using the heel of the delivering hand to exert pressure on the perineum and the fingers below the woman's anus to extend the fetal head to hasten delivery and maintain station between contractions may be performed. This procedure tends to lead to greater perineal lacerations, but is effective during a prolonged deceleration to effect delivery.

Once the head of the infant is delivered, the mouth and upper airway are bulb suctioned. After suctioning is complete, the infant's neck is checked for a wrapped umbilical cord. If such a nuchal cord exists, an attempt is made to reduce the cord over the infant's head. If it is too tight, two options exist. If the clinician is extremely confident that delivery will be accomplished shortly, the cord is clamped and cut at this point. If a shoulder dystocia is suspected, an attempt is made to deliver the infant with the nuchal cord intact.

Delivery of the rest of the infant follows first with delivery of the anterior shoulder by exerting direct downward pressure on the infant's head. Once the anterior shoulder is visualized, a direct upward pressure is exerted to deliver the posterior shoulder (Fig. 4-13). After this, exertion of gentle traction will deliver the torso and the rest of the infant. At this point, the cord is clamped and cut and the infant passed either to the labor nurse and mother or to the waiting pediatricians.

Episiotomy

An **episiotomy** is an incision made in the perineum to facilitate delivery. Indications for episiotomy include need to hasten delivery and impending or ongoing shoulder dystocia. A relative contraindication for episiotomy is the assessment that there will be a large perineal laceration as episiotomies have been associated with higher risk of severe perineal lacerations. Once the episiotomy is cut, great care should be taken to support the perineum around the episiotomy to avoid extension into the rectal sphincter or rectum itself. In the past, episiotomies were used routinely in the setting of spontaneous and operative vaginal deliveries. However, evidence suggests that the rate of third- and fourth-degree lacerations increases with the use of routine midline episiotomy.

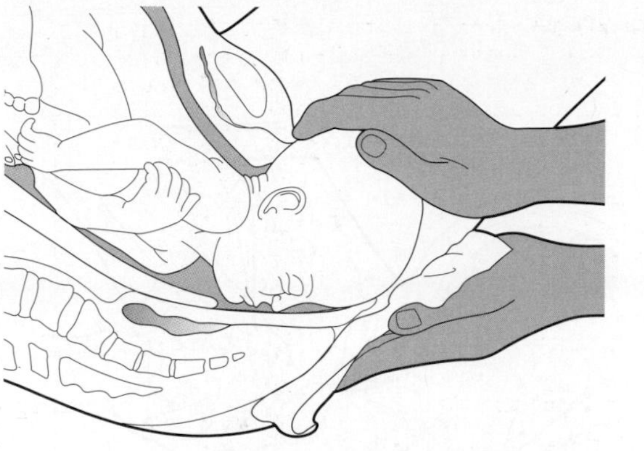

Figure 4-12 • Near completion of the delivery of the fetal head by the modified Ritgen maneuver. Moderate upward pressure is applied to the fetal chin by the posterior hand covered with a sterile towel while the suboccipital region of the fetal head is held against the symphysis.

There are two common types of episiotomies: median (or midline) and mediolateral (Fig. 4-14). The median episiotomy, the most common type used in the United States, uses a vertical midline incision from the posterior fourchette into the perineal body. The mediolateral episiotomy is an oblique incision made from either the 5- or 7-o'clock position on the perineum and cut laterally. It is used less frequently and reportedly causes more pain and wound infections. However, mediolateral episiotomies are thought to lead to fewer third- and fourth-degree extensions, particularly in patients with short perineums or with operative deliveries.

Operative Vaginal Delivery

In the case of a prolonged second stage, maternal exhaustion, or the need to hasten delivery, an operative vaginal delivery may be indicated. The two possibilities are forceps delivery or vacuum-assisted delivery. Both are effective methods to facilitate vaginal delivery and have similar indications. The decision of which method to choose depends upon clinician's preference and experience, though they carry slightly different risks of maternal and neonatal complications.

Forceps Delivery

Forceps (Fig. 4-15) have blades that are placed around the fetal head and are shaped with a cephalic curve to accommodate the head. In addition, most have a pelvic curve that conforms to the maternal pelvis. The blade of each forceps is at the end of a shank that is connected to a handle. The two forceps are connected at the lock between the shank and the handle. Once the forceps are placed around the fetal head, the operator uses varying vector forces on the handles to aid maternal expulsive efforts and guide the fetal head through the curvature of the pelvis (Table 4-2).

The conditions necessary for safe application of forceps include full dilation of the cervix, ruptured membranes, engaged head and at least +2 station, absolute knowledge of fetal position, no evidence of CPD, adequate anesthesia, empty bladder, and—most important—an experienced operator. In some institutions, mid-forceps applications (fetal station between 0 and +2) and rotational forceps (fetal head more than 45 degrees from either direct OA or OP position) are also used. An experienced operator is, again, the most important component of these deliveries. Using high forceps with the fetal vertex above 0 station is no longer considered a safe obstetric procedure. Complications from forceps application include bruising on the face and head, lacerations to the fetal head, cervix, vagina, and perineum, facial nerve palsy, and, rarely, skull fracture and/or intracranial damage.

Vacuum Extraction

The **vacuum extractor** consists of a vacuum cup that is placed on the fetal scalp and a suction device that is connected to the cup to create the vacuum. Conditions for the safe use of the vacuum extractor are identical to that of forceps. Vacuum should never be chosen because position is unknown or the station is too high. Exertion on the cup and consequently on the fetal scalp is made parallel to the axis of the maternal pelvis concomitant with maternal bearing-down efforts and uterine contractions. The most common complications of use of the vacuum are scalp laceration and cephalohematoma. However, a rare complication from the vacuum extractor is the subgaleal hemorrhage, which can be a neonatal emergency.

Forceps versus Vacuum

There is great debate between clinicians as to which of these forms of operative delivery are safer. In several studies that compare the two modes of operative vaginal delivery, the rates of severe neonatal complications such as intracranial hemorrhage are not statistically different. However, vacuums are associated with a higher rate of cephalohematomas and shoulder dystocias, whereas forceps are associated with a higher rate of facial nerve palsies. With respect to maternal complications, forceps are associated with higher rates of third- and fourth-degree perineal lacerations. Some of the differences between these instruments are related to design. The forceps are applied around the fetal head and the tips of the blades lie on the fetal cheek, thus are more likely to cause compression of the facial nerve. The vacuum exerts its entire force on the fetal scalp, thus fetal cephalohematomas are a common complication. Because of the higher placement and their rigidity, forceps can be used to generate greater downward force on both the fetus and concomitantly the maternal anatomy. This may lead to a lower rate of shoulder dystocia, but higher rates of maternal lacerations. In the end, the most important factor in the use of these instruments is operator experience. Because either of these instruments may be the tool of choice in different given situations, it is important for obstetricians to be trained in the use of both.

Stage 3

Stage 3 begins once the infant has been delivered and is completed with the delivery of the placenta. Placental separation usually occurs within 5 to 10 minutes of delivery of the infant; however, up to 30 minutes is usually considered within normal limits. With the abrupt decrease in intrauterine cavity size after the delivery of the fetus, the placenta is mechanically sheared from the uterine wall with contractions. Classically, the use of oxytocin was contraindicated during stage 3. However, this was established prior to the use of ultrasound out of concern for causing abruption in the case of an undiagnosed twin. If here is no doubt about completion of stage 2, oxytocin can be used during the stage 3 to strengthen uterine contractions to decrease both placental delivery time and blood loss.

The three signs of placental separation include cord lengthening, a gush of blood, and uterine fundal rebound as the placenta detaches from the uterine wall. No attempt to deliver the placenta should be made until all these signs are noted. The placenta is delivered by gentle traction on

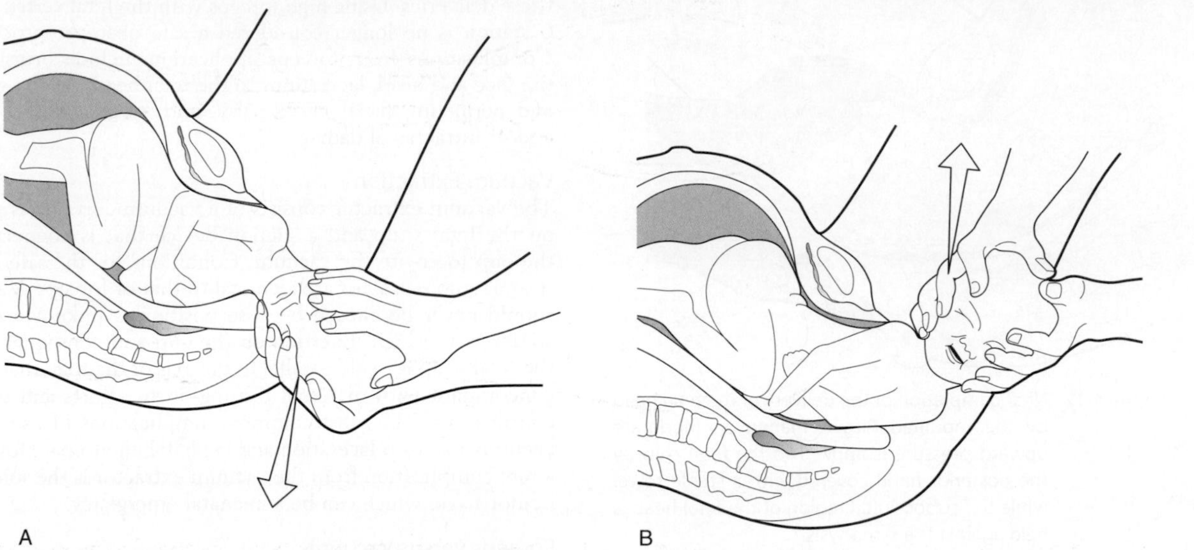

Figure 4-13 • **(A)** Delivery of the anterior shoulder. **(B)** Delivery of posterior shoulder.

the cord. It is important not to use too much traction because the cord may avulse or uterine inversion may occur. When the patient begins bearing down for delivery of the placenta, it is imperative that one of the examiner's hands is applying suprapubic pressure to keep the uterus from inverting or prolapsing (Fig. 4-16). When the placenta is evident at the introitus, the delivery should be controlled to avoid both further perineal trauma and tearing of any of the membranes that often trail the placenta at delivery.

Retained Placenta

The diagnosis of retained placenta is made when the placenta does not deliver within 30 minutes after the infant. Retained placenta is common in preterm deliveries, particularly previable deliveries. However, it is also a sign of placenta accreta,

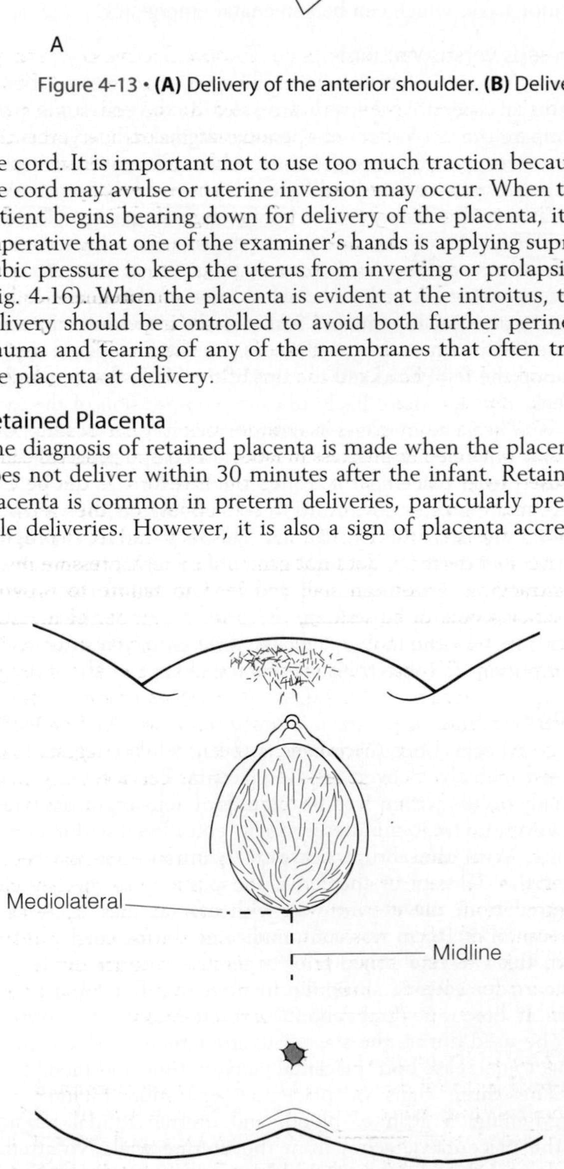

Figure 4-14 • Placement of mediolateral and midline episiotomy.

where the placenta has invaded into or beyond the endometrial stroma. The retained placenta may be removed by manual extraction. A hand is placed in the intrauterine cavity and the fingers used to shear the placenta from the surface of the uterus (Fig. 4-17). If the placenta cannot be completely extracted manually, curettage is performed to ensure no products of conception (POC) are retained.

Laceration Repair

Lacerations are usually repaired after placental delivery. A thorough examination of the perineum, labia, periurethral area, vagina, anus, and cervix is performed to assess lacerations. The most common lacerations are perineal lacerations, which are described by the depth of tissues they involve (Fig. 4-18). A first-degree laceration involves the mucosa or skin. Second-degree lacerations extend into the perineal body but do not involve the anal sphincter. Third-degree lacerations extend into or completely through the anal sphincter. A fourth-degree tear occurs if the anal mucosa itself is entered. A rectal examination should always be performed as occasionally a "buttonhole" fourth-degree laceration will be noted. This is a laceration through the rectal mucosa into the vagina, but with the sphincter still intact.

Repair of any superficial lacerations, including first-degree perineal tears, is usually accomplished with interrupted sutures. A second-degree laceration is repaired in layers. The apex of the laceration, which often lies beyond the hymenal ring, is located and a suture is anchored at the apex. This suture is then run down to the level of the hymenal ring, bringing together the vaginal tissue. This suture is then passed beyond the hymenal ring and used to bring together the perineal body. Sometimes a separate suture is used to place a "crown stitch," which brings together the perineal body. Finally, the skin of the perineum is closed with a subcuticular closure (Fig. 4-19).

Third-degree lacerations require repair of the anal sphincter with several interrupted sutures and then the rest of the repair is completed as in a second-degree repair. Fourth-degree repairs are begun with repairing the anal mucosa. Mucosal repair is performed meticulously to prevent fistula formation. Once

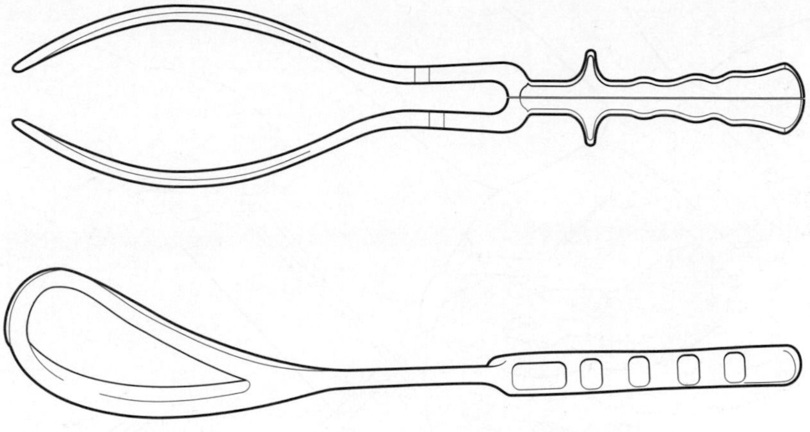

Figure 4-15 • Forceps.

the rectum is repaired, a fourth-degree laceration is completed just as a third-degree repair.

Cesarean Delivery

Cesarean delivery or cesarean section has been used effectively throughout the 20th century and is one of the most common operations performed today. The cesarean rate in the United States in 2009 had increased to 32.9%—a 50% rise over the last 15 years and an absolute rise of about 1% per year over the last several years. It is not entirely clear why the cesarean delivery rate is rising so rapidly, but it is likely multifactorial including (1) biologic reasons such as higher rates of multiple gestations, an older population with more medical disorders, and higher rates of overweight and obesity; (2) patient preferences toward elective cesarean also known as cesarean delivery on maternal request (CDMR); and (3) clinician preferences related to the escalating medical–legal environment and inadequate economic incentives to encourage clinician patience. Although maternal mortality from cesarean section is low, approximately 0.01% to 0.02%, it is still higher than from vaginal delivery. Further, the morbidity from infections, thrombotic events, wound dehiscence, and recovery time is greater than that of vaginal delivery. In addition, the risk in subsequent pregnancies from having a prior cesarean delivery is an important aspect to consider when performing the first cesarean. These include the need for future cesareans and the risk of future placenta previa and accreta.

The most common indication for primary cesarean delivery is that of failure to progress in labor. Failure to progress can be caused by problems with any of the three Ps. If the pelvis is too small or the fetus too large (depending on the viewpoint taken), the diagnosis is CPD, which leads to failure to progress. If the uterus simply does not generate enough pressure during contractions, labor can stall and lead to failure to progress. If labor seems to be stalling, there are a number of measures that can be taken to augment it, such as oxytocin or ROM. Commonly, 2 hours without cervical change in the setting of adequate uterine contractions in the active phase of labor is deemed failure to progress or active phase arrest often leading to cesarean delivery. However, a recent study suggests that it is reasonable to wait at least 4 hours for cervical stage in the active phase of labor, leading to a vaginal delivery in the majority of these patients.

Other common indications for primary cesarean section (Table 4-3) are breech presentation, transverse lie, shoulder presentation, placenta previa, placental abruption, fetal intolerance of labor, nonreassuring fetal status, cord prolapse, prolonged second stage, failed operative vaginal delivery, or active herpes lesions. Overall, the most common indication for cesarean section is a previous cesarean section.

TABLE 4-2 Classification of Forceps Delivery According to Station and Rotation

Type of Procedure	Classification
Outlet forceps	1. Scalp is visible at the introitus without separating the labia 2. Fetal skull has reached pelvic floor 3. Sagittal suture is in anteroposterior diameter or right or left occiput anterior or posterior position 4. Fetal head is at or on perineum 5. Rotation does not exceed 45 degrees
Low forceps	Leading point of fetal skull is at station 2 or greater, but not on the pelvic floor Rotation <45 degrees (left or right occiput anterior to occiput anterior, or left or right occiput posterior to occiput posterior) Rotation >45 degrees
Mid forceps	Station above +2 cm but head engaged
High forceps	Not included in classification

From Cunningham FG, Gant NF, Leveno KJ, et al. *Williams Obstetrics*, 19th ed. Norwalk, CT: Appleton & Lange; 1993:557.

Vaginal Birth after Cesarean

Vaginal birth after cesarean (VBAC) can be attempted if the proper setting exists. This includes an in-house obstetrician, anesthesiologist, surgical team, and informed patient consent. The prior hysterotomy needs to be either a Kerr (low transverse incision) or Kronig (low vertical incision) without

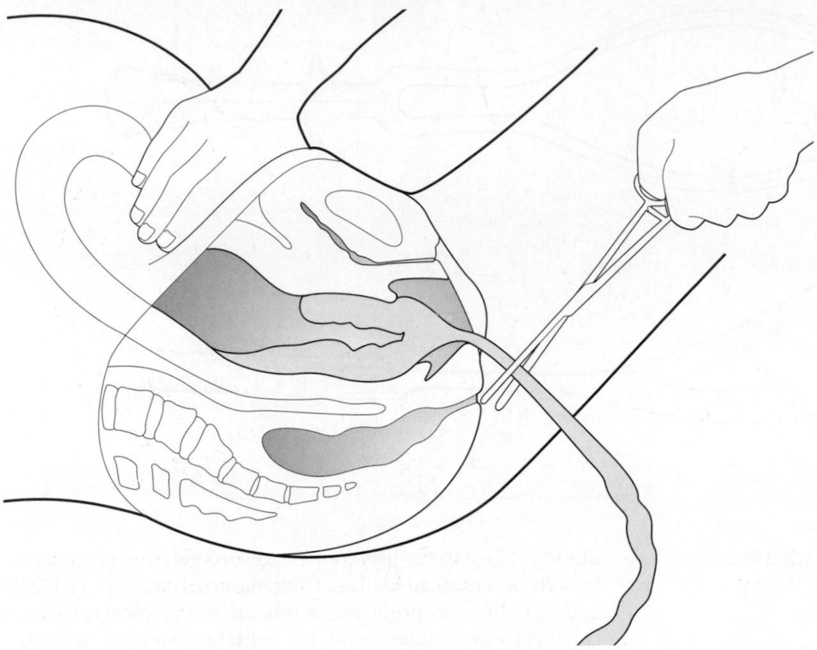

Figure 4-16 • Delivery of the placenta with traction on the cord and suprapubic pressure on the uterus to prevent uterine inversion.

any extensions into the cervix or upper uterine segment. The greatest risk during a trial of labor after cesarean (TOLAC) is that of rupture of the prior uterine scar, which occurs approximately 0.5% to 1.0% of the time. Prior classical hysterotomies, or vertical incisions through the thick upper segment of the uterine corpus, are at a higher risk for uterine rupture in labor and women who have had this type of cesarean are not usually allowed to attempt a trial of labor. Similarly, multiple prior cesarean deliveries increase the risk of uterine rupture and are a relative contraindication. Unfortunately, induction of labor has been associated with higher rates of uterine rupture, thus women with a medical indication for induction of labor need to be counseled and consented again regarding the risks and benefits of a trial of labor when they present for an induction.

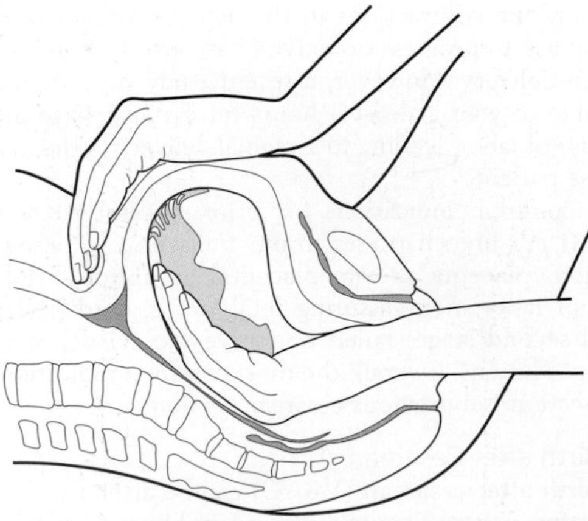

Figure 4-17 • Manual removal of placenta. The fingers are alternately abducted, adducted, and advanced until the placenta is completely detached.

Other factors associated with success or failure of a TOLAC and with uterine rupture are listed in Table 4-4. Common signs of rupture include abdominal pain, FHR decelerations or bradycardia, sudden decrease of pressure on an IUPC, and maternal sensation of a "pop." Therefore, the patient needs to be monitored closely in labor and delivered emergently if uterine rupture is suspected. Over the last decade, the rate of VBAC in the United States has plummeted from as high as 40% to 50% in some populations to below 10%. Because of medical–legal issues, many hospitals no longer sanction trial of labor after cesarean. These trends have contributed to the overall rising cesarean delivery rate. Because of lack of access to in-hospital TOLAC, some patients have opted to attempt VBAC at home.

OBSTETRIC ANALGESIA AND ANESTHESIA

Natural Childbirth

Certainly a component of the discomfort during labor comes from the anticipation of pain and the apprehension that accompanies this event. The concept behind natural childbirth is to educate patients regarding the experiences of labor and delivery in order to prepare them for the event. In addition, a variety of relaxation techniques, showers, and massage are used to help patients cope with the pain from uterine contractions. These practices have been formalized in a variety of characterized techniques, such as the Lamaze method, which involves a series of classes for both the patient and a birthing coach that teach relaxation and breathing techniques.

Systemic Pharmacologic Intervention

Either narcotics or sedatives can be useful in the first stage of labor to relax patients and decrease pain. These commonly include fentanyl, Nubain, and Stadol. Early in labor, IM

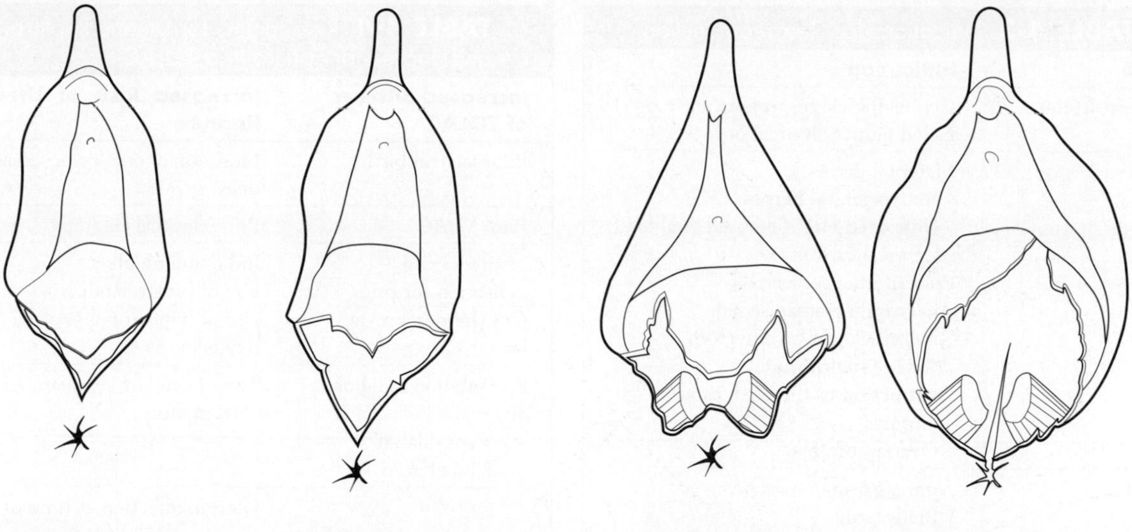

Figure 4-18 • Perineal tears.

morphine sulfate is commonly used to achieve patient pain relief and rest. Sedating medications should not be used close to the time of expected delivery because they cross the placenta and may result in a depressed infant. Other complications of these medications are maternal respiratory depression and increased risk of aspiration.

Pudendal Block

The pudendal nerve travels just posterior to the ischial spine at its juncture with the sacrospinous ligament. With the pudendal block, anesthetic is injected at that site, bilaterally, to give perineal anesthesia. A pudendal block is commonly used in the case of operative vaginal delivery with either forceps or vacuum. It may be combined with local infiltration of the perineum to ensure perineal anesthesia (Fig. 4-20).

Local Anesthesia

In patients without anesthesia who are going to require an episiotomy, local infiltration with an anesthetic is used. Local anesthetic is also used before repair of vaginal, perineal, and periurethral lacerations.

Epidural and Spinal Anesthesia

Epidurals are commonly administered to patients who wish to have anesthesia throughout the active phase and delivery of the infant. Many patients worry about nerve damage and

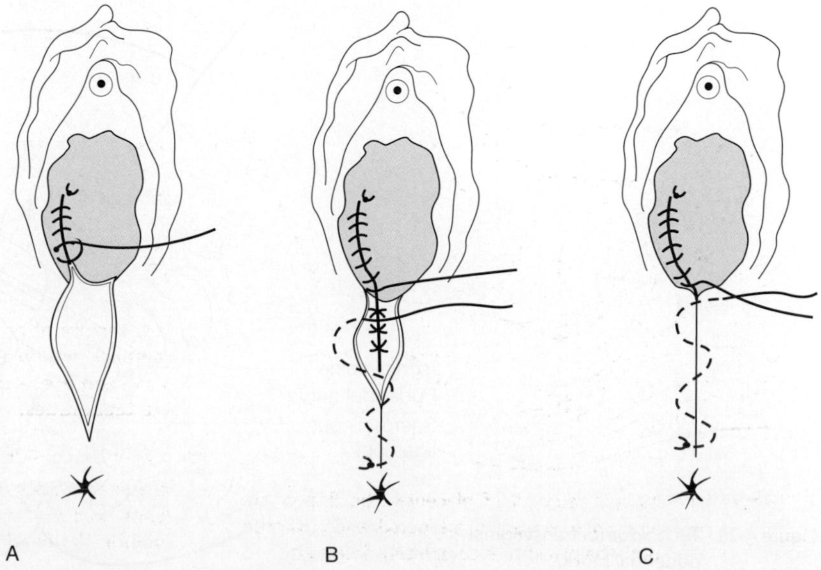

Figure 4-19 • Repair of a second-degree laceration. **(A)** The vaginal mucosa is repaired down to the level of the hymenal ring. **(B)** The subcutaneous tissue of the perineum is then brought together. **(C)** Finally, the skin of the perineum is reapproximated in a subcuticular fashion.

TABLE 4-3 Indications for Cesarean Section

Type	Indication
Maternal/fetal	Cephalopelvic disproportion Failed induction of labor
Maternal	Maternal diseases Active genital herpes Untreated HIV (elevated viral load) Cervical cancer Prior uterine surgery Classical cesarean section Full-thickness myomectomy Prior uterine rupture Obstruction to the birth canal Fibroids Ovarian tumors
Fetal	Nonreassuring fetal testing Bradycardia Absence of FHR variability Scalp pH <7.20 Cord prolapse Fetal malpresentations Breech, transverse lie, brow Multiple gestations Nonvertex first twin Higher-order multiples Fetal anomalies Hydrocephalus Osteogenesis imperfecta
Placental	Placenta previa Vasa previa Abruptio placentae

TABLE 4-4 Risk Factors for Uterine Rupture and Success or Failure in a TOLAC

Increased Success of TOLAC	Increased Risk of Uterine Rupture
Prior vaginal birth	More than one prior cesarean delivery
Prior VBAC	Prior classical cesarean
Nonrecurring indication for prior C/S (herpes, previa, breech)	Induction of labor Use of prostaglandins Use of high amounts of oxytocin
Presentation in labor at: >3 cm dilated >75% effaced	Time from last cesarean <18 months
	Uterine infection at time of last cesarean
Decreased Success of TOLAC	**Decreased Risk of Uterine Rupture**
Prior C/S for cephalopelvic disproportion	Prior vaginal birth
Induction of labor	

the pain of the epidural itself. An early consult with an anesthesiologist to help answer questions about the epidural can be reassuring. The epidural catheter is placed in the L3–L4 interspace when the patient requires analgesia, although usually not until labor is deemed to be in the active phase. Once the catheter is placed, an initial bolus of anesthetic is given and a continuous infusion is started. Again, the epidural does not commonly remove all sensation and can actually be detrimental to the ability to push during the second stage if it does so. However, if the patient requires cesarean delivery, a bolus of epidural can be given and this usually provides adequate anesthesia.

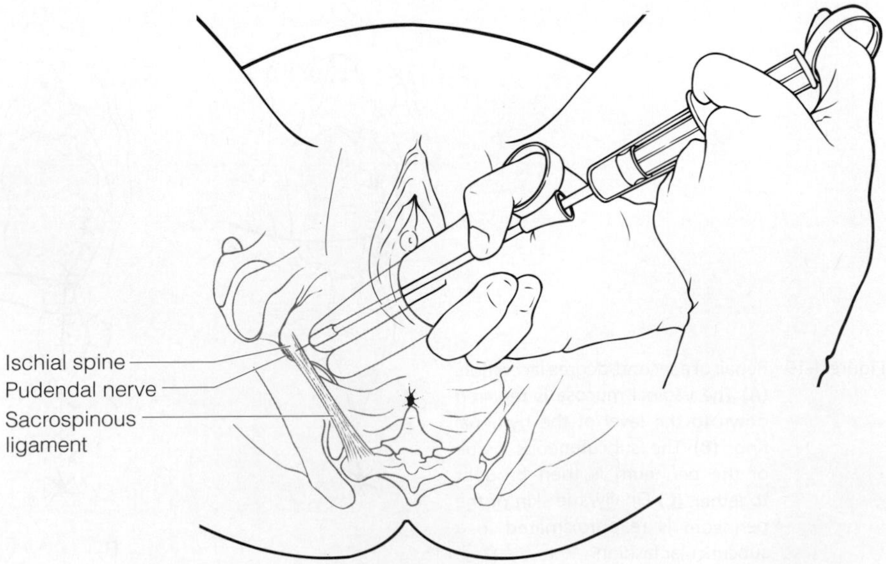

Figure 4-20 • Technique for transvaginal pudendal block.

Spinal anesthesia provides anesthesia over a region similar to that of an epidural, but differs in that it is given in a one-time dose directly into the spinal canal leading to more rapid onset of anesthesia. It is used more commonly for cesarean section than for vaginal delivery. A common complication of both forms of anesthesia is maternal hypotension secondary to decreased systemic vascular resistance, which can lead to decreased placental perfusion and fetal bradycardia. A more serious complication can be maternal respiratory depression if the anesthetic reaches a level high enough to affect diaphragmatic innervation. A spinal headache due to the loss of cerebrospinal fluid is a postpartum complication seen in less than 1% of patients.

General Anesthesia

Although general anesthesia is rarely used for vaginal delivery, it may be used for cesarean delivery, particularly in the emergent setting. For less urgent cesarean sections, epidural or spinal anesthesia is usually preferred. The two principal concerns of general anesthesia are the risk of maternal aspiration and the risk of hypoxia to mother and fetus during induction. Thus, when choosing the route of anesthesia for a cesarean section, the urgency of the delivery must be assessed. Common reasons for an emergent cesarean section are abruption, fetal bradycardia, umbilical cord prolapse, uterine rupture, and hemorrhage from a placenta previa.

KEY POINTS

- The physical examination of a pregnant woman in labor and delivery often includes Leopold maneuvers, a sterile speculum examination, and a cervical examination.
- It is important to determine both the presentation of the fetus and the status of the cervix. The cervical examination includes dilation, effacement, station, consistency, and position.
- Labor can be induced or augmented with prostaglandins, oxytocin, laminaria, Foley bulb, and artificial ROM.
- The fetus can be monitored in labor with external fetal monitoring, fetal scalp electrode, ultrasound, and fetal scalp pH.
- Labor is divided into three stages: the first stage extends until complete cervical dilation, the second stage extends until delivery of the infant, and the third stage extends until delivery of the placenta.
- Forceps delivery and vacuum extraction are two forms of operative vaginal delivery that are used to expedite vaginal delivery.
- Cesarean delivery has multiple indications and is the most common operation performed in the United States.
- Because the most common indication for cesarean delivery is a prior cesarean delivery, attempts should be made to achieve vaginal delivery in the first pregnancy.
- Obstetric anesthesia allows for more patient comfort throughout labor.
- Epidurals are commonly used during labor, whereas spinals are used more often for cesarean section.
- Epidural anesthesia leads to a longer second stage of labor, but offers better control during crowning.
- Occasionally, general anesthesia is used in the emergent setting.

C Clinical Vignettes

Vignette 1

A 31-year-old G1P0 woman at 39 weeks and 4 days presents to labor and delivery unit, with regular contractions occurring every 3 to 5 minutes. Her contractions last 30 to 90 seconds. She not sure if she's been leaking any fluid from her vagina. You take her history and conduct a physical examination.

1. ROM would be supported by which of the following?
   a. Nitrazine paper remaining orange when exposed to fluid in the vagina
   b. A negative fern test
   c. An ultrasound with a normal AFI
   d. A negative tampon test
   e. Speculum examination with evidence of pooling in the vagina

2. You determine her membranes have ruptured and admit her for active management of labor. The first stage of labor
   a. includes an active and latent phase
   b. begins when the cervix has completely dilated
   c. is considered prolonged if its duration is longer than 2 hours in a nulliparous woman
   d. begins with the onset of Braxton Hicks contractions
   e. is commonly associated with repetitive early and variable decelerations

3. On examination you attempt to determine the presentation of the fetus. Which of the following presentations and positions would be most favorable to achieve a vaginal delivery?
   a. Breech
   b. Transverse
   c. Vertex with occiput posterior
   d. Vertex with occiput anterior
   e. Vertex with occiput transverse

4. The patient dilates without difficulty to 10 cm and the second stage of labor begins. She is pushing effectively, but during contractions you notice decelerations on fetal heart tracings. Which of the following would be most concerning?
   a. Isolated early decelerations
   b. Repetitive variable decelerations that resolve quickly after each contraction
   c. Repetitive early decelerations and variable decels
   d. Repetitive late decelerations and loss of variability between contractions
   e. Absence of decelerations

5. She pushes the head to the perineum and you deliver the head and shoulders without complication. The cord is clamped and the placenta delivered. You examine her for lacerations. A second-degree laceration
   a. involves the anal mucosa
   b. is commonly associated with buttonhole lacerations
   c. involves the mucosa or the skin only
   d. will heal well without repair
   e. extends into the perineal body, but does not involve the anal sphincter

Vignette 2

A 26-year-old G2P2001 woman at 40 weeks and 2 days is seen in clinic for prenatal care. She is experiencing occasional contractions and has a sense of pressure in her vagina, but does not feel like she is in labor (as she experienced in her first delivery). Her first child was born at 41 weeks following an induction, resulting in a normal spontaneous vaginal delivery. She's interested in an induction for this pregnancy as well. You perform a cervical examination and discuss options with her.

1. Which of the following cervical examinations is the most favorable for induction of labor?
   a. Cervix closed, posterior, firm with 0% effacement
   b. Cervix soft, midposition, 3 cm dilated, 50% effaced with −2 station
   c. Cervix soft, anterior, 4 cm dilated, 80% effaced with −1 station
   d. Cervix medium, posterior, consistence, 2 cm dilated, 30% effaced
   e. Cervix soft, midposition, 3 cm dilated, 50% effaced with −3 station

2. For women undergoing induction of labor with a Bishop score of 5 or less, which of the following is a commonly used first step?
   a. Nonstress test
   b. Oxytocin drip
   c. Cervical application of prostaglandin E2
   d. Cesarean section
   e. Attempts at induction should be avoided at a Bishop score of less than 5

3. Which of the following is not a contraindication to use of prostaglandins in labor induction?
   a. Maternal asthma
   b. Nonreassuring fetal testing
   c. A prior cesarean section

d. Maternal glaucoma
e. Maternal SLE

4. Once the patient is in active labor and 6 cm dilated, you notice that on two subsequent examinations she is failing to make progress. Which of the following would be appropriate for evaluating the adequacy of contractions?
   a. Fetal scalp electrode
   b. Intrauterine pressure catheter
   c. Abdominal ultrasound
   d. Speculum examination
   e. Serum oxytocin levels

Vignette 3

A 34-year-old G3P2002 woman at 38 weeks and 6 days was admitted to labor and delivery unit for active management of labor after it was determined that her membranes had ruptured and she was dilated to 3 cm. Her cervix has been steadily dilating and now she is at 6 cm. She is very uncomfortable and finds her contractions very painful. Her partner is also very concerned that she needs pain relief.

1. You advise your patient that
   a. narcotics are available, but should be reserved for closer to the time of delivery when her pain will be greatest
   b. if she continues with natural childbirth and eventually needs a cesarean section she will require general anesthesia
   c. spinal anesthesia is her best option because it gives a constant infusion of medicine over a long period of time
   d. she cannot have an epidural yet because she is not yet in the active phase of labor
   e. a variety of relaxation techniques can be incorporated into her labor in addition to pain medication

2. With adequate pain control she dilates to 10 cm and second stage begins. Which of the following is the correct order of the cardinal movements of labor?
   a. Internal rotation, engagement, descent, flexion, external rotation
   b. Engagement, descent, internal rotation, flexion, external rotation
   c. Internal rotation, descent, engagement, flexion, external rotation
   d. Engagement, descent, flexion, internal rotation, external rotation
   e. Engagement, descent, internal rotation, flexion, external rotation

3. An uncomplicated vaginal delivery typically includes which maneuver?
   a. Perineal support to decrease perineal trauma
   b. An episiotomy to hasten delivery
   c. Vacuum extraction if the fetal station is low
   d. Forceps to aid maternal efforts
   e. The McRoberts maneuver

4. Stage 3 begins following the delivery of the infant and typically involves which of the following?
   a. Placental separation
   b. Stopping oxytocin drips if they were used during stage 2
   c. An abrupt increase in the size of the intrauterine cavity
   d. Uterine prolapse
   e. A delay of 60 minutes before the placenta is delivered

Vignette 4

A 24-year-old G2P1001 woman at 39 weeks and 3 days is seen in clinic. She has been experiencing more frequent contractions and thinks she might be in labor. Her last pregnancy ended with a cesarean delivery after a stage 1 arrest. There was no evidence of cephalopelvic disproportion. Earlier in the course of her current pregnancy she had desired a scheduled repeat cesarean, but now that she might be in labor she would like to try and delivery vaginally.

1. What would be a contraindication to a trial of labor after cesarean (TOLAC)?
   a. Prior classical hysterotomy
   b. Prior Kerr hysterotomy
   c. Small for gestational age fetus
   d. Oligohydramnios
   e. GBS + mother

2. After counseling and consent, the patient agrees to a trial of labor and after dilating to 10 cm, she begins to push. After 1 hour of pushing, the fetal heart tracing has absent variability and a baseline that has risen to the 180 beats per minute. The baby's station is low enough to consider using either forceps or vacuum. Which of the following is not required for forceps delivery?
   a. Adequate anesthesia
   b. Evidence of cephalopelvic disproportion
   c. Full dilation of the cervix
   d. At least 2 station and engaged head
   e. Knowledge of fetal position

3. You decide to attempt vacuum extraction. Which of the following is the most common complication of vacuum extraction?
   a. Fetal facial nerve palsy
   b. Maternal perineal laceration
   c. Cephalohematoma
   d. Fetal skull fracture
   e. Prolonged stage 3

A Answers

Vignette 1 Question 1
Answer E: Diagnosis of ROM is suspected with a history of a gush or leaking of fluid from the vagina. It can be confirmed by the pool, nitrazine, and fern tests. If tests are equivocal, an ultrasound examination can evaluate the amount of fluid around the fetus. The tampon tests is used in situations where accurate diagnosis is necessary and involves using amniocentesis to inject dilute indigo carmine dye and looking for leaking of the blue fluid from the cervix onto a tampon.

Vignette 1 Question 2
Answer A: The first stage of labor includes an active and latent phase. Braxton Hicks are irregular contractions that do not result in cervical change, which is common in the third trimester of pregnancy. The other answer choices are associated with the second stage of labor.

Vignette 1 Question 3
Answer D: Fetal position in the vertex position depends on the relationship of the fetal occiput to the maternal pelvis. Occiput transverse and occiput posterior can lead to a prolonged labor and a higher rate of cesarean delivery. Breech and transverse presentations are also associated with prolonged labor, and when identified, are treated by either external cephalic version, and if that fails, by cesarean delivery in most labor wards in the United States. Breech vaginal delivery is still offered at some labor units, but even in that setting, the risk of cesarean delivery is still higher than in vertex presentations.

Vignette 1 Question 4
Answer D: Repetitive early and variable decelerations that resolve quickly between contractions are common in the second stage. Repetitive late decelerations bradycardias, and loss of variability are all signs of nonreassuring fetal status.

Vignette 1 Question 5
Answer E: Second-degree lacerations extend into the perineal body, but do not involve the anal sphincter, whereas first-degree lacerations only involve the mucosa or skin and fourth-degree lacerations can occasionally be button-hole, wherein the rectal mucosa is torn but the sphincter is intact. All but shallow first-degree lacerations are typically repaired after placental delivery.

Vignette 2 Question 1
Answer C: The Bishop score is a method of evaluating the cervix and associated points for fetal station and for cervical dilation, effacement, consistency and position. The higher the Bishop score, the greater the likelihood for successful vaginal delivery following induction of labor. Soft is the best consistency, anterior the best position, and greater dilation and effacement are more favorable.

Vignette 2 Question 2
Answer C: A Bishop score of 5 or less may lead to a failed induction as often as 50% of the time. In these patients, prostaglandin E2 (PGE2) gel, PGE2 pessary (Cervidil), or PGE1M (misoprostol) is often used to "ripen" the cervix. Oxytocin is used to induce labor with a Bishop score greater than 5.

Vignette 2 Question 3
Answer E: There are both maternal and obstetric contraindications for the use of prostaglandins. Maternal reasons include asthma and glaucoma, whereas obstetric reasons include having had a prior cesarean section and nonreassuring fetal testing. All of these are relative contraindications that allow individual clinicians to decide depending on the specific clinical situation. Because PGE2 gel cannot be turned off with the ease of oxytocin, there is a risk of uterine hyperstimulation and tetanic contractions.

Vignette 2 Question 4
Answer B: The intrauterine pressure catheter (IUPC) is inserted into the uterine cavity to directly measure the pressure changes during contractions and can evaluate the adequacy of contractions. A fetal scalp electrode can directly monitor fetal heart rate and variability. Abdominal ultrasound and speculum examinations are not used to assess adequacy of contractions. Serum oxytocin levels are not routinely measured.

Vignette 3 Question 1
Answer E: A variety of relaxation techniques, including the Lamaze method, have been developed to ease the pain of labor. She is in active labor now that she has dilated past 4 cm and is therefore eligible for an epidural. Spinal anesthesia is given as a one-time bolus. Narcotics should not be used close to the time of delivery, as they may lead to decreased respiratory drive in the infant. General anesthesia is only rarely used in emergent situations for cesarean deliveries.

Vignette 3 Question 2
Answer D: The correct order of the cardinal movements of labor is engagement, descent, flexion, internal rotation, and external rotation.

Vignette 3 Question 3
Answer A: Perineal support is usually provided with the fingers of the deliverer's hand keeping pressure on the perineum to prevent a sudden, uncontrolled delivery to minimize the extent and depth of the perineal laceration. Episiotomy is used to hasten delivery particularly in the case of impending or ongoing shoulder dystocia.

Forceps and vacuum extractors are both forms of operative delivery used commonly in the case of prolonged second stage or to hasten delivery. The McRoberts maneuver is used in the setting of shoulder dystocia.

Vignette 3 Question 4

Answer A: Placental separation occurs secondary to mechanical shearing due to an abrupt decrease in intrauterine cavity size after delivery of the fetus. This is perceived by the provider as a gush of blood, cord lengthening, and uterine fundal rebound. Uterine prolapsed can be a serious complication and so provider should apply suprapubic pressure when the patient begins bearing down for placental delivery. Oxytocin is used in the third stage to decrease placental delivery time and blood loss.

Vignette 4 Question 1

Answer A: A prior classical hysterotomy or other vertical uterine incision is an absolute contraindication to TOLAC given the increased risk of uterine rupture. Prior Kerr (low horizontal) or Kronig (low vertical) incisions are required for TOLAC. GBS + mothers should receive prophylactic antibiotics during labor, but may proceed with TOLAC. Oligohydramnios and SGA fetus are not contraindications to TOLAC.

Vignette 4 Question 2

Answer B: Adequate anesthesia, full dilation of the cervix, station 2 or lower with an engaged head, and knowledge of the fetal position are all required for forceps delivery. Evidence of cephalopelvic disproportion is a contraindication to forceps.

Vignette 4 Question 3

Answer C: Facial nerve palsy, maternal laceration, and skull fracture are associated with forceps delivery. Prolonged stage 3 is commonly seen in preterm deliveries and in placenta accrete and is not associated with mode of delivery. Cephalohematoma and scalp lacerations are the most common complications of vacuum extraction.

ANSWERS

Chapter

5 Antepartum Hemorrhage

Obstetric hemorrhage is a leading cause of maternal death in the United States and one of the leading causes of perinatal morbidity and mortality. In 2005, hemorrhage was the third leading cause of maternal deaths due to obstetric factors in the United States. Bleeding during pregnancy has different etiologies depending on the trimester. As discussed in Chapter 2, first-trimester bleeding is associated with spontaneous abortion, ectopic pregnancy, and even normal pregnancies. Third-trimester vaginal bleeding occurs in 3% to 4% of pregnancies and may be obstetric or nonobstetric (Table 5-1). Hemorrhage can occur antepartum or postpartum (Chapter 12), with the major causes of antepartum hemorrhage including placenta previa (20%) and placental abruption (30%).

PLACENTA PREVIA

PATHOGENESIS

Placenta previa is defined as abnormal implantation of the placenta over the internal cervical os (Fig. 5-1). **Complete previa** occurs when the placenta completely covers the internal os. **Partial previa** occurs when the placenta covers a portion of the internal os. **Marginal previa** occurs when the edge of the placenta reaches the margin of the os. A **low-lying placenta** is implanted in the lower uterine segment in close proximity but not extending to the internal os. Rarely, a fetal vessel may lie over the cervix; this is known as a **vasa previa** (discussed later in this chapter).

It is unclear why some placentas implant in the lower uterine segment rather than in the fundus. Uterine scarring may predispose to placental implantation in the lower uterine segment. With the progression of pregnancy, more than 90% of these low-lying placentas identified early in pregnancy will appear to move away from the cervix and out of the lower uterine segment. Although the term **placental migration** has been used, most experts do not believe the placenta actually moves. The apparent movement of the placenta is most likely due to the development of the lower uterine segment. Additionally, it may be that the placenta grows preferentially toward a better vascularized fundus (trophotropism), whereas the placenta overlying the less well-vascularized cervix may undergo atrophy. In some cases, this atrophy leaves vessels running through the membranes, unsupported by placental tissue or umbilical cord. If this occurs over the cervix, it is termed a **vasa previa**. In cases where the atrophy is incomplete, leaving a placental lobe discrete from the rest of the placenta, it is termed a **succenturiate lobe**.

Bleeding from a placenta previa results from small disruptions in the placental attachment during normal development and thinning of the lower uterine segment during the third trimester. This bleeding may stimulate further uterine contractions, which in turn stimulates further placental separation and bleeding. Although they may be a reason for hospitalization, these initial bleeds are rarely a major problem. In labor, as the cervix dilates and effaces, there is usually placental separation and unavoidable bleeding. As a result, profuse hemorrhage and shock can occur, leading to significant maternal and fetal morbidity and mortality. Maternal mortality is estimated to occur in 0.03% of cases of placenta previa in the United States. Although the maternal and perinatal mortality from placenta previa has dropped rapidly in the United States over the past few decades, the perinatal mortality rate is still 10 times higher than in the general population. Most risk to the fetus comes from premature delivery, which is responsible for 60% of perinatal deaths. Other fetal risks associated with placenta previa are listed in Table 5-2.

Placenta previa may also be complicated by an associated placenta accreta (placenta previa accreta). **Placenta accreta** is defined as the superficial attachment of the placenta to the uterine myometrium. An **increta** occurs when the placenta invades the myometrium. A **percreta** occurs when the placenta invades through the myometrium to the uterine serosa. In some cases, this may lead to invasion of other organs such as the bladder anteriorly or the rectum posteriorly.

Placenta accreta causes an inability of the placenta to properly separate from the uterine wall after the delivery of the fetus. This can result in profuse hemorrhage and shock with substantial maternal morbidity and mortality, such as need for hysterectomy, surgical injury to the ureters, bladder, and other viscera, adult respiratory distress syndrome, renal failure, coagulopathy, and death. The average blood loss at delivery in women with placenta accreta is 3,000 to 5,000 mL. Historically, the most frequent indication for a peripartum hysterectomy has been uterine atony. Recent literature suggests that this may be shifting, as abnormal placentation is increasingly becoming a more common reason for peripartum hysterectomy. With the increasing cesarean section rate, as well as a decrease in vaginal birth after cesarean section, this number is likely to further increase in the future. Indeed, in several centers, placenta accreta has become the leading reason for cesarean hysterectomy.

Two-thirds of women with both a placenta previa and an associated accreta require a hysterectomy at the time of delivery (**peripartum hysterectomy**). Rarely, placenta accreta may lead to spontaneous uterine rupture in the second or third trimester, resulting in intraperitoneal hemorrhage, a life-threatening emergency. Minor degrees of placenta accreta may occur, which may lead to slightly heavier postpartum bleeding, but may not require the aggressive management that is often

TABLE 5-1 Differential Diagnosis of Antepartum Bleeding

Obstetric causes	
Placental	Placenta previa, placental abruption, vasa previa
Maternal	Uterine rupture
Fetal	Fetal vessel rupture
Nonobstetric causes	
Cervical	Severe cervicitis, polyps, cervical dysplasia/cancer
Vaginal/vulvar	Lacerations, varices, cancer
Other	Hemorrhoids, congenital bleeding disorder, abdominal or pelvic trauma, hematuria

Adapted from Hacker N, Moore JG. *Essentials of Obstetrics and Gynecology*. Philadelphia, PA: WB Saunders; 1992:155.

percreta: can invade bladder or rectum

accreta: 3-5L blood lost

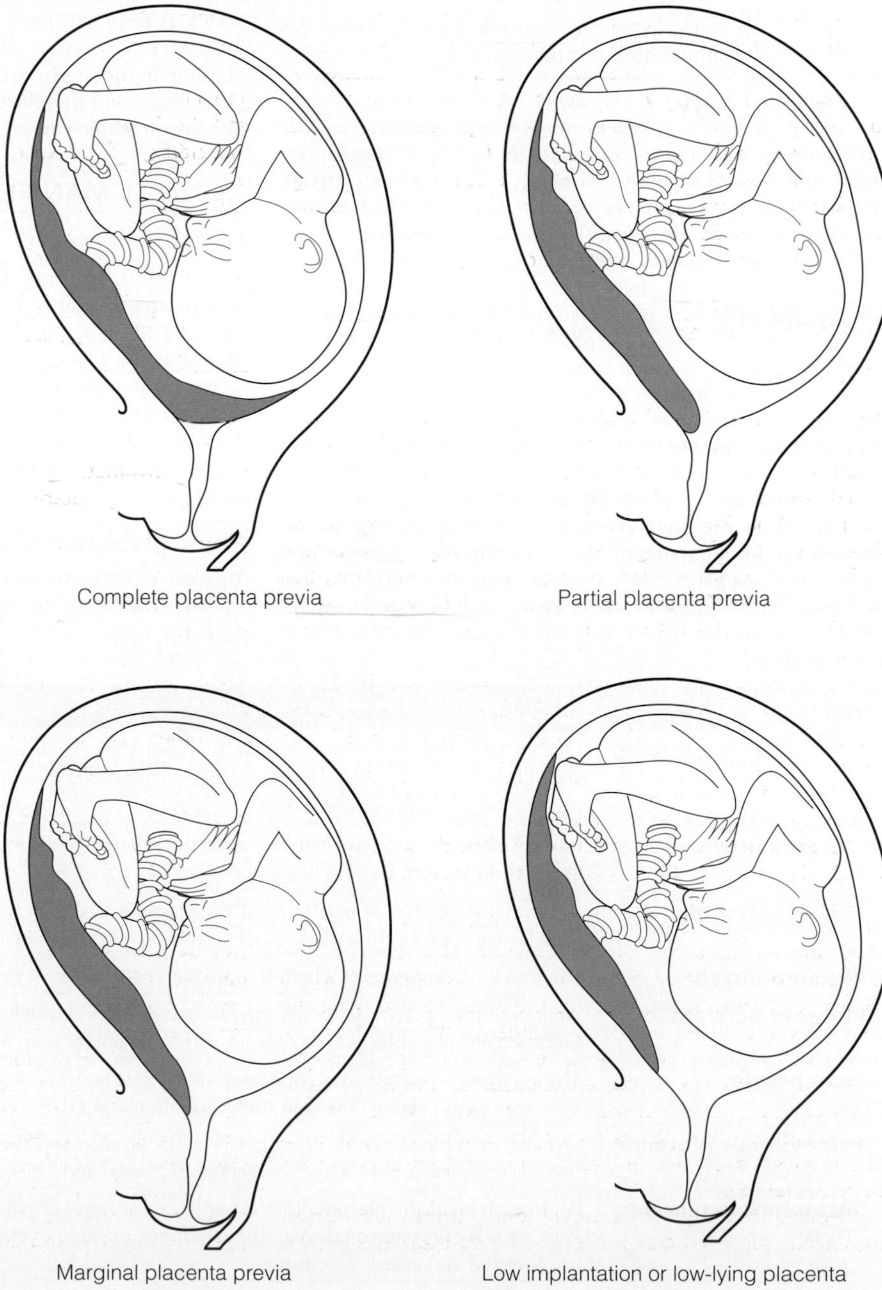

Figure 5-1 • Classifications of placenta previa.

c/s : ↑ previa

■ **TABLE 5-2** Fetal Complications Associated with Placenta Previa

Preterm delivery and its complications
Preterm premature rupture of membranes
Intrauterine growth restriction
Malpresentation
Vasa previa
Congenital abnormalities

Adapted from Hacker N, Moore JG. *Essentials of Obstetrics and Gynecology.* Philadelphia, PA: WB Saunders; 1992:155.

employed with more extensive placenta accreta. Table 5-3 summarizes the abnormalities of placentation.

EPIDEMIOLOGY

previa : 15%

Placenta previa occurs in approximately 0.5% of pregnancies (1:200 births) and accounts for nearly 20% of all antepartum hemorrhage. Previa occurs in as many as 1% to 4% of women with a prior cesarean section. Because a bleeding previa often results in delivery, which may occur preterm, it is a common indication for preterm delivery. Placenta previa can also be complicated by an associated placenta accreta (placenta previa accreta) in approximately 5% of cases. The risk of placenta accreta is increased in women with placenta previa in the setting of prior cesarean delivery. It has been seen in 15% to 30% of women with one prior cesarean section, 25% to 50% of women with two prior cesarean sections, and in 29% to 67% of women with three or more prior cesarean sections.

Abnormalities in placentation are the result of events that prevent normal migration of the placenta during normal progressive development of the lower uterine segment during pregnancy (Table 5-4). Previous placental implantations and prior uterine scars are thought to contribute to abnormal

PTL

previa & accretia

15-30% 25-50% 29-67%

placentation in subsequent pregnancies. Thus, the risk of placenta previa is increased in patients with other prior uterine surgery such as myomectomy, uterine anomalies, multiple gestations, multiparity, advanced maternal age, smoking, and previous placenta previa. The likelihood of placenta previa increases significantly with each additional cesarean delivery, putting those women with repeat cesarean section at significant risk with each additional pregnancy. Of note, because many patients receive a routine obstetric ultrasound, marginal previa or low-lying placenta is commonly diagnosed in the second trimester. Most resolve on repeat ultrasound by "moving" up and away from the cervix during the third trimester as the lower uterine segment develops. The later in pregnancy that placenta previa is diagnosed, the higher the likelihood of persistence to delivery. Women who at 20 weeks have a low-lying placenta that does not overlie the internal os will not have a placenta previa at term and need no further sonographic examinations for placental location. However, the presence of a low-lying placenta in the second trimester is a risk factor for developing a vasa previa, and therefore, in these cases, an ultrasound should be performed later in pregnancy to exclude that condition.

unlikely to have previa but can get vasa previa

CLINICAL MANIFESTATIONS

History

Patients with placenta previa classically present with sudden and profuse **painless vaginal bleeding**. The first episode of bleeding—the "sentinel" bleed—usually occurs after 28 weeks of gestation. During this time, the lower uterine segment develops and thins, disrupting the placental attachment and resulting in bleeding. Placenta accreta (and increta) is usually asymptomatic. On rare occasions, however, a patient with a percreta into the bladder or rectum may present with hematuria or rectal bleeding.

28 wk

Physical Examination

Vaginal examination is contraindicated in placenta previa because the digital examination can cause further separation

■ **TABLE 5-3** Abnormalities of Placentation

Circumvallate placenta	Occurs when the membranes double back over the edge of the placenta, forming a dense ring around the periphery of the placenta. Often considered a variant of placental abruption, it is a major cause of second-trimester hemorrhage
Placenta previa	Occurs when the placenta develops over the internal cervical os Types include complete, partial, and marginal
Placenta accreta	Abnormal adherence of part or all of the placenta to the uterine wall May be associated with a placenta in normal locations, but incidence increases in placenta previa
Placenta increta	Abnormal placentation in which the placenta invades the myometrium
Placenta percreta	Abnormal placentation in which the placenta invades through the myometrium to the uterine serosa Occasionally, placentas may invade into adjacent organs such as the bladder or rectum
Vasa previa	Occurs when a velamentous cord insertion causes the fetal vessels to pass over the internal cervical os Also seen with velamentous and succenturiate placentas
Velamentous placenta	Occurs when blood vessels insert between the amnion and the chorion, away from the margin of the placenta, leaving the vessels largely unprotected and vulnerable to compression or injury
Succenturiate placenta	An extra lobe of the placenta that is implanted at some distance away from the rest of the placenta Fetal vessels may course between the two lobes, possibly over the cervix, leaving these blood vessels unprotected and at risk for rupture

false positive on u/s over belly.

■ **TABLE 5-4** Predisposing Factors for Placenta Previa
Prior cesarean section and uterine surgery (e.g., myomectomy)
Multiparity
Multiple gestation
Erythroblastosis
Smoking
History of placenta previa
Increasing maternal age

of the placenta and trigger catastrophic hemorrhage. Because many women have an ultrasound examination that can diagnose placenta previa, diagnosis by digital examination of the placenta previa is uncommon today. However, in the rare patient that is undiagnosed, the cervical examination may reveal soft, spongy tissue just inside the cervix. Because of the increased vascularity, there may be notable varices in the lower uterine segment or cervix, which can be visualized on speculum examination or palpated. A marginal previa can be palpated at the edge of, or quite near, the internal os.

DIAGNOSTIC EVALUATION

u/s 95%.

The diagnosis of placenta previa can be made via ultrasonography with a sensitivity of greater than 95% (Fig. 5-2). If made before the third trimester in pregnancy, a follow-up ultrasound is often obtained in the third trimester to determine if the previa has resolved. Although transabdominal sonography is frequently used for placental location, this technique lacks some precision in diagnosing placenta previa. Numerous studies have demonstrated the accuracy and superiority of transvaginal sonography for the diagnosis of placenta previa. One study of 131 women believed to have a placenta previa by transabdominal sonography found that anatomic landmarks crucial for the accurate diagnosis were poorly recognized in 50% of cases. In 26% of the cases of suspected placenta previa, the initial diagnosis was changed after transvaginal sonography demonstrated the diagnosis to be incorrect.

The superiority of transvaginal sonography over transabdominal sonography can be attributed to several factors:

1. If a transabdominal ultrasound is performed with a full maternal bladder, placenta previa may be overdiagnosed. Compression of the anterior and posterior walls of the lower uterine segment with bladder filling can result in the perception of a longer cervix. Consequently, a normally situated placenta may falsely appear to be a previa. Therefore, it is important to have the bladder entirely emptied before this portion of the ultrasound is performed if a previa is a possibility.
2. Vaginal probes are closer to the region of interest, and typically of higher frequency, and therefore obtain higher resolution images than transabdominal probes.
3. The internal cervical os and the lower placental edge frequently cannot be imaged adequately by the transabdominal approach. The position of the internal os is assumed rather than actually seen.
4. The fetal head may obscure views of the lower placental edge when using the transabdominal approach, and a posterior placenta previa may not be adequately imaged.

The improved accuracy of transvaginal sonography over transabdominal sonography means that fewer false-positive diagnoses are made. Thus, the rate of placenta previa is significantly lower when using transvaginal sonography as compared to using transabdominal sonography. A recent study found that the incidence of placenta previa is considerably lower (1.1%) when routine transvaginal sonography is performed at 15 to 20 weeks, versus the previously reported incidence (15 to 20%) in the second trimester when using transabdominal sonography.

Numerous studies have demonstrated the safety of transvaginal sonography for the diagnosis of placenta previa. Importantly, this imaging technique does not lead to an increase in bleeding. The two main reasons for this are (1) the vaginal probe is introduced at an angle that places it against the anterior fornix and anterior lip of the cervix and (2) the optimal distance for visualization of the cervix is 2 to 3 cm away from the cervix, so the probe is generally not advanced sufficiently to make contact with the placenta. Nonetheless, the examination should be performed by personnel experienced in transvaginal sonography, and the transvaginal probe should always be inserted carefully, with the examiner looking at the monitor to avoid putting the probe in the cervix.

Translabial sonography has been suggested as an alternative to transvaginal sonography, and it has been shown to be superior to transabdominal sonography for placental location. However, because transvaginal sonography appears to be accurate, safe, and well tolerated, it should be the imaging modality of choice.

Of note, it is important to make the diagnosis of placenta accreta prenatally because this allows effective planning and management to minimize morbidity. This diagnosis is usually made by ultrasonography or MRI. Placenta accreta should be suspected in women who have both a placenta previa and a history of cesarean delivery or other uterine surgery. Close surveillance is particularly indicated when the placenta is anterior and overlies the cesarean scar.

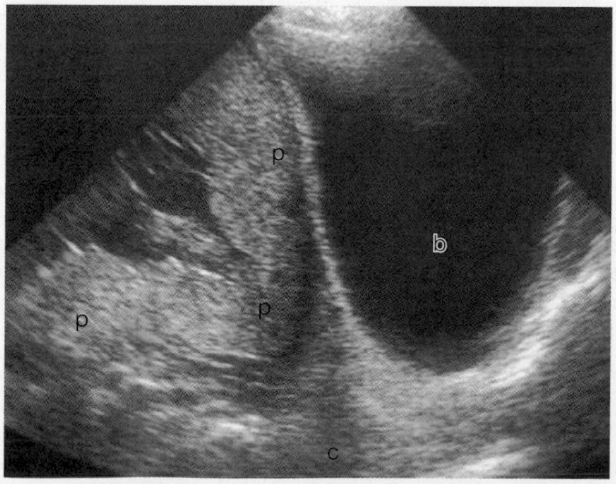

Figure 5-2 • Complete placenta previa. *p*, placenta; *c*, cervix; *b*, bladder.

TREATMENT

Management of patients with placenta previa varies between providers. Although there are minimal data to support the efficacy of avoidance of intercourse and excessive activity, antepartum patients with a placenta previa are commonly managed with strict pelvic rest (i.e., no intercourse) and modified bed rest. However, some clinicians will not institute this conservative management until the patient presents with a sentinel bleed. Similarly, some clinicians prescribe hospitalized bed rest after the sentinel bleed, whereas others wait until the patient has a large bleed by history, examination, or a drop in hematocrit of at least three points. Inpatient versus outpatient management remains an area of controversy. In one of the few prospective randomized studies dealing with placenta previa, 53 women with placenta previa at gestational ages between 24 and 36 weeks, who had been initially stabilized in hospital after a bleeding event, were randomized to inpatient or outpatient management. The investigators found no significant difference in clinical outcomes between the two groups. Thus, women who are stable and asymptomatic, and who are reliable and have quick access to the hospital, may be considered for outpatient management.

Unstoppable labor, fetal distress, and life-threatening hemorrhage are all indications for immediate cesarean delivery regardless of gestational age. There is consensus that patients with complete or partial placenta previa require delivery by cesarean. However, patients with a low-lying placenta or marginal previa (>2 cm from the internal os) may generally be allowed to deliver vaginally as long as there is no evidence of fetal distress or excessive hemorrhage. Some authors suggest that women with placenta previa should have a transvaginal ultrasound in the late third trimester, and that those with a placental edge less than 2 cm from the internal os should be delivered by cesarean. Of note, there is potential for postpartum hemorrhage in women with a placenta that extends into the noncontractile lower uterine segment and have a vaginal delivery. In case of preterm pregnancy, if the bleeding is not profuse, fetal survival can be enhanced by aggressive expectant management. However, 70% of patients with placenta previa have a recurring bleeding episode and will require delivery before week 36. For patients who make it to week 36, typical management involves amniocentesis to determine fetal lung maturity and delivery by cesarean section between 36 and 37 weeks after confirmation of fetal lung maturity. If the amniocentesis does not demonstrate lung maturity, many physicians will deliver the women by elective cesarean at 38 weeks, without repeating the amniocentesis, if they remain stable, or earlier if bleeding occurs or the patient goes into labor.

A recent decision analysis suggested that delivery as early as 34 weeks of gestation and no later than 37 weeks may be optimal, and that amniocentesis for determination of fetal lung maturity does not improve outcomes and is not recommended (*Obstet Gynecol.* 2010;116:835–842). Advanced planning and interdisciplinary collaboration are fundamental, and as gestational age increases, so does the risk of emergent bleeding. It is reasonable to say that patients with suspected placenta previa and/or accreta should be delivered between 34 and 37 weeks with minimal benefit gained by confirming fetal lung maturity.

The following should be the course of action in the case of vaginal bleeding and suspected placenta previa and/or placenta accreta:

1. **Stabilize the patient.** Every patient with vaginal bleeding and a known or suspected previa should be hospitalized, placed on continuous fetal monitoring, and have IV access established. If the patient presents with a particularly large bleed, two large-bore IV catheters will commonly be placed. Laboratory evaluation includes hematocrit, type and cross, and, if considerable bleeding or coagulopathy is suspected, PT, PTT, D-dimer or fibrin split products, and fibrinogen. For an Rh-negative woman, a Kleihauer-Betke test should be performed to determine the extent of any fetomaternal transfusion so that the appropriate amount of RhoGAM can be administered to prevent alloimmunization.
2. **Prepare for catastrophic hemorrhage.** Expectant management in the stabilized patient includes hospitalization, bed rest, hematocrit monitoring, and consideration of limiting any oral intake. Two or more units of blood should be typed, cross-matched, and made available. Transfusions are usually given to maintain a hematocrit of 25% or greater.
3. **Prepare for preterm delivery.** Generally, at the time of admission, women between 24 and 34 weeks of gestation with vaginal bleeding should be given steroids to promote fetal lung maturity. The patient and her family should have a neonatology consultation so that the management of the infant after birth may be discussed. In women who have a history of cesarean delivery or uterine surgery, detailed ultrasonography should be performed to exclude placenta accreta. Because prematurity is the main cause of perinatal mortality associated with placenta previa, it is desirable to prolong the pregnancy as long as safely possible. Therefore, before 32 weeks of gestation, moderate to severe bleeding without maternal or fetal compromise may be managed aggressively with blood transfusions, rather than moving toward delivery. Cautious use of tocolytics in women with placenta previa who are having contractions appears reasonable to assist in prolonging the pregnancy up to 34 weeks of gestation, as long as both mother and fetus are stable. Occasionally, tocolysis is used past week 34 to help control bleeding.

Following are additional considerations for suspected placenta accreta/increta/percreta:

1. **Plan for total abdominal hysterectomy at the time of cesarean section.** It is generally accepted that placenta accreta is ideally treated by total abdominal hysterectomy. In addition, there is almost universal consensus that the placenta should be left in place; attempts to detach the placenta frequently result in massive hemorrhage. However, the physician should be aware that focal placenta accreta may exist, which may not require such aggressive therapy.
2. **Schedule delivery at 34 to 37 weeks of gestation.** A study comparing emergency with elective peripartum hysterectomy found that women in the emergency hysterectomy group had greater intraoperative blood loss, were more likely to have intraoperative hypotension, and were more likely to receive blood transfusions than women who had elective obstetric hysterectomies.
3. **Plan ahead and have back-up available.** The patient should be counseled regarding hysterectomy and blood transfusion. The patient should be type and crossed for blood products and these should be readily available at the time of cesarean section. Urology, urogynecology, and/or gynecologic oncology should be aware of the patient in the event of percreta or catastrophic blood loss.

abruption

50%, 15%, 30% →

30wk labor delivery

PLACENTAL ABRUPTION

PATHOGENESIS

Placental abruption (abruptio placentae) is the premature separation of the normally implanted placenta from the uterine wall, resulting in hemorrhage between the uterine wall and the placenta. Fifty percent of abruptions occur before labor and after 30 weeks of gestation, 15% occur during labor, and 30% are identified only on placental inspection after delivery. Large placental separations may result in premature delivery, uterine tetany, disseminated intravascular coagulation (DIC), and hypovolemic shock.

The primary cause of placental abruption is unknown, although it is associated with a variety of predisposing and precipitating factors (Table 5-5). These factors include maternal hypertension, prior history of placental abruption, maternal cocaine use, external maternal trauma, and rapid decompression of the overdistended uterus. Abnormal placental vasculature, thrombosis, and reduced placental perfusion are some of the mechanisms that have been proposed to explain the pathogenesis of placental separation and that these anomalies might have some genetic basis.

At the initial point of separation, nonclotted blood courses from the injury site. The enlarging collection of blood may cause further separation of the placenta. In 20% of placental separations, bleeding is confined within the uterine cavity and is referred to as a **concealed hemorrhage** (Fig. 5-3). In the remaining 80% of placental separations, the blood dissects downward toward the cervix, resulting in a **revealed** or **external hemorrhage**. Because there is an egress for the blood, revealed hemorrhages are less likely to result in larger retroplacental clots, which are associated with fetal demise. The result of hemorrhage from torn placental vessels can vary from maternal

20% blood stays in uterine cavity
80% blood workes out cervix → less clot/fetal demise

■ **TABLE 5-5** Predisposing and Precipitating Factors for Placental Abruption
Predisposing factors
Hypertension
Previous placental abruption
Advanced maternal age
Multiparity
Uterine distension
Multiple pregnancy
Polyhydramnios
Vascular deficiency
Diabetes mellitus
Collagen vascular disease
Cocaine use
Methamphetamine use
Cigarette smoking
Alcohol use (>14 drinks/wk)
Circumvallate placenta
Short umbilical cord
Precipitating factors
Trauma
External/internal version
Motor vehicle accident
Abdominal trauma
Sudden uterine volume loss
Delivery of first twin
Rupture of membranes with polyhydramnios
Preterm premature rupture of membranes

leak 80% better

Apparent bleeding

concealed, stays in uterine cavity 20%

clot

Concealed bleeding

Relatively concealed bleeding

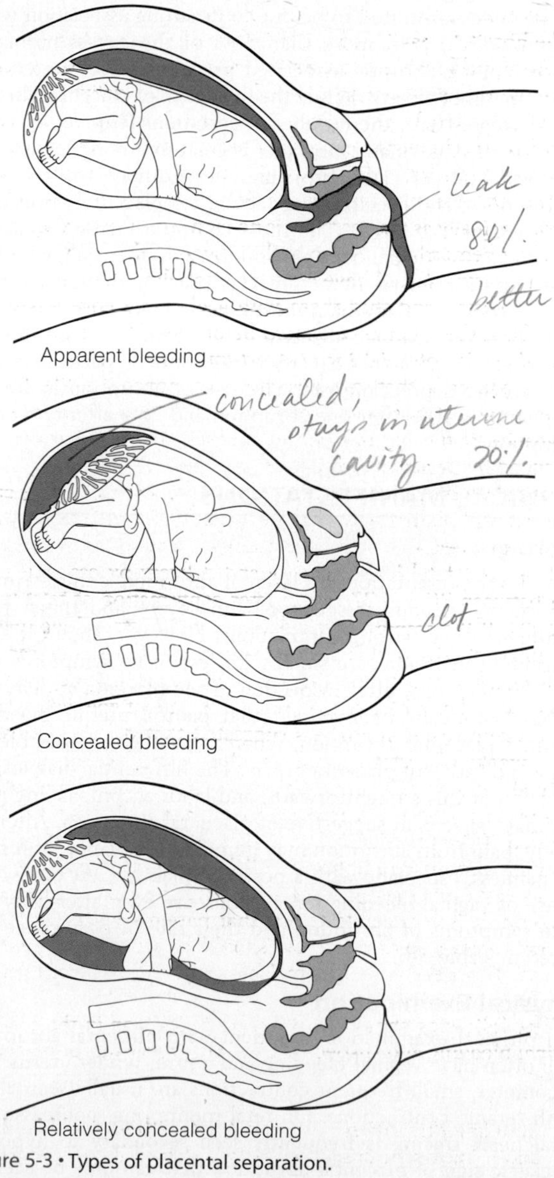

Figure 5-3 • Types of placental separation.

anemia in mild cases to shock, acute renal failure, and maternal death in severe cases.

Global maternal mortality from placental abruption varies from 0.5% to 5.0%. Most deaths are due to hemorrhage, cardiac failure, or renal failure. Fetal mortality occurs in about 35% of all clinically relevant antepartum placental abruptions and can be as high as 50% to 80% in cases of severe placental abruption. The cause of fetal demise is usually due to hypoxia resulting from decreased placental surface area and maternal hemorrhage.

EPIDEMIOLOGY

Placental abruption occurs in about 0.5% to 1.5% of pregnancies and is responsible for 30% of cases of third-trimester bleeding and 15% of perinatal mortality. Abruption occurs in about 0.7% to 1.0% of singleton births and in twins the incidence ranges from 1% to 2%. Although relatively uncommon, placental abruption is a major cause of fetal and neonatal mortality. The high mortality associated with abruptio placentae has been demonstrated to be due to its strong association with preterm birth, with more than 50% of the excess perinatal deaths among abruptio-associated pregnancies accounted for by premature delivery. While the incidence of placental abruption increases with the number of gestations (triplets > twins > singletons), perinatal mortality is greatest among singletons, followed by twins, and surprisingly least among triplets. The predisposing and precipitating factors for placental abruption are listed in Table 5-5. The most common factor associated with increased incidence of abruption is hypertension, whether it is chronic, the result of preeclampsia, or maternal ingestion of cocaine or methamphetamine. In cases of abruptions that are severe enough to cause fetal death, 50% are due to hypertension: 25% of these are from chronic hypertension and 25% are from preeclampsia. The risk of abruption in future pregnancy is 10% after one abruption and 25% after two prior abruptions.

CLINICAL MANIFESTATIONS

History

The classic presentation of placental abruption is third-trimester vaginal bleeding associated with severe abdominal pain and/or frequent, strong contractions. However, about 30% of placental separations are small with few or no symptoms and are identified only after inspection of the placenta at delivery. It has historically been taught that **painful** uterine bleeding signifies placental abruption, whereas **painless** uterine bleeding is indicative of placenta previa. The differential diagnosis is usually not this straightforward, and labor accompanying previa may cause pain suggestive of placental abruption. Alternatively, pain from abruption may mimic normal labor, or it may be painless, especially with a posterior placenta. At times, the cause of vaginal bleeding remains obscure even after delivery. The symptoms of abruption and their rate of occurrence are listed in Table 5-6.

TABLE 5-6 Presentation of Abruptio Placentae

Symptom	Occurrence (%)
Vaginal bleeding	80
Uterine tenderness/abdominal or back pain	67
Abnormal contractions/increased uterine tone	34
Fetal distress	50
Fetal demise	15

Physical Examination

On physical examination, a patient with placental abruption will often have vaginal bleeding and a firm, tender uterus. On tocometer, small frequent contractions are usually seen along with tetanic contractions. On fetal monitoring, nonreassuring fetal heart tracing is frequently seen secondary to hypoxia. A classic sign of placental abruption that can only be seen at the time of cesarean delivery is the Couvelaire uterus, which is a life-threatening condition and occurs when there is enough blood from the abruption that markedly infiltrates the myometrium to reach the serosa, especially at the cornua, that it gives the myometrium a bluish purple tone that can be seen on the surface of the uterus.

DIAGNOSTIC EVALUATION

The diagnosis of placental abruption is primarily clinical. Only 2% to 25% of abruptions are diagnosed by ultrasound (evidenced by a retroplacental clot). However, because abruption can present clinically in a similar fashion to placenta previa with vaginal bleeding, ultrasonography is routinely performed to rule out previa in cases of suspected abruption. Importantly, negative findings on ultrasound examination do **NOT** exclude placental abruption. The diagnosis of abruption may be confirmed by inspection of the placenta at delivery. The presence of a retroplacental clot with overlying placental destruction confirms the diagnosis.

ADDITIONAL CLINICAL FINDINGS

Hypovolemic Shock

One study showed that in women with abruption severe enough to kill the fetus, blood loss often amounted to at least half of the pregnant blood volume. Conversely, neither hypotension nor anemia is obligatory even with extreme concealed hemorrhage. Oliguria from inadequate renal perfusion that is observed in these circumstances is responsive to vigorous IV fluid and blood infusion.

Consumptive Coagulopathy

Placental abruption is one of the most common causes of clinically significant consumptive coagulopathy in obstetrics. In approximately one-third of women with an abruption severe enough to kill the fetus, there are measurable changes in coagulation factors. Specifically, clinically significant hypofibrinogenemia (i.e., plasma levels <150 mg/dL) is found. This is coupled with elevated levels of fibrinogen–fibrin degradation products and/or D-dimers, which are specific degradation products of fibrin. Other coagulation factors are also variably decreased. Consumptive coagulopathy is more likely with a concealed abruption. In cases where the fetus survives, severe coagulation defects are seen less commonly. In general, if serious coagulopathy develops, it is usually evident by the time abruption symptoms appear.

The major mechanism of consumptive coagulopathy in the setting of abruption is activation of intravascular coagulation with varying degrees of defibrination. Procoagulants are also consumed in the retroplacental clots, although the amounts recovered are insufficient to account for all of the missing fibrinogen. An important consequence of intravascular coagulation is the activation of plasminogen to plasmin, which lyses fibrin microemboli to maintain microcirculatory patency. With placental abruption severe enough to kill the fetus, there are always pathological levels of fibrinogen–fibrin degradation products and/or D-dimers in maternal serum. Overt thrombocytopenia may or may not accompany severe hypofibrinogenemia initially, but commonly becomes evident after repeated blood transfusions.

TREATMENT

The potential for rapid deterioration (e.g., hemorrhage, DIC, fetal hypoxia) necessitates delivery in some cases of placental abruption. However, most abruptions are small and noncatastrophic, and do not therefore necessitate immediate delivery. Treatment of placental abruption varies depending on gestational age and the status of the mother and fetus. Emergency cesarean delivery is chosen by most clinicians if vaginal delivery is not imminent and the fetus is of viable gestational age. With massive external bleeding, intensive resuscitation with blood products, crystalloid fluids, and prompt delivery to control hemorrhage are lifesaving for the mother and, hopefully, for the fetus. If the diagnosis is uncertain and the fetus is alive but without evidence of compromise, then close observation can be practiced in facilities capable of immediate intervention.

The following should be done in case of suspected placental abruption:

1. **Stabilize the patient.** When placental abruption is known or suspected, the patient should be hospitalized with continuous fetal monitoring and IV access gained (ideal to have two large-bore IV catheters). Laboratory evaluation should include CBC, type and cross, PT/PTT, fibrinogen, and D-dimer or fibrin split products. For an Rh-negative woman, RhoGAM should be administered to prevent alloimmunization. The anesthesiologist should be notified of the patient's condition in case emergent cesarean delivery is indicated.
2. **Prepare for the possibility of future hemorrhage.** Standard antishock measures should be taken, including placement of large-bore IV catheters, infusion of lactated Ringer's solution, and preparation of units of crossed-matched blood (whole or packed RBCs). Blood loss due to placental abruption is commonly grossly underestimated because of to concealed bleeding. If cross-matched blood is not available, "code gray" (O-negative) blood may be given in an emergency to help prevent massive blood loss and development of a consumptive coagulopathy/DIC. Additionally, patients should also be transfused fresh frozen plasma and occasionally cryoprecipitate in similar ratios as found in massive transfusion protocols for trauma (i.e., 2 units of packed RBCs: 1 unit FFP) to improve maternal outcomes.
3. **Prepare for preterm delivery.** In the preterm pregnancy, betamethasone may be given to promote fetal lung maturity and some providers tocolyze to assist in prolonging the pregnancy to week 34 for pregnancies complicated by suspected abruption with no evidence of fetal compromise. Others view abruption as a contraindication to tocolysis.
4. **Deliver if bleeding is life threatening or fetal testing is nonreassuring.** Delivery should be performed in patients with a life-threatening hemorrhage. This is a clinical determination, but any patient whose vital signs are unstable or has a coagulopathy should be delivered regardless of gestational age and steroid administration. Vaginal delivery is preferred as long as bleeding is controlled and there are no signs of fetal distress. Vaginal delivery is also preferred in the case of intrauterine fetal demise in the setting of severe placental abruption. Because the uterus is typically hyperactive and persistently hypertonic in patients with an abruption, a rapid labor and delivery should be expected. If the fetal heart rate tracing is nonreassuring, delivery should occur for fetal indications.

UTERINE RUPTURE

PATHOGENESIS

Uterine rupture represents a potential obstetric catastrophe and can lead to both maternal and fetal death. Most complete uterine ruptures occur during the course of labor. More than 90% of all uterine ruptures are associated with a prior uterine scar either from cesarean section or other uterine surgery. Uterine ruptures without a prior uterine scar may be related to an abdominal trauma (e.g., auto accidents, external or internal version procedures), associated with labor or delivery (e.g., improper oxytocin use or excessive fundal pressure), or spontaneously initiated (e.g., placenta percreta, multiple gestation, grand multiparity, invasive mole, or choriocarcinoma).

The primary maternal complications from a ruptured uterus include hemorrhage and hypovolemic shock. The overall maternal mortality for uterine rupture is less than 1%, but if rupture occurs in the antepartum patient at home, it is likely to be higher. The perinatal mortality for uterine rupture ranges from 1% to 15%, again depending on where the patient is when the uterine rupture occurs.

EPIDEMIOLOGY

Uterine rupture is rare, occurring in an estimated 1 in 15,000 to 20,000 deliveries of patients with no prior uterine surgery. In women with a prior low transverse cesarean delivery, it is estimated to occur in 0.5% to 0.1% of deliveries. However, in women with a prior classical cesarean delivery (vertical uterine incision), the incidence of uterine dehiscence or rupture is estimated to be 6 to 12%. Risk factors for uterine rupture are conditions that predispose to a weakened uterine wall, including uterine scars, overdistension, inappropriate and aggressive use of uterotonic agents, maternal congenital uterine anomalies, and abnormal placentation (Table 5-7).

TABLE 5-7 Risk Factors for Uterine Rupture
Prior uterine surgery/uterine scar
Injudicious use of oxytocin
Grand multiparity
Marked uterine distension
Abnormal fetal lie
Large fetus
External version
Trauma

CLINICAL MANIFESTATIONS

The presentation of uterine rupture is highly variable. Typically, it is characterized by the sudden onset of intense abdominal pain. Vaginal bleeding, if present, may vary from spotting to severe hemorrhage. Nonreassuring fetal testing, abnormal abdominal contour, cessation of uterine contractions, disappearance of fetal heart tones, and regression of the presenting fetal part are other signs of uterine rupture.

TREATMENT

Management of uterine rupture requires immediate laparotomy and delivery of the fetus. If feasible, the rupture site should be repaired and hemostasis obtained. In cases of large rupture extensions, repair may not be feasible and the patient may require a hysterectomy. Patients are usually discouraged to attempt future pregnancies given the high risk of recurrent rupture. Trial of labor would be avoided in any subsequent pregnancy, and the patient would commonly be delivered via repeat cesarean section either at week 36 after confirmation of fetal lung maturity or at 37 weeks with out testing for fetal lung maturity.

FETAL VESSEL RUPTURE

PATHOGENESIS

Most pregnancies complicated by rupture of a fetal vessel are due to **velamentous cord insertion**, where the blood vessels insert between the amnion and chorion away from the placenta instead of inserting directly into the chorionic plate (Table 5-3). Because the vessels course unprotected through the membranes before inserting on the placental margin, they are vulnerable to rupture, shearing, or laceration. In addition, these unprotected vessels may cross over the internal cervical os (**vasa previa**), making them vulnerable to compression by the presenting fetal part or to being torn when the membranes are ruptured. Although vasa previa is rare, perinatal mortality is high (approximately 40% to 60%) and increases if the membranes are also ruptured. The condition is important because, when the membranes rupture, spontaneously or artificially, the fetal vessels running through the membranes have a high risk of concomitant rupture, frequently resulting in fetal exsanguination and death. Because the fetal blood volume is only about 80 to 100 mL/kg, loss of even small amounts of blood could prove disastrous to the fetus. Additionally, pressure on the unprotected vessels by the presenting fetal part could lead to fetal asphyxia and death.

Unprotected fetal vessels and vasa previa may occur with a **succenturiate lobe** of the placenta. In this case, the bulk of the placenta is implanted in one portion of the uterine wall, but a small lobe of the placenta is implanted in another location. The vessels that connect these two portions of the placenta are unprotected and may course over the cervix and present as a vasa previa.

EPIDEMIOLOGY

Only 0.1% to 0.8% of pregnancies are complicated by the rupture of a fetal vessel. The incidence of vasa previa is 1:2,500 to 1:5,000 pregnancies. Risk factors for fetal vessel rupture include abnormal placentation leading to a succenturiate lobe as well as multiple gestations that increase the risk of velamentous insertion. Although the rate of velamentous insertion is only 1% in singleton gestations, it increases up to as high as 4% to 12% for twin gestations (4% to 7% for dichorionic twins and 10% to 12% for monochorionic twins), and 28% to 50% for triplet gestations. There is an increased incidence of both velamentous cord insertion and vasa previa in pregnancies that result from in vitro fertilization, particularly in twin pregnancies.

CLINICAL MANIFESTATIONS

In fortunate cases of unknown vasa previa, the fetal vessels are palpated and recognized through the dilated cervix. More commonly, the presentation of a fetal vessel rupture is vaginal bleeding associated with a sinusoidal variation of the FHR indicative of fetal anemia. Whenever bleeding accompanies rupture of the membranes in labor, especially if there are associated fetal heart rate decelerations, fetal bradycardia, or a sinusoidal fetal heart rate pattern, the obstetrician should have a high index of suspicion for a ruptured vasa previa.

DIAGNOSIS

Unfortunately, diagnosis is often made after a large bleed and fetal compromise have already occurred. With advancing capabilities of ultrasound, velamentous insertion of the umbilical cord and succenturiate placental lobes can be diagnosed in the antepartum period. Further, with the use of color Doppler, vasa previa may also be diagnosed antepartum, but the sensitivity and specificity of these diagnoses are yet to be determined and are likely related to the experience of the sonographer and/or sonologist and ultrasound equipment available. However, several small prospective studies have demonstrated that the majority of cases of vasa previa in asymptomatic women can be diagnosed prenatally through a policy of routinely evaluating the placental cord insertion when an ultrasound examination is performed, and considering vaginal sonography with color Doppler if the placental cord insertion cannot be identified, or if there is a low-lying placenta or a suspected succenturiate placental lobe. These studies found that sonographic identification of placental cord insertion was accurate, sensitive, and added little or no extra time to the duration of the obstetric sonographic examination. In the prenatally diagnosed cases, the neonatal survival of infants without congenital malformations was approximately 97%. This is dramatic when compared to the 45% neonatal survival rate when the diagnosis was not made prenatally.

Diagnosis at the time of vaginal bleeding can be accomplished by the **Apt test** or examination of the blood for nucleated (fetal) RBCs. The Apt test involves diluting the blood with water, collecting the supernatant, and combining it with 1% NaOH. If the resulting mixture is pink, it indicates fetal blood; a yellow-brown color is seen with maternal blood. However, when acute bleeding occurs from a ruptured vasa previa, emergent delivery is frequently indicated, and there may be no time to test for fetal blood cells.

TREATMENT

Given the high risk of fetal exsanguination and death (the vascular volume of the term fetus is <250 mL), the treatment of a ruptured fetal vessel is emergent cesarean delivery. Even when the neonate has lost considerable blood, immediate transfusion may be lifesaving. Now that vasa previa can occasionally be diagnosed antepartum, these patients are often given the option of elective cesarean delivery, although there are few data as to the fetal risk with expectant management. One study suggests that women with prenatally diagnosed vasa previa be offered elective delivery by cesarean at about 35 weeks of gestation, or earlier, if fetal lung maturity is documented. This is earlier than the 39 weeks that is generally recommended for elective cesarean delivery. The mean age of delivery for the cases *not* diagnosed prenatally in this series was approximately 38 weeks. In these cases, perinatal mortality was 56%. The risks associated with prematurity at 35 weeks of gestation must be weighed against the risk of a dismal outcome should the membranes rupture, especially because approximately 8% of women at term will have ruptured membranes before the onset of labor. Unfortunately, membrane rupture, even in a hospital, often results in infants with low Apgar scores and who require transfusions, suggesting significant morbidity. If patients with known vasa previa elect to undergo a trial of labor, artificial rupture of membranes is contraindicated.

NONOBSTETRIC CAUSES OF ANTEPARTUM HEMORRHAGE

Nonobstetric causes of antepartum hemorrhage are listed in Table 5-1. Patients with these conditions usually present with spotting rather than frank bleeding. Typically, there are no uterine contractions or abdominal pain. The diagnosis is usually made by speculum examination, Papanicolaou test, cultures, or colposcopy as indicated. Other than advanced maternal neoplasia, which is associated with poor maternal outcome, most nonobstetric causes of antepartum hemorrhage require relatively simple management and have good outcomes. Vaginal lacerations and varices can be located and repaired. Infections may be treated with appropriate agents, cervical polyps can be removed, and benign neoplasms usually require simple treatment.

KEY POINTS

- Placenta previa accounts for 20% of antepartum hemorrhage and is associated with placenta accreta in up to 5% of cases without prior cesareans and in 15% to 67% of cases with prior cesarean deliveries.
- Previa occurs more often in patients with prior placenta previa, uterine scars, or multiple gestations.
- The classic presentation of placenta previa is **painless** vaginal bleeding in the third trimester and it is usually diagnosed via ultrasound.
- Placenta previa is associated with antepartum hemorrhage, preterm delivery, preterm premature rupture of membranes (PPROM), intrauterine growth restriction (IUGR), and increases the risk of puerperal hysterectomy.
- Patients are delivered by cesarean section in the case of unstoppable preterm labor, large hemorrhage, nonreassuring fetal testing, or at week 36 with mature lung indices.
- Placenta accreta is the abnormal attachment of the placenta to the uterus. When the placenta invades into the myometrium, it is known as placenta increta, whereas when it invades through the myometrium and to the serosa, it is known placenta percreta.
- Placental abruption accounts for 30% of all third-trimester hemorrhages and is seen more often in women with chronic hypertension, with preeclampsia, using cocaine or methamphetamines, or with a history of abruption.
- Women with placental abruption usually present with vaginal bleeding, painful contractions, and a firm, tender uterus; 20% of patients present with no bleeding (concealed hemorrhages).
- Placental abruption can be complicated by hypovolemic shock, DIC, and preterm delivery. Women can be delivered vaginally if they are stable; cesarean delivery is necessary in the unstable patient or when fetal testing is nonreassuring.
- Uterine rupture is a rare obstetric catastrophe, but is seen in 1 in 200 laboring women with a prior cesarean delivery.
- Maternal and fetal morbidity and mortality are increased in the setting of uterine rupture.
- Uterine rupture requires immediate laparotomy, delivery of the fetus, and either repair of the rupture site or hysterectomy.
- Fetal vessel rupture is a rare obstetric complication and is usually associated with multiple gestation and/or a velamentous cord insertion.
- Fetal vessel rupture is associated with a perinatal mortality of up to 60% of cases.
- Patients may present with vaginal bleeding and a sinusoidal FHR pattern, which requires emergent cesarean delivery.
- Nonobstetric causes of antepartum hemorrhage include cervical and vaginal lacerations, hemorrhoids, infections, and neoplasms.
- Nonobstetric causes of antepartum hemorrhage generally require simple management and have good outcomes.

C Clinical Vignettes

Vignette 1

A 30-year-old G3P2002 Asian woman at 28 weeks 0 days by LMP consistent with a 7-week ultrasound presents for her follow-up ultrasound. At 20 weeks' gestation, she had a complete previa on ultrasound. No concerns today. No vaginal bleeding, leakage of fluid, no discharge, just starting to feel fetal movement. No significant past medical history (PMH). Past surgical history was significant for two prior low-transverse cesarean sections at term, first cesarean section for breech at 39 weeks secondary to failed external cephalic version in 2007 and second for repeat cesarean section at 39 weeks in 2009. On ultrasound, the fetus is noted to have normal anatomy, normal amniotic fluid index, and an anterior placenta that is noted to be completely covering the internal os of the cervix. Transvaginal ultrasound confirms complete anterior placental previa.

1. What is this patient most at risk for at delivery given her history and ultrasound findings?
   a. Preterm labor
   b. Placenta abruption
   c. Intrauterine fetal demise
   d. Placenta accreta
   e. Preeclampsia
2. What care precautions should be given to this patient?
   a. Complete bed rest for the remainder of the pregnancy or until previa resolves
   b. Complete pelvic rest for the remainder of the pregnancy or until previa resolves
   c. No special precautions necessary
   d. Bed rest and pelvic rest for the remainder of the pregnancy or until previa resolves
   e. Limited activity but pelvic rest is unnecessary
3. What further imaging, if any, might be helpful in the diagnosis of placenta accreta in this patient?
   a. No further imaging would be helpful
   b. Noncontrast CT of the abdomen/pelvis
   c. Noncontrast MRI of the abdomen/pelvis
   d. Cystoscopy by urologist
   e. Continue with serial ultrasound but no additional imaging
4. What is the most appropriate management plan if this patient continues to labor?
   a. Attempt to tocolyze the patient and give a steroid course for fetal lung maturity
   b. Cesarean section with manual extraction of the placenta, followed by hysterectomy
   c. Cesarean section, leaving the placenta in situ, followed by hysterectomy
   d. Expectant management and spontaneous vaginal delivery if she continues to labor

Vignette 2

A 32-year-old G1P0 Caucasian woman presents for her anatomy ultrasound at 18 weeks by in vitro fertilization (IVF) dating. On ultrasound, the fetus is noted to have an anterior placenta with a posterior succenturiate lobe. She has no concerns. Her pregnancy is otherwise uncomplicated at this time.

1. What does the finding an anterior placenta with a posterior succenturiate lobe on ultrasound put this patient at risk for?
   a. Placenta previa
   b. Placental abruption
   c. Cervical incompetence
   d. Vasa previa
   e. Preterm labor
2. What is the preferred mode of delivery in patients with this finding?
   a. Emergent cesarean delivery
   b. Scheduled cesarean delivery
   c. Induction of labor, including artificial rupture of membranes
   d. Spontaneous vaginal delivery, including spontaneous rupture of membranes
   e. None of the above
3. What does the sinusoidal pattern on the fetal monitoring strip suggest?
   a. Fetal anemia
   b. Uteroplacental insufficiency
   c. Cord compression
   d. Head compression
   e. Normal tracing for twin gestation

Vignette 3

A 24-year-old G2P1001 Hispanic woman at 38 weeks by LMP consistent with 10 week ultrasound presents to labor and delivery (L & D) triage, complaining of painful uterine contractions every 4 to 5 minutes. She has no significant PMH. Her obstetrical history is significant for one prior low-transverse cesarean section for breech at 39 weeks' gestation. On sterile vaginal examination, the patient is initially found to be 2 cm dilated, 50% effaced, and −3 station. The patient strongly desires to have a vaginal delivery if at all possible.

1. What is the best initial management for this patient?
   a. Close observation in triage with continuous fetal monitoring and repeat sterile vaginal exam in 2 to 4 hours
   b. Discharge home and follow-up in 1 week at clinic
   c. Admission to L & D triage and repeat cesarean delivery without a trial of labor
   d. Admission to L & D triage, continuous fetal monitoring, and start oxytocin augmentation

2. What is next best step?
   a. Admission to L & D triage, continuous fetal monitoring, counsel patient regarding trial of labor after cesarean (TOLAC), proceed with expectant management of labor if she desires to proceed with TOLAC
   b. Discharge home and follow-up in 1 week at clinic
   c. Admission to L & D triage and repeat cesarean delivery without a trial of labor
   d. Admission to L & D triage, continuous fetal monitoring, counsel patient regarding TOLAC, and start oxytocin augmentation if she desires to proceed with TOLAC

3. What is the best explanation for these findings?
   a. Placental abruption
   b. Fetal head compression
   c. Umbilical cord compression
   d. Uterine rupture
   e. None of the above

4. What is the most appropriate next step?
   a. Stop the oxytocin and observe expectantly
   b. Place an intrauterine pressure catheter and start an amnioinfusion
   c. Administer tocolysis to stop the uterine contractions
   d. Proceed to the operating room for emergent cesarean delivery
   e. None of the above

Vignette 4

A 22-year-old G1P0 African American woman at 36 weeks by LMP consistent with 12-week ultrasound with limited prenatal care presents via ambulance to the L & D triage unit complaining of severe abdominal pain and profuse vaginal bleeding. The patient is unstable and unable to communicate coherently. The EMT reports that initially her BP was 180/100 mm Hg and pulse rate was 110 bpm, but she has lost at least 500 mL blood in route. On examination her BP is 90/50 mm Hg, pulse rate is 120 bpm, she appears to be in significant pain, is unable to answer questions, and her abdomen feels rigid.

1. What is the most likely diagnosis in this patient?
   a. Placenta previa
   b. Normal labor
   c. Vasa previa
   d. Cervical tear after intercourse
   e. Placental abruption

2. What is the best next step?
   a. Sterile speculum examination, followed by sterile vaginal examination
   b. Abdominal ultrasound
   c. Stabilize the patient, obtain two large-bore IV catheters, and start IV fluid bolus while checking for fetal heart tones
   d. Emergent cesarean section
   e. Transvaginal ultrasound

3. The nurse attempts to find FHTs and they seem to be about 70 bpm but the nurse is unsure. You quickly do a bedside ultrasound and confirm that FHTs are 70 bpm. What is the best next step?
   a. Proceed immediately to the OR for emergent cesarean delivery
   b. Sterile vaginal examination to see if the patient is in labor
   c. Transfuse two units of packed RBCs while continuously monitoring the fetus
   d. Expectant management
   e. None of the above

4. What is the most important laboratory test to order for this patient emergently?
   a. Type and cross
   b. CBC
   c. Urine drug screen
   d. Chemistry
   e. PT, PTT, INR

5. What does this patient now have as a result of her abruption and significant blood loss?
   a. Anemia
   b. Thrombocytopenia
   c. Hypovolemia
   d. Consumptive coagulopathy
   e. All of the above

A Answers

Vignette 1 Question 1

Answer D: If the patient's placenta previa persists into the third trimester, then she is most at risk for placenta accreta in the presence of an anterior placenta previa and a history of two previous cesarean sections. With the progression of pregnancy, more than 90% of low-lying placentas identified early in pregnancy will appear to move away from the cervix and out of the lower uterine segment. However, placenta previa occurs in as many as 1% to 4% of women with a prior cesarean section. If placenta previa persists, it can be complicated by an associated placenta accreta (placenta previa accreta) in approximately 5% of cases. The risk of placenta accreta is increased in women with placenta previa in the setting of one or more prior cesarean deliveries: estimated 15% to 30% of women with one prior cesarean section, 25% to 50% of women with two prior cesarean sections, and 29% to 67% of women with three or more prior cesarean sections. While Asian women are at a higher risk for having a placenta previa than are Caucasian women, there is no known association between placenta accreta and race. The patient is at increased risk of preterm labor and preterm delivery if she has an antepartum hemorrhage as a result of her placenta previa but her risk of placenta accreta is likely higher given her two prior cesarean deliveries. She does not have any other risk factors for preterm labor/preterm delivery. This patient is not at increased risk from the general population for placenta abruption or preeclampsia. She does not have any significant risk factors for intrauterine fetal demise.

Vignette 1 Question 2

Answer B: It is recommended for patients with a complete or partial previa to have complete pelvic rest, meaning no intercourse, in order to prevent significant vaginal bleeding. If significant bleeding occurs, it can lead to both maternal and fetal anemia and potentially preterm labor. There is no evidence that complete bed rest will help prevent vaginal bleeding or preterm labor in patients with complete or partial placenta previa. The special precautions regarding placenta previa are complete pelvic rest and close observation. Although it is reasonable to limit the patient's activity, particularly if they experience preterm contractions or bleeding, it is more important for them to observe pelvic rest.

Vignette 1 Question 3

Answer C: Because this patient has had two prior cesarean sections, has an anterior placenta previa, and because the sonographer cannot distinguish the placenta from the bladder, it is might be helpful to get further imaging to rule out a placenta accreta, increta, or percreta. MRI is the imaging modality of choice to evaluate for the myometrial and/or bladder invasion of the placenta, particularly when it is not clear on ultrasound. Further imaging to rule out placenta accreta (or increta/percreta) can be helpful in cases such as this where the diagnosis is unclear on ultrasound. CT is not the modality of choice in this case as MRI is far superior to evaluate the muscular planes of the uterine wall and bladder. Although it may be necessary for the patient to have cystoscopy by an urologist or urogynecologist at some point, it is more helpful to get an MRI of the abdomen and pelvis first. Cystoscopy is often indicated if there is evidence of accreta/increta/percreta on ultrasound or MRI, or if the patient has significant hematuria develop. Although it is important to continue performing serial ultrasounds of the fetus and placenta in order to evaluate fetal growth and fluid, cervical length, and the placenta, additional imaging with MRI can be helpful and should be considered.

Further imaging reveals complete anterior previa with evidence of placental invasion into the bladder. Four weeks later, at 32 weeks' gestation, the patient presents to labor and delivery triage complaining of passing two large blood clots with continued spotting. She denies contractions but on the tocometer is noted to have contractions every 2 to 4 minutes. A sterile speculum examination is performed and her cervix is dilated to approximately 2 cm. The patient also reports noting blood in her urine over the last few days. Of note, she does not desire future fertility and would like a tubal ligation after delivery, if possible.

Vignette 1 Question 4

Answer A: The most appropriate management plan if the patient continues to labor would be to tocolyze her so as to prolong the pregnancy long enough to administer a steroid course to improve prior to completion of the steroid course. fetal lung maturity in the event that she continues to labor. It is reasonable to attempt to tocolyze at this early gestation as long as the patient remains hemodynamically stable with minimal vaginal bleeding. However, if the patient bleeds significantly, she may need to be delivered prior to completion of the steroid course. Although in some cases it is reasonable to allow a patient to have a trial of labor after two cesarean sections, it is not appropriate in a patient with a complete placenta previa, as it would result in significant hemorrhage and likely both maternal and fetal compromise. Because the patient has had two prior cesarean sections, has complete placenta previa, and is now experiencing hematuria, this is concerning for a placenta percreta with invasion into the bladder. If she indeed has a percreta documented by cystoscopy or MRI, the mode of delivery would be a cesarean section, often followed by hysterectomy. A hysterectomy outright without removal of the placenta will minimize hemorrhage.

However, because of the challenges of making certain diagnoses, if the patient desires future fertility, then some clinicians will attempt placental removal in an attempt to avoid hysterectomy. If she does have complete previa and placenta percreta, the most common delivery plan is to proceed with a cesarean section (often a high vertical or transverse hysterotomy to avoid the placenta), deliver the fetus, leave the placenta in situ (rather than extraction), and to proceed with hysterectomy. By leaving the placenta in situ, closing the hysterotomy, and proceeding with hysterectomy, the surgeon avoids the significant bleeding that can occur from the placenta bed after manual extraction of the placenta. In this patient's case, because she does not desire future fertility and was planning on a tubal ligation, the more appropriate choice would be to leave the placenta in situ so as to minimize blood loss during the procedure.

Vignette 2 Question 1

Answer D: There is an increase incidence of vasa previa when there is a succenturiate lobe, particularly when this lobe is noted to be some distance from the rest of the placenta. A succenturiate lobe is an accessory placental lobe. In this case, the bulk of the placenta is implanted in one portion of the uterine wall, but a small lobe of the placenta is implanted in another location. The vessels that connect these two portions of the placenta are unprotected and may course over the cervix and present as a vasa previa. When a vasa previa is present in the case of a succenturiate lobe, these unprotected vessels may cross over the internal cervical os, making them vulnerable to compression by the presenting fetal part or to being torn when the membranes are ruptured. In this case, the bulk of the placenta is anterior and the succenturiate lobe is posterior so it is possible that the vessels connecting the two lobes could course over the internal os of the cervix resulting in a vasa previa. There is no significant increase in the incidence of placenta previa, placental abruption, cervical incompetence, or preterm labor as a result of a succenturiate posterior lobe of the placenta.

On transvaginal ultrasound, color Doppler demonstrates that there are vessels from the anterior placental lobe coursing over the internal os to connect to the posterior succenturiate placenta lobe. The fetus is noted to be in the vertex presentation. Otherwise, the pregnancy continues to be uncomplicated.

Vignette 2 Question 2

Answer B: In patients with a known vasa previa diagnosed on ultrasound, generally a cesarean delivery is the preferred mode of delivery so as to decrease the risk of rupture of the fetal vessels. There are very few studies on this; however, because a ruptured fetal vessel leads to catastrophic neonatal outcomes of cognitive injury and death, when a vasa previa is diagnosed, most clinicians recommend a cesarean delivery. There is a significantly higher neonatal survival rate in those infants who have a vasa previa diagnosed prenatally, most likely because when it is not diagnosed prenatally, the diagnosis is usually made at the time of fetal vessel rupture, which in turn leads to significant fetal anemia and often death. Ideally, cesarean delivery should be scheduled before the patient goes in to labor and/or spontaneously ruptures in order to prevent fetal vessel rupture at the time of the rupture of membranes. This is commonly done at 36 weeks' gestation, though some clinicians have even recommended earlier. Although not preferable, if the patient does desire to have a vaginal delivery and there is evidence of fetal anemia on continuous fetal monitoring, emergent cesarean delivery would then be necessary. Also, if the patient does choose to undergo a vaginal delivery (induction or spontaneous), artificial rupture of membranes is contraindicated, as the risk of fetal vessel rupture is higher than with spontaneous rupture of membranes.

The patient presents to L & D triage at 34 weeks and complains of leakage of fluid, vaginal bleeding, and contractions. On sterile speculum examination, the patient appears to have preterm premature rupture of membranes and to be 4 cm dilated. There appears to be a sinusoidal pattern on the continuous fetal monitoring tracing strip.

Vignette 2 Question 3

Answer A: A sinusoidal pattern on continuous fetal heart rate monitoring indicates fetal anemia. Although this can sometimes be confused with a pseudosinusoidal pattern, when there is a true sinusoidal pattern, it is considered to be nonreassuring because it indicates fetal anemia. Given the small fetal blood volume, a sinusoidal pattern should prompt an emergent delivery (as fast as possible) by the obstetrician. Fetal anemia in this case was most likely caused by rupture of the fetal vessels (vasa previa) upon rupture of the membranes. Uteroplacental insufficiency is not associated with a sinusoidal fetal heart rate tracing. Late decelerations are the typical fetal tracing finding when uteroplacental insufficiency occurs. These can be subtle or overt but if they are recurrent with every contraction for more than three contractions, the obstetrician should undertake immediate intervention. Cord compression causes variable decelerations, rather than a sinusoidal pattern. This can usually be resolved with an intraamniotic infusion using an intrauterine pressure catheter. By instilling the uterus with fluid, the cord has more protection from compression during uterine contractions. Head compression during labor is usually associated with early decelerations that start before a contraction and recover by the end of the contraction. A true sinusoidal tracing is never normal and is indicative of nonreassuring fetal status.

Vignette 3 Question 1

Answer A: Because the patient is 2 cm dilated, 50% effaced, and −3 station, with painful contractions every 4 to 5 minutes, and has a known uterine scar (from her previous cesarean delivery), the most appropriate initial course of action is to continue close observation with continuous fetal monitoring, and reevaluate in 2 to 4 hours (or earlier if clinically necessary). Although the patient does not seem to be in active labor and is only 2 cm dilated, the patient is painfully contracting and is at risk of uterine rupture so she needs to be adequately ruled out for active labor before being sent home. It is not appropriate to proceed immediately to repeat cesarean delivery at this stage, as it is not clear that she is laboring and there is no other indication for cesarean section at this time. A prospective, randomized, contronlled trial showed that in the setting of latent labor admission and augmentation led to a higher risk of uterine rupture. Therefore, admission to L & D triage for labor augmentation is not indicated. In general, in the setting of TOLAC, the patient is at increased risk of uterine rupture with oxytocin augmentation and so oxytocin should not be started unless it necessary.

The patient is expectantly managed in L & D triage for 2 hours. On repeat vaginal examination, she is found to have changed to 6 cm dilated, 75% effaced, and −1 station. She is now contracting painfully every 1 to 2 minutes. The fetal heart rate tracing is reactive with no decelerations.

Vignette 3 Question 2

Answer A: The next best step now that the patient has changed from 2 to 6 cm, that is, active labor, is to admit her to L & D triage, to continue with fetal monitoring, and to counsel her regarding the risks, benefits, alternatives, and indications for TOLAC versus repeat cesarean delivery. If after counseling the patient considers the risks of TOLAC and desires to have a vaginal delivery (vaginal birth after cesarean, or VBAC), then most physicians would expectantly manage her active labor. Because oxytocin augmentation has been shown to double the risk of uterine rupture, it is more appropriate to follow expectant management than to immediately start oxytocin augmentation on admission to L & D triage. It is better to wait to start oxytocin until it is clear she is not continuing to change her cervix or contract regularly after 4 hours (provider dependent). It is not appropriate to send an actively laboring patient with a prior cesarean section, and who is dilated to 6 cm, home with follow-up. Given the risk of uterine rupture, at the very least the patient needs to be expectantly managed with continuous fetal monitoring. It is an option to proceed immediately to repeat cesarean delivery if there is concern for uterine rupture, fetal distress, or if the patient desires a repeat cesarean after being counseled regarding the risks, benefits, alternatives and indications for TOLAC and repeat cesarean delivery.

The patient labors spontaneously without an epidural but after 4 hours her cervical examination is unchanged. The fetal heart rate tracing continues to be reactive with no late decelerations noted. Oxytocin augmentation is started. Two hours later the patient is found to be 8 cm dilated, 90% effaced, and 0 station. Approximately 1 hour later, the nurse calls you to the room because the patient is complaining of severe abdominal pain with and without contractions. On SVE, the patient is now noted to be 8 cm dilated, 90% effaced, but station has changed from 0 to −3. You note that there had been several recurrent deep variable decelerations with each contraction on the fetal heart rate tracing that now shows fetal bradycardia.

Vignette 3 Question 3

Answer D: The most likely explanation for these findings in this clinical scenario is uterine rupture of the prior cesarean scar. The rupture of the scar disrupts uterine blood flow to the placenta, resulting in uteroplacental insufficiency, which in turns causes late decelerations. Additionally, the umbilical cord or fetal parts can be extruded into the patient's abdomen leading to cord compression and severe variable decelerations or frank bradycardia. Severe abdominal pains with loss of station of the fetal head on vaginal examination are classic findings in a uterine rupture, especially when associated with a nonreassuring fetal status on the continuous fetal monitoring. While placental abruption can result in recurrent late decelerations as a result of uteroplacental insufficiency and can occur with a uterine rupture, it is unlikely in this situation as there is minimal bleeding noted. Additionally, loss of station is not generally found on a placental abruption unless it occurs concurrently with uterine rupture. Fetal head compression causes early decelerations, not late decelerations, and does not result in the loss of station on vaginal examination. Umbilical cord compression is not generally associated with pain worse than usual with contractions, causes variable decelerations, and does not cause loss of station of the fetal head.

Vignette 3 Question 4

Answer D: Uterine rupture is an obstetrical emergency. It can result in placental abruption, or if the fetus is delivered through the uterine dehiscence into the abdomen, it can result in significant fetal hypoxic injury because of complete cord compression. Additionally, there is risk for significant maternal blood loss; thus, immediate delivery via cesarean section is imperative. Once the neonate is delivered, the surgeon should then assess the uterine rupture site for the feasibility of repair and to obtain hemostasis. If it cannot be repaired or hemostasis cannot be obtained, peripartum hysterectomy is indicated. While intuitively it is important to stop the oxytocin augmentation when one suspects uterine rupture, expectant management would not be appropriate. An amnioinfusion is not appropriate in this clinical situation, as there is no evidence of cord compression. While there may be uterine tetany as a result of excess oxytocin, once the uterus has dehisced, tocolysis is neither appropriate nor helpful in this situation.

Vignette 4 Question 1

Answer E: Given the patient's hemodynamic instability, significant vaginal bleeding resulting in profound blood loss, and rigid abdomen, along with severe abdominal pain, the most likely clinical diagnosis is placental abruption. Normal labor does not cause significant blood loss with cervical change except in the instance of placenta previa. While patients who labor with a placenta previa can have pain from the contractions and profuse vaginal bleeding, they are not usually hemodynamically unstable nor are they usually in severe pain with a rigid abdomen. Also, the initial elevated BP of 180/100 mm Hg suggests preeclampsia or superimposed preeclampsia, which is a known risk factor for placental abruption. Vasa previa can lead to profuse vaginal bleeding if a patient ruptures her membranes and the fetal vessels also rupture, but it does not result in maternal hemodynamic instability. A cervical tear from intercourse can cause significant pain and vaginal bleeding but does not fit with this clinical scenario.

Vignette 4 Question 2

Answer C: Typically when a patient in this scenario presents to the emergency department or obstetrics triage unit, multiple steps are undertaken at the same time. However, the best next step is to start stabilizing the patient and to assess the fetal status. Given the patient's hemodynamic instability (hypotension, tachycardia, profuse bleeding), two large-bore IV catheters should be placed, a bolus of IV fluids (normal saline or lactated ringer's) should be given, while another nurse or clinician is attempting to assess the fetal status. This is important to do immediately, as it determines the speed with which the team must mobilize the patient to the operating room (OR) for an emergent cesarean section. If the fetus is dead, the team's sole focus can be placed on the mother's status before addressing the fetus and delivery planning. If the fetal status cannot be determined with external fetal monitoring quickly, an abdominal ultrasound is the next step but should not supersede gaining IV access and fetal Doppler. Often in these cases, the fetal heart tones (FHTs) are difficult to determine as they are usually bradycardic (and/or similar to maternal heart rate). Ultrasound becomes critical to determine the fetal status, as it can be used to visualize the fetal heart rate, particularly in the setting of terminal bradycardia as is often found in these cases. Ultrasound is also important to determine the location of the placenta if there is any concern for a placenta previa. Given this patient's limited prenatal care and profuse vaginal bleeding, ultrasound is important in this situation but, again, should not supersede obtaining maternal IV access and starting her stabilization. Sterile vaginal examination and/or speculum examination are important steps in the evaluation process but should not come before IV access or assessing the fetal status and location of the placenta. Often it is not necessary at all in the setting of placental abruption as most proceed to emergent cesarean delivery if the fetus has a documented heart rate. Emergent cesarean delivery should follow shortly after obtaining maternal vital signs, IV access, fetal assessment, and ultrasound if placental abruption is strongly suspected and there is fetal bradycardia or nonreassuring fetal status on external fetal monitoring. Transvaginal ultrasound should come later if the patient stabilizes and needs further assessment of placental location because placenta previa is suspected.

Vignette 4 Question 3

Answer A: In the setting of suspected placental abruption, once the fetus is determined to have a heart rate and to be in distress, emergent cesarean delivery is indicated. Unless the patient appears to be laboring with delivery imminent, when FHTs are about 50 beat per minute, it is best to proceed with emergent cesarean delivery. Often there is time in the OR to do a vaginal examination to assess cervical dilation. If delivery is imminent, then the patient can begin pushing, but otherwise one should proceed with emergent cesarean section. While the patient should be transfused two units of packed RBCs during the cesarean delivery, it is not appropriate to wait for the blood transfusion to proceed to the OR for cesarean delivery in the setting of terminal fetal bradycardia. Expectant management is similarly not appropriate.

Vignette 4 Question 4

Answer A: While all the above laboratory tests are important and should be ordered as soon as possible, the most important laboratory test to send immediately is a type and cross because it will allow you to start preparing blood and FFP to transfuse for the patient. While the patient can be given O-negative ("code grey") blood in this type of emergency, in the case of placental abruption, the patient will likely need multiple units of packed RBCs, platelets, FFP, and cryoprecipitate as patients frequently lose more than 2 L of blood and can develop consumptive coagulopathy. A CBC is important to assess the patient's baseline Hgb/Hct and platelet count. A urine drug screen is important because placental abruption frequently occurs in the setting of cocaine abuse and this patient in particular is high risk for cocaine abuse. A chemistry and coagulation laboratory test results (PT/PTT, INR) are also important to establish the patient's baseline renal function and clotting ability, particularly if the patient develops a consumptive coagulopathy.

The patient undergoes delivery with Apgar scores of 1 and 5, at 5 and 10 minutes, respectively. The placenta is removed easily and 500 mL clot follows the delivery of the placenta. Total estimated blood loss (EBL) from cesarean sectionis 1,500 mL (2,500 mL EBL estimated including blood lost in the field). Intraoperative hematocrit is 20%, platelet count 70,000, fibrinogen level 50, INR value 3, and creatinine level 1.5.

Vignette 4 Question 5

Answer E: In addition to patient's obvious anemia, thrombocytopenia, hypofibrinogenemia, elevated INR, hypovolemia, and acute renal failure, the patient appears to have consumptive coagulopathy caused by the massive hemorrhage from the placental abruption. Consumptive coagulopathy is commonly associated with placental abruption, particularly in the setting of preeclampsia. It can be fatal if adequate resuscitation is not administered in a timely fashion. It is important to anticipate profound blood loss and coagulopathy with placental abruption. Consumptive coagulopathy often occurs when the patient's blood loss is underestimated and she is under-resuscitated, particularly if she is given packed RBCs without FFP in a ratio of at least 4:1. Recent literature suggests these patients should be managed more like a trauma patient and transfused with a ratio of 2:1 or 1:1 (PRBCs to FFP). It is also important to follow fibrinogen and platelets and to transfuse platelets and cryoprecipitate as needed. Acute renal failure as a result of acute tubular necrosis is common in this scenario and usually resolves with adequate resuscitation.

Chapter

6 Complications of Labor and Delivery

PRETERM LABOR

Labor that occurs before week 37 is called **preterm labor** (PTL). Many patients present with preterm contractions, but only those who have cervical change as measured on cervical examination are diagnosed as having PTL. It differs from **cervical insufficiency**, which is a silent, painless dilation, and effacement of the cervix. Both can result in preterm delivery, which is the leading cause of fetal morbidity and mortality in the United States. The incidence of preterm delivery in the United States reached a peak in 2005 to more than 12% of all births, which is higher than that in 2000 where the rate was 11.6%. Although since 2006 the preterm birth rate has declined, it is still higher than that in 2000. Approximately a half of a million babies are born preterm each year, though only approximately 80,000 of these are before 32 weeks' gestation.

PRETERM DELIVERY

Infants born before 37 weeks' gestation are termed **preterm**. Infants born weighing less than 2,500 g are termed **low-birth-weight** (LBW) infants. Infants who have not grown appropriately for their gestational age have **intrauterine growth restriction** (IUGR) or are **small for gestational age** (SGA). Thus, an IUGR infant can be born after week 37 but still be LBW. Morbidity and mortality of preterm infants are dramatically affected by gestational age and birth weight. Prematurity puts infants at increased risk of respiratory distress syndrome (RDS) or hyaline membrane disease, intraventricular hemorrhage, sepsis, and necrotizing enterocolitis. Infants born on the cusp of viability at 24 weeks' gestation have a greater than 50% mortality rate, whereas infants born after week 34 have a mortality rate that is only slightly higher than that of full-term neonates.

ETIOLOGY AND RISK FACTORS

The defining physiologic mechanism that causes the onset of labor is unknown. However, various risk factors have been associated with PTL. These include preterm rupture of membranes; chorioamnionitis; multiple gestations; uterine anomalies such as a bicornuate uterus; previous preterm delivery; maternal prepregnancy weight less than 50 kg; placental abruption; maternal disease including preeclampsia, infections, intra-abdominal disease or surgery; and low socioeconomic status.

TOCOLYSIS

Tocolysis is the attempt to prevent contractions and the progression of labor. Many tocolytics are used in the United States, but only ritodrine—a beta-mimetic agent—is FDA approved for this purpose. It is difficult to conduct placebo-controlled studies of new tocolytics because most patients and clinicians are unwilling to allow contractions to proceed without some tocolytic therapy. Thus, many of the current trials compare currently used tocolytics to other tocolytics. Because the evidence for which of the tocolytic agents may be the most effective is unclear, institutions and practitioners vary widely in practice.

Studies have demonstrated that tocolytics prolong gestation for only 48 hours. The principal benefit from gaining 48 hours in a pregnancy is to allow treatment with steroids to enhance fetal lung maturity and reduce the risk of complications associated with preterm delivery. **Betamethasone**, a glucocorticoid, has been shown to reduce the incidence of RDS and other complications from preterm delivery. Prior to 34 weeks of gestation, the advantages of treating with steroids need to be weighed against the risks of prolonging the pregnancy. There are many situations in which PTL should be allowed to progress. Chorioamnionitis, nonreassuring fetal testing, and significant placental abruption are absolute indications to allow labor to progress and often to hasten delivery. With many other issues such as maternal disease—particularly preeclampsia or poor placental perfusion—an assessment of the severity of the situation, the precipitous nature of the complication, and the risks from prematurity all contribute to the decision of whether or not to tocolyze.

TOCOLYTICS

The goal of a tocolytic is to decrease or halt the cervical change resulting from contractions. In the case of preterm contractions without cervical change, hydration can often decrease the number and strength of the contractions. This operates along the principle that a dehydrated patient has increased levels of vasopressin or **antidiuretic hormone** (ADH), the octapeptide synthesized in the hypothalamus along with oxytocin. Because ADH differs from oxytocin by only one amino acid, it may bind with oxytocin receptors and lead to contractions. Thus, hydration, which decreases the level of ADH, may also decrease the number of contractions. For patients who do not respond to hydration or whose cervices are actively changing, a variety of tocolytics may be used.

Beta-mimetics

Uterine myometrium is composed of smooth muscle fibers. The contraction of these fibers is regulated by myosin light chain kinase (MLK), which is activated by calcium ions through their interaction with calmodulin (Fig. 6-1). By increasing the level of cAMP, calcium is sequestered in the sarcoplasmic reticulum, causing a decrease in the level of free calcium ions and a decrease in uterine contractions. Conversion of ATP to cAMP is increased by β-agonists that bind and activate β_2 receptors on myometrial cells.

The two **beta-mimetics** historically used for PTL are ritodrine and terbutaline. Although both are certainly effective in halting preterm contractions, randomized controlled studies in which patients were truly in PTL showed that β-agonists increased gestation an average of only 24 to 48 hours further over hydration and bed rest alone. Side effects of these drugs include tachycardia, headaches, and anxiety. More seriously, pulmonary edema may occur and, in rare cases, maternal death. Ritodrine is given as continuous IV therapy, whereas terbutaline is usually given as 0.25 mg SC, loaded Q 20 min × 3 dosages, and then Q 3 to 4 h maintenance. Because terbutaline may cause maternal death and cardiac events, including tachycardia, transient hyperglycemia, hypokalemia, cardiac arrhythmias, pulmonary edema, and myocardial ischemia, the FDA has now added a black box warning to the use of terbutaline IV beyond 24 to 48 hours. Additionally, oral terbutaline is not recommended because studies have not shown it to be an effective tocolytic beyond the 48-hour window. Subcutaneous terbutaline is still used to acutely stop contractions in obstetric triage when ruling out PTL and with uterine hypertonus leading to an abnormal fetal heart tracing.

Magnesium Sulfate

Magnesium decreases uterine tone and contractions by acting as a calcium antagonist and a membrane stabilizer. Although magnesium can stop contractions, in small placebo-controlled trials, it has not been shown to change gestational age of delivery. In larger trials, the efficacy of magnesium did not vary significantly from that of beta-mimetics. Side effects such as flushing, headaches, fatigue, and diplopia are seen, but they

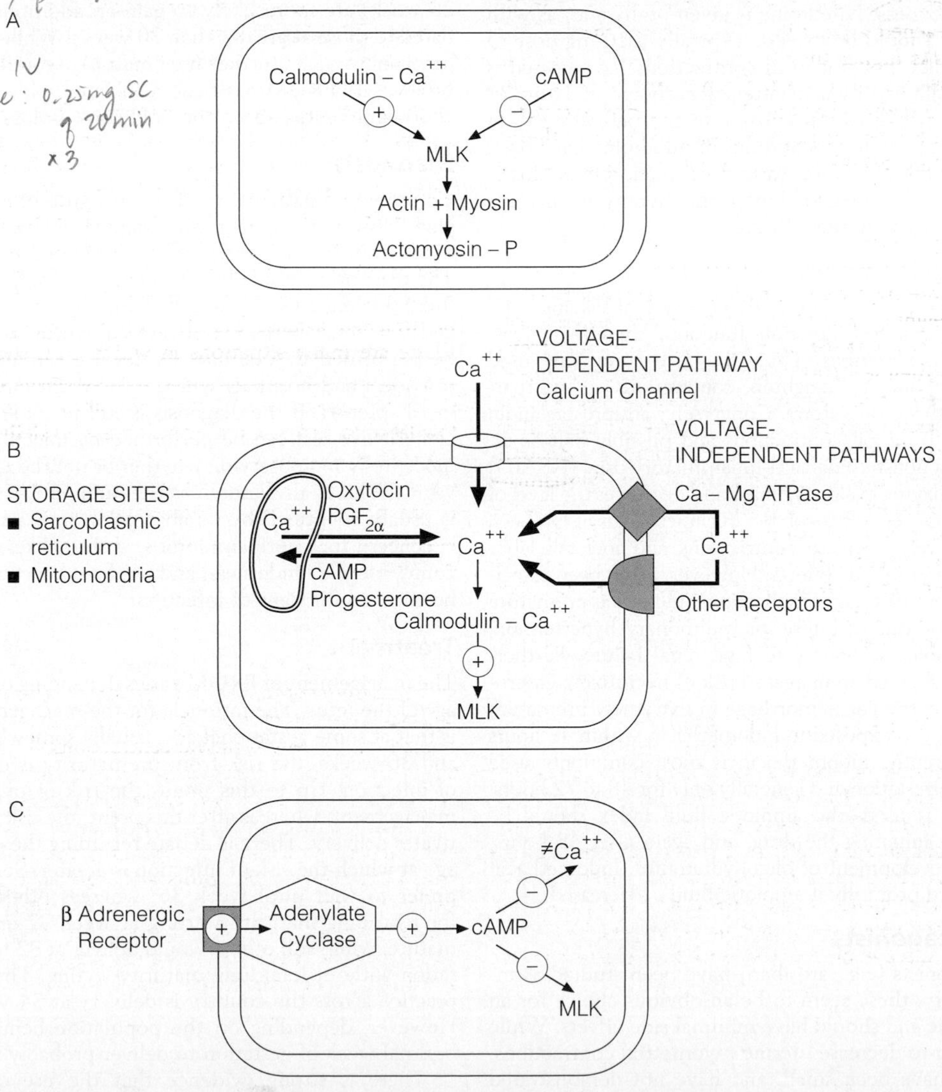

Figure 6-1 • Control of myometrial contractility: myosin light-chain kinase (MLK) is the key enzyme.

are generally considered to be less severe than those seen with ritodrine and terbutaline. At toxic levels of magnesium (> 10 mg/dL), respiratory depression, hypoxia, and cardiac arrest have been seen. Deep tendon reflexes (DTRs) are depressed at magnesium levels less than 10 mg/dl. Therefore, a reliable and quick assessment for magnesium toxicity can be achieved with serial DTR exams. Pulmonary edema has also been seen in women treated with magnesium sulfate, although it may be secondary to the concomitant IV fluid given to patients in PTL. Generally, magnesium sulfate should be loaded as a 6-g bolus over 15 to 30 minutes, and then maintained at a 2- to 3-g/hour continuous infusion. A slower infusion should be used in the case of renal insufficiency because magnesium is cleared via the kidneys.

Calcium Channel Blockers

Calcium channel blockers decrease the influx of calcium into smooth muscle cells, thereby diminishing uterine contractions. In vitro they have been shown to decrease myometrial contractions. In clinical trials, **nifedipine** has been the principal drug studied, and it seems to have comparable efficacy to that of ritodrine and magnesium. Side effects include headaches, flushing, and dizziness. Nifedipine is given orally and, as with other tocolytics, should be loaded. Typically a 10 mg dose Q 15 min for the first hour or until contractions have ceased is given. This is followed by a maintenance dosage of 10 to 30 mg Q 4 to 6 h as tolerated according to the patient's BP. In small studies, long-acting preparations of nifedipine have been shown to have efficacy similar to that of quick-release doses, and therefore can be used for long-term therapy to increase compliance and decrease side effects.

Prostaglandin Inhibitors

Prostaglandins increase the intracellular levels of calcium and enhance myometrial gap junction function, thereby increasing myometrial contractions. Thus, they are commonly used to induce labor and to heighten contractions in postpartum patients with uterine atony. Conversely, antiprostaglandin agents are used to inhibit contractions and possibly halt labor. **Indomethacin**—a nonsteroidal anti-inflammatory drug (NSAID) that blocks the enzyme cyclooxygenase and decreases the level of prostaglandins—is used as a tocolytic. In clinical trials, it has been shown to effectively decrease contractions and forestall labor with minimal maternal side effects. However, it has been associated with a variety of fetal complications, including premature constriction of the ductus arteriosus, pulmonary hypertension, and oligohydramnios secondary to fetal renal failure. Furthermore, one study showed an increased risk of necrotizing enterocolitis and intraventricular hemorrhage in extremely premature fetuses that had been exposed to indomethacin within 48 hours of delivery. Currently, indomethacin is most commonly used before 32 weeks' gestation and generally only for 48 to 72 hours. If indomethacin is used, the amniotic fluid index should be checked prior to initiating the drug, and again after 48 hours, to monitor for development of oligohydramnios. Indomethacin should be stopped promptly if amniotic fluid is decreased.

Oxytocin Antagonists

Oxytocin antagonists (e.g., atosiban) have been studied as tocolytics. In theory, these seem to be an obvious choice for an effective tocolytic and should have minimal side effects. While they have shown to decrease uterine myometrial contractions, clinical studies have been small, and have not demonstrated an improvement in outcomes. Current use has been limited to experimental trials that have shown no clinical difference from the other commonly used tocolytics.

PRETERM AND PREMATURE RUPTURE OF MEMBRANES

Rupture of membranes (ROM) occurring before week 37 is considered **preterm rupture of the membranes**, whereas ROM occurring before the onset of labor is termed **premature rupture of the membranes** (PROM). If the two occur together it is termed **preterm premature rupture of the membranes** (PPROM). Anytime ROM lasts longer than 18 hours before delivery, it is described as **prolonged rupture of membranes**.

PRETERM ROM

Spontaneous rupture of the fetal membranes before week 37 is a common cause of PTL, preterm delivery, and chorioamnionitis. Without intervention, approximately 50% of patients who have ROM will go into labor within 24 hours and up to 75% will do so within 48 hours. These rates are inversely correlated to gestational age at ROM; thus, patients with ROM prior to 26 weeks are more likely to gain an additional week as compared to those at greater than 30 weeks. While maintaining the pregnancy to gain further fetal maturity would seem beneficial, prolonged PPROM has been associated with increased risk of chorioamnionitis, abruption, and cord prolapse.

Diagnosis

Commonly, a patient complains of a gush of fluid from the vagina. However, any increased vaginal discharge or complaints of stress incontinence should be evaluated to rule out ROM. The diagnosis is made by obtaining a history of leaking vaginal fluid, pooling on speculum examination, and positive nitrazine and fern tests. If these tests are equivocal, an ultrasound can be performed to examine the level of amniotic fluid. Some providers and hospitals will use the Amnisure test (discussed in Chapter 4). If the diagnosis is still unconfirmed, an amniocentesis dye test can be performed by injecting a dye via amniocentesis and observing whether or not the dye leaks into the vagina. This is also known as the **tampon test** because the dye is usually identified by its absorption into a tampon. If there is concern for chorioamnionitis, maternal temperature, WBC count, uterine tenderness, and the fetal heart tracing should all be checked for signs of infection.

Treatment

The management of PROM varies depending on the gestational age of the fetus. The rationale for the management of PPROM is that at some gestational age, usually somewhere between 32 and 36 weeks, the risk from prematurity is equal to the risk of infection. Up to this point, the risk of prematurity drives management, whereas after this point, the risk of infection motivates delivery. There is debate regarding the exact gestational age at which the risk of infection is greater. Some practitioners prefer to wait until week 36, whereas others prefer to test for fetal lung maturity starting at week 32 and deliver when mature, while still others would deliver at 32 to 34 weeks' gestation without fetal lung maturity testing. The most common practice across the country is delivery at 34 weeks' gestation. However, depending on the population being cared for, the optimal week of gestation to deliver probably varies.

There is strong evidence that the use of antibiotics in PPROM leads to a longer latency period prior to the onset of labor. Thus, ampicillin with or without erythromycin is recommended in the setting of PPROM. There is debate surrounding the use of tocolysis and corticosteroids in the setting of PPROM. Tocolysis seems to add little, if any, benefit in PPROM and may even be harmful in the setting of chorioamnionitis. However, at many institutions tocolysis is used for 48 hours, particularly at earlier gestational ages, in order to gain time to administer a course of corticosteroids. Currently, the recommendation is to use corticosteroids in the setting of PPROM because of the fetal benefits, despite any concern regarding immunosuppression.

PREMATURE RUPTURE OF THE MEMBRANES

The most common concern of PROM is that of chorioamnionitis, the risk of which increases with the length of ROM. Antibiotics are recommended for women with prolonged ROM and women with unknown group B streptococcus (GBS) status. Commonly, labor is induced/augmented if ROM occurs anytime after 34 to 36 weeks. Some patients may elect to bear the risk of increased infection to await the onset of spontaneous labor. However, the risks of infection with prolonged PROM should be discussed with patients before any decision is made. One large, randomized, controlled trial demonstrated that there is no difference in length of labor or mode of delivery with immediate induction/augmentation of PROM, but the rate of chorioamnionitis is higher among those with expectant management.

OBSTRUCTION, MALPRESENTATION, AND MALPOSITION

Although the most common form of delivery is the spontaneous vertex vaginal delivery, other presentations and deliveries also occur. Many of the malpresentations lead to cesarean delivery.

CEPHALOPELVIC DISPROPORTION

One of the most common indications for cesarean section is failure to progress (FTP) in labor, most often caused by **cephalopelvic disproportion** (CPD). The three "Ps"—pelvis, passenger, and power—are primarily responsible for a vaginal delivery. If the pelvis is too small, the fetal presenting part is too large, or the contractions are inadequate, there will be FTP. The strength of uterine contractions can be measured with an intrauterine pressure catheter (IUPC) and augmented with oxytocin, but little can be done about the other two factors that contribute to CPD.

Diagnosis

The maternal pelvis is described as one of four dominant types: **gynecoid**, **android**, **anthropoid**, and **platypelloid** (Fig. 6-2). Many pelvises have characteristics from more than one of these types. Common measurements of the pelvis include those of the pelvic inlet, the midpelvis, and the pelvic outlet. The **obstetric conjugate** is the distance between the sacral promontory and the midpoint of the symphysis pubis, and the shortest anteroposterior diameter of the pelvic inlet. The anteroposterior diameter of the pelvic outlet is the distance from the tip of the sacrum to the inferior margin of the pubic symphysis and usually ranges from 9.5 to 11.5 cm. These measurements are performed with both clinical and X-ray pelvimetry, but it is rare to assume CPD based on measurements alone.

The fetal skull is composed of the face, the base, and the vault. The face and base are composed of fused bones that do not change during labor; however, the bones of the vault are not fused and can undergo molding to conform to the maternal pelvis. The vault is composed of five bones: two frontal, two parietal, and one occipital. The spaces between the bones are known as sutures; the two places where the sutures intersect

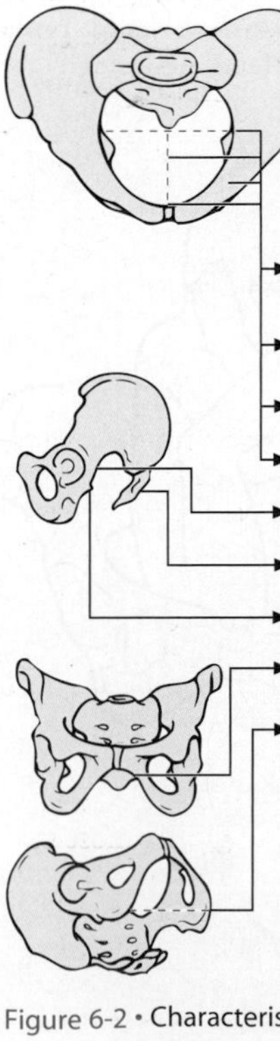

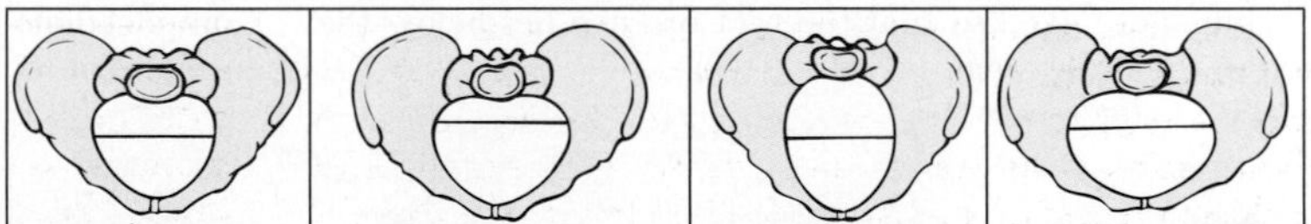

	Gynecoid	Android	Anthropoid	Platypelloid
Widest transverse diameter of inlet	12 cm	12 cm	<12 cm	12 cm
Anteroposterior diameter of inlet	11 cm	11 cm	>12 cm	10 cm
Side walls	Straight	Convergent	Narrow	Wide
Forepelvis	Wide	Narrow	Divergent	Straight
Sacrosciatic notch	Medium	Narrow	Backward	Forward
Inclination of sacrum	Medium	Forward (lower 1/3)	Wide	Narrow
Ischial spines	Not prominent	Not prominent	Not prominent	Not prominent
Suprapubic arch	Wide	Narrow	Medium	Wide
Transverse diameter of outlet	10 cm	<10 cm	10 cm	10 cm
Bone structure	Medium	Heavy	Medium	Medium

Figure 6-2 • Characteristics of four types of pelvises.

are the **anterior** and **posterior fontanelles**. How the fetal head presents to the maternal pelvis is important in accomplishing a vaginal delivery. There is great variation in the diameter of the skull at various levels and with various inclinations. When the fetal skull is properly flexed, the suboccipitobregmatic diameter presenting to the pelvis averages 9.5 cm in a term infant. When the sagittal suture is not located midline in the pelvis (asynclitism), the diameter of the skull being accommodated is effectively increased.

Treatment

Even if CPD is suspected, it is still often worthwhile to attempt a trial of labor. In the case of fetal macrosomia, elective induction of labor may be chosen before the opportunity for vaginal delivery passes. This practice leads to a similar rate of cesarean delivery, but as a result of failed induction rather than CPD.

BREECH PRESENTATION

Breech presentation, or buttocks first, occurs in 3% to 4% of all singleton deliveries. Factors associated with breech presentation include previous breech delivery, uterine anomalies, polyhydramnios, oligohydramnios, multiple gestation, PPROM, hydrocephaly, and anencephaly. Persistent breech presentation is also associated with placenta previa and fetal anomalies. Complications of a vaginal breech delivery include prolapsed cord and entrapment of the head.

Types of Breech

There are three categories of the breech presentation (Fig. 6-3): **frank**, **complete**, and **incomplete** or **footling**. The frank breech has flexed hips and extended knees, and thus the feet are near the fetal head. The complete breech has flexed hips, but one or both knees are flexed as well, with at least one foot near the breech. The incomplete or footling breech has one or both of the hips not flexed so that the foot or knee lies below the breech in the birth canal.

Diagnosis

The breech presentation may be diagnosed in several ways. With abdominal examination using the Leopold maneuvers, the fetal head can be palpated near the fundus while the breech is palpated in the pelvis. With vaginal examination, the breech can be palpated using common landmarks such as the gluteal cleft and the anus or, in the case of an incomplete breech, the fetal lower extremity. Diagnosis is often made or confirmed with ultrasound. On ultrasound, it is easy to confirm breech and then to determine the type of breech. With bedside Doppler, the fetal heart beat is often heard in the upper part of the uterus.

Treatment

How a breech presentation is managed depends on the experience of the obstetrician and the patient's wishes. The three management options are external cephalic version of the breech, trial of breech vaginal delivery, and elective cesarean delivery. External version consists of manipulation of the breech infant into a vertex presentation. It is rarely performed before 36 to 37 weeks' gestation because of the potential for spontaneous version before this point and the risk of delivery after version secondary to abruption or ROM. External version is usually attempted without anesthesia, and if successful, the patient can continue the pregnancy with a 5% to 10% risk of the fetus reverting back to breech presentation. If the version is not successful, a second attempt is often made under epidural anesthesia at 39 weeks of gestation. If successful, then either labor can be induced or the patient can continue the pregnancy. If the second attempt fails, often the patient will then have a cesarean delivery.

Trial of breech vaginal delivery can be attempted in the proper setting, but is becoming increasingly rare in the United States because a prospective randomized trial found higher rate of neonatal morbidity and mortality with trial of labor. Complications of breech deliveries include cord prolapse, entrapment of the fetal head, and fetal neurologic injury.

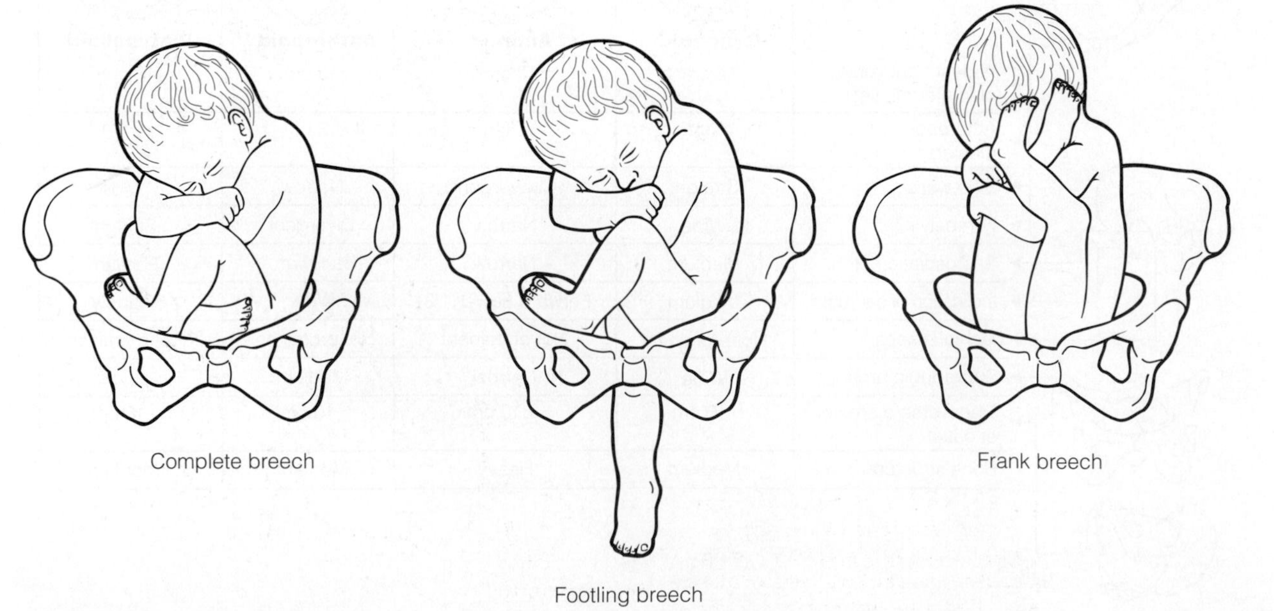

Figure 6-3 • Types of breech presentations.

A favorable pelvis (by clinical examination, pelvic radiograph, MRI, or CT pelvimetry), a flexed head, estimated fetal weight between 2,000 and 3,800 g, and frank or complete breech are common criteria used for trial of labor of breech presentation. Relative contraindications include nulliparity, estimated fetal weight greater than 3,800 g, and incomplete breech presentation. Patients with these contraindications are usually recommended to undergo cesarean delivery. However, if a patient wishes to attempt vaginal delivery, careful monitoring of the fetus and progress of labor is imperative.

OTHER MALPRESENTATION

Malpresentation can occur even in the setting of a cephalic or vertex presentation. The face, brow, or a compound presentation with a fetal upper extremity can complicate the cephalic presentation. Additionally, the shoulder can present in the setting of a transverse lie.

Face

The diagnosis of face presentation (Fig. 6-4) can be made with vaginal examination and palpation of the nose, mouth, eyes, or chin (mentum). If the fetus is mentum anterior, vaginal delivery will often ensue. However, with a mentum posterior or transverse, the fetus must rotate to mentum anterior to deliver vaginally. Augmentation is used only sparingly with a face presentation as the pressure on the face leads to edema. Of note, many anencephalic fetuses have a face presentation.

Brow

Brow presentation (Fig. 6-5) occurs when the portion of the fetal skull just above the orbital ridge presents. With the brow presenting, a larger diameter must pass through the pelvis. Therefore, unless the fetal head is particularly small (e.g., preterm) or the pelvis is particularly large, the brow presentation must convert to vertex or face to deliver.

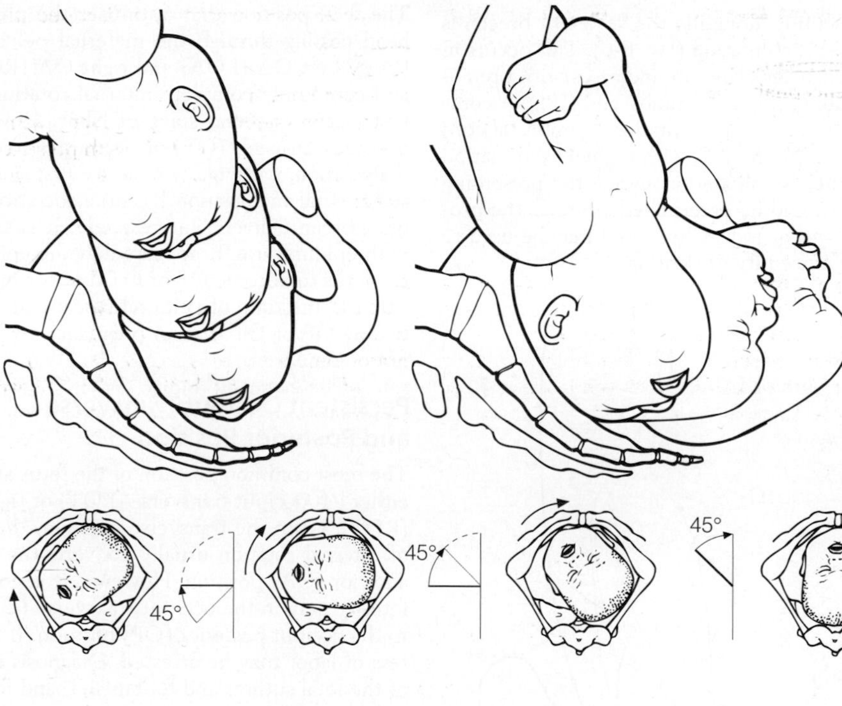

A

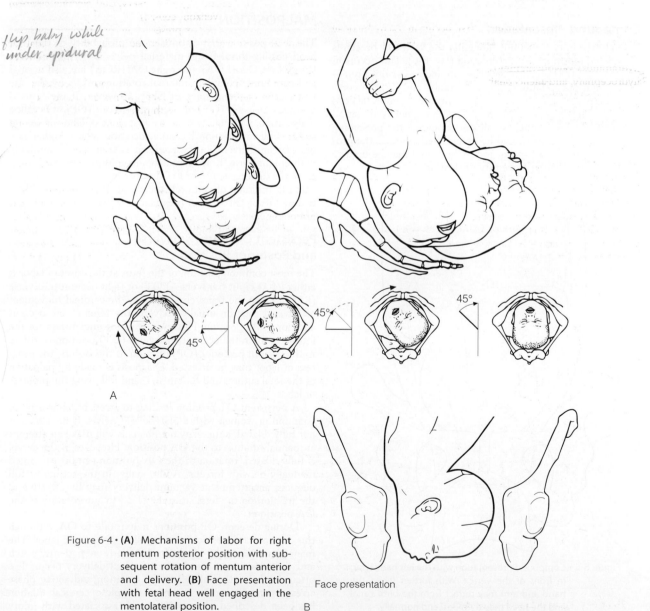

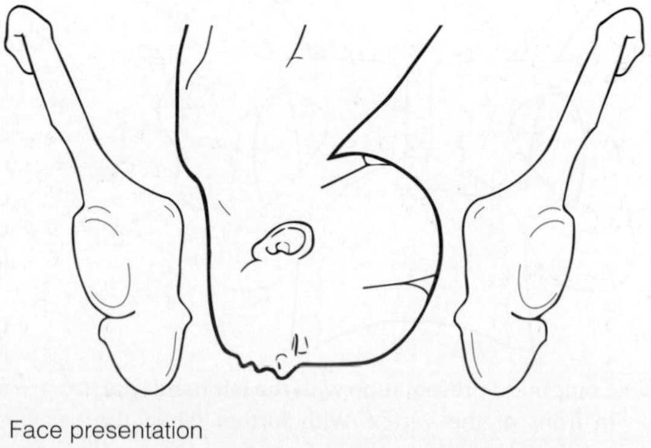

B

Figure 6-4 • **(A)** Mechanisms of labor for right mentum posterior position with subsequent rotation of mentum anterior and delivery. **(B)** Face presentation with fetal head well engaged in the mentolateral position.

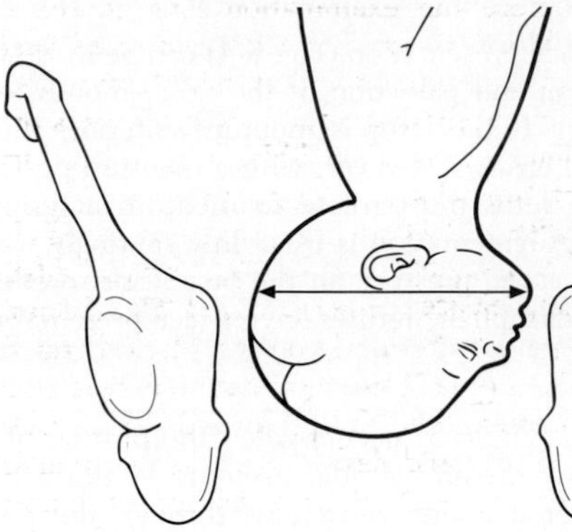

Brow presentation

Figure 6-5 • Brow presentation with mentovertex diameter presenting.

Compound Presentation

A fetal extremity presenting alongside the vertex or breech is considered a compound presentation (Fig. 6-6). This occurs in less than 1:1,000 pregnancies. The rate increases with prematurity, multiple gestations, polyhydramnios, and CPD. A common complication of compound presentation is umbilical cord prolapse. The diagnosis is often made with vaginal examination when the fetal extremity is palpated alongside the presenting part. At this point, it should be determined whether the prolapsed fetal part is a hand or foot. Ultrasound may be used to determine the type of extremity presenting.

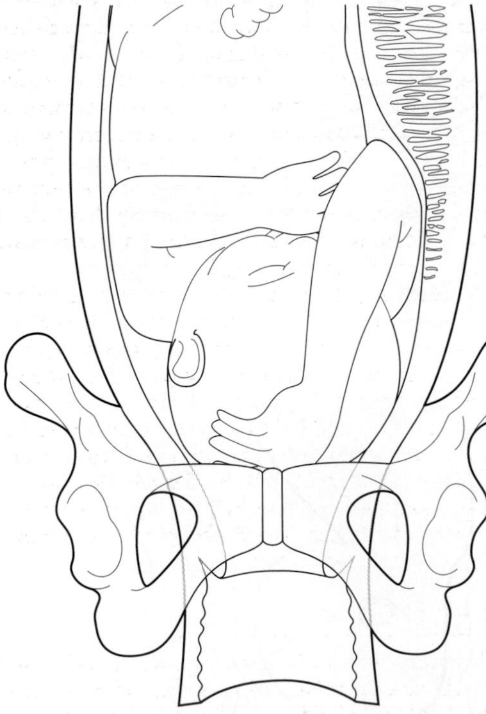

Figure 6-6 • Compound presentation with the left hand lying in front of the vertex. With further labor, the hand and arm may retract from the birth canal and the head may then descend normally.

Often, if an upper extremity is presenting alongside the vertex, the part may be gently reduced. However, prolapse of a lower extremity in vertex presentation is far less likely to deliver vaginally. Compound presentation of a lower extremity with a breech is considered a footling or incomplete breech presentation and calls for cesarean section. In all cases of compound presentation, umbilical cord prolapse should be suspected and careful monitoring with continuous fetal heart tracings and frequent vaginal examinations should ensue.

Shoulder

If the fetus is in a transverse lie, often the shoulder is presenting to the pelvic inlet. Diagnosis of this malpresentation can be made with abdominal or vaginal examination and ultrasound confirmation. Unless there is spontaneous conversion to vertex, shoulder presentations are delivered via cesarean section because of the increased risk of cord prolapse, increased risk for uterine rupture, and the difficulty of vaginal delivery.

MALPOSITION

The fetal position that optimizes the probability of the fetal head passing through the maternal pelvis is occiput anterior (OA). Left OA (LOA) and right OA (ROA) are also normal and commonly complete internal rotation to OA by the late first stage or second stage of labor. However, if the fetus is occiput transverse (OT) or occiput posterior (OP), it is called malposition, particularly in active first stage of labor or second stage. Fetal malposition has an association with a higher rate of cesarean delivery. Interestingly, it is seen more commonly with epidural use. It appears that the epidural does not cause the fetus to become OP or OT, but for those in OP or OT position at the time of epidural placement, they are more likely to stay OP or OT than in pregnancies where an epidural was not obtained.

Persistent Occiput Transverse and Posterior Position

The most common position of the fetus at the onset of labor is either left occiput transverse (LOT) or right occiput transverse (ROT). From the transverse position, the cardinal movement of internal rotation usually converts the fetus to the occiput anterior (OA) position. However, it is not uncommon for the fetus to stay in the occiput transverse (OT) position or rotate to the occiput posterior (OP) position. If this occurs, the progress of labor may be arrested. Diagnosis is made by palpation of the fetal sutures and fontanelles, and following the progress of labor.

A persistent OT position leading to arrest of labor is more common in women with a platypelloid pelvis. If the cervix is not fully dilated, a minority of clinicians will make an attempt at manual rotation to the OA position. However, if the cervix is fully dilated, rotation to the OA position can be attempted manually or with forceps. Additionally, in the setting of full dilation, an attempt at vacuum delivery may be effective as the traction on the fetal scalp may lead to autorotation to the OA position.

During descent, OP positions may rotate to OA, although this does not always occur and can slow progress in labor. The management is similar to that for OA position: patiently watch and wait. However, spontaneous vaginal delivery occurs less often. In the setting of OP or OT position and active phase arrest, manual rotation prior to complete cervical dilation has been described, though it may be associated with injury to the cervix. If the second stage of labor is prolonged, the options include delivery of the fetus with forceps or vacuum in the OP position, rotation with forceps, or manual rotation. In either the OT or OP position, if the attempt at rotation or operative vaginal delivery fails, cesarean delivery is commonly required. While OP position fetuses deliver vaginally in about 50% of cases, OT position fetuses rarely deliver vaginally in the OT position and must rotate to either OA or OP to deliver vaginally.

OBSTETRIC EMERGENCIES

FETAL BRADYCARDIA

One of the most common events in labor and delivery that leads to anxiety among both the practitioners and the patients is fetal heart rate (FHR) bradycardia. Any time the fetal heart rate is below 100 to 110 bpm for longer than 2 minutes, it is called a **prolonged deceleration**. Longer than 10 minutes is termed **bradycardia**. Older terminology deemed a deceleration lasting longer than 2 minutes a bradycardia, and so this term is commonly used in labor and delivery in the setting of prolonged decelerations. Either way, these FHR decelerations are associated with a number of complications such as placental abruption, cord prolapse, uterine tetanic contraction, uterine rupture, pulmonary embolus (PE), amniotic fluid embolus (AFE), and seizure. They have also been associated with poor fetal outcome.

The etiology of prolonged FHR decelerations can be considered to be preuterine, uteroplacental, or postplacental. Preuterine issues would be any event leading to maternal hypotension or hypoxia. These would include seizure, AFE, PE, MI, respiratory failure, or recent epidural or spinal placement leading to hypotension. Uteroplacental issues include placental abruption, infarction, and hemorrhaging previa, as well as uterine hyperstimulation. Postplacental etiologies include cord prolapse, cord compression, and rupture of a fetal vessel such as vasa previa.

Diagnosis

FHR decelerations are usually not subtle. However, the FHR can easily be confused with the maternal heart rate, which is commonly between 60 to 100 bpm, and therefore, these should be differentiated. This can be done by placing a fetal scalp electrode (FSE) on the fetal scalp and concomitantly an O_2 saturation monitor on the mother. In facilities without access to these tools, palpation of the maternal pulse while listening to the FHR can usually help differentiate between the two.

Diagnosis of the etiology of the bradycardia is often more important than the diagnosis of bradycardia, which is relatively straightforward in the era of continuous fetal monitoring. A simple algorithm to diagnose the etiology of bradycardia is as follows:

1. Look at the mother for signs of respiratory compromise or change in mental status. This should commonly diagnose seizures, PE, and AFE.
2. While putting on a glove for a cervical examination, assess the maternal BP and heart rate. This will diagnose maternal hypotension, commonly seen after epidural placement and a potential cause of FHR decelerations. This will also aid in determining whether the FHR being recorded could be maternal.
3. Immediately before the examination look to see how much vaginal blood is passing. With increased vaginal bleeding, placental abruption and uterine rupture should be considered. If placentation is unknown, placenta previa is also a possibility. Rarely, vaginal bleeding is secondary to rupture of a fetal vessel as in vasa previa.
4. Examine the patient with one hand on the maternal abdomen and one hand vaginally feeling for cervical dilation, fetal station, and prolapsed umbilical cord. The abdominal hand should feel for uterine hyperstimulation and fetal parts outside the uterus. If the fetal station is dramatically lower than expected, then the prolonged FHR deceleration may be due to rapid descent and vagal stimulation. If the fetal station is much higher than expected, uterine rupture should be suspected. If the cervix is fully dilated and the fetus in the pelvis, operative vaginal delivery can be performed if the FHR decelerations do not resolve in a timely fashion.

Treatment

In the setting of prolonged FHR deceleration, the initial management is standardized. The patient is moved to left or right lateral decubitus position to resolve a FHR deceleration secondary to compression of the inferior vena cava (IVC), leading to decreased preload or, more commonly, a compressed umbilical cord by the fetus. Oxygen by face mask is commonly administered to the mother in case hypoxia is an issue. The examination is performed as described above, and the individual etiologies are diagnosed and treated appropriately. In the setting of maternal hypotension, the patient can be given aggressive IV hydration and ephedrine. The management of seizure, AFE, uterine rupture, are discussed later in the current chapter, and PE is discussed in Chapter 11. Tetanic uterine contraction is treated with nitroglycerin, usually administered via a sublingual spray, and/or terbutaline (a β-agonist tocolytic). If umbilical cord prolapse is identified, there have been case reports of replacement into the uterus; but most commonly this requires an emergent cesarean delivery, performed with the examining clinician lifting the fetal head to avoid compression of the prolapsed cord. In the setting of previa, cesarean delivery should be expedited. If abruption is suspected, and the patient is remote from delivery, cesarean section may be necessary.

It is imperative that the timing of these events is followed very closely. Clinicians need to know the capabilities of their labor and delivery units and the rapidity of response of the anesthesiologists. Commonly, a patient is moved from the labor room to the OR after 4 to 5 minutes of FHR deceleration. If the FHR is checked in the OR (at this time, usually 8 minutes) and the bradycardia persists, plans for emergent cesarean delivery should proceed. The rapidity of this delivery may not allow all of the most common sterile techniques typically employed because delivery of the fetus within the next 2 to 4 minutes is the goal.

SHOULDER DYSTOCIA

Once the head of the fetus is delivered, the difficulty in delivering the shoulders, particularly because of impaction of the anterior shoulder behind the pubic symphysis, is termed **shoulder dystocia**. Risk factors for shoulder dystocia include fetal macrosomia (weight over 4,000 g), preconceptional and gestational diabetes, previous shoulder dystocia, maternal obesity, postterm pregnancy, prolonged second stage of labor,

0.15% → 1.7%

and operative vaginal delivery. The incidence of shoulder dystocia has been reported to be between 0.15% and 1.7% of all vaginal deliveries. Increased morbidity and mortality are associated with shoulder dystocia. Fetal complications include fractures of the humerus and clavicle, brachial plexus nerve injuries (Erb palsy), phrenic nerve palsy, hypoxic brain injury, and death.

① fx humerus, clavicle
② hypoxic brain
③ Erb ⑤ death
④ phrenic n.

Diagnosis

The actual diagnosis of a shoulder dystocia is made when routine obstetric maneuvers fail to deliver the fetus. When antepartum risk factors are present, shoulder dystocia can be predicted, prepared for, and possibly even prevented. Preparation for a shoulder dystocia includes placing the patient in the dorsal lithotomy position, having adequate anesthesia, and having several experienced clinicians present at the birth. At the time of delivery, suspicion is increased with prolonged crowning of the head and then with the "turtle" sign of either incomplete delivery of the head or the chin tucking up against the maternal perineum. When a fetus is suspected to weigh over 4,500 g, elective cesarean section should be offered. → *c/s*

Treatment

As with any obstetric emergency, it is important to have all members of the health care team effectively working together. Once a shoulder dystocia is identified, the labor and delivery alert should be sounded and the pediatric team should be called. Similar to a code, someone needs to be running the shoulder dystocia emergency; in a teaching hospital this is usually the attending or chief resident, and in a private hospital, this is usually the delivering obstetrician. Someone should be assigned to keep track of time as a shoulder dystocia can lead to entrapment and complete compression of the umbilical cord, thus delivery in less than 5 minutes is imperative. Two individuals should be assigned to hold the patient's legs and one person assigned to give suprapubic pressure. ✳

The specific series of maneuvers for delivering an infant with a shoulder dystocia are as follows:

- **McRoberts maneuver**—sharp flexion of the maternal hips that decreases the inclination of the pelvis increasing the AP diameter can free the anterior shoulder (Fig. 6-7).
- **Suprapubic pressure**—pressure applied just above the maternal pubic symphysis at an oblique angle to dislodge the anterior shoulder from behind the pubic symphysis (Fig. 6-8).
- **Rubin maneuver**—pressure on an either accessible shoulder toward the anterior chest wall of the fetus to decrease the bisacromial diameter and free the impacted shoulder (Fig. 6-9). *squish: Rubin*

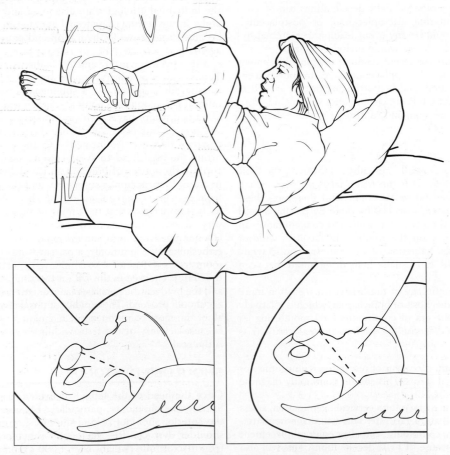

Figure 6-7 • Sharp flexion of both maternal hips (McRoberts maneuver) brings the pelvic inlet and outlet into a more vertical alignment, facilitating delivery of the fetal shoulders.

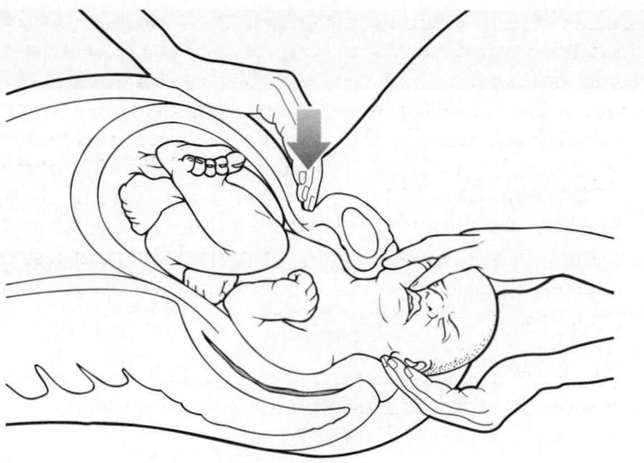

Figure 6-8 • Moderate suprapubic pressure is often the only additional maneuver necessary to free the anterior fetal shoulder.

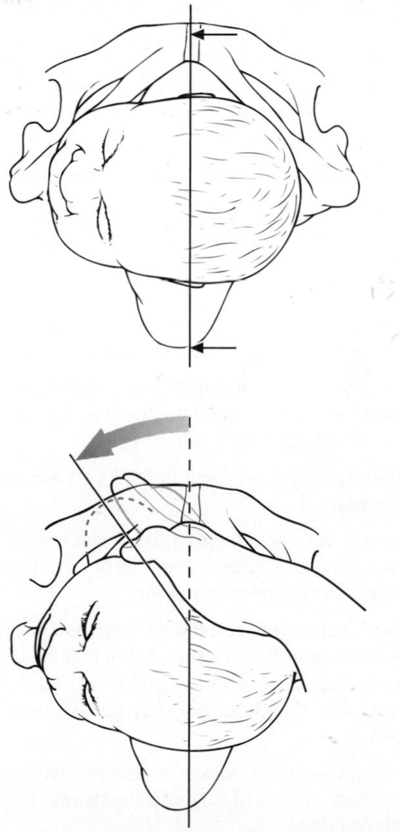

A

B

Figure 6-9 • Rubin maneuver. **(A)** The shoulder-to-shoulder diameter is shown as the distance between the two small arrows. **(B)** The most easily accessible fetal shoulder (the anterior is shown here) is pushed toward the anterior chest wall of the fetus. Most often, this results in abduction of both the shoulders, reducing the shoulder-to-shoulder diameter, and freeing the impacted anterior shoulder.

- **Wood's corkscrew maneuver**—pressure behind the posterior shoulder to rotate the infant and dislodge the anterior shoulder.
- **Delivery of the posterior arm/shoulder**—delivery of the posterior arm by sweeping the posterior arm across the chest to allow the bisacromial diameter to rotate to an oblique diameter of the pelvis and the anterior shoulder to be freed.

If these maneuvers are unsuccessful, they may be performed again. If the infant is still undelivered, there are several other maneuvers that can be performed. A generous episiotomy may provide more room to deliver the posterior arm/shoulder, or the cutting or fracturing the fetal clavicle can disimpact the anterior shoulder. If these maneuvers fail, the **Zavanelli** maneuver, which involves placing the infant's head back into the pelvis and performing cesarean delivery, can be attempted. Additionally, symphysiotomy, cutting the maternal pubic symphysis, will often release the infant; however, this is a morbid procedure often complicated by infection, healing difficulties, and chronic pain. Thus, it should be reserved for the true emergency, and in the United States, most clinicians would simply do a cesarean and attempt to facilitate delivery abdominally before performing a symphysiotomy.

UTERINE RUPTURE

Uterine rupture is seen in 1 in 10,000 to 20,000 deliveries in patients with unscarred uteri. Associated complications in these patients include uterine fibroids, uterine malformations, obstructed labor, and the use of uterotonic agents such as oxytocin and prostaglandins. In patients who have had a prior uterine scar from myomectomy or cesarean delivery, the risk of uterine rupture is theoretically 0.5% to 1.0%. The risk is increased in patients who have more than one cesarean scar, have a "classical" or high vertical scar, undergo labor induction, and/or are treated with uterotonic agents.

Uterine rupture is suspected in the setting of FHR decelerations in patients with prior scars on their uterus. Patients may feel a "popping" sensation or experience sudden abdominal pain. On physical examination, the fetus may be palpable in the extrauterine space, there may be vaginal bleeding, and commonly the fetal presenting part is suddenly at a much higher station than previously. If a uterine rupture is strongly suspected, the patient should be taken to the OR for immediate cesarean delivery and exploratory laparotomy.

MATERNAL HYPOTENSION

Pregnant patients commonly have BPs around 90/50 mm Hg. BPs much lower than the 80/40 mm Hg range is unusual and can lead to poor maternal and uterine perfusion. Common etiologies of maternal hypotension include vasovagal events, regional anesthesia, overtreatment with antihypertensive drugs, hemorrhage, anaphylaxis, and AFE. Most of these events can be differentiated quickly by the clinical scenario.

Treatment of maternal hypotension may vary depending on the etiology, but the mainstays are aggressive IV hydration and adrenergic medications to constrict peripheral vessels, and increase both the preload and the afterload. If the event occurs in close proximity to medication administration, Benadryl and epinephrine should be considered for a possible anaphylactic reaction. If the patient has an AFE, the mortality rate is quite high. The definitive diagnosis of AFE is the finding of fetal cells in the pulmonary vasculature at autopsy.

SEIZURE

Seizures on labor and delivery are usually quite startling and can be dangerous. In patients with a history of a seizure disorder as well as those with preeclampsia, careful observation for particular seizure precursors is maintained. However, many patients who seize on labor and delivery have no history and may be normotensive.

Many vasovagal events are misdiagnosed as a seizure because the patient may have several tonic–clonic movements. One of the key ways to differentiate between the two is the presence of a postictal period after the event. To help sort out the etiology, patients should have a full preeclamptic workup, toxicology panel, chemistry panel, and, when it is safe for the patient to leave the unit, obtain a head CT. A neurology consult is also indicated. Acutely, the patients should be managed with the ABCs of resuscitation and with antiseizure medications (Table 6-1). In pregnancy, magnesium sulfate is the antiseizure medication of choice.

TABLE 6-1 Management of a Pregnant Patient with Seizures or in Status Epilepticus

Assess and establish airway and vital signs including oxygenation
Assess FHR or fetal status
Bolus magnesium sulfate, or give 10 g IM
Bolus with lorazepam 0.1 mg/kg, 5.0–10.0 mg at no more than 2.0 mg/min
Load phenytoin 20 mg/kg, usually 1–2 g at no more than 50 mg/min
If not successful, load phenobarbital 20 mg/kg, usually 1–2 g at no more than 100 mg/min
Laboratory tests include CBC, metabolic panel, AED levels, and toxicology screen
If fetal testing is not reassuring, move to emergent delivery

KEY POINTS

- Preterm delivery occurs in greater than 10% of all pregnancies.
- PTL is treated with tocolytics including β-agonists, magnesium, calcium channel blockers, and NSAIDs.
- Current tocolytics are only marginally effective, but may buy time for a course of betamethasone to accelerate fetal lung maturity.
- Preterm rupture of membranes is when ROM occurs before 37 weeks of gestation; premature rupture of membranes (PROM) is ROM that occurs before the onset of labor.
- The latency period prior to the onset of labor is inversely correlated with gestational age in PPROM.
- Once ROM is confirmed, the therapeutic course depends on gestational age, risk of infection, and fetal lung maturity; any patient who shows signs of infection or fetal distress needs delivery.
- If the fetal head is too large to pass through the maternal pelvis, it is deemed CPD.
- Unless ultrasound and CT have been used to document a fetal head larger than the maternal pelvis, in the case of suspected CPD, a trial of labor is often attempted.
- There are three types of breech: frank, complete, and incomplete or footling.
- Breech presentations may be managed by external version to vertex, cesarean delivery, and less frequently a trial of labor. The complications of labor and delivery of breech presentation include cord prolapse and entrapment of the fetal head.
- Vertex malpresentations include face, brow, compound, and persistent OP. These presentations will often deliver vaginally but need closer monitoring and sometimes require different maneuvers.
- Prolonged fetal heart rate decelerations may have a variety of etiologies and can be thought of as preuterine, uteroplacental, and postplacental.
- A quick examination and verification of vital signs will often determine the etiology of a prolonged deceleration.
- If there is no sign of resolution of the FHR deceleration in 4 to 5 minutes, the patient should either be delivered vaginally or moved to the OR for cesarean.
- Shoulder dystocias can result in fetal fractures, nerve damage, and hypoxia.
- Risk factors for shoulder dystocia include fetal macrosomia, diabetes, previous dystocia, maternal obesity, postterm deliveries, and prolonged stage 2 of labor.
- The maneuvers to reduce a shoulder dystocia include McRoberts maneuver, suprapubic pressure, Rubin maneuver, Wood's corkscrew maneuver, delivery of posterior arm, episiotomy, fracture or cutting the clavicle or pubic symphysis, and the Zavanelli maneuver.
- Uterine rupture is uncommon in patients with no prior uterine scar; it is seen in 0.5% to 1.0% of patients who labor with a prior cesarean delivery.
- Maternal hypotension may have a variety of etiologies including regional anesthesia, hemorrhage, vasovagal events, AFE, and anaphylaxis.
- The first-line treatment of patients with seizures in pregnancy is IV or IM magnesium sulfate.

C Clinical Vignettes

Vignette 1

A 29-year-old G3P1102 woman at 29 weeks 3 days presents to labor and delivery triage for evaluation of abdominal pain. Her pain started 2 hours ago and comes and goes every 5 minutes. She denies any leaking fluid, change in vaginal discharge, or vaginal bleeding. Her baby has been active. Her pregnancy is complicated by a history of a urinary tract infection at 10 weeks with GBS and a history of preterm birth at 31 weeks with her last child. She is currently taking progesterone injections weekly and a prenatal vitamin. On vaginal examination, her cervix is closed, 25% effaced, and −3 station. Uterine contractions are noted every 4 to 5 minutes with a category 1 tracing. A fetal fibronectin test returns positive. Repeat examination after 1 hour shows dilation of 1 cm, 50% effacement, and −2 station. The team decides to start her on magnesium sulfate for tocolysis and administers the first dose of betamethasone.

1. Which of the following is the mechanism of action of magnesium sulfate on cellular calcium?
   a. Increases conversion of ATP to cAMP, which results in decreased levels of free calcium ions through sequestration in the sarcoplasmic reticulum
   b. Antagonizes calcium and stabilizes cell membranes
   c. Decreases influx of calcium into cells
   d. Blocks cyclooxygenase and decreases levels of prostaglandins

2. What side effects or complications should you counsel your patient that she might experience from magnesium sulfate?
   a. Flushing, diplopia, headache
   b. Headache, tachycardia, anxiety
   c. Headache, flushing, dizziness
   d. Constriction of the ductus arteriosis in the neonate

3. Magnesium sulfate has potential for serious complications such as respiratory depression, hypoxia, cardiac arrest, and even death. Which of the following clinical tests is most useful to monitor patients who are receiving magnesium sulfate infusions?
   a. Serum magnesium levels every 4 hours
   b. Serum magnesium levels every 2 hours
   c. Serial BP measurements
   d. Serial deep tendon reflex examination
   e. Serial pulmonary examination

4. What is the next best step in clinical management of this patient?
   a. NICU consult
   b. Penicillin G 5 million units loading dose, followed by 2.5 million units every 4 hours
   c. Fetal ultrasound for growth
   d. CBC, type and screen, urine dip

5. What is the next best step in management?
   a. Recommend cesarean section for placental abruption remote from delivery
   b. Continue expectant management, bleeding is likely from the cervix
   c. Send a CBC, type and screen, Kleihauer-Betke (KB) test, and place a second IV
   d. Consent the patient for transfusion of PRBCs
   e. Place fetal scalp electrode and IUPC to better monitor fetus and contractions

Vignette 2

A 35-year-old G2P1001 woman at 40 weeks 6 days presents to labor and delivery triage with a 5-hour history of painful contractions. Monitoring reveals contractions every 3 minutes and cervical examination on arrival is 3 cm dilated, 50% effaced, and −2 station. Her pregnancy has been complicated by A1 gestational diabetes and 45 lb weight gain in pregnancy (BMI 24). In her first pregnancy, she presented at 2 cm dilation and 90% effacement. Her labor progressed slowly with dilation of 1 cm every 3 hours until labor arrested at 7 cm. A healthy baby girl weighing 4,200 g was delivered by cesarean section after arrest at 7 cm for 4 hours. Today your patient requests a trial of labor after cesarean section. You recheck her cervix 2 hours later and find that it is 4 cm dilated, 90% effaced, and −1 station. The estimated fetal weight by Leopold's is 9 lb. A recent ultrasound preformed at 38 weeks estimated the fetal weight at 3,900 g. You admit the patient to labor and delivery for expectant management.

1. Which of the following factors was least likely to result in her prior failure to progress?
   a. Obstetric conjugate diameter of the pelvis greater than 11.5 cm
   b. Inadequate strength of uterine contractions
   c. Fetal size or position
   d. Maternal pelvis shape

2. Which of the following factors places the patient at greatest risk for shoulder dystocia?
   a. Gestational diabetes

b. Prior failure to progress
c. 45 lb weight gain in pregnancy
d. Suspected fetal macrosomia
e. Prior fetus weighing 4,200 g

3. What is the name of the maneuver used to relieve the shoulder dystocia?
a. McRobert maneuver
b. Wood's corkscrew maneuver
c. Rubin maneuver
d. Zavanelli maneuver

4. What is the most common fetal complication of shoulder dystocia?
a. No complication
b. Erb's palsy
c. Humerus fracture
d. Hypoxic brain injury
e. Clavicle fracture

Vignette 3

A 32-year-old G3P2002 woman presents for routine prenatal care at 37 weeks. Her pregnancy is complicated by Rh-negative status, depression, and a history of LSIL Pap smear with normal colposcopy in the first trimester. Today she reports good fetal movement and denies leaking fluid or contractions. During your examination you measure the fundal height at an appropriate 37 cm, and find fetal heart tones located in the upper aspect of the uterus. A bedside ultrasound reveals frank breech presentation.

1. Which of the following is the next best step in management of this patient?
a. Schedule a cesarean delivery for 39 weeks
b. Return visit in 1 week to reassess fetal position
c. Schedule an external cephalic version
d. Offer a trial of vaginal breech delivery

2. Prior to discharging the patient from labor and delivery triage after her successful external cephalic version, which of the following should you do first?
a. Schedule induction for 39 weeks
b. Place abdominal binder to help hold fetus in cephalic presentation
c. Prescribe tocolytic
d. Give RhoGAM
e. Check fetal position with ultrasound

3. Which of the following findings would deter you from offering this patient a trial of breech delivery?
a. Frank breech presentation
b. Fetal weight of 3,200 g
c. Complete breech presentation
d. Fetal weight of 4,100 g

4. Which of the following is not associated with increased risk for breech presentation?
a. Fetal anencephaly
b. Uterine anomalies
c. Polyhydramnios
d. Chorioamnionitis

Vignette 4

You are working in the emergency department when an 18-year-old Caucasian woman arrives via ambulance. EMS reports that she was found seizing in a local drug store approximately 10 minutes ago. She appears to be 7 to 8 months pregnant. She had no family or friends with her, but police have contacted family who are on the way to the emergency department. Here vital signs on arrival are as follows: BP, 180/116 mm Hg; heart rate, 76 bpm; respiratory rate, 16 bpm; oxygen saturation, 98%. Her pants are soiled and she is not responding to questions at this time. Bedside ultrasound demonstrates fetal cardiac activity in the 130s. Quick bedside biometry estimates gestation age to be 32 weeks 1 day.

1. What is the best first step in managing this patient?
a. Obtain formal fetal ultrasound for gestational age
b. Obtain CBC, metabolic panel, serum toxicology screening
c. Order CT head
d. Emergent cesarean section
e. Begin empiric magnesium sulfate therapy

2. What is the most appropriate next step in management?
a. Intubation to protect airway
b. IV labetalol
c. Head CT
d. Lumbar puncture to rule out infection
e. Delivery

3. What do you recommend next?
a. Load phenytoin for seizure control
b. Begin induction of labor
c. Give betamethasone for fetal lung maturity
d. Lumbar puncture to rule out meningitis and encephalitis
e. Cesarean section

4. At what stage of pregnancy is eclampsia most likely to occur?
a. First trimester
b. Second trimester
c. Third trimester
d. Immediately postpartum within 48 hours of delivery
e. Postpartum period between 48 hours and 4 weeks

A Answers

Vignette 1 Question 1

Answer B: Uterine myometrium is composed of smooth muscle fibers whose contraction is regulated by MLK, which is activated by calcium ions. Magnesium decreases uterine tone and contractions by acting as a calcium antagonist and a membrane stabilizer. Terbutaline acts by increasing conversion of ATP to cAMP, which decreases free calcium ions through sequestration in the sarcoplasmic reticulum. Calcium channel blockers decrease intracellular calcium, which reduces uterine contractility. Indomethacin blocks the enzyme cyclooxygenase and decreases the level of prostaglandins, which decreases intracellular levels of calcium and therefore decreases myometrial contractions.

Vignette 1 Question 2

Answer A: Flushing, diplopia, and headache are common side effects of magnesium sulfate. Women taking terbutaline often note headache, tachycardia, and anxiety. Calcium channel blockers such as nifedipine can cause headache, flushing, and dizziness. Lastly, indomethacin has been associated with the premature closure of the ductus arteriosis in the neonate.

Vignette 1 Question 3

Answer D: The most effective test to monitor patients for magnesium toxicity is through serial deep tendon reflex (DTR) examination. DTRs are diminished and then lost with magnesium serum levels below 10 mg/dL. Toxic levels of magnesium (>10 mg/dL) result in respiratory depression, hypoxia, and cardiac arrest. Serial DTR examination is therefore a cost-effective screening test for magnesium toxicity. Serum levels are not necessary unless there is concern for absent DTRs or patients show symptoms of respiratory depression. Serial pulmonary examination and BP monitoring are useful tests when monitoring patients with preeclampsia who are being treated with magnesium sulfate to prevent eclampsia, but not the most effective monitoring method.

Vignette 1 Question 4

Answer B: Early in pregnancy this patient had a urinary tract infection, which demonstrated GBS bacteriuria. Patients with GBS bacteriuria are colonized and should be treated with penicillin if in labor or threatened PTL. As a result, it is important to treat this patient with GBS prophylaxis as long as labor is threatened. The goals of GBS prophylaxis are to have antibiotics in the mother 4 hours prior to ruptured membranes or delivery. Antibiotics are discontinued when labor is no longer threatened. In a patient without a history of GBS bacteriuria, a GBS culture swab is collected on presentation and diagnosis of PTL and antibiotics are continued until the results either return negative for GBS or labor is no longer threatened. A NICU consult should be obtained for the family so they can gather information on the risks of delivery of a preterm fetus. Fetal ultrasound, if not performed in the previous 4 weeks, can provide additional information on the well-being of the fetus. Routine CBC, type and screen, and urine dip should also be collected but are not as important as starting GBS prophylaxis.

The nurse calls you to the patient's room to evaluate her vaginal for bleeding. You look at the tocometer and see that uterine contractions are every 2 minutes. The fetal heart tracing shows a baseline of 135 bpm with moderate variability and accelerations. There are occasional early decelerations. You examine the cervix and find 5 cm dilation, 100% effacement, and −1 station. There is a moderate amount of bright red blood on your glove.

Vignette 1 Question 5

Answer C: This scenario describes the development of placental abruption. The description of the fetal monitoring and maternal status tells us that the situation is not emergent and trial of vaginal delivery can continue. However, it is important to be prepared for worsening vaginal bleeding or need for emergent delivery should the fetal status or maternal status deteriorate. Therefore, you should check the maternal blood counts, prepare for transfusion, evaluate for fetal–maternal exposure of blood, and place a second IV in case blood products or fluids need to be administered for resuscitation. Cesarean delivery is not necessary at this time. You could discuss blood transfusion at this time, but it is not the best answer choice. Lastly, the question does not suggest that fetal or contraction monitoring is difficult and therefore fetal scalp electrode or internal contractions monitoring with an IUPC is not indicated.

Vignette 2 Question 1

Answer A: Failure to progress is commonly associated with the 3 Ps—power, passenger, and pelvis. Power refers to the strength of uterine contractions. Contraction strength is most commonly measured by the Montevideo unit and data is collected from an IUPC. Montevideo units are a measure of average uterine strength of contractions in millimeters of mercury multiplied by the number of contractions in 10 minutes, and 200 to 250 Montevideo units define adequate labor in the active phase of labor. Optimal uterine contractions are believed to be necessary for vaginal birth and are also measured by cervical dilation and effacement. The second P, the passenger or fetus, can be too large to deliver or be malpositioned for delivery. Lastly, the pelvic outlet may not be the right shape or size, in combination with the fetal position, to allow delivery. Generally, an obstetric conjugate of 11.5 cm should be adequate to deliver a cephalic fetus because the suboccipitobregmatic diameter presenting to the pelvis averages 9.5 cm.

Vignette 2 Question 2

Answer D: Shoulder dystocia is reported to occur in 0.15% to 1.7% of all vaginal deliveries. Traditionally, shoulder dystocia is associated with fetal macrosomia, but up to one-half of shoulder dystocia events occur in neonates weighing less than 4,000 g. However, an 11-fold increased relative probability of shoulder dystocia has been found in pregnancies where the neonate weighed over 4,000 g. Approximately 7% of neonates will weigh over 4,000 g and 2% will weigh over 4,500 g. In those deliveries where neonates weighed over 4,500 g, the relative probability of shoulder dystocia during delivery was 22-fold. With fetal macrosomia, the trunk and chest grow larger relative to the fetal head. Macrosomia is more common in gestational diabetes but also occurs in prolonged pregnancies. Maternal obesity, previous fetus weighing over 4,000 g, prolonged second stage of labor, prolonged deceleration phase (8 to 10 cm), and prior shoulder dystocia all appear to be related to fetal macrosomia. Some studies have shown increased maternal age and excess maternal weight gain in pregnancy to be associated with shoulder dystocia.

Over the course of the next 6 hours, the patient progresses to 8 cm dilation. Her progress slows and she does not make any change over the next 2 hours. You place an IUPC and Montevideo units are 160. Pitocin is started. Three hours later she is completely dilated, 100% effaced, and 0 station. She has a strong urge to push so you begin pushing. Two hours into pushing she is at +2 station. An hour later, the fetus is crowning and you see the turtle sign. You immediately announce, "I have a shoulder dystocia," and call for additional help from nursing, anesthesia, and neonatology. You ask the patient to stop pushing. The time of the shoulder dystocia is noted. You ask to have the patients hips flexed, and ask another nurse to apply pressure just above the maternal pubic symphysis directed obliquely. The anterior fetal shoulder remains trapped. Next you place your hand inside the vagina and attempt to put pressure on the posterior shoulder to decrease the biacromial diameter and facilitate the anterior shoulders delivery. The maneuver works, and the fetus delivers and is handed to the awaiting neonatology team. The shoulder dystocia lasted 65 seconds.

Vignette 2 Question 3

Answer C: Rubin maneuver. This maneuver involves pressure on either fetal shoulder to diminish the biacromial diameter in effort to free the anterior shoulder and allow delivery of the fetus. In this scenario, McRobert maneuver is described first and involves flexing the maternal hips, which results in ventral rotation of the maternal pelvis and an increase in the size of the pelvic outlet. It is the least invasive of maneuvers. Next, suprapubic pressure is applied by directing force just above the pubic symphysis in an oblique direction. The goal of this maneuver is to disimpact the anterior shoulder. It is very important that pressure be applied obliquely to free the shoulder, as downward pressure will not change the biacromial diameter. Wood's cork maneuver involves placing a hand behind either the anterior or posterior fetal shoulder and rotating the fetus in 180 degrees to lead to descent and delivery of the shoulders. Lastly, if all other attempts are unsuccessful and approximately 4 to 5 minutes time has passed, consideration should be given to Zavanelli maneuver and emergent cesarean section. Zavanelli involves replacement of the fetal head by reversing the cardinal movements of labor.

Vignette 2 Question 4

Answer A: In 90% to 95% cases of shoulder dystocia, there is no long-term sequelae. Depending on the type of maneuver used to deliver the baby, clavicle or humerus fracture may be more likely. This is true for delivery of the posterior arm. Erb's palsy results from brachial plexus injury. This injury is due to traction on the anterior shoulder, as it is trapped behind the pubic symphysis. It is important that the mother does not push while the shoulder is impacted, as this can worsen risk for injury. Brachial plexus injuries can occur without shoulder dystocia and are thought to be due to uterine forces on the fetus while delivering. Hypoxic brain injury occurs when a shoulder dystocia is prolonged. This risk increases after 3 minutes but is highly variable, and depends on the reserve of the fetus prior to the shoulder dystocia. This is the rarest of complications from shoulder dystocia and the most severe apart from fetal demise.

Vignette 3 Question 1

Answer C: Given her gestational age prior to 39 weeks, it would be best to try an external cephalic version. If unsuccessful, a second trial of version at 39 weeks with epidural or spinal anesthesia should be offered. If the version is successful prior to 39 weeks, the patient is followed expectantly with routine prenatal care. If the version is accomplished after 39 weeks, she may be induced at that time. If the version is unsuccessful on second attempt with anesthesia, delivery by cesarean section is recommended. External cephalic versions carry the risk of cord compression and placental abruption. It is critically important to monitor the fetus for a period of time after the procedure. Occasionally, an emergent delivery is indicated by cesarean following a trial of version due to nonreassuring fetal testing. If the patient declines a trial of version, she should be scheduled for an elective cesarean section after 39 weeks' gestation. In a select population, trial of vaginal breech delivery can be attempted but requires stringent criteria be met.

Vignette 3 Question 2

Answer D: Because the patient is Rh negative, she should receive a dose of RhoGAM prior to discharge. External cephalic version carries the risk of placental abruption and also the possibility of maternal exposure to fetal blood through disruption in the placental interface. In Rh-negative mothers, this could lead to formation of antibodies against Rh factor if the fetus is Rh positive. In future pregnancy with an Rh-positive fetus, maternal antibodies can cross the placenta and destroy fetal blood cells resulting in anemia and fetal hydrops. A dose of RhoGAM can prevent this problem. Other risk factors of external cephalic version include fetal distress, failed rotation, and need for urgent cesarean section. Induction is generally scheduled at 39 to 40 weeks and abdominal binders are commonly used to prevent the fetus from returning to breech presentation but theses are not the best answers. There is no role for use of tocolytics at this stage of pregnancy. Lastly, rechecking the fetal position is possible and reasonable especially if the mother describes a large fetal movement, but it is not necessary or the best answer choice.

Vignette 3 Question 3

Answer D: Fetal weight over 4,100 g is a relative contraindication to offering a trial of breech delivery. The criteria recommended to offer a trial of breech labor include an adequate pelvis as determined by pelvimetry and imaging (generally X-ray, CT, or MRI), frank or complete breech, a flexed fetal head, and estimated fetal weight of 2,500 to 3,800 g. Relative contraindications to offering a vaginal breech trial of labor include weight over 3,800 g, nulliparity, and incomplete breech such as footling breech presentation.

Vignette 3 Question 4

Answer D: Breech presentation is associated with fetal anomalies such as anencephaly and hydrocephaly as well as uterine anomalies. Both oligohydramnios and polyhydramnios are also associated with risk of breech presentation. Prior breech delivery, multifetal gestation, and PPROM are also associated risk factors. Chorioamnionitis is not a direct cause of breech presentation but can occur as a result of PPROM or be the cause of PPROM.

Vignette 4 Question 1

Answer E: Any pregnant woman with a seizure is presumed to have eclampsia until proven otherwise. Treatment begins with a 6 g bolus of magnesium given over 15 to 20 minutes, followed by 2 to 3 g/hour. The goal of treatment with magnesium sulfate in eclampsia is to prevent recurrent convulsions. However, approximately 10% of women with eclampsia will have a second convulsion after treatment with magnesium, and a second bolus of 2 g can be given over 3 to 5 minutes. Other antiepileptic medications can be given as well, such as lorazepam, phenytoin, and phenobarbital in status epilepticus. Fetal age is important but you already have an estimate and fetal age will not change management of eclampsia at this time. CBC, metabolic panel, serum toxicology should be obtained but are not as important as preventing future convulsions. If focal deficits are suspected, CT head may be warranted but again, this is not as critical as starting magnesium sulfate. Delivery is ultimately the treatment of eclampsia but not the first step in management.

Vignette 4 Question 2

Answer B: On arrival BP is reported to be elevated at 180/116 mm Hg. The second step in management of eclampsia is to control severe hypertension. The goal of treating severe hypertension in eclampsia is to avoid loss of cerebral autoregulation and prevent congestive heart failure without compromising cerebral or placental perfusion, which can be reduced in women with eclampsia. Treatment is usually given IV and labetalol or hydralazine are appropriate agents. Target BP is between 140 and 160 mm Hg systolic, and 90 and 110 mm Hg diastolic. Because she has normal oxygen saturation and is therefore protecting her airway, intubation is not warranted at this time. Again, unless focal deficits are noted on examination, CT head is not as important as controlling BP. While infection is a common cause of seizure in the general population, it is less likely the etiology in a pregnant woman. Delivery is reasonable but not the best answer. Ultimately, delivery is the treatment of eclampsia but will not improve her condition as acutely as BP control.

Family arrives and informs you of the patient's due date, making her 33 weeks 2 days. They also reveal that the patient has been feeling unwell for the past 2 days. She has had a severe frontal headache associated with visual changes, which she described as blurry vision. She has also been nauseated and had worsening swelling in her legs. She missed her last doctor's appointment and has not been seen in over 5 weeks. Her medical history is significant only for asthma and this is her first pregnancy. It has been 20 minutes since her first seizure. The patient develops a glazed look on her face and twitching. She then begins having another tonic–clonic seizure. A repeat bolus of 2 g magnesium sulfate is given and the seizure subsides within 2 minutes.

Vignette 4 Question 3

Answer E: At this point in management, cesarean section is indicated. The patient is remote from delivery and the definitive treatment of eclampsia is delivery. There is no time to begin induction of labor or wait to give betamethasone for fetal lung maturity. Treatment with phenytoin to prevent additional seizures is reasonable but not the best answer. Lastly, an LP is not the best answer because all signs and symptoms point to eclampsia as the etiology of her seizures.

Vignette 4 Question 4

Answer C: Eclampsia can occur antepartum, intrapartum, or postpartum. Antepartum eclampsia occurs in 38% to 53%, while postpartum eclampsia ranges from 11% to 44% and most cases occur in the immediate postpartum period within 48 hours. Late postpartum eclampsia after 48 hours is rare but does occur. Reviewing the intrapartum history will often reveal that these women had preeclampsia and were treated with magnesium sulfate. Almost all cases of eclampsia occur in the third trimester (91%), 7.5% of cases will occur in the second trimester, and approximately 1.5% cases in the first trimester. Eclampsia in the first trimester is often associated with a molar or hydropic degeneration of the placenta.

Chapter

7 Fetal Complications of Pregnancy

DISORDERS OF FETAL GROWTH

Newborns with birth weight less than the 10th percentile or greater than the 90th percentile are easily identified. However, the accuracy of antepartum estimates of fetal weight can vary. Ultrasound is the most commonly used modality to estimate fetal weight. Fetuses whose estimated fetal weight (EFW) is less than the 10th percentile are termed **small for gestational age** (SGA). Fetuses whose EFW is greater than the 90th percentile are termed **large for gestational age** (LGA). SGA fetuses are further described as either symmetric or asymmetric. *Symmetric* implies that the fetus is proportionally small. *Asymmetric* implies that certain organs of the fetus are disproportionately small. Classically, an asymmetric infant will have wasting of the torso and extremities while preserving the brain. Thus, the skull will be at a greater percentile than the rest of the body. Screening for disorders of fetal growth is done during routine prenatal care. Once the fetus is at or greater than 20 weeks' gestational age, the uterine fundal height (in centimeters) should be approximately equal to the gestational age (in weeks). Fetal growth can therefore be followed by serial examinations of the fundal height. Before making the diagnosis of either SGA or LGA, it is imperative that accurate dating of the pregnancy is ascertained. If the fundal height varies by more than 3 cm from the gestational age, ultrasound is usually obtained. Of note, while birth percentiles are useful in identifying small neonates, they fail to distinguish between infants who reached their growth potential and those with disproportionate growth. For example, a small infant may have normally grown due to his/her genetic potential, while another may be small due to genetic disease.

FETAL GROWTH REGULATION

Regulation of fetal growth begins early in the first trimester when the placental cytotrophoblast villi anchor to the uterine decidua. As vascular connections form between the maternal circulation and the intervillous spaces, endocrine and paracrine signaling promote adaptation of the maternal circulation, which provides both oxygen and nutrients to the developing fetus. Placental growth is supported by increased substrate delivery and perfusion, which is critical to its intricate function. As the site of maternal–fetal exchange, the placenta provides active transport to glucose, amino acids, and free fatty acids, which is facilitated by its low resistance and high capacitance vascular network. By term, 600 mL/min of maternal cardiac output will pass through the placental exchange network, which has an area up to 12 m^2. The ultimate growth potential of the fetus is felt to be predetermined genetically. When the expected regulatory processes occur in the fetus, mother, and placenta, normal growth ensues. However, fetal growth regulation can be impacted both positively and negatively depending on genetic potential, maternal diet, pathophysiology, and placental function.

SMALL FOR GESTATIONAL AGE

SGA refers to a neonate with signs of fetal growth disruption but in whom the causative factor for small size is unknown. SGA infants are associated with higher rates of mortality and morbidity for their gestational age. Even within the SGA category, infants with birth weight less than 5th percentile or even less than 3rd percentile have even worse outcomes. However, SGA infants do better than infants with the same weight delivered at earlier gestational ages. For example, an SGA neonate born at 34 weeks that weighs the same as a 28-week neonate will have lower morbidity and mortality rates. Factors that can result in infants being SGA can be divided into those that lead to **decreased growth potential** and those that lead to **intrauterine growth restriction** (IUGR) (Table 7-1).

Decreased Growth Potential

Congenital abnormalities account for approximately 10% to 15% of SGA infants. Trisomy 21 (Down syndrome), trisomy 18 (Edward syndrome), and trisomy 13 (Patau syndrome) all lead to SGA babies. Turner syndrome (45,XO) leads to a decrease in birth weight. Infants with osteogenesis imperfecta, achondroplasia, neural tube defects, anencephaly, and a variety of autosomal recessive syndromes may all be SGA.

Many intrauterine infections—particularly **cytomegalovirus** (CMV) and **rubella**—lead to SGA infants. These probably account for 10% to 15% of all SGA babies. Exposure to **teratogens**, most chemotherapeutic agents, and other drugs during pregnancy can also lead to decreased growth potential. The two most common teratogens causing SGA are alcohol and cigarettes. Up to 10% of SGA fetuses are constitutionally small based purely on parental stature or their genetic potential, and this appears to vary by race/ethnicity.

Intrauterine Growth Restriction

Fetal growth can be divided into two phases: Prior to 20 weeks of gestation, growth is primarily hyperplastic (increasing number of cells); after 20 weeks, it is primarily hypertrophic (increasing cell size). As a consequence of this, an insult occurring prior to 20 weeks will most likely result in symmetric growth restriction, whereas an insult occurring after 20 weeks, in a prolonged fashion, will most likely result in asymmetric growth. Asymmetric growth is presumably caused by decreased nutrition and oxygen being transmitted across the placenta, which is then shunted to the fetal brain. Two-thirds of the time growth restriction is asymmetric and can be identified by increased head-to-abdominal measurements.

■ **TABLE 7-1** Risk Factors for SGA Infants
Decreased growth potential
Genetic and chromosomal abnormalities
Intrauterine infections
Teratogenic exposure
Substance abuse
Radiation exposure
Small maternal stature
Pregnancy at high altitudes
Female fetus
Intrauterine growth restricted (IUGR)
Maternal factors including hypertension, anemia, chronic renal disease, malnutrition, and severe diabetes
Placental factors including placenta previa, chronic abruption, placental infarction, multiple gestations

small maou
hyprexra

Maternal risk factors include baseline hypertension, anemia, chronic renal disease, antiphospholipid antibody syndrome, systemic lupus erythematosus (SLE), and severe malnutrition. Severe diabetes with extensive vascular disease may also lead to IUGR. Placental factors leading to diminished placental

blood flow may lead to IUGR. These factors include placenta previa, marginal cord insertion, and placental thrombosis with or without infarction. Multiple gestations often lead to lower birth weights because of earlier delivery and SGA infants.

Diagnosis

The risk of having an SGA neonate increases in mothers with a previous SGA neonate or with any of the above etiologies. The intrauterine growth of these fetuses should be followed carefully. Fundal height is measured at each prenatal visit. Oligohydramnios and SGA fetuses tend to have fundal heights less than expected. Anytime a fundal height is 3 cm less than expected, fetal growth should be estimated via ultrasound. Of note, the use of fundal height as a screening tool for either SGA or LGA is quite poor with sensitivities well below 50% and positive predictive values below 50% as well. Thus, with concern in the setting of the risk factors listed previously, ultrasound to evaluate fetal growth is common even without abnormal fundal height measurements.

If SGA is suspected, the accuracy of the pregnancy's dating should be verified. Any infant at risk for IUGR or being SGA is followed with serial ultrasound scans for growth every 2 to 3 weeks. A fetus with decreased growth potential will usually start small and stay small, whereas one with IUGR will progressively fall off the growth curve. Another test to differentiate IUGR fetuses is Doppler investigation of the umbilical artery. Normal flow through the umbilical artery is higher during systole, and decreases only 50% to 80% during diastole (Fig. 7-1). The flow during diastole should never be absent

u/s q 2-3 wk

IUGR - prog. fall

SGA - stays sm-

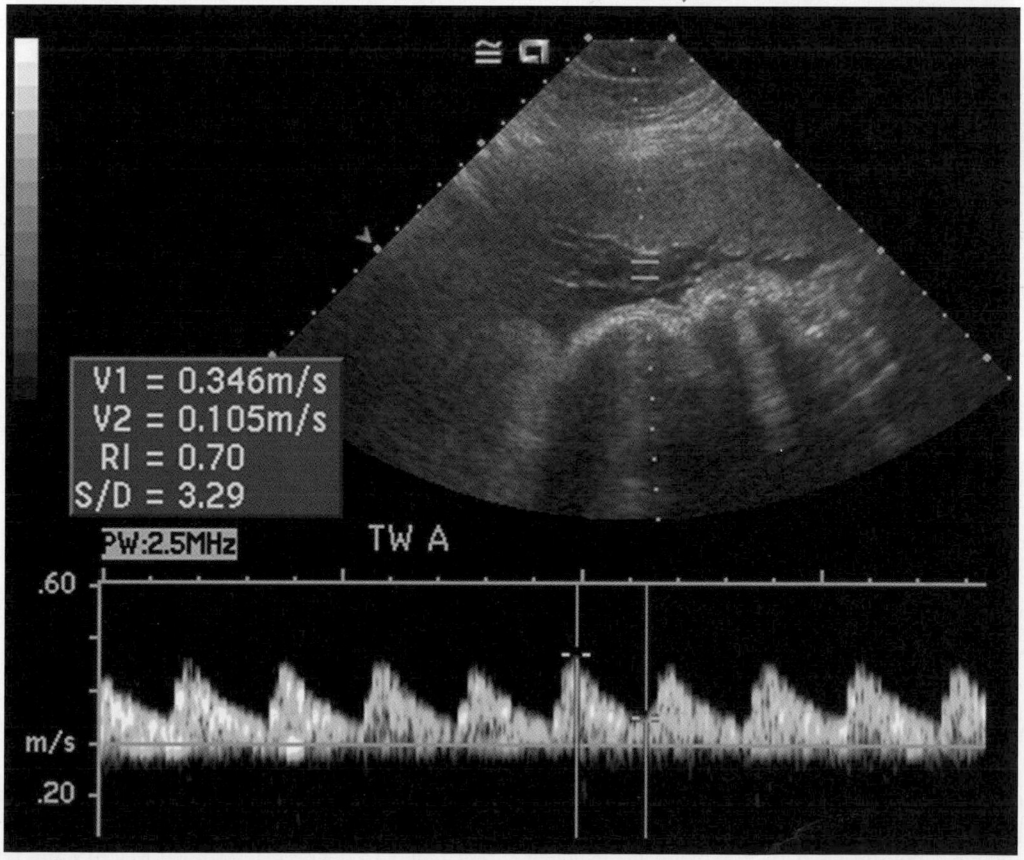

Figure 7-1 • Normal umbilical artery Doppler. Note that the ratio between systolic peak and diastolic trough is 3.29:1.

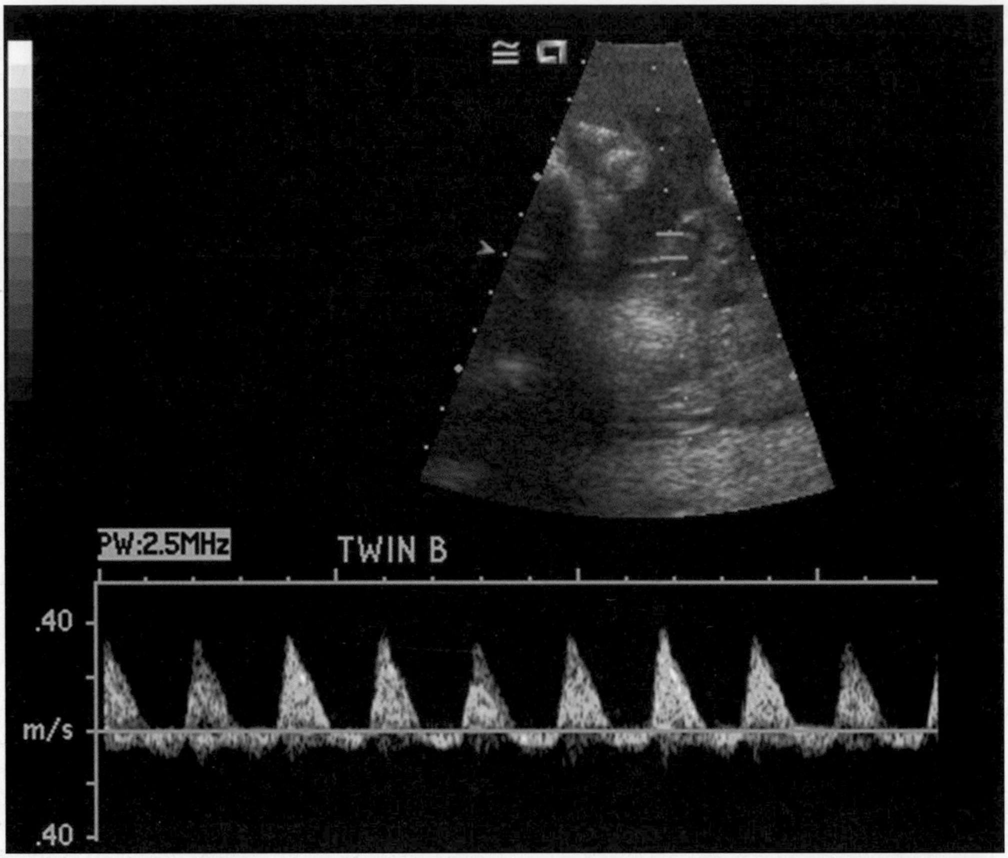

Figure 7-2 • Reversed diastolic flow on umbilical artery Doppler in the setting of IUGR.

or reversed (Fig. 7-2). However, in the setting of increased placental resistance, which can be seen with a thrombosed or calcified placenta, diastolic flow decreases or even becomes absent or reversed. Reversed diastolic flow is particularly concerning and is associated with a high risk of intrauterine fetal demise. Thus, while an SGA fetus with normal Dopplers is often expectantly managed to term, those with abnormal Doppler values are often delivered early.

Treatment

For patients with a history of SGA infants, the underlying etiology should be explored. If malnutrition or drugs like alcohol or cigarettes were issues in a prior pregnancy, these should be dealt with at each prenatal visit. Patients with a history of placental insufficiency, preeclampsia, collagen vascular disorders, or vascular disease are often treated with low-dose aspirin. Patients with prior placental thrombosis, thrombophilias, or antiphospholipid antibody syndrome have been treated with heparin and corticosteroids as well, with mixed results.

There is no indication to expedite delivery in SGA fetuses who have consistently been small throughout the pregnancy. However, the neonatal risk of delivery is likely to be lower than that of remaining in the intrauterine environment for some SGA fetuses in the late preterm and early term period who have fallen off the growth curve. This risk is assessed with fetal testing such as a nonstress test (NST), oxytocin challenge test (OCT), biophysical profile (BPP), and umbilical Doppler velocimetry. With increasing placental resistance due to calcifications or thromboses, the umbilical arterial diastolic flow will decrease, halt, and occasionally reverse. Doppler investigation of the fetal umbilical cord is particularly useful because of the high predictive value of poor outcomes in the setting of absent or reversed end diastolic flow. If fetal testing is nonreassuring, the fetus should be delivered. The decision of whether to deliver SGA fetuses remote from term is based on how the infant will do in a neonatal intensive care unit versus how it will be maintained in the intrauterine environment. For those left undelivered, frequent antenatal testing with NSTs, OCTs, and BPPs; weekly ultrasounds for fetal growth; antenatal corticosteroids to accelerate fetal lung maturity; and, possibly, admission to the hospital for continuous monitoring may be indicated.

LARGE FOR GESTATIONAL AGE AND FETAL MACROSOMIA

An LGA fetus is defined as having an EFW greater than the 90th percentile. While LGA identifies neonates with increased growth at a particular gestational age, it is considered less important than the diagnosis of fetal macrosomia, which is better correlated to identifying fetuses at higher risk for birth trauma or cesarean delivery. Although definitions of macrosomia vary, the American College of Obstetricians and Gynecologists uses **a birth weight greater than 4,500 g**. Birth weights of greater than 4,000 or 4,200 g are also used by many clinicians and researchers to define macrosomia. Macrosomic fetuses have a higher risk of shoulder dystocia and birth trauma with resultant brachial plexus injuries with vaginal deliveries. Other neonatal risks include low Apgar scores, hypoglycemia, polycythemia, hypocalcemia, and jaundice. LGA infants are at a higher risk for childhood leukemia, Wilms tumor, and osteosarcoma.

Mothers with LGA or macrosomic fetuses are at increased risk for cesarean delivery, perineal trauma, and postpartum hemorrhage. There is a higher rate of cesarean delivery in women with macrosomic infants due to failure to progress in labor. In addition, some women with suspected fetal macrosomia elect to have a cesarean delivery out of concern for increased risk for shoulder dystocia and the possibility of neonatal injury. Clinicians are obligated to offer such elective cesareans with an estimated fetal weight of 5,000 gms or greater in women without gestational diabetes and 4,500 gms or greater in women with gestational diabetes.

Etiology

The most classically associated risk factor for fetal macrosomia is preexisting or gestational diabetes mellitus. **Maternal obesity**, with a BMI greater than 30 or weight greater than 90 kg, is also correlated with an increased risk for fetal macrosomia as is increased maternal weight gain in pregnancy. This association is seemingly independent of maternal stature and gestational diabetes. Any woman who has previously delivered an LGA infant is at increased risk in ensuing pregnancies for fetal macrosomia. **Postterm pregnancies** have an increased rate of macrosomic infants. **Multiparity** and **advanced maternal age** are also risk factors (Table 7-2), but these are mostly secondary to the increased prevalence of diabetes and obesity.

Diagnosis

Upon routine prenatal care, patients with macrosomic infants will more often be of a size greater than dates on measurement of the fundal height and, by the late third trimester, Leopold's examination reveals a fetus that seems large. Patients whose fetuses are a size greater than dates by 3 cm or more are referred to ultrasound for EFW. Again, as noted under the SGA section, fundal height screening has a relatively poor sensitivity and specificity for fetal growth disorders. Unfortunately, ultrasound is not particularly accurate for the identification of LGA fetuses either. Ultrasound uses the biparietal diameter, femur length, and abdominal circumference to estimate fetal weight. These estimates are usually accurate to within 10% to 15%; however, with estimates beyond the 90th percentile, the positive predictive value of the weight being greater than or equal to that predicted is less than 50%. As with SGA fetuses, pregnancy dating should be verified. At many institutions, any patient with diabetes or a previous LGA infant merits an EFW by ultrasound in the late third trimester.

TABLE 7-2 Risk Factors for Macrosomic Infants

Diabetes
Maternal obesity
Postterm pregnancy
Previous LGA or macrosomic infant
Maternal stature
Multiparity
AMA
Male infant
Beckwith-Wiedemann syndrome (pancreatic islet cell hyperplasia)

Treatment

Management of LGA and macrosomic infants includes prevention, surveillance, and—in some cases—induction of labor before the attainment of macrosomia. The key to prevention of LGA in the broad obstetric population is counseling women about the goals for gestational weight gain including specific counseling about diet and exercise in pregnancy. Women with type 1 and 2 pregestational diabetes or gestational diabetes are at increased risk of LGA fetuses, and will benefit from tight control of blood glucose during pregnancy. Well-controlled blood glucose has been shown to decrease the incidence of macrosomic infants in this population. Specifically, studies of gestational diabetes have demonstrated a decrease in birth weight when women maintained good control of blood glucose.

Maternal obesity is an independent risk factor for LGA infants. With the epidemic of obesity in the United States, approximately one-third of pregnant women are obese and another third are overweight. Preconceptual counseling should be incorporated into the annual well women examination of all reproductive age women, whether they receive care from an obstetrician gynecologist or another primary care provider. Obese patients must be encouraged to lose weight before conception and offered specific programs to help them do so. Once pregnant, these patients should be advised to gain less weight (but never to lose weight) than the average patient, and they should be referred to a nutritionist for assistance in maintaining adequate nutrition, with some control of caloric intake.

Given the risk for birth trauma and failure to progress in labor secondary to cephalopelvic disproportion, LGA pregnancies are often induced before the fetus can attain macrosomic status. The risks of this course of action are thought to be an increased rate of cesarean section for failed induction, and potentially neonatal complications of prematurity in a poorly dated pregnancy. Thus, induction should be used primarily when there is either excellent dating or lung maturity as assessed via amniocentesis. For induction in the setting of an unfavorable cervix, prostaglandins and mechanical means should be used to achieve cervical ripening, and this can often take several days to accomplish. Interestingly, prospective studies of the practice of induction for impending macrosomia have not demonstrated an increase in cesarean delivery rates, but do appear to lead to lower rates of macrosomia. Vaginal delivery of the suspected macrosomic infant involves preparing for a shoulder dystocia, and counseling patients on the risks and treatment options. Operative vaginal delivery with forceps or vacuum is generally not advised in the setting of known macrosomia because of the increased risk of shoulder dystocia; however, this decision is one to be made in a setting of shared decision making with the patient.

DISORDERS OF AMNIOTIC FLUID

The amniotic fluid reaches its maximum volume of about 800 mL at about 28 weeks. This volume is maintained until close to term when it begins to fall to about 500 mL at week 40. The balance of fluid is maintained by production of the fetal kidneys and lungs and resorption by fetal swallowing and the interface between the membranes and the placenta. A disturbance in any of these functions may lead to a pathologic change in amniotic fluid volume.

Ultrasound can be used to evaluate the amniotic fluid volume. The classic measure of amniotic fluid is the **amniotic fluid index** (AFI). The AFI is calculated by dividing the maternal abdomen into quadrants, measuring the largest vertical pocket of fluid in each quadrant in centimeters, and summing them. An AFI of less than 5 is considered **oligohydramnios**. An AFI greater than 20 or 25 is used to diagnose **polyhydramnios**, depending on gestational age.

OLIGOHYDRAMNIOS

Oligohydramnios in the absence of rupture of membranes (ROM) is associated with a 40-fold increase in perinatal mortality. This is partially because without the amniotic fluid to cushion it, the umbilical cord is more susceptible to compression thus leading to fetal asphyxiation. It is also associated with congenital anomalies, particularly of the genitourinary system, and growth restriction. In labor, nonreactive nonstress tests, fetal heart rate (FHR) decelerations, meconium, and cesarean delivery due to nonreassuring fetal testing are all associated with an AFI of less than 5.

Etiology

The cause of oligohydramnios can be thought of as either decreased production or increased withdrawal. Amniotic fluid is produced by the fetal kidneys and lungs. It can be resorbed by the placenta, swallowed by the fetus, or leaked out into the vagina. Chronic uteroplacental insufficiency (UPI) can lead to oligohydramnios because the fetus likely does not have the nutrients or blood volume to maintain an adequate glomerular filtration rate. UPI is commonly associated with growth-restricted infants.

Congenital abnormalities of the genitourinary tract can lead to decreased urine production. These malformations include renal agenesis (Potter syndrome), polycystic kidney disease, or obstruction of the genitourinary system. The most common cause of oligohydramnios is ROM. Even without a history of leaking fluid, the patient should be examined to rule out this possibility.

Diagnosis

Oligohydramnios is diagnosed when AFI is less than 5 as measured by ultrasound. Some centers use the deepest vertical pocket of amniotic fluid less than 2 cm as diagnostic for oligohydramnios. Patients screened for oligohydramnios include those measuring size less than dates, with a history of ruptured membranes, with suspicion of IUGR, and who have a postterm pregnancy. Once the diagnosis of oligohydramnios is made, the etiology needs to be determined prior to creating a management plan.

Treatment

Management of oligohydramnios is entirely dependent on the underlying etiology. In pregnancies that are IUGR, a host of other data should be considered, including the rest of the biophysical profile (BPP), umbilical artery Doppler flow, gestational age, and the cause of the IUGR. Labor is usually induced in the case of a pregnancy at term or postdate, In the case of a fetus with congenital abnormalities, the patient should be referred to maternal–fetal medicine care for conversations regarding genetic counseling and prenatal diagnosis. A plan for delivery should be made in coordination with the pediatricians and pediatric surgeons. Severely preterm patients with no other etiology are usually managed expectantly with frequent antenatal fetal testing.

Labor is induced in patients with ROM at term if they are not already in labor. If there is meconium or frequent decelerations in the FHR, an amnioinfusion may be performed to increase the AFI. Traditionally, amnioinfusion has been performed to dilute any meconium present in the amniotic fluid, and therefore decrease the risk of meconium aspiration syndrome. However, in a large, multinational, randomized trial, amnioinfusion in the setting of meconium did not improve neonatal outcomes, and it is decreasingly used for this indication. In the setting of recurrent variable decelerations, there is evidence to suggest that amnioinfusion does decrease the number of variable decelerations caused by cord compression, and it is still used commonly for this indication, despite less clear evidence for neonatal benefit. Preterm premature rupture of membranes (PPROM) has already been discussed in Chapter 6.

2 - 3% oligio AFI <5
poly AFI >20

POLYHYDRAMNIOS

Polyhydramnios, defined by an AFI greater than 20 or 25, is present in 2% to 3% of pregnancies. Fetal structural and chromosomal abnormalities are more common in polyhydramnios. It is associated with maternal diabetes and malformations such as neural tube defects, obstruction of the fetal alimentary canal, and hydrops.

Etiology

Polyhydramnios is not as ominous a sign as oligohydramnios. However, it is associated with an increase in congenital anomalies. It is also more common in pregnancies complicated by diabetes, hydrops, and multiple gestation. An obstruction of the gastrointestinal tract (e.g., tracheoesophageal fistula, duodenal atresia) may render the fetus unable to swallow the amniotic fluid, leading to polyhydramnios. Just as in other diabetic patients, the increased levels of circulating glucose can act as an osmotic diuretic in the fetus leading to polyhydramnios. Hydrops secondary to high output cardiac failure is generally associated with polyhydramnios. Monozygotic multiple gestations can lead to twin-to-twin transfusion syndrome with polyhydramnios around one fetus and oligohydramnios around the other.

Diagnosis *u/s*

Polyhydramnios is diagnosed by ultrasound in patients being scanned for size greater than dates, routine screening of diabetic or multiple gestation pregnancies, or as an unsuspected finding on an ultrasound performed for other reasons.

Treatment

As in oligohydramnios, the particular setting of polyhydramnios dictates the management of the pregnancy. Patients with polyhydramnios are at risk for malpresentation and should be carefully evaluated during labor. There is an increased risk of cord prolapse with polyhydramnios. Thus, ROM should be performed in a controlled setting if possible and only if the head is truly engaged in the pelvis. Upon spontaneous ROM, a sterile vaginal examination should be performed to verify fetal presentation and rule out cord prolapse.

Rh INCOMPATIBILITY AND ALLOIMMUNIZATION

If a woman is Rh negative and her fetus is Rh positive, she may be sensitized to the Rh antigen and develop antibodies. These IgG antibodies cross the placenta and cause hemolysis of fetal RBCs. The incidence of Rh negativity varies among

TABLE 7-3 Prevalence of Rh Negativity by Race and Ethnicity

Race and Ethnicity	Percent Rh Negative
Caucasian	15
African American	8
African	4
Native American	1
Asian	<1

race (Table 7-3), with the highest incidence of 30% seen among individuals in the Basque region of Spain. Commonly, most individuals become sensitized only during pregnancy and blood transfusion. In the United States, the incidence of sensitization is decreasing because of both careful management of transfusions and the use of Rh immunoglobulin (RhoGAM) in pregnancy. Interestingly, because there is some transplacental passage of fetal cells in all pregnancies, ABO incompatibility actually decreases the risk of Rh sensitization as a result of destruction of these fetal cells by anti-A or anti-B antibodies.

In sensitized patients with Rh-positive fetuses, the antibodies cross the placenta and cause hemolysis leading to disastrous complications in the fetus. The anemia caused by hemolysis leads to increased extramedullary production of fetal red cells. **Erythroblastosis fetalis**, or fetal hydrops (see Color Plate 1), a syndrome that includes a hyperdynamic state, heart failure, diffuse edema (Fig. 7-3), ascites (Fig. 7-4), and pericardial effusion, is the result of serious anemia. Fetal hydrops is defined as accumulation of fluid in the extracellular space in at least two body compartments. Bilirubin, a breakdown product of

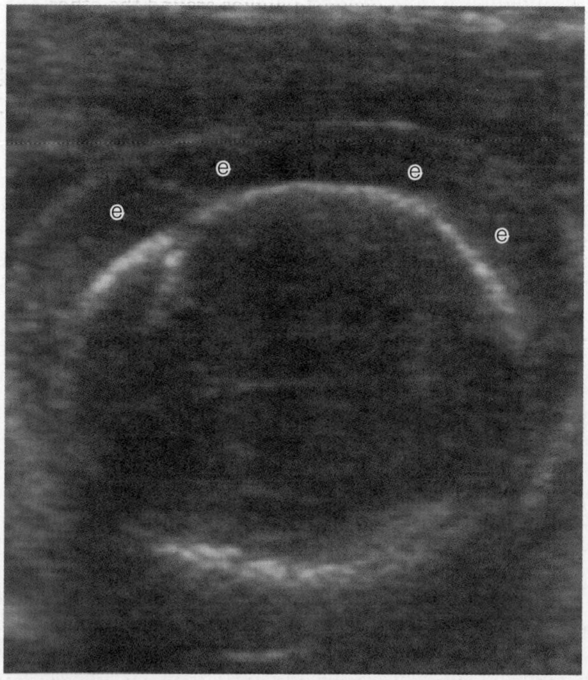

Figure 7-3 • Scalp edema (e).

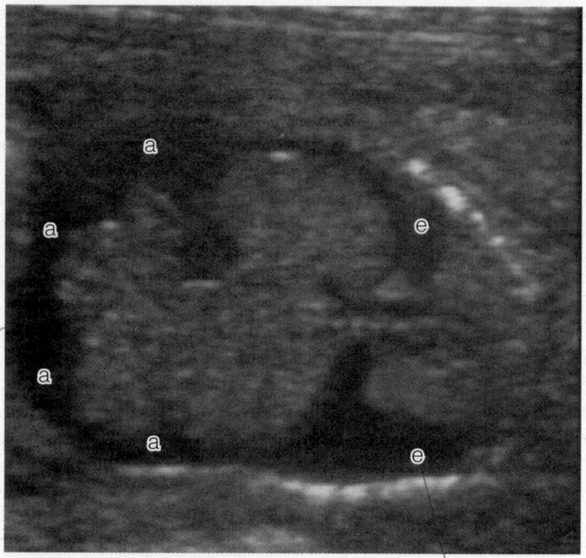

Figure 7-4 • Note the large ascites (a) and pleural effusions (e) in this fetus with hydrops.

RBCs, is cleared by the placenta before birth but can lead to jaundice and neurotoxic effects in the neonate.

THE UNSENSITIZED Rh-NEGATIVE PATIENT

If a patient is Rh negative but has a negative antibody screen, the goal during pregnancy is to keep her from becoming sensitized. Any time during the pregnancy if there is a possibility that a patient may be exposed to fetal blood (in the form of intact cells or free DNA), such as during amniocentesis, miscarriage, vaginal bleeding, abruption, and delivery, she should be given RhoGAM, an anti-D immunoglobulin (Rh IgG). An antibody screen is performed at the initial visit to detect prior sensitization. RhoGAM should be administered at 28 weeks and postpartum if the neonate is Rh positive.

A standard dose of RhoGAM, 0.3 mg of Rh IgG, will eradicate 15 mL of fetal RBCs (30 mL of fetal blood with a hematocrit of 50). This dose is adequate for a routine pregnancy. However, in the setting of placental abruption or any antepartum bleeding, a Kleihauer-Betke test for the amount of fetal RBCs in the maternal circulation can be sent. If the amount of fetal RBCs is more than can be eliminated by the single RhoGAM dose, additional dosages can be given.

THE SENSITIZED Rh-NEGATIVE PATIENT

If the antibody screen for Rh comes back positive during the initial prenatal visit, the titer is checked as well. Antibody titers of 1:16 and greater have been associated with fetal hydrops. If paternity is not in question, blood type can be performed on the father of the baby to determine whether the fetus is at risk. However, because approximately 5% of all pregnancies have unknown or incorrect paternity, the safest course is to treat all pregnancies as if the fetus is at risk.

Throughout pregnancy, the antibody titer is followed approximately every 4 weeks. As long as it remains less than 1:16, the pregnancy can be managed expectantly. However, if it becomes 1:16 or greater, serial amniocentesis is begun as early as 16 to 20 weeks. At the first amniocentesis, fetal cells can be collected and analyzed for the Rh antigen to determine fetal Rh status. If negative, the pregnancy can be followed expectantly. However, if the fetus is Rh positive, fetal anemia is screened for using fetal middle cerebral artery (MCA) Doppler measurements. It was demonstrated more than a decade ago that in anemic fetuses there is greater blood flow to the brain, thus the MCA Doppler measures peak systolic velocity (PSV). In fetuses with greater PSV measurements, concern for fetal anemia merits more invasive testing and potentially treatment.

Historically, prior to the use of MCA Doppler, the evaluation of Rh-positive fetus in a Rh-negative woman with positive titers 1:16 or greater was done with serial amniocenteses to assess the amniotic fluid by a spectrophotometer. Because the breakdown products of hemoglobin include bilirubin, which discolors the amniotic fluid, the light absorption (ΔOD_{450}) by bilirubin will increase, as it is concentrated in the amniotic fluid with increasing fetal hemolysis. These measurements are plotted on the Liley curve (Fig. 7-5), which predicts the severity of disease. The curve is divided into three zones.

Zone 1 is suggestive of a mildly affected fetus, and follow-up amniocentesis can be performed approximately every 2 to 3 weeks. Zone 2 is suggestive of a moderately affected fetus, and amniocentesis should be repeated every 1 to 2 weeks. The severely affected fetus will fall into zone 3. Once in zone 3, it is likely that the fetus has anemia.

Because most centers currently screen for fetal anemia with MCA Doppler measurements of blood flow, amniocentesis has been reserved for those with questionable results or in the setting of a positive MCA Doppler screen prior to intervention. A potentially enormously beneficial procedure, percutaneous umbilical blood sampling (PUBS) and intrauterine transfusion (IUT) is the treatment of fetal anemia. PUBS can be used to obtain a fetal hematocrit to verify fetal anemia and to perform an IUT. If a PUBS or IUT cannot be performed, fetal intraperitoneal transfusion may be performed. While the risk of immediate delivery may be as high as 3%, this risk is preferred to worsening fetal anemia, hydrops, and likely fetal death.

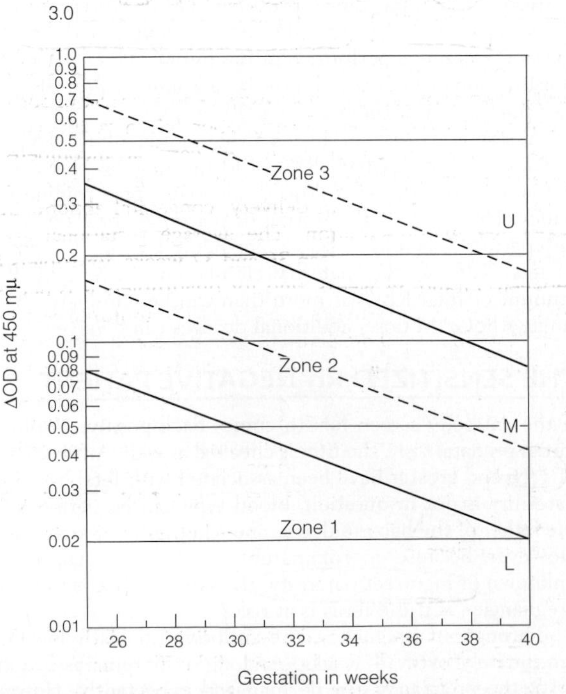

Figure 7-5 • Liley curve used to predict severity of fetal hemolysis with red cell isoimmunization.

OTHER CAUSES OF IMMUNE HYDROPS

There are a variety of other RBC antigens including the **ABO** blood type, antigens CDE in which D is the Rh antigen, **Kell**, **Duffy**, and **Lewis**. Some may cause fetal hydrops (e.g., Kell and Duffy), whereas others may lead to a mild hemolysis but not severe immune hydrops (e.g., ABO, Lewis). With the advent of treatment with RhoGAM, the incidence of Rh isoimmunization has decreased, and the other causes of immune-related fetal hydrops now account for a greater percentage of cases. Sensitized patients are managed similarly to Rh-negative patients with antibody titers, MCA Doppler measurements, PUBS, and transfusions. While most of the RBC antigens lead to a hemolytic anemia alone, anti-Kell antibodies lead also to suppression of the marrow and decreased RBC production. Thus, the advent of MCA Doppler screening has made an enormous difference in the management of such patients.

FETAL DEMISE

Intrauterine fetal demise (IUFD) is a rare but disastrous occurrence, occurring in approximately 0.5% to 1% of pregnancies overall and approximately 1:1,000 term births. The risk of IUFD increases with a variety of medical and obstetric complications of pregnancy including abruption, congenital abnormalities, infection, and postterm pregnancy. Chronic placental insufficiency secondary to rheumatologic, vascular, or hypertensive disease may lead to IUGR and eventually IUFD. When there is no explanation for a fetal demise, it is usually attributed to as "cord accident." A retained IUFD greater than 3 to 4 weeks can lead to hypofibrinogenemia secondary to the release of thromboplastic substances from the decomposing fetus. In some cases, full-blown disseminated intravascular coagulation (DIC) can result.

DIAGNOSIS

Early in pregnancy, before 20 weeks, the diagnosis of fetal death (missed abortion) is suspected by lack of uterine growth or cessation of symptoms of pregnancy. Diagnosis is confirmed with serially falling human chorionic gonadotropin (hCG) and ultrasound documentation. After week 20, fetal death is suspected with absence of fetal movement noted by the mother or absence of uterine growth. Diagnosis can be confirmed by ultrasound. Given the importance of making an appropriate, accurate diagnosis, the absence of fetal heart motion is usually verified by two clinicians.

TREATMENT

Because of the risk of DIC with retained IUFD, the best treatment is delivery. Early gestations can be evacuated from the uterus by dilation and evacuation or with mifepristone and misoprostol in some cases. After 20 weeks, the pregnancy is usually terminated by induction of labor with prostaglandins or high-dose oxytocin. Helping patients understand what may have caused the fetal death is imperative to helping them cope with the situation. Tests for causes of fetal death include screening for collagen vascular disease or hypercoagulable state, fetal karyotype, and often TORCH titers (i.e., toxoplasmosis,

RPR, CMV, and HSV). Because the cells of an IUFD will often not grow to obtain karyotype, recent studies have examined performing microarray studies of the fetal or placental genome to both look for aneuploidy, in addition to, other genetic abnormalities such as copy number variants. It is also extremely important to get an autopsy on the fetus, which can contribute valuable information. Despite this extensive battery of tests, the etiology of fetal demise will likely remain unknown in the majority of cases.

POSTTERM PREGNANCY

A postterm pregnancy is defined as one that goes beyond 42 weeks' gestational age or greater than 294 days past the last menstrual period (LMP). As many women are induced at 41 weeks of gestation, this gestation is occasionally labeled as prolonged, but 42 weeks continues to be how we define postterm pregnancy. It is estimated that 3% to 10% of all pregnancies will go postterm. This is an important obstetric issue because of the increased risk of macrosomic infants, oligohydramnios, meconium aspiration, intrauterine fetal death, and dysmaturity syndrome. There is also greater risk to the mother because of a greater rate of cesarean delivery (approximately doubled) and delivery of large infants. With improved dating, there are an increasing number of studies that show these complications of pregnancy may increase after 40 or 41 weeks of gestation.

ETIOLOGY

The most common reason for the diagnosis of postterm pregnancy is inaccurate dating; accurate dating is therefore imperative. Postterm pregnancy appears to be more common in overweight and obese women as well. Because the physiologic basis for the onset of labor is poorly understood, the mechanisms for preterm or postterm labor are also unclear. There are a few rare conditions of the fetus associated with postterm pregnancy. These include anencephaly, fetal adrenal hypoplasia, and absent fetal pituitary. All are notable for diminished levels of circulating estrogens.

DIAGNOSIS

Again, the diagnosis is made by accurate dating. Because ultrasound can be off by as much as 3 weeks near term, this cannot be used to confirm dating. Accurate dating is made by a certain LMP consistent with a first or second trimester ultrasound. Dating by a third-trimester ultrasound or unsure LMP is more suspect.

TREATMENT

The varying approaches to the postterm pregnancy generally involve more frequent visits, increased fetal testing, and plans for eventual induction. A typical plan for following a postterm pregnancy is outlined as follows:

Patients whose pregnancies go past 40 weeks of gestation usually receive an NST during the 41st week of pregnancy. Induction is indicated with nonreassuring fetal testing. During the 42nd week (between 41 and 42 weeks of gestation), the patient should be seen twice for antenatal testing. Alternatively, many practitioners use the modified BPP (an NST and AFI) for fetal testing at each visit past the due date. Because oligohydramnios is a marker for worsening placental function and would likely be seen prior to an abnormal NST, the advantage of this test is that it may improve the sensitivity for fetuses at risk for IUFD. Induction is indicated with nonreassuring fetal testing or electively with an inducible cervix (Bishop score > 6). After 42 weeks of gestation, the patient is offered induction of labor regardless of cervical examination.

In most practices, patients are offered induction of labor at 41 weeks of gestation, as a result of improved dating by ultrasound, patient demand, as well as the risk-averse environment of obstetrics. Several randomized trials have demonstrated that induction of labor at 41 weeks of gestation as compared to expectant management leads to lower rates of cesarean delivery (even with an unfavorable cervix) as well as lower rates of meconium aspiration syndrome in the neonate. The lower rate of cesarean delivery with induction of labor is counterintuitive to most clinicians and patients. However, this makes sense when one considers that the common indications for cesarean delivery (a fetus that is too big for the maternal pelvis or a nonreassuring fetal tracing) increase with increasing gestational age at term. The key is to allow active labor to ensue in an induction of labor, which can take longer than in spontaneous labor. Recent evidence suggests that active labor does not begin until at least 6 cm in induced labor.

MULTIPLE GESTATIONS

If a fertilized ovum divides into two separate ova, monozygotic, or "identical," twins result. If ovulation produces two ova and both are fertilized, dizygotic twins result. Without assisted fertility, the rate of twinning is approximately 1:80 pregnancies, with 30% of those monozygotic. The rate of dizygotic twinning varies between races and is influenced by maternal age and parity. By race/ethnicity, the frequency of dizygotic twins is lowest in Asians, intermediate in Caucasians, and higher in African Americans. The rate of naturally occurring triplets is approximately 1:7,000 to 8,000 pregnancies. However, with ovulation-enhancing drugs and in vitro fertilization (IVF), the incidence of multiple gestations is increasing.

COMPLICATIONS OF MULTIPLE GESTATIONS

Multiple gestations result in an increase in a variety of obstetric complications including preterm labor, placenta previa, cord prolapse, postpartum hemorrhage, cervical incompetence, gestational diabetes, and preeclampsia. The fetuses are at increased risk for preterm delivery, congenital abnormalities, SGA, and malpresentation. The average gestational age of delivery for twins is between 36 and 37 weeks, for triplets it is between 33 and 34 weeks, and for quadruplets it is between 28 and 29 weeks. Neonates delivered from multiple gestations weigh less than their singleton counterparts and have a greater overall mortality rate as a result of prematurity and low birth weight. Monochorionic (one placenta), diamnionic (two amniotic sacs) twins, also referred to as Mo-Di twins, often have placental vascular communications and can develop **twin-to-twin transfusion syndrome** (TTTS). Monochorionic, monoamnionic (Mo-Mo) twins have an extremely high mortality rate (reported as high as 40% to 60%) secondary to cord accidents from entanglement.

Pathogenesis

Monozygotic twinning results from division of the fertilized ovum or cells in the embryonic disk. If separation occurs before the differentiation of the trophoblast, two chorions and two amnions (Di-Di) result (Fig. 7-6). After trophoblast differentiation and before amnion formation (days 3 to 8),

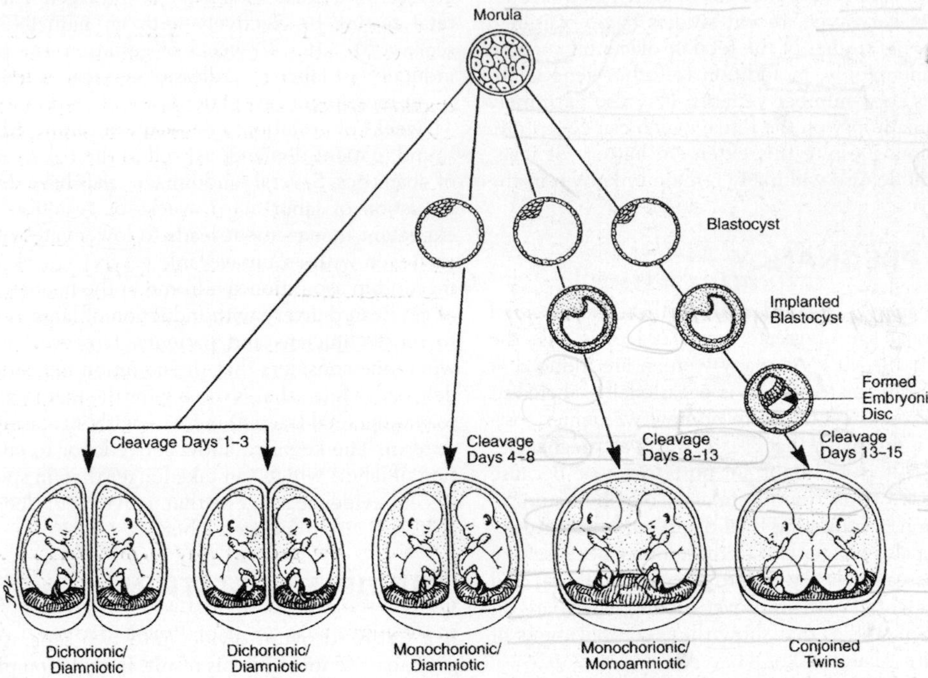

Figure 7-6 • The relationship between the timing of cleavage and the resulting amnionicity/chorionicity in monozygotic twinning.

separation leads to a single placenta, one chorion, and two amnions (Mo-Di). Division after amnion formation leads to a single placenta, one chorion, and one amnion (Mo-Mo) (days 8 to 13) and, rarely, conjoined or "Siamese" twins (days 13 to 15). Division of cells beyond day 15 or 16 will result in a singleton fetus. Monozygotic twinning does not follow any inheritable pattern and, historically, the only risk factor ever identified is a slight increase with advancing maternal age. In the 1990s it was determined that assisted reproductive techniques, while increasing the risk of dizygotic twins, also increase the risk of monozygotic twins to as high as 5%.

Dizygotic twins primarily result from fertilization of two ova by two sperm. There are varying risk factors associated with dizygotic twinning. Dizygotic twins tend to run in families and are more common in people of African descent. Globally, the rate of dizygotic twins ranges from 1:1,000 in Japan to 1:20 in several Nigerian tribes. The rate of all multiple gestations has increased sharply since the onset of medical treatment of infertility. Clomiphene citrate, a fertility-enhancing drug, increases the rate of dizygotic twinning up to 8%. The use of multiple embryos in IVF to improve the pregnancy rates also leads to increased rates of twinning and higher order multiple gestations in 30% to 50% of these pregnancies.

Diagnosis

Multiple gestations are usually diagnosed by ultrasound. Multiple gestations are indicated by rapid uterine growth, excessive maternal weight gain, or palpation of three or more fetal large parts (cranium and breech) on Leopold's. Family history and use of reproductive technology also raise suspicion for multiples. The level of β-hCG, human placental lactogen (HPL), and maternal serum a-fetoprotein (MSAFP) are all elevated for gestational age. Rarely, diagnosis will be made after delivery of the first fetus with palpation of the aftercoming fetus(es). Differentiation between Di-Di and Mo-Di twins is easier, the earlier the ultrasound is performed. For example, quite early in pregnancy, one can see a single chorion and two amniotic sacks (Fig. 7-7) indicative of Mo-Di twins. Later in pregnancy, sonologists rely on the thickness of the membrane and the "twin peak" sign (Fig. 7-8), which is formed by the two placentae fusing together in the setting of Di-Di twins. Mo-Mo twins are usually easiest as they should have no intertwin membrane.

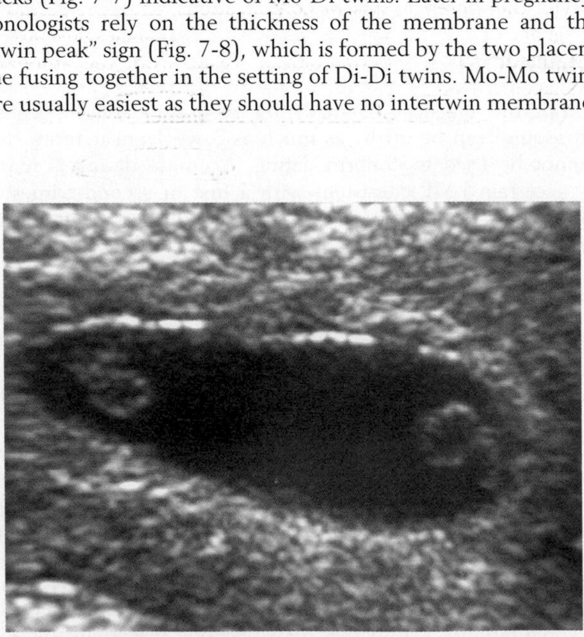

Figure 7-7 • Monochorionic–diamniotic (Mo-Di) twins. Note the single chorion, but two developing amniotic sacs.

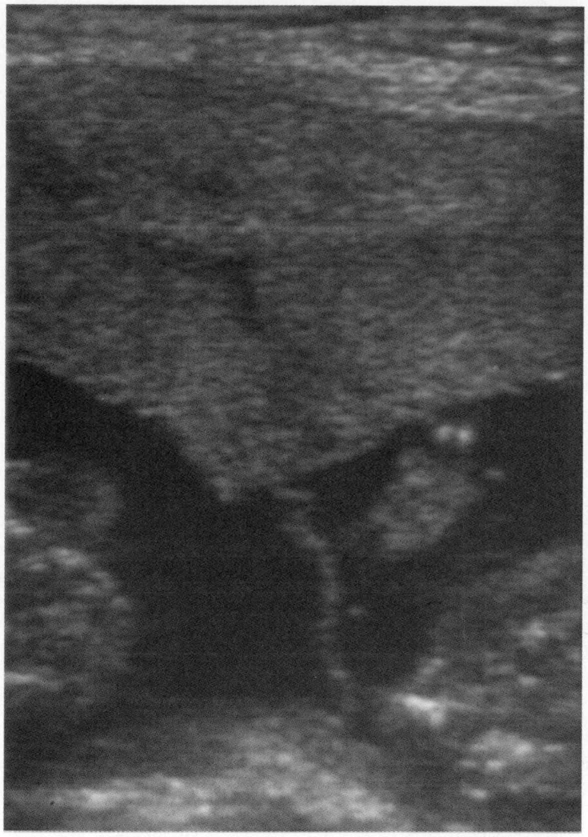

Figure 7-8 • The fused chorionic and amniotic membranes lead to the "twin peak" sign in the middle of image in Di-Di twins.

Treatment

Given the increased risk of complications, multiple-gestation pregnancies are managed as high-risk pregnancies, usually in conjunction with a perinatologist. Aside from the antenatal management of the complications, the principal issue in twin gestations is mode of delivery. With higher order multiple gestations, triplets and above, selective reduction down to twins or even a singleton, is commonly recommended. While there is a chance of losing the entire pregnancy in the setting of selective reduction, if successful, the chances of delivering a severely premature infant is also dramatically reduced. However, the question of the risks and benefits of selective reduction from twins to a singleton gestation is unanswered at this time.

TWIN-TO-TWIN TRANSFUSION SYNDROME

Polyhydramnios-oligohydramnios (poly-oli) sequence or TTTS has been described for several centuries and results in a small, anemic twin and a large, plethoric, polycythemic, and occasionally hydropic twin. The etiology of TTTS appears to be secondary to unequal flow within vascular communications between the twins in their shared placenta, leading to one twin becoming a donor, and the other a recipient of this unequal blood flow. This can result in one fetus with hypervolemia, cardiomegaly, glomerulotubal hypertrophy, edema, and ascites, and the other with hypovolemia, growth restriction, and oligohydramnios. Given the risk of this syndrome in Mo-Di twins, serial ultrasounds examining the amniotic fluid and fetal growth should be obtained every 2 weeks after diagnosis. The syndrome can present at any gestational age; however, earlier diagnosis is associated with worse outcomes.

TTTS has historically been managed with serial amnio reduction, which can reduce preterm contractions secondary to uterine distension and maternal symptoms, but only occasionally actually cures the fetal syndrome. More recently, as these vascular connections have been identified as the etiology of the syndrome, coagulating these vessels has been proposed as the treatment of choice in more severe cases. This is accomplished by fetal surgeons using a fetoscopically placed laser to coagulate the vessels. Risks of the procedure include maternal risks, loss of the pregnancy entirely, and eventual preterm delivery. Because TTTS leads to an extremely high rate of poor pregnancy outcomes, the procedure appears to be beneficial to these patients. However, because of the potential risks, pregnancy termination should always be offered as an option as well.

MO-MO TWINS

Given the risk of cord entanglement and IUFD, Mo-Mo twins are often managed with frequent antenatal testing and early delivery. Unfortunately, frequent antenatal testing has not, in and of itself, appeared to make a difference in the rate of IUFD in these cases. As a result, some patients are offered admission to the hospital and continuous electronic fetal monitoring from weeks 28 to 34, during which time delivery is performed via cesarean section. Mo-Mo and conjoined twins are almost always delivered via cesarean section.

DELIVERY OF TWINS

There are four possibilities for twin presentation: both vertex (40%), both breech, vertex then breech (40%), and breech then vertex. When deciding mode of delivery, all breech-presenting twins (20%) are considered together. Patients should be thoroughly counseled on all possible presentations and delivery options.

Vertex/vertex twins should undergo a trial of labor with cesarean section reserved for the usual indications. Vertex/nonvertex twins can also undergo a trial of labor if the twins are concordant or the presenting twin is larger. Generally, the twins should be between 1,500 and 3,500 g, though there is scant data that breech extraction between 500 and 1,500 g leads to any worse outcomes. Breech extraction for delivery of the second twin has advantages over a vertex second twin because the twin Bs lower extremity can be grasped and delivery expedited quickly. In the setting of a vertex second twin, occasionally, placental abruption occurs necessitating a rapid delivery. However, if the cervix is no longer fully dilated or the fetal vertex is above 0 station, a cesarean delivery may be necessary. External cephalic version and internal podalic version have also been used for delivery of the second twin, but in small studies lower Apgar scores have been found as compared to breech extraction. Further, the chances of failure of such maneuvers is higher. Nonvertex presenting twins are usually delivered via cesarean.

DELIVERY OF TRIPLETS

Most triplet gestations are delivered via cesarean section. Rarely, triplets will be concordant, with vertex presenting, all greater than 1,500 to 2,000 g, and a vaginal delivery can be attempted. Multiple gestations beyond triplets are all delivered via cesarean.

KEY POINTS

- Fetuses whose EFW is less than the 10th percentile are considered SGA, though the rate of poor neonatal outcomes rises significantly below the 5th and 3rd percentiles.
- Common causes of decreased growth potential include congenital abnormalities, drugs, infections, radiation, and small maternal stature.
- IUGR infants are commonly born to women with systemic diseases leading to poor placental blood flow.
- An LGA fetus has an EFW greater than the 90th percentile at any particular gestational age.
- Both 4,000 and 4,500 g have been used as the threshold for defining fetal macrosomia.
- LGA and macrosomic fetuses are at greater risk for birth trauma, hypoglycemia, jaundice, lower Apgar scores, and childhood tumors.
- Increased size in the fetus is seen with maternal diabetes, maternal obesity, increased maternal height, postterm pregnancies, multiparity, advanced maternal age, and male sex.
- Oligohydramnios is defined by an AFI of less than 5 and can be caused by decreased placental perfusion, decreased fluid production by the fetus, and ROM.
- Pregnancies at term complicated by oligohydramnios should be delivered.
- Polyhydramnios is diagnosed by an AFI greater than 20 on ultrasound and is associated with diabetes, multiple gestations, hydrops, and congenital abnormalities.
- Obstetric management of polyhydramnios should include careful verification of presentation and close observation for cord prolapse.
- Rh-sensitized women with Rh-positive fetuses have antibodies that cross the placenta, leading to hemolysis and anemia in the fetuses. If the anemia is severe enough, hydrops develops with edema, ascites, and heart failure.
- Rh-negative patients who are not sensitized should be treated with antepartum RhoGAM to prevent sensitization. Postpartum, they should receive another dose of RhoGAM if the fetus is Rh positive.
- Rh-negative patients undergoing miscarriage, abruption, amniocentesis, ectopic pregnancy, and vaginal bleeding should also be given RhoGAM.
- Rh-negative patients who are sensitized are followed closely with serial MCA Doppler velocities and ultrasound. If fetal anemia is suspected, PUBS and IUT can be performed.
- While IUFD is more common with disorders of the placenta, the actual cause of most IUFDs is usually unknown and is often attributed to cord accidents.
- Retained IUFD can lead to DIC; thus, delivery soon after diagnosis is indicated.
- Postterm pregnancy is defined as greater than 42 weeks' gestational age.
- Postterm pregnancies are at increased risk for fetal demise, macrosomia, meconium aspiration, and oligohydramnios.
- Increased fetal surveillance and labor induction are the most common management options for postterm pregnancies.
- Monozygotic twins carry identical genetic material, whereas dizygotic twins are from separate ova and sperm.
- Multiple gestations are at increased risk for preterm labor and delivery, placenta previa, postpartum hemorrhage, preeclampsia, cord prolapse, malpresentation, and congenital abnormalities.
- There is a genetic predisposition for dizygotic twinning, whereas the rate of monozygotic twinning is the same throughout all races and families.
- Monozygotic twins are at risk for TTTS and should have frequent ultrasound examinations to diagnose this early.
- Vaginal delivery of vertex/vertex presenting twins is preferred and is possible with vertex/nonvertex twins under the right circumstances. Nonvertex presenting twins are delivered by cesarean section.

C Clinical Vignettes

Vignette 1

A 23-year-old G1P0 woman at 30 weeks 3 days presents to clinic for routine prenatal care. Her pregnancy is dated by LMP consistent with a 10-week ultrasound. She has had three prenatal visits and her pregnancy has been complicated by vaginal bleeding in the first trimester and the development of heartburn at 25 weeks. She has no complaints today. She continues to smoke half a pack of cigarettes daily, which has decreased from one pack per day at the beginning of her pregnancy. Her medical history is significant for asthma. Ultrasound at 20 weeks' gestation showed no evidence of fetal abnormality, posterior placenta, AFI of 10.6, and fetal growth in the 20th percentile. Her current weight is 130 lb and her height is 5 ft 6 in. She has gained 10 lb so far in pregnancy. Urine dip is negative for protein, glucose, ketones, and leukocytes. BP is 112/64 mm Hg and heart rate is 80 bpm. Fetal heart tones are in the 130s. Fundal height measures 25 weeks. Of note, at her last visit at 25 weeks, fundal height measured 23 weeks and she had a normal glucose tolerance test and CBC.

1. Which of the following is the next best step in managing this patient's pregnancy?
   a. Nonstress test
   b. Fetal ultrasound
   c. Group B streptococcus culture
   d. TORCH titers
   e. Amniocentesis

2. Which of the following is the most likely risk factor for this patient's SGA fetus?
   a. Congenital anomaly such as cardiac anomaly
   b. Congenital cytomegalovirus infection
   c. Tobacco abuse
   d. History of chemotherapy exposure as a child
   e. Genetic potential

3. Ultrasound demonstrates that the fetus measures less than the 10th percentile for head circumference, femur length, and abdominal circumference. Doppler velocimetry of the fetal umbilical artery were normal. AFI was 11.2. Which of the following is the most appropriate component of the treatment strategy at this time?
   a. Induction of labor
   b. Continue routine prenatal care
   c. Fetal ultrasound every 2 to 3 weeks
   d. Admission to the hospital for daily NST and BPP
   e. Daily Doppler velocimetry

4. The patient has a repeat ultrasound preformed at 33 weeks gestation. Fetal growth is noted to be at the 4th percentile with intermittently elevated umbilical cord Dopplers, and an AFI of 8.4. What do you recommend at this time?
   a. Repeat growth ultrasound in 4 to 6 weeks
   b. Amniocentesis for fetal lung maturity and delivery if mature
   c. Admission to hospital for continuous fetal monitoring until delivery
   d. Induction of labor
   e. Betamethasone administration

5. The patient is admitted to the antepartum service for inpatient monitoring. Repeat ultrasound on hospital day 5 is notable for AFI of 4.3 and umbilical Doppler is elevated with absent end-diastolic flow. NST is nonreactive and a biophysical profile is six out of eight. The decision is made to induce labor. Bishop score is 2 and a Foley bulb is placed for cervical ripening. Which of the following is not a complication commonly associated with oligohydramnios in labor?
   a. Meconium amniotic fluid
   b. Cesarean delivery
   c. Fetal heart rate decelerations
   d. Cord prolapse
   e. Nonreactive fetal tracing

Vignette 2

A 38-year-old G3P2002 woman presents at 40 weeks 3 days with contractions to labor and delivery triage. Contractions started 1 hour ago and are very painful. The patient denies leaking fluid but did notice blood and mucus on her underwear. The baby has not been particularly active since contractions started. Her pregnancy has been complicated by A2GDM. Fasting blood glucose are usually between 80 and 90 mg/dL with 1-hour postprandial values between 120 and 140 mg/dL. Her prepregnancy weight was 130 lb and she is 5 ft 5 in (BMI 21.6). She has gained 30 lb this pregnancy (BMI 26.6). Hemoglobin A1C is 6.0%. Fetal ultrasound at 20 weeks demonstrated normal fetal anatomy. Repeat ultrasound for growth at 38 weeks demonstrated fetus with weight in the 90th percentile and an EFW of 4,350 g. Her last pregnancy was complicated by A1GDM and she delivered a 4,200 g infant without complications. Initial cervical examination reveals dilation of 6 cm, 50% effacement, and −1 station. Two hours later the nurse calls you to the room after the patient's water breaks. Examination shows complete dilation and effacement, and fetus at +1 station. The patient has a strong urge to push and begins pushing.

The delivery is complicated by a second=degree perineal laceration and a postpartum hemorrhage of 600 mL. Fetal weight is 4,560 g and the Apgar scores are 6, 8.

1. What neonatal risks are most commonly present in macrosomic fetuses?
1. Jaundice
2. Hypoglycemia
3. Hyperglycemia
4. Birth trauma
5. Asthma
6. Hypocalcemia

a. 1, 2, 4, 6
b. 1, 3, 4, 5
c. 3, 4, 5
d. 1, 3, 5, 6
e. 2, 4, 5, 6

2. Which of the following is most likely the cause of fetal macrosomia in this case?
a. Maternal weight gain in pregnancy
b. Gestational diabetes
c. Poor glycemic control
d. Advanced maternal age
e. Postterm pregnancy

3. The patient returns to your clinic for her 6-week postpartum visit. You ask her about contraception, and she states that she would like to have one more child in the near future. She is breastfeeding and it is going well. What do you also recommend as part of her postpartum care in this setting?
a. Immediate weight loss to 20% under prepregnancy weight
b. RPR
c. Continue insulin regimen postpartum
d. Start metformin
e. Perform a 2-hour glucose tolerance test

4. The patient returns 2 years later to your office. She is now 8 weeks 3 days pregnant by certain LMP. She weighs 160 lb (BMI 26.6). She has been very nauseated this pregnancy and is eating frequent small snacks. She has not seen a physician since her last postpartum visit with you during her last pregnancy. What test in particular do you recommend performing, in addition to, routine prenatal laboratory studies?
a. Preeclampsia panel (creatinine, AST, BUN, platelets, uric acid)
b. 24-hour urine protein collection
c. Referral for eye examination to evaluate for retinopathy
d. Glucose tolerance test
e. Hemoglobin A1C

Vignette 3

A 35-year-old woman with a history of primary infertility presents with her partner for initial prenatal visit. They had been attempting pregnancy for the past 3 years and have now conceived through IVF. She had one embryo transferred 7 weeks ago. The patient's medical history is significant for rheumatoid arthritis and polycystic ovarian syndrome. She is overweight. In reviewing their family history, she tells you that her grandmother was a twin and there is no family history of congenital abnormalities or known genetic disorders in their family. Today she reports nausea and vomiting, which is worse in the morning. She has not had any vaginal bleeding or cramping. You perform a transvaginal ultrasound and notice not one but two embryos. There appears to be a thin dividing membrane between the two. Heart rate for each embryo is around 150 bpm.

1. At what stage of division in the embryonic disc does monochorionic–diamniotic twining occur?
a. Before the differentiation of the trophoblast
b. After trophoblast differentiation and before amnion formation
c. After amnion formation
d. Not until after day 15 of development

2. During your visit with the couple, you explain to them that you will be monitoring fetal growth of their twins closely because they are at risk for SGA and twin-to-twin transfusion syndrome. You also explain that multiple gestations are at risk for preterm labor, preterm birth, placental abnormalities, cesarean section due to malpresentation, preeclampsia, and gestational diabetes. In twin-to-twin transfusion syndrome, the recipient twin may suffer from which of the following complications?
a. Fetal hydrops
b. Anemia
c. Growth restriction
d. Oligohydramnios
e. Hypovolemia

3. The couple returns for routine prenatal care at 30 weeks. The patient has been feeling well. She reports mild low back pain and fatigue. The babies are very active. The last ultrasound showed only 12% discordance in fetal weights, with baby A estimated to be 200 g larger than baby B. Baby A is currently cephalic and baby B is frank breech. The couple would like a trial of labor. You begin counseling them on the risks and benefits of vaginal birth with twins, including breech extraction, and cesarean section. In which of the following pairs would trial of labor not be recommended?
a. Twin A 2,800 g cephalic; twin B 2,650 g cephalic
b. Twin A 2,850 g cephalic; twin B 3,775 g breech
c. Twin A 3,150 g cephalic; twin B 3,010 g frank breech
d. Twin A 3,440 g cephalic; twin B 3,220 g footling breech
e. Twin A 1,645 g cephalic; twin B 1,550 g cephalic

Vignette 4

A 33-year-old G8P5116 woman with fundal height of 39 cm presents for initial prenatal visit in your clinic. She is currently an inmate at a local jail. She is imprisoned on charges of marijuana possession. She has had no prenatal care. She is unsure of her last period but reports that she started feeling the baby move approximately 5 months ago. She denies vaginal bleeding, leaking fluid, or contractions during the pregnancy. She reports using marijuana nearly daily throughout the pregnancy. She has not been taking any medications in pregnancy and has had no other exposures. The father of the baby is not involved. She does not have custody of her other children and has an open DHS case. She hopes to regain custody and is interested in drug rehabilitation. Ultrasound performed in your clinic shows gestational age to be approximately 40 weeks 3 days.

1. What is the most common cause of a diagnosis of postterm pregnancy?
a. Inaccurate dating
b. Fetal anomaly
c. Delayed presentation to prenatal care
d. Advanced maternal age
e. Multiparity

2. In a routine pregnancy, NST should be started during which week of pregnancy to monitor for fetal well-being?
a. 38
b. 39

c. 40
d. 41
e. 42

3. Postterm pregnancy is associated with all the following except
a. Transient tachypnea of the newborn
b. Oligohydramnios
c. Macrosomia
d. Meconium aspiration
e. Intrauterine fetal demise

4. You receive a call from the infirmary nurse at the jail at 4:30 PM. Your patient reports decreased fetal movement for the past 2 days. She is now 41 weeks 2 days. She had monitoring 3 days ago and fetal testing was reassuring. The nurse reports that the patient denies any contractions, leaking fluid, or vaginal bleeding. She last felt the baby move once this morning and only felt the baby move twice yesterday. What do you recommend to the nurse?
a. Perform kick counts and phone back if less than 10 movements in 2 hours
b. Schedule NST with BPP for first thing tomorrow morning
c. Schedule induction of labor tomorrow morning
d. Evaluation on labor and delivery triage as soon as possible
e. Schedule patient for evaluation in clinic first thing tomorrow morning

A Answers

Vignette 1 Question 1

Answer B: Fetal ultrasound to evaluate growth is the next best step in management. At each routine prenatal visit after 20 weeks gestation, the fundal height is measured to evaluate fetal growth. For each week of gestation over 20 weeks, the corresponding fundal height should match in centimeters. For example, at 28 weeks this patient's fundal height should be close to 28 cm. When the fundal height and gestational age are discordant by 3 or more centimeters, a fetal ultrasound is indicated to better assess fetal growth. It is also very important to reevaluate the patients' dating criteria to ensure that the growth discrepancy is not related to dating error. Fetal nonstress tests can be used to evaluate fetal well-being but not to determine fetal growth, which is most concerning at this time. Group B streptococcus cultures are collected around 35 to 36 weeks gestation or sooner if preterm birth is suspected. Intrauterine infection can lead to SGA fetuses. TORCH titers are commonly collected in the evaluation of the SGA fetus; "To" stands for toxoplasmosis, "R" for Rubella, "C" for cytomegalovirus, and "H" for herpes. Toxoplasmosis is acquired either by consuming infected undercooked meat or through contact with infected cat feces. One third of women have antibodies to toxoplasmosis indicating previous exposure. The frequency of seroconversion during pregnancy is approximately 5%. In women who are exposed to toxoplasmosis for the first time in pregnancy, rates of fetal infection are 10% to 15% in the first trimester, 25% in the second trimester, and 60% in the third trimester. While increasing gestational age is associated with increased risk of infection, the severity diminishes. Fifty-five percent to 85% infants will develop sequela to infection with toxoplasmosis, which includes IUGR, microcephaly, chorioretinitis, intracranial calcifications, hearing loss, mental retardation, hepatosplenomegaly, ascites, periventricular calcifications, ventriculomegaly and seizures. Fetal rubella infection depends on gestational age and is worse if acquired in early gestation. Fetal growth retardation is the most common effect, followed by sensorineural hearing loss, cardiac lesions and eye defects. These findings are generally only seen in fetuses infected in the first 12 weeks of gestation. Primary maternal infection with cytomegalovirus complicates 0.7% to 4% of pregnancies and results in mental retardation, microcephaly, chorioretinitis, and cerebral calcifications. It is the most common congenital infection in pregnancy. Congenital herpes virus is rare and is associated with growth restriction, eye disease, microcephaly, or hydranencephaly. Amniocentesis can be performed to evaluate for fetal chromosomal abnormalities or intrauterine infection. It is not indicated at this point in the evaluation for SGA.

Vignette 1 Question 2

Answer C: Tobacco abuse causes IUGR by directly effecting fetal growth. Tobacco use reduces uterine blood flow to the placenta and impairs fetal oxygenation. It is a major cause of growth restriction in women who are tobacco smokers. It is imperative to counsel women who smoke on the risks of IUGR and provide support for smoking cessation in pregnancy. Congenital anomalies are a cause for IUGR but are unlikely to be a major source for IUGR in this patient who had a normal ultrasound at 20 weeks. Congenital cytomegalovirus infection is less likely to be the cause of IUGR in this case. Seroconversion in the mother is more common in daycare workers, individuals of lower socioeconomic status, as well as those with increased parity, abnormal Pap smear history, and multiple sexual partners. Chemotherapy exposure during pregnancy is a known risk for IUGR. Prior history of chemotherapy should not directly impact a pregnancy. Genetic potential refers to the fetus's inherent growth potential. In this mother, we know that she is of average height and weight. Poor nutritional status can contribute to IUGR. There is not enough information to gather what the fetus's growth potential may be otherwise, and therefore, this is not the best answer.

Vignette 1 Question 3

Answer C: While no one answer is perfect; the best answer is fetal ultrasound every 2 to 3 weeks. It is important to monitor the fetus for interval growth and assure that fetal growth continues. Ultrasound is usually combined with fetal testing such as NST or BPP with AFI on a weekly or twice weekly basis. At 30 weeks of gestation, NST is not a great modality because it may be more commonly false negative (falsely nonreassuring), but it is commonly used in this setting. Induction of labor is not yet indicated at this time. Delivery is warranted when the benefits of the intrauterine environment are outweighed by the risks to the fetus. Fetal testing done with NST or BPP suggests a compromised intrauterine environment when testing indicates acidemia. A reactive NST displaying two accelerations in 20 minutes reassures the provider that the fetus is not acidotic. Similarly, an abnormal BPP can help predict the pH in an IUGR fetus. Before induction of labor of a 30-week fetus, the mother should receive betamethasone to improve fetal outcomes after birth. Given the fetus' poor growth, this patient's care is no longer routine and will require additional testing and monitoring. Admission to the hospital for daily NST and BPP is not the best answer. While this may be an option for management, it is more common to start with twice weekly testing with NST and once weekly BPP and Doppler's. If abnormal testing develops, it may become appropriate to admit the patient to the hospital for more frequent monitoring such as daily NST, twice weekly BPP, AFI and Doppler's. Doppler velocimetry is a valuable tool to try to predict placental dysfunction. Decreased oxygen delivery to the fetus can trigger changes in the vascular smooth muscle tone of the fetus. Changes in the flow resistance through the umbilical artery can be measured and used to predict fetal well-being and placental dysfunction. Late signs of dysfunction such as reversed end-diastolic flow suggest fetal acidemia and delivery is warranted. Frequent Doppler testing is only preformed when abnormalities have been identified on prior testing. In that scenario, repeat testing is done to help guide delivery planning.

Vignette 1 Question 4

Answer E: This scenario describes IUGR. Elevated Doppler of the umbilical artery and declining weight raise the concern for fetal well-being. It is possible that this patient may require premature delivery if fetal condition deteriorates further. To improve outcomes in the neonate, betamethasone should be administered at this time. Ultrasound should be repeated in 2 to 3 weeks to assess growth. Even with fetal lung maturity documented, one would not deliver on this basis alone. The decision to deliver in this setting would be based on nonreassuring fetal testing, for example, a worsening Doppler ultrasound of the umbilical artery or a nonreassuring BPP. If fetal status changes, such as absent or reversed Doppler flow, delivery will be indicated regardless of fetal lung maturity.

Vignette 1 Question 5

Answer D: Cord prolapse is not a direct consequence of oligohydramnios, nor is it strongly associated with oligohydramnios. It is seen more commonly in women with polyhydramnios. Meconium, cesarean section, fetal heart rate decelerations, and nonreactive fetal tracing are all associated with oligohydramnios in labor.

Vignette 2 Question 1

Answer A: Macrosomic neonates are most at risk for neonatal jaundice, hypoglycemia, birth trauma, hypocalcemia, and childhood cancers such as leukemia, osteosarcoma, or Wilms tumor. Asthma has not been shown to be associated with fetal macrosomia. Hypoglycemia is thought to be due to maternal hyperglycemia resulting in fetal hyperglycemia and hyperinsulinemia. Beta-cell hyperplasia also occurs, and immediately after birth when the umbilical cord is clamped, the neonate experiences a sudden drop in blood glucose likely due to an exaggerated insulin release after delivery. In macrosomic infants, as many as 50% can experience hypoglycemia and this rate is lowered to 5% to 15% when tight glucose control is achieved in the later half of pregnancy as well as during the labor process. Neonatal jaundice occurs in approximately 25% to 50% pregnancies complicated by GDM. The pathogenesis is unclear but may be related to polycythemia. Birth trauma is directly related to the risk of shoulder dystocia in mothers with diabetes and macrosomic infants. Birth injury can be a transient palsy to permanent neurologic deficits or even death.

Vignette 2 Question 2

Answer B: This mother has gestational diabetes. Fetal macrosomia complicates as many as 50% of pregnancies in women with gestational diabetes, including women treated with intensive glycemic control. The Pedersen hypothesis proposes that maternal hyperglycemia results in fetal hyperglycemia and hyperinsulinemia, which in turn results in excessive fetal growth. Although the patient gained 35 lb, it is still within the recommended weight gain guidelines of 25 to 35 lb for a women with a normal prepregnancy BMI. She actually achieved good glucose control during the pregnancy. Target fasting levels are less than 90; 1-hour postprandial values should be less than 140 and 2-hour postprandial values less than 120. However,

even with reasonable control, women with GDM are at increased risk of having a fetus with macrosomia. Advanced maternal age has been found to be associated with macrosomia but may be related due to an increased rate of diabetes in older women. Postterm pregnancies are at increased risk for fetal macrosomia due to the additional time in utero that the fetus has to grow. However, postterm is beyond 42 weeks' gestation.

Vignette 2 Question 3

Answer E: Perform a 2-hour glucose tolerance test. Women who develop GDM are at increased risk of developing type 2 diabetes later in life. All women with GDM should have a 2-hour glucose challenge test at or around their 6-week postpartum visit. It is best to actually give the patient the laboratory slip to obtain the test prior to the 6-week follow-up visit so that the results can be discussed at the visit. This test helps to identify those women who either have type 2 diabetes or who remain at high risk due to insulin insensitivity. Education, diet, and exercise are mainstay treatments to improve insulin sensitivity. While this patient should eventually lose weight down to and even slightly below her prepregnancy weight, this does not need to occur immediately. She does not need to lose 20% of her body weight, which would potentially make her underweight. Weight loss can be challenging after childbirth and breastfeeding is a very effective way for women to return toward their prepregnancy weight in the postpartum period. The RPR is often obtained twice during pregnancy, but not needed postpartum. Once the placenta is delivered, the patient's insulin demands decline dramatically. For type 1 and type 2 diabetic patients, prepregnancy doses of insulin are resumed. For patients with gestational diabetes, all medications are stopped. It is not standard of care to continue GDM patients on anti-hyperglycemic medications unless there is a suspicion for type 2 diabetes or they have a diagnostic 2-hour glucose tolerance test.

Vignette 2 Question 4

Answer D: In patients with a history of gestational diabetes, it is valuable to perform an early glucose tolerance test to evaluate for type 2 diabetes. Because she has not had any routine health care in the past 2 years, she has not been screened for development of diabetes. Early diagnosis improves outcomes because patients can be educated on diet and started on insulin-lowering medications if indicated. If the patient has elevated blood glucose values that suggest type 2 diabetes, then answer options a, b, c, and e should be performed for the patient at that time. In patients with type 2 diabetes, eye examination is recommended to evaluate for retinopathy, which can worsen in pregnancy. *2-3d dicho*

2-3d dichо
3-8d monodiordiam
8-15d mono mon.

Vignette 3 Question 1

Answer B: Monochorionic–diamniotic twinning results from cleavage between 3 and 8 days and occurs after placental differentiation has occurred but prior to amnion formation. This leads to the formation of a single placenta but two amnions. Dichorionic–diamniotic twins result from cleavage of the fertilized ovum during the first 2 to 3 days. Cleavage at this stage occurs before cells are differentiated to form the trophoblast. As a result, two placentas (chorions) and two amnions develop. Embryo cleavage between days 8 and 13 again occurs after differentiation of the trophoblast but also after formation of the amnion. This results in a monochorionic and monoamniotic gestation. After day 15 of development, only a singleton pregnancy will result.

Vignette 3 Question 2

Answer A: TTTS is characterized by one twin who is the donor and the other who is the recipient. The placenta has shared vascular connections between monochorionic twins and in some gestations these connections are markedly unequal and result in one twin receiving more blood flow than the other. The donor twin is typically smaller, anemic, and has less amniotic fluid, which can lead to hypovolemia, growth restriction, and oligohydramnios. The recipient twin is generally larger, polycythemic, and occasionally hydropic as the result of hypervolemia. Cardiomegaly and glomerulotubal hypertrophy, edema, and ascites result. Monitoring for development of TTTS is recommended early in the gestation and ultrasounds to assess fetal growth should occur every 2 weeks starting around 16 weeks. About 15% monochorionic twins will develop TTTS. The earlier it is diagnosed, the poorer the prognosis. The mainstay of treatment of severe cases of TTTS today is laser ablation of placental anastomoses with perinatal survival rates between 53% and 69%. Other treatments include serial reduction amniocentesis and amniotic septostomy. Anemia, growth restriction, oligohydramnios, and hypovolemia are all findings in the donor twin.

Vignette 3 Question 3

Answer B: In this answer, twin A is 925 g smaller than twin B, so more than 20% discordant (925/3,775). For twins, if both are cephalic, vaginal delivery is usually reasonable to attempt. However, with vertex/breech twins, the second twin should not be more than 20% discordant; if the second twin is significantly larger than the first, then there can be head entrapment during the breech extraction. In fact, some clinicians are uncomfortable with offering breech extraction of the second twin if it is even slightly larger than the first. In all cases, counseling and informed consent should include discussion of the possible need for an emergent cesarean delivery of the second twin should cord prolapse, fetal distress, or placental abruption occur and delivery not be imminent. Answer options a, c, d, and e are appropriate scenarios for a trial of labor.

Vignette 4 Question 1

Answer A: The most common reason for postterm pregnancy is inaccurate dating. It is very common for a woman to be uncertain of the first date of her LMP. As a result, we must rely on ultrasound for dating the pregnancy and ultrasound is not without errors. Ultrasound dating is best when performed in the first trimester and may have up to a 1 week error in either direction of the proposed due date. For pregnancies dated during the second trimester, the error may be as great at 2 weeks and in the third trimester, as much as 3 weeks. Fetal anomaly is occasionally a cause of postterm pregnancy but is not the most common cause. Delayed presentation to prenatal care is a problem that contributes to delayed and inaccurate dating, but is not the most specific answer in this case. AMA and multiparity do not contribute to postterm pregnancy.

Vignette 4 Question 2

Answer D: NSTs are generally not indicated in a routine pregnancy until the pregnancy goes into the 41st week. Therefore, in a routine pregnancy, a patient is usually scheduled for an NST during the 41st week, which is between the 40 0/7 and 41 0/7 weeks' gestation. If the pregnancy continues into the 42nd week, in other words between 41 and 42 weeks, the patient should receive an NST twice during that week as well as a biophysical profile on one of the visits. If nonreassuring testing is identified, induction of labor is initiated.

Vignette 4 Question 3

Answer A: Postterm pregnancy is not associated with transient tachypnea of the newborn, which is seen more commonly in cesarean deliveries and in early term births at 37 and 38 weeks of gestation. Oligohydramnios, macrosomia, meconium aspiration, and intrauterine fetal demise are all risks associated with postterm pregnancy.

Vignette 4 Question 4

Answer D: The patient should be seen on labor and delivery triage as soon as possible. Given her gestational age and risk for adverse pregnancy outcome, it is best to perform monitoring this evening. Delayed care could have disastrous consequences. In patients less than 40 weeks, it may be acceptable to have them perform kick counts at home prior to presentation. Kick counts involve the women resting in a quiet room and counting fetal movements over time. In general, 6 movements in the first hour or 10 movements in 2 hours suggest reassuring fetal status. However, while widely used, there is not strong evidence to support the use of kick counts in predicting fetal well-being. Answer options b, c, and e all delay presentation and evaluation of fetal well-being and are therefore not the best answer choices. At 41 2/7 weeks, even if the fetal testing were reassuring, it would be reasonable to recommend induction of labor in this setting.

Hypertension and Pregnancy

Invasion of trophoblast into myometrium.

↑ thromboxane ↓ prostacyclin form not as much

Blood pressure (BP) routinely decreases during pregnancy. As a result of decreased systemic vascular resistance, the BP decreases in the latter half of the first trimester, reaching its nadir in the mid-second trimester. During the third trimester, BP will slowly increase back to baseline, but should not be higher than that during prepregnancy. The categories of hypertension in pregnancy are stratified between chronic hypertension and hypertension specific to pregnancy. Chronic hypertension is seen increasingly in pregnancy and is associated with a number of complications of pregnancy. Alternatively, hypertension may be caused by the pregnancy as with gestational hypertension (GH), preeclampsia, and eclampsia (Table 8-1). Liver injury is seen in a small percentage of patients with preeclampsia and is associated with two diseases in pregnancy with high morbidity and mortality: HELLP syndrome (hemolysis, elevated liver enzymes, low platelets) and acute fatty liver of pregnancy (AFLP). Complications from these disorders are consistently among the leading causes of maternal death in both developed and developing countries. Because treatment is delivery, these disorders are also the leading causes of premature delivery.

HELLP AFLP

PREECLAMPSIA

PATHOGENESIS

Historically, preeclampsia was diagnosed by the presence of nondependent edema, hypertension, and proteinuria in the pregnant woman. While this triad is typically how women present, nondependent edema is no longer a component of the diagnosis. The classic presentation is of a nulliparous woman in her third trimester. Although no definitive cause for preeclampsia has been determined, it is well-accepted that the underlying pathophysiology involves a generalized arteriolar constriction (vasospasm) and intravascular depletion secondary to a generalized transudative edema that can produce symptoms related to ischemia, necrosis, and hemorrhage of organs. Thus, one of the fundamental aspects of the disease is vascular damage and an imbalance in the relative concentrations of prostacyclin and thromboxane. It is theorized that this is primarily related to circulating antibodies or antigen—antibody complexes (not unlike systemic lupus erythematosus) that damage the endothelial lining of vessel walls leading to exposure of the underlying collagen structure. The hyperdynamic state of pregnancy has also been proposed to cause this underlying vascular injury rather than an immunogenic phenomenon.

As outlined in Table 8-2, major fetal complications of preeclampsia are due to prematurity. Also, the generalized vasoconstriction of preeclampsia can result in decreased blood flow to the placenta. This may manifest as acute uteroplacental insufficiency, resulting in abruption or fetal hypoxia. The uteroplacental insufficiency may also be chronic in nature and result in an intrauterine growth restricted (IUGR) fetus.

Maternal complications associated with preeclampsia (Table 8-3) are related to the generalized arteriolar vasoconstriction that affects the brain (seizure and stroke), kidneys (oliguria and renal failure), lungs (pulmonary edema), liver (edema and subcapsular hematoma), and small blood vessels (thrombocytopenia and disseminated intravascular coagulation [DIC]). Severe preeclampsia is diagnosed with severely elevated BPs, defined as systolic blood pressure (SBP) greater than 160 mm Hg or diastolic blood pressure (DBP) greater than 110 mm Hg, or the presence of any of the above clinical findings.

About 10% of patients with severe preeclampsia develop HELLP syndrome. HELLP syndrome is a subcategory of preeclampsia in which the patient presents with hemolysis, elevated liver enzymes, and low platelets. Hypertension and proteinuria may be minimal in these patients. HELLP syndrome is uncommon, but patients who experience it decline rapidly, resulting in poor maternal and fetal outcomes. Despite careful management, HELLP syndrome results in a high rate of stillbirth (10% to 15%) and neonatal death (20% to 25%).

EPIDEMIOLOGY *6%*

Preeclampsia occurs in 5% to 6% of all live births and can develop any time after the 20th week, but is most commonly seen in the third trimester near term. When hypertension is seen early in the second trimester (14 to 20 weeks), a hydatidiform mole or previously undiagnosed chronic hypertension should be considered. Unlike other preeclamptic patients, the patient with HELLP is more likely to be less than 36 weeks' gestation at the time of presentation. Although 80% of patients develop HELLP after being diagnosed with preeclampsia (30% with mild preeclampsia; 50% with severe preeclampsia), 20% of patients with HELLP have no previous history of hypertension before their diagnosis and will present merely with the symptom of right upper-quadrant (RUQ) pain. Thus, any patient who presents with RUQ pain, epigastric pain, or nausea and vomiting in the third trimester should be seen immediately to rule out HELLP.

RISK FACTORS

Risk factors for preeclampsia fall essentially into two categories: those related to the manifestations of the disease (like chronic hypertension or renal disease) and those related to the immunogenic nature of preeclampsia (Table 8-4). African American race has been put into the disease manifestations category, as these women are more likely to have chronic hypertension, obesity, and type 2 diabetes, all of which are

■ **TABLE 8-1** Hypertensive States of Pregnancy
GH (or pregnancy-induced hypertension)
Preeclampsia
Severe preeclampsia
Chronic hypertension
Chronic hypertension w/superimposed preeclampsia
HELLP syndrome
AFLP

■ **TABLE 8-3** Maternal Complications of Preeclampsia
Medical manifestations
Seizure
Cerebral hemorrhage
DIC and thrombocytopenia
Renal failure
Hepatic rupture or failure
Pulmonary edema
Obstetric complications
Uteroplacental insufficiency
Placental abruption
Increased premature deliveries
Increased cesarean section deliveries

underdiagnosed and associated with preeclampsia. The risk factors posited to be immunogenic are particularly interesting. For example, it has been shown that in addition to a family history in the parturient, if the mother of the father of her baby (mother-in-law) had preeclampsia, the patient is at greater risk of developing preeclampsia. Further, it has been demonstrated that parental ethnic discordance slightly increases the risk of developing preeclampsia. While multiparous women who have not had preeclampsia in the past have a decreased risk, if a woman conceives with a new father of her baby, her risk increases back to that of a nullipara. A tolerance effect is seen in women who cohabitate with the father of the baby longer than 1 year prior to conceiving in comparison to women who conceive sooner. These risk factors support the theory that preeclampsia has an alloimmunogenic pathophysiology. Interestingly, smoking appears to be associated with a decreased risk of preeclampsia, a phenomenon which has not been explained.

CLINICAL MANIFESTATIONS AND DIAGNOSES

Gestational Hypertension

BPs elevated above 140/90 mm Hg are necessary to diagnose GH (formerly known as pregnancy-induced hypertension [PIH]). BPs should be elevated on at least two occasions 4 to 6 hours apart and taken while the patient is seated. The patient's position is important while a patient is being evaluated because when patients lie in the supine position on their side, this lowers their BP. While this might seem helpful to manage the patient's hypertension, it is not appropriate in the assessment of hypertension as the BP should be taken in the seated position to obtain the most accurate reading. In the past, an increase of 30 mm Hg above prepregnancy systolic BP or 15 mm Hg above prepregnancy diastolic BP was utilized to identify GH, in addition to a SBP greater than 140 mmHg or a DBP greater than 90 mmHg. This distinction is no longer recognized as diagnostic but should still be documented as it is clinically important. If the patient's 24-hour urinary protein total is less than 300 mg, then preeclampsia is ruled out and the patient can be managed expectantly. Because it is believed that preeclampsia is part of a continuum from GH through severe disease, these patients are at risk for developing preeclampsia and should be followed closely with frequent BP checks, laboratory tests, and antenatal fetal testing.

■ **TABLE 8-2** Fetal Complications of Preeclampsia
Complications related to prematurity (if early delivery is necessary)
Acute uteroplacental insufficiency
Placental infarct and/or abruption
Intrapartum fetal distress
Stillbirth (in severe cases)
Chronic uteroplacental insufficiency
Asymmetric and symmetric SGA fetuses
IUGR
Oligohydramnios

■ **TABLE 8-4** Risk Factors for Preeclampsia
Primarily disease related
Chronic hypertension
Chronic renal disease
Collagen vascular disease (e.g., SLE)
Pregestational diabetes
African American
Maternal age (<20 or >35)
Primarily immunogenic related
Nulliparity
Previous preeclampsia
Multiple gestation
Abnormal placentation
New paternity
Family history
Female relatives of parturient
Mother-in-law
Cohabitation <1 y

Mild Preeclampsia

As shown in Table 8-5, mild preeclampsia is classically defined as a third-trimester BP greater than 140 mm Hg systolic or 90 mm Hg diastolic on two occasions, at least 6 hours apart, accompanied by proteinuria greater than 300 mg/24 hours and nondependent edema (face and/or hands). It has been determined that edema is not essential to the diagnosis of preeclampsia, but the occurrence of hypertension and proteinuria is diagnostic. If a diagnosis is being made in the acute setting, proteinuria of 1+ or greater on a clean catch urine dipstick on two occasions has also been used to diagnose proteinuria. Of note, women with 2+ or greater have been demonstrated to have significant proteinuria, greater than 300 mg/24 hours, well above 90% of the time. While an abnormal urine dip for protein is concerning for preeclampsia, a negative urine dip should be less reassuring in the setting of hypertension. In one study, more than two-thirds of patients with elevated BPs and negative or trace on urine dip had greater than 300 mg of protein on a 24 hour urine collection of urine protein and all patients with 3+ and 4+ protein on urine dip had significant proteinuria on a 24 hour urine protein. A better predictor of significant proteinuria than the urine clean catch dip is a spot urine protein-to-creatinine ratio. Because creatinine excretion is relatively constant, this ratio gives a rough estimate of the amount of protein that will be excreted over a 24-hour period. A spot urine P/C ratio of 0.2 to 0.3 is concerning for preeclampsia and should prompt further evaluation, including a 24 hour urine protein collection.

TABLE 8-5 Criteria for Diagnosis of Gestational Hypertension, Preeclampsia, and Eclampsia

Gestational hypertension
BP: SBP >140 mm Hg or DBP >90 mm Hg
Mild preeclampsia
BP: SBP >140 mm Hg or DBP >90 mm Hg
Proteinuria: >300 mg/24 h or >1 to 2> on dipstick
Severe preeclampsia (by systems)
Neuro: severe headache (not relieved by acetaminophen)
Visual changes; scotomata
Cardiovascular: SBP ≥160 mm Hg or DBP ≥110 mm Hg
Pulmonary: Pulmonary edema
Renal: Acute renal failure with rising creatinine
Oliguria <500 mL/24 h
Proteinuria: 24-h urine protein of ≥5 g or >3+ on dipstick
GI: RUQ pain
Elevation of transaminases, AST and ALT
Heme: hemolytic anemia
Thrombocytopenia: <100,000 platelets/mL
DIC
Fetal: IUGR, abnormal umbilical Dopplers
Eclampsia
Seizure

Severe Preeclampsia

Criteria for severe preeclampsia (Table 8-5) include: BP greater than 160 mm Hg systolic or 110 mm Hg diastolic on two occasions at least 6 hours apart, accompanied by proteinuria greater than 5 g/24 hours (or 3 to 4+ protein on dipstick on two occasions), or signs/symptoms of severe preeclampsia. Signs and symptoms of severe preeclampsia include: altered consciousness, headache or visual changes, epigastric or RUQ pain, significantly impaired liver function (greater than two times normal), oliguria (< 400 mL in 24 hour), pulmonary edema, and significant thrombocytopenia (< 100,000/mm^3). Thus, if a patient with mild preeclampsia by BP and laboratory parameters develops any of these signs or symptoms, she should be considered to have severe preeclampsia and managed accordingly. Many clinical manifestations of preeclampsia are explained by vasospasm leading to necrosis and hemorrhage of organs.

HELLP Syndrome

The disorder is characterized by rapidly deteriorating liver function and thrombocytopenia. In addition, a number of patients will develop DIC. The criteria for diagnosis and relevant laboratory tests are outlined in Table 8-6. Liver capsule distension produces epigastric pain, often with progressive nausea and vomiting and can lead to hepatic rupture. Patients with HELLP syndrome who present with frank hepatic failure should be screened for acute fatty liver of pregnancy (AFLP).

Acute Fatty Liver of Pregnancy

It is unclear whether AFLP is truly in the spectrum of preeclamptic syndromes or an entirely separate entity with similar signs and symptoms. More than 50% of patients with AFLP will also have hypertension and proteinuria. It presents in approximately 1 in 10,000 pregnancies and has a high mortality rate. Interestingly, it has been found that a number of AFLP patients will have fetuses with long-chain hydroxyacyl-CoA dehydrogenase (LCHAD) deficiency. To differentiate AFLP from HELLP, laboratory tests associated with liver failure such as an elevated ammonia level, blood glucose less than 50 mg/dL, and markedly reduced fibrinogen and antithrombin III levels have been associated with AFLP. Management of these patients is supportive and, while liver transplant has been used, some studies have reported that AFLP can be treated in many patients without requiring this aggressive intervention.

TABLE 8-6 Diagnosis of HELLP Syndrome

Hemolytic anemia
Schistocytes on peripheral blood smear
Elevated lactate dehydrogenase
Elevated total bilirubin
Elevated liver enzymes
Increase in aspartate aminotransferase
Increase in alanine aminotransferase
Low platelets
Thrombocytopenia

TREATMENT

Mild Preeclampsia

Because delivery is the ultimate treatment of preeclampsia, induction of labor is the treatment of choice for pregnancies at term, unstable preterm pregnancies, or pregnancies where there is evidence of fetal lung maturity. In these cases, vaginal delivery may be attempted with the assistance of prostaglandins, Foley bulb, oxytocin, or amniotomy as needed. Cesarean delivery need only be performed for obstetric indications. For stable preterm patients, bed rest and expectant management is the most commonly employed management plan until effecting delivery at 37 weeks' gestation or until delivery is otherwise indicated. Expectant management most commonly takes place in the hospital setting, though for very stable patients outpatient management, with frequent laboratory and fetal testing, is an option. Betamethasone is given to enhance fetal lung maturity. Patients with mild preeclampsia are often, though not always, started on magnesium sulfate therapy for seizure prophylaxis during labor and delivery, and should be continued for 12 to 24 hours after delivery. A large, multinational study demonstrated excellent seizure prophylaxis with a 4 g load and 1 g/hour maintenance, however, some institutions still use a 4 or 6 g load and 2 g/hour maintenance regimen.

Severe Preeclampsia

The goals of treatment in severe preeclampsia are to prevent eclampsia, control maternal BP, and deliver the fetus. However, management varies depending on gestational age. Initially, patients with severe preeclampsia should be stabilized using magnesium sulfate for seizure prophylaxis and hydralazine (a direct arteriolar dilator) or labetalol (beta and alpha blockade) for BP control. Once the patient is stabilized, if the gestational age is between 24 and 32 weeks, expectant management to allow time for treatment with betamethasone and further fetal maturity is often used. Beyond 32 weeks of gestation or in a severe preeclamptic patient with signs of renal failure, pulmonary edema, hepatic injury, HELLP syndrome, or DIC, delivery should ensue immediately.

Even though delivery is the cure for preeclampsia, patients can have lingering effects for up to several weeks. In fact, some patients will worsen acutely in the immediate postpartum period, possibly due to the increased placental antigen exposure during labor and delivery. Because of this, seizure prophylaxis is usually continued 24 hours postpartum or until the patient improves markedly. In the setting of chronically elevated BPs, antihypertensive medications (most commonly labetalol and nifedipine) should be used and, in some cases, patients may need to continue medications for several weeks after release to home. Patients with HELLP syndrome may have worsening thrombocytopenia, and it has been shown that corticosteroid treatment can decrease the amount of time until the nadir and return to normal levels.

Follow-Up

Women who develop preeclampsia during their first pregnancy will have a 25% to 33% recurrence rate in subsequent pregnancies. In patients with both chronic hypertension and preeclampsia, the risk of recurrence is 70%. Low doses of aspirin prior to and during subsequent pregnancies to decrease the risk of preeclampsia, IUGR, and preterm deliveries have been studied. While this appeared to be a promising treatment in smaller, nonrandomized studies, larger studies have shown mixed outcomes. Calcium supplementation has also been associated with decreased rates of subsequent preeclampsia, but one large randomized controlled trial found no difference between calcium and placebo.

ECLAMPSIA

Eclampsia is the occurrence of grand mal seizures in the preeclamptic patient that cannot be attributed to other causes (Table 8-5). Although patients with severe preeclampsia are at greater risk for developing seizures, 25% of women with eclampsia were originally found to have only mild preeclampsia before the onset of seizures. Of note, eclampsia may also occur without proteinuria. Complications of eclampsia include cerebral hemorrhage, aspiration pneumonia, hypoxic encephalopathy, and thromboembolic events.

CLINICAL MANIFESTATIONS

Seizures in the eclamptic patient are tonic—clonic in nature and may or may not be preceded by an aura. These seizures may develop before labor (25%), during labor (50%), or after delivery (25%). Most postpartum seizures occur within the first 48 hours after delivery, but will occasionally occur as late as several weeks after delivery.

TREATMENT

Treatment strategies for eclamptic patients include seizure management, BP control, and prophylaxis against further convulsions. Seizure management should always start with the ABCs (airway, breathing, circulation), though the majority of seizures are unwitnessed by clinicians and will resolve spontaneously without major morbidity. Hypertension management can usually be achieved using hydralazine to lower the BP. For seizure control and prophylaxis, eclamptic patients are treated with magnesium sulfate ($MgSO_4$) to decrease hyperreflexia and prevent further seizures by raising the seizure threshold. In prospective, randomized studies, magnesium has been found to be as good as or better than phenytoin, carbamazepine, and phenobarbital in the prevention of recurrent seizures in eclamptic patients. In eclampsia, $MgSO_4$ therapy is initiated at the time of diagnosis and continued for 12 to 24 hours after delivery. The goal of magnesium sulfate therapy is to reach a therapeutic level while avoiding toxicity through careful clinical monitoring (Table 8-7). In the case of overdose, 10 mL

TABLE 8-7 Clinical Response to Serum Magnesium Sulfate Concentrations

Serum Concentration $MgSO_4$ (mg/mL)	Clinical Response
4.8–8.4	Therapeutic seizure prophylaxis
8	CNS depression
10	Loss of deep tendon reflexes
15	Respiratory depression/ paralysis
17	Coma
20–25	Cardiac arrest

10% calcium chloride or calcium gluconate should be rapidly administered intravenously for cardiac protection.

Delivery should be initiated only after the eclamptic patient has been stabilized and convulsions have been controlled. It is common for prolonged fetal heart rate decelerations to occur in the setting of an eclamptic seizure. The most appropriate way to treat the fetus is to stabilize the mother by establishing adequate maternal oxygenation and cardiac output. Occasionally, the fetal heart rate abnormalities will not resolve and emergent cesarean delivery will be necessary. Otherwise, cesarean delivery should be reserved for obstetric indications and such patients can undergo an induction of labor after they are stabilized.

CHRONIC HYPERTENSION

PATHOGENESIS

Chronic hypertension is defined as hypertension present before conception, before 20 weeks' gestation, or persisting more than 6 weeks postpartum. For women who present without prenatal care prior to 20 weeks of gestation, this can be difficult to differentiate from GH. Approximately one-third of patients with chronic hypertension in pregnancy will develop superimposed preeclampsia. Because of poor vascular development, the fetus may suffer from IUGR and the mother is at increased risk for superimposed preeclampsia, premature delivery, and abruptio placentae.

TREATMENT

Treatment of mild chronic hypertension is controversial. However, patients with controlled BPs tend to have fewer complications in pregnancy. Patients with chronic hypertension whose BPs in early pregnancy are consistently 140/90 mm Hg or less can be managed expectantly. Antihypertensives are used in patients with persistently elevated BPs or in those who were already on medications prior to pregnancy. The two most common medications used are labetalol (a beta-blocker with concomitant alpha blockade) and nifedipine (a peripheral calcium channel blocker). In retrospective studies, beta-blocker use has been associated with decreased birth weight. However, these studies are likely biased by the severity of disease. Methyldopa (a central alpha-adrenergic agonist) has been the drug of choice in such patients for several decades. It has not been shown to effectively manage BP or change outcomes, so its use has decreased.

Because these patients are at risk for other complications of chronic hypertension, a baseline 24-hour urine collection for creatinine clearance and protein should be obtained. This will also help differentiate superimposed preeclampsia from chronic renal disease later in pregnancy. It also important to get a baseline ECG in patients with chronic hypertension to ensure that there is no current cardiac compromise requiring further evaluation. Low-dose aspirin may decrease the risk of developing superimposed preeclampsia and is used by some practitioners.

Superimposed Preeclampsia

One-third or more of patients with chronic hypertension will develop superimposed preeclampsia. Because the hypertension is longstanding, complications such as IUGR and placental abruption are more common. The diagnosis can sometimes be difficult to make because many of these patients will have concomitant renal disease at baseline. An increase in the SBP of 30 mm Hg or in the SBP of 15 mm Hg over prepregnancy BP is also indicative of superimposed preeclampsia, but experts disagree on how to use BP changes in the diagnosis of superimposed preeclampsia. If a 24-hour urine protein becomes elevated greater than 300mg/24 hours, the diagnosis is clearly super-imposed preeclampsia; if not, then the BP can be managed with increasing dosages of medications. In patients who have baseline renal disease as well, an elevated uric acid above 6.0 to 6.5 is sometimes used to differentiate preeclampsia from exacerbation of hypertension. Of course, if any of the severe preeclampsia signs and symptoms are present, this points to a diagnosis of severe superimposed preeclampsia.

KEY POINTS

- Preeclampsia is the presence of hypertension (>140/90 mm Hg) and proteinuria (> 300 mg/24 hours).
- Preeclampsia has an incidence of 5% to 6% of all live births and occurs most commonly in nulliparous women in their third trimester.
- Preeclampsia is characterized by generalized multiorgan vasospasm that can lead to seizure, stroke, renal failure, liver damage, DIC, or fetal demise.
- Risk factors for preeclampsia include nulliparity, multiple gestation, and chronic hypertension.
- Preeclampsia is ultimately treated with delivery, but seizures can be prevented with magnesium sulfate and BPs can be controlled with antihypertensive medications.
- Eclampsia is the occurrence of grand mal seizures in the preeclamptic patient that cannot be attributed to other causes.
- Patients present with eclamptic seizures occurring before labor (25%), during labor (50%), or after delivery (25%).
- Eclampsia is treated with seizure management and prophylaxis with magnesium sulfate, hypertension management with hydralazine, and delivery only after the patient has been stabilized.
- Chronic hypertension is defined as hypertension occurring before conception, before 20 weeks' gestation, or persisting more than 6 weeks postpartum.
- Chronic hypertension leads to superimposed preeclampsia in one-third of patients.
- Chronic hypertension is generally treated with antihypertensives, commonly nifedipine or labetalol.
- A baseline ECG and 24-hour urine collection for protein and creatinine should be performed.

C Clinical Vignettes

Vignette 1

A 36-year-old G2P1001 woman at 12 weeks' gestation presents to clinic for routine prenatal visit. She reports her nausea has resolved and denies vaginal bleeding. Her pregnancy has been uncomplicated. Her prior pregnancy 2 years ago was complicated by the diagnosis of GH that led to an induction of labor and cesarean delivery. She has no other medical history. On examination her BP is 138/84 mm Hg, her body mass index (BMI) is 36 kg/m, and a urine dip shows trace protein.

1. Given her history of gestational hypertension (GH) and the BP today, what diagnosis is most likely?
   a. Gestational diabetes
   b. GH
   c. Preeclampsia
   d. Chronic hypertension
   e. HELLP syndrome

2. Which of the following laboratory tests should be ordered today?
   a. Quad screen
   b. 24-hour urine protein collection
   c. HgbA1c
   d. LDL
   e. HSV titer

3. Which of the following pregnancy complications is not associated with chronic hypertension?
   a. Superimposed preeclampsia
   b. Placental abruption
   c. Placenta previa
   d. Preterm delivery
   e. Intrauterine growth restriction

4. The patient's 24-hour urine shows 100 mg of protein. You counsel the patient on the pregnancy complications associated with chronic hypertension as well as management. What is the next best step in her management?
   a. Expectant management with close observation for early signs of preeclampsia and fetal growth restriction
   b. Start antihypertensive therapy
   c. Hospitalization for further maternal and fetal testing
   d. Bed rest
   e. Recommend termination of pregnancy

Vignette 2

A 17-year-old G1P0 woman presents at 25 weeks' gestation complaining of headache for the past 36 hours. She has had regular prenatal visits going back to her first prenatal visit at 8 weeks' gestation. A 20-week ultrasound redated her pregnancy by 2 weeks as it was 15 days earlier than her LMP dating. She has a BP of 155/104 mm Hg.

1. Which of the following is the most important question to ask on history?
   a. Do you have heartburn?
   b. Do you have low back pain?
   c. Are you constipated?
   d. Do you have pain in your right upper abdomen?
   e. Do you have urinary frequency?

2. Which of the following would NOT help to determine her diagnosis?
   a. Baseline or prepregnancy BP
   b. Bilirubin levels
   c. Urine dip for protein
   d. CBC
   e. AST and ALT

3. You review her medical record and determine that she does not have chronic hypertension. The patient denies having RUQ pain but because of your high suspicion of severe preeclampsia you order a CBC, liver enzymes, renal function test, and a 24-hour urine protein collection. Her laboratory test results reveal a normal platelet count and liver enzymes but a slightly elevated creatinine and proteinuria of 550 mg in 24 hours. Her headache has resolved after a dose of acetaminophen. What is the next best step in her management?
   a. Give her a prescription for labetalol and have her follow-up in clinic in 2 weeks
   b. (a) plus bed rest
   c. Hospitalization for further evaluation and treatment
   d. Immediate delivery
   e. Begin induction of labor

4. Over the next 12 hours, her SBPs rise above 160 mm Hg on several occasions, most notably to 174/102 mm Hg 2 hours after admission and to 168/96 mm Hg 9 hours after admission. Her headache does not return and she has no RUQ pain

or visual symptoms. A set of repeat laboratory test results are unchanged and by increasing her labetalol dose to 400 mg TID, her BPs decrease to 140s–150s/70–90 mm Hg. She is also started on magnesium sulfate. What change in physical or laboratory examination do you observe that would indicate delivery?

a. Another BP of 174/102 mm Hg
b. Headache returning
c. Double vision
d. Platelets of 108
e. AST of 265

5. Forty-eight hours later, she has completed the course of betamethasone, her magnesium sulfate is stopped, and her, laboratory test results have been stable, and she has had no further headaches. Your next plan of care is:

a. Discharge home for expectant management
b. Discharge home on bedrest
c. Continue to expectantly manage in hospital on modified bedrest and monitoring
d. remain in hospital for 48 more hours and then consider discharge home on bedrest
e. Continue to expectantly manage in hospital for 48 more hours and then move towards delivery

Vignette 3

A 26-year-old G1P0 woman presents for a prenatal visit at 34 weeks' gestation. She complains of some mild nausea and vomiting over the past 3 days. She has no headache and no visual changes. Her BP is 142/83 mm Hg. On examination, she has 2+ lower extremity pitting edema, and 3+ reflexes bilaterally with four beats of clonus. A urinalysis dip has 1+protein.

1. Which of the following questions would be helpful?

a. Do you have double vision?
b. Do you have pain radiating down your legs?
c. Are you constipated?
d. Do you have pain in your right upper abdomen?
e. Do you have ringing in your ears?

2. Which of the following laboratory tests would NOT be helpful at this point?

a. Platelets
b. WBC
c. LFTs
d. LDH
e. Obstetric ultrasound

3. The laboratory test results come back with elevated LFTs, low platelets, a normal hematocrit (Hct), and an elevated LDH. What is her diagnosis?

a. Preeclampsia
b. Eclampsia
c. Chronic hypertension
d. HELLP syndrome
e. GH

4. The next step in her management is:

a. betamethasone
b. expectant management until severe preeclampsia
c. IV hydralazine
d. induction of labor
e. immediate cesarean delivery

Vignette 4

A 17-year-old G1P0 woman presents to labor and delivery complaining of contractions at 38 weeks' gestation. Her initial BP was 90/60 mm Hg. She has gained 46 lb throughout pregnancy (10 lb in the past 4 weeks). Her BP is 134/86 mm Hg. A urine dip is 1+ protein. On examination, her cervix is 3 cm dilated, 90% effaced, -1 station.

1. What is the next step in her management?

a. Magnesium sulfate
b. Betamethasone
c. Send laboratory tests
d. Artificial rupture of the membranes
e. Send home until in active labor

2. While you are writing a note, the patient's nurse calls out of the room that the patient is having a seizure. As you run to the patient's room, you plan your next step, which is:

a. IV magnesium sulfate
b. IV midazolam
c. IV phenytoin
d. Check the fetal heart rate
e. Assess the patient's airway

3. The patient's seizure is self-limited and she is in a postictal state. Her BP is 145/96 mm Hg, O_2 saturation 96%, FHR 160s, minimal variability after a 4 minute prolonged deceleration. The IV is in and you begin a bolus of magnesium sulfate. All of the labor rooms are full, so she remains in triage. Thirty minutes later, you evaluate the fetal heart tracing. There are contractions every minute, accompanied by late decelerations with most of the contractions. The fetal heart tracing demonstrates another prolonged late deceleration down to the 60 beats/minute, and you:

a. wait for 4 to 5 minutes, given that the last FHR deceleration resolved
b. move immediately to the operating room
c. perform an emergency cesarean in triage
d. rebolus the magnesium sulfate
e. look up her laboratory test results

A Answers

Vignette 1 Question 1

Answer D: This patient's age, BMI, history of GH, and BP indicate that the patient most likely has a diagnosis of chronic hypertension. Chronic hypertension complicates 1% to 5% of pregnancies in the United States. Its prevalence varies depending on the woman's age, race, and BMI. With the increasing prevalence of advanced maternal age mothers and obesity in the United States, there has been an increase in chronic hypertension during pregnancy. In pregnant women, chronic hypertension is defined as hypertension that is present before pregnancy, sustained hypertension before 20 weeks' gestation, or hypertension persisting for more than 6 weeks postpartum. As is the case with this patient, the diagnosis may be difficult in women with previously undiagnosed chronic hypertension because of the physiologic decrease in BP that usually begins in the latter half of the first trimester. This decrease may result in normal BP readings (systolic < 140 mm Hg and diastolic <90 mm Hg), which will eventually increase in the third trimester. Subsequently, these women are more likely to be misdiagnosed with GH. Gestational diabetes is impairment in glucose metabolism that first presents during pregnancy. While the patient is obese, she has no other risk factors for or history to suggest that she has gestational diabetes. GH is defined as elevated BPs (> 140/90 mm Hg) after 20 weeks' gestation. While GH is on the differential, this patient's elevated BPs in the first trimester make chronic hypertension more likely. While the patient could have superimposed preeclampsia and/or HELLP syndrome, in addition to chronic hypertension, again these diagnoses are made after 20 weeks' gestation and we need more laboratory data to make those diagnoses.

Vignette 1 Question 2

Answer B: The initial evaluation of women with chronic hypertension includes assessing for the presence of other medical complications and target end-organ damage associated with chronic hypertension. A baseline 24-hour urine collection should be done to assess protein and creatinine clearance. In addition to establishing a baseline, this will help to differentiate between chronic renal disease and superimposed preeclampsia later in the pregnancy. A baseline ECG is important to obtain in order to determine the patient's baseline cardiac status. A quad screen is a maternal blood screening test that looks at the levels of alpha fetoprotein (AFP), beta-human chorionic gonadotropin (HCG), estradiol, and inhibin A to assess the probability of potential genetic abnormalities. Quad screens are usually performed in the second trimester between 15 and 18 weeks, assuming the patient desires genetic testing. Hemoglobin A1c, LDL, and HSV titers are not evaluated unless there is an indication. Women with pregestational diabetes may have their HgbA1c measured to assess their glucose control. LDL levels are not routinely tested as they tend to increase in pregnancy and then return to normal after delivery. HSV titers may be checked to differentiate between a primary and secondary infection if a woman has an outbreak during pregnancy. On the basis of the information given, there are no indications to test her HgbA1c, LDL, or HSV titer.

Vignette 1 Question 3

Answer C: Pregnant women with chronic hypertension do not have an increased risk of placenta previa. However, they are at increased risk of superimposed preeclampsia, placental abruption, preterm delivery, and small-for-gestational age infants. Depending on the severity of disease,.one-third or more of pregnant women with chronic hypertension will develop superimposed preeclampsia. The diagnosis is made by the presence of new onset proteinuria (>300 mg/24 hours) after 20 weeks' gestation. In women with proteinuria before 20 weeks, the diagnosis is confirmed if there is a sudden increase in proteinuria or BP, or if the patient develops HELLP syndrome. In addition to pregnancy complications, these women are also at increased risk of maternal complications such as pulmonary edema, cerebral hemorrhage, and acute renal failure.

Vignette 1 Question 4

Answer A: While treatment of mild chronic hypertension is controversial, women who are early in pregnancy with mild chronic hypertension without superimposed preeclampsia are usually managed expectantly. Although most are not treated with antihypertensives, these women are stilled monitored closely for signs of superimposed preeclampsia and fetal growth restriction by scheduled ultrasounds and regular laboratory tests. Those who develop severe hypertension may be hospitalized for further maternal and fetal testing and then started on antihypertensive medications such as labetalol or nifedipine.Women who develop severe persistent hypertension and/or superimposed preeclampsia may be hospitalized and managed expectantly with bed rest and antihypertensives until 32 weeks' gestation when delivery is indicated.While this patient is at increased risk of pregnancy complications, there would be no reason to recommend termination of pregnancy.

Vignette 2 Question 1

Answer D: This patient's BP and headache are concerning for severe preeclampsia. While her BP may not meet severe criteria (SBP >160 mm Hg or DBP > 110 mm Hg), severe preeclampsia can also be diagnosed in patients who develop other associated conditions. These include oliguria (< 500 mL of urine in 24 hours), cerebral or visual disturbances, pulmonary edema or cyanosis, epigastric or RUQ pain, impaired liver function (greater than two times normal), thrombocytopenia, or intrauterine growth restriction. It is important to evaluate for these conditions when severe preeclampsia is suspected. It is thought that the pathophysiology of preeclampsia involves vasospasm, hemoconcentration, and capillary leakage, resulting in ischemia and hemorrhage of maternal organs such as a hepatic subscapular hematoma leading to RUQ pain. Heartburn, low back pain, constipation, and urinary frequency are common complaints associated with routine problems of pregnancy. While these are important issues to address, the concern for severe preeclampsia takes precedent due to the increased risk of maternal and fetal mortality.

Vignette 2 Question 2

Answer B: Bilirubin levels are not part of the criteria for diagnosing severe preeclampsia. Prepregnancy BP is important in differentiating severe preeclampsia from superimposed preeclampsia in a woman who has chronic hypertension as the two diseases are managed differently and they have different prognoses. The diagnosis of severe preeclampsia is made when one or more of the following criteria is met: SBP greater than 160 mm Hg or DBP greater than 110 mm Hg on two separate occasions at least 6 hours apart; proteinuria greater than 5 g/24 hours or greater than 3+ protein on dipstick on two separate occasions at least 4 hours apart; cerebral or visual disturbances; pulmonary edema or cyanosis; epigastric or RUQ pain; impaired liver function (elevation in AST and ALT); oliguria (< 500 mL of urine in 24 hours); thrombocytopenia; or fetal growth restriction.

Vignette 2 Question 3

Answer C: Although the patient does not yet meet criteria for severe preeclampsia at this point since her BPs are not severe and her head has resolved, her clinical picture at 25 weeks is very concerning for impending severe preeclampsia. Because this patient is at signficant risk of developing severe preeclampsia at such an early gestational age, she should be hospitalized for close observation and monitoring. Management in this situation includes: modified bedrest, antihypertensive medications (labetalol or nifedipine), ultrasound to assess fetal growth, daily NSTs, and at least daily preeclampsia laboratory tests (CBC, liver enzymes, basic metabolic panel, and uric acid). Additionally, betamethasone should be given to facilitate fetal maturation, particularly the pulmonary system. While she does not formally meet the diagnosis of severe preeclampsia, one might consider seizure prophylaxis with magnesium for 48 hours as well.

Vignette 2 Question 4

Answer E: At this gestational age, there are few clinical scenarios that force one's hand to deliver at 25 weeks' gestational age. Rapidly worsening HELLP syndrome is one of those situations. An AST of 265 is markedly elevated, far above the reference range. Elevated BPs are expected and can be managed by maxing out the first antihypertensive agent and then adding a second agent. If the headache returns, it may be due to the high BPs, so it may resolve with better BP control. Further, her previous dose of acetaminophen was several hours ago and she can be given another dose. Double vision is common with magnesium sulfate and while double vision is not concerning, if the patient develops scotomata in the setting of HELLP, that is concerning for worsening end organ damage and vasospasm. Platelets of 108 are not normal as low platelet counts are seen in 8% to 9% of pregnancies, and so not considered to be an indication for a 25 week delivery.

Vignette 2 Question 5

Answer C: Because of her elevated BPs, this patient carries a diagnosis of severe preeclampsia. Severe preeclampsia is ideally and typically not managed at home. The only patient with severe BPs who could potentially be managed at home is a reliable patient with chronic hypertension who is being closely monitored and treated with antihypertensives. Thus, she should not be discharged. Rather, she should be managed expectantly with at least daily fetal and laboratory testing. Further, because she is still quite early in gestation, she should be managed expectantly until she reaches term (37 weeks' gestation), evidence of HELLP syndrome, uncontrollable/severe BPs, eclampsia, or severe symptoms of headache, scotomata, or significantly elevated liver enzymes.

Vignette 3 Question 1

Answer D: While one might ask any of the questions on review of systems, the question about RUQ pain is important when evaluating a patient who signs/symptoms concerning for preeclampsia. In a pregnant patient with nausea and vomiting in the third trimester, it is important to know about right upper quadrant (RUQ) pain has it can be related to severe preeclampsia and/or HELLP syndrome. Of note, another cause of nausea, vomiting, and RUQ pain common in pregnancy is cholelithiasis. Women in pregnancy can occasionally get gall bladder symptoms even without stones from, gall bladder sludge in the setting of a fatty meal.

Vignette 3 Question 2

Answer B: While one frequently orders a WBC as part of a CBC, it is not particularly useful in the setting of preeclampsia. Platelets, LFTs, LDH, Cr, hematocrit, and uric acid are all useful in determining whether the patient has preeclampsia. An obstetric ultrasound would be useful to assess fetal growth and, in the setting fetal growth restriction, if growth restricted to assess Doppler flow of the umbilical artery.

Vignette 3 Question 3

Answer D: HELLP syndrome is **h**emolysis, **e**levated **l**iver enzymes, and **l**ow **p**latelets. This is a severe form of preeclampsia that is typically not managed expectantly. Before 28 to 32 weeks' gestation, expectant management of HELLP syndrome has been employed in order to administer a course of betamethasone to improve fetal lung maturity. In order to manage this disease expectantly, the patient needs to be fully informed as expectant management is more dangerous to the mother than the fetus. When expectant management of HELLP is employed, if the patient develops severe symptoms, has worsening of the laboratory test results, or when the patient completes the bethamethasone course, the patient should then be delivered.

Vignette 3 Question 4

Answer D: HELLP syndrome is a subtype of severe preeclampsia, and both necessitate delivery at 32 to 34 weeks (this is an area of some controversy). While some clinicians opt to delivery via cesaran in the setting of severe preeclampsia or HELLP syndrome, there is little data to suggest that cesarean delivery is necessary or better than attempting induction and a trial of labor as long as the fetal status remains reassuring. The patient's BPs are not severely elevated, so she does not need IV hydralazine. Because she is beyond 34 weeks' gestation, most clinicians would not use betamethasone in this setting.

Vignette 4 Question 1

Answer C: This patient does not have a diagnosis of preeclampsia. However, since her initial BP was 90/60 mm Hg, she does meet the previous diagnostic criteria of a rise in SBP of greater than 30 mm Hg. While a rise in SBP greater than 30 mmHg is no longer part of the criteria for diagnosis of GH or preeclampsia, it should cause the astute clinician to be concerned. In order to fully evaluate this patient, serial BPs, particularly between contractions when she is in less pain, would be helpful. Additionally, a set of preeclamptic laboratory tests should be ordered.

Vignette 4 Question 2

Answer E: With seizures, ABCs are first–airway, breathing, circulation. The vast majority of eclamptic seizures are self-limited, thus, there will be no need for emergent antiseizure medications. However, this is not always true and so a basic understanding of an antiseizure algorithm is always good to know. With eclampsia, magnesium sulfate should be given IV or IM. In this patient who is unlikely to have an IV as of yet, 10 g of IM $MgSO_4$ (two separate 5 g IM doses) is the ideal way to load the patient to prevent future seizures. However, her initial seizure does not stop, often the fastest way to break her seizure is do with an IV benzodiazepine such as midazolam. Once the patient has been stabilized, it is important to determine the fetal heart rate. It is common for the fetal heart rate to have a deceleration during the seizure and to return to baseline after the seizure activity has resolved. If it does not, an emergent cesarean delivery may be indicated, thus the operating room should be notified and all other key staff notified of a potential emergent cesarean delivery.

Vignette 4 Question 3

Answer B: First, it is not appropriate to leave a patient with presumed eclampsia in triage. They should be placed in a labor room with 1:1 nursing if at all possible. Given the frequent contractions, it is likely that she is having a placental abruption, thus this late deceleration may be a prolonged bradycardia necessitating an emergent delivery. By moving her to the operating room you are better prepared to perform an emergent cesarean delivery if necessary. It is inappropriate in this setting to wait 4 to 5 minutes to see if the fetal bradycardia resolves. It is important to remember that it typically takes at least 5 minutes to move a patient to the operating room and assemble the necessary staff to start an emergent cesarean. It will take time to consent the patient in the postictal state, for the anesthesiologist to evaluate the patient, and to get the patient prepped for a cesarean. Thus, moving her to the operating room should be your top priority in this situation. Another option would have been to perform a cervical examination. If she was complete, one could perform an emergent forceps delivery. She could also have had a cord prolapse or a tetanic uterine contraction, both of which can be diagnosed by cervical examination. This should happen as one prepares to move the patient to the operating room. She is not having another seizure; there is no need for rebolusing the magnesium sulfate. Her laboratory test results are of interest, and if the anesthesiologist is planning to attempt to perform regional anesthesia, her platelet count is important to know. However, this is all secondary to moving the patient emergently to the operating room.

Chapter 9 Diabetes During Pregnancy

Diabetes during pregnancy encompasses a range of disease entities that includes gestational diabetes and overt diabetes mellitus (Table 9-1). In the nonpregnant state, diabetic patients are subgrouped into two types based on the pathophysiology of their disease, whereas during pregnancy, diabetes is usually characterized as pregestational or gestational diabetes. Patients with pregestational diabetes include all those diagnosed with type 1 and type 2 diabetes mellitus prior to pregnancy. Patients with gestational diabetes are those diagnosed with carbohydrate intolerance during pregnancy. Because of a lack of routine screening for diabetes in many nonpregnant women, this latter group may occasionally include women with undiagnosed pregestational diabetes mellitus.

GESTATIONAL DIABETES MELLITUS

True **gestational diabetes mellitus** (GDM) is an impairment in carbohydrate metabolism that first manifests during pregnancy. These patients may have borderline carbohydrate metabolism impairment at baseline or be entirely normal in the nonpregnant state. However, during pregnancy, human chorionic somatomammotropin (a.k.a. human placental lactogen) and other hormones produced by the placenta act as anti-insulin agents leading to increased insulin resistance and generalized carbohydrate intolerance. This increased insulin resistance occurs in all pregnant women, but those in whom the balance between insulin function and resistance is tipped beyond a usual carbohydrate metabolism state will have elevated postprandial and occasionally fasting glucose. Because this balance between insulin production and insulin sensitivity appears to be important, it has also been hypothesized that beta cell function in the pancreas may also play a part. In particular, in animal models, it appears that there is beta cell hypertrophy that occurs in the first half of pregnancy that enables enough insulin production to overcome the increased insulin resistance produced by the placental hormones.

Because these placental hormones increase in volume with the size and function of the placenta, the carbohydrate metabolism abnormalities usually are not apparent until the late second trimester or early third trimester. Thus, women with GDM generally are not at increased risk for congenital anomalies like women with pregestational diabetes. They do, however, carry an increased risk of fetal macrosomia and birth injuries as well as neonatal hypoglycemia, hypocalcemia, hyperbilirubinemia, and polycythemia like those with pregestational diabetes. Further, these women have a 4- to 10-fold increased risk of developing type 2 diabetes mellitus (T2DM) during their lifetime.

EPIDEMIOLOGY

The incidence of GDM ranges from 1% to 12% of pregnant women depending on the population. In the United States, it often has been reported to range between 5% and 8%. Higher rates of GDM are seen in women of Hispanic/Latina, Asian/Pacific Islander, and Native American descent. There is also evidence to suggest that paternal race/ethnicity in these three groups is associated with GDM. Initial studies found higher rates of GDM among African American women. However, subsequent studies controlling for maternal BMI have found little difference in incidence between African Americans and Caucasians. Other risk factors include increasing maternal age, obesity, family history of diabetes, history of a previous infant weighing more than 4,000 g, and previous stillborn infant.

DIAGNOSTIC EVALUATION

The best time to screen for diabetes during pregnancy is at the end of the second trimester between 24 and 28 weeks' gestation in women with low risk for GDM. However, to identify women with preexisting T2DM, patients with one or more risk factors for developing GDM should be screened at their first prenatal visit as part of initial prenatal laboratory tests. If such a testing is negative, patients are screened for GDM in the early third trimester (24 to 28 weeks' gestation).

There are a variety of proposed methods of screening for diabetes during pregnancy (Table 9-2). In the United States, the most common laboratory screening test consists of giving a 50-g glucose load and then measuring the plasma glucose 1 hour later. If the 1-hour glucose level is greater than 130 or 140 mg/dL, then the test is considered positive and a glucose tolerance test (GTT), which often consists of a 100-g glucose load, is indicated. Recently, screening thresholds of 130 or 135 mg/dL have been proposed; this would increase the sensitivity of the test but at a cost of a larger proportion of women who will screen positive and thus need subsequent confirmatory testing. Thus, the optimal screen-positive threshold that maximizes sensitivity and costs is still under intense research and requires further elucidation.

Women with a positive screening test are diagnosed with a 100-g, 3-hour oral GTT to evaluate their carbohydrate metabolism (Table 9-3). To conduct the GTT, the patient is given 100 g of oral glucose after an 8-hour overnight fast preceded by a 3-day special carbohydrate diet. Glucose levels are measured immediately before glucose administration (fasting) and again at 1, 2, and 3 hours after the load. If two or more of the four values are elevated, a diagnosis of GDM is made. The values shown in Table 9-3 reflect recently lowered values that will increase the number of women diagnosed with GDM.

TABLE 9-1 White Classification for Diabetes During Pregnancy

Classification	Description
Class A_1	Gestational diabetes; diet controlled
Class A_2	Gestational diabetes; insulin controlled
Class B	Onset: age 20 or older Duration: <10 y
Class C	Onset: age 10–19 Duration: 10–19 y
Class D	Onset: before age 10 Duration: >20 y
Class F	Diabetic nephropathy
Class R	Proliferative retinopathy
Class RF	Retinopathy and nephropathy
Class H	Ischemic heart disease
Class T	Prior renal transplantation

More recently, the American Diabetes Association (ADA), the World Health Organization (WHO), and the International Association of Diabetes in Pregnancy Study Group (IADPSG) have recommended that women in pregnancy be screened and diagnosed with a single test similar to that for nonpregnant individuals. The test would be a fasting blood glucose followed by a 75-g load and then a 1-hour and a 2-hour blood glucose assessments. The diagnosis of GDM would be made with one out of the three values being elevated. These recommendations are in part based upon the findings from the Hyperglycemia and Pregnancy Outcomes (HAPO) study. In the HAPO study, women with either an elevated fasting blood glucose, 1-hour postprandial glucose, or 2-hour postprandial glucose all had higher risks of a wide range of neonatal complications. Thus, those groups recommending the lower threshold, single test justify the change because of this prior work. Of note, a benefit in treating these patients has not, specifically, been demonstrated. The downside of this change in care would be an estimated 17% of the pregnant population being diagnosed with GDM and how to care for them all.

TREATMENT

Once the diagnosis of GDM is made, the patient is usually started on a diet recommended for patients with diabetes. The American Diabetes Association (ADA) diet plan of 2,200 calories per day is recommended for all patients with diabetes during pregnancy, although the total carbohydrate intake is more important. The recommended intake is approximately 200 to 220 g of carbohydrates per day. In addition, both the timing and content of meals are important; therefore, a meal plan based on intake of 30 to 35 kcal/kg of ideal body weight is suggested. Patients are taught to count carbohydrates and meals are designed to contain between 30 and 45 g of carbohydrates at breakfast, 45 to 60 g of carbohydrates for lunch and dinner, and 15 g of carbohydrates for snacks. While on this diet, the patient also monitors her blood glucose levels four times per day, which includes a fasting and three postprandial values. In addition to diet, mild exercise, usually postprandial walking, is encouraged as well. The best way for walking to enhance postprandial blood glucose control is to have the woman walk for 15 minutes about 30 to 40 minutes after the meal.

TABLE 9-2 Glucose Screening Tests During Pregnancy

	Normal Glucose Test Level (mg/dL)
Fasting	<105
1 h after a 50-g glucose load	<140

TABLE 9-3 Three-Hour Glucose Tolerance Test: Venous and Plasma Criteria for GDM[a]

Timing of Glucose Measurement	Normal Venous Blood Glucose (mg/dL)	Normal Whole Plasma Glucose (mg/dL)
Fasting	90	105
1 h	165	190
2 h	145	165
3 h	125	145

[a]Results reflect upper limits of normal. Diagnosis of gestational diabetes is made if fasting value or any two values are exceeded.

If the recommended diet plus exercise controls the blood glucose levels within target range (fasting values < 90 mg/dL and 1-hour postprandial values < 140 mg/dL or 2-hour postprandial values < 120 mg/dL), then this management is continued throughout the pregnancy. These patients are classified as class A_1 or diet-controlled gestational diabetic patients in the **White classification of GDM**. This classification is used as a prognostic tool to determine the likely severity of a woman's diabetes and its interaction with pregnancy; it was originally designed to predict perinatal survival. However, if more than 25% to 30% of a patient's blood glucose values are elevated, medication—usually insulin or an oral hypoglycemic agent—is indicated. These individuals are then considered class A_2 or medication-controlled gestational diabetic patients.

In true gestational diabetic patients, fasting values are commonly normal, while postprandial values are elevated. This is because the pathophysiology is related to metabolism of large carbohydrate boluses rather than carbohydrate intolerance at baseline. These patients can be started on short-acting insulin in combination with an intermediate-acting insulin in the morning (to cover breakfast and lunch) and a short-acting insulin at dinner. Commonly, the short-acting insulin is Humalog (lispro) or NovoLog and the intermediate-acting insulin is NPH. Regular insulin had long been the mainstay of diabetic management; however, it has been replaced by Humalog because of the latter's faster onset of action and shorter length of action. Humalog's profile better represents normal physiology and leads to better control of postprandial blood glucose with less hypoglycemia.

Historically, the oral hypoglycemic agents were not used in pregnancy due to concerns regarding fetal hypoglycemia.

However, recent studies indicate that in some patients, adequate blood glucose control can be achieved without particular harm to the fetus. Because of the ease of patient administration and possibly improved compliance, oral agents such as glyburide or metformin are now being used by some clinicians. With respect to glyburide, there have been only three relatively small randomized prospective trials and these were not adequately powered to examine all important neonatal outcomes, and long-term results are not yet available. However, one of the studies did find an improvement in several neonatal outcomes in those treated with insulin as compared to glyburide. A recent randomized trial comparing metformin and insulin demonstrated no differences in outcomes. At this time, ACOG still considers the use of oral hypoglycemic agents during pregnancy to be experimental.

FETAL MONITORING

In A_2 GDM patients who are started on insulin or an oral hypoglycemic agent, fetal monitoring via nonstress test (NST) or modified biophysical profile (BPP) is typically begun between 32 and 36 weeks' gestation and continued until delivery on a weekly or biweekly basis. Because of the increased risk of macrosomia, these patients commonly receive an obstetric ultrasound for an estimated fetal weight (EFW) between 34 and 37 weeks. It is not common to offer fetal monitoring to A_1 GDM patients who are well-controlled on diet alone. The decision to offer these patients an ultrasound for EFW varies among practitioners.

DELIVERY MANAGEMENT

The intrapartum management of diet-controlled gestational diabetic patients does not differ from that of nondiabetic women, provided that a random glucose check on admission does not reveal significant hyperglycemia that requires correction to avoid neonatal hypoglycemia. It is unclear whether well-controlled gestational diabetic patients have any particular increased risk for peripartum complications other than the theoretical risk of macrosomia. A closer evaluation of fetal weight at term may be prudent in patients whose pregnancy extends beyond their due date.

Scheduled delivery (typically via induction of labor) at 39 weeks of gestation is common in patients on insulin or a hypoglycemic agent (class A_2 GDM). One concern about allowing their pregnancies to proceed is that there may be an increased risk of hypoglycemia as their placental function decreases toward the end of pregnancy. These patients are commonly brought in to labor and delivery at 39 weeks for induction, where their long-acting hypoglycemic agents are discontinued and blood glucose monitored every hour. Dextrose and insulin drips are used if necessary to maintain blood glucose within reference limits (<120 mg/dL). Patients with poor glycemic control are offered delivery between weeks 37 and 39 after verification of fetal lung maturity. Patients who have an estimated fetal weight above 4,000 g have increased risks of shoulder dystocia and their labor curves should be followed closely. Some clinicians offer these patients an elective cesarean birth but, more commonly, elective cesarean delivery is offered to those with an EFW greater than 4,500 g.

At the time of delivery, forceps and vacuum are generally not used if macrosomia is suspected because of the increased risk of shoulder dystocia, except in the case of true outlet forceps for nonreassuring fetal monitoring. To prepare for a possible shoulder dystocia, there should be at least one experienced obstetrician in the delivery room and usually several extra nurses/assistants. This allows one individual to perform suprapubic pressure, two others to perform McRoberts maneuver, while another can be available to time events and function as an assistant.

FOLLOW-UP

Among patients with GDM, over 50% will experience GDM in subsequent pregnancies and 25% to 35% will go on to develop overt diabetes within 5 years. Women with GDM should be screened for T2DM at the postpartum visit and every year thereafter, most commonly with a fasting serum blood glucose or a 75 g, 2-hour GTT. The infants of patients with GDM have an increased incidence of childhood obesity and T2DM during early adulthood and later in life. Unfortunately, only a minority of patients actually obtain the recommended GTT follow-up test postpartum. However, there are several small intervention studies that find that scheduling such follow-up testing or sending reminders by a nurse improves test completion rates.

PREGESTATIONAL DIABETES

Diabetes during pregnancy can have devastating effects on both the mother (Table 9-4) and the fetus (Table 9-5). Women with diabetes are four times more likely to develop preeclampsia or eclampsia than women without diabetes. They are also twice as likely to have a spontaneous abortion. In addition, the risks of infection, polyhydramnios, postpartum hemorrhage, and cesarean delivery are all increased for diabetic mothers. Similarly, diabetes can have adverse effect on the

TABLE 9-4 Maternal Complications of Diabetes During Pregnancy

Obstetric complications
Polyhydramnios
Preeclampsia
Miscarriage
Infection
Postpartum hemorrhage
Increased cesarean section
Diabetic emergencies
Hypoglycemia
Ketoacidosis
Diabetic coma
Vascular and end organ involvement
Cardiac
Renal
Ophthalmic
Peripheral vascular
Neurologic
Peripheral neuropathy
Gastrointestinal disturbance

TABLE 9-5 Fetal Complications of Diabetes Mellitus

Macrosomia
Traumatic delivery
Shoulder dystocia
Erb palsy
Delayed organ maturity
Pulmonary
Hepatic
Neurologic
Pituitary–thyroid axis
Congenital malformations
Cardiovascular defects
Neural tube defects
Caudal regression syndrome
Situs inversus
Duplex renal ureter
IUGR
Intrauterine death

fetus, including a fivefold increase in perinatal death and a two- to threefold increase in the risk of congenital malformations, depending on glycemic control.

Control of maternal glucose levels in overtly diabetic women is a particularly important factor in determining fetal outcome. In older studies, with minimal glycemic management in gravid diabetic women, the perinatal mortality was as high as 30%. However, with careful management by specialists, this risk can be reduced to less than 1%. The fetuses of diabetic mothers are more likely to develop congenital anomalies, including both cardiac anomalies and neural tube defects, and most dramatically, caudal regression syndrome. The fetus is also at risk for fetal growth abnormalities and sudden intrauterine fetal demise (IUFD).

EPIDEMIOLOGY

Less than 1% of pregnant women have pregestational diabetes. However, with improved management of type 1 diabetes mellitus (T1DM) and increased rates of T2DM in the setting of the obesity epidemic, the number of women with pregestational diabetes who become pregnant is increasing.

RISK FACTORS

The White classification system was originally designed to prognosticate perinatal survival; with changing management of diabetes as a chronic disease, it has, however, become less applicable. The length of illness used to differentiate classes B, C, and D has little predictive value at this point because there are likely some class B patients with poor control and many class D patients with excellent control, and thus less likely to be at risk of perinatal complications. However, the severity of illness as reflected by classes R (retinopathy), F (nephropathy), and H (heart disease) is certainly predictive of worsened perinatal outcomes in these patients. Along with the White classification, other prognostic factors include hypertension, pyelonephritis, ketoacidosis, and poor glycemic control. Glycemic control is often measured by $HgbA_1c$, which gives an estimate of the average blood glucose control over the prior 8 to 12 weeks. Patients with an $HgbA_1c$ less than 6.5% generally have good outcomes, whereas patients with an $HgbA_1c$ greater than or equal to 12% are estimated to have a 25% rate of congenital anomalies.

TREATMENT

The goals of managing the diabetic patient include thorough patient education, control of maternal glucose, as well as careful maternal and fetal monitoring and testing. To achieve these goals, tight glycemic control should be maintained prior to conception and throughout pregnancy. Studies now show that stricter control of serum glucose levels during pregnancy can decrease the rate of maternal and neonatal complications. To achieve euglycemia, diet, insulin, and exercise must all be regulated.

Diabetic patients have become increasingly aware of the differences that tight control can make as well as the importance of this management during pregnancy. Ideally, these patients should be seen prior to conception to discuss the risks and benefits of pregnancy. In these visits, a diabetic woman can be counseled regarding the risks to her health, particularly in the setting of chronic renal disease that has been shown to worsen during pregnancy. The patient can also be counseled about the risk of congenital anomalies in the fetus based on her $HgbA_1c$. If she is not in optimal control, this can be tightened to prepare for pregnancy. Because these patients are at higher risk of neural tube defects, they are also placed on 4 mg of folate daily.

It has been standard for patients to follow the ADA diet plan of 2,200 calories per day. More recently, however, the focus on diabetic diet management has focused on total carbohydrate intake rather than caloric intake. Generally, patients keep their carbohydrate intake at 30 to 45 g for breakfast, and at 45 to 60 g for lunch and dinner, and at 15 g for snacks. Patients can increase or decrease protein and fat depending on whether they need more or fewer calories to gain or maintain weight. These carbohydrate-focused diets should be maintained during pregnancy, although the total caloric intake is usually about 300 kcal higher than for nonpregnant patients.

TYPE 1 DIABETES MELLITUS

Historically, patients with T1DM had extremely poor maternal and perinatal outcomes, many of which can be attributed to long-standing disease and difficulty in maintaining euglycemia. Nowadays many T1DM patients are checking their blood glucose seven or more times per day, doing carbohydrate counting, and maintaining their $HgbA_1c$ below 6.0% to 6.5%. When patients are able to maintain tight control prior to and during their pregnancies, the risks of microvascular disease, renal disease, and hypertension are significantly decreased. These lower rates of baseline disease lead to fewer complications during pregnancy.

Because of the correlation of outcome with prepregnant disease, patients are extensively screened at their first visit (if not preconceptionally). Routinely, patients should obtain an ECG, particularly those with longstanding disease, hypertension, advanced maternal age (AMA), or renal disease. A 24-hour urine collection for creatinine clearance and protein should be sent to assess baseline renal function. An $HgbA_1c$ is ordered to assess baseline glucose management as well as thyroid function tests (TSH and free T4) since these patients are at risk for other autoimmune endocrinopathies. In addition, a referral to an ophthalmologist should be made to check for baseline retinopathy.

Because patients with T1DM require insulin, they are usually very experienced at managing their disease. However, this experience may not be applicable during pregnancy, when glycemic control can be dramatically different. During the first half of pregnancy, the patient's prior dosing regimen is usually increased slightly, but can increase substantially during the latter half of pregnancy as insulin resistance increases. If patients have been managed on an insulin pump, this practice should be continued. In fact, because an insulin pump can help maintain patients in tight control, it is often begun either preconception for patients planning to conceive or after the first trimester in patients who are becoming increasingly difficult to manage with NPH and Humalog insulin shots. Some patients will have excellent control prepregnant with Lantus (glargine insulin). This insulin is a slow-release insulin that gives a very flat steady-state level of insulin for 24 hours. Unfortunately, the experience in pregnancy is minimal. Although generally not recommended during pregnancy at this time, it is being used increasingly by clinicians who care for preconceptional diabetic patients during pregnancy.

Table 9-6 demonstrates the relationship between the time of insulin dose, the time of glucose testing, and the target blood glucose levels. When adjusting a patient's dosing schedule, it is important to consider other factors that may alter insulin requirements, such as diet, exercise, stress, and infection. When insulin changes become necessary, there are a few simple rules that aid in the process (Table 9-7). In addition to the schedules given in Tables 9-6 and 9-7, patients on insulin pumps should also check premeal glucose values throughout the day to get a sense of how well blood glucose levels are being managed at baseline.

Because the level of physical activity affects the plasma glucose level, consistent levels of physical activity are suggested. Keep in mind that a hospitalized patient who achieves euglycemia in the context of relatively low activity may encounter bouts of hypoglycemia when discharged home on the same insulin regime because her physical activity level increases at home, thus lowering the need for insulin. Physical activity can also be used to help manage blood glucose. If a patient consistently has an elevated postmeal blood glucose, the premeal insulin or postmeal activity can be increased. It is also important to consider differences between weekday and weekend activity. Some patients will require entirely different insulin regimens on the weekends.

TABLE 9-6 Glucose Monitoring and Insulin Dosing During Pregnancy

Insulin Type and Dose Time	***Time Impact Seen***	***Target Glucose Level (mg/dL)***
Evening NPH	Fasting	70–90
Morning Humalog	Postbreakfast	100–139
Morning NPH	Postlunch	100–139
Evening Humalog	Postdinner	100–139

TABLE 9-7 Instructions for Adjusting Insulin Dosage

1. Establish a fasting glucose level between 70 and 90 mg/dL
2. Adjust only one dosing level at a time
3. Do not change any dosage by more than 20% per day
4. Wait 24 h between dosage changes to evaluate the response

TYPE 2 DIABETES MELLITUS

The pathophysiology of T2DM differs from T1DM. Patients with T1DM have had autoimmune destruction of their pancreatic islet cells, resulting in diminished or absent insulin production, whereas patients with T2DM have peripheral insulin resistance. Many type 2 diabetic patients are managed prior to pregnancy with oral hypoglycemic agents or diet alone. However, in pregnancy, most will require insulin. Oral hypoglycemic agents have not generally been used during pregnancy because of concerns regarding fetal hypoglycemia or potential teratogenicity, but recent studies have not demonstrated any particular association with congenital anomalies and patients are often initially maintained on these medications during pregnancy. However, eventually, most of these patients will be hyperglycemic even on the maximum doses of the oral agents and need to be switched to insulin.

When oral hypoglycemic agents do not adequately maintain glucose control during pregnancy, insulin can be substituted or supplemented. In general, insulin is started as NPH at bedtime to control fasting blood glucose and in the morning to provide a longer-acting substrate throughout the day. A short-acting insulin, usually Humalog or lispro, is used at meals to control immediate carbohydrate intake. Once patients are started on insulin, management is very similar to that of type 1 diabetic patients, although the doses are often higher depending on the patient's degree of insulin resistance. Again, although regular insulin has been used traditionally, it is a poor substitute for the newer fast-acting insulins for postprandial blood glucose control.

Fetal Testing and Delivery

In the patient with pregestational diabetes, antenatal testing to evaluate the growth and well-being of the fetus usually begins at 32 weeks. Earlier testing is recommended in the setting of poor glycemic control. Testing regimens vary, but may resemble the following: antenatal fetal assessment consisting of weekly NSTs until 36 weeks, during which time biweekly testing is implemented, including weekly NST alternating with weekly modified BPP to assess amniotic fluid measurement as well. In addition to the weekly testing, an ultrasound to assess fetal growth is usually obtained between 32 and 36 weeks' gestation.

In general, well-controlled pregestational insulin-dependent diabetic patients with no complications are offered induction of labor at 39 weeks' gestation. This is a change from older management plans that delivered such patients at 37 or 38 weeks' gestation given a reassuring amniocentesis for fetal lung maturity. Thus, expectant management beyond 37 weeks is acceptable, but the clinician needs to follow the patient closely beyond that point. Indications for earlier delivery include nonreassuring fetal testing, poor glycemic control, worsening or uncontrolled hypertension, worsening renal disease, or poor fetal growth.

Blood glucose levels can be extremely difficult to manage in the laboring diabetic woman. The physical effort of labor and delivery decreases the overall insulin requirements. Patients are usually begun on dextrose and insulin drips to maintain blood glucose between 100 and 120 mg/dL. If the blood glucose level increases above 120 mg/dL, the insulin can be increased. Conversely, if the blood glucose level drops to between 80 and 100 mg/dL, an infusion of dextrose can be started or increased.

After delivery, maternal insulin requirements decrease significantly because of the removal of the placenta, which contains many insulin antagonists. In fact, insulin requirements may go below prepregnant levels during the puerperium, particularly in breastfeeding women. Type 2 diabetic patients may require no insulin during this period. However, type 1 diabetic patients should always be maintained on at least a small amount of insulin because they do not produce any endogenously.

Follow-Up

In the puerperal period, pregestational diabetic patients should resume their prepregnancy regimens. Patients who were on oral hypoglycemic agents, however, are often not advised to resume their use if breastfeeding because of concerns regarding neonatal hypoglycemia. This complication is more theoretical as it has not been documented in any large case series or cohort studies. In patients with preexisting renal disease, a 24-hour urine collection for creatinine clearance and protein is usually done at 6 weeks postpartum to assess worsening of disease. In addition, an ophthalmologic appointment is usually scheduled 12 to 14 weeks postpartum. After 6 to 8 weeks postpartum, management of the patient's diabetes should be transferred back to her primary provider or endocrinologist.

KEY POINTS

- GDM occurs in 1% to 12% of pregnant women.
- Risk factors for GDM include Hispanic, Asian American, Native American, and African American ethnicity, obesity, family history of diabetes, and prior pregnancy complicated by GDM, macrosomia, shoulder dystocia, or fetal death.
- All pregnant women should be screened for diabetes between weeks 24 and 28. High-risk women should also be screened at their first prenatal visit.
- Fetal complications of GDM include macrosomia, shoulder dystocia, and neonatal hypoglycemia.
- Pregnancy management should include frequent health care visits, thorough patient education, ADA diet plan, glucose monitoring, fetal monitoring, and insulin or an oral hypoglycemic agent as indicated.
- Patients should generally be induced between 39 and 40 weeks' gestation. Intrapartum insulin and dextrose are used to maintain tight control during delivery. Cesarean section is offered if fetal weight is over 4,500 g.
- Maternal complications of diabetes during pregnancy include hyperglycemia, hypoglycemia, urinary tract infection, worsening renal disease, hypertension, and retinopathy.
- Fetal complications of diabetes during pregnancy include spontaneous abortion, congenital anomalies, macrosomia, IUGR, neonatal hypoglycemia, respiratory distress syndrome, and perinatal death.
- Pregnancy management is optimized by a preconceptional visit, early prenatal care, thorough patient education, tight glucose monitoring and management with insulin, fetal monitoring, and thoughtful plan for delivery.
- Motivated type 1 diabetic patients can usually maintain tighter control on an insulin pump. Management in labor and delivery usually requires an insulin drip; however, insulin requirements decrease dramatically postpartum.

C Clinical Vignettes

Vignette 1

A 32-year-old G0 woman with type 1 diabetes mellitus (T1DM) presents for a preconception visit. She was diagnosed with T1DM at age 4, and other than some challenges with glucose control during her teen age years, she generally has good control per her report. She uses a subcutaneous insulin pump. She has no history of retinopathy, renal disease, heart disease, proteinuria, peripheral neuropathy, or any other medical conditions. On examination, she is 5′6″ tall and weighs 122 lb. Her BP is 128/76 mm Hg.

1. During your counseling, which of the following do you NOT mention that she or her fetus is at increased risk for during pregnancy?
   - a. Preeclampsia
   - b. Congenital abnormalities
   - c. Breech presentation
   - d. Cesarean delivery
   - e. Fetal macrosomia

2. You order a laboratory test and her $HgbA_1c$ returns at 11. You advise her which of the following?
   - a. She should go ahead and start trying to get pregnant
   - b. She should aggressively try to lower her $HgbA_1c$ to less than 9 to reduce the risk of preterm birth
   - c. She should aggressively lower her $HgbA_1c$ to less than 5 in order to reduce her risk of preeclampsia
   - d. She should aggressively lower her $HgbA_1c$ to less than 7 to reduce her risk of congenital anomalies
   - e. She should go ahead and start trying to get pregnant, but also slowly reduce her blood glucoses with a $HgbA_1c$ target of less than 9

3. In addition to the above, what other tests/recommendations do you make?
   - a. Perform a 24-hour urine collection for protein and creatinine clearance
   - b. Obtain a baseline ECG
   - c. Obtain a baseline ophthalmology examination
   - d. Check a thyroid test—TSH
   - e. All of the above

4. She returns 6 months later with a positive pregnancy test and an LMP that was 6 weeks ago. You check that her $HgbA_1c$ is now 8.6. Given her baseline medical history, what is her White classification?
   - a. Class A
   - b. Class B
   - c. Class C
   - d. Class D
   - e. Class F

5. You review her blood glucose levels with her. Her fasting blood glucose levels range from 102 to 188 mg/dL; preprandial values range from 102 to 168 mg/dL, and postprandial values range from 120 to 179 mg/dL. Given these values and her current $HgbA_1c$ of 8.6, what management do you recommend?
   - a. Add glyburide to the medical management
   - b. Add metformin to the medical management
   - c. Increase her basal insulin throughout the day and night
   - d. Increase her insulin boluses at mealtimes
   - e. No changes at this time to avoid hypoglycemia

Vignette 2

A 29-year-old G2P1 woman with obesity, a history of GDM in the prior pregnancy, and a strong family history for type 2 diabetes mellitus (T2DM) presents at 7 weeks' gestation by LMP. In her previous pregnancy, she required insulin therapy. She delivered at 39 weeks and her baby boy weighed 4,300 g (or approximately 9½ lb).

1. In addition to the routine prenatal laboratory tests, what other testing do you also obtain at this point?
   - a. A glucose challenge test with fasting blood glucose
   - b. An ultrasound to estimate fetal weight
   - c. Anti-insulin antibodies
   - d. No testing at this point; we would get a glucose challenge test at 24 weeks' gestation
   - e. No other testing needed; we assume she has GDM

2. Laboratory test results return, and her fasting blood glucose is 145 mg/dL. An ultrasound reveals the pregnancy to be 7 weeks and 2 days, consistent with LMP, and anti-insulin antibodies are negative. Her diagnosis is:
   - a. A_1 GDM
   - b. A_2 GDM
   - c. T1DM
   - d. T2DM
   - e. no diabetes in pregnancy

3. In order to reduce her risk of congenital anomalies, you start her on:
   - a. glyburide
   - b. metformin
   - c. Humalog insulin with meals only
   - d. NPH insulin and Humalog insulin
   - e. Lantus insulin only

4. Her pregnancy progresses without complication. At 34 weeks' gestation, she begins antenatal testing with nonstress tests and amniotic fluid indices twice weekly. This is done in order to:
   a. prevent preterm birth
   b. prevent preeclampsia
   c. prevent macrosomia
   d. prevent shoulder dystocia
   e. prevent stillbirth

Vignette 3

A 36-year-old Hispanic G1P0 woman presents for consultation after undergoing a 50 g glucose loading test, which returned with a value of 168 mg/dL. She carries a diagnosis of asthma, but her pregnancy has been otherwise uncomplicated with routine first and second prenatal laboratory tests. She is 5'2" and weighs 150 lb. Her mother has T2DM.

1. What is the next step in management?
   a. Begin dietary management of GDM
   b. Begin insulin treatment
   c. Further glucose testing
   d. No need for further management—routine prenatal care
   e. Begin treatment with glyburide
2. What in her history increases her risk for GDM?
   a. Maternal weight
   b. Maternal age
   c. Maternal race/ethnicity
   d. Family history of diabetes
   e. History of asthma
3. Once she is diagnosed with GDM, the next step in management is to:
   a. begin low-fat diet
   b. exercise three times per week
   c. have blood glucose checks on the glucometer four times per day
   d. begin insulin
   e. begin glyburide

Vignette 4

A 28-year-old G1P0 woman presents to the diabetes clinic at 28 weeks with a recent diagnosis of GDM. On the 3-hour test, she had two elevated values. Her pregnancy has otherwise been uncomplicated. She undergoes counseling with a nutritionist who discusses carbohydrate counting and the need for between-meal snacks. She is also given a glucometer to check some blood glucose values.

1. As part of her routine counseling, you mention that she is at increased risk of all of the following except:
   a. preeclampsia
   b. fetal macrosomia
   c. her baby having jaundice
   d. her baby having a shoulder dystocia
   e. her baby having a cardiac defect
2. She returns in 1 week with blood glucose values ranging from 75 to 85 mg/dL fasting (threshold goal <90 mg/dL), postbreakfast values ranging from 120 to 142 mg/dL (threshold goal values <140 mg/dL), postlunch values ranging from 128 to 148 mg/dL (threshold goal values <140 mg/dL), and postdinner values ranging from 124 to 152 mg/dL (threshold goal values <140 mg/dL). Your next step in management is to:
   a. continue checking blood glucose values
   b. discuss exercise plan, including walking after each meal
   c. begin insulin
   d. begin glyburide
   e. begin metformin
3. By 37 weeks' gestation, she has been started on medical treatment with insulin before each meal. The insulin dosing has increased until 36 weeks when her glycemic control was excellent with all values below threshold. You schedule her for induction of labor at:
   a. 37 weeks
   b. 38 weeks
   c. 39 weeks
   d. 40 weeks
   e. 41 weeks

A Answers

Vignette 1 Question 1

Answer C: Women with preexisting diabetes mellitus, both type 1 and type 2, are at increased risk for a number of complications in pregnancy. First, because of elevated blood glucose during the first trimester, there is increased risk of congenital anomalies including cardiac and a pathognomonic finding of caudal regression sequence. Throughout the rest of the pregnancy, there is an increased risk of preterm birth, preeclampsia, induction of labor, cesarean delivery, and hyperglycemia, which can lead to fetal macrosomia and predispose to a shoulder dystocia at vaginal delivery. Neonate delivered from women with pregestational diabetes are at increased risk of hyperbilirubinemia, respiratory distress syndrome, and hypoglycemia, but are not particularly at increased risk for malpresentation.

Vignette 1 Question 2

Answer D: In pregnancy, the goal is to get the $HgbA_1c$ as low as possible, within reason. Commonly, less than 7 or less than 6 may be used as targets. With an $HgbA_1c$ of 11, her risk of a congenital anomaly is in the 20% to 30% range, which would be reduced to less than 5% with $HgbA_1c$ less than 7. Thus, it is worth delaying attempting to get pregnant for a few months in order to improve glycemic control. While getting the $HgbA_1c$ even lower to less than 6 may further improve outcomes, being too aggressive to get $HgbA_1c$ less than 5 may lead to too many hypoglycemic events and is not encouraged. Further, it does not appear that lowering $HgbA_1c$ levels necessarily reduces the risk of either preterm birth or preeclampsia.

Vignette 1 Question 3

Answer E: Yes, all of these are things one would get on a preconceptional diabetic patient. Some clinicians would obtain only an ECG on women 35 years or older, but in this women who has had diabetes for more than 30 years, it seems like a good idea. The 24-hour urine collection is to establish baseline renal function, and the baseline ophthalmology examination is to look for diabetic retinopathy. Because women with T1DM are more likely to have autoimmune thyroid disease, a TSH screening test is always good to obtain. One would also start this patient on folate supplementation to lower the risk of neural tube defects, and make tight glycemic control recommendations.

Vignette 1 Question 4

Answer D: The White classification of diabetes in pregnancy relies on the number of years an individual has had diabetes and the number of medical complications of diabetes she has. Class A is gestational diabetes (A_1, diet controlled; A_2, medically controlled). Classes B, C, and D are all related to either the amount of time the patient has had diabetes or their age of onset of diabetes, whichever leads to the higher class. By years of disease, less than 10 years is Class B, 10 to 20 years is Class C, and 20 years or greater is Class D. By age of onset, older than 20 years is Class B, age 10 to 20 years is Class C, and age younger than 10 years is Class D. Because she was diagnosed at age 4, that makes her Class D, and because she has had the disease for 28 years, that makes her D as well. Class F is for nephropathy, Class R is for retinopathy, and Class H is for heart disease.

Vignette 1 Question 5

Answer C: She has increased basal and preprandial blood glucose levels. Thus, she needs greater amounts of basal insulin overnight and through the day. While her postprandial blood glucose levels are also elevated, the reference range for the mealtime glucose excursion is about 20 to 40 mg/dL and her excursions seem reasonable. Thus, if we lower her preprandial blood glucose levels, her postprandial glucose levels should improve as well. Women with true T1DM do not take glyburide or metformin. Glyburide stimulates the beta cells in the pancreas to release more insulin, but a T1DM patient with the disease for 28 years would not have any beta cell function. Metformin decreases insulin resistance, but most T1DM patients will have minimal insulin resistance because they do not get exposed to chronic hyperglycemic diets like T2DM patients do.

Vignette 2 Question 1

Answer A: A patient such as this with obesity, prior history of GDM, and a family history of T2DM is at relatively high risk of having T2DM. Thus, one would obtain testing at the very first prenatal visit. Such a test could simply be the standard 75-g load with fasting and a 2-hour blood glucose that is done to diagnose T2DM. Others clinicians go for the pregnancy 50-g load and 1-hour blood glucose check; in such a case, it is advisable to obtain a fasting blood glucose as well. Anti-insulin antibodies can be seen in women with T1DM, which seems less likely in this setting. Despite her being a high-risk patient, most clinicians will still do GDM testing in such a patient because as many as one-third will not have GDM in a subsequent pregnancy.

Vignette 2 Question 2

Answer D: Until recently, women with elevated blood glucose values in pregnancy were not given a formal diagnosis of T2DM during pregnancy. They had to wait until 6 weeks postpartum to do a no-pregnant glucose challenge test with the 75-g load to receive a diagnosis. Recently, this was changed, as it was realized that, particularly early on, there should only be mild elevations in blood glucose values so that women who exceeded the standards commonly used, greater than 125 mg/dL on a fasting blood glucose or greater than 200 mg/dL

2 hours after a 75-g load, should be diagnosed with T2DM. If this woman had GDM, we would not know whether it was A_1 or A_2 until we followed some blood glucose levels.

Vignette 2 Question 3

Answer D: In this patient with T2DM, some clinicians will manage with either glyburide or metformin. It is likely that either of those medications will not adequately control a patient with T2DM in pregnancy and she will eventually require insulin. However, in this setting, in particular with a need to rapidly control her blood glucose to reduce the risk of congenital anomalies, a combination of long-acting and short-acting insulin is indicated. Often, in this setting, such a patient will be admitted to the hospital and placed on an insulin drip for 24 hours to assess the potential total need for insulin. However, with a reliable patient, it is reasonable to give a dose of 0.7 units/kg split between long- and short-acting insulin and frequently revise the dosages based on the glucometer values. We would recommend doing so every 1 to 2 days for the first week in order to rapidly titrate the dosing.

Vignette 2 Question 4

Answer E: Women with pregestational diabetes are at increased risk of having an IUFD or stillbirth. This is thought to be due to the elevated blood glucose values, the wide swings in glucose values, or the effect of diabetes on placental function. Antenatal testing including nonstress tests and biophysical profiles are performed to identify any fetal complications before they occur, in particular to decrease the risk of stillbirth. It would not do any of the other four options given. Treatment of diabetes in pregnancy by controlling blood glucose does seem to lower the risk of complications such as preterm birth, preeclampsia, macrosomia, and shoulder dystocia.

Vignette 3 Question 1

Answer C: This patient has an elevated GLT. Thresholds for the GLT that have been used include 140, 135, or 130 mg/dL. This patient has a positive screen by any measure. However, the GLT is just a screening test and a follow-up diagnostic test is indicated. There are some clinicians who will not do any further testing for GLT values greater than 200 mg/dL, but will instead consider such values diagnostic of GDM and start blood glucose monitoring at that point. This patient with a value of 168 mg/dL on GLT should undergo the 3-hour, 100-g load test to confirm the diagnosis of GDM. Once she is diagnosed, we could move forward with answer option a or b.

Vignette 3 Question 2

Answer E: There are a number of risk factors for developing GDM. These include maternal risk factors such as an elevated BMI, increased maternal age, family history of T2DM, or maternal race ethnicity including Asian/PI, Hispanic, or Native American. African American race has also been noted to be a risk factor in some studies. Maternal history of a macrosomic baby or a history of GDM also increases the risk of GDM. Asthma is not known as a risk factor for GDM. However, an asthma patient who is on chronic systemic steroids can, occasionally, be diagnosed and need to be treated for GDM.

Vignette 3 Question 3

Answer C: Once diagnosed with GDM, the next step in the care is to check the patient's blood glucose values four times per day. At the same time, she should begin a carbohydrate-controlled diet with 30 g of carbohydrates in the morning, 45 g for lunch and dinner, and 15 g for snacks between meals. Daily exercise, particularly exercise after each meal, can help to control blood glucose values. Although three times per week exercise (or more) is a great part of a baseline of healthy exercise, it is the frequent, postprandial activity that makes a larger difference on blood glucose control.

Vignette 4 Question 1

Answer E: While all of these complications can be seen in pregestational diabetic patients, women with GDM do not have an appreciable increased risk in congenital anomalies.

Vignette 4 Question 2

Answer B: In this patient with only slight postprandial elevations, walking after each meal is likely to reduce her blood glucose values into the reference range. Given that conservative management has only been tried for 1 week, reviewing dietary plan and reinforcing exercise, particularly after meals, is important with follow-up in another week. It is not yet time to begin medical therapy with hypoglycemic agents.

Vignette 4 Question 3

Answer C: Women with well-controlled pregestational diabetes and A_2 GDM are usually induced at 39 weeks' gestation. This allows enough time for the fetus to reach full maturity and minimize fetal metabolic complications, but prevents stillbirth and overgrowth that would occur in subsequent weeks' gestation. A_1 GDM patients are usually managed expectantly until 40/41 weeks' gestation. Finally, pregestational or A_2 GDM patients who have poor glycemic control are commonly delivered earlier, typically 36 to 38 weeks' gestation.

Chapter 10

Infectious Diseases in Pregnancy

As with other diseases in pregnancy, one must think about the effect of an infectious disease on the pregnant woman and the fetus, as well as on the pregnancy outcome. In this chapter we discuss common infections that increase or whose complications increase in pregnancy, infections specific to pregnancy, and infections that can affect the fetus (Table 10-1). The infectious complications that are common to the puerperium (postpartum period), such as endomyometritis and wound infections, are discussed in Chapter 12.

URINARY TRACT INFECTIONS

Urinary tract infection (UTI) is one of the most common medical complication of pregnancy. UTIs occur in up to 20% of pregnancies and account for as many as 10% of antepartum hospitalizations. The incidence of UTIs increases during pregnancy. The prevalence of asymptomatic bacteriuria (i.e., >100,000 colonies on culture) in pregnant women ranges from 2% to 11%, with the majority of studies reporting 4% to 7%. An increased prevalence of bacteriuria in women has been associated with lower socioeconomic status, diminished availability of medical care, and increased parity. Although this prevalence is similar to that in the nonpregnant population, women with asymptomatic bacteriuria (ASB) in early pregnancy are at a 20- to 30-fold increased risk of developing acute pyelonephritis during pregnancy as compared to pregnant women without bacteriuria. ASB in pregnancy is further associated with preterm birth and low-birth-weight infants. A recent meta-analysis demonstrated a significant association between bacteriuria and preterm delivery and showed a statistically significant reduction in the incidence of low-birth-weight infants among bacteriuric women treated in eight placebo-controlled treatment trials. Untreated ASB will progress to cystitis or pyelonephritis in 25% to 40% of pregnant patients. Before the advent of universal screening for ASB in early pregnancy, the reported rate of acute pyelonephritis in pregnancy was 3% to 4%; afterward, it was 1% to 2%. Of the cases of pyelonephritis, up to 15% may be complicated by bacteremia, sepsis, or adult respiratory distress syndrome (ARDS). In pregnant women with sickle cell disease, the rate of ASB doubles to 10%, although recently it was shown that there is no increase risk in sickle cell trait carriers.

PATHOGENESIS

Women are 14 times more likely to develop UTIs compared to men. Presumably, this women predominance is the result of several factors, including (1) a shorter urethra in women, (2) continuous contamination of the external one-third of the urethra by pathogenic bacteria from the vagina and rectum, (3) failure of women to empty their bladders as completely as men, and (4) movement of bacteria into the female bladder during sexual intercourse. A number of factors can contribute to a higher incidence of cystitis and pyelonephritis in pregnancy. During pregnancy, the smooth muscle relaxation effects of progesterone decrease bladder tone and cause ureteral and renal pelvis dilation, as well decreased ureteral peristalsis, resulting in physiologic hydronephrosis of pregnancy. In addition, mechanical compression from the enlarged uterus can cause obstruction of the ureters, leading to stasis. Changes in the bladder also occur in pregnancy, including decreased tone, increased capacity, and incomplete emptying, all of which predispose pregnant women to vesicoureteral reflux. Hypotonia of the vesicle musculature, vesicoureteral reflux, and dilation of the ureters and renal pelves result in static columns of urine in the ureters, facilitating the ascending migration of bacteria to the upper urinary tract after bladder infection is established. The hypokinetic collecting system reduces urine flow and urinary stasis occurs, predisposing to infection.

DIAGNOSIS

UTIs are diagnosed with clinical signs and symptoms of dysuria, urinary frequency, and urinary urgency in conjunction with a positive urine culture. Because urine cultures may take 3 to 4 days to become positive, a urinalysis is often used as a proxy during initial evaluation. The urinalysis may be positive for leukocyte esterase, nitrates, or hematuria, and the urine sediment will have elevated WBCs and bacteria. Acute cystitis is a distinct syndrome characterized by urinary urgency, frequency, dysuria, and suprapubic discomfort (tenderness on palpation) in the absence of systemic symptoms such as high fever and costovertebral angle tenderness. Gross hematuria may be present; the urine culture is invariably positive for bacterial growth. The gold standard for diagnosing acute cystitis has been a quantitative culture containing at least 100,000 CFU/mL.

TREATMENT

Escherichia coli accounts for greater than 70% of all ASB and UTIs, and the remaining are caused by gram-negative enterobacteria (e.g., *Klebsiella*, *Proteus*) and gram-positive bacteria such as coagulase-negative *Staphylococcus*, group B *Streptococcus* (GBS), and *Enterococcus*. Because most UTIs are caused by *E. coli*, initial treatment of ASB is usually with amoxicillin, nitrofurantoin (Macrodantin), trimethoprim/sulfamethoxazole (Bactrim), or cephalexin. Treatment duration consists of a 3- to 7-day course of antibiotics, although many authorities prefer 7-day treatment course for pregnant women. Single-dose therapy is not recommended in pregnancy. Symptomatic UTIs and cystitis are also treated in

TABLE 10-1 Infectious Diseases in Pregnancy

Infections whose complications increase during pregnancy
UTIs
Bacterial vaginosis
Surgical wound
Group B streptococcal
Infections more common in pregnancy and the puerperium
Pyelonephritis
Endomyometritis
Mastitis
Toxic shock syndrome (TSS)
Infections specific to pregnancy
Chorioamnionitis
Septic pelvic thrombophlebitis
Episiotomy or perineal lacerations
Infections that affect the fetus
Neonatal sepsis (e.g., Group B *Streptococcus, Escherichia coli*)
HSV
VZV
Parvovirus B19
CMV
Rubella
HIV
Hepatitis B and C
Gonorrhea
Chlamydia
Syphilis
Toxoplasmosis

this fashion, with adjustment of medication depending on culture-sensitivity results. Because ASB may persist, a test of cure culture should be obtained 1 to 2 weeks after completion of therapy. If the test of cure is positive, a different regimen should be initiated. Continuous nightly antibiotic prophylaxis is recommended for women who have two or more UTIs during pregnancy. Either Macrodantin or Bactrim can be used for prophylaxis. In addition to treating the infection, in patients with dysuria or bladder pain, phenazopyridine (Pyridium), which is concentrated in the urine and acts as a local anesthetic to reduce the pain, is commonly used for symptomatic relief. Of note, patients should be counseled that Pyridium will cause the urine to turn bright orange.

PYELONEPHRITIS

The most common complication of a lower UTI is an ascending infection to the kidneys, or **pyelonephritis**. Pyelonephritis is estimated to complicate as many as 1% to 2.5% of pregnancies despite recommendations for universal screening for ASB. Recurrence during the same pregnancy is frequent, occurring in 10% to 18% of cases. The major risk factors for developing pyelonephritis are previous pyelonephritis and ASB. Among pregnant women not receiving antibiotic prophylaxis to prevent acute pyelonephritis in pregnancy, recurrence has been noted to be up to 60%; conversely, in pregnant women on suppressive therapy, recurrence is less than 10%. Although ASB is not more frequent in pregnant women, pyelonephritis is a much more frequent complication. The pathogenesis for this phenomenon is the same as described for increased acute cystitis in pregnancy, including the effects of progesterone on the bladder and ureters as well as external compression caused by the uterus leading to hydronephrosis, vesicoureteral reflux, stasis, and ascending infections. The most common organisms associated with acute antepartum pyelonephritis are similar to those in ASB and acute cystitis: *E. coli* (70%), *Klebsiella–Enterobacter* (3%), *Proteus* (2%), and gram-positive bacteria, including GBS (10%).

DIAGNOSIS

Acute pyelonephritis is characterized by fever, chills, flank pain, dysuria, urgency, and frequency. It is sometimes associated with nausea and vomiting. On physical examination, fever and costovertebral angle tenderness are often present. Laboratory abnormalities include pyuria, bacteriuria, and elevated WBC count. WBC casts are highly associated with pyelonephritis and the diagnosis can be confirmed on urine culture. Onset of symptoms is often abrupt and fever is universally present.

Pyelonephritis is not only a risk factor for preterm labor but also has particularly serious associated maternal complications including septic shock and ARDS. Up to 20% of pregnant women with acute pyelonephritis develop multiorgan system involvement secondary to endotoxemia resulting in sepsis. Endotoxin release results in increase capillary permeability and decreased perfusion of vital organs. ARDS, the most severe complication of severe sepsis, develops in 2% to 8% of pregnant women with acute pyelonephritis. ARDS should be suspected in patients who present with hypoxemia, dyspnea, tachypnea, and radiographic evidence of pulmonary edema or ARDS.

TREATMENT

Because of the associated risks, pyelonephritis during pregnancy is usually treated aggressively with hospital admission, intravenous (IV) hydration, and IV antibiotics—often cephalosporins (cefazolin, cefotetan, or ceftriaxone) or ampicillin and gentamicin—until the patient is afebrile and asymptomatic for 24 to 48 hours. Aggressive IV hydration is imperative as there is often transient renal dysfunction in patients with pyelonephritis. The patient is then transitioned to an oral antibiotic regimen. Given the high incidence of resistance by *E. coli* to ampicillin and first-generation cephalosporins (cephalexin or cefazolin), these agents are not recommended. Small trials have examined the possibility of treating these patients with a single dose of IV or IM antibiotics, such as ceftriaxone, followed by outpatient oral antibiotic regimen. While these treatments seem to be effective in certain groups, consideration of appropriate patient criteria, including absence of signs of sepsis, compliance, ability to tolerate oral medications, and gestational age (GA), is imperative. Treatment duration for pyelonephritis consists of a total of 10 to 14 days of combined IV and oral antibiotics. If the patient is not improving on IV antibiotics, a renal ultrasound should be performed to evaluate for a perinephric or renal abscess. Pregnant women with one episode of pyelonephritis or two or more episodes of ASB and/or cystitis are generally placed on antimicrobial prophylaxis, usually Macrodantin or Bactrim nightly, for the remainder of the duration of the pregnancy.

BACTERIAL VAGINOSIS IN PREGNANCY

Several large studies have demonstrated that **bacterial vaginosis** (BV) increases the risk for preterm premature rupture of membranes (PPROM), preterm delivery, and puerperal infections, including chorioamnionitis and endometritis. Because of this, it has been proposed that patients with BV be treated and followed up with a test of cure to decrease their risk of preterm delivery. Several studies have also demonstrated a reduction of preterm births when high-risk asymptomatic pregnant women (those with prior preterm delivery or PPROM) were treated for BV with an oral agent. However, the largest, prospective randomized trial of screening and treating asymptomatic women did not demonstrate benefit. Therefore, screening for BV in asymptomatic women is not routinely recommended. Treatment of symptomatic women who are diagnosed in pregnancy is recommended.

DIAGNOSIS AND TREATMENT

Common symptoms of BV include a malodorous discharge or vaginal irritation, although many patients with BV may be asymptomatic. Diagnosis can be made with three of the four following findings (Amsel's criteria): (1) presence of thin, white or gray, homogeneous discharge coating the vaginal walls; (2) an amine (or "fishy") odor noted with addition of 10% KOH ("whiff" test); (3) pH of greater than 4.5; (4) presence of more than 20% of the epithelial cells as "clue cells" (squamous epithelial cells so heavily stippled with bacteria that their borders are obscured) on microscopic examination. There are generally few leukocytes and less lactobacilli than usual on wet mount. Gram stain with examination of bacteria in the vaginal discharge is considered the gold standard for BV diagnosis. Common BV organisms include *Gardnerella vaginosis*, *Bacteroides*, and *Mycoplasma hominis*. Oral metronidazole (Flagyl) for 1 week is recommended for treatment of BV in pregnancy. Clindamycin (as oral dose) for 1 week may also be used. Because a majority of studies have demonstrated adverse perinatal events when intravaginal forms of clindamycin were used for treatment of BV, an oral form is preferred for pregnant women. In pregnancy, because of high rates of asymptomatic infection and because treatment of high-risk patients may prevent adverse perinatal outcomes, a test of cure may be considered 1 month after treatment completion.

GROUP B *STREPTOCOCCUS*

GBS is commonly responsible for UTIs, chorioamnionitis, and endomyometritis during pregnancy. It is also a major pathogen in neonatal sepsis, which has severe implications. Although early-onset neonatal sepsis occurs in 2 to 3 per 1,000 live births, the mortality rate with GBS sepsis ranges from 2% to 50%, depending on GA at the time of delivery. One recent study showed an overall mortality rate of 4%, 2% in term infants, and 16% in preterm infants. Various studies have demonstrated a wide range of asymptomatic colonization in pregnant women, from 10% to 35%. To protect infants from GBS infections, widespread screening programs have been implemented utilizing a rectovaginal culture for GBS colonization between 35 and 37 weeks. Large prospective studies have demonstrated that these screening programs do indeed decrease the rate of neonatal sepsis from GBS. Of note, there are concerns that the increase in prophylactic antibiotics given to these patients will increase widespread antibiotic resistance. Another concern is that by focusing clinical attention on GBS, the incidence of *E. coli* sepsis, which has an even higher mortality rate, will increase.

DIAGNOSIS AND TREATMENT

GBS screening is performed by a culture of the vagina and rectum between 35 and 37 weeks of gestation. Women with positive GBS cultures (including GBS bacteriuria) are subsequently treated with IV penicillin G at the time of labor or rupture of membranes (ROM). Women with an unknown GBS status and experiencing labor before 37 weeks of gestation or those with an unknown status and have ROM greater than 18 hours are also treated with penicillin G until delivery depending on specific risk factor criteria. In the case of labor or ROM before 37 weeks with "significant risk of imminent preterm delivery," patients should be screened for GBS and treated empirically until delivery or a negative culture result. For cesarean delivery before ROM and labor, GBS prophylaxis is not indicated. Because of the difficulty of obtaining the correct dosage of penicillin G, ampicillin is commonly used instead. However, ampicillin is a broader-spectrum antibiotic than penicillin, and some authorities feel that its use should be discouraged because of the risk of developing resistance. For GBS-colonized women with an allergy to penicillin but low risk for anaphylaxis to (i.e., rash allergy), cefazolin (Ancef) is used for prophylaxis during labor. In women with a significant penicillin allergy (i.e., high risk for anaphylaxis), clindamycin is the drug of choice but it can be used only if the GBS susceptibilities are known. In patients with a severe penicillin allergy where GBS is resistant to clindamycin or of unknown susceptibility, vancomycin is the drug of choice for GBS prophylaxis.

CHORIOAMNIONITIS

Chorioamnionitis is an infection of the membranes and amniotic fluid surrounding the fetus. It is frequently associated with preterm and prolonged ROM but can also occur without ROM. Clinical chorioamnionitis occurs in 0.5% to 10% of pregnancies, while histologic chorioamnionitis is present in up to 20% of term deliveries and more than 50% of preterm deliveries. Chorioamnionitis is the most common precursor of neonatal sepsis, which has a high rate of neonatal mortality. There is increasing evidence that intrauterine infection is associated with increased risk of neonatal respiratory distress, pneumonia, meningitis, periventricular leukomalacia, and cerebral palsy. Additionally, it has maternal sequelae of uterine atony, postpartum hemorrhage, need for cesarean delivery, endomyometritis and, in some cases, septic shock.

DIAGNOSIS

The clinical diagnosis of chorioamnionitis requires a high index of suspicion. Diagnosis is typically made based on maternal fever (body temperature >100.4°F or 38°C), elevated maternal WBC count (>15,000/mL), uterine tenderness, maternal tachycardia and/or fetal tachycardia (>160 bpm), and foul-smelling amniotic fluid. Because chorioamnionitis is so significant and necessitates delivery, other physiologic events that may have similar signs and symptoms should be excluded. Other loci of maternal infection may cause maternal fever, elevated WBC count, as well as fetal tachycardia. Elevations in maternal temperature have been seen in patients undergoing labor induction with prostaglandins as well as in those patients with epidurals. Fetal tachycardia may be congenital. Thus, a prior baseline fetal heart rate (FHR) can be useful. Fetal tachycardia can also be caused by medications administered to the mother, such as β-agonist tocolytic agents and promethazine. The maternal WBC count is elevated in pregnancy and further elevated with the onset of labor. The WBC count is also increased when corticosteroids are given.

In patients at term, if the constellation of the above signs exists without any other etiology, the diagnosis of chorioamnionitis should be presumed and treatment started. In preterm patients whose fetuses would benefit from remaining in utero for more time, a more aggressive means to reach the diagnosis can be taken if there is any doubt. The gold standard for diagnosis of chorioamnionitis is a culture of the amniotic fluid, which can be obtained via amniocentesis. At the same time, the amniotic fluid can be sent for glucose, WBC count, protein, and Gram stain. Unfortunately, these tests have a sensitivity that ranges from 40% to 70%. In patients with suspected chorioamnionitis, low amniotic fluid glucose concentrations are a good predictor of a positive amniotic fluid culture but a poor predictor of clinical chorioamnionitis. The infected fetus has been described to experience a fetal immune response syndrome (FIRS), which results in the release of cytokines. This has led to research that shows that an elevated interleukin 6 (IL-6) level in the amniotic fluid is the most sensitive and specific marker for predicting a positive amniotic fluid culture. This screening test is still used only in experimental protocols at most institutions.

TREATMENT

When acute chorioamnionitis is strongly suspected, most experts agree that prompt initiation of IV antibiotics and delivery of the fetus are required. Commonly, the causative organisms are those that colonize the vagina and rectum. Thus, broad-spectrum coverage should be used, most commonly a second- or third-generation cephalosporin or ampicillin and gentamicin. Multiple studies have shown that there are decreased rates of neonatal sepsis and maternal morbidity if antibiotics are begun intrapartum, rather than immediately postpartum. In addition to antibiotics, delivery should be hastened with induction and augmentation by vaginal delivery, or, in the case of a nonreassuring fetal tracing, by cesarean delivery.

INFECTIONS THAT AFFECT THE FETUS

HERPES SIMPLEX VIRUS

Herpes simplex virus (HSV) is a DNA virus that has two subtypes: HSV-1 and HSV-2. Genital herpes infections are primarily caused by HSV-2; however, there are extragenital HSV-2 infections and genital HSV-1 infections. Among women with serologic test results that indicate susceptibility to HSV infection, the incidence of new HSV-1 or HSV-2 infection during pregnancy is approximately 2%. Approximately 10% of women who are HSV-2 seronegative have partners who are seropositive and are at risk for transmission of HSV-2 during the pregnancy. Consistent with nonpregnant patients, most new infections in pregnant patients are asymptomatic. The timing of infection is relatively evenly distributed, with approximately one-third of women becoming infected in each trimester. Among women with recurrent genital HSV, approximately 75% can expect at least one recurrence during pregnancy, and approximately 14% of patients will have prodromal symptoms or clinical recurrence at delivery.

All suspected herpes virus infections should be confirmed through viral or serological testing. A diagnosis of genital herpes based on the clinical presentation alone has a sensitivity of 40% and specificity of 99% and a false-positive rate of 20%. The tests used to confirm the presence of HSV infection can be divided into two basic groups: (1) viral detection techniques and (2) antibody detection techniques. Primary viral DNA testing techniques are viral culture and HSV antigen detection by PCR. The antibody detection techniques include the use of serologic tests to detect the presence of antibodies to either HSV-1 or HSV-2. With viral detection techniques, negative results do not rule out the presence of infection. The diagnosis of HSV should be confirmed either serologically or with viral culture. For patients who do not present with active lesions or whose lesions have negative culture or PCR test results, accurate type-specific serologic assays that accurately distinguish between HSV-1 and HSV-2 antibodies are now commercially available. The sensitivity of these assays varies from 93% to 100% and specificity from 93% to 98%. In a high-risk population, the positive predictive value for the ELISA test results is 80% to 94%. Because HSV-2 is an uncommon cause of oral infection, detection of HSV-2 antibodies is virtually diagnostic of genital HSV infection. Conversely, detection of HSV-1 antibodies alone may represent orolabial infection or may be indicative of genital infection. Correlation with direct viral identification techniques and the patient's symptoms is important.

Patients with a history of herpes should have a thorough perineal examination for lesions when presenting in labor because of the risk of vertical transmission of HSV to the fetus during vaginal delivery. If lesions are present, cesarean delivery is recommended by leading authorities to be the optimal mode of delivery for prevention of vertical transmission, although data demonstrating a clear benefit of cesarean delivery in prevention of neonatal HSV during a recurrent maternal infection is limited. According to one large cohort study, women who had given birth by cesarean delivery were much less likely to transmit HSV infection to their infants. Among women with HSV detected at delivery, neonatal herpes occurred in 1% of infants delivered by cesarean delivery compared with 8% of infants delivered vaginally. However, cesarean delivery does not completely prevent vertical transmission to the neonate. Transmission has been documented in the setting of cesarean delivery performed before membrane rupture. Cesarean delivery is not indicated in women with a history of HSV in the absence of active genital lesions or prodromes.

At the time of an initial outbreak in a pregnant woman, antiviral treatment with acyclovir or valacyclovir may be administered orally to pregnant women to reduce the duration and the severity of the symptoms as well as to reduce the duration of viral shedding. In patients who have severe disease, oral treatment can be extended for more than 10 days if lesions are incompletely healed at that time. Acyclovir may be administered intravenously to pregnant women with severe genital HSV infection or with disseminated herpetic infections. Case reports have associated significant improvement in expected survival with acyclovir treatment in cases of pregnant women with disseminated HSV, herpes pneumonitis, herpes hepatitis, and herpes encephalitis.

Patients with an HSV genital outbreak during their pregnancies are also offered acyclovir prophylaxis from week 36 until delivery to prevent recurrent lesions. Women with a history of genital HSV, but without an outbreak in pregnancy are more controversial, though the majority of clinicians also recommend acyclovir prophylaxis beyond 36 weeks of gestation. Asymptomatic shedding during the antepartum period does not predict asymptomatic shedding at delivery. Thus, routine antepartum genital HSV cultures in asymptomatic patients with recurrent disease are not recommended. Additionally, since a large proportion of women who are infected with HSV are unaware of their status, universal screening for HSV in pregnancy has been proposed as well. Currently this practice is dissuaded as it is an expensive venture with no demonstrated benefit and may lead to anxiety in a great many women and their partners.

Primary genital herpes infection during pregnancy constitutes a higher risk for perinatal (fetal and neonatal) transmission than does recurrent infection. The risk of vertical transmission to the neonate when a primary outbreak occurs at the time of delivery is approximately 30% to 60%. Several factors likely contribute to the increased risk of transmission. First, when women have acquired infection near the time of delivery, there is either reduced or no transplacental passage of protective HSV specific antibodies. Higher titers of neutralizing antibodies in the neonate have been associated with a reduced risk of neonatal infection. Second, neonatal exposure to the virus in the genital tract may be increased. The genital viral shedding in women with primary infection is of higher concentration and longer duration than shedding that occurs with recurrent episodes. Women with primary herpes that is untreated have a mean duration of viral shedding of 15 days. In addition, cervical shedding has been detected by viral culture in 90% of women with primary infection. Among women with recurrent lesions at the time of delivery, the rate of transmission is estimated to range between less than 1% and 3%. For women with a history of recurrent disease and no visible lesions at delivery, the transmission risk has been estimated to be 2/10,000. The low risk is in part attributed to the presence and transplacental passage of anti-HSV antibodies. A primary infection can be differentiated from a secondary one by checking maternal antibody titers. A previously infected mother will have circulating IgG antibodies. Thus, to determine whether an HSV lesion is primary or secondary, IgM and type-specific IgG HSV antibodies may be ordered.

HSV can cause severe infections in the neonate. Neonatal herpes usually is acquired during the intrapartum period through exposure to the virus in the genital tract, though rarely in utero and postnatal infections can also occur. Approximately 80% of infected infants are born to mothers with no reported history of HSV infection. Risk of transmission to the infant is up to 50% in a primary maternal infection and less than 1% in a recurrent maternal infection. Additionally, primary infection acquired near the time of labor is associated with the highest risk of transmission to the neonate during delivery. Although the actual incidence is unknown because neonatal herpes infection is not a reportable disease, estimates suggest that approximately 1,200 to 1,500 cases occur each year in the United States. Approximately one-third to one-half of cases of neonatal herpes are caused by HSV-1. Infection in the neonate can be diagnosed by viral cultures of the herpetic lesions, oropharynx, or eyes. Neonatal HSV infections can be classified as disseminated disease (25%); CNS disease (30%); and disease limited to the skin, eyes, or mouth (45%) (see Color Plate 2). The infection in the neonate can progress to a viral sepsis, pneumonia, and herpes encephalitis, which can lead to neurologic devastation and death. Infected infants are treated with IV acyclovir as soon as infection is suspected. Mortality has decreased substantially over the past two decades, decreasing to 30% for disseminated disease and 4% for CNS disease. Approximately 20% of survivors of neonatal herpes have long-term neurologic sequelae.

VARICELLA ZOSTER VIRUS

Varicella zoster virus (VZV) is a highly contagious DNA herpes virus that is transmitted by respiratory droplets or close contact and causes chicken pox. It can later reactivate to cause herpes zoster or shingles. The attack rate among susceptible contacts is 60% to 90% after exposure. The incubation period after infection is 10 to 20 days, with a mean of 14 days. The period of infectivity begins 48 hours before the rash appears and lasts until the vesicles crust over. The primary infection causes chicken pox, which is characterized by fever, malaise, and a maculopapular pruritic rash that becomes vesicular. After the primary infection, VZV remains dormant in sensory ganglia and can be reactivated to cause a vesicular erythematous skin rash known as herpes zoster (or shingles). The antibody to VZV develops within a few days after the onset of infection, and prior infection with VZV confers lifelong immunity.

Because it is primarily a disease of childhood, more than 90% of adults are immune to VZV infection. Severe complications, such as encephalitis and pneumonia, are more common in adults than in children; VZV pneumonia in pregnancy is a risk factor for maternal mortality. Varicella infection is uncommon in pregnancy (occurring in 0.4 to 0.7 per 1,000 patients) because of the high prevalence of natural immunity. Varicella titers may be evaluated during pregnancy for those patients who are unsure about exposure history. Women who present preconceptionally can be screened for VZV titers and, if negative, be immunized prior to conceiving. The varicella vaccine (Varivax) is a live virus vaccine that is highly immunogenic and therefore contraindicated in pregnancy to avoid transmission to the fetus. The CDC guidelines indicate that the vaccine may be considered in breastfeeding mothers, although there is little information about whether the vaccine virus is excreted in breast milk. Vaccine recipients pose minimal risk of transmitting infection to susceptible contacts if no rash develops after the vaccination. If a rash does develop, there is a very small risk of transmission to susceptible contacts. Pregnancy complicated by maternal varicella infection is associated with untoward maternal, fetal, and neonatal effects. Vertical transmission occurs transplacentally. More recent large studies do not demonstrate an increased risk of spontaneous abortion during maternal VZV infection in the first trimester. Investigations have shown that the frequency of fetal anomalies was less than 1% when maternal infection occurred in weeks 1 through 12 of pregnancy and 2% or less when infection occurred in weeks 13 through 20. However, VZV is associated with congenital malformations characterized as congenital varicella syndrome (see Color Plate 3) in approximately 0.5% to 2% of cases, resulting predominantly when mothers are infected between 8 and 20 weeks of gestation. Congenital varicella syndrome is characterized by skin scarring, limb hypoplasia, chorioretinitis, and microcephaly. Neonatal VZV infection is associated with a high neonatal death rate when maternal disease develops from 5 days before delivery up to 48 hours postpartum as a result of the relative immaturity of the neonatal immune system and the lack of protective maternal antibody. Infections near term may lead to a postnatal infection that may range from a benign course (like chicken pox) to a fulminant disseminated infection, leading to death. In the absence of timely antiviral chemotherapy, up to 30% of infected infants die of complications of neonatal varicella. Other infants may show no signs of infection at birth; however, they will develop shingles (recurrent herpes zoster outbreaks) at some point later in childhood. Infants of mothers who develop varicella disease within 5 days before delivery or 2 days after should also receive VZIG and/or treatment with antiviral agents such as acyclovir or valacyclovir. Of note, maternal herpes zoster, recurrent VZV outbreaks, is not associated with congenital anomalies.

If a susceptible pregnant patient is exposed to someone with varicella, she should be treated within 72 to 96 hours with one of two agents to prevent active infection. Varicella zoster immune globulin (VZIG) may ameliorate maternal disease but does not prevent transmission of the disease to the fetus. Therefore, any patient without a history of chicken pox with an exposure in pregnancy should receive VZIG within 96 hours of exposure. However, the US company that manufactured this agent has discontinued its production, and securing the product through international manufacturers is problematic. An alternative method of prophylaxis is to administer oral acyclovir (800 mg, five times daily for 7 days) or oral valacyclovir (1,000 mg, three times daily for 7 days). Pregnant women who develop varicella despite immunoprophylaxis should be treated with oral acyclovir or valacyclovir in the same dose as outlined for prophylaxis. Patients who have evidence of pneumonia, encephalitis, or disseminated infection and those who are immunosuppressed should be hospitalized and treated with IV acyclovir.

PARVOVIRUS

Parvovirus B19 is a DNA virus that causes erythema infectiosum (fifth disease). The virus is transmitted primarily by respiratory droplets and infected blood products. Immunity to parvovirus increases progressively throughout childhood and young adult life. Approximately 50% to 60% of women of reproductive age have evidence of prior infection, and immunity is long-lasting. Erythema infectiosum is usually manifested by a low-grade fever, malaise, myalgias, arthralgias, and a red macular "slapped cheek" facial rash. An erythematous, lace-like rash also may extend onto the torso and upper extremities. In children, parvovirus infection also can cause transient aplastic crisis. This same disorder may occur in adults who have an underlying hemoglobinopathy.

Erythema infectiosum usually resolves with minimal intervention. In pregnancy, however, there is concern for maternal–fetal transmission, which has been noted to cause fetal infection and death. First-trimester infections have been associated with miscarriage, but midtrimester and later infections are associated with fetal hydrops. The risk of hydrops is directly related to the GA at which maternal infection occurs. If infection develops during the first 12 weeks of gestation, the risk of hydrops varies from less than 5% to approximately 10%. If infection occurs during weeks 13 through 20, the risk of infection decreases to 5% or less. If infection occurs beyond the 20th week of gestation, the risk of fetal hydrops is 1% or less. When maternal parvovirus infection occurs during pregnancy, the virus can cross the placenta and infect RBC progenitors in the fetal bone marrow. The virus attaches to an antigen on RBC stem cells and suppresses erythropoiesis, thereby resulting in severe anemia and high-output congestive heart failure. This same antigen also is present on fetal myocardial cells, and, in some fetuses, the viral infection causes a cardiomyopathy that further contributes to heart failure (i.e., hydrops).

The incubation period for parvovirus is 10 to 20 days. If parvovirus exposure is suspected in the mother, acute infection can be diagnosed by checking parvovirus IgM and IgG levels. If IgM is negative and IgG is positive then the patient has prior immunity and is protected against a second infection. If IgM and IgG are both negative, then the patient does not have an acute infection but is susceptible to future infections. However, if studies indicate an acute parvovirus infection (positive IgM and positive or negative IgG) beyond 20 weeks of gestation, then the fetus should undergo serial ultrasounds, up to 8 to 10 weeks after maternal infection is suspected to have occurred. However, by the time sonographic evidence of hydrops is present, the fetal hematocrit is likely to be less than 20%. Therefore, a more precise way to detect evolving fetal anemia is to use Doppler velocimetry to examine the peak systolic velocity of the middle cerebral artery (MCA). Increases in peak systolic velocity are associated with fetal anemia. If velocimetry indicates fetal anemia, a cordocentesis should be performed to determine the fetal hematocrit. If anemia is confirmed, an intrauterine blood transfusion should be performed. Because the fetal anemia in the setting of parvovirus is due to marrow suppression rather than hemolysis, this screening test offers the ability to identify patients at risk prior to the development of hydrops. Because of the risk of fetal anemia, serial ultrasounds and management with fetal transfusion, when there is evidence of hydrops, have been recommended by some perinatologists. Management of parvovirus infection with intrauterine blood transfusion can correct fetal anemia and may reduce the mortality of parvovirus infection significantly. While this intervention has not been studied in large populations, there are several studies that have shown that timely intrauterine blood transfusion in cases of severe hydrops in patients who are infected prior to 20 weeks' gestation decreases the risk of stillbirth. A few cases of spontaneous resolution of hydrops due to parvovirus infection have been described. Most clinicians choose to proceed with transfusion when the fetal blood sample shows anemia, even if there is already evidence of recovery of erythropoiesis by a high reticulocyte count. Because of the rarity of the disease and ethical considerations, a randomized trial to find the best policy is unlikely ever to be performed.

CYTOMEGALOVIRUS

Cytomegalovirus (CMV) is a DNA virus in the herpes virus family. CMV is not highly contagious; close personal contact is required for infection to occur. Horizontal transmission may result from infected blood, sexual contact, or contact with contaminated saliva or urine. Vertical transmission may occur as a result of transplacental infection, exposure to contaminated genital tract secretions during delivery, or breastfeeding. The incubation period of CMV ranges from 28 to 60 days. CMV infections in the mother usually cause either a subclinical or mild viral illness. Only rarely will it lead to hepatitis or a mononucleosis-like syndrome. Thus, maternal infections are rarely diagnosed. After the initial infection, CMV remains latent in host cells; recurrent infection can occur following reactivation of latent virus. In rare cases, recurrent CMV infection can occur by infection with a new strain of virus. Approximately 50% to 80% of adult women in the United States have serologic evidence of past CMV infection. However, the presence of antibodies is not perfectly protective against either reinfection or vertical transmission of infection from mother to fetus. Therefore, pregnant women with either recurrent or primary infection pose a risk to their fetus.

Diagnosis of CMV infection in adults is usually confirmed by serologic testing. Serum samples collected 3 to 4 weeks apart, tested in parallel for anti-CMV IgG, are essential for the diagnosis of primary infection. Seroconversion from negative to positive or a significant increase (greater than fourfold, e.g., from 1:4 to 1:16) in anti-CMV IgG titers is evidence of infection. The presence of CMV-specific IgM is a useful but not completely reliable indication of a primary infection. IgM titers may not be positive during an acute infection, or they may persist for months after the primary infection.

Congenital CMV may be suspected prenatally after a documented maternal primary infection or, more typically, after detection of ultrasound findings suggestive of infection. The most sensitive and specific test for diagnosing congenital CMV infection is the identification of CMV in amniotic fluid by either culture or PCR. Identification of the virus in amniotic fluid by culture or PCR does not necessarily indicate the severity of fetal injury. The principal sonographic findings suggestive of serious fetal injury are microcephaly, ventriculomegaly, intercerebral calcification, fetal hydrops, growth restriction, and oligohydramnios. Less common findings include fetal heart block, echogenic bowel, meconium peritonitis, renal dysplasia, ascites, and pleural effusions. Fetuses that demonstrate abnormalities, particularly if they involve the CNS, generally have a much poorer prognosis.

CMV is the most common congenital infection, occurring in approximately 1% to 2% of all neonates, and is the leading cause of congenital hearing loss. Vertical transmission may occur at any stage of pregnancy, with the overall risk of infection greatest when the infection occurs during the third trimester. However, more serious fetal sequelae occur after maternal CMV infection during the first trimester. With primary maternal CMV infection, the risk of transmission to the fetus is 30% to 40%. Approximately 5% to 15% of infants who develop congenital CMV infection as a result of primary maternal infection are symptomatic at birth. The incidence of severe fetal infection is much lower after recurrent maternal infection than after primary infection. Vertical transmission after a recurrent infection is 0.15% to 2%. Infants infected after maternal CMV reactivation generally are asymptomatic at birth. Congenital hearing loss is typically the most severe sequela of secondary infection, and congenital infection following recurrent infection is unlikely to produce multiple sequelae. CMV infection acquired as a result of exposure to infected cervical secretions or breast milk is typically asymptomatic and is not associated with severe neonatal sequelae. Infants who are symptomatic can develop cytomegalic inclusion disease manifested by a constellation of findings including hepatomegaly, splenomegaly, thrombocytopenia, jaundice, cerebral calcifications, chorioretinitis, and interstitial pneumonitis (see Color Plate 4). The most common clinical manifestations of severe neonatal infection are hepatosplenomegaly, intracranial calcifications, jaundice, growth restriction, microcephaly, chorioretinitis, hearing loss, thrombocytopenia, hyperbilirubinemia, and hepatitis. Approximately 30% of severely infected infants die, and 80% of survivors have severe neurologic morbidity such as mental retardation, sensorineural hearing loss, and neuromuscular disorders. Among the 85% to 90% of infants with congenital CMV infection who are asymptomatic at birth, 10% to 15% subsequently develop hearing loss, chorioretinitis, or dental defects within the first 2 years of life, while 85% will have no sequelae of the infection.

Currently, there is no treatment or prophylaxis for the disease. Studies reporting use of IV hyperimmune globulin and antiviral medications have been published and these treatments are supported by some clinicians. In particular, the use of IVIG demonstrated improvement in outcomes, but large randomized trials demonstrating decrease in fetal infection are still lacking. A vaccine for the prevention of disease in the mother is also being investigated.

RUBELLA VIRUS

Rubella (also called "German measles") is caused by an RNA virus. With licensure of an effective vaccine in 1969, the frequency of rubella declined markedly. In 1999, the incidence of rubella was 0.1 per 100,000. Persistence of this infection appears to be caused by failure to vaccinate susceptible individuals rather than by a lack of immunogenicity of the vaccine. Rubella infection in adults leads to a mild illness with a widely disseminated, nonpruritic, erythematous maculopapular rash, arthritis, arthralgias, and a diffuse lymphadenopathy that lasts 3 to 5 days. Postauricular adenopathy and mild conjunctivitis also are common. The infection can be transmitted to the fetus and cause congenital rubella infection, which may lead to **congenital rubella syndrome**. Rubella virus crosses the placenta by hematogenous dissemination, and the frequency of congenital infection is critically dependent on the time of exposure to the virus. The fetus is not at risk from infection before the time of conception. However, approximately 50% to 80% of infants exposed to the virus within 12 weeks after conception will manifest signs of congenital infection. The rate of congenital infection declines sharply with advancing GA so that very few fetuses are affected if infection occurs after 18 weeks of gestation. The maternal–fetal transmission rate is highest during the first trimester, as are the rates of congenital abnormalities. However, transmission may occur at any time during pregnancy.

The four most common anomalies associated with congenital rubella syndrome (CRS) are deafness (affecting 60% to 75% of fetuses), eye defects such as cataracts or retinopathy (10% to 30%), CNS defects (10% to 25%), and cardiac malformations (10% to 20%). The most common cardiac abnormality is patent ductus arteriosus, although supravalvular pulmonic stenosis is perhaps the most pathognomonic. Other possible abnormalities include microcephaly, mental retardation, pneumonia, fetal growth restriction, hepatosplenomegaly, hemolytic anemia, and thrombocytopenia. Specifically, if maternal rubella infection occurs during the period of organogenesis, any fetal organ system may be affected. There are a variety of latent sequelae including the delayed onset of diabetes, thyroid disease, deafness, ocular disease, and growth hormone deficiency. The prognosis for infants with CRS is guarded. Approximately 50% of affected individuals have to attend schools for the hearing-impaired. An additional 25% require at least some special schooling because of hearing impairment, and only 25% are able to attend mainstream schools.

The diagnosis of maternal rubella infection is made with serology studies. IgM titers will result from primary infection and reinfection with rubella. Because IgM does not cross the placenta, IgM titers in the infant are indicative of infection. IgG titers that are elevated over time support the diagnosis of CRS in an infant as well. Fetal blood, obtained by cordocentesis, can be used to determine the total and viral-specific IgM concentration. However, cordocentesis technically is difficult before 20 weeks' gestation, and fetal immunoglobulins usually cannot be detected before 22 to 24 weeks. Chorionic villi, fetal blood, and amniotic fluid samples all can be tested via PCR for rubella antigen. Because of its lower complication rate, amniocentesis is the procedure of choice. Although these tests can demonstrate that rubella virus is present in the fetal compartment, they do not indicate the degree of fetal injury. Furthermore, the possibility of false-positive test results cannot be excluded. Accordingly, detailed ultrasound examination is the best test to determine whether serious fetal injury has occurred as a result of maternal rubella infection. Possible anomalies detected by ultrasound include growth restriction, microcephaly, CNS abnormalities, and cardiac malformations.

Currently, there is no treatment of rubella. The incidence of CRS in the United States has declined dramatically. Fewer than 50 cases of congenital rubella occur each year. However, approximately 10% to 20% of women in the United States remain susceptible to rubella, and their fetuses are at risk for serious injury should infection occur during pregnancy. Ideally, women of reproductive age should have a preconception appointment when they are contemplating pregnancy. At that time, they should be evaluated for immunity to rubella. If serologic testing demonstrates that they are susceptible, they should be vaccinated with rubella vaccine before conception occurs. If preconception counseling is not possible, patients should have a test for rubella at the time of their first prenatal appointment. Women who are susceptible to rubella should be counseled to avoid exposure to other individuals who may have viral exanthems. If a susceptible woman subsequently is exposed to rubella, serologic tests should be obtained to determine whether acute infection has occurred. If acute infection is documented by identification of IgM antibody, the patient should be counseled about the risk of CRS. The diagnostic tests for detection of congenital infection should be reviewed, and the patient should be offered the option of pregnancy termination, depending on the assessed risk of serious fetal injury. In pregnancy, the rubella titer is checked during the first trimester. Because of theoretic risk of transmission of the live virus in the vaccine, patients do not receive the measles, mumps, and rubella (MMR) vaccine until postpartum, and patients are advised to avoid pregnancy for 1 month following vaccination.

HUMAN IMMUNODEFICIENCY VIRUS

In the United States approximately 7,000 infants are born annually to mothers who are infected with **human immunodeficiency virus** (HIV). Perinatal transmission is the most common cause of HIV infection in infants and children in the United States, responsible for more than 90% of pediatric AIDS cases and almost all new HIV infections in preadolescent children. In the absence of interventions, the reported frequency of mother-to-child transmission varies widely across the globe with rates ranging from 10% to 60%. This range reflects differences in patterns of breastfeeding, viral loads, and obstetric practices. It is estimated that 70% of mother-to-child transmission occur at delivery, and about 30% of transmissions occur in utero. About two of three in utero transmissions occur in the last 14 days before delivery. Increased transmission can be seen with higher viral burden or advanced disease in the mother, rupture of the membranes, and invasive procedures during labor and delivery that increase neonatal exposure to maternal blood. In 1994, Pediatric AIDS Clinical Trials Group (PACTG) protocol 076 demonstrated that a three-part regimen of zidovudine (ZDV) administered during pregnancy and labor and to the newborn could reduce the risk of perinatal transmission by two-thirds (from approximately 25% down to 8%). Before the PACTG HIV treatment regimen gained purchase as a standard approach in the United States, as many as 2,000 children each year were infected through birth. However, subsequent to the use of routine antiviral prophylaxis, only 174 pediatric AIDS cases were reported in the year 2000. Additionally, with the use of highly active antiretroviral therapy (HAART) to further decrease viral load with potent regimens, the rate of transmission can be further decreased to less than 1% to 2% with an undetectable viral load (mother-to-child transmission rates are linked to viral loads) and rates start to climb well before viral loads of 55,000 copies are reached. As discussed below, cesarean deliveries are recommended for women whose viral loads exceed 1,000 copies. For both those reasons, pregnant women should be informed of the advantages of initiating HAART (usually a three-drug regimen) whenever their viral loads are above 1,000 copies/mL. Even women whose counts are below 1,000 copies/mL will have lower rates of transmission if they take antiretroviral therapy during gestation, though in that circumstance, the advantage of HAART over the simpler PACTG 076 zidovudine regimen is less clear. However, even in that circumstance, HAART might lower the likelihood (already relatively low in women with undetectable virus) of development of resistance. Trials of HAART versus zidovudine in the setting of counts under 1,000 have not been undertaken to date. All HIV-infected women should be monitored with (1) viral loads every month until the virus is undetectable and then every 2 to 3 months, (2) CD4 counts (absolute number or percent) each trimester, and (3) resistance testing if they have recently seroconverted or if the therapy failed. The goal in pregnancy should be to bring the viral load to levels that are undetectable. All pregnant women should receive antiretroviral therapy. In the vast majority of circumstances that therapy should be a highly active regimen that includes zidovudine. If a woman has a low viral load that would not require therapy if she were not pregnant (e.g., <1,000 copies), then use of monotherapy can be considered with the understanding that there may be a small risk of the development of resistance.

Cesarean delivery has been shown to lower transmission rates by roughly two-thirds compared to vaginal delivery in patients on no therapy and particularly without onset of labor or ROM or in the setting of high viral load. However, in women with viral loads of less than 1,000 copies/mL, there does not appear to be any additional benefit of cesarean delivery versus vaginal delivery in HIV perinatal transmission. Therefore, scheduled cesarean delivery should be considered only in HIV-infected pregnant women with viral loads of greater than 1,000 copies/mL and without long-standing onset of labor or ROM. During labor, every precaution should be taken to minimize contact between the infant's skin and mucous membranes and contaminated maternal blood and genital tract secretions. Specifically, amniotomy, scalp monitoring, scalp pH assessment, episiotomy, and instrumental delivery should be avoided if at all possible.

Because of the effective interventions in HIV-positive women to decrease vertical transmission, it is recommended that HIV screening be offered to all pregnant women at their first prenatal visit on an informed "opt-out" basis and again in the third trimester if the woman has specified risk factors for HIV infection (i.e., other sexually transmitted infections diagnosed during pregnancy). Testing should be performed in the intrapartum and/or neonatal periods if serostatus has not been previously determined. Despite the increasingly simple and straightforward approach recommended for prenatal testing, because approximately 15% of HIV-infected women receive no or minimal care and 20% do not initiate care until the third trimester, a number of women will still arrive in labor and delivery suites with unknown serostatus. In some circumstances, despite adequate care, women will not have been offered the test. There are compelling data to suggest that intrapartum and early neonatal prophylaxis, even in the absence of antepartum therapy, can reduce the risk of mother-to-child transmission. Therefore, efforts should be made during labor to rapidly discern the serostatus of those women whose results were not previously known. Although the current generation of rapid tests (often using a single enzyme-linked immunosorbent assay) are not as reliable as the standard approach used for prenatal testing (one or two enzyme-linked immunosorbent assays followed by a confirmatory Western blot), they are still sufficiently sensitive to identify women who should be offered therapy while confirmatory tests are pending. Patients should be informed that if the confirmatory tests turn out to be negative (which they often will in low-prevalence communities), then treatment of the infant would be discontinued. Women identified as HIV infected in labor should be treated with either (1) zidovudine—in labor intravenously and 6 weeks to the neonate; (2) nevirapine—as a single dose to the mother in labor and as a single dose to the neonate; (3) zidovudine–lamivudine—in labor and to the neonate for 1 week; or (4) both nevirapine as above and the zidovudine regimen as above.

Furthermore, in resource-rich nations where safe bottle-feeding alternatives are available, breastfeeding is contraindicated in HIV-infected woman, as virus is found in breast milk and can lead to HIV transmission to the infant. Postnatal HIV transmission from breast milk at 2 years may be as high as 15%. Furthermore, studies are lacking regarding the efficacy of maternal antiretroviral therapy for prevention of transmission of HIV through breast milk and the toxicity of antiretroviral exposure of the infant via breast milk. Conversely, randomized controlled trials of breast- versus bottle-feeding in Africa have shown that the advantage of bottle-feeding in reducing neonatal deaths from AIDS is counterbalanced by increases in neonatal deaths from other illnesses, malnutrition, and dehydration.

Neisseria Gonorrhoeae

Gonococcal infections are associated with pelvic inflammatory disease in early pregnancy, as well as preterm delivery, PPROM, and puerperal infections throughout pregnancy duration. Studies have shown an association between untreated maternal endocervical gonorrhea and perinatal complications, including PROM, preterm delivery, chorioamnionitis, neonatal sepsis, and maternal postpartum sepsis. The amniotic infection syndrome is an additional manifestation of gonococcal infection in pregnancy. This condition is characterized by placental, fetal membrane, and umbilical cord inflammation that occurs after PROM and is associated with infected oral and gastric aspirate, leukocytosis, neonatal infection, and maternal fever. Preterm delivery is common, and perinatal morbidity may be significant. The prevalence of gonorrhea in pregnancy ranges from 0% to 10%, with marked variations according to risk status and geographic locale. The infection is transmitted during passage of the neonate through the birth canal. Neonatal infection can affect the eye, oropharynx, external ear, and anorectal mucosa. These infections can furthermore become disseminated, causing arthritis and meningitis. Untreated gonococcal ophthalmia can rapidly progress to corneal ulceration, resulting in corneal scarring and blindness.

Screening for gonorrhea should be performed for pregnant women with risk factors in the first prenatal visit and again in the third trimester. Screening for gonorrhea during pregnancy is clearly cost-effective if the prevalence exceeds 1%. Therefore, the CDC recommends that all pregnant women at risk for gonorrhea, as well as those living in an area where the prevalence of *N. gonorrhoeae* is high, be tested for *N. gonorrhoeae* at their first prenatal visit. The CDC and the ACOG recommend that at-risk women be rescreened for *N. gonorrhoeae* during the third trimester. A recent study demonstrated the value of a repeat screen in the third trimester for *N. gonorrhoeae* among at-risk women who had an initial negative early pregnancy screen. In this study, approximately one-third of at-risk women tested positive for *N. gonorrhoeae* only on the repeat third-trimester screen. The diagnosis is made by nucleic acid amplification tests (NAAT) or culture. Treatment can be with IM ceftriaxone, oral cefixime, or IM spectinomycin in cases where cephalosporins cannot be tolerated. Patients should be treated with azithromycin or amoxicillin for presumed chlamydial infection as well because the two diseases often cooccur.

Chlamydia Trachomatis

Chlamydial infection during pregnancy is associated with several adverse maternal outcomes, including preterm delivery, premature rupture of the membranes, low birth weight, and neonatal death. Untreated *C. trachomatis* infection also may result in neonatal conjunctivitis or pneumonia or both. The infection is transmitted during delivery from the genital tract to the infant. Infants born to women with a chlamydial infection of the cervix are at a 60% to 70% risk of acquiring the infection during passage through the birth canal. Approximately 25% to 50% of exposed infants acquire conjunctivitis in the first 2 weeks of life, and 10% to 20% develop pneumonia within 3 or 4 months.

Asymptomatic infection is common. The prevalence of *C. trachomatis* infection among pregnant women is about 2% to 3%, but may be higher in certain high-risk populations. In the Preterm Prediction Study of the National Institute of Child Health and Human Development Maternal-Fetal Medicine Units Network, the overall prevalence of *C. trachomatis* among pregnant women was found to be 11%. Therefore many authorities recommend that all pregnant women should be screened in the first prenatal visit and, if deemed as high risk, again in the third trimester. Because tetracycline and doxycycline are not advised in pregnancy, the treatment of choice for chlamydial infection in pregnancy is azithromycin, amoxicillin, or erythromycin. In 2006, azithromycin, as a single 1-g dose, was added to the list of recommended regimens for treatment of chlamydial infection during pregnancy. Single-dose therapy with azithromycin definitely improves patient compliance. Repeat testing (preferably by NAATs) 3 weeks after completion of therapy is recommended for all pregnant women to ensure cure, in light of the sequelae that can occur in the mother and newborn infant if chlamydial infection persists. Sex partners should be referred for evaluation, testing, and treatment.

HEPATITIS B

Viral hepatitis caused by the **hepatitis B** DNA virus can be acquired from sexual contact, exposure to blood products, and transplacentally. The clinical manifestations of the disease range from mild hepatic dysfunction to fulminant liver failure and death (<1%). It can be diagnosed using a variety of antibody and antigenic markers. Acute hepatitis B occurs in 1 or 2 of every 1,000 pregnancies in the United States. The chronic carrier state is more frequent, occurring in 6 to 10 of 1,000 pregnancies (approximately 10% of those infected). Worldwide, more than 400 million individuals are chronically infected with hepatitis B virus. In the United States alone, approximately 1.25 million people are chronically infected.

During the prenatal period, all patients are screened for hepatitis B surface antigen (HBsAg). Those with a positive HBsAg test are likely to have chronic disease and are at risk for transmission to the fetus. In order to confirm an active hepatitis B infection, hepatitis B core antibody and hepatitis B surface antibody IgM and IgG should also be checked. Patients with acute hepatitis B are positive for the HBsAg and positive for IgM antibody to the core antigen. Patients with chronic hepatitis B are positive for the surface antigen and positive for IgG antibody to the core antigen. Acutely or chronically infected patients may or may not be positive for the hepatitis B e antigen. If this latter antigen is present, it denotes active viral replication and a high level of infectivity. In the absence of intervention, approximately 20% of mothers who are seropositive for hepatitis B surface antigen will transmit infection to their neonates. Approximately 90% of mothers who are positive for both the surface antigen and the e antigen transmit infection. Fortunately, excellent immunoprophylaxis for prevention of perinatal transmission of hepatitis B infection is now available. Neonates delivered to seropositive mothers should receive hepatitis B immune globulin within 12 hours after birth. Before their discharge from the hospital, these infants also should begin the hepatitis B vaccination series. The CDC now recommends universal vaccination of all infants for hepatitis B. In addition, the vaccine should be offered to all women of reproductive age.

SYPHILIS

Syphilis is caused by infection with the spirochete *Treponema pallidum* and is usually transmitted via sexual contact or transplacentally to the fetus. Vertical transmission can occur at any time during pregnancy and while *T. pallidum* can cross the placenta and infect the fetus as early as 6 weeks' gestations, clinical manifestations are not apparent until after 16 weeks of gestation when fetal immunocompetence develops. Transmission may also occur intrapartum via contact with active genital lesions in the mother. Women with primary or secondary syphilis are more likely to transmit infection to their offspring than are women with latent disease. Maternal primary syphilis and secondary syphilis are associated with a 50% probability of congenital syphilis and a 50% rate of perinatal death; early latent syphilis, with a 40% risk of congenital syphilis and a 20% mortality rate; and late latent syphilis, with a 10% risk of congenital syphilis. More than 70% of infants born to mothers with untreated syphilis will be infected (with a 40% perinatal death rate and 40% developing congenital syphilis), compared with 1% to 2% of infants born to women who received adequate treatment during pregnancy. Despite prenatal screening and readily available treatment, there are still several hundred cases of congenital syphilis annually in the United States.

Syphilis during pregnancy that results in vertical transmission may lead to a late abortion, intrauterine fetal demise, hydrops, preterm delivery, neonatal death, early congenital syphilis, and the classic stigmata of late congenital syphilis. The most severe adverse pregnancy outcomes occur with primary or secondary syphilis. Pregnant women diagnosed with syphilis are usually in the latent stage and have had the disease for longer than 1 year. Consequently, about two-thirds of infants with early congenital syphilis are asymptomatic at birth and do not develop evidence of active disease for 3 to 8 weeks. Chancres do not occur unless the disease is acquired at the time of passage through the birth canal. Neonates with early congenital syphilis (onset at younger than 2 years of age) present with a systemic illness accompanied by a maculopapular rash, snuffles (a flu-like syndrome associated with a nasal discharge), hepatomegaly, splenomegaly, hemolysis, lymphadenopathy, jaundice, pseudoparalysis of Parrot due to osteochondritis, chorioretinitis, and iritis. Diagnosis of congenital syphilis can be made by identification of IgM antitreponemal antibodies, which do not cross the placenta. If early congenital syphilis is untreated, manifestations of late congenital syphilis can develop including saber shins, mulberry molars (see Color Plate 5), Hutchinson's teeth, saddle nose, and neurologic manifestations (eighth nerve deafness, mental retardation, hydrocephalus, optic nerve atrophy, and Clutton joints).

All pregnant women should be screened at the initial prenatal visit using nonspecific antibody tests including either the Venereal Disease Research Laboratory (VDRL) test or the rapid plasma reagin (RPR) test. If the test is positive, a titer is sent. Treponema-specific tests are employed for confirming the diagnosis of syphilis in patients who have reactive VDRL or RPR results. All positive results must then be confirmed with FTA-Abs, as there are false positives with both RPR and VDRL. There are several conditions that can cause false-positive RPR, including systemic lupus erythematosus and antiphospholipid antibody syndrome. Confirmatory tests include the fluorescent treponemal antibody absorption (FTA-ABS) test and the *T. pallidum* particle agglutination (TP-PA) test. Once reactive, specific treponemal tests usually remain positive for life. In pregnancy, it is best to consider all seropositive women as infected unless an adequate treatment history is documented and sequential serologic antibody titers have declined. High-risk patients should be rescreened at 28 weeks of gestation. In areas with high rates of congenital syphilis, rescreening at admission in labor is also recommended.

Penicillin remains the only treatment with sufficient evidence demonstrating efficacy for treating maternal infection, preventing maternal syphilis transmission to the fetus, and for treating fetal infection. Therefore, if a pregnant patient diagnosed with syphilis is penicillin allergic, she must undergo desensitization and then be treated with penicillin. A high maternal VDRL titer at the time of diagnosis, unknown duration of infection, treatment within 4 weeks of delivery, and ultrasound signs of fetal syphilis (e.g., hepatomegaly, fetal hydrops, placentomegaly) are associated with failure to prevent congenital syphilis. It is important to distinguish whether a patient has primary, secondary, latent, or tertiary syphilis in order to determine the length of treatment. If the patient has primary syphilis, one dose of 2.4 million units benzathine penicillin G is sufficient. However, if the patient has secondary or latent syphilis, the patient will require weekly treatments of 2.4 million units of benzathine penicillin G for 3 consecutive weeks. Syphilis can involve the CNS during any stage of disease. Therefore, any patient with syphilis who demonstrates clinical evidence of neurologic involvement should have a lumbar puncture to assess the cerebrospinal fluid for evidence of neurosyphilis. Patients with neurosyphilis should be treated with high doses of aqueous penicillin G. For primary and secondary syphilis, patients should be reexamined clinically and serologically at 6 and 12 months after treatment. A two-dilution (fourfold) decline in the nontreponemal titer at 1 year after treatment is used to define response.

TOXOPLASMOSIS

Toxoplasma gondii is a common protozoan parasite that can be found in humans and domestic animals. *T. gondii* has three distinct life forms: trophozoite, cyst, and oocyst. The life cycle of this organism is dependent on wild and domestic cats, which are the only known host for the oocyst. The oocyst is formed in the intestine of the cat and subsequently is excreted in feces. Mammals, such as cows, ingest the oocyst, which is disrupted in the animal's intestine, releasing the invasive trophozoite. The trophozoite then is disseminated throughout the body, ultimately forming cysts in brain and muscle. Human infection occurs when infected meat is ingested or oocysts are ingested via contamination by cat feces. Infection rates are highest in areas of poor sanitation and crowded living conditions. Stray cats and domestic cats that eat raw meat are most likely to carry the parasite. The cyst is completely destroyed by heating.

Approximately half of all adults in the United States have antibody to this organism. Immunity is usually long-lasting except in immunosuppressed patients. The prevalence of antibody is highest in lower socioeconomic classes. The frequency of seroconversion during pregnancy is approximately 5%, and about 3 in 1,000 infants show evidence of congenital infection. Clinically significant infection occurs in only 1 in 8,000 pregnancies. Clinical manifestations of infection are the result of direct organ damage and the subsequent immunologic response to parasitemia and cell death. Immunity to this infection is mediated primarily through T lymphocytes. The infections in immunocompetent hosts are often subclinical. Occasionally, a patient will develop fevers, malaise, lymphadenopathy, and a rash as with most viral infections. A pregnant woman who is infected can transmit the disease transplacentally to the fetus. Approximately 40% of neonates born to mothers with acute toxoplasmosis have evidence of infection. Transmission is more common when the disease is acquired in the third trimester, although neonatal manifestations are usually mild or subclinical. Infections acquired in the first trimester are transmitted less commonly; however, the infection has far more serious consequences in the fetus.

Severe congenital infection can involve fevers, seizures, chorioretinitis, hydro- or microcephaly, hepatosplenomegaly, and jaundice (see Color Plate 6). The usual clinical manifestations of congenital toxoplasmosis include a disseminated purpuric rash, enlargement of the spleen and liver, ascites, chorioretinitis, uveitis, periventricular calcifications, ventriculomegaly, seizures, and mental retardation. Chronic or latent infection in the mother is unlikely to be associated with serious fetal injury. Thus, the differential diagnosis for this infection includes nearly all other commonly acquired intrauterine infections. Diagnosis of toxoplasmosis in the neonate can be made with detection of IgM antibodies, but lack of the antibodies does not necessarily rule out infection.

Because women with previous *Toxoplasma* exposure are likely to be protected from further infections, high-risk patients can be screened with titers for IgG to ascertain whether or not they are at risk for infection. Pregnant women are advised to avoid contact with cat litter boxes and significant gardening without glove and mask protection during pregnancy, as the organism is found in cat feces and soil that may be contaminated with animal feces. Toxoplasmosis in pregnancy can be diagnosed maternally with IgM and IgG titers. Because IgM may persist for years, presence of IgM antibody cannot confirm an acute infection. Given the wide variability of IgM assays, diagnosis of an acute infection should be confirmed by a reference laboratory. If maternal diagnosis is made or suspected early in pregnancy, evaluation of amniotic fluid with DNA PCR for *T. gondii* via amniocentesis at least 4 weeks after maternal infection is the recommended procedure for evaluation of fetal infection. Fetal blood evaluation via percutaneous umbilical blood sampling (PUBS) is discouraged given the low sensitivity, as absence of fetal IgM does not completely rule out fetal infection and in turn has the potential of transplacental fetal infection. Once amniocentesis has confirmed toxoplasmic infection, targeted ultrasound examination is indicated to look for specific findings suggestive of severe fetal injury. Diagnosis may influence the decision of whether to terminate a pregnancy in the first two trimesters. When acute toxoplasmosis occurs during pregnancy, treatment is indicated because maternal therapy reduces the risk of congenital infection and decreases the late sequelae of infection. Maternal disease can be treated with spiramycin. Spiramycin is preferable in pregnant women because no teratogenic effects are known. However, because spiramycin does not cross the placenta, it is not effective in treatment of fetal infection. Therefore, pyrimethamine and sulfadiazine are recommended for treatment of documented fetal infection. Pyrimethamine is not recommended for use during the first trimester of pregnancy because of possible teratogenicity. Folic acid is concurrently administered due to the bone marrow suppression effects of pyrimethamine and sulfadiazine, given their folate antagonist effects. Aggressive early treatment of infants with congenital toxoplasmosis is indicated and consists of combination therapy with pyrimethamine, sulfadiazine, and leucovorin for 1 year. Early treatment reduces, but does not eliminate, the late sequelae of toxoplasmosis such as chorioretinitis. Early treatment of the neonate appears to be comparable in effectiveness to in utero therapy.

KEY POINTS

- Five percent of pregnant women have ASB and are at increased risk for cystitis and pyelonephritis.
- Lower UTIs can be treated with oral antibiotics, whereas pyelonephritis in pregnancy is usually treated initially with IV antibiotics, with change to oral regimen once afebrile for 24 to 48 hours.
- Pyelonephritis may be complicated by septic shock and ARDS.
- Symptomatic BV is associated with preterm delivery.
- BV treatment in pregnancy consists of oral metronidazole for 7 days.
- Screening and treatment of BV in asymptomatic high-risk pregnant women may be considered.
- GBS has traditionally been a leading cause of neonatal sepsis.
- Screening for GBS and using prophylactic antibiotics in labor has been shown to decrease GBS neonatal sepsis.
- GBS screening is performed between 35 and 37 weeks of gestation.
- Chorioamnionitis is diagnosed by maternal fever, uterine tenderness, elevated maternal WBC count, and fetal tachycardia.
- Although the infection is often polymicrobial, GBS colonization has a high correlation with both chorioamnionitis and neonatal sepsis.
- Chorioamnionitis is treated by IV antibiotics and delivery.
- It is important to differentiate between infections that are transmitted transplacentally and those that are acquired from passage through the birth canal.
- Infections during the first trimester during organogenesis are more likely to cause congenital abnormalities and spontaneous abortions.
- Congenital infections can lead to serious infections in the neonatal period, often with severe long-term sequelae, including mental retardation, blindness, and deafness.

C

Clinical Vignettes

Vignette 1

A 27-year-old G1P0 woman at 9 weeks' GA presents to your office to initiate prenatal care. She has no significant medical or surgical history. She has mild nausea throughout the day, but on review of systems, has no other concerns. You explain to her recommendations for prenatal screening tests at the first visit.

1. Which of the following are not recommended as part of routine prenatal laboratory test screening?
a. Urine culture
b. Herpes simplex antibody screen
c. Chlamydia PCR
d. HIV antibody screen
e. Rubella immune status

2. The screening urine culture returns with 100,000 colony forming units of *E. coli*. Which of the following are not complications of ASB in pregnancy?
a. Pyelonephritis
b. Preterm labor
c. Low-birth-weight infants
d. UTI
e. Oligohydramnios

3. You prescribe a 7-day course of Macrodantin. Two days later the sensitivities return and the *E. coli* is resistant to Macrodantin and sensitive to ciprofloxacin, amoxicillin, and cephalexin. Of these antibiotics, which would you avoid in the first trimester?
a. Ciprofloxacin
b. Amoxicillin
c. Cephalexin
d. None

4. You prescribe a 7-day course of amoxicillin to treat the *E. coli* bacteriuria. She does not fill the amoxicillin and continues to take the Macrodantin. She presents to the emergency department 1 week later with fever, urinary frequency, and right flank pain. She is mildly tachycardic and has a fever of 38.4°C. Her examination is significant for right-sided costovertebral angle tenderness. A urinalysis shows moderate leukocyte esterase, large nitrites, and many WBCs. In addition to hospital admission, what is the best initial treatment for this patient?
a. Direct admission to the ICU and aggressive IV fluid hydration
b. IV vancomycin
c. IV ceftriaxone
d. Oral amoxicillin
e. Oral Keflex

5. What is the most concerning complications of pyelonephritis during pregnancy?
a. Nephrolithiasis
b. Pneumonia
c. Acute respiratory distress syndrome (ARDS)
d. Chorioamnionitis
e. Oligohydramnios

Vignette 2

A 28-year-old G2P1001 woman at 39 and 4/7 weeks' GA presents to labor and delivery. Her contractions started 10 hours ago and now have increased in frequency to every 5 minutes. She reports a spontaneous gush of fluid, which was clear, just before the contractions started. She has continued to leak clear fluid and denies any vaginal bleeding. Her vital signs are significant for maternal heart rate of 110 bpm. You put her on the monitor and note the fetal heart rate to be in the 170s and reactive. You perform a sterile speculum examination and confirm ROM and note the fluid is cloudy with a foul odor. An abdominal examination confirms cephalic presentation but is notable for mild uterine tenderness.

1. What additional information would help you confirm the diagnosis?
a. Maternal fever greater than 38°C
b. Decreased maternal WBC
c. Decreased amniotic fluid
d. Blood cultures
e. Urine culture

2. You diagnose her with chorioamnionitis and admit her for IV antibiotics and augmentation of her labor. What is the most common causative organism(s)?
a. Listeria monocytogenes
b. Gardnerella vaginosis
c. Polymicrobial infection of rectovaginal organisms
d. Group B Streptococcus (GBS)
e. Enterococcus

3. Which of the following is one of the recommended antibiotic regimens?
a. IV penicillin
b. IV vancomycin
c. IV ceftriaxone

d. IV ampicillin and gentamicin
e. IV clindamycin

4. Which of the following is not a complication of chorioamnionitis?
a. Endomyometritis
b. Maternal sepsis
c. Postpartum hemorrhage
d. Neonatal pneumonia
e. Pyelonephritis

Vignette 3

A 28-year-old G1P0 woman at 28 weeks' GA comes to your office for a routine prenatal visit. She works as a kindergarten teacher and one of her students was recently sent home with a rash and fever. She states that the child had a rash on both cheeks and the pediatrician said it was a viral infection called fifth disease. She relates the baby is moving well and denies any vaginal bleeding, abnormal vaginal discharge, or contractions. She wonders if she needs any more testing to see if she has been affected.

1. What is the most likely causative organism of the child's infection?
a. Parvovirus
b. Varicella
c. CMV
d. Toxoplasmosis
e. Listeriosis

2. You send serologies for the agent above and they come back showing the patient has a positive IgM and negative IgG consistent with an acute infection. What is the most common fetal/neonatal complication of this infection during pregnancy?
a. Fetal anemia
b. Preterm labor
c. Premature preterm ROM
d. Fetal anomalies
e. Oligohydramnios

3. You perform an ultrasound of the fetus to evaluate for fetal anemia and hydrops. The ultrasound shows elevated MCA Doppler peak systolic velocity measurements consistent with fetal anemia. There is no evidence of fetal hydrops. What is the mechanism by which parvovirus infection causes fetal anemia?
a. Hemolysis
b. Bone marrow suppression
c. Sequestration of RBCs in the spleen
d. Fetal intracranial hemorrhage
e. Fetomaternal hemorrhage

Vignette 4

A 24-year-old G2P0010 woman at 8 weeks' GA presents for an initial prenatal visit. Her pregnancy is complicated by a history of IV drug use as a teenager and HIV. She had never been on HAART medication prior to this pregnancy. You order a viral load and it returns at 10,000. Her CD4 count is normal (>500). She is otherwise healthy and has no other significant medial history.

1. When would you recommend she start HAART?
a. At this visit
b. At 37 weeks in preparation for delivery
c. At the beginning of the second trimester
d. Immediately after delivery
e. Only if it is medically indicated for maternal health

2. She returns at 14 weeks and you start her on a three-drug HAART regimen of zidovudine, lamivudine, and lopinavir/ritonavir, which she tolerates well for the remainder of her pregnancy. Her viral load in the second trimester decreases to 5,000 and you consult an infection disease specialist to consider adjusting her medications. A repeat viral load at 38 weeks has decreased to 1,250. At 39 weeks she is admitted to labor and delivery in active labor. What would you recommend to her in order to further decrease neonatal transmission?
a. Early artificial ROM for labor augmentation
b. Placement of a fetal scalp electrode to monitor for signs of fetal distress
c. Assisted vaginal delivery with vacuum or forceps
d. Stopping all antiviral therapy to decrease risk of neonatal resistance
e. Cesarean delivery

3. The patient has an uncomplicated delivery of a vigorous female infant. Mother and baby are transferred to the postpartum ward. Which of the following activities would increase the risk of transmission to her baby?
a. Breastfeeding
b. Treatment of the infant on zidovudine prophylaxis
c. Treatment of the infant with zidovudine + nevirapine
d. Continuation of maternal HAART
e. Encouraging good hand washing and standard precautions at home

A Answers

Vignette 1 Question 1

Answer B: Herpes simplex antibody screening is not recommended for routine prenatal screening in the first visit. It is not recommended to screen for this infection, as there has been no demonstrated benefit in decreasing rates of vertical transmission to neonates.

It is recommended to screen for asymptomatic bacteriuria (ASB) with a urine culture at the initial prenatal visit given the risk of progression to a UTI or pyelonephritis. ASB is also associated with preterm birth and low-birth-weight infants. Screening is used to provide early treatment to decrease these risks.

Asymptomatic infection with Chlamydia is common and therefore, the CDC recommends that all pregnant women be screened at the beginning of pregnancy.

Given the proven benefit of antiretroviral therapy to decrease vertical transmission of HIV to 1% to 2%, it is recommended that all women be screened at the onset of pregnancy in order to diagnose those that would benefit from this intervention.

Rubella infection during pregnancy can lead to significant congenital malformations. Screening at the beginning of pregnancy is recommended in order to counsel women to avoid possible exposures. In addition, it is recommended that women who are rubella non-immune receive vaccination postpartum.

Vignette 1 Question 2

Answer E: Oligohydramnios is unrelated to maternal UTIs. Some factors that may lead to oligohydramnios include chromosomal abnormalities, uteroplacental insufficiency, hypertension, postterm pregnancy, twin–twin transfusion syndrome.

There is a risk of approximately 25% to 40% that ASB will progress to cystitis or pyelonephritis. Treatment should be initiated shortly after confirming the diagnosis and a test of cure should be performed to prove adequate treatment. Bacteriuria has also been associated with preterm birth and low-birth-weight infants.

Vignette 1 Question 3

Answer A: Ciprofloxacin has been associated with renal anomalies in the fetus, particularly in the first-trimester exposure. Because some fetal complications have been associated with ciprofloxacin even in later exposure, this medication is generally not given in pregnancy. Amoxicillin and Keflex are thought to be safe in pregnancy; both are category B, which means there were no adverse outcomes in animal reproduction studies.

Vignette 1 Question 4

Answer C: Pyelonephritis is estimated to complicate as many as 1% to 2% of pregnancies and has particularly serious associated complications including septic shock and ARDS. Because of these risks, pyelonephritis during pregnancy is usually treated aggressively with hospital admission, IV hydration, and IV antibiotics—often cephalosporins (cefazolin, cefotetan, or ceftriaxone) or ampicillin and gentamicin—until the patient is afebrile and asymptomatic for 24 to 48 hours. The patient is then transitioned to an oral antibiotic regimen. Small trials have examined the possibility of treating these patients with a single dose of IV or IM antibiotics, such as ceftriaxone, followed by outpatient oral antibiotic regimen. While these treatments seem to be effective in certain groups, consideration of appropriate patient criteria, including absence of signs of sepsis, compliance, ability to tolerate oral medications, and GA, is imperative. Treatment duration for pyelonephritis consists of a total of 10 to 14 days of combined IV and oral antibiotics.

Vignette 1 Question 5

Answer C: Pyelonephritis has significant morbidity during pregnancy and is associated with high rates of ICU admission and ARDS. Because of this, it is recommended that pregnant women be admitted to the hospital for observation and treatment. IV fluids should be used judiciously given the risk of pulmonary edema and ARDS. Pregnant women are also at increased risk for urosepsis and septic shock. Initial antibiotic choice is usually ceftriaxone. Women should improve after 24 to 48 hours if therapy and once afebrile for 48 hours can be transitioned to oral therapy based on sensitivities. Oral antibiotics should be continued for total course of 10 to 14 days. For the remainder of the pregnancy, it is recommended the patient takes prophylactic antibiotics, usually 100 mg Macrobid daily.

Pyelonephritis has not been shown to cause nephrolithiasis. However, UTIs with *Proteus mirabilis* and other urea-splitting bacteria are commonly associated with struvite kidney stones. These stones are usually found in patients who are predisposed to UTIs, such as those with spinal cord injury or neurogenic bladder syndromes.

Pneumonia is not a common complication of pyelonephritis. However, pyelonephritis can lead to pulmonary edema from the release of endotoxin that causes increased vascular and alveolar capillary permeability.

Pyelonephritis may lead to urosepsis, but the placenta serves as a barrier and there is no increased risk of intra-amniotic infection. In addition, placental function is unchanged and as a result there is no increased risk of oligohydramnios.

Vignette 2 Question 1

Answer A: Chorioamnionitis is a clinical diagnosis that complicates 2% to 4% of term pregnancies. Research criteria require a maternal fever of greater than 38°C and at least two of the following signs: elevated maternal WBC count, maternal tachycardia, uterine tenderness, fetal tachycardia, and foul-smelling amniotic fluid. The gold standard for diagnosis of chorioamnionitis is a culture of the amniotic fluid, which can be obtained via amniocentesis. At the same time, the amniotic fluid can be sent for glucose, WBC count, protein, and Gram stain. Amniocentesis is most commonly used in preterm patients whose fetuses would benefit from remaining in utero for more time and where a more aggressive means to reach the diagnosis can be taken if there is any doubt.

Vignette 2 Question 2

Answer C: Chorioamnionitis at term is most commonly caused by polymicrobial infections of bacteria from the vagina and rectum. In some studies, almost 60% had more than one organism present from amniotic fluid culture. The most common organisms regardless of GA are genital *mycoplasma* species (*ureaplasma* and *mycoplasma*). Other common organisms include *Gardnerella vaginosis*, *E. coli*, *Enterococcus*, *Bacteroides* species, and GBS.

Vignette 2 Question 3

Answer D: When chorioamnionitis is suspected, the patient should be admitted and IV antibiotics started. Because chorioamnionitis is a polymicrobial infection caused by organisms that colonize the vagina and rectum, broad-spectrum coverage should be used. Most commonly treatment is with cefoxitin (or other second- or third-generation cephalosporin) or ampicillin and gentamicin. In addition to antibiotics, delivery should be hastened with induction and augmentation by vaginal delivery, or, in the case of a nonreassuring fetal tracing, by cesarean delivery.

The patient's initial cervical examination was 7 cm dilation, 100% effacement, and 0 station. After starting IV fluids, ampicillin and gentamicin and giving Tylenol, the maternal fever resolves and the fetal tachycardia improves. You start oxytocin for augmentation and the fetal heart tracing remains reassuring. She progresses to complete dilation and delivers a vigorous infant. The neonatal resuscitation team is in attendance and due to the risk of neonatal sepsis they recommend that the baby be admitted to the NICU for blood cultures and IV antibiotics.

Vignette 2 Question 4

Answer E: Chorioamnionitis is the most common precursor of neonatal sepsis, which has a high rate of fetal mortality. Other neonatal complications include pneumonia and meningitis. Neonatal morbidity and mortality appears to be increased for infants and earlier GAs. The most common maternal complications include dysfunctional labor and need for cesarean section, uterine atony, and postpartum hemorrhage. Other maternal complications include endomyometritis, bacteremia, adult acute respiratory distress syndrome, and septic shock. With early initiation of IV antibiotics, the more severe complications of ARDS and sepsis are quite rare.

Vignette 3 Question 1

Answer A: Parvovirus B19 causes erythema infectiosum (fifth disease). Classically, this mild infection presents with a low-grade fever and a red macular rash giving the "slapped cheek" appearance, and usually resolves with minimal intervention. Approximately one-third to one-half of pregnant women have IgG to the virus and are immune from a prior infection. Among pregnant women who do not have immunity, the incidence of acute parvovirus infection during pregnancy is around 3%. If parvovirus exposure is suspected in the mother, acute infection can be diagnosed by checking parvovirus IgM and IgG levels.

Vignette 3 Question 2

Answer A: Acute parvovirus infections during pregnancy may be transmitted through the placenta to the fetus. First-trimester infections have been associated with miscarriage, but midtrimester and later infections are associated with fetal anemia and hydrops. If studies indicate an acute parvovirus infection (positive IgM and positive or negative IgG) beyond 20 weeks of gestation, then the fetus should undergo serial ultrasounds, up to 8 to 10 weeks after maternal infection. Currently, Doppler ultrasound to examine the peak systolic velocity of the MCA is frequently used identify fetal anemia. Small studies have shown a benefit of fetal transfusion for fetal anemia leading to hydrops; however, these studies also reported fetal deaths from complications related to transfusion so this procedure is likely to be reserved for the most severe cases.

Vignette 3 Question 3

Answer B: Parvovirus B19 causes fetal anemia by bone marrow suppression. The virus is cytotoxic to RBC precursors, leading to decreased production. Severe anemia can lead to high output cardiac failure, hydrops, and fetal death. Parvovirus can also lead to pancytopenia in the fetus, and this has important clinical implications as fetal thrombocytopenia can increase the risk of exsanguination and fetal death during attempts at intrauterine transfusion. It is also important to note that this mechanism for fetal anemia is different from that of Rh alloimmunization, which leads to fetal anemia via hemolysis.

Vignette 4 Question 1

Answer C: Currently, antiretroviral therapy in pregnancy includes a three-drug regimen generally started in the second trimester with a goal of viral suppression by the third trimester. This is started regardless of need for antiretrovirals for maternal health indication. With improved antiretroviral treatment during pregnancy, rates of perinatal transmission have decreased from 1,650 in 1991 to less than 240 per year in 2002 (CDC). Transmission occurs in utero (one-third) generally late in pregnancy or during labor and delivery (two-third). In 1994, Pediatric AIDS Clinical Trials Group (PACTG) protocol 076 demonstrated that a three-part regimen of zidovudine (ZDV) administered during pregnancy and labor and to the newborn could reduce the risk of perinatal transmission by two-thirds. Additionally, with the use of HAART to further decrease viral load with potent regimens, the rate of transmission can be further decreased to less than 1% to 2% with an undetectable viral load. Increased transmission can be seen with higher viral burden or advanced disease in the mother, rupture of the membranes, and invasive procedures during labor and delivery that increase neonatal exposure to maternal blood.

Vignette 4 Question 2

Answer E: Cesarean delivery has been shown to lower transmission rates by roughly two-thirds compared to vaginal delivery in patients on no therapy and particularly without onset of labor or ROM or in the setting of high viral load. However, in women with viral loads of less than 1,000 copies/mL, there is no additional benefit of cesarean delivery versus vaginal delivery in HIV perinatal transmission. Therefore, cesarean delivery should be considered in HIV-infected pregnant women with viral loads greater than 1,000 copies/mL and without long-standing onset of labor or ROM.

Vignette 4 Question 3

Answer A: In resource-rich nations where safe bottle-feeding alternatives are available, breastfeeding is contraindicated in HIV-infected women as virus is found in breast milk and responsible for HIV transmission to the infant. Postnatal HIV transmission from breast milk at 2 years may be as high as 15%. Furthermore, studies are lacking regarding the efficacy of maternal antiretroviral therapy for prevention of transmission of HIV through breast milk and the toxicity of antiretroviral exposure of the infant via breast milk. In resource-poor nations, breastfeeding is encouraged because of increased risk of neonatal mortality from diarrheal diseases, pneumonia, and other infectious diseases. In resource-rich nations, infants are placed on a 6-week course of zidovudine or zidovudine + nevirapine to further decrease the risk of vertical transmission. Standard precautions and good hand washing behavior should always be encouraged because they may not lower the risk of transmission but would not increase the risk either.

Chapter

11 Other Medical Complications of Pregnancy

The previous three chapters discussed hypertension, diabetes, and infectious disease in the context of the pregnant patient. In this chapter, a variety of the other common medical complications of pregnancy are discussed. Pregnancy affects every physiologic system in the body as well as many disease states. Disease management in pregnancy requires consideration of any potential fetal effects of treatment or imaging modalities.

HYPEREMESIS GRAVIDARUM

Nausea and vomiting in pregnancy, or "morning sickness," are common. Seen in 88% of pregnancies, morning sickness usually resolves by week 16. Various etiologies have been proposed, including elevated levels of human chorionic gonadotropin, thyroid hormone, or the intrinsic hormones of the gut. There seems to be a disordered motility of the upper gastrointestinal tract that contributes to the problem. Despite the nausea and vomiting, patients are usually able to maintain adequate nutrition. However, patients occasionally become dehydrated and potentially develop electrolyte abnormalities. The diagnosis of **hyperemesis gravidarum** is made when a woman has persistent vomiting, weight loss of greater than 5% of prepregnancy body weight, and ketonuria. In particular, hyperemesis is common in the setting of molar pregnancies (likely since HCG levels can be very high) and a viable IUP should always be documented in patients with hyperemesis.

TREATMENT AND PROGNOSIS

For patients with true hyperemesis gravidarum, symptoms may persist into the third trimester and, rarely, until term. The goal of therapy is to maintain adequate nutrition. First-line antiemetic therapy is usually with Phenergan, followed by addition of Reglan, Compazine, and Tigan. If these fail, droperidol and Zofran can also be used safely in pregnancy. Persistent nausea and vomiting during pregnancy can also be treated with vitamin B_6 and doxylamine (Unisom). Ginger and supplementation with vitamin B_{12} have also been shown to be effective adjuncts to antiemetic therapy. If symptoms persist to dehydration, patients should be rehydrated and electrolyte abnormalities corrected. Since a hypochloremic alkalosis often results from extensive vomiting, normal saline with 5% dextrose is commonly used for IV hydration. In the acute setting, antiemetics should be given intravenously, intramuscularly, or as suppositories because oral medications may be vomited prior to systemic absorption.

Long-term management of hyperemesis includes maintaining hydration, adequate nutrition, and symptomatic relief from the nausea and vomiting. Many patients respond to antiemetics and IV hydration. Once they are rehydrated, they can use the antiemetic to control nausea so that they are able to maintain oral intake. In addition, since hypoglycemia may contribute to the symptom of nausea, frequent small meals can help maintain more stable blood glucose and decrease nausea.

Rarely patients will not respond to antiemetics and recurrent rehydration. In these cases, treatment with corticosteroids has been shown to decrease symptoms. Other alternative treatments shown to decrease nausea include acupuncture, acupressure, hypnotherapy, and nerve stimulation. A small percentage of patients for whom the treatment fails will require feeding tubes or even parenteral nutrition for the course of the pregnancy. As long as hydration and adequate nutrition are maintained, pregnancy outcomes are usually good.

SEIZURE DISORDERS

Approximately 20,000 women with seizure disorders give birth each year. Concerns during these pregnancies include risk of fetal malformations, miscarriage, perinatal death, and increased seizure frequency. Women with epilepsy appear to have a greater baseline risk of fetal malformations that is further increased with the use of antiepileptic drugs (AEDs). Concerns regarding fetal effects lead to decreased compliance with AEDs. Additionally, normal physiologic changes of pregnancy include increased volume of distribution (V_D) and increased hepatic metabolism of AEDs. The combination of these factors is thought to contribute to increased seizure frequency in 17% to 33% of pregnancies. When managing these women in pregnancy, the risks of increased seizures versus use of AEDs need to be weighed carefully.

SEIZURE FREQUENCY

There are a variety of possible etiologies proposed for the increase in seizure frequency seen in some pregnancies. Increased levels of circulating estrogen during pregnancy in turn increase the function of the P_{450} enzymes, which leads to more rapid hepatic metabolism of AEDs. In addition, renal function increases during pregnancy with a 50% rise in creatinine clearance that affects the metabolism of carbamazepine, primidone, and the benzodiazepines. The increase in total blood volume and concomitant rise in the V_D leads to decreased levels of circulating AEDs. Hormonal changes, added stress, and decreased sleep during pregnancy likely lower seizure threshold and have been shown to increase seizure frequency in nonpregnant patients. Finally, many women may have decreased compliance with AEDs because of concerns regarding fetal effects.

Increased levels of estrogen and progesterone may both have direct effects on seizure activity during pregnancy. Estrogen has been shown to be epileptogenic, decreasing seizure threshold. Thus, rising estrogen levels in pregnancy that peak in the third trimester may have some impact on the observed increase in seizure frequency. Conversely, progesterone seems to have an antiepileptic effect. It has been observed that women with seizure disorders have fewer seizures during the luteal phase of the menstrual cycle.

FETAL CONGENITAL ABNORMALITIES AND ADVERSE OUTCOMES

The earliest reports of congenital malformations associated with AEDs occurred in the 1960s. Since then, unique malformations and syndromes have been ascribed to phenytoin, phenobarbital, primidone, valproate, carbamazepine, and trimethadione. However, there are similarities between most of the congenital abnormalities caused by the AEDs (Table 11-1). There is evidence that epileptic women have an increased risk of fetal malformations even without AED use. While some studies suggest monotherapy does not increase that baseline risk, there are other studies that do show evidence of an increase in fetal malformations with AED polytherapy.

Specific increases in congenital abnormalities seen in infants born to epileptic mothers include a fourfold increase in cleft lip and palate and a three- to fourfold increase in cardiac anomalies. There is also an increase in the rate of neural tube defects (NTDs) seen in the offspring of epileptic patients who are using carbamazepine or valproic acid. Long-term studies on neurodevelopment show higher rates of abnormal EEG findings, higher rates of developmentally delayed children, and lower IQ scores. There are specific findings that are attributed to particular AEDs.

MECHANISMS OF TERATOGENICITY

The mechanisms of teratogenicity of AEDs have not been fully characterized. Phenobarbital, primidone, and phenytoin act as folate antagonists. Certainly, it appears that folate deficiency can lead to an increase in congenital malformations, particularly NTDs. Folate prior to conception has therefore been recommended for prophylaxis. Since all AEDs have a similar central mechanism to control seizures, there may be a common pathway—disrupted during embryogenesis—that leads to the similarities in the syndromes described. This may explain why there is an additive effect in polytherapy.

Recent studies in teratogenesis—particularly in the fetal hydantoin syndrome—point to a genetic predilection for the generation of epoxides. Specifically, children whose enzyme activity of epoxide hydrolase is one-third less than normal have an increased rate of fetal hydantoin syndrome. Anomalies have also been observed in children exposed to carbamazepine with low epoxide hydrolase activity.

CLINICAL MANAGEMENT

Because exposure to multiple AEDs seems to be more teratogenic than monotherapy, patients are advised to switch to a single AED prior to conception and taper down to the lowest possible dose. Patients who have been seizure-free for 2 to 5 years may wish to attempt complete withdrawal from AEDs prior to conception. Because there is particular evidence that high peak plasma levels of valproic acid may be more teratogenic than constant steady-state levels, it should be dosed three to four times per day rather than the standard twice per day dosing. However, epileptic patients should be counseled that they are still at a greater risk (4% to 6% vs. 2% to 3%) for fetal

TABLE 11-1 Fetal Anomalies Associated with Antiepileptic Drugs

Fetal Anomaly	Phenytoin	Phenobarbital	Primidone	Valproate	Carbamazepine	Trimethadione
NTD				X	X	
IUGR	X					X
Microcephaly					X	X
Low IQ	X		X			
Distal digital hypoplasia	X	X	X			
Low-set ears	X	X				X
Epicanthal fold	X	X		X	X	X
Short nose	X	X		X	X	
Long philtrum			X		X	
Lip abnormalities	X	X	X	X		
Hypertelorism	X	X				
Developmental delay		X			X	X
Other	Ptosis	Ptosis	Hirsutism of forehead		Hypoplastic nails	Cardiac anomalies

anomalies than the baseline population. Folate has been shown to decrease NTDs in patients without epilepsy. Therefore patients should be advised to take supplemental folate prior to conception, particularly those using either valproic acid or carbamazepine. There are a number of new AEDs (levetiracetam, lamotrigine, felbamate, topiramate, and oxcarbazepine) that have not demonstrated the same frequency of congenital anomalies as the older AEDs, but these medications have not been formally studied beyond small case series, so it is difficult to truly determine the safety at this time.

Because of the increased risk of anomalies, a level II fetal survey at 19 to 20 weeks of gestation should be performed with careful attention to the face, CNS, and heart (Table 11-2). Because of the increased risk of NTDs, a maternal serum α-fetoprotein (MSAFP) screening test should be offered. The decision to perform an amniocentesis routinely for AFP and acetylcholinesterase is controversial. Since the sensitivity of amniocentesis is higher than either MSAFP or ultrasound for NTDs, many practitioners recommend amniocentesis in the setting of a family history of NTDs or with use of valproic acid or carbamazepine.

Recent studies of seizure frequency show less of an increase than older studies, which suggests that the practice of closer monitoring of AED dosing and levels may have some effect on the number of seizures during pregnancy. A recent study shows that 38% of pregnant patients with epilepsy require changes in their AED dosing to achieve seizure control. Assuming that monotherapy with one of the AEDs has been achieved preconceptionally, total and free serum levels of the AED should be obtained on a monthly basis (see Table 11-2).

LABOR AND DELIVERY

Management of the epileptic patient on labor and delivery should involve preparation and close monitoring. All care providers—obstetricians, neurology, nursing, anesthesia, and pediatrics—should be informed about an epileptic patient in labor and delivery. AED levels should be checked upon admission. If the level is low, patients may be given extra dosing or switched to IV benzodiazepines or phenytoin, bearing in mind that benzodiazepines can cause respiratory depression in both the mother and newborn. Since trauma and hypoxia from a seizure can put both the mother and fetus at risk, treatment of seizures should be discussed a priori with the group of practitioners caring for the patient. Management of seizures on labor and delivery is discussed in Chapter 6. One difference is that the drug of choice in patients with a known seizure disorder is usually phenytoin compared to magnesium used in preeclamptic patients.

There have been reports of increased risk of spontaneous hemorrhage in newborns because of the inhibition of vitamin K–dependent clotting factors (i.e., II, VII, IX, X) secondary to increased vitamin K metabolism and inhibition of placental transport of vitamin K by AEDs. While the risk is small, conservative management is to overcome this theoretical vitamin K deficiency by aggressive supplementation with vitamin K toward the end of pregnancy. The benefit of this treatment is theoretical as it is not clear if vitamin K actually crosses the placenta. Upon delivery, clotting studies can be performed on the cord blood and vitamin K administered to the infant. If the cord blood is deficient in clotting factors, fresh frozen plasma may be required to protect the newborn.

TABLE 11-2 Management of Women with Epilepsy During Pregnancy

Check total and free levels of antiepileptic drugs on a monthly basis
Consider early genetic counseling
Check MSAFP
Level II ultrasound for fetal survey at 19 to 20 wks' gestation
Consider amniocentesis for α-fetoprotein and acetylcholinesterase
Supplement with oral vitamin K 20 mg QD starting at 37 wks until delivery (optional)

MATERNAL CARDIAC DISEASE

The cardiovascular system undergoes a number of dramatic changes in pregnancy with a 50% increase in blood volume, decrease in systemic vascular resistance, increase in cardiac stroke volume, and actual remodeling of the myocardium to accommodate some of these changes. Recent studies demonstrate that cardiac disease is leading to an increasing proportion of maternal mortality in the United States. When caring for patients with cardiac disease preconceptionally or during pregnancy, these changes are paramount when counseling them regarding their options and managing their disease. In particular, patients with primary pulmonary hypertension, Eisenmenger physiology, severe mitral or aortic stenosis, and Marfan syndrome are at a high risk of maternal mortality in pregnancy (reportedly ranging from 15% to 70% in small case series). In patients with cardiac disease and an increased risk of maternal mortality, the option to terminate the pregnancy should always be offered and discussed at length with the patient. Unfortunately, since such women often may not be able to adopt because of their illness, they may think of their own pregnancy as the only way to have children.

PRINCIPLES OF MANAGEMENT

Cardiac diseases vary widely but the principles of management are similar. Many of the diseases are stable prior to pregnancy with medical management, but during pregnancy can become quite unstable in response to the physiologic changes. Additionally, medications used during pregnancy may be different from those used outside of pregnancy. In particular, many of the newest antihypertensives and antiarrhythmics have been sparsely studied in pregnant women, and are thus commonly avoided. Of the more common agents, ACE inhibitors, diuretics, and warfarin (Coumadin) have all been associated with congenital anomalies and other fetal effects and are usually discontinued in pregnancy. The 2007 American Heart Association Guidelines state that routine vaginal delivery and cesarean section are not indications for subacute bacterial endocarditis (SBE) prophylaxis. However, SBE prophylaxis may be considered for women with high-risk lesions (mechanical or prosthetic valves, unrepaired cyanotic lesions, etc.) and an infection that could cause bacteremia (chorioamnionitis or pyelonephritis).

Patients who would benefit from surgical repair of a lesion as in mitral or aortic stenosis should undergo surgical repair a year or more before becoming pregnant. Because of high maternal risk, those who become pregnant before surgical repair should be offered termination of the pregnancy as the first line of management. It is important that patients and their families are aware of the risks of disabling morbidity and mortality if they decide to continue the pregnancy. Management and early intervention during labor and delivery can help reduce risk for cardiac patients. Early epidural analgesia to control pain can minimize the cardiac stress of labor and delivery. Likewise, an assisted vaginal delivery (using forceps or vacuum) can diminish the potential detrimental cardiac effect of Valsalva while pushing. In addition, careful fluid monitoring should be maintained, possibly with a central venous pressure monitor and arterial line. After delivery, massive fluid shifts make the immediate postpartum period a particularly dangerous transition for women with congenital heart disease. These fluid shifts have two main sources. First, postpartum women have increased venous return because they no longer have an enlarged uterus compressing the vena cava. Second, the uterus clamps down after placental expulsion and demands less circulation, leading to an effective autotransfusion of its blood supply (approximately 500 cc).

CARDIOVASCULAR DISEASE

Rising average maternal age in pregnancy means there will be an increasing number of patients with a history of a myocardial infarction (MI) who become pregnant. Small case series show that, if optimally managed, these patients do relatively well in pregnancy. A baseline ECG and adjustment of medications, if necessary, should be performed at the initial visit. Throughout pregnancy and during labor and delivery, it is important to minimize increased demand on the heart.

EISENMENGER SYNDROME AND PULMONARY HYPERTENSION

Patients with right-to-left shunts and pulmonary hypertension (PH) are among the sickest pregnant women, with mortality rates estimated at 50% and higher. The most common right-to-left shunts are patent ductus arteriosus (PDA) and ventricular septal defect (VSD), which have reversed as a result of Eisenmenger syndrome. In Eisenmenger syndrome, an initial left-to-right shunt overfills the right heart. This, in turn, leads to increased flow through the pulmonary vasculature, pulmonary capillary damage, and the formation of scar tissue. As a result, patients develop right ventricular hypertrophy and pulmonary hypertension and eventually a right-to-left shunt.

These patients are chronically hypoxic secondary to the mixing of deoxygenated blood and are encouraged to terminate their pregnancies. Patients who elect to continue are followed with serial echocardiograms to measure the pulmonary pressures and cardiac function. Some have been managed with inhaled nitric oxide, but this has not been shown to significantly improve the measured clinical indicators of disease or the outcomes. These patients often decompensate in the third trimester of pregnancy. Labor and assisted vaginal delivery are preferable to elective cesarean delivery. Perhaps the greatest concentrated risk of morbidity and mortality is in the postpartum period for approximately 2 to 4 weeks after delivery. It has been hypothesized that this risk is secondary to the sudden changes in hormones. Unfortunately, attempts to counter these changes with progesterone and estrogen supplementation have had little success.

VALVULAR DISEASE

While the manifestations of the different valvular diseases vary, they are similar in that surgical treatment or repair prior to becoming pregnant is preferred for moderate or severe disease carrying increased risk of maternal mortality. Patients with aortic stenosis and aortic insufficiency require a decreased afterload to maintain cardiac output, and thus initially may have diminished symptoms in response to the decreased systemic vascular resistance seen in pregnancy. Patients with mitral stenosis may be unable to meet the increased demands of pregnancy and experience a backup into the pulmonary system leading to congestive heart failure (CHF). Patients with pulmonary stenosis who elect to continue their pregnancy may actually undergo valvuloplasty during the pregnancy if they have severe disease.

MARFAN SYNDROME

Patients with Marfan syndrome have a deficiency in their elastin that can lead to a number of valvular cardiac complications as well as dilation of the aortic root. During pregnancy, the hyperdynamic state can increase the risk of aortic dissection and/or rupture, particularly in those patients with an aortic root diameter greater than 4 cm. In order to decrease some of the pressure on the aorta, patients are advised to maintain a sedentary lifestyle and are often placed on beta-blockers to decrease cardiac output.

PERIPARTUM CARDIOMYOPATHY

A small percentage of patients will be found to have heart failure secondary to a dilated cardiomyopathy immediately before, during, or after delivery. Some of these patients likely have a baseline mild cardiomyopathy, whereas others have a postinfectious dilated cardiomyopathy. However, the epidemiology supports the idea that, at least in some cases, **peripartum cardiomyopathy** (PPCM) is specifically caused by pregnancy. Patients present with classic signs and symptoms of heart failure and on echocardiogram have a dilated heart with an ejection fraction far below normal in the 20% to 40% range.

Patients with PPCM should be managed according to the GA of the fetus. Beyond 34 weeks' GA, the risks to the mother of remaining pregnant are usually greater than those of premature delivery of the fetus. At earlier GAs, however, betamethasone should be administered to promote fetal lung maturity, and the patient delivered accordingly. The patient's heart failure is managed similarly to other patients with heart failure using diuretics, digoxin, and vasodilators. Well over half of the patients with PPCM have excellent return to baseline of their cardiac activity within several months of delivery.

MATERNAL RENAL DISEASE

Chronic renal disease can be divided into mild (Cr < 1.5), moderate (Cr from 1.5 to 2.8), and severe (Cr > 2.8), although other thresholds have been used. Renal blood flow and creatinine clearance increase during pregnancy in patients without renal disease, and this is also true initially in patients with renal disease. In fact, patients with mild renal disease will usually experience improvement in renal function throughout much of pregnancy. Moderate and severe patients, however, may experience decreasing renal function in the latter half of pregnancy that may persist postpartum in as many as half of pregnancies. Because of this, it is important to counsel these patients preconceptionally regarding the risks to them from pregnancy—in particular, the increased risk of requiring dialysis and its concomitant morbidities.

CRD Patients with chronic renal disease have increased risk of preeclampsia, preterm delivery, and intrauterine growth restriction (IUGR) in addition to worsening renal disease, and therefore, they should be screened at least once per trimester with a 24-hour urine for creatinine clearance and protein. Patients who present in early pregnancy should be counseled regarding these risks and offered termination of pregnancy, particularly for the mother's health. Because of the risk to the fetus, antenatal fetal testing usually begins at 32 to 34 weeks' gestation. For patients who have baseline proteinuria and hypertension, the diagnosis of preeclampsia can be difficult to make. In these patients, a baseline uric acid is assessed and, if normal at baseline, can be used in the setting of worsening BPs to help diagnose preeclampsia. An increase in BP of 30/15 mm Hg above prepregnancy BPs can also be used, though experts disagree on its utility.

An interesting subgroup of women are those who are status post renal transplant. It seems that such women will have outcomes similar to women with similar creatinine clearance. However, there are several issues. Commonly, these women will be on immunosuppressants such as cyclosporine, tacrolimus, prednisone, and Imuran. Because of increased metabolism and volume of distribution, dosages of these medications may need to be increased during pregnancy. If this is not done, the risk of acute rejection increases due to undertreatment. Similarly, because women may be concerned about the effects of these medications on the developing fetus, they may stop taking the medications and be at increased risk for rejection. Medication levels, creatinine, and creatinine clearance are commonly checked monthly in such women.

COAGULATION DISORDERS

Pregnancy is generally considered a "hypercoagulable" state. The pathogenesis of this state has not been elucidated, but several mechanisms have been proposed, including increased coagulation factors, endothelial damage, and venous stasis (Virchow's triad). The risk for superficial vein thrombosis, deep vein thrombosis, and pulmonary embolus is further increased postpartum, and pulmonary embolus remains one of the leading causes of maternal mortality. Additionally, women with a preexisting thrombophilia may get pregnant. These women, in particular, are at high risk for developing deep vein thrombosis or pulmonary embolus.

PATHOGENESIS

No single cause of the hypercoagulability of pregnancy has been found, but there are several possible mechanisms hypothesized. The first is that there is an intrinsic increase in coagulability of the serum itself. In pregnancy, the production of all clotting factors is increased except for II, V and IX. Turnover time for fibrinogen is also decreased during pregnancy and there are increased levels of fibrinopeptide A, which is cleaved from fibrinogen to make fibrin. Additionally, there are increased levels of circulating fibrin monomer complexes. These levels increase further at the time of delivery and immediately postpartum. Finally, it has been hypothesized that the placenta synthesizes a factor that decreases fibrinolysis, but there is minimal evidence for this.

Another proposed source of hypercoagulability is increased exposure to subendothelial collagen as a result of increased endothelial damage during pregnancy, although no mechanism has been proposed. It has also been hypothesized that endothelial damage in the venous system during parturition increases the amount of thrombogenesis postpartum. This seems feasible, particularly as the etiology of pelvic vein thrombosis, but it does not account for the hypercoagulability throughout pregnancy.

Venous stasis may also account for some of the increase in venous thromboses during and after pregnancy. There are two principal causes for venous stasis in pregnancy. The first is decreased venous tone during pregnancy, which may be related to the smooth muscle relaxant properties of this high progesterone state. Second, the uterus, as it enlarges, compresses the inferior vena cava, the iliac, and pelvic veins. This compression, in particular, likely contributes to the increase in pelvic vein thromboses.

SUPERFICIAL VEIN THROMBOSIS

Although **superficial vein thrombosis** (SVT) is a painful complication of hypercoagulability, it is believed to be unlikely to lead to emboli. The diagnosis is usually obvious with a palpable, usually visible, venous cord that is quite tender, with local erythema and edema. Because of the low risk of emboli from SVT, it is not routinely treated other than symptomatically with warm compresses and analgesics. However, the patient should be informed of the signs and symptoms of DVTs and PEs because she may be at an increased risk for either.

DEEP VEIN THROMBOSIS

Diagnosis of **deep vein thrombosis** (DVT) is often made clinically with confirmation by Doppler studies or venography. The typical patient presents with unilateral lower extremity pain and swelling. On examination, patients will often have edema, local erythema, tenderness, venous distension, and a palpable cord underlying the region of pain and tenderness. When clinical suspicion is high, the patient is usually sent for noninvasive lower extremity studies with the Doppler ultrasound for confirmation of a venous obstruction. Rarely, venography, the gold standard, will be used.

Treatment of DVT during pregnancy involves the use of adjusted dose low-molecular-weight heparin (enoxaparin 1 mg/kg BID) or unfractionated heparin (goal aPTT of 1.5 to 2.5 times normal). Low-molecular-weight heparin has become the preferred option because levels do not need to be checked and it is also thought to be safer due to a lower risk of heparin-induced thrombocytopenia. When using unfractionated heparin, the initial treatment is with IV heparin, which is later transitioned to subcutaneous heparin throughout the remainder of the pregnancy and postpartum. Warfarin therapy is contraindicated in pregnancy because it is teratogenic. When given in the first trimester, it causes warfarin embryopathy, a combination of nasal hypoplasia and skeletal abnormalities. In addition, warfarin appears to cause diffuse CNS abnormalities, including optic atrophy, when given during pregnancy.

PULMONARY EMBOLUS

Pulmonary embolus (PE) results when emboli from DVTs travel to the right side of the heart and then lodge in the pulmonary arterial system, leading to **pulmonary hypertension**, **hypoxia**, and, depending on the extent of the emboli,

right-sided heart failure and **death**. Clinical suspicion of pulmonary embolus is raised whenever a patient presents with acute onset of shortness of breath, simultaneous onset of pleuritic chest pain, hemoptysis or tachycardia, and/or concomitant signs of DVT.

The diagnosis of PE usually depends on the clinical picture correlated with a variety of diagnostic tests. A chest X-ray may be entirely normal. However, when abnormal, two common signs on chest X-ray are the abrupt termination of a vessel as it is traced distally and an area of radiolucency in the region of lung beyond the PE. An ECG may also be entirely normal or simply show sinus tachycardia. On occasion, however, it will show signs of right-heart strain with right-axis deviation, nonspecific ST changes, and peaked T-waves. Spiral CT scan is the most common diagnostic tool for PE in both the pregnant and nonpregnant patient. The risk of radiation exposure must be weighed against the suspected risk of a PE and the dangers that a PE poses to a pregnant woman's health. As with other life-threatening medical conditions, the woman's health should be the primary consideration and she should receive the same standard-of-care as a nonpregnant patient. Previously more common, ventilation/perfusion (V/Q) scanning is now used less frequently. The V/Q scan is a radionuclide scan that first allows visualization of lung perfusion by detecting a radioisotope in the pulmonary circulation (Fig. 11-1). An entirely normal perfusion scan rules out PE. However, if there is a defect in perfusion, a ventilation scan is performed. Mismatched defects in the ventilation and perfusion scans are suggestive of PE. Pulmonary angiography is the gold standard for diagnosis of PE. The pulmonary artery is catheterized and a radiopaque dye is injected. Diagnosis is made by the presence of intraluminal filling defects or if sharp vessel cutoffs are seen (Fig. 11-2).

Treatment of mild PE is similar to the treatment of DVT, with low-molecular-weight heparin (enoxaparin) being the preferred choice in hemodynamically stable patients. In the hypotensive or unstable patient, IV heparin is the recommended option. Massive PE leading to an unstable hypoxic patient is often treated with streptokinase for thrombolysis in addition to supportive measures. Enoxaparin has a long half-life and is thus sometimes switched for unfractionated heparin at 36 weeks of gestation. This allows women the option of regional anesthesia (e.g., epidural) without an increased risk for epidural hematoma.

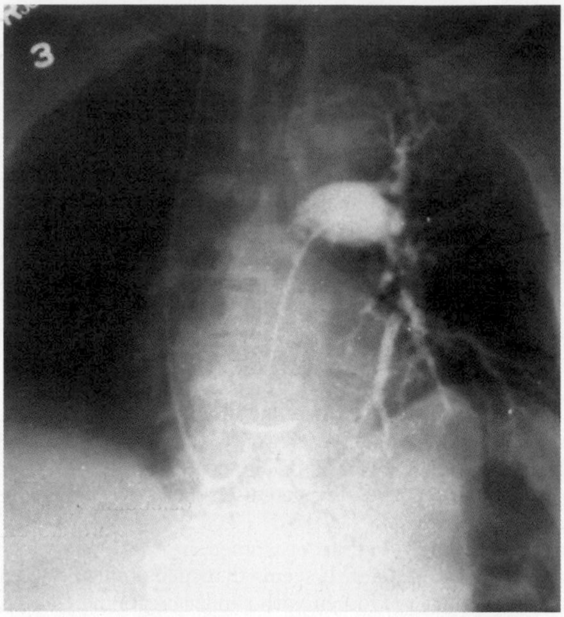

Figure 11-2 • Arteriogram of the left pulmonary artery showing filling defects and an unperfused segment of lung as demonstrated by the absence of contrast dye.

(Reproduced with permission from Clark SL, Cotton DB, Hankins GDV, Engel EL. *Critical Care Obstetrics*, 2nd ed. Cambridge: Blackwell Science; 1991:162.)

In the postpartum period, warfarin can be used as well, though some women choose to remain on enoxaparin because of the need for serial blood draws to check PT/PTT and INR on warfarin. Patients are usually treated for a minimum of 6 months.

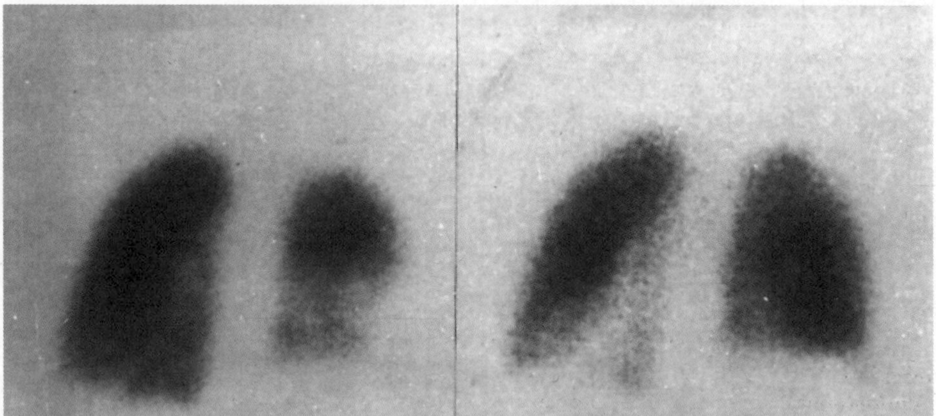

Figure 11-1 • In these posterior views, the perfusion lung scan (left) reveals segmental defects that are not matched in the normal ventilation scan (right). This is consistent with a high probability of pulmonary embolism.

(Reproduced with permission from Clark SL, Cotton DB, Hankins GDV, Engel EL. *Critical Care Obstetrics*, 2nd ed. Cambridge: Blackwell Science; 1991:162.)

MATERNAL THYROID DISEASE IN PREGNANCY

Management of thyroid disease changes in pregnancy because of the V_D, increased circulating thyroid binding globulin, and sex hormone binding globulin (SHBG), which also binds thyroid hormone. Each of these lead to decreased availability of thyroid hormone. Additionally, because metabolic demands increase in pregnancy, thyroid-stimulating hormone (TSH) and FT4 levels are commonly followed every 6 to 8 weeks.

HYPERTHYROIDISM

The most common cause of hyperthyroidism is **Graves disease**. Patients with medically managed Graves disease can continue their **propylthiouracil** (PTU) or methimazole, which decrease the production of the T4 moiety, and in the case of PTU, block its peripheral conversion to T3. Since Graves disease is the result of thyroid-stimulating immunoglobulins (TSI), TSI levels are checked at the initial visit. If levels are elevated, the fetus is at risk of developing a fetal goiter and should undergo a fetal survey at 18 to 20 weeks of gestation as well as an ultrasound in the third trimester to look for fetal goiter. Antenatal testing with serial NSTs is also recommended given the risk of fetal hyperthyroidism, which can be diagnosed with fetal tachycardia. Finally, PTU and methimazole can cross the placenta and can lead to fetal goiter as well. Thus, during pregnancy, it is best to use the minimum dosage possible. Occasionally, patients with Graves disease can be tapered off of their medications.

Given these issues, it is important to follow both symptoms of hyperthyroidism and the thyroid function laboratory test results closely. While in the general population, TSH should be kept between 0.5 and 2.5, in pregnancy, it should be kept closer to 0.5 than 2.5 if possible.

HYPOTHYROIDISM

The most common etiology for hypothyroidism is **Hashimoto thyroiditis**, and the second is ablation or removal of the thyroid after Graves disease or cancer. Several physiologic changes in pregnancy increase demand for thyroid hormone including increased V_D, increased binding globulin (in particular, SHBG), increased clearance, and increased basal metabolic rate. As a result, all women on levothyroxine (Synthroid) supplementation should have their dose increased from 25% to 30%. TSH levels should be kept low normal by increasing levothyroxine supplementation throughout pregnancy and following the TSH level. In women with a history of thyroid cancer, TSH levels should be kept below the reference range of TSH to prevent recurrence of disease.

SYSTEMIC LUPUS ERYTHEMATOSUS

Systemic lupus erythematosus (SLE) and other associated collagen vascular disorders (CVD) such as Sjögren syndrome, scleroderma, and antiphospholipid antibody syndrome can be particularly worrisome in pregnancy. There is particular concern in patients with concomitant hypertension or renal disease because these patients bear an even greater risk of developing preeclampsia, IUGR, and having preterm deliveries than women with SLE without these manifestations. The natural history of SLE in pregnancy follows the one-third rule; that is, one-third improve, one-third worsen, and one-third remain unchanged. In general, it also seems that patients who are without flares immediately prior to pregnancy have a better course. Medications such as aspirin and corticosteroids are continued in pregnancy, whereas cyclophosphamide and methotrexate are not.

EARLY PREGNANCY COMPLICATIONS

Patients with SLE and, in particular, antiphospholipid antibody syndrome, have a high risk of early pregnancy loss in both the first and second trimesters. The pathophysiology of these losses is placental thrombosis. The high rate of second-trimester losses is a hallmark of these diseases, and they will often show symmetric IUGR by 18 to 20 weeks' gestation. Treatment and prophylaxis with low-dose aspirin, heparin, and corticosteroids have been tried with some improvement in prognosis.

LATER PREGNANCY COMPLICATIONS

Just as in the early pregnancy losses, the placenta can become thrombosed in the third trimester as well, leading to IUGR and intrauterine fetal demise (IUFD). Because of this risk, frequent antenatal testing is performed, usually starting at week 32. SQ heparin or Lovenox prophylaxis and low-dose aspirin have also been used, each exhibiting some improvement in prognosis. However, even on these agents, the risks are still higher than those of the baseline population. Patients are also at increased risk of developing preeclampsia.

LUPUS FLARES VERSUS PREECLAMPSIA

One of the most difficult differential diagnoses to sort out is that of a lupus flare versus preeclampsia in the pregnant lupus patient. Both diseases are likely mediated by circulating antigen–antibody complexes or tissue-specific antibodies that cause a vasculitis. The similarity between the two diseases is remarkable (Table 11-3). One method of differentiating between the two is checking complement levels. Patients having a lupus flare will have reduced C3 and C4, whereas patients with preeclampsia should have normal levels. In addition, lupus flares are often accompanied by active urine sediment, whereas preeclampsia is not. Differentiating between the two

TABLE 11-3 Lupus Flare Versus Severe Preeclampsia

Organ System	Lupus Complication	Severe Preeclampsia
Neuro	Lupus cerebritis, seizures	Seizures, visual changes
CV	Hypertension	Hypertension
Pulmonary	Pulmonary edema	Pulmonary edema
Renal	Worsening renal disease	Significant proteinuria, oliguria, renal failure
GI	Hepatitis	Liver dysfunction, ↑ transaminases, hepatic edema
Heme	Thrombocytopenia	Thrombocytopenia, hemolytic anemia
	Hemolytic anemia	DIC

conditions is important because the management for each is distinct. A lupus flare is managed with high-dose corticosteroids and, if unresponsive, cyclophosphamide. Worsening preeclampsia, in contrast, is managed by delivery.

NEONATAL LUPUS

As with other maternal diseases, lupus can affect the fetus and neonate. There are two complications of interest. The first is a lupus syndrome related to maternal antigen–antibody complexes that have crossed the placenta and cause lupus in the neonate. These flares can be quite severe. The other complication seen is that of irreversible congenital heart block. SLE patients (and more commonly Sjögren syndrome patients) can produce antibodies called anti-Ro (SSA) and anti-La (SSB) that are tissue-specific to the fetal cardiac conduction system. Because these antibodies damage the AV node in particular, congenital heart block is seen in 5% of patients. Of these antibodies, anti-Ro is more likely than anti-La to cause heart block. Patients are screened for these antibodies at the first prenatal visit and treatments include corticosteroids, plasmapheresis, and IVIG. It is unclear whether any of these interventions improves outcomes and because these treatments have complications and are quite expensive, many clinicians use serial screening for the fetuses at risk of heat block. Such screening includes serial fetal monitoring and serial fetal echocardiogram to identify cases of potential heart block early in the process.

SUBSTANCE ABUSE IN PREGNANCY

Substance abuse in pregnancy contributes to maternal and fetal morbidity and mortality in both the antepartum and postpartum periods. The most commonly used substances are alcohol and cigarettes, both of which contribute to poor outcomes of pregnancy. The two most common illicit drugs used in pregnancy are cocaine and opiates, each of which has associated problems for the infant. Finally, even when infants are born with minimal effects from the intrapartum insult, substance abuse is an indicator for other social problems that may contribute to a poor environment for child rearing.

ALCOHOL

A constellation of abnormalities in the infants born to women who abuse alcohol during pregnancy have been included in the diagnosis of **fetal alcohol syndrome** (FAS). The syndrome has a spectrum of increasing severity in children of women who drink more heavily (two to five drinks per day) during pregnancy. However, there is no safe amount of alcohol in pregnancy that confers no risk. FAS, which includes growth retardation, CNS effects, and abnormal facies, is estimated to occur in approximately 1 in 2,000 live births. Many milder cases may go unrecognized. Diagnosis is made by a history of alcohol abuse in the mother combined with the constellation of infant abnormalities. Other teratogenic effects of alcohol include almost every organ system. Cardiac defects are particularly associated with alcohol abuse.

Treatment

Several studies show that aggressive counseling programs for expectant mothers have led to a significant decrease in alcohol intake in greater than 50% of participants. For patients who are at risk for alcohol withdrawal, barbiturates are often used for withdrawal symptoms because of the potential teratogenicity of benzodiazepines. Because alcoholics are at higher risk for nutritional deficiencies, special care should be taken to ensure adequate nutrition during pregnancy.

CAFFEINE

Caffeine is found in coffee (30 to 170 mg/cup), tea (10 to 100 mg/cup), and caffeinated soft drinks (30 to 60 mg/12 oz). It is the most commonly used drug during pregnancy, with almost 80% of all pregnant women being exposed in the first trimester. Studies on rats show teratogenicity at high levels of caffeine exposure. However, these studies have not been duplicated with humans. There does appear to be an increased risk of first- and second-trimester miscarriages with consumption of greater than 150 mg/day of caffeine. Patients should be advised of this risk and to reduce caffeine consumption during pregnancy to less than 150 mg/day.

CIGARETTES

Cigarette smoking in pregnancy has been correlated with increased risk of spontaneous abortions, preterm births, abruptio placentae, and decreased birth weight. Further, infants exposed to cigarette smoking in the womb are at an increased risk for sudden infant death syndrome (SIDS) and respiratory illnesses of childhood. A dose–response effect has been noted for many of these outcomes. In the Ontario Perinatal Mortality Study, smokers were divided into those having less than one pack per day (PPD) and those having more than one PPD. A 20% increase in the risk of fetal death was found in those pregnancies in which patients smoked less than one PPD while a 35% increase was found in the more than one PPD group.

Treatment

There is no demonstrated safe amount of smoking. But because of the demonstrated dose–response effect of smoking, patients should be counseled on the increased risks for the fetus and advised, at minimum, to decrease cigarette use. Several studies show that smoking cessation programs targeting pregnant patients are more effective than those for nonpregnant patients. Further, primary care providers of women of childbearing age should begin this counseling prior to pregnancy.

COCAINE

Cocaine use in pregnancy is correlated with abruptio placentae, IUGR, and an increased risk for preterm labor and delivery. The adverse events related to cocaine use during pregnancy are consistent with the physiologic effects of cocaine, which include vasoconstriction and hypertension. Mounting evidence shows that children who were exposed to cocaine in utero are also at increased risk for CNS complications, including developmental delay.

Treatment

Patients who admit to cocaine use should be advised of its risks to both mother and fetus. Social services should be involved in prenatal care, and patients who continue to abuse the drug should be encouraged to enter a detoxification center.

OPIATES

The most common narcotics used in pregnancy are oxycodone, heroin, and methadone. There are no known teratogenic effects of narcotics. In fact, there is some evidence that opioid withdrawal may pose a greater risk to the fetus than chronic narcotic use. Risks of opiod withdrawal include miscarriage, preterm delivery, and fetal death. Patients using narcotics in pregnancy should therefore be enrolled in methadone programs rather than advised to quit outright. A new medication for opiate maintenance, buprenorphine (Suboxone), is also being used during pregnancy and some data suggest fetal benefit in using this medication compared to standard methadone treatment. Once infants are delivered, they require careful monitoring and slow withdrawal from their narcotic addiction using tincture of opium. An aggressive effort should be made to taper their methadone postpartum.

KEY POINTS

- Nausea and vomiting in pregnancy are common; however, patients with hyperemesis gravidarum will not be able to maintain adequate hydration and nutrition.
- Acute management of hyperemesis gravidarum involves IV hydration, electrolyte repletion, and antiemetics; chronic management includes antiemetics and occasionally tube feeding or parenteral nutrition.
- The increase in seizure frequency may be related to increased metabolism of AEDs, decreased patient compliance, lower seizure threshold, and/or hormonal changes in pregnancy; patients should be followed frequently in pregnancy with monthly AED level.
- While patients with seizure disorders have an increased baseline risk for congenital anomalies, this risk is likely increased with the use of AEDs, particularly in cases of polytherapy. Because of the risk for congenital anomalies, all patients should have a targeted ultrasound/fetal survey.
- The changes in cardiac physiology during pregnancy can have an enormous impact on cardiac disease. Common aspects of management include offering termination of pregnancy, medical stabilization, surgical or valvuloplasty repair if necessary, and consideration of the changes of pregnancy.
- On labor and delivery, cardiac patients are commonly given an early epidural, careful fluid monitoring, and an assisted vaginal delivery to minimize maternal stress and strain. The most risky period of time for cardiac patients is during labor, delivery, and the puerperium.
- Patients with mild renal disease suffer minimal effects, but may carry an increased risk of preeclampsia and IUGR, which is associated with the underlying diagnosis.
- Patients with moderate or severe renal disease are at risk for preeclampsia and IUGR, as well as worsening renal disease during and after the pregnancy. Careful monitoring of the patient's renal function and of fetal status are hallmarks of the management of these patients during pregnancy.
- Pregnancy is a hypercoagulable state with increased clotting factors, endothelial damage, and venous stasis.
- Pulmonary embolus is the leading cause of maternal death. DVT and PE may be treated with enoxaparin or unfractionated heparin. Thrombolysis may be necessary for the unstable patient.
- In pregnancy, there are particular changes to the thyroid system including increased V_D and metabolism.
- In hyperthyroidism, TSIs should be screened for and, if elevated, fetal surveillance initiated to screen for fetal goiter and IUGR.
- In hypothyroidism, increased Synthroid requirements are common.
- Patients with SLE are at risk of developing complications throughout pregnancy. Prophylaxis against pregnancy loss, preeclampsia, and IUGR has been tried with low-dose aspirin, heparin, and corticosteroids, all of which have some possible benefit.
- Lupus flares and preeclampsia can be differentiated on the basis of complement levels.
- Mothers with anti-Ro and anti-La antibodies are at risk of having a fetus with congenital heart block.
- Alcohol abuse in pregnancy is correlated with FAS, which includes a constellation of growth restriction, CNS effects, and abnormal facies. Alcohol has also been correlated with other teratogenic effects, particularly cardiac defects.
- Caffeine use greater than 150 mg/day has been correlated with an increased risk of spontaneous abortions.
- Cigarette use during pregnancy has been correlated with growth restriction, abruptions, preterm delivery, and fetal death. Patients should be strongly encouraged to forgo its use during pregnancy.
- Cocaine use has been correlated with abruptio placentae and CNS effects in children. Patients should be advised to quit outright.
- Narcotic abusers should be enrolled in methadone or Suboxone programs because the acute withdrawal effects of narcotics are more dangerous to the fetus than chronic use.

C Clinical Vignettes

Vignette 1

A 28-year-old G2P1001 woman who is 18 weeks pregnant presents to the ED with increasing left lower extremity swelling, redness, and pain. She first noticed these symptoms 2 days ago and has tried elevation and warm compresses, which have not helped. She has no personal or family history of blood clots. She is otherwise healthy and her only medication is a prenatal vitamin. In the ED, her vital signs are normal. Physical examination is significant for left lower extremity edema, calf tenderness, and erythema. You suspect she has a lower extremity DVT and you plan to start her on anticoagulation therapy.

1. Which of the following is the most important test to confirm your diagnosis?
   a. Venography
   b. D-dimer
   c. Left lower extremity venous Doppler ultrasound
   d. MRI of the left lower extremity
   e. No further testing is indicated

2. The lower extremity Doppler studies show a filling defect in the left popliteal vein. What is the best initial treatment for this patient?
   a. Coumadin
   b. IV heparin
   c. Subcutaneous low-molecular-weight heparin
   d. Placement of an inferior vena cava filter
   e. Thrombolytic therapy

3. You start her on 1 mg/kg Lovenox therapy twice daily and discharge her to follow-up with you next week. She returns to the emergency department later that evening with increasing shortness of breath, chest pain, and a small amount of blood when she coughs. Her examination is significant for sinus tachycardia and the left lower extremity edema and erythema. You are concerned that she has developed a PE. Which of the following tests would be most likely to confirm the diagnosis?
   a. Chest X-ray
   b. Pulse oximetry
   c. Echocardiogram
   d. V/Q study
   e. Spiral chest CT

4. The spiral CT shows evidence of a large filling defect in the left pulmonary artery. You admit her for observation and continued treatment. On admission to the medical ward, her heart rate is 105, BP is 80/54 mm Hg, her SaO_2 is 89%, and she is becoming increasingly short of breath. You decide to transfer to the ICU. What is the best treatment at this time for the PE?
   a. Continue subcutaneous Lovenox 1 mg/kg BID
   b. Start IV heparin unstable patient
   c. Start Coumadin
   d. Start subcutaneous unfractionated heparin
   e. Embolectomy

5. The patient improved in the ICU on IV heparin and is transferred back to the general medical ward on hospital day number 2. She is transitioned back to subcutaneous Lovenox and discharged to home on hospital day number 5. You see her for follow-up a few days later and she asks why you think she had the DVT. Which of the following is not a risk factor for venous thromboembolism during pregnancy?
   a. Increased serum clotting factors
   b. Decreased levels of circulating fibrin
   c. Uterine compression of the IVC
   d. Progesterone-induced decreased venous tone
   e. None of the above

Vignette 2

A 27-year-old G2P0010 woman at 8 weeks' GA comes to your clinic for an initial prenatal visit. A medical history reveals a diagnosis of lupus 2 years ago. She was initially well-controlled with aspirin and cyclophosphamide. When she started trying to conceive, the cyclophosphamide was discontinued and she has continued the daily aspirin. She has had no lupus flares for over a year. The remainder of her medical history is normal. A physical examination is normal. Her BP today in clinic is 110/60 mm Hg and she has trace proteinuria. You draw her basic prenatal laboratory tests and perform a Pap smear and GC/CT test. You also order a complete metabolic panel, baseline preeclampsia laboratory tests, complement levels, and antidouble stranded DNA antibodies.

1. What additional test should you order to determine appropriate management during pregnancy?
   a. Anti-Ro (SSA) and anti-La (SSB)
   b. Chest X-ray
   c. 1-hour GTT
   d. Thrombophilia testing (factor V Leiden, prothrombin, etc.)
   e. Coagulation panel

2. You recommend she continue the daily aspirin and prenatal vitamin. You counsel her regarding healthy diet and exercise in pregnancy, normal weight gain, and when to call the clinic. You

also counsel her regarding the increased risk of complications during this pregnancy due to lupus. Which of the following is not a maternal complication of this condition during pregnancy?

a. Recurrent miscarriage
b. Intrauterine growth restriction (IUGR)
c. Preeclampsia
d. Stillbirth
e. Placental abruption

3. Her laboratory test results are notable for an initial creatinine of 1.0, a 24-hour urine protein total of 190 mg, positive anti-Ro (SSA), and negative anti-La (SSB) antibodies. Complement levels were normal. She does well through the first and second trimester. She had a normal ultrasound and fetal echocardiogram. At 32 weeks you started twice weekly NSTs, which have been reactive. At 36 weeks, you see her in the office and she has 2+ proteinuria and a BP of 165/88 mm Hg. You admit her to labor and delivery triage unit for further evaluation. What finding can help you diagnose her with preeclampsia and not a lupus flare?

a. Elevated uric acid
b. BP greater than 140/90 mm Hg
c. Thrombocytopenia
d. Increasing urine protein
e. Normal C3 and C4 levels

4. You diagnose her with severe preeclampsia based on persistently elevated BPs in the severe range and normal complement levels. You start her on IV magnesium for seizure prophylaxis and misoprostol for cervical ripening. Her labor is uncomplicated and she has a successful SVD of a vigorous male infant. Mother and baby do well and are transferred to the postpartum ward. What is the most significant neonatal complication of maternal lupus?

a. Congenital abnormalities
b. Neonatal heart block
c. Neonatal thrombosis
d. Acute respiratory distress syndrome (ARDS)
e. Feeding difficulties

Vignette 3

A 26-year-old G3P2002 woman at 9 weeks' GA comes to clinic for an initial prenatal care visit. She has a history of thyroid cancer and had a total thyroidectomy 5 years ago. She has no evidence of recurrent disease. She has been maintained on 50 mcg of Synthroid for the past 3 years and has no symptoms of hypothyroidism. Her other pregnancies occurred prior to the diagnosis of her thyroid cancer so she is concerned about how this pregnancy might be managed differently.

1. How would you manage her dose of Synthroid at this initial visit?

a. Increase Synthroid dose by 25%
b. Triple her Synthroid dose
c. Decrease Synthroid dose to 25 mcg
d. Stop Synthroid
e. No changes

inc to 25% ⊕ hy 5% to T4

2. You increase her Synthroid dose to 62.5 mcg daily. What is your goal TSH?

a. TSH < 0.5
b. TSH 1.0
c. TSH 3.0
d. TSH 5.0
e. TSH > 5.0

3. You see another patient in your office who had a thyroidectomy from Graves disease. She is now hypothyroid and on Synthroid replacement. You monitor her TSH and keep it between 0.5 and 2.5. You increase her Synthroid each trimester and her TSH remains around 2.0 during the entire pregnancy. In addition to monitoring her TSH, what other additional testing should you perform during her pregnancy?

a. Amniocentesis to determine if the fetus is affected by Graves disease
b. A detailed fetal ultrasound at 18 to 20 weeks and again in the third trimester should be performed given the increased risk of fetal goiter
c. Fetal echocardiogram to evaluate for cardiac abnormalities
d. Umbilical Dopplers to monitor for placental dysfunction
e. MCA Dopplers to monitor for fetal anemia

Vignette 4

You see a patient for preconception counseling. She is a 24-year-old G3P0020 woman and her medical history is significant for IgA glomerulonephritis and a recent creatinine of 2.0. She is otherwise healthy.

1. What can you tell her to expect regarding her kidney function if she were to get pregnant?

a. It will improve
b. It will stay the same
c. It will get worse
d. It is unlikely she will need dialysis by the end of pregnancy
e. She will need kidney transplant in order to have a successful pregnancy

2. She returns 6 months later and is 8 weeks pregnant. Her creatinine at this time is 1.8. Her baseline 24-hour urine protein is 1,200 mg and she has a mildly impaired creatinine clearance. You again counsel that this is a high-risk pregnancy and will need close monitoring. Which of the following is she not at risk for during this pregnancy?

a. Preeclampsia
b. Preterm delivery
c. IUGR
d. Fetal cardiac malformations
e. Worsening renal disease

3. She decides to continue the pregnancy. She has an uncomplicated course during the first and second trimester. She has baseline proteinuria and dips 3 to 4+ protein on most clinic visits. In the third trimester, her kidney function worsens and her creatinine rises to 2.8. A screening 24-hour urine protein at 32 weeks is significant for an increased value of 5,000 mg. She does not require dialysis. You see her in your clinic at 35 weeks and she has a new onset increase in her BP. She has been mildly hypertensive during most of the pregnancy with values ranging between 130/90s and 140/90s mm Hg. Today, her BP is 170/110 mm Hg and you send her to labor and delivery triage unit for further evaluation. What clinical data is most likely to help you make the diagnosis of preeclampsia?

a. Proteinuria of 5,000 mg at 32 weeks
b. An increase in BP of 30/15 mm Hg above prepregnancy values
c. Elevated uric acid
d. Increased creatinine to 3.0
e. Proteinuria of 7,000 mg at 35 weeks

CLINICAL VIGNETTES

A Answers

Vignette 1 Question 1

Answer C: Diagnosis of DVT is often made clinically with confirmation by compression Doppler studies of the suspected extremity. The diagnosis is made by the following ultrasound findings: abnormal compressibility of the vein, abnormal color Doppler flow, the presence of an echogenic band, and abnormal change in diameter of the vessel. Venography, the gold standard, is rarely used because of the invasive nature of test and questionable improved sensitivity. D-dimer levels are elevated during pregnancy and so are not helpful to diagnose DVT in this population. MRI of the left lower extremity is thought to be as accurate as venography to diagnose DVT; however, due to the high cost of MRI it is unlikely at this time to replace Doppler ultrasound.

Vignette 1 Question 2

Answer C: Treatment of DVT during pregnancy involves the use of adjusted dose low-molecular-weight heparin (enoxaparin 1 mg/kg BID) or unfractionated heparin (goal aPTT of 1.5 to 2.5 times normal). Low-molecular-weight heparin has become the preferred option because you do not need to check levels and it is also thought to be safer due to a lower risk of heparin-induced thrombocytopenia.
IV heparin is difficult to administer and requires hospitalization and frequent blood draws to confirm adequate treatment levels. It is also associated with increased risk of bleeding complications and would not be first-line therapy in this scenario. Warfarin (Coumadin) therapy is contraindicated in pregnancy secondary to evidence of fetal abnormalities caused by warfarin. When given in the first trimester, it causes warfarin embryopathy, which causes nasal hypoplasia and skeletal abnormalities. In addition, warfarin appears to cause diffuse CNS abnormalities, including optic atrophy, when given during pregnancy. Placement of an inferior vena cava filter is an invasive procedure that is generally used in situations where the patient has a contraindication to anticoagulation. The use of thrombolytic therapy for DVT is controversial and not recommended as first-line treatment at this time.

Vignette 1 Question 3

Answer E: The diagnosis of PE usually involves the clinical picture correlated with a variety of diagnostic tests. Spiral CT scan has become the first-line diagnostic tool for PE in both the pregnant and nonpregnant patient. The risk of radiation exposure must be weighed against the suspected risk of a PE and the dangers that this poses to a pregnant woman's health. As with other life-threatening medical conditions, the woman's health should be considered first and foremost and she should be evaluated and treated just as any nonpregnant patient would be in a similar condition.

A chest X-ray may be entirely normal and is not likely to confirm the diagnosis. If abnormal, two common signs are the abrupt termination of a vessel, as it is traced distally, and an area of radiolucency in the area of the lung beyond the PE. Hypoxemia on pulse oximetry can raise clinical suspicion for PE, but is not diagnostic. An ECG may also be entirely normal or simply show sinus tachycardia. V/Q studies are recommended as the first-line diagnostic test only in institutions that have limited experience with spiral CT.

Vignette 1 Question 4

Answer B: In the hypotensive or unstable patient, IV heparin is the recommended option. It is also the recommended option if you are concerned about subcutaneous absorption or considering thrombolytics.

Low-molecular-weight heparin (enoxaparin) is the preferred choice in hemodynamically stable patients. Subcutaneous unfractionated heparin is also an option, but is associated with increased risk of heparin induced thrombocytopenia and bleeding complications. Coumadin is contraindicated in pregnancy (see previous question). Embolectomy is reserved only for severe cases where thrombolytics are indicated but are either not effective or contraindicated.

Vignette 1 Question 5

Answer B: Actually, levels of circulating fibrin monomer complexes are increased in pregnancy and thought to be a contributing factor in the hypercoagulability of pregnancy. These levels increase further at the time of delivery and immediately postpartum.

The etiology of the hypercoagulability of pregnancy is thought to be multifactorial. In pregnancy, the production of all clotting factors is increased except for II, V, and IX. Also noted in pregnancy is that the turnover time for fibrinogen is decreased and that there are increased levels of fibrinopeptide A, which is cleaved from fibrinogen to make fibrin. It has also been hypothesized that the placenta synthesizes a factor that decreases fibrinolysis, but there is minimal evidence for this. Another proposed source of hypercoagulability is increased exposure to subendothelial collagen secondary to increased endothelial damage during pregnancy, although no mechanism has been proposed. Venous stasis may also account for some of the increase in venous thromboses during and after pregnancy. There are two principal causes for venous stasis in pregnancy. The first is decreased venous tone during pregnancy, which may be related to the smooth muscle relaxant properties of this high progesterone state. Second, the uterus, as it enlarges, compresses the inferior vena cava, the iliac, and pelvic veins. This compression, in particular, likely contributes to the increase in pelvic vein thromboses.

Vignette 2 Question 1

Answer A: SLE patients (and more commonly Sjögren syndrome patients) can produce antibodies called anti-Ro (SSA) and anti-La (SSB) that are tissue-specific to the fetal cardiac conduction system. Because these antibodies damage the AV node in particular, congenital heart block is seen in 5% of patients. Of these antibodies, anti-Ro is more likely than anti-La to cause heart block. Patients are screened for these antibodies at the first prenatal visit, and treatments include corticosteroids, plasmapheresis, and IVIG. It is unclear whether any of these interventions improves outcomes and because these treatments have complications and are quite expensive, many clinicians use serial screening for the fetuses at risk of heart block. Such screening includes serial fetal monitoring and serial fetal echocardiogram to identify cases of potential heart block early in the process.

Chest X-ray, early diabetes screening, thrombophilia, and a coagulation panel are not routine screening tests for lupus.

Vignette 2 Question 2

Answer E: Placental abruption has not been found to be associated with lupus. Patients with SLE and, in particular, antiphospholipid antibody syndrome, have a high risk of early pregnancy loss both in the first and second trimester. The pathophysiology of these losses is placental thrombosis. The high rate of second-trimester losses is a hallmark of these diseases, and they will often show symmetric IUGR by 18 to 20 weeks' gestation.

Just as in the early pregnancy losses, the placenta can become thrombosed in the third trimester as well, leading to IUGR and IUFD (stillbirth). Because of this risk, frequent antenatal testing is performed, usually starting at week 32. SQ heparin, Lovenox prophylaxis, or low-dose aspirin have also been used, each exhibiting some improvement in prognosis. However, even on these agents, the risks are still much higher than those of the baseline population. Patients are also at increased risk of developing preeclampsia.

Vignette 2 Question 3

Answer E: One of the most difficult differential diagnoses to sort out is that of a lupus flare versus preeclampsia in the pregnant lupus patient. Both diseases are likely mediated by circulating antigen–antibody complexes or tissue-specific antibodies that cause a vasculitis. One method of differentiating between the two is checking complement levels. Patients having a lupus flare will have reduced C3 and C4, whereas patients with preeclampsia should have normal levels. Differentiating between the two conditions is important because the management for each highly differs. A lupus flare is managed with high-dose corticosteroids and, if unresponsive, cyclophosphamide. Worsening preeclampsia, on the other hand, is managed by delivery.

Elevated uric acid, hypertension, thrombocytopenia, and increasing urine protein can be present in both preeclampsia and lupus flares.

Vignette 2 Question 4

Answer B: One of the most significant neonatal complications is that of irreversible congenital heart block. SLE patients (and more commonly Sjögren disease patients) can produce antibodies, called anti-Ro (SSA) and anti-La (SSB), that are tissue-specific to the fetal cardiac conduction system and can cause fetal/neonatal heart block. These neonates may need to have a pacemaker placed and will usually require a pacemaker for life.

Maternal lupus can also cause a neonatal lupus syndrome related to maternal antigen–antibody complexes that have crossed the placenta and cause lupus in the neonate. These flares can be quite severe. Maternal lupus has not been associated with congenital abnormalities, neonatal thrombosis, ARDS, or feeding difficulties.

Vignette 3 Question 1

Answer A: Because the demands on thyroid hormone are going to increase in pregnancy due to increased volume of distribution, increased binding globulin (in particular, SHBG), increased clearance, and increased basal metabolic rate, all women on levothyroxine (Synthroid) supplementation should have their dosage increased 25% to 30% at the beginning of the pregnancy.

Tripling the dose is more likely to cause side effects of hyperthyroidism like agitation, anxiety, and palpitations. Decreasing or stopping the Synthroid dose may lead to subacute hypothyroidism, which is associated with abnormal neuropsychological development. Subacute hypothyroidism may also be caused by not making changes to her dose at this initial visit.

Vignette 3 Question 2

Answer B: The levels of TSH should be kept low normal (0.5 to 2.5) by increasing levothyroxine supplementation throughout pregnancy and following the TSH level each trimester. For women with a history of thyroid cancer, like this patient, TSH levels should be kept below the reference range of TSH (closer to 1.0) to prevent recurrence of disease.

Vignette 3 Question 3

Answer B: Fetal goiter is a complication of maternal hyperthyroidism from Graves disease and placental transfer of TSI to the fetal circulation, not maternal hypothyroidism. Fetal goiter is a serious complication, and if severe, can lead to compression of the fetal trachea and difficulty with respiration at the time of birth. If present, consultation with a pediatric ENT physician is warranted prior to delivery to determine if intubation or an EXIT procedure is needed at the time of birth. In addition to ultrasound, weekly NSTs should be performed later in pregnancy to monitor for fetal tachycardia, which could be evidence of placental transfer of TSI to the fetal circulation.

Maternal Graves disease is not associated with fetal congenital abnormalities, placental dysfunction, or fetal anemia. Amniocentesis is not indicated because there is no associated test that can determine if the fetus is affected by Graves disease.

Vignette 4 Question 1

Answer C: Chronic renal disease can be divided into mild (Cr $<$ 1.5), moderate (Cr from 1.5 to 2.8), and severe (Cr $>$ 2.8), although other thresholds have been used. Renal blood flow and creatinine clearance increase during pregnancy in patients without renal disease, and this is also true initially in patients with renal disease. Patients with mild renal disease will usually experience improvement in renal function throughout much of pregnancy. Moderate and severe patients, however, may experience decreasing renal function in the latter half of pregnancy that may persist postpartum in as many as half of pregnancies. It is not uncommon for patients with moderate to severe renal dysfunction to require dialysis at some point during the pregnancy or postpartum period.

Vignette 4 Question 2

Answer D: Patients with chronic renal disease have increased risk of preeclampsia, preterm delivery, and IUGR in addition to worsening renal disease. There is no data that suggests an increased risk of fetal malformations, including cardiac abnormalities. Because of the above risks, these patients should be screened at least once per trimester with a 24-hour urine for creatinine clearance and protein. Patients who present in early pregnancy should be counseled regarding these risks and offered termination of pregnancy, particularly for the mother's health. Because of the risk to the fetus, antenatal fetal testing usually begins at 32 to 34 weeks' gestation.

Vignette 4 Question 3

Answer B: For patients who have baseline proteinuria and hypertension, the diagnosis of preeclampsia can be difficult to make.

An increase in BP of 30/15 mm Hg above prepregnancy BPs can be used, though some experts disagree on its utility. In this situation, your patient has a significant increase in her BP from baseline and this is most likely due to preeclampsia.

Increasing proteinuria is expected and a value of 5,000 mg at 32 weeks with other evidence of preeclampsia is not diagnostic. In addition, a value of 7,000 at 35 weeks would raise your suspicion for preeclampsia but is not diagnostic. An elevated uric acid is not specifically associated with preeclampsia and may be present with worsening kidney function. In addition her kidney function is expected to worsen and a creatinine of 3.0 is not unexpected. In isolation, each of the other answers is not diagnostic of preeclampsia.

Chapter 12 Postpartum Care and Complications

ROUTINE POSTPARTUM CARE

The puerperium, or postpartum period, is defined as the first 6 weeks after delivery. While still in the hospital, the patient often needs instruction about care of the neonate, breastfeeding, and her limitations during the ensuing weeks. The patient needs emotional support during the period of adjustment to the new member of the family and to her own physiologic changes. Given that the risk of postpartum complications can extend past the average patient's hospital stay, partners and family should be included in any maternal or child care counseling as available.

VAGINAL DELIVERY

Routine medical issues in patients after vaginal delivery include pain control and perineal care. Usually, pain can be reduced with nonsteroidal anti-inflammatory drugs (NSAIDs) or acetaminophen. Low-dose opioids are occasionally required for adequate patient comfort, particularly at the hour of sleep. For patients with vaginal deliveries that involved either episiotomies or lacerations, perineal care is particularly important. Ice packs around the clock for the first 24 hours can be beneficial for both pain and edema in the perineum and labia. When inspecting the perineum of a postpartum patient, it is important to ensure that the perineal repair is intact and that no hematomas have developed. It is also important to note whether the patient has hemorrhoids, which are common in pregnancy and postpartum, particularly after a long second stage of labor. These should resolve with time, but patients' symptoms may be ameliorated with over-the-counter hemorrhoidal medications, stool softeners, and ice packs.

CESAREAN DELIVERY

As more than 30% of deliveries are now by cesarean, wound care and pain management in these women are a common component of postpartum care. Local wound care and observation for signs of wound infection or separation are part of routine care. Wound infections include cellulitis or a wound abscess. Wound separations can be at the level of the skin or subcutaneous tissue or deeper at the level of the rectus fascia, also known as a *wound dehiscence*. Pain is usually managed with opioids that can contribute to a postoperative ileus or constipation. Patients on opioids should therefore be prescribed stool softeners and occasionally laxatives. NSAIDs should be used concomitantly for the cramping pain caused by uterine involution. Patients have usually received a first- or second-generation cephalosporin during the cesarean section as prophylaxis against infection. Although it is routine in many institutions to give additional dosages, this has never been shown to further decrease the risk of infection.

BREASTFEEDING AND BREAST CARE

While there are rare contraindications such as infections that may lead to an increase in vertical transmission to the infant or in the case of mothers on medications or using recreational drugs that could be dangerous to a newborn, the vast majority of new mothers should be encouraged to breastfeed. There are various beliefs and racial/cultural differences regarding the practice of breastfeeding, but regardless, the health benefits to babies and mothers are being increasingly identified. Oxytocin release from the pituitary gland with breastfeeding stimulates postpartum uterine contractions, thereby increasing uterine tone and decreasing the risk of bleeding. Numerous studies have demonstrated a decrease in childhood infectious diseases in newborns and infants of breastfeeding mothers attributed to the passive immunity transmitted via immunoglobulins in the breast milk. Women who breastfeed are more likely to lose the weight they have gained during pregnancy. Further, women who have breastfed appear to have a lower long-term risk of developing type 2 diabetes and its associated morbidities.

Despite all of these benefits, breastfeeding is challenging, particularly for the primipara, that is, the first-time mother. Historically, women would have likely learned about breastfeeding from female relatives and family, but in today's society in the United States, many women have not had such experiences. Thus, while they may be interested in breastfeeding, many women do not recognize the inherent difficulties and discomforts. A number of barriers to breastfeeding, both iatrogenic and natural, can be introduced in the birthing process and initial postpartum period. In a variety of complicated births such as a preterm birth, emergency birth, or simply a cesarean delivery, the initial skin-to-skin contact that has been shown to initiate breastfeeding in the neonate is interrupted. Further, while breastfeeding is natural, it is often not instinctive or intuitive to many women. Since they have expectations that breastfeeding should be easier, any delay or drawback can be interpreted as a failure. This misalignment of expectations and reality coupled with concerns about providing adequate nutrition of the neonate leads many women to give up breastfeeding for formula feeding only a few days postpartum. Reassurance that breastfeeding can be challenging and uncomfortable (even painful) but that it should become easier and less uncomfortable can help women to get through the initial weeks of breastfeeding.

All postpartum patients need breast care, regardless of whether or not they are breastfeeding. Patients usually experience the onset of lactation, engorgement or "letdown," approximately 24 to 72 hours postpartum. When this occurs, the breasts usually become uniformly warmer, firmer, and tender. Patients often complain of pain or warmth in the breasts and may experience fever. For patients not breastfeeding, ice packs, a tight bra, analgesics, and anti-inflammatory medications are all useful. Patients who are breastfeeding obtain relief from the breastfeeding itself, although this can lead to its own difficulties, such as tenderness and erosions around the nipple. While protective creams and barriers can help symptomatically for sore nipples/breasts, providers should also assess breastfeeding positions and the infant's latch onto the breast. If the provider does not have this expertise, referral to a lactation consult is recommended.

POSTPARTUM PREVENTATIVE MEDICATIONS

Previously it was thought that those who were exposed to pertussis or were vaccinated as children received lifelong immunity. However, recent findings suggest that immunity may only last up to 20 years. Consequently, many women in their childbearing years run the risk of contracting pertussis in the postpartum period and transmitting the disease to their infants prior to their scheduled immunizations at 2 months of age. With a general rise in the incidence of pertussis, routine postpartum immunization of women with Tdap is essential if they have not received the vaccine within the 10 years previous to pregnancy. Caregivers who will be in close contact to the infant should also be vaccinated to create an immunologic cocoon. Mothers found to have low Rubella antibody titers in their prenatal laboratory test results should receive a measles, mumps, and rubella (MMR) vaccine postpartum as well. The vaccine is a mixture of three attenuated live viruses that cannot be given during pregnancy.

If a woman is found to be Rh negative at the time of her prenatal laboratory tests or a type and screen, it is necessary that she receive an intramuscular injection of Rhogam within 72 hours postpartum. Rhogam contains antibodies to the Rh D factor such that any Rh-positive fetal cells that mix with maternal blood during the time of delivery will be removed from the circulation, prior to sensitizing the mother's own immune system. Maternal sensitization would lead to the creation of antibodies that result in hemolytic disease of the newborn when maternal antibodies pass into fetal circulation in future Rh-positive pregnancies. Newborns routinely have their blood typed and screened at birth; only if the infant is found to be Rh negative will the mother not need to receive Rhogam.

POSTPARTUM CONTRACEPTION

Most patients are advised to have pelvic rest until the 6-week follow-up visit. However, many women resume sexual activity prior to this time. Thus, contraception is an important issue to begin addressing during the prenatal period and continue while patients are still in the hospital postpartum. Because most states require women to consent to a postpartum tubal ligation (PPTL) at least 30 days prior to their EDD, this should be brought up early in the third trimester. For women who desire permanent sterilization, PPTL is an extremely effective form of sterilization. Poor surgical candidates who desire sterilization may consider sterilization of the male partner by means of vasectomy, with equally effective results.

For those women who have not undergone or do not desire PPTL, counseling regarding other options is important. For patients interested in hormonal modes of contraception and who are breastfeeding, the progesterone-only mini-pill, Depo-Provera, or implantable progestogenic agents are the usual recommended options. Combination estrogen–progesterone OCPs in some studies have been shown to decrease milk production so are usually recommended only to those patients who are not interested in breastfeeding or have excellent milk production (not usually known during the first week postpartum). Progesterone-only contraceptives may decrease milk production as well, but this has not been demonstrated to be clinically significant. They are therefore preferable to combination OCPs for patients who are dedicated to breastfeeding and interested in hormonal forms of birth control. An alternative course of action for those women who are interested in using combination OCPs is to establish breastfeeding and then begin the combination OCPs at 3 to 6 weeks postpartum. If their milk production is adequate, they can then continue on this form of contraception. Women should be counseled against starting their combined OCPs until after 3 weeks postpartum, at which point the benefits of contraception and pregnancy prevention outweigh the risks of venous thromboembolism (VTE) in the puerperium. Early initiation of combination OCPs should not be recommended to patients with risk factors for VTE, such as age ≥35 years, previous VTE, thrombophilia, immobility, transfusion at delivery, BMI ≥30, postpartum hemorrhage, post-Cesarean delivery, preeclampsia, or active smoking. After 6 weeks, the risk of VTE decreases to that seen in the non-pregnant state.

For patients interested in nonhormonal methods, condoms are particularly good because of the prevention against sexually transmitted infections. The other barrier methods—the diaphragm and cervical cap—should be avoided until 6 weeks postpartum when the cervix has returned to its normal shape and size. Intrauterine devices (IUDs) may be inserted postpartum. Uptake of the progesterone-eluting IUD (Mirena) has steadily increased over the past decade. Prior concerns about infections from IUDs in the 1970s or the increased volume and length of menses from the copper IUD are alleviated by the Mirena. Because of the low release of local progesterone, the use of the Mirena can actually lead to lighter, shorter menses and even amenorrhea in 15% to 20% of users. However, the IUD has a higher rate of expulsion in the immediate postpartum period. Because of the dilated cervix, placement usually is done at the 6-week postpartum appointment. In women who are less likely to follow up or for whom contraception is paramount, placement postpartum with several follow-up visits to verify that it is still in situ may be considered.

DISCHARGE INSTRUCTIONS

Hospital stay after delivery is short, and while insurance companies have been mandated to cover up to 2 days after a vaginal delivery and 4 days after a cesarean delivery, many hospitals still discharge patients after 1 and 3 days, respectively. After a vaginal delivery, the above issues of perineal care, contraception, and breast care are discussed with the patient. Further, a discussion regarding how common the postpartum "blues" can be as well as the availability of professionals to talk the patient through any problems as she transitions to home can be of help. Patients who have a cesarean delivery should be counseled regarding wound care and activity in addition to the above. With Pfannenstiel incisions that were stapled closed, the staples can be removed prior to discharge. Patients are often advised to avoid heavy lifting ("nothing heavier than your baby") and vigorous activities including driving. Before patients drive, it is recommended that they try to slam on the brakes as an experiment to be sure they are comfortable enough to drive.

POSTPARTUM COMPLICATIONS

The primary complications that arise postpartum include postpartum hemorrhage, endomyometritis, wound infections and separations, mastitis, and postpartum depression (Table 12-1).

TABLE 12-1 Complications of Vaginal and Cesarean Deliveries

	Vaginal Delivery	Cesarean Delivery
Common complications	Postpartum hemorrhage	Postpartum hemorrhage
	Vaginal hematoma	Surgical blood loss
	Cervical laceration	Wound infection
	Retained POCs	Endomyometritis
	Mastitis	Mastitis
	Postpartum depression	Postpartum depression
Rare complications	Endomyometritis	Wound separation
	Episiotomy infections	Wound dehiscence
	Episiotomy breakdown	

Postpartum hemorrhage usually occurs during the first 24 hours, while the patient is still in the hospital. However, it can also occur in patients with retained products of conception (POCs) for up to several weeks postpartum. Endomyometritis and wound complications typically occur in the first week to 10 days postpartum, and mastitis typically occurs 1 to 2 weeks after delivery but may present anytime during breastfeeding. Postpartum depression can occur at any time during the puerperium and beyond and is probably grossly underdiagnosed.

POSTPARTUM HEMORRHAGE

Postpartum hemorrhage is defined as blood loss exceeding 500 mL in a vaginal delivery and greater than 1,000 mL in a cesarean section. If the hemorrhage occurs within the first 24 hours, it is deemed early postpartum hemorrhage; after 24 hours, it is considered late or delayed postpartum hemorrhage. Common causes of postpartum bleeding include uterine atony, retained POCs, placenta accreta, cervical lacerations, and vaginal lacerations (Tables 12-2 and 12-3). While the cause of the hemorrhage is being investigated, the patient is simultaneously started on fluid resuscitation and preparations are made for blood transfusions. With blood loss greater than 2 to 3 L, patients may develop a consumptive coagulopathy and require coagulation factors and platelets. In rare cases, if patients become hypovolemic and hypotensive, Sheehan syndrome, or pituitary infarction, may occur. Sheehan syndrome may manifest with the absence of lactation secondary to the lack of prolactin or failure to restart menstruation secondary to the absence of gonadotropins. Each of the etiologies of postpartum hemorrhage is discussed sequentially; the obstetrician often has to consider and/or attempt to treat several etiologies simultaneously.

Vaginal Lacerations and Hematomas

Vaginal lacerations with uncontrolled bleeding should be considered in the case of postpartum hemorrhage. Initially after a delivery, the perineum, labia, periurethral area, and deeper aspects of the vagina are examined for lacerations. These should be repaired at that time. However, deep sulcal tears or vaginal lacerations behind the cervix may be quite difficult to visualize without careful retraction. Occasionally, these lacerations will involve arteries and arterioles and lead to a significant postpartum hemorrhage. Adequate anesthesia, an experienced obstetrician, and assistance with retraction are all necessary to perform an adequate exploration and repair of these lacerations.

TABLE 12-2 Risk Factors for Postpartum Hemorrhage

Prior Postpartum Hemorrhage
Abnormal placentation
Placenta previa
Placenta accreta
Hydatidiform mole
Trauma during labor and delivery
Episiotomy
Complicated vaginal delivery
Low- or midforceps delivery
Sulcal or sidewall laceration
Uterine rupture
Cesarean delivery or hysterectomy
Cervical laceration
Uterine atony
Uterine inversion
Overdistended uterus
Macrosomic fetus
Multiple gestation
Polyhydramnios
Exhausted myometrium
Rapid labor
Prolonged labor
Oxytocin or prostaglandin stimulation
Chorioamnionitis
Coagulation defects—intensify other causes
Placental abruption
Prolonged retention of demised fetus
Amnionic fluid embolism
Severe intravascular hemolysis
Severe preeclampsia and eclampsia
Congenital coagulopathies
Anticoagulant treatment

Occasionally, the trauma of delivery will injure a blood vessel without disrupting the epithelium above it. This leads to the development of a hematoma. If a patient has a larger than expected drop in hematocrit, an examination should be performed to rule out a vaginal wall hematoma. A hematoma can be managed expectantly unless it is tense or expanding, in which case it should be opened, the bleeding vessel ligated, and the vaginal wall closed. Rarely, a patient will develop a retroperitoneal hematoma that can lead to a large blood loss

TABLE 12-3 Etiology of Postpartum Hemorrhage in Vaginal and Cesarean Deliveries

Vaginal Delivery	Cesarean Delivery
Vaginal lacerations	Uterine atony
Cervical lacerations	Surgical blood loss
Uterine atony	Placenta accreta
Placenta accreta	Uterine rupture
Vaginal hematoma	
Retained POCs	
Uterine inversion	
Uterine rupture	

into this space. Patients usually complain of low back or rectal pain and there will be a large drop in hematocrit. Diagnosis is made via ultrasound or CT. If the patient is stable without a falling hematocrit, expectant management may be followed. However, if the patient demonstrates continued bleeding with evidence of expansion of the hematoma or a further drop in hematocrit, interventional radiology can use embolization techniques in order to treat such bleeding. Because these clinicians are rarely in house, early notification of the potential for such an intervention is necessary. If the patient becomes unstable, surgical exploration and ligation of the disrupted vessels may be required.

Cervical Lacerations

Cervical lacerations can cause a brisk postpartum hemorrhage. Commonly, they are a result of rapid dilation of the cervix during the stage 1 of labor or maternal expulsive efforts prior to complete dilation of the cervix. If a patient is bleeding at the level of the cervix or above, a careful exploration of the cervix should be performed. The patient should have adequate anesthesia via epidural, spinal, or pudendal block. The walls of the vagina are retracted so the cervix can be well visualized. When the anterior lip of the cervix is seen, it is grasped with a ring forcep. Then another ring forcep can be used to grasp beyond the first and in this fashion the cervix should be "walked" around its entirety so that no lacerations, particularly on the posterior aspect, are missed. If any lacerations are seen, they are usually repaired with either interrupted or running absorbable sutures.

Uterine Atony

Uterine atony is the leading cause of postpartum hemorrhage. Patients are at a higher risk for uterine atony if they have chorioamnionitis, exposure to magnesium sulfate, multiple gestations, a macrosomic fetus, polyhydramnios, prolonged labor, a history of atony with any prior pregnancies, or if they are multiparous, particularly a grand multipara (more than five deliveries). Uterine abnormalities or fibroids may also interfere with uterine contractions leading to and increasing bleeding. The diagnosis of atony is made by palpation of the uterus, which is soft, enlarged, and boggy. Occasionally, the uterine fundus is well contracted, but the lower uterine segment, which has less contractile tissue, will be less so.

Atony is initially treated with IV oxytocin (Pitocin), which is usually given prophylactically after delivery of the infant. While the oxytocin is being administered, strong uterine massage should be performed to assist the uterus in contracting. If atony continues, the next step is methylergonovine (Methergine), which is contraindicated in hypertensive patients. If the uterus is still atonic, the next step is to give Hemabate (also known as Prostin or PGF_2), which is contraindicated in asthma patients. The prostaglandin is thought to be more effective if injected directly into the uterine musculature, either transabdominally or transcervically, although this has not been demonstrated in studies. Misoprostol, a PGE1 analog traditionally used for the treatment of gastric ulcers, may also be used off-label for its uterotonic properties. Administered sublingually or rectally, misoprostol is an effective method for decreasing blood loss associated with atony when patients are without IV access. Its shelf-stability makes it suitable for settings that lack electricity, as Pitocin, Hemabate, methylergonovine all require refrigeration.

If atony continues despite maximal medical management, the patient is brought to the OR for a **dilation and curettage** (D&C) to rule out possible retained POCs. Patients with uterine atony unresponsive to these conservative measures, but bleeding at a rate that can tolerate some watchful waiting, may benefit from uterine packing with an inflatable tamponade (Bakri balloon) or occlusion of pelvic vessels (uterine artery embolization) by interventional radiology to prevent the necessity of a hysterectomy. If this is unsuccessful, exploratory laparotomy with ligation of pelvic vessels and possible hysterectomy is required.

Retained Products of Conception

Careful inspection of the placenta should always be performed. However, with vaginal delivery, it can often be difficult to determine whether a small piece of the placenta has been left behind in the uterus. Usually the retained fetal membranes or placental tissue pass in the lochia. However, they occasionally lead to endomyometritis and postpartum hemorrhage. If suspicion is high for retained POCs, the uterus should be explored either manually if the cervix has not contracted down or by ultrasound. If there is evidence of a normal uterine stripe, the probability of retained products is much lower. However, if clinical suspicion is high, a D&C would be next for both diagnostic and therapeutic measures. If hemorrhage continues even after ascertaining that there are no further POCs via exploration, placenta accreta should be suspected.

Accreta

Placenta accreta, increta, and percreta are discussed briefly in Chapter 5 with antepartum hemorrhage. These conditions are the result of abnormal attachment of placental tissue to the uterus that may invade into or beyond the uterine myometrium, leading to incomplete separation of the placenta postpartum and postpartum hemorrhage. Risk factors for developing placenta accreta include placenta previa and prior uterine surgery, including cesarean delivery and myomectomy. Often the third stage will have been longer than usual and the placenta may have delivered in fragments. Accreta involves bleeding that is unresponsive to uterine massage and contractile agents such as oxytocin, ergonovines, and prostaglandins. Patients with accreta are taken to the operating room for surgical management via exploratory laparotomy.

Uterine Rupture

Uterine rupture is estimated to occur in 0.5% to 1.0% of patients with prior uterine scars and in about 1:15,000 to 20,000 women with an unscarred uterus. It is an intrapartum complication but may lead to postpartum bleeding. It is rare for rupture to occur in a nulliparous patient. Risk factors include previous uterine surgery, breech extraction, obstructed labor, and high parity. Symptoms usually include abdominal pain and a popping sensation intra-abdominally. Treatment involves laparotomy and repair of the ruptured uterus. If hemorrhage cannot be controlled, hysterectomy may be indicated.

Uterine Inversion

Uterine inversion may occur in 1:2,500 deliveries. Risk factors include fundal implantation of the placenta, uterine atony, placenta accreta, and excessive traction on the cord during the third stage. Diagnosis is made by witnessing the fundus of the uterus attached to the placenta on placental delivery. Uterine inversion can be an obstetric emergency if hemorrhage occurs. Additionally, patients often experience an intense vasovagal response from the inversion and may require stabilization with the aid of an anesthesiologist before manual replacement of the uterus can be attempted, which should be the first step in treatment (Fig. 12-1). Uterine relaxants such as nitroglycerin or general anesthesia with halogenated agents may be given to aid uterine relaxation and replacement. If this is unsuccessful, laparotomy is required to surgically replace the uterus.

Operative Management of Postpartum Hemorrhage

In the case of vaginal delivery, the management of postpartum hemorrhage is as described above. A differential diagnosis is created and a rapid physical examination is performed to establish the likely etiology. If vaginal and cervical lacerations have been ruled out and the patient is unresponsive to uterotonic agents and massage, the patient should be moved to an operating room and a D&C performed. If this fails to stop the bleeding, placement of an inflatable balloon in the uterine cavity may limit further hemorrhage; if these measures fail, a laparotomy is performed.

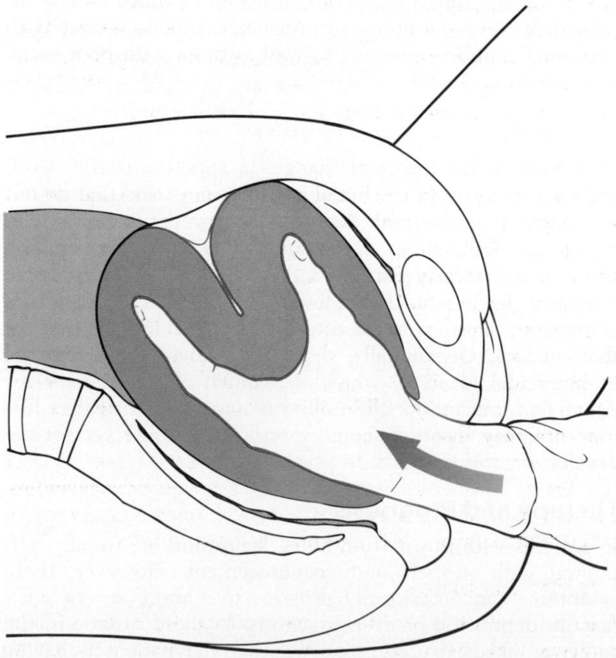

Figure 12-1 • Manual replacement of an inverted uterus.

On entering the abdomen, the surgeon should note whether there is blood in the abdomen, which would indicate a uterine rupture. Unless the patient is unstable and coagulopathic secondary to excessive blood loss, the first surgical procedure is usually bilateral O'Leary sutures to tie off the uterine arteries. The second is ligation of the hypogastric, or internal iliac, arteries, which requires considerable skill and experience. If uterine atony is the cause of hemorrhage, B-Lynch sutures can be placed in an attempt to compress the uterus and achieve hemostasis. A uterine incision must first be made, through which a suture is looped around the uterus and used to tamp it back into place. If these measures fail to provide hemostasis, often the patient requires a puerperal hysterectomy (known as cesarean hysterectomy if that has been the mode of delivery).

If the patient has been delivered via cesarean section and there is evidence of accreta, the first step is usually to place hemostatic sutures in the placental bed. If these fail, or the patient has no focal site of bleeding, O'Leary sutures can be placed next with the uterus still open to watch the bleeding. If this fails, often the next step is to close the uterus with or without packing it and proceed to hypogastric artery ligation. If this fails, hysterectomy is the definitive procedure.

If a patient is not bleeding too briskly, with either vaginal or cesarean delivery, packing the uterus and obtaining an interventional radiology consult for uterine artery embolization is possible. This is reserved for those patients who are truly stable and desire future fertility.

ENDOMYOMETRITIS

Endomyometritis is a polymicrobial infection of the uterine lining that often invades the underlying muscle wall. It is most common after cesarean section but may occur after vaginal deliveries as well, particularly in cases of manual extraction of the placenta. Risk factors include meconium, chorioamnionitis, and prolonged rupture of membranes.

Diagnosis is made in the setting of fever, elevated WBC count, and uterine tenderness, with a higher suspicion after cesarean. Endomyometritis commonly occurs 5 to 10 days after delivery but may be suspected when all other sources of infection have been ruled out for several weeks after delivery. Because retained POCs can be the etiology of infection, an ultrasound is often obtained to examine the intrauterine contents.

Endomyometritis is usually treated with broad-spectrum IV antibiotics, or triple antibiotics, though in some institutions a second-generation cephalosporin is used. If retained POCs are identified on ultrasound, a D&C is performed. Because the postpartum uterus is at greater risk for perforation, great care should be taken during dilation, using blunt rather than sharp curettage and ultrasound guidance to limit complications. Antibiotics are continued until the patient is afebrile for 48 hours, uterine pain and tenderness are absent, and the WBC count normalizes.

WOUND COMPLICATIONS

Wound Infections

Wound infections include cellulitis and abscess. While such infections of the cesarean skin incision are seen in 1% to 5% of cases, these can also be seen in the perineal laceration or episiotomy site. Cellulitis is suspected with local erythema around the surgical site. If the erythema is tender and particularly warm, the level of suspicion is usually high enough to diagnose cellulitis. If these two symptoms are not present, often a line is drawn around the erythema and if it expands over 12 to 24 hours, this also makes a diagnosis of cellulitis. Cellulitis can be treated with broad-spectrum antibiotics with a focus on covering skin flora. In the case of a cellulitis not responding to antibiotics and with increasing fever, evidence of pus from the wound, or a palpable collection within the incision, an abscess should be suspected. Wound abscesses need to be treated surgically with incision and drainage, wound cleaning, and packing. Often, antibiotics are continued until 48 hours afebrile. Anytime a wound abscess is suspected, it should either be ruled out with an imaging study or definitively by opening the wound. Delay in treating a wound abscess may lead to necrotizing fasciitis. One hallmark sign of necrotizing fasciitis is the loss of initial pain from cellulitis caused by nerve injury without change in the visual appearance of the cellulitis. Necrotizing fasciitis requires surgical resection of the necrotic tissue and often repair of the fascia with grafts.

Perineal cellulitis or abscesses are treated similarly to abdominal wound infections. However, the diagnosis is often more difficult to make as the area can be more difficult to readily inspect and women can confuse the infection with normal postpartum perineal pain. Similar treatment with broad-spectrum antibiotics for cellulitis and opening the wound in the setting of an abscess is performed. If such an abscess occurs in the setting of third- or fourth-degree perineal laceration, usually the infection is treated and a long-delayed closure by a specialist, for example, a urogynecologist or rectal surgeon, is performed. Of note, perineal infections in the setting of third- and fourth-degree lacerations may be decreased by the use of prophylactic antibiotics.

Wound Separations

Even in the absence of an infection, wounds may not heal by primary intention after their first closure. Fluid collections of either serum (seroma) or blood (hematoma) can increase the chances of wound separation by preventing tissue apposition. Thus, continued leaking of either fluid or blood from a wound can signal a seroma or hematoma. Usually the skin of a transverse incision has adequately healed to remove staples on postoperative day 3 and for a vertical incision by postoperative day 6 or 7. If, when the staples are removed, the skin separates, this is considered a wound separation. In this setting, it is important to make sure it is just a superficial separation and the wound should be probed to verify that the fascia is still intact. If the fascia is also separated, this is termed a *wound dehiscence*.

With a superficial wound separation, there are two options. The first is to simply let the wound heal by secondary intention. The wound may be packed with gauze or Sorbsan and changed once to twice per day. More recently, wounds have been treated with a wound vacuum. By applying negative pressure to the wound, serous fluid is removed, local blood supply to the area improved, and wound edges mechanically reapproximated, thus decreasing wound healing time. Another alternative is that if the wound is not infected, it can be simply closed by primary intention again. As many postcesarean wounds are complicated by seromas from the surrounding tissue edema, these reattempts at primary closure will often be unsuccessful. For a complete wound dehiscence, the fascia is usually closed and the skin incision above treated in either fashion detailed above.

MASTITIS

Mastitis is a regional infection of the breast, commonly caused by the patient's skin flora or the oral flora of breastfeeding infants. The organisms enter an erosion or cracked nipple and proliferate, leading to infection. Lactating women will often have bilaterally warm, diffusely tender, and firm breasts, particularly at the time of engorgement or milk letdown. This should be differentiated from focal tenderness, erythema, and differences in temperature from one region of the breast to another, which are classic signs of mastitis. The diagnosis can be made with physical examination, fever, and an elevated WBC count. Mastitis can be complicated by formation of an abscess, which then requires treatment by incision and drainage (I&D).

Mastitis can be treated with oral antibiotics; dicloxacillin is the treatment of choice. In addition, patients should be encouraged to breastfeed, which prevents intraductal accumulation of infected material. Those who are not breastfeeding should breast pump in the acute phase of the infection. Women who are unresponsive to oral antibiotics are admitted for IV antibiotics until afebrile for 48 hours. If there is no response to IV antibiotics, a breast abscess should be suspected and an imaging study obtained.

POSTPARTUM DEPRESSION

More than half of all women will experience postpartum changes in their mood. Many patients have the postpartum blues, experiencing rapid mood swings from elation to sorrow, and changes in appetite, concentration, and sleep. These postpartum changes generally occur within 2 to 3 days after delivery, peaking at the 5th and resolving within 2 weeks. Symptoms of sadness and disinterest that persist may point toward a diagnosis of true postpartum depression, complicating more than 5% of pregnancies. The pathophysiology of depression is poorly understood, but may be due to the rapid changes in estrogen, progesterone, and prolactin in postpartum patients. It also may be related to the lack of sleep in the postpartum period as well as the psychosocial stress of caring for a newborn. Although all women experience hormonal fluctuation after delivery, some may be more sensitive to these changes and thereby predisposed to the development of postpartum depression. Such patients include those with a history of or family history of depression or other mental illness, depressive symptoms in pregnancy, mood changes with hormonal contraceptive use, as well as those with poor social support networks.

Diagnosis

Most patients have normal changes in appetite, energy level, and sleep patterns in the initial postpartum period that do not necessarily indicate frank depression. However, patients who experience low energy level, anhedonia, anorexia, apathy, sleep disturbances, extreme sadness, and other depressive symptoms for greater than a few weeks may have postpartum depression. These patients often feel incapable of caring for their infants. Occasionally, depressed patients have suicidal or homicidal ideation, which is a much clearer marker for depression and merits close observation. Patients with a history of bipolar disorder should specifically be observed for the development of postpartum psychosis.

Therapy and Prognosis

In patients with postpartum blues, symptoms are usually self-limited with support and encouragement. However, these symptoms can occasionally progress to a more severe postpartum depression or even psychosis. In these situations, the caregiver needs to determine whether the patient is having suicidal or homicidal ideation. A social worker and professional counselor should be involved, as should the immediate family and any other individuals who are close to the patient and can provide support. While an episode of postpartum blues may resolve quite readily, depression and psychosis should be treated with medications. SSRIs have been used for postpartum depression with good efficacy and compatibility with breastfeeding. Most patients without a history of depression or other mental illness improve, usually to their prepregnant state.

KEY POINTS

- Two central issues in the immediate postpartum period, regardless of the mode of delivery, are pain management and wound care.
- Condoms with a spermicidal foam or gel can be used by anyone postpartum.
- Diaphragms and cervical caps need to be refitted at 6 weeks. IUDs are best placed at 6 weeks as well.
- Depo-Provera, Implanon, the progesterone-releasing IUD, or the progesterone-only mini-pill are the hormonal contraceptives of choice in the puerperium because they are less likely to decrease milk production in breastfeeding patients and affect risk of venous thromboembolism.
- Discharge instructions should include discussion of medical issues such as contraception and wound care. Instructions to both patient and partner on social issues such as the transition to home with the newborn, how to deal with some of the changes related to the delivery, and care of the baby are also needed.
- Causes of postpartum hemorrhage include uterine atony, uterine rupture, uterine inversion, retained POCs, placenta accreta, and cervical or vaginal lacerations.
- Treatment of PPH may require use of blood products including fresh frozen plasma, cryoprecipitate, and platelets in patients who develop a consumptive coagulopathy.
- Surgical management of PPH ranges from D&C to exploratory laparotomy, uterine artery ligation, hypogastric artery ligation, and, if these fail, hysterectomy.
- In PPH patients for whom there is enough time, an alternative to exploratory laparotomy is uterine artery embolization by interventional radiology.
- Endomyometritis is more common in patients with cesarean section than vaginal delivery, although patients with manual removal of the placenta are also at increased risk.
- Diagnosis of endomyometritis is clinical with fever, elevated WBC count, and uterine tenderness; treatment is with broad-spectrum antibiotics and D&C for retained POCs.
- Cesarean incisions may be complicated by cellulitis, wound abscess, wound separation, or frank dehiscence. Wound healing is improved by blood glucose control and smoking cessation.
- Mastitis is differentiated from engorgement by focal tenderness, erythema, and edema, and treatment is usually with oral antibiotics. Breastfeeding/pumping is compatible with mastitis and encouraged.
- Changes in appetite, sleep patterns, and energy level are common in the first few weeks postpartum.
- Postpartum depression is common and probably underdiagnosed. In most patients, the depressive symptoms resolve on their own, but occasionally antidepressants are required.

C Clinical Vignettes

Vignette 1

You are seeing a 20-year-old single G1P1 who is postpartum day 2 after a normal spontaneous vaginal delivery of a healthy female infant. Her pregnancy and delivery were uncomplicated. She is notable for being teary and anxious when you begin providing her discharge instructions. She explains that she has been unable to get any sleep between her baby crying, breastfeeding every 3 hours, and her constant worries about whether she will be able to handle a baby at home by herself. She is particularly bothered by pervasive thoughts that her daughter could roll onto her stomach and be unable to breathe or that she could choke while breastfeeding without her mother recognizing it because of her inexperience and sleep deprivation. She is concerned about the overwhelming responsibility of raising a baby by herself and that she may never be able to go back to school; she expresses that "this may all have been a bad idea." She denies any history of depression.

1. Which of the following is the most important next step in evaluating the patient?
   a. Reassure the patient that she is likely experiencing a common condition called "the baby blues"
   b. Contact the father of the baby to ensure the patient will have an alternative source of childcare when she needs to care for herself
   c. Offer a prescription sleep aid to help the patient get a full night's rest
   d. Prescribe the patient an SSRI for a new diagnosis of postpartum depression
   e. Tell the patient that she likely has postpartum depression and should be seen by a counselor while in the hospital

2. The patient sees you again 6 weeks later for her postpartum appointment and still reports difficulty coping with her new baby. She's still having difficulty with sleep, but is now unable to stay asleep even when the baby has been sound asleep. She has been avoiding phone calls from her friends because she does not want them to see her in this state. She has a limited appetite, decreased interest in her normal sources of entertainment, and she reports just generally being sad since the baby was born. Although she has taken her baby to the pediatrician as needed and notes interval weight gain, she reports having ignored her crying baby on more than one occasion over the last few weeks. Which of the following is the most important next step in evaluating the patient?
   a. Tell the patient that she likely has postpartum depression and should be seen by a counselor as soon as can be arranged
   b. Prescribe the patient an SSRI for a new diagnosis of postpartum depression
   c. Provide careful reassurance and arrange for follow-up appointment in 2 weeks to assess for resolution of symptoms
   d. Contact the Department of Human Services for your concerns regarding child neglect
   e. Assess the patient for any current or historical thoughts of harming herself or her baby

3. After extensive counseling the patient agrees to pharmacologic therapy for her postpartum depression. In which of the following cases would an SSRI not be recommended for her?
   a. The patient is currently breastfeeding
   b. She reports a family history of bipolar disease
   c. The patient is unlikely to be compliant with a daily medication
   d. She desires to become pregnant again in the near future
   e. She reports having a glass of wine every other day

Vignette 2

A 36-year-old G7P50015 woman has just delivered a 4,500 g female infant at 39 weeks gestation. She underwent induction of labor with oxytocin for severe preeclampsia diagnosed with systolic BPs elevated to 160 mm Hg. Her pregnancy was complicated by uncontrolled gestational diabetes and resultant polyhydramnios. She was placed on magnesium throughout her induction for seizure prophylaxis. She had an epidural placed during the first stage of labor and remained on a normal labor curve throughout. Her second stage of labor lasted 3½ hours; she was, however, able to deliver vaginally with preemptive McRoberts maneuvers and steady traction. The third stage of labor lasted 10 minutes and the placenta was delivered intact. Immediately after the third stage her bleeding was significant with the expulsion of blood clots and a fundus that was notable for bogginess.

1. Which of the following are not risk factors for postpartum hemorrhage?
   a. Advanced maternal age
   b. Grand multiparity
   c. Prolonged use of oxytocin during labor
   d. Polyhydramnios
   e. Prolonged exposure to magnesium during labor

2. Which of the following medications would be contraindicated in the treatment of uterine atony in this patient?
   a. Methylergonovine (Methergine)
   b. Carboprost (Hemabate, PGF2-alpha)
   c. Intramuscular Pitocin
   d. Misoprostol (PGE1)
   e. Calcium gluconate

3. Prompt use of a 250 mcg IM injection of carboprost manages to increase the tone of her uterus stop the bleeding; however, you continue to notice a steady stream of blood descending from the vagina. What is the most appropriate next step in the evaluation of this patient's bleeding?
   a. Perform a bedside ultrasound for retained products of conception
   b. Perform a bedside ultrasound to look for blood in the abdomen significant for uterine rupture
   c. Perform a manual exploration of the uterine fundus and exploration for retained clots or products
   d. Examine the perineum and vaginal sulci for tears sustained during delivery
   e. Consult interventional radiology for uterine artery embolization

4. The patient was noted to have a third-degree perineal laceration (affected the external anal sphincter) that was repaired in normal standard fashion. Which of the following considerations in the treatment and counseling of these patients is false?
   a. You should provide a rectal examination to ensure that the mucosa is intact
   b. She should be on regular stool softeners throughout the postpartum period
   c. She should be given narcotic medications for pain control on a PRN basis
   d. She should be counseled about her risk of anal sphincter defect and incontinence
   e. She should undergo anal endosonography and/or anal manometry in 1 year to evaluate for sphincter defects

5. You are examining the patient's postpartum hematocrit and note a drop from her antepartum measurement from 33% to 24%. Her estimated blood loss from her vaginal delivery and perineal laceration repair was 400 mL. The nurse reports that the patient has had minimal vaginal bleeding overnight. What is the next best step in her evaluation/treatment?
   a. Reassurance and offer iron supplementation postpartum
   b. Offer a blood transfusion for palliation of symptoms of anemia
   c. Request a procedure room for dilation and curettage of the uterus
   d. Request an abdominal ultrasound for blood in the uterine or abdominal cavity
   e. Examine the site of her laceration repair for hematoma

Vignette 3

A 22-year-old G3P1021 woman recently delivered and is now attempting to breastfeed her baby. Her pregnancy and delivery were uncomplicated. She denies any medical history or social history significant for drug use. She is frustrated by her lack of volume, worried that her son will not gain weight, and is now requesting a bottle and prepared formula.

1. Which of the following statements about the benefits of breastfeeding is false?
   a. Breast-fed children are more resistant to disease and infection early in life than formula-fed children
   b. Breastfeeding women have a lower risk of breast, uterine, and ovarian cancer if they have breastfed for at least 2 years cumulatively
   c. Children who are breast-fed are significantly less likely to become obese later in childhood
   d. Oxytocin released during breastfeeding causes the uterus to return to its normal size more quickly
   e. None. All of the above are true statements

2. Your patient is convinced of the benefits of breastfeeding and continues to try, successfully breastfeeding by the end of postpartum day 1. The following morning, however, she develops a low-grade fever of 38.0°C, for which your nurse alerts you. She complains about the pain associated with the engorgement of her breasts bilaterally and very sharp, recurrent pelvic pains. Her vital signs are otherwise normal. What is the most likely explanation for these findings?
   a. Lactation fever
   b. Mastitis
   c. Breast abscess
   d. Endometritis
   e. Chorioamnionitis

3. Which of the following would be an appropriate form of contraception for this breastfeeding patient?
   a. Progesterone-eluting IUD
   b. Combined oral contraceptive pills
   c. Contraceptive vaginal rings
   d. Contraceptive patch
   e. None of the above

4. Your patient is admitted to the hospital 2 weeks later with rigors and chills and complaint of a swollen and reddened right breast. She has been breastfeeding throughout the last 2 weeks. Her vitals are significant for a fever up to 38.4°C and tachycardia with pulse of 112; all other vital signs are normal. Her physical examination is significant for cracked nipples and engorged breasts bilaterally; her right breast is particularly tense, notable for erythema and increased temperature compared to the left breast without masses. What is the appropriate therapy for the above condition?
   a. Dicloxacillin × 10 to 14 days
   b. Dicloxacillin until afebrile for 48 hours
   c. Reassurance, ice, breast support, and breast pumping
   d. Protective nipple shields and soothing ointments
   e. Ultrasound-guided localization of abscess and aspiration

Vignette 4

A 28-year-old G1P1 woman is being discharged from the hospital on postoperative day 4 after having received a primary low transverse cesarean section for breech presentation, with an estimated blood loss of 700 mL. Her pregnancy was otherwise uncomplicated and her hospital course was also uncomplicated.

1. Which of the following discharge considerations is accurate?
   a. She should have her staples removed as an outpatient at 7 to 10 days postpartum
   b. She should avoid vaginal intercourse and tub bathing for 1 to 2 weeks
   c. She should not lift anything weighing more than 10 lb or the weight of her baby until her postpartum appointment
   d. She should be on strict bed rest for the first week following her cesarean

2. One week after hospital discharge the patient ends up in the emergency department complaining of severe abdominal pain.

Her vitals are significant for a fever of 39°C and tachycardia. Her physical examination reveals acute fundal tenderness beneath a low transverse skin incision that is well-healed, clean, dry, and intact. She received preoperative antibiotics prior to her procedure. Her staples were removed prior to discharge. She endorses residual vaginal bleeding with a slight odor that is confirmed by speculum examination. What is the most appropriate next step in your treatment of this patient?

a. Wound exploration
b. Abdominal and pelvic ultrasound
c. Dilation and curettage
d. Outpatient antibiotics
e. Inpatient antibiotics

3. Two weeks after her cesarean section the patient presents to you with a chief complaint of serous drainage from a 1 cm area of skin separation. The borders of the skin are mildly painful, but nonerythematous. Which of the following would be the best approach for the described condition?

a. The patient's skin separation is a result of infection, requiring immediate administration of antibiotics
b. She is at risk for necrotizing fasciitis. She should be admitted to the hospital and undergo wound debridement and reapproximation
c. Skin separation at the incision with serous drainage is normal and need only be managed by application of a bandage
d. Skin separation should be evaluated further with a probe to examine whether the fascial layer below it is intact
e. Skin separation should be closed tightly with suture to prevent recurrence

4. The patient sees you at her 6 week postpartum visit and thanks you for your careful attention to her health; however, she is now thinking about the future and worries about her risk of uterine rupture with subsequent pregnancy. What is this patient's risk of uterine rupture with subsequent trial of labor?

a. 1%
b. 5%
c. 10%
d. 20%
e. 50%

A Answers

Vignette 1 Question 1
Answer A: More than 75% of new mothers experience some degree of emotional disturbance after delivering their babies. Their feelings do not always meet their expectations of how they would feel while pregnant, with many feeling sad, tired, fragile, anxious, isolated, or even regretful. These feelings may sometimes also be manifested as agitation and anger toward their baby or their caregivers. These feelings however, are normal and are called the postpartum blues, a period of emotional and hormonal lability following childbirth. They begin approximately 2 to 3 days after birth and resolve within 2 weeks without treatment. Postpartum blues can be alleviated through a team approach where family and friends continue to support and reassure the patient once outside the hospital; however, contacting the father of the baby may not be the correct approach without any further information about their relationship or a history of domestic violence or sexual abuse. Although it may seem like most of the patient's concerns may stem from her tiredness, a pharmacologic sleep aid would not ease her anxieties about motherhood.

Vignette 1 Question 2
Answer E: This patient has developed postpartum depression with symptoms persisting and worsening for more than 2 weeks after childbirth. Although she has no history of depression, postpartum depression can and should be treated like a major depressive episode with a combination of psychotherapy and antidepressant medications. There is no consistent evidence that any one class of antidepressant is superior; patients with a history of depression and treatment should be placed back on the medications that they had responded to previously. Prior to treatment, however, it is more important to assess the severity of her current state; any mention of suicide or infanticide needs to be taken seriously and counseled appropriately, with scheduling of close follow-up. Although it is concerning the patient has ignored her baby, we can be reassured that the baby has been taken to the pediatrician and has good interval weight gain, indicating that the neglect may not be pervasive and persistent.

Vignette 1 Question 3
Answer B: A number of studies have shown benefit with the use of SSRIs to treat postpartum depression, including sertraline, paroxetine, venlafaxine, and fluvoxamine. SSRIs are generally well tolerated and have a low–side-effect profile compared to other antidepressants available. Sertraline and paroxetine are most often recommended for breastfeeding mothers. Although psychotropic medications pass through the breast milk, studies have shown that they are not subsequently detected in infant serum at appreciable levels. Paroxetine should not be prescribed if a woman is planning on becoming pregnant again, as it has been associated with congenital heart defects and persistent pulmonary hypertension. Other SSRIs, however, have been found to be safe in pregnancy and can be prescribed as needed. MAO-inhibitors should not be taken while drinking alcohol because of the risk of serotonin syndrome; this, however, does not apply to SSRIs. As family history is one of the strongest predictors of bipolar disorder, it is possible that the use of an antidepressant could trigger mania in a yet undiagnosed, underlying bipolar disorder. In these cases, a mood stabilizer would be the best treatment.

Vignette 2 Question 1
Answer A: Postpartum hemorrhage in the context of vaginal delivery is defined as an estimated blood loss greater than 500 mL. Most of all postpartum hemorrhages results from uterine atony, the failure of uterine muscles to contract normally after the second and third stages of labor. Without muscular contraction, severed vessels of the placental bed will continue to bleed. Any factor that might cause uterine muscle exhaustion or distend and distort the muscle can cause atony. These factors allow prediction of PPH and preparation of uterotonic medications prior to delivery. Advanced maternal age is not associated with postpartum hemorrhage, though it can be associated with multiparity and the development of preeclampsia requiring magnesium.

Vignette 2 Question 2
Answer A: Methylergonovine should NOT be used to treat her atony, as it works by causing systemic vasoconstriction, which would increase her BP even further than it may already be elevated by her preeclampsia. Carboprost, Pitocin, and misoprostol would be suitable options. Carboprost is contraindicated in patients with asthma as the prostaglandin is a bronchoconstrictor. Calcium gluconate may be able to reverse the effects of magnesium, thereby allowing the uterus to better contract; however, it is indicated only in life-threatening cases of hypermagnesemia and in the setting of preeclampsia would leave the patient without any seizure prophylaxis.

Vignette 2 Question 3
Answer D: The second most common cause of postpartum hemorrhage is genital tract laceration or trauma. Lacerations of the cervix or vagina are common in precipitous deliveries and in deliveries assisted with the vacuum or forceps. Shoulder dystocia can also cause lacerations. In this case, a thorough examination of the vagina should be performed, and if no source is found, a subsequent examination

of the cervix would be the correct procedure to evaluate the source of bleeding. Retained products of conception or clots would prevent full contraction of the uterus and present as atony. Uterine rupture is rare, especially in women without a history of cesarean, occurring in 1/2,000 deliveries. Uterine artery embolization is used infrequently, reserved as a last resort after attempting to stop bleeding by conventional procedures such as dilation and curettage and intrauterine balloon tamponade.

Vignette 2 Question 4

Answer E: Although anal incontinence is one of the reported consequences of vaginal deliveries affected by a third- or fourth-degree laceration and repair, it occurs in women who report having never had a laceration as well. The likelihood of these disorders can be dependent upon the provider's ability to provide a reinforcing repair and the patient's ability to prevent further disruption of the repair with good bowel habits and such patients are put on around the clock stool softeners for 2 to 3 weeks to prevent constipation. Postpartum pain control is important and NSAIDs are first-line treatment option, with opioids being used PRN to prevent associated constipation as well. Routine anal endosonography and manometry are not currently the standard of care for all women affected by deep lacerations.

Vignette 2 Question 5

Answer E: An examination should be performed to rule out a hematoma from either her wound site or an occult hematoma from any blood vessels injured beneath the vaginal mucosa during delivery. Hematomas can often be managed expectantly, but should be observed for their enlargement or any increase in tension of the wall of the hematoma. In such cases, the hematoma should be opened, the bleeding vessel ligated, and the vaginal wall closed. A hemogram should be repeated for further drop in hematocrit. Retained products often present with continued vaginal bleeding. Although a blood transfusion may be a part of this patient's ultimate management, it would not be indicated until a source of bleeding has been identified. Reassurance as well should not be given until a source of bleeding has been identified.

Vignette 3 Question 1

Answer E: All of the above responses are reasons to endorse breastfeeding. Breast milk, especially during its initial production (colostrums), is enriched with immunoglobulins that help to protect the infant from disease such as gastroenteritis, otitis media, and lower respiratory tract infection. Children who are breast-fed have a lower likelihood of obesity and even developing type 1 diabetes. In cases of exclusive breastfeeding, women are able to suppress ovulation, believed to thereby decrease the risk of ovarian cancer. The reduction of endogenous estrogen exposure and cycling also contributes to the decreased risk of both breast and endometrial cancers.

Vignette 3 Question 2

Answer A: For the first 24 hours after the initiation of lactation, it is not uncommon for the breasts to become firm, distended, and associated with a rise in temperature. Fevers can be as high as 39°C, but rarely do they last for more than 24 hours. They often self-resolve with breastfeeding/pumping and can be treated with a supportive bra, the application of ice, and antiinflammatory medications. Mastitis and abscesses tend to present unilaterally. The pelvic pain she is having is associated with the release of oxytocin with breastfeeding, causing the uterus to contract. This is normal; nevertheless infection must always be excluded prior to giving a diagnosis of lactation fever.

Vignette 3 Question 3

Answer A: Any estrogen-containing form of contraception would be contraindicated in a woman attempting to establish breastfeeding. Estrogens have been known to reduce the quantity and quality of breast milk. Estrogen-containing methods may also increase the risk of venous thromboembolism during the first 6 weeks postpartum. Progesterone-only methods such as the IUD, implant, intramuscular Depo, and progesterone-only contraceptive pills would be better options. Although the IUD is often not recommended for insertion until after the uterus involutes at 6 weeks postpartum, it can be used in contraceptive-needing patients whose follow-up cannot be guaranteed.

Vignette 3 Question 4

Answer A: The patient has a diagnosis of mastitis, which is caused by infection of the breast most commonly by *Staphylococcus aureus* entering the broken skin sometimes caused by the infant's suckling. Abscess should not be suspected unless an isolated mass is felt in the affected breast that does not resolve with pumping and in cases where the fever is refractory to at least 48 to 72 hours of antibiotics. Treatment is with dicloxacillin to complete a full 10- to 14-day course, even though symptoms may dramatically resolve within 48 hours. Patients should be encouraged to breastfeed through the infection, with counseling on how to improve their baby's latch and avoid further trauma to the nipple.

Vignette 4 Question 1

Answer C: Women who have had a cesarean section will have their staples removed in the hospital, before discharge on postoperative day 3 or 4 as long as they have had a low transverse skin incision. Women who have had a vertical incision will often have to wait to have their staples removed on days 7 to 10. The incision is considered water tight at 48 hours, at which point the patient can shower. Full immersion in a bath should wait, however, until 4 to 6 weeks. Sex should also be delayed for 6 weeks to prevent the introduction of infection from an open cervix and/or continued uterine bleeding. Women who have had a cesarean section are encouraged to walk as soon as possible to decrease their risk of deep vein thrombosis.

Vignette 4 Question 2

Answer B: The patient's presentation is most likely significant for endomyometritis. Her wound is well-healed and nonerythematous, making a cellulitis unlikely. Were that patient's symptoms to be observed in the hospital during the immediate postoperative period, a simple endomyometritis could be suspected and treated with antibiotics with the expectation that involution of the uterus would be sufficient to expel any residual intrauterine contents. In this case, however, the patient continues to have a malodorous discharge that may be significant for retained products that should be evaluated by ultrasound. Failing to perform an ultrasound and performing a dilation and curettage without an understanding of expected findings may lead to more vigorous curettage that results in uterine perforation, especially in the setting of a fragile, infected uterine wall. Patients will receive antibiotics after evacuation of uterine contents, which will continue until 48 hours after their last fever.

Vignette 4 Question 3

Answer D: Any skin separation may look innocuous superficially, but should be evaluated by a physician to ensure that the fascial layer below it is intact. Any fascial dehiscence could leave the patient prone to the development of a hernia later in life. Skin separation likely stems from the pressurized accumulation of serous fluid in the subcutaneous tissue that ultimately prevents healing. Although the inclination might be to resuture the skin tightly, doing so would prevent a collection of serous fluid from exiting the wound, thereby leaving a nidus for infection. Given that the patient is not showing any signs of skin erythema, it is unlikely that she has a cellulitis. No prophylactic antibiotics are given for cases of skin separation.

Vignette 4 Question 4

Answer A: Uterine rupture is estimated to occur in 0.5% to 1.0% of patients with prior uterine scars and about 1:15,000 to 20,000 women with an unscarred uterus. This risk varies based on a variety of risk factors. For example, the risk appears to be 0.5% or lower in women in spontaneous labor, but 1% to 2% in those who are induced. Women with more than one prior cesarean have an increased risk of subsequent uterine rupture as compared to those with only one. Women with a prior vaginal delivery have a lower risk of uterine rupture as compared to those with no prior vaginal delivery. Additionally, it appears that a two-layered uterine closure is at decreased risk of uterine rupture as compared to a one-layer closure.

Part II Gynecology

Chapter 13 Benign Disorders of the Lower Genital Tract

BENIGN LESIONS OF THE VULVA, VAGINA, AND CERVIX

This chapter encompasses an overview of the many congenital anomalies, epithelial disorders, and benign cysts and tumors of the vulva, vagina, and cervix. Infections of these structures are covered in Chapter 16, and premalignant and malignant lesions are covered in Chapter 27 (vulva and vagina) and Chapter 28 (cervix).

CONGENITAL ANOMALIES OF THE VULVA AND VAGINA

A variety of congenital defects occur in the external genitalia, vagina, and cervix including but not limited to labial fusion, imperforate hymen, transverse vaginal septum, longitudinal vaginal septum, vaginal atresia, and vaginal agenesis. Congenital anomalies of the female genital tract are associated with concomitant **anomalies in the upper reproductive tract** as well as **anomalies in the genital urinary (GU) tract** such as unilateral renal agenesis, pelvic or horseshoe kidneys, or irregularities in the collecting system.

LABIAL FUSION

Labial fusion is associated with excess androgens. Most commonly, the etiology is the result of **exogenous androgen exposure** but may also be due to an enzymatic error leading to increased androgen production. The most common form of enzymatic deficiency is **21-hydroxylase deficiency** (Chapter 23) leading to **congenital adrenal hyperplasia**. This may be phenotypically demonstrated in the neonate with **ambiguous genitalia**, hyperandrogenism with salt wasting, hypotension, hyperkalemia, and hypoglycemia. The neonates often present in adrenal crisis with salt wasting seen approximately 75% of the time. This autosomal recessive trait occurs in roughly 1 in 40,000 to 50,000 pregnancies. The diagnosis is made by elevated **17α-hydroxyprogesterone** or urine 17-ketosteroid with decreased serum cortisol.

Because cortisol is not being made in the adrenal cortex, the treatment for this disorder is **exogenous cortisol**. The exogenous cortisol then negatively feeds back on the pituitary to decrease the release of adrenocorticotropic hormone (ACTH), thus inhibiting the stimulation of the adrenal gland that is shunting all steroid precursors into androgens. If salt wasting is documented, a mineralocorticoid (usually fludrocortisone acetate) is also given. Labial fusion and other forms of ambiguous genitalia often require **reconstructive surgery**.

IMPERFORATE HYMEN

The hymen is at the junction between the urogenital sinus and the sinovaginal bulbs (Fig. 13-1). Before birth, the epithelial cells in the central portion of the hymenal membrane degenerate, leaving a thin rim of mucous membrane at the vaginal introitus. This is known as the **hymenal ring**. When this degeneration fails to occur, the hymen remains intact. This is known as an **imperforate hymen**. It occurs in 1 in 1,000 female births. Other congenital abnormalities of the hymen are shown in Figure 13-2. These can result from incomplete degeneration of the central portion of hymen.

An **imperforate hymen** results in an obstruction to the outflow tract of the reproductive system. This can lead to a buildup of secretions in the vagina behind the hymen (hydrocolpos or **mucocolpos**) similar to that seen with a transverse vaginal septum (Fig. 13-3). If not identified at birth, an imperforate hymen is often diagnosed at puberty in adolescents who present with **primary amenorrhea** and **cyclic pelvic pain**. These symptoms are due to the accumulation of menstrual flow behind the hymen in the vagina (**hematocolpos**) and uterus (**hematometra**). In these patients, the physical examination may be notable for the absence of an identifiable vaginal lumen, a tense bulging hymen, and possibly increasing lower abdominal girth. Treatment of imperforate hymen and other hymenal abnormalities is with **surgery** to excise the extra tissue, evacuate any obstructed material, and create a normal-sized vaginal opening (Color Plate 7).

TRANSVERSE VAGINAL SEPTUM

The **upper vagina** is formed as the paramesonephric (Müllerian) ducts elongate and meet in the midline. The internal portion of each duct is canalized and the remaining septum between them dissolves (Fig. 13-1A). The caudal portion of the Müllerian ducts develops into the uterus and

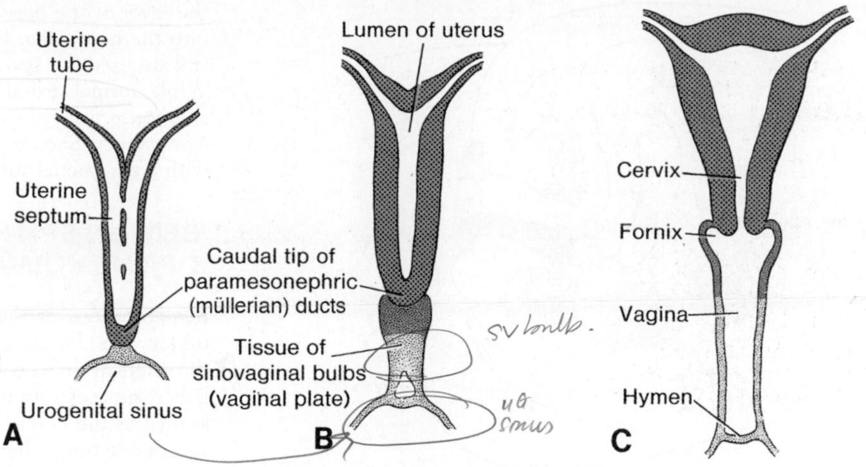

Figure 13-1 • Embryonic formation of the vagina and uterus.
(From Sadler T. *Langman's Medical Embryology*, 9th ed. Baltimore, MD: Lippincott Williams & Wilkins; 2003.)

upper vagina (Fig. 13-1B and C). The **lower vagina** is formed as the urogenital sinus evaginates to form the sinovaginal bulbs (Fig. 13-1B). These then proliferate to form the vaginal plate. The lumen of the lower vagina is then formed as the central portion of this solid vaginal plate degenerates (Fig. 13-1C). This process is known as canalization or vacuolization.

The vagina is formed as the Müllerian system from above joins the sinovaginal bulb–derived system from below. This takes place at the **Müllerian tubercle** (Fig. 13-1B). The Müllerian tubercle must be canalized for a normal vagina to form. If this does not occur, the tissue may be left as a **transverse vaginal septum**. These septa often lie near the junction between the lower two-thirds and **upper one-third** of the vagina (Fig. 13-3) but can be found at various levels in the vagina. This occurs in approximately 1 in 30,000 to 1 in 80,000 women. Similar to the imperforate hymen, diagnosis is usually made at the time of puberty in adolescents who present with **primary amenorrhea** and **cyclic pelvic pain** accompanied by menstrual symptoms. On physical examination, patients typically have normal external female genitalia and a short vagina that appears to end in a blind pouch. The transverse vaginal septa are usually less than 1 cm thick and may have a central perforation. **Ultrasound and MRI** can be used to characterize the thickness and location of the septum and to confirm the presence of other parts of the reproductive tract. **Surgical correction** is the only form of treatment.

VAGINAL ATRESIA

Vaginal atresia (also known as agenesis of the lower vagina) is often confused with imperforate hymen or transverse vaginal septum. It occurs when the **lower vagina fails to develop** and is replaced by fibrous tissue. **The ovaries, uterus, cervix, and upper vagina are all normal.** Developmentally, vaginal atresia results when the urogenital sinus fails to contribute the lower portion of the vagina (Fig. 13-1). It presents during adolescence with **primary amenorrhea** and **cyclic pelvic pain**. Physical examination reveals the absence of an introitus and the presence of a **vaginal dimple**. Pelvic imaging with ultrasound and/or MRI may show a large **hematocolpos** and confirm the presence of a normal upper reproductive tract. **Surgical correction** can be achieved by incising the fibrous tissue and dissecting it until the normal upper vagina is identified. Any accumulated blood or materials can be evacuated and the normal upper vaginal mucosa is then brought down to the introitus and sutured to the hymenal ring. This is known as a **vaginal pull-through procedure**.

VAGINAL AGENESIS

Vaginal agenesis, also known as **Mayer-Rokitansky-Kuster-Hauser** syndrome (MRKH), occurs in 1 to 2.5 per 10,000 female births. It is characterized by the congenital **absence of the vagina** (Color Plate 8) and **the absence or hypoplasia of**

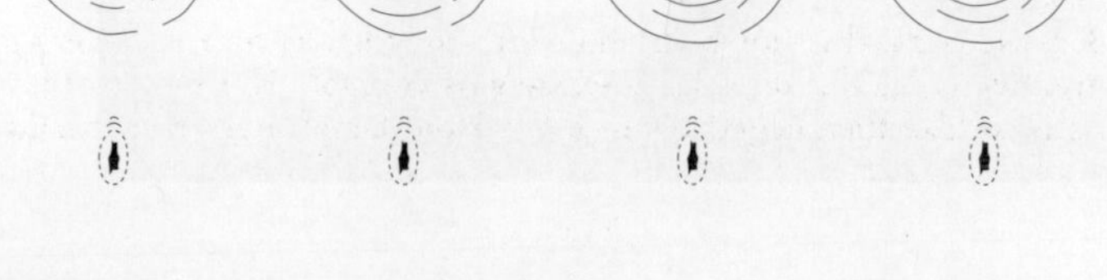

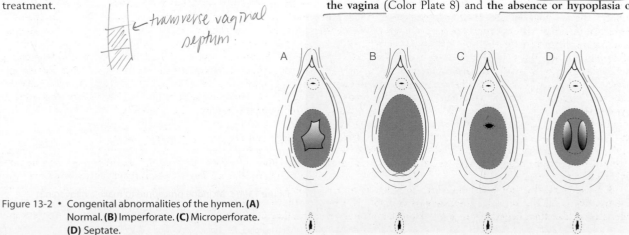

Figure 13-2 • Congenital abnormalities of the hymen. **(A)** Normal. **(B)** Imperforate. **(C)** Microperforate. **(D)** Septate.

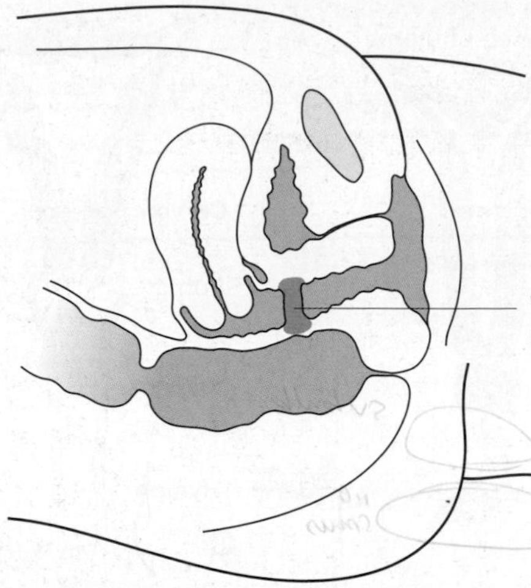

Figure 13-3 • Transverse vaginal septum.

all or part of the cervix, uterus, and fallopian tubes. These patients typically have normal external genitalia, normal secondary sexual characteristics (breast development, axillary, and pubic hair), and normal ovarian function. These patients are **phenotypically and genotypically female** with normal 46,XX karyotypes. These patients typically present in adolescence with primary amenorrhea. Pelvic imaging with **ultrasound and MRI** can be used to assess the vagina, uterus, ovaries, and kidneys because these patients will often have associated urologic and skeletal anomalies.

Treatment for patients with vaginal agenesis involves a combination of **psychosocial support**, counseling, and **nonsurgical and surgical correction** individualized to the patient. In motivated patients, a vagina can be created using **serial vaginal dilators** pressed into the perineal body (Frank and Ingram procedures). This can take 4 months to several years depending on the patient. If this nonsurgical approach fails, a variety of vaginal, laparoscopic, and abdominal procedures are available to **create a neovagina**. The most commonly used is the **McIndoe** procedure. In this procedure a split-thickness skin graft is taken from the buttocks and is placed over a silicone mold to create a tube with one closed end (Fig. 13-4). A transverse incision is then made at the vaginal dimple and the fibrous tissue in the location of the normal vagina. The tissue is then dissected to the level of the peritoneum. The mold and graft are inserted into the neovagina. Once the mold is removed, dilators must still be used for several months to maintain vaginal patency. While **normal sexual intercourse** is possible after these surgical and nonsurgical procedures, the patient will be unable to carry a pregnancy. She can, however, have her eggs harvested for use with a gestational surrogate.

BENIGN EPITHELIAL DISORDERS OF THE VULVA AND VAGINA

Benign lesions of the mucosa of the vulva and vagina come under this broad category. The **nonneoplastic epithelial disorders** of the vulva, including lichen sclerosis, lichen planus, lichen simplex chronicus, and vulvar psoriasis, were formerly known as the vulvar dystrophies. "Dystrophy" is no longer an acceptable term; the 2006 International Society for the Study of Vulvar Disease classification system now lists the specific dermatologic disorders (Table 13-1). These lesions often **require histologic examination** (Table 13-2) to identify and treat the disorder and to differentiate the lesion from vulvar and vaginal intraepithelial neoplasia and cancer (Chapter 27).

Lichen sclerosis is an inflammatory dermatosis that can be found on the vulva of women of all age groups, but has major significance in **postmenopausal women**, where it is associated with a 3% to 4% risk of vulvar skin cancer. The etiology is unknown, but several mechanisms have been proposed including immunologic, genetic, hormonal, and infectious mechanisms. The resulting atrophy can cause resorption of the labia minora, labial fusion, occlusion of the clitoris, contracture of the vaginal introitus, thinning of the vulvar skin, and skin fragility (Fig. 13-5).

Lichen planus is an uncommon inflammatory skin condition that can affect the nails, scalp and skin mucosa. Vulvar lichen planus is characterzed by papular or erosive lesions of the vulva that may also involve the vagina. The etiology is unknown, but several mechanisms have been proposed including immunologic, genetic, hormonal, and infectious mechanisms. This inflammatory dermatosis results in chronic eruption of shiny purple **papules** with white striae on the vulva. Similar lesions are often found on the flexor surfaces, and mucous membrane of the oral cavity. Lichen planus can be associated with **vaginal adhesions** and with erosive vaginitis. It generally occurs in women in their 50s or 60s and it is associated with a 3% to 4% risk of vulvar skin cancer.

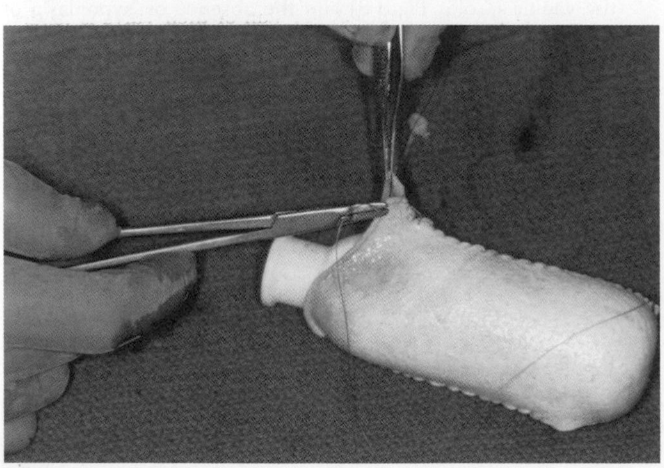

Figure 13-4 • McIndoe procedure to make a neovagina. The skin graft is sewn around a mold.
(Image from Emans J. *Pediatric & Adolescent Gynecology*, 5th ed. Philadelphia, PA: Lippincott Williams & Wilkins; 2004.)

TABLE 13-1 Pathological Subsets and Their Clinical Correlates

Lichenoid pattern (and dermal homogenization/ sclerosis pattern)
Lichen sclerosus
Lichen planus
Acanthotic pattern (formerly squamous cell hyperplasia)
Psoriasis
Lichen simplex chronicus
Primary (idiopathic) acanthosis
Secondary (superimposed on lichen sclerosus, lichen planus, or other vulvar disease)
Spongiotic pattern
Atopic dermatitis
Allergic contact dermatitis
Irritant contact dermatitis
Vesiculobullous pattern
Pemphigoid, cicatricial type
Linear IgA disease
Vasculopathic pattern
Aphthous ulcers
Behcet disease
Plasma cell vulvitis
Acantholytic pattern
Hailey-Hailey disease
Darier disease
Papular genitocrural acantholysis
Granulomatous pattern
Crohn disease
Melkersson-Rosenthal syndrome
Intraepithelial neoplasia
VIN, usual type
a. VIN, warty type
b. VIN, basaloid type
c. VIN, mixed (warty/basaloid) type
VIN, differentiated type

Lynch PJ, Moyal-Barrocco M, Bogliatto F, Micheletti L, Scurry J. 2006 ISSVD classification of vulvar dermatoses: pathologic subsets and their clinical correlates. *J Reprod Med*; 2007:52(1):3–9.

Vulvar psoriasis may be a feature of psoriasis—a very common skin rash that affects up to 2% of the population. There are several different types but the usual form appears as silvery-red scaly patches over the elbows and knees. Other areas of the skin can be affected including the scalp and nails. Psoriasis can occur on the genital skin as part of more general disease but in some people, it affects only this area. The etiology is unknown.

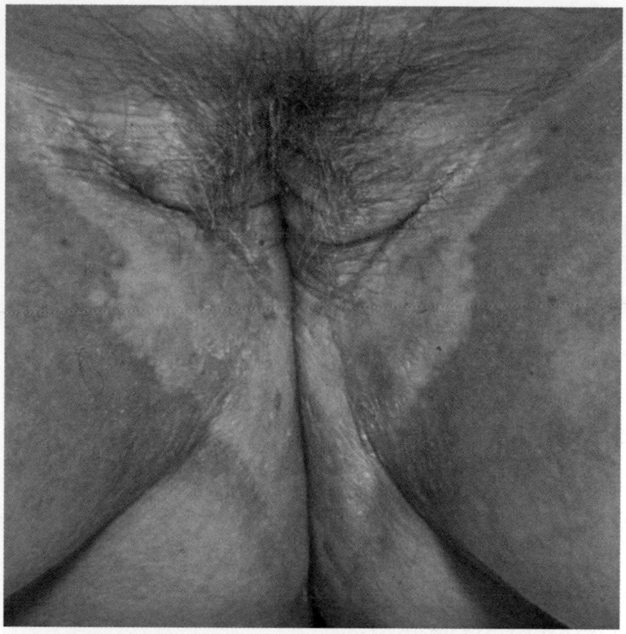

Figure 13-5 • A late case of lichen sclerosis. Note the thin, white, atrophic epithelium and the labial fusion.
(From Rubin E, Farber JL. *Pathology*, 3rd ed. Philadelphia, PA: Lippincott Williams & Wilkins; 1999.)

Lichen simplex chronicus is characterized by thickened skin with accentuated skin markings and excoriations due to chronic itching and scratching. The intense pruritis may be due to atopic dermatitis, psoriasism, neuropathic pain, or psychologic disorders. This skin disorder leads to a scratch–itch cycle; it may begin with something that rubs, irritates, or scratches the skin, such as clothing. This may cause the person to rub or scratch the affected area. Constant scratching causes the skin to thicken. The thickened skin itches, causing more scratching, which causes more thickening.

Clinical Manifestations

History

Patients with benign lesions of the vulva and vagina present with a variety of complaints including vulvar itching, irritation, and burning. They may also report dysuria, dyspareunia, and vulvar pain and feel that the skin of their vulva is tender, bumpy, irritated, or thickened.

Physical Examination

These disorders range in appearance from erythematous plaques to hyperkeratotic white plaques to erosions and ulcers (Table 13-2). Occasionally, petechiae and/or ecchymoses are present as a result of trauma from scratching.

Diagnostic Evaluation

Diagnosis of these disorders may be made clinically. Often histologic confirmation is sought, and biopsy of vulvar lesions is appropriate (Fig. 13-6) for identification purposes and to rule or premalignant and malignant disease. Indications for **definite biopsy** include ulceration, unifocal lesions, uncertain suspicion of lichen sclerosus, unidentifiable lesions, and lesions or symptoms that recur or persist after conventional therapy. Vulvar and vaginal lesions can be evaluated with a colposcope and this will aid directed biopsy.

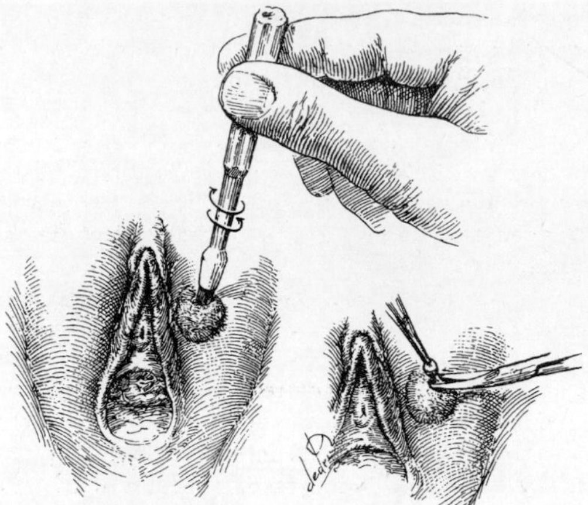

Figure 13-6 • Vulvar biopsy.
(From Beckman CRB, Ling FW, Laube DW, et al. *Obstetrics and Gynecology*, 4th ed. Baltimore, MD: Lippincott Williams & Wilkins; 2002.)

Differential Diagnosis

The differential diagnosis of benign lesions of the vulva and vagina includes disorders such as aphthous ulcers, Behçet syndrome, Crohn disease, erythema multiforme, bullous pemphigoid, and plasma cell vulvitis. The differential diagnosis also includes carcinomas such as squamous cell, basal cell, melanoma, sarcoma, and Paget disease of the vulva. Biopsies should therefore be performed whenever there is uncertainty.

Treatment

For all of these lesions, **healthy vulvar and vaginal hygiene practices** are of recommended. Patients should avoid tight-fitting clothes; pantyhose; panty liners; scented soaps and detergents; bubble baths; washcloths; and feminine sprays, douches, and powders. Patients should wear loose-fitting cotton underwear and **loose-fitting clothing**. They should use **unscented detergents and soaps** such as Neutrogena or Dove, and take morning and evening tub baths without additives.

High-potency **topical steroids** such as clobetasol can be used to treat lichen sclerosus or lichen planus and severe lichen simplex chronicus, and low- to medium-potency steroids should be used for mild cases of dermatoses (Table 13-2). The frequency of use ranges from once per week to one to two times a day. Treatment of lichen simplex chronicus and atopic dermatitis is often limited. However, lichen sclerosus and lichen planus are chronic conditions and require long-term maintenance with topical steroid application, one to three times per week.

In general, there is **no role for topical estrogens or testosterone** in the treatment of these disorders; however, low-dose vaginal estrogen is an effective treatment for concomitant postmenopausal vulvovaginal atrophy. Similarly, surgical management is generally not indicated in treatment of these disorders. An exception is cases of lichen planus, where postinflammatory sequelae can include vaginal adhesions and introital stenosis. Likewise, surgical procedures to enlarge the introitus and open adhesions in lichen sclerosus may be necessary if attempts at intercourse have been unsuccessful following conservative measures.

BENIGN CYSTS AND TUMORS OF THE VULVA AND VAGINA

A variety of cysts and tumors can arise on the vulva and vagina. Cysts can originate from occlusion of pilosebaceous ducts, sebaceous ducts, and apocrine sweat glands. Treatment of benign cystic and solid tumors is needed only if the lesions become symptomatic or infected.

EPIDERMAL INCLUSION CYSTS

Epidermal inclusion cysts are the **most common tumor found on the vulva**. These cysts usually result from occlusion of a pilosebaceous duct or a blocked hair follicle. They are lined with squamous epithelium and contain tissue that would normally be exfoliated. These solitary lesions are normally small and asymptomatic; however, if these become superinfected and develop into abscesses, incision and drainage or complete excision is the treatment.

TABLE 13-2 Benign Epithelial Disorders of the Vulva and Vagina

	Physical Findings	Symptoms	Treatment Options
Lichen sclerosis	Symmetric white, thinned skin on labia, perineum, and perianal region; shrinkage and agglutination of labia minora	Usually pruritus or dyspareunia, often asymptomatic	High-potency topical steroids (clobetasol or halobetasol 0.05%) 1–2×/d for 6–12 wk, then a maintenance schedule of topical steroid
Lichen planus	Multiple shiny, flat, red-purple papules, usually on the inner aspects of the labia minora and vestibule with lacy white changes; often erosive	Pruritus with mild inflammation to severe erosions	High-potency topical steroids (clobetasol or halobetasol 0.05%) 1–2×/d for 6–12 wk, then a maintenance schedule of topical steroid
Lichen simplex chronicus	Localized thickening of the vulvar skin, slight scaling	Chronic pruritus	Medium- to high-potency topical steroid 2×/d for 6 or more weeks
Vulvar psoriasis	Red moist lesions, sometimes scaly	Asymptomatic or sometimes pruritus	Topical steroids, UV light

SEBACEOUS CYSTS

When the duct of a sebaceous gland becomes blocked, a sebaceous cyst forms. The normally secreted sebum accumulates in this cyst. Cysts are often multiple and asymptomatic. As with any cyst, these can become superinfected with local flora and require treatment with incision and drainage.

APOCRINE SWEAT GLAND CYSTS

Sweat glands are found throughout the mons pubis and labia majora. They can become occluded and form cysts. **Fox-Fordyce disease** is an infrequently occurring chronic pruritic papular eruption that localizes to areas where apocrine glands are found. The etiology of Fox-Fordyce disease currently is unknown. **Hidradenitis suppurativa** is a skin disease that most commonly affects areas bearing apocrine sweat glands or sebaceous glands, such as the underarms, breasts, inner thighs, groin, and buttocks. As in the axillary region, if these cysts become infected and form multiple abscesses, excision or incision and drainage are the treatments of choice. If an overlying cellulitis is present, antibiotics are often used as well.

SKENE'S GLAND CYSTS

Skene's glands, or **paraurethral glands**, are located next to the urethra meatus (Fig. 13-7). Chronic inflammation of the Skene's glands can cause obstruction of the ducts and result in cystic dilation of the glands.

BATHOLIN'S DUCT CYST AND ABSCESS

The Bartholin's glands are located bilaterally at approximately **4-o'clock and 8-o'clock** positions on the posterior-lateral aspect of the vaginal orifice (Fig. 13-7). They are mucus-secreting glands with ducts that open just external to the hymenal ring. Obstruction of these ducts leads to **cystic dilation of the Bartholin's duct** while the gland itself is unchanged (Fig. 13-8). If the cyst remains small (1 to 2 cm) and is asymptomatic, it can be left untreated and will often resolve on its own or with sitz baths. When a Bartholin's duct cyst first presents in a woman older than 40 years, a biopsy should be performed to rule out the rare possibility of **Bartholin's gland carcinoma**.

While many Bartholin's cysts will resolve with minimal treatment, some cysts can become quite large and cause pressure symptoms such as local pain, dyspareunia, and difficulty walking. If these cysts do not resolve, they can become infected and lead to a **Bartholin's gland abscess**. These abscesses are the result of polymicrobial infections, but they are also occasionally associated with sexually transmitted diseases. These abscesses can become quite large, causing exquisite pain and tenderness and associated cellulitis. Bartholin's abscesses or symptomatic cysts should be treated like any other abscess: by **incision and drainage**. However, simple incision and drainage can often lead to recurrence; therefore, one of the two methods can be used.

Word catheter placement is commonly performed in the emergent setting or in the office. This method involves making a small incision (5 mm) to drain and irrigate the abscess. Then a Word catheter with a balloon tip is placed inside the remaining cyst and inflated to fill the space. The balloon is left in place for 4 to 6 weeks, being serially reduced in size, while epithelialization of the cyst and tract occurs (Fig. 13-9).

Marsupialization is usually done for recurrent Bartholin's duct cysts or abscesses. The entire abscess or cyst is incised and the cyst wall is sutured to the vaginal mucosa to prevent reformation of the abscess (Fig. 13-10).

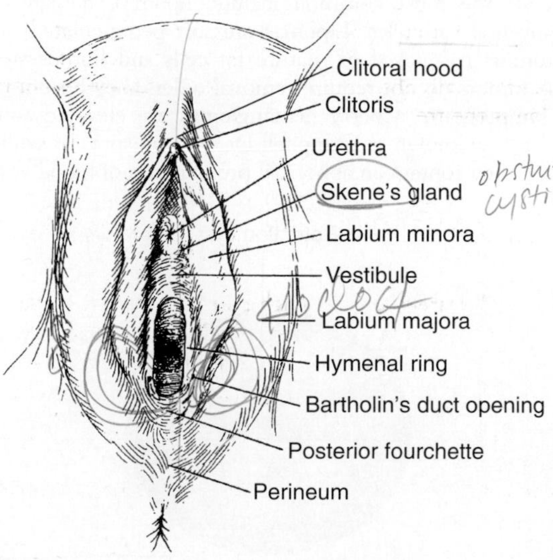

Figure 13-7 • **Vulvar and perineal anatomy.**
(From Beckman CRB, Ling FW, Laube DW, et al. *Obstetrics and Gynecology*, 4th ed. Baltimore, MD: Lippincott Williams & Wilkins; 2002.)

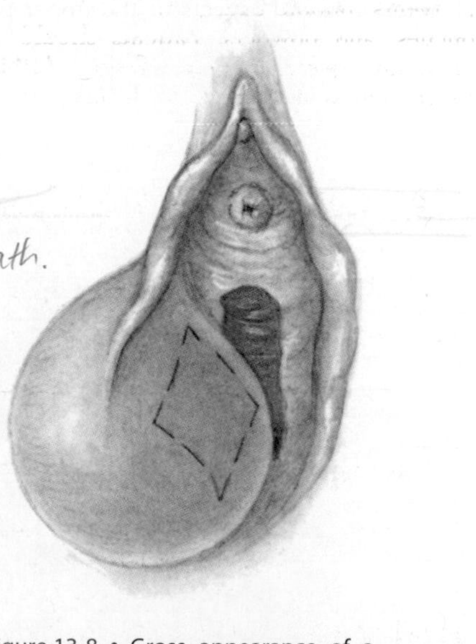

Figure 13-8 • **Gross appearance of a Bartholin's cyst of the vulva.**
(From LifeART image copyright © 2006 Lippincott Williams & Wilkins. All rights reserved.)

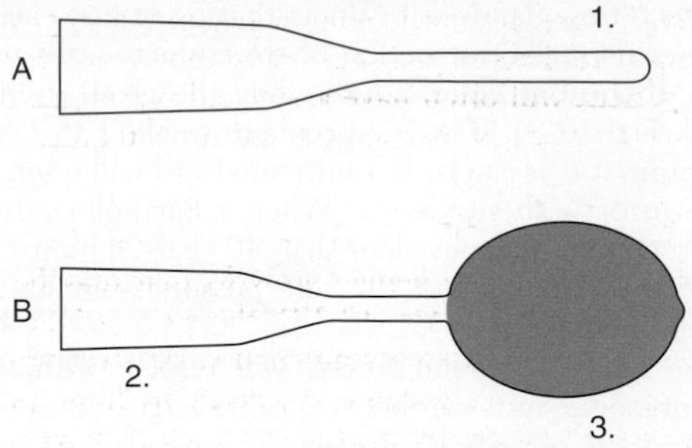

Figure 13-9 • Word catheter (A) before inflation and (B) after inflation. 1. The balloon-tipped end is placed into the incision site on the Bartholin's cyst. 2. A small-gauge needle is inserted into the opposite end and 2 to 4 mL of water is injected. 3. The inflated balloon remains inside the cyst for 4 to 6 weeks until an epithelialized tract is formed to prevent blockage of the duct to recur.

With either treatment, warm sitz baths several times per day are recommended both for pain relief and to decrease healing time. Adjunct antibiotic therapy is only recommended when the drainage is cultured for *Neisseria gonorrhoeae*, which occurs approximately 10% of the time. Concomitant cellulitis or an abscess that seems refractory to simple surgical treatment should also be treated with antibiotics that cover skin flora, primarily *Staphylococcus aureus*.

GARTNER'S DUCT CYSTS

Gartner's duct cysts are **remnants of the mesonephric ducts** of the Wolffian system. They are found most commonly in the **anterior lateral** aspects of the upper part of the vagina.

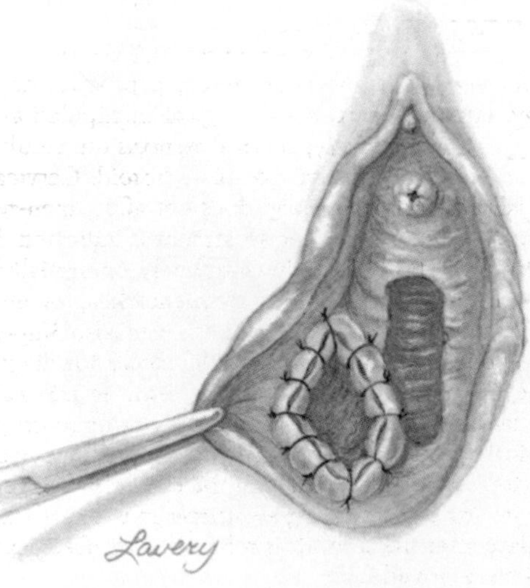

Figure 13-10 • Incision, drainage, and marsupilization of a Bartholin's abscess.
(From LifeART image copyright © 2006 Lippincott Williams & Wilkins. All rights reserved.)

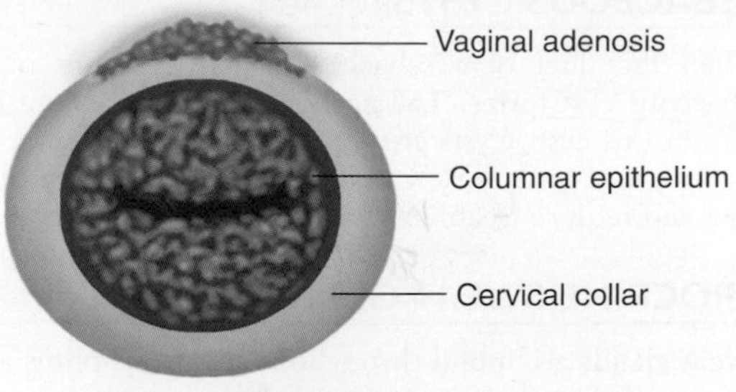

Figure 13-11 • Congenital cervical abnormalities due to in utero DES exposure. Other characteristic DES-associated cervical anomalies include cervical ectropion, cervical ridges, and hypoplastic cervix.
(From Bickley LS, Szilagyi P. *Bates' Guide to Physical Examination and History Taking*, 8th ed. Philadelphia, PA: Lippincott Williams & Wilkins; 2003.)

Most are **asymptomatic**. However, patients may present in adolescence with dyspareunia or difficulty inserting a tampon. These cysts are typically treated by excision. When removal is necessary, an IVP and cystoscopy should be performed preoperatively to locate the position of the bladder and ureters relative to the cyst. Urethral diverticula, ectopic ureters, and vaginal and cervical cancer should be ruled out. Because of the potential for significant bleeding during excision, vasopressin may be used to maintain hemostasis during the procedure.

BENIGN SOLID TUMORS OF THE VULVA AND VAGINA

There are many benign solid tumors of the vulva and the vagina. Some of the most common include lipomas, hemangiomas, and urethral caruncles. **Lipomas** are soft pedunculated or sessile tumors composed of mature fat cells and fibrous strands. These tumors do not require removal unless they become large and symptomatic. Cherry **hemangiomas** are elevated soft red papules, also known as Campbell De Morgan spots or senile angiomas; they contain an abnormal proliferation of blood vessels.

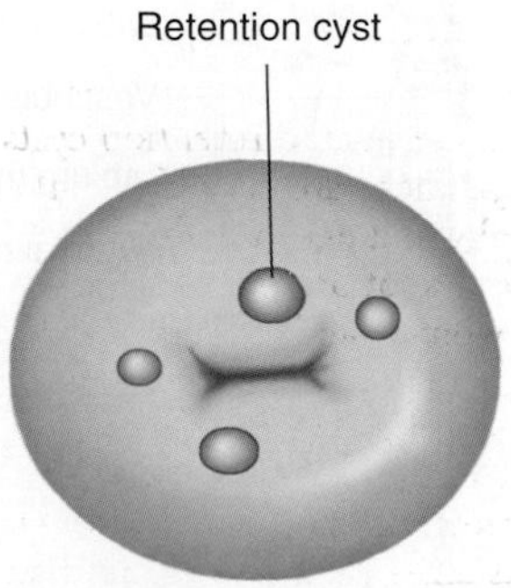

Figure 13-12 • Nabothian cysts of the cervix.
(From Bickley LS, Szilagyi P. *Bates' Guide to Physical Examination and History Taking*, 8th ed. Philadelphia, PA: Lippincott Williams & Wilkins; 2003.)

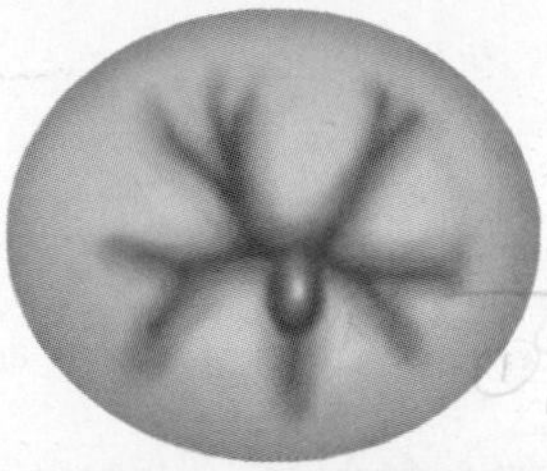

Figure 13-13 • Cervical polyp. (From Bickley LS, Szilagyi P. *Bates' Guide to Physical Examination and History Taking*, 8th ed. Philadelphia, PA: Lippincott Williams & Wilkins; 2003.)

Urethral caruncles and **urethral prolapse** present as small, red, fleshy tumors found at the distal urethral meatus. These occur almost exclusively in postmenopausal women as a result of vulvovaginal atrophy. This results in formation of an ectropion at the posterior urethral wall. These lesions are usually asymptomatic and no treatment is required. When bloody spotting results, a short course of topical estrogen is appropriate. Rarely, surgical excision may be needed.

BENIGN CERVICAL LESIONS

CONGENITAL ANOMALIES

Isolated congenital anomalies of the cervix are rare. In case of a uterine didelphys with a double vagina, a **double cervix** (bicollis) may be found, but this does not arise in isolation. However, 25% of women who were exposed **in utero to diethylstilbestrol** (DES) have an associated abnormality of the cervix. These benign abnormalities include cervical hypoplasia, cervical collars (Fig. 13-11), cervical hoods, cock's comb cervix, and pseudopolyps. These women are also at increased risk of **cervical insufficiency** in pregnancy. Women who have been exposed to DES in utero are also at increased risk of a very rare **clear cell adenocarcinoma** of the cervix and vagina. This cancer is seen in young women under the age of 20 but only occurs in 0.1% of DES-exposed patients.

CERVICAL CYSTS

Most cervical cysts are dilated retention cysts called **nabothian cysts** (Fig. 13-12). These are caused by intermittent blockage of an endocervical gland and usually expand to no more than 1 cm in diameter. Nabothian cysts are more commonly found in menstruating women and are usually asymptomatic. Most often, nabothian cysts are discovered on routine gynecologic examination and require no treatment.

Cervical cysts can also be **mesonephric cysts**. These are remnants of the mesonephric (wolffian) ducts that can become cystic. These cysts differ from nabothian cysts in that they tend to lie deeper in the cervical stroma and on the external surface of the cervix.

Finally, in rare instances, **endometriosis** can implant on or near the cervix. These cysts tend to be red or purple in color and the patient will often have associated symptoms of endometriosis such as cyclic pelvic pain and dyspareunia.

CERVICAL POLYPS

True cervical polyps are benign growths that may be pedunculated or broad-based (Fig. 13-13); these can arise anywhere on the cervix and are often **asymptomatic**. When symptomatic, cervical polyps usually cause **intermenstrual or postcoital spotting** rather than pain. Although cervical polyps are not usually considered a premalignant condition, they are generally removed to decrease the likelihood of masking irregular bleeding from another source such as cervical cancer, fibroids, adenomyosis, endometrial polyps, endometrial hyperplasia, and endometrial cancer. Removal of pedunculated cervical polyps is typically quick and easily performed in the office. However, sessile (broad-based) polyps or larger polyps may require removal with electrocautery in the office or the operating room. Hysteroscopy may also be helpful in distinguishing cervical polyps from endometrial polyps.

CERVICAL FIBROIDS

Leiomyomas (myomas or fibroids) are common benign tumors of the uterine corpus but may also arise in the cervix or prolapse into the cervical canal from the endometrial cavity. Leiomyomas can cause symptoms of **intermenstrual bleeding** similar to both uterine fibroids and cervical polyps. Depending on their location and size, these can also cause **dyspareunia** and bladder or rectal pressure. Fibroids of the cervix can cause **problems in pregnancy** and may lead to hemorrhage, poor dilation of the cervix, malpresentation, or obstruction of the birth canal. When evaluating an asymptomatic cervical fibroid, the possibility of cervical cancer should be ruled out, and then the fibroid can be followed with routine gynecologic care. Symptomatic fibroids can be surgically removed but, depending on their location, hysterectomy rather than myomectomy may be required.

CERVICAL STENOSIS

Cervical stenosis can be congenital, a product of **infection, atrophy, or scarring** (cervical surgical manipulation or radiotherapy). Less frequently, cervical stenosis can result from obstruction with a neoplasm, polyp, or fibroid. Cervical stenosis is typically **asymptomatic** and **does not affect menstruation or fertility**. In these settings, no treatment is indicated. However, if egress from the uterus is completely or partially blocked, oligomenorrhea, amenorrhea, dysmenorrhea, or an enlarged uterus may result. Cervical stenosis can also impede access to the endocervical and endometrial canals for diagnostic and therapeutic procedures. And, it can result in cervical dystocia during labor. When symptoms are present or access to the endocervical or endometrial canals are needed, cervical stenosis can be treated by **gently dilating the cervix**. Prolonged patency can be improved by leaving a catheter in the cervical canal for a few days after the stenosis is relieved. Any obstructive lesions should be removed.

KEY POINTS

- Labial fusion may be the result of excess androgen exposure or an enzymatic deficiency, most commonly 21-hydroxylase deficiency leading to congenital adrenal hyperplasia and ambiguous external genitalia.
- Patients with imperforate hymen and transverse vaginal septa commonly present with primary amenorrhea at puberty and cyclic abdominal pain. Both can be repaired surgically.
- Vaginal agenesis is seen in patients with MRKH who have an absent vagina and partial uterus and tubes. Patients are genetically female with normal ovarian function and normal secondary sexual characteristics.
- Vulvar itching and lesions can be secondary to a variety of atopic and atrophic skin changes, irritants, and allergens. Lesions can become hypertrophic secondary to chronic irritation and pruritus.
- Diagnosis of vulvar lesions is made by palpation, visualization, magnified vulvoscopy, and biopsy. Cancer should always be excluded by biopsy.
- Treatment involves hygiene practices, avoidance of irritants, and use of medium- to high-potency topical steroids. There is a limited role for vaginal estrogens and surgery in the treatment of these disorders.
- A variety of cysts can arise on the vulva and vagina from occlusion of pilosebaceous ducts, sebaceous ducts, and apocrine sweat glands.
- Treatment of benign cystic and solid skin tumors is only needed if the lesions become symptomatic or infected. This can generally be achieved with incision and drainage or excision.
- Bartholin's cysts and abscesses are located at 4-o'clock and 8-o'clock positions on the labia majora. Cysts are usually asymptomatic and resolve on their own.
- When a Bartholin's cyst first appears in a woman older than 40 years, the cyst wall should be biopsied to rule out the rare possibility of Bartholin's gland carcinoma.
- Large symptomatic Bartholin's cysts and Bartholin's abscesses should be appropriately drained along with placement of a Word catheter or marsupialization. Antibiotics are generally not indicated.
- Congenital anomalies of the cervix are rare and may be associated with abnormalities of the upper genital tract and/or in utero exposure to DES.
- Cervical polyps and fibroids are typically benign and can be removed if symptomatic.
- Cervical stenosis may be congenital or idiopathic and may result from scarring from infection or surgical manipulation. When symptomatic, the stenosis can be treated with gentle dilation of the cervical canal.

C Clinical Vignettes

Vignette 1

A 26-year-old G0 patient comes in with a problem visit for a complaint of an intermittent painless mass on her vulva near the introitus. It seems to be aggravated by intercourse, but usually goes away on its own. She's had two lifetime sexual partners and has been with her last partner for 5 years. She has always had normal periods and Pap smears and has never had an STI. You examine her and find a 3 cm nontender mass in the area described.

1. What type of abnormality is this most likely to be?
   a. Skene's gland cyst
   b. Gartner's duct cyst
   c. Bartholin's duct cyst
   d. Cystocele
   e. Epidermal inclusion cyst
2. What treatment would you recommend for this patient?
   a. Expectant management
   b. Word catheterization
   c. I&D
   d. Marsupialization
   e. Excision
3. Two years later she comes in with a recurrent cyst. This time it is tender, red, and growing. She is having difficulty sitting at work, and has not been able to exercise for 3 days due to pain. She denies fever or chills. What treatment do you recommend?
   a. Expectant management
   b. Word catheterization
   c. I&D
   d. Marsupialization
   e. Excision
4. If this patient had been 46 years old at the first onset of her cyst, what would be required?
   a. Biopsy of the cyst wall
   b. Word catheterization
   c. I&D
   d. Marsupialization
   e. Excision of the cyst

Vignette 2

Your next patient is a 65-year-old G2P2 new patient who has been referred from her primary care provider for recurrent yeast vaginitis. Review of her outside medical records reveals five episodes of vulvar pruritus that were treated with oral and vaginal antifungal medication. The patient says these helped minimally but her intense pruritus has been persistent for more than a year. She was married for 35 years but is now widowed and has not been sexually active in 3 years. You examine her and find a thin white atrophic epithelium and a contracted, small introitus. There is loss of the normal architecture of the labia minora. An area of hypopigmentation surrounds the labia and the anus in a figure-of-eight pattern. Wet prep shows a pH of 5.5, rare pseudohyphae, no lactobacilli, no WBC or RBC, and rare clue cells.

1. What would you do next?
   a. Collect fungal cultures
   b. Screen for gonorrhea and chlamydia
   c. Prescribe a longer course of oral fluconazole (Diflucan)
   d. Check a fasting glucose level
   e. Perform a vulvar biopsy
2. Most likely the diagnosis is:
   a. atrophic change
   b. lichen simplex
   c. lichen sclerosis
   d. lichen planus
   e. vulvar psoriasis
3. How would you counsel this patient regarding her treatment options?
   a. Expectant management
   b. Topical estrogen
   c. Topical high-potency steroids
   d. Oral steroids
   e. Surgical excision

Vignette 3

While on call you are paged to the emergency department to see a 16-year-old G0 adolescent girl with cyclic pelvic pain. She has never had a menstrual cycle. She denies any history of intercourse. She is afebrile and her vital signs are stable. Her pregnancy test is negative. On physical examination, she has age-appropriate breast and pubic hair development and normal external genitalia. However, when attempting the pelvic examination, you are unable to locate a vaginal introitus. You obtain a transabdominal ultrasound, which reveals a hematocolpos and hematometra.

1. What is the most likely diagnosis?
   a. Transverse vaginal septum
   b. Vertical vaginal septum
   c. Imperforate hymen

d. Vaginal agenesis (MRKH)
e. Bicornuate uterus

2. You explain to the patient and her mother that further evaluation is needed. Evaluation would most likely include all except which of the following?
a. IVP
b. Ultrasound
c. MRI
d. Removal of streak ovaries
e. Karyotyping

3. What are the treatment options for this condition?
a. Patient education
b. Vaginal dilators
c. Creation of a neovagina
d. Psychological support
e. All of the above

Vignette 4

Your next patient is a 13-year-old adolescent girl who presents with cyclic pelvic pain. She has never had a menstrual cycle. She denies any history of intercourse. She is afebrile and her vital signs are stable. On physical examination, she has age-appropriate breast and pubic hair development and normal external genitalia. However, you are unable to locate a vaginal introitus. Instead, there is a tense bulge where the introitus would be expected. You obtain a transabdominal ultrasound, which reveals a hematocolpos and hematometra.

1. What is the most likely diagnosis?
a. Transverse vaginal septum
b. Longitudinal vaginal septum
c. Imperforate hymen
d. Vaginal atresia (MRKH)
e. Bicornuate uterus

2. Symptoms that support this include:
a. absent vaginal lumen
b. tense bulging hymen
c. cyclic pelvic pain
d. increasing abdominal girth blood
e. all of the above

3. Appropriate treatment option is:
a. I&D
b. high-dose steroid application
c. topical estrogen application
d. excision of the extra tissue and evacuation of accumulated material
e. creation of a neovagina when ready for intercourse

A Answers

Vignette 1 Question 1

Answer C: This describes the classic location of the Bartholin's glands. These glands, located at 4-o'clock and 8-o'clock positions near the introitus provide lubrication of the vagina. The ducts of Bartholin's glands can become blocked resulting in a cyst formation. The Skene's glands can be identified as small openings on either side and just below the urethral meatus. Gartner's duct cysts are remnants of wolffian system. They are found in the upper one-third of the vagina on the anterior vaginal wall. A cystocele is a prolapse of the bladder into the vagina. It typically appears as a midline protrusion of the anterior vaginal wall into the vagina and, if severe, through the introitus. Cystoceles and other pelvic organ prolapse occur most commonly in older women and in women who have had multiple vaginal deliveries. This patient has neither of those traits. The mass could represent an epidermal inclusion cyst. However, these are the most common cause of cutaneous cysts and are typically small and solitary. They can be asymptomatic or become enlarged or inflamed.

Vignette 1 Question 2

Answer A: In this case where the cyst is largely asymptomatic and there is no sign of abscess or super-infection, expectant management is appropriate.

Vignette 1 Question 3

Answer B: Expectant management is appropriate for an asymptomatic Bartholin's duct cysts. However, for a painful, large Bartholin's, a Word catheter is placed to relieve the obstruction. Leaving the Word catheter in place for several weeks gives the new tract time to reepithelialize hopefully resulting in a means of long-term drainage. I&D is insufficient for the management of a symptomatic Bartholin's duct cyst or of an abscess. Marsupialization is typically reserved for patients in whom the Word catheter has failed. Excision of the entire gland is rarely indicated.

Vignette 1 Question 4

Answer A: When a patient over 40 years of age presents with a new onset Bartholin's duct cyst, a biopsy of the cyst wall is necessary to rule out the rare possibility of Bartholin's cyst carcinoma. If benign, treatment would then depend on the status of the cyst. As above, Word catheter is most commonly used. For recurrent symptomatic cysts, marsupialization may be necessary. Excision of the Bartholin's gland is rarely indicated and often complicated by bleeding from the many venous complexes in the vulvar tissue.

Vignette 2 Question 1

Answer E: While yeast infections are a common cause of vaginitis in women, this patient has been adequately treated for yeast vaginitis but still has persistent symptoms. Her wet prep also does not support the diagnosis of yeast infection because minimal pseudohyphae are found. Therefore, it would not be reasonable to check fungal futures, prescribe a long course of antifungal, or to check a fasting glucose level to look for diabetes as a reason for recurrent yeast infections. Instead, this patient needs a vulvar biopsy to determine the source of her pruritus. This would be the best way to look for a source of the pruritus and to also rule out VIN (vulvar intraepithelial neoplasia) and cancer. She has not been sexually active in 3 years and her primary complaint is vulvar pruritus so is unlikely to have chlamydial infection or gonorrhea.

Vignette 2 Question 2

Answer C: Although this patient was diagnosed with recurrent yeast infections, it's likely that she was misdiagnosed. The findings noted are consistent with lichen sclerosis. Lichen sclerosis is a chronic and progress benign condition characterized by vulvar inflammation and epithelial thinning. Symptoms include intense pruritus, pain, and anogenital hypopigmentation (whitening—often in a "keyhole" fashion around the perineum and anal region). When left untreated, it can result in distortion of vulvar architecture (loss of labia minora, constriction of the introitus, fissures, labial fusion, scarring). Despite its benign nature, vulvar biopsy is still required to rule out underlying atypia or malignancy.

Vignette 2 Question 3

Answer C: The treatment of lichen sclerosis includes patient education, vulvar hygiene, cessation of scratching, and high-potency topical corticosteroid use (e.g., clobetasol). The goal of treatment is to reduce the symptoms (itching, burning, and irritation) and to avoid progression of the disease, which could result in loss of vulvar architecture, introital constriction, labial fusion, and scarring. Of note, the classic whitening or hypopigmentation of the skin, atrophy, and scarring are often permanent and should not be used as a measurement of treatment success. Expectant management is not appropriate as treatment is needed to avoid progression of the disease even in asymptomatic patients. Surgical resection of lichen sclerosis is rarely indicated. Vaginal estrogen is used to treat atrophic vaginitis.

Vignette 3 Question 1

Answer D: Vaginal agenesis, also known as Mayer-Rokitansky-Küster-Hauser (MRKH) syndrome, is the congenital absence of the vagina along with some variable uterine development. Transverse vaginal septum is also obstructive but a normal introitus is usually identifiable. The imperforate hymen typically presents with a tense vaginal bulge at birth or during menarche. A bicornuate uterus is nonobstructing and may be diagnosed only during pregnancy or incidental imaging.

Vignette 3 Question 2

Answer D: In addition to absence of the vagina, MRKH patients can also have agenesis of the cervix and most (95%) will have a rudimentary nonfunctioning uterus. Because most (75%) will have normal ovaries, normal female karyotype, and normal ovarian function. Patients typically have normal secondary sex characteristics. Many (25% to 50%) will have associated genitourinary anomalies such as horseshoe kidney, pelvic kidney, duplication of the collecting system, and bladder exstrophy. Evaluation most typically involves a full physical examination, pelvic/abdominal ultrasound, and MRI for better delineation of the anatomy. The genitourinary system can be evaluated with KUB, ultrasound, MRI, and IVP if needed. Streak ovaries are generally found in cases of gonadal dysgenesis (most commonly Turner syndrome) and sometimes in cases of ambiguous genitalia and premature ovarian failure. They are not typically seen in patients with MRKH.

Vignette 3 Question 3

Answer E: Treatment of MRKH is often multifaceted involving gynecologic, urologic, plastics surgery, and psychiatric specialists. When correction is desired, a neovagina can be created using nonsurgical (vaginal dilators) or, least commonly, surgical techniques (vaginoplasty). Psychological support and education are critical components of treatment plans for any congenital malformation.

Vignette 4 Question 1

Answer C: In this young patient with a tense perineum, hematocolpos, and hematometra, the most likely diagnosis is imperforate hymen. MRKH can present similarly, but these patients have a congenitally absent vagina (vaginal atresia) therefore their clinical presentation does not include a hematocolpos or bulging perineum. A transverse vaginal septum and bicornuate uterus are typically nonobstructing malformations. The blood is able to escape so you do not see a hematocolpos or hematometra. This also explains why these diagnoses are made comparatively later—most typically at the start of pelvic examinations (vaginal septum) or when pregnancy is desired (bicornuate uterus).

Vignette 4 Question 2

Answer E: An imperforate hymen can be diagnosed in the newborn period if the infant is noted to have a bulging introitus. This can develop if maternal estrogen stimulates production of vaginal secretions in the infant resulting in a mucocolpos. If the imperforate hymen is not diagnosed in infancy, the mucus is reabsorbed and the patient is asymptomatic until menarche. At this time, if the hymen is completely imperforate, blood cannot escape from the upper reproductive system. This can result in all of the signs and symptoms mentioned in the question. Other symptoms can include chronic pelvic pain and primary amenorrhea.

Vignette 4 Question 3

Answer D: The treatment of imperforate hymen is surgical repair under anesthesia. This involves excising the membrane, evacuating the obstructed materials, and suturing the vaginal mucosa to the hymenal ring. This can be performed at any age but the repair is improved if done when the tissue has been estrogenized—in the newborn, postpubertal, or premenarchal periods. I&D is not an appropriate treatment for an imperforate hymen. Vaginal estrogen would be used to treat vaginal atrophy. High-potency steroid trials are often given for benign epithelial disorders like lichen sclerosis or lichen planus. Creation of a neovagina is reserved for cases of vaginal agenesis (MRKH) or agenesis of the lower vagina.

ovaries - genital ridge, lower 1/3 vagina

CONGENITAL MÜLLERIAN ANOMALIES

PATHOGENESIS

All reproductive structures arise from the müllerian system except the ovaries (which arise from the genital ridge) and the lower one-third of the vagina (which arises from the urogenital diaphragm). Specifically, the superior vagina, cervix, uterus, and fallopian tubes are formed by fusion of the **paramesonephric (müllerian) ducts** (see Fig. 13-1). Uterine anomalies arise during embryonic development, generally as a result of incomplete fusion of the ducts, incomplete development of one or both ducts, or degeneration of the ducts (müllerian agenesis). These anomalies (Table 14-1) can vary in scope and severity from the presence of simple septa to bicornuate uterus to complete duplication of the entire female reproductive system (Fig. 14-1). Of the disorders not related to drugs, the most common condition is the **septate uterus** due to malfusion of the paramesonephric ducts. Many anatomic uterine abnormalities may also be associated with **inguinal hernias** and **urinary tract anomalies** (unilateral renal agenesis, pelvic or horseshoe kidneys, or irregularities in the collecting system) (Fig. 14-2).

EPIDEMIOLOGY

Anatomic anomalies of the uterus are extremely rare. Several years ago, the incidence was estimated to be 0.5% (1 in 201) of the female population. There is an increased incidence of müllerian anomalies in women who were exposed in utero to **diethylstilbestrol** (DES) from 1940 to 1971 (Fig. 14-3). DES was a synthetic nonsteroidal estrogen that was indicated for gonorrheal vaginitis, atrophic vaginitis, menopausal symptoms, postpartum lactation, miscarriage prevention, and for advanced prostate and breast cancer.

CLINICAL MANIFESTATIONS

History

Most congenital anomalies are discovered incidentally in the workup for common obstetrical and gynecologic complaints at the onset of menache, onset of coitus, or attempts at childbearing. Some uterine anomalies are asymptomatic and may never be discovered. Some symptoms associated with anomalies of the uterus include menstrual abnormalities, dysmenorrhea, dyspareunia, cyclic and noncyclic pelvic pain, infertility, and recurrent miscarriage.

Uterine septa are positioned vertically and can vary in length and thickness (Fig. 14-1). They are primarily composed of collagen fibers and often lack an adequate blood supply to facilitate placentation and maintain a growing pregnancy. Thus, 25% of women with uterine septa may suffer from recurrent first-trimester **pregnancy loss**. A **bicornuate uterus** (Fig. 14-1), however, is more commonly complicated by the limited size of the uterine horn (similar to a unicornuate uterus) rather than by blood supply. As such, bicornuate and unicornuate uteri are associated with **second-trimester pregnancy loss**, malpresentation, and **preterm labor** and delivery. Müllerian agenesis or hypoplasia (Mayer-Rokitansky-Kuster-Hauser syndrome) results in absence of the vaginal with variable uterine development and presents as primary amenorrhea (Chapter 13). *uterine septa 1st tri loss*
bicornuate 2nd tri loss

Diagnostic Evaluation

The primary investigative tools for uterine abnormalities are pelvic ultrasound, CT, MRI, sonohistogram, hysterosalpingogram, hysteroscopy, and laparoscopy. Keep in mind that uterine septa and bicornuate uteri may appear identical on hysteroscopic evaluation (Fig. 14-4). The two can be better distinguished using MRI or laparoscopy to evaluate the uterine fundus. Because there is an increased incidence of renal anomalies (unilateral renal agenesis, pelvic or horseshoe kidneys, or irregularities in the collecting system), additional radiologic evaluation should be pursued in the setting of a congenital Müllerian anomaly.

Treatment

Many uterine anomalies **require no treatment**. However, when the defect causes significant symptoms such as pain, menstrual irregularities, or infertility, treatment options should be explored. Uterine septa can be excised with operative hysteroscopy once bicornuate uterus has been ruled out. Many women with a bicornuate uterus are able to carry a pregnancy to fruition, although preterm labor and delivery is a significant risk. When a viable pregnancy cannot be achieved in a patient with a bicornuate uterus, viable pregnancies have been achieved with surgical unification procedures. These patients will require delivery via cesarean section to decrease the risk of uterine rupture.

TABLE 14-1 Classification of Müllerian Anomalies

Class I. Segmented müllerian agenesis or hypoplasia
A. Vaginal
B. Cervical
C. Fundal
D. Tubal
E. Combined
Class II. Unicornuate uterus
A. With a rudimentary horn
1. With a communicating endometrial cavity
2. With a noncommunicating cavity
3. With no cavity
B. Without any rudimentary horn
Class III. Uterus didelphis
Class IV. Bicornuate uterus
A. Complete to the internal os
B. Partial
C. Arcuate
Class V. Septate uterus
A. With a complete septum
B. With an incomplete septum
Class VI. Uterus with internal luminal changes

UTERINE LEIOMYOMA

Uterine leiomyomas, also called *fibroids* or *uterine myomas,* are benign **proliferations of smooth muscle cells** of the myometrium. Fibroids typically occur in women of childbearing age and then regress during menopause. These benign tumors constitute the **most common indication for surgery** for women in the United States. Approximately one-third of all hysterectomies performed are for uterine fibroids. Most fibroids, however, cause no major symptoms and **require no treatment**. Generally, fibroids become problematic only when their location results in heavy or irregular bleeding or reproductive difficulties. Fibroids may also be identified when they become large enough to cause a mass effect on other pelvic structures resulting in pelvic pain and pressure, urinary frequency, or constipation.

PATHOGENESIS

The cause of uterine leiomyomas is unclear. Fibroids are benign **monoclonal tumors**, with each tumor resulting from propagation of a single muscle cell. The normal myocytes are transformed to abnormal myocytes which are then stimulated to grow into tumors. Genetic predisposition, steroid hormone factors, growth factors, and angiogenesis may all play a role in the formation and growth of uterine fibroids.

Fibroids can vary in size from microscopic to the size of a full-term pregnancy. Fibroids are also **hormonally responsive to both estrogen and progesterone** but the relationship is complex. In reproductive age women individual fibroids can grow and shrink at differing rates in the same woman. During menopause, the tumors usually stop growing and may atrophy in response to naturally lower endogenous estrogen levels.

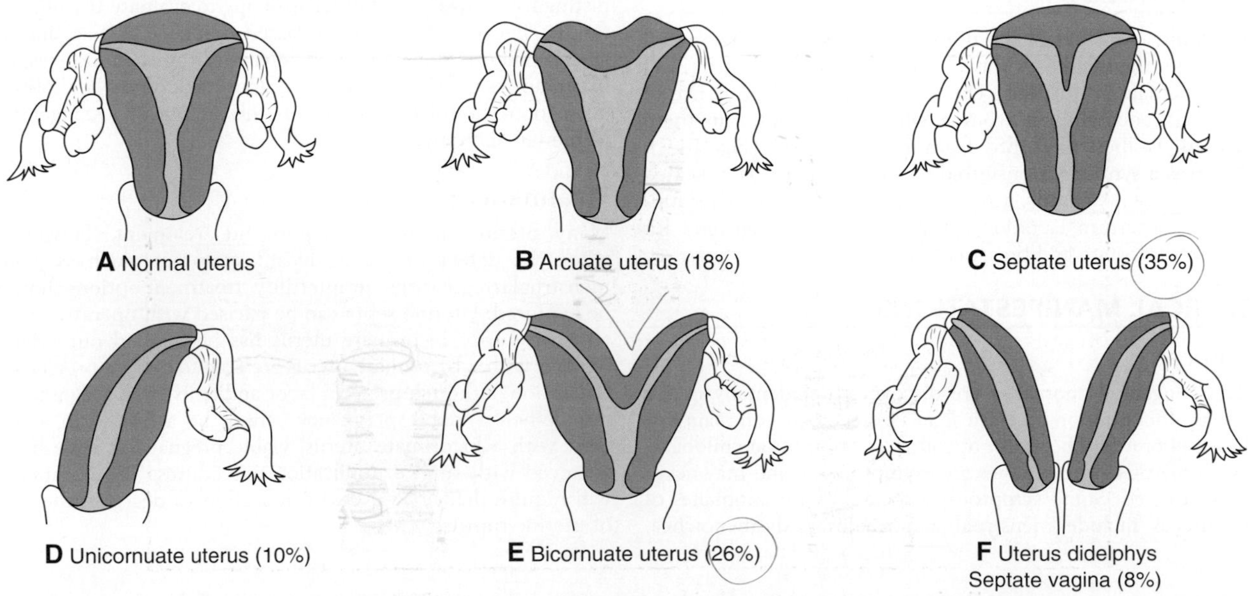

Figure 14-1 • Examples of anatomic anomalies of the uterus. **(A)** Normal uterus. The most common uterine anomalies include **(B)** arcuate uterus, **(C)** septate uterus (failure of dissolution of the septum), **(D)** unicornuate uterus (failure of formation of one müllerian duct), **(E)** bicornuate uterus (failure of fusion of the mid-müllerian ducts), and **(F)** uterine didelphys (complete failure of fusion).

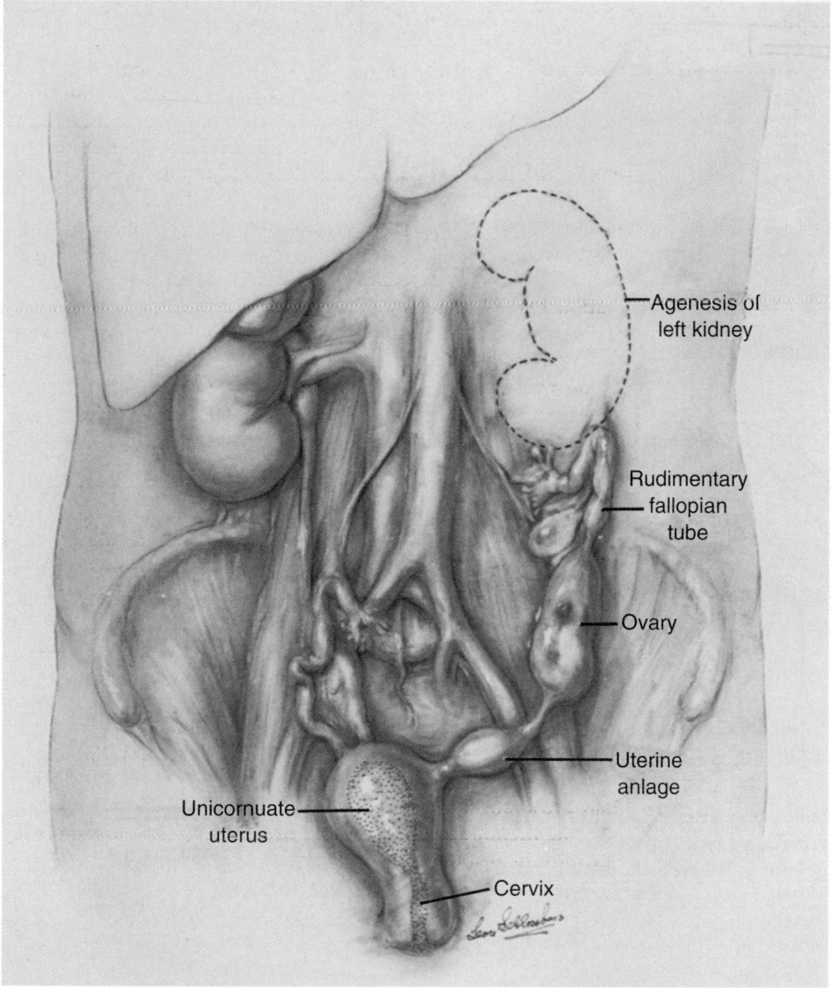

Figure 14-2 • A congenital uterine anomaly (unicornuate uterus) and associated renal anomaly (agenesis of the kidney on the left).
(Image from Rock J, Jones H. *TeLinde's Operative Gynecology*, 10th ed. Philadelphia, PA: Lippincott Williams & Wilkins; 2008.)

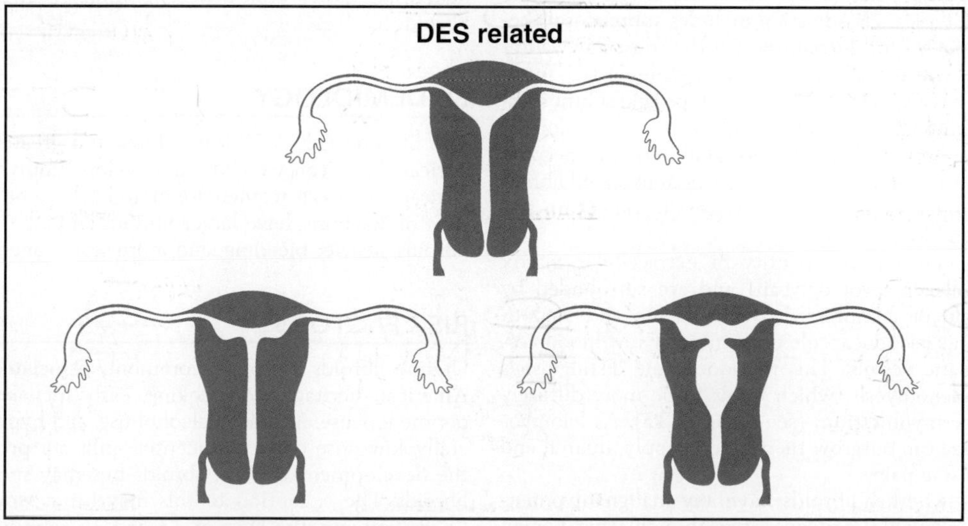

Figure 14-3 • Uterine anomalies associated with in utero diethylstilbestrol (DES) exposure. Others include hypoplastic uterine cavity, shortened upper uterine segment, and transverse septa. The classic anomaly is a T-shaped uterus.
(From Speroff L, Fritz M. *Clinical Gynecologic Endocrinology and Infertility*, 7th ed. Philadelphia, PA: Lippincott Williams & Wilkins; 2005.)

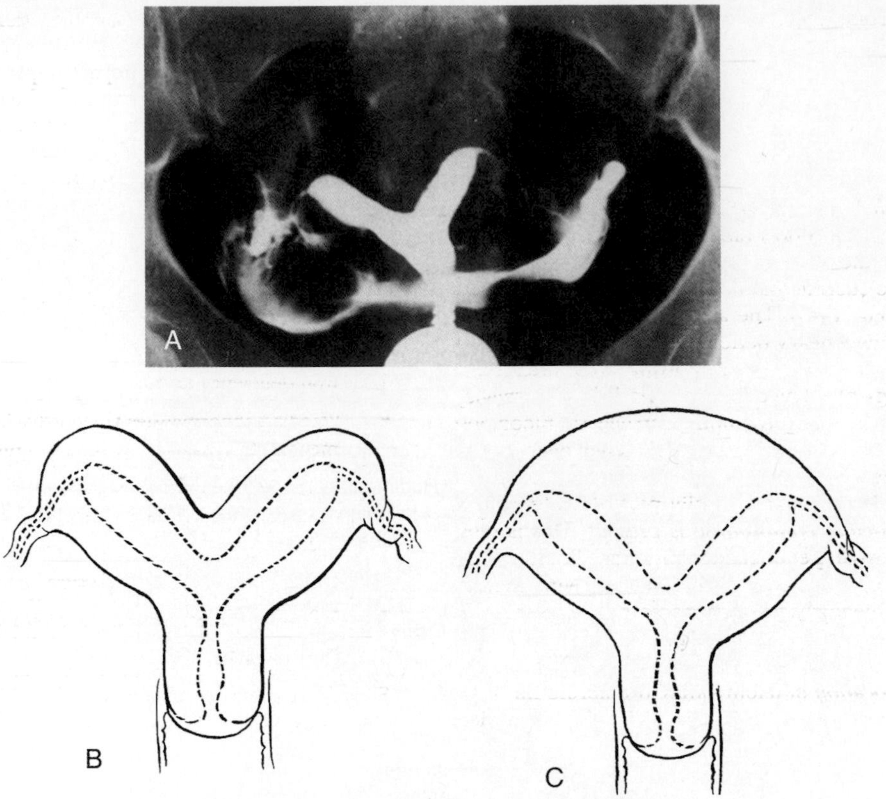

Figure 14-4 • (A) A hysterosalpingogram of a double uterus. (B) A bicornuate uterus and (C) a septate uterus are types of double uteri. Visualization of the fundus is required to determine the type of uterine anomaly.
(Image from Rock J, Jones H. *TeLinde's Operative Gynecology*, 10th ed. Philadelphia, PA: Lippincott Williams & Wilkins; 2008.)

Uterine fibroids are classified by their location in the uterus (Fig. 14-5). The typical classification includes **submucosal** (beneath the endometrium), **intramural** (in the muscular wall of the uterus), and **subserosal** (beneath the uterine serosa). **Intramural** leiomyomas are the most common type, and submucosal fibroids are commonly associated with heavy or prolonged bleeding. Both submucosal and subserosal fibroids may become **pedunculated**. A **parasitic** leiomyoma is a pedunculated fibroid that becomes attached to the pelvic viscera or omentum and develops its own blood supply.

Fibroids contain a large quantity of extracellular matrix (fibronectin, collagen, proteoglycan) and are surrounded by a **pseudocapsule** of compressed areolar tissue and smooth muscle cells. This pseudocapsule contains very few blood vessels and lymphatic vessels. This pseudocapsule distinguishes fibroids from adenomyosis, which tends to be more diffusely organized in the myometrium (see Chapter 15). As leiomyomas enlarge, they can outgrow their blood supply, infarct, and degenerate, causing pain.

It is unclear whether fibroids have any malignant potential. From the available evidence, it is thought that benign leiomyomas and leiomyosarcomas coexist in the same uterus but with rare exception, they are **independent entities**. Leiomyosarcomas are thought to represent separate new neoplasias rather than a degeneration of an existing benign fibroid.

EPIDEMIOLOGY

The lifetime risk is 70% in whites and **greater than 80% of African American women** will develop leiomyoma by age 50. African American women are more likely to be younger at the time of diagnosis, have larger fibroids and a greater number of fibroids, heavier bleeding, and more severe anemia.

RISK FACTORS

Uterine fibroids are more commonly associated with African American heritage, nonsmoking, early menarche, nulliparity, perimenopause, increased alcohol use, and hypertension. Generally, low-dose oral contraceptive pills are protective against the development of new fibroids but may stimulate existing fibroids. The exception to this may be in women who start OCPs between the ages of 13 and 16. The use of hormone replacement in postmenopausal women with fibroids is associated with fibroid growth but typically does not result in clinical symptoms.

The risk of fibroids decreases with increasing parity, with oral contraception use, and injectable depot medroxyprogesterone acetate use.

CLINICAL MANIFESTATIONS

History

Most women with fibroids (50% to 65%) have **no clinical symptoms**. Of those who do (Table 14-2), **abnormal uterine bleeding** is by far the most common symptom. This is due most commonly to submucosal fibroids impinging on the endometrial cavity (Fig. 14-5). The abnormal bleeding typically presents as increasingly heavy periods of longer duration (**menorrhagia**). Fibroids can also cause spotting after intercourse (postcoital spotting), bleeding between periods (metrorrhagia), or heavy irregular bleeding (menometrorrhagia). Blood loss from fibroids can lead to **chronic iron-deficiency anemia**, dizziness, weakness, and fatigue.

In general, pelvic pain is not usually part of the symptom complex unless vascular compromise is present. This is most common in subserosal pedunculated fibroids. Patients may, however, experience **secondary dysmenorrhea** with menses, particularly when menorrhagia or menometrorrhagia are present. **Pressure-related symptoms** (pelvic pressure, constipation, hydronephrosis, and venous stasis) vary depending on the number, size and location of leiomyomas. If a fibroid impinges on nearby structures, patients may complain of constipation, urinary frequency, or even urinary retention as the space within the pelvis becomes more crowded.

Submucosal fibroids can impact implantation, placentation, and ongoing pregnancy. Resection of submucosal fibroids in patients diagnosed with infertility does lead to increased conception rates. Intramural and subserosal fibroids are unlikely to affect conception or pregnancy loss except when multiple fibroids are present. The vast majority of women with fibroids, however, are

TABLE 14-2 Clinical Symptoms of Uterine Leiomyomas (Mnemonic: FIBROIDS)

F	Frequency and retention of urine, hydronephrosis
I	Iron deficiency anemia
B	Bleeding abnormalities (menorrhagia, metrorrhagia, menometrorrhagia, postcoital spotting), bloating
R	Reproductive difficulties (dysfunctional labor premature labor/delivery, fetal malpresentation, increased need for cesarean delivery)
O	Obstipation and rectal pressure
I	Infertility (failed implantation, spontaneous abortion)
D	Dysmenorrhea, dyspareunia
S	Symptomless (most common)

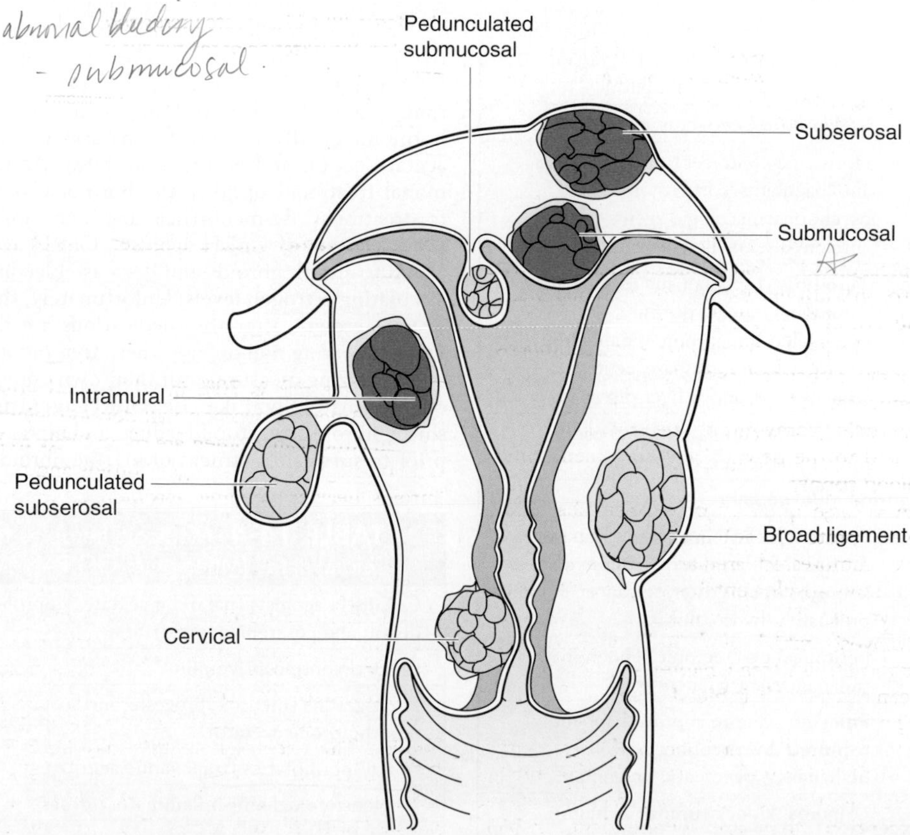

Figure 14-5 • Common locations of uterine fibroids.

able to conceive without any difficulties. When fibroids multiple, large (5-10cm) or located behind the placenta, they may contribute to increased rates of preterm labor and delivery, fetal malpresentation, dysfunctional labor, and Cesarean delivery. The antepartum and intrapartum complication rate is 10% to 40%.

Physical Examination

Depending on their location and size, uterine leiomyomas can sometimes be palpated on bimanual pelvic examination or on abdominal examination. Bimanual examination often reveals a **nontender irregularly enlarged uterus** with "lumpy-bumpy" or cobblestone protrusions that feel firm or solid on palpation.

DIAGNOSTIC EVALUATION

The differential diagnosis for uterine leiomyoma depends on the patient's symptoms (Table 14-3). Because most women with leiomyomas are **asymptomatic**, the diagnosis is sometimes made only as an incidental finding.

Pelvic ultrasound is the most common means of diagnosis. Fibroids can be seen as areas of hypoechogenicity among normal myometrial material. Hysterosalpingogram (**HSG**), saline infusion sonogram (**sonohysterogram**), and **hysteroscopy** are additional tools for imaging the location and size of uterine fibroids. These tools can be valuable in identifying submucosal fibroids and in distinguishing fibroids from polyps within the uterine cavity. **MRI** is especially helpful in distinguishing fibroids from adenomyosis (Chapter 15) as well as for surgical planning.

TABLE 14-3 Differential Diagnosis of Uterine Fibroids[a]

Abnormal bleeding	
Structural	Adenomyosis, endometrial polyps, endometrial hyperplasia Cancer: endometrial cancer, cervical cancer, vaginal cancer
Endocrinopathies	Thyroid disease, hyperprolactinemia, polycystic ovarian syndrome, Cushing's disease
Anovulation or oligo-ovulation	Idiopathic, stress, exercise, obesity, rapid weight changes, polycystic ovarian syndrome, or endocrinopathy
Infections	Endometritis, cervicitis, vaginitis
Drugs	Hormonal contraception, progestins, anticoagulants, corticosteroids, psychopharmacologic agents, anticonvulsants digitalis, chemotherapy
Coagulopathies	Thrombocytopenia (due to idiopathic thrombocytopenic purpura, hypersplenism, chronic renal failure), von Willebrand's disease, acute leukemia, advanced liver disease
Trauma	Sexual intercourse, sexual abuse, foreign bodies, pelvic trauma
Pelvic mass or uterine enlargement	
Gynecologic	Pregnancy, adenomyosis, ovarian cyst, ovarian neoplasm, tubo-ovarian abscess, leiomyosarcoma, uterine cancer, ectopic pregnancy, hydrosalpinx
Abdominal	peritoneal cyst, ectopic (abdominal) pregnancy, aortic aneurysm
Gastrointestinal	Phlegmon due to ruptured appendix, ruptured diverticulum, bowel malignancy, pancreatic phlegmon
Genitourinary	Urinoma, kidney tumor (including pelvic kidney)

[a]Any of these conditions can coexist with fibroids.

TREATMENT

Most cases of uterine fibroids do not require treatment, and **expectant management** is appropriate. However, the diagnosis of leiomyoma must be unequivocal. Other pelvic masses should be ruled out, and the patient with actively growing fibroids should be followed every 6 months to monitor the size and growth.

When leiomyomas result in severe pain, heavy or irregular bleeding, infertility, or pressure symptoms, treatment should be considered. When fibroids show evidence of postmenopausal or extremely rapid growth, surveillance should be initiated and treatment should be considered. The choice of treatment depends on the patient's age, pregnancy status, desire for future pregnancies, and size and location of the fibroids.

There are **multiple medical therapies** for leiomyomas (Table 14-4). **Nonhormonal options,** which include nonsteroidal anti-inflammatory drugs and anti-fibrinolytics (tranexamic acid), are limited at treating symptoms of dysmenorrhea and heavy, prolonged bleeding, and anemia.

Hormonal options include combined oral contraceptive pills, progestins (medroxyprogesterone acetate, Mirena IUD, norethindrone acetate), mifepristone, androgenic steroids (danazol and gestrinone), and gonadotropin-releasing hormone (GnRH) agonists (nafarelin acetate, leuprolide acetate depot, and goserelin acetate). As with the nonhormonal treatment options, the hormonal options are limited to treatment dysmenorrhea and abnormal bleeding with the exception of GnRH agonists. GnRH agonists have been found to shrink fibroids and decrease bleeding by **decreasing circulating estrogen levels.** Unfortunately, the tumors usually resume growth after the medications are discontinued. For women nearing menopause, these treatments may be used as a temporizing measure until their own endogenous estrogens decrease naturally. Likewise, **GnRH agonists** may be used to shrink fibroid size, stop bleeding, and increase the hematocrit prior to surgical treatment of uterine fibroids.

TABLE 14-4 Medical Therapies for Uterine Leiomyomas (Mnemonic: GO PAN AM)

G: GnRH agonists (nafarelin acetate, leuprolide acetate depot, and goserelin acetate)
O: Oral contraceptive pills
P: Progestins (medroxyprogesterone acetate, Mirena IUD, norethindrone acetate)
A: Antifibrinolytics (tranexamic acid)
N: Nonsteroidal anti-inflammatory drugs
A: Androgenic steroids (danazol and gestrinone)
M: Mifepristone

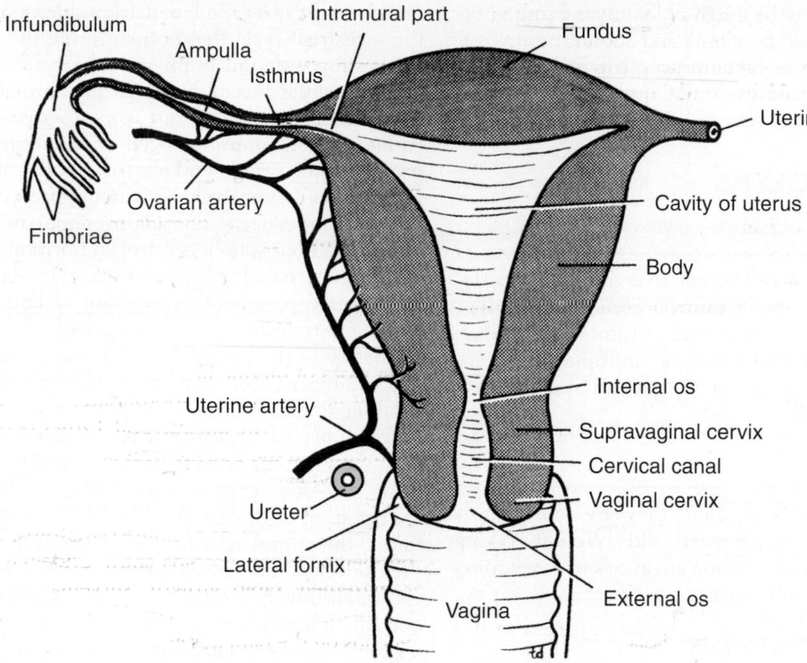

Figure 14-6 • Uterine artery embolization (UAE) for the treatment of uterine fibroids. The uterine artery, shown here, can be catheterized through a femoral approach under fluoroscopy. The catheter is guided to the uterine artery, where polyvinyl alcohol (PVA) microspheres are injected. As a result, there is decreased blood flow to the fibroids, causing necrosis and devascularization of the fibroids.

Uterine artery embolization (UAE) is being used with greater frequency as a less invasive surgical approach for treating symptomatic fibroids. The procedure is usually preformed by an interventional radiologist who catheterizes the femoral artery under local anesthesia in order to inject an embolizing agent into each uterine artery (Fig. 14-6). The goal is to decrease the blood supply to the fibroid, thereby causing ischemic necrosis, degeneration, and reduction in fibroid size. Because the therapy is not specific to a given fibroid, the blood supply to the uterus and/or ovaries can be compromised. UAE should not be used in women who are planning to become pregnant after the procedure. This treatment option is not recommended for large and pedunculated fibroids.

One of the newest options for uterine fibroids is the use of **MRI-guided high-intensity ultrasound** (e.g., ExAblate 2000). This uses MRI to locate individual fibroids that are then thermoablated with high-intensity ultrasound waves. The technique is typically reserved for premenopausal women who have completed childbearing and wish to retain their uterus. The procedure can be performed in an outpatient setting but is **expensive and not widely available** at this time.

The indications for surgical intervention for fibroids are listed in Table 14-5. A **myomectomy** is the surgical resection of one or more fibroids from the uterine wall. Myomectomy is usually reserved for patients with symptomatic fibroids who wish to preserve their fertility or who choose not to have a hysterectomy. Myomectomics can be performed hysteroscopically, laparoscopically with and without robotic assistance, or abdominally. The primary disadvantage of myomectomy is that fibroids **recur in more than 60% of patients in 5 years** and adhesions frequently form that may further complicate pain and infertility.

TABLE 14-5 Indications for Surgical Intervention for Uterine Leiomyomas

Abnormal uterine bleeding, causing anemia
Severe pelvic pain or secondary amenorrhea
Uterine size (>12 wk) obscuring evaluation of adnexa
Urinary frequency, retention, or hydronephrosis
Growth after menopause
Recurrent miscarriage or infertility
Rapid increase in size

Hysterectomy is the definitive treatment for leiomyomas. Vaginal and laparoscopic hysterectomy can be performed for small myomas and abdominal hysterectomy is generally required for large or multiple myomas. If the ovaries are diseased or if the blood supply has been damaged, then oophorectomy should be performed as well. Otherwise, the ovaries should be preserved in women younger than 45 years with normal-appearing ovaries. Because of the **potential for hemorrhage**, surgical intervention should be avoided during pregnancy, although myomectomy or hysterectomy may be necessary at some point after delivery.

FOLLOW-UP

When hysterectomy is not indicated for a patient with leiomyomas, careful follow-up should take place to monitor the size and location of the tumors. Rapid growth of a tumor in postmenopausal women may be a sign of leiomyosarcoma (extremely rare) or other pelvic neoplasia and should be investigated immediately. **Low-dose oral contraceptives** and hormone replacement therapy at low doses do not appear to pose a risk of recurrence to the patient.

ENDOMETRIAL POLYPS

PATHOGENESIS

Endometrial polyps are localized benign overgrowths of **endometrial glands and stroma** over a vascular core. These polyps vary in size from millimeters to several centimeters and may be pedunculated or sessile and single or multiple. They are generally within the endometrial cavity but can also prolapse through the endocervical canal.

EPIDEMIOLOGY

The incidence increases with age and they are found most commonly in women **40 to 50 years old**. Women taking **tamoxifen** for breast cancer prevention are at risk of developing endometrial polyps, cysts, and cancer.

CLINICAL MANIFESTATIONS

History

Women with endometrial polyps most commonly present with abnormal vaginal bleeding. Premenopausal women can present with bleeding between periods (metrorrhagia) but may also have increasingly heavy menses (menorrhagia), heavy irregular bleeding (menometrorrhagia), or postcoital bleeding. Any bleeding in a postmenopausal woman merits investigation. Endometrial polyps account for a quarter of all causes of postmenopausal bleeding.

Diagnostic Evaluation

Ultrasound, sonohysterogram, and hysteroscopy are the best means of evaluation for the presence, size, and number of polyps. The added benefit of hysteroscopy is the possibility of immediate treatment. As with any other etiology for abnormal bleeding, women 45 or older with abnormal bleeding from endometrial polyps should be evaluated with endometrial biopsy prior to removal.

TREATMENT

Although the majority of polyps are benign, they can be **malignant or premalignant** in approximately 5% of postmenopausal women and 1% to 2% of premenopausal women. In addition, endometrial polyps can mask bleeding from another sources such as endometrial hyperplasia (25%) or endometrial cancer (<1%). For this reason, it is generally recommended that any polyp be removed in postmenopausal patients. Premenopausal women require removal of symptomatic polyps and asymptomatic polyps for those at risk of infertility, endometrial hyperplasia, and endometrial cancer.

ENDOMETRIAL HYPERPLASIA

PATHOGENESIS

Endometrial hyperplasia is clinically important because it is a **source of abnormal uterine bleeding** and because of its link to endometrial cancer. Endometrial proliferation is a normal part of the menstrual cycle that occurs during the follicular (proliferative) estrogen-dominant phase of the cycle. Simple proliferation is an overabundance of histologically normal endometrium.

When the endometrium is exposed to **continuous endogenous or exogenous estrogen stimulation in the absence of progesterone**, simple endometrial proliferation can advance to endometrial hyperplasia. This unopposed estrogen stimulation may be from exogenous or endogenous sources. The most common exogenous source is estrogen hormone replacement without progesterone. In obese women, excess adipose tissue results in increased **peripheral conversion of androgens** (androstenedione and testosterone) to estrogens (estrone and estradiol) by aromatase in the adipocytes. This excess endogenous estrogen stimulation can then stimulate overgrowth of the endometrium resulting in endometrial hyperplasia and even cancer.

Endometrial hyperplasia is the abnormal proliferation of both the **glandular and stromal elements** of the endometrium. In its earliest stages, the stimulation results in changes to the organization of the glands (Fig. 14-7). In its later, more severe forms, the stimulation results in atypical changes in the cells themselves. The changes do not necessarily involve the entire endometrium, but rather may develop **focal patches** among normal endometrium. If left untreated, endometrial hyperplasia can progress to **endometrial carcinoma** (Fig. 14-7) and can also coexist alongside endometrial carcinoma.

The histologic variations of endometrial hyperplasia and their rates of progression to cancer are outlined in Table 14-6. When only **architectural changes** (changes in the complexity and crowding of the glandular components of the endometrium) are present, the hyperplasia is known as either simple or complex. When **cytologic atypia** (changes in the cellular structure of the endometrial cells) is present, then the hyperplasia is said to be either ***atypical* simple or *atypical* complex hyperplasia**. These cytologic changes include large nuclei with lost polarity, increased nuclear-to-cytoplasmic ratios, prominent nuclei, and irregular clumped chromatin. As noted in Table 14-6, atypical hyperplasia carries a higher risk of **progression to endometrial cancer** and may have **coexistent endometrial cancer** as often as 17% to 52% of the time.

1. Simple hyperplasia is the simplest form of hyperplasia. It represents an abnormal proliferation of both the stromal and glandular endometrial elements. Less than 1% of these lesions progress to carcinoma.

TABLE 14-6 Classification of Endometrial Hyperplasia and Progression to Endometrial Cancer

Architectural Type	Cytologic Atypia	Progression to Endometrial Cancer (in %)
Simple hyperplasia	Absent	1
Complex hyperplasia	Absent	3
Atypical simple hyperplasia	Present	10
Atypical complex hyperplasia	Present	30

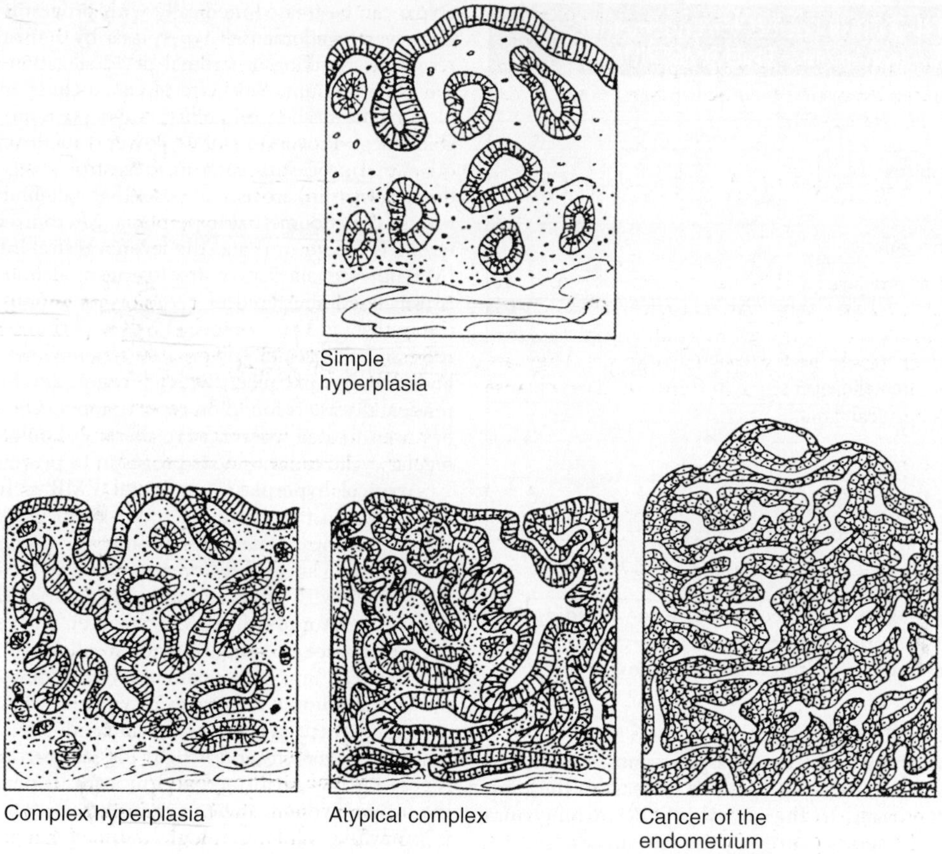

Figure 14-7 • Endometrial histology: hyperplasia to carcinoma. Simple hyperplasia without atypia and complex hyperplasia without atypia both represent architectural changes in the endometrium (e.g., crowding of glands), whereas simple or complex hyperplasia with atypia and endometrial carcinoma both demonstrate cytologic (cellular) abnormalities as well as architectural changes.
(From Beckmann C, Ling F. *Obstetrics & Gynecology*, 5th ed. Philadelphia, PA: Lippincott Williams & Wilkins; 2006.)

2. **Complex hyperplasia** consists of abnormal proliferation of the glandular endometrial elements without proliferation of the stromal elements. In these lesions, the glands are crowded in a back-to-back fashion and are of varying shapes and sizes, but **no cytologic atypia is present**. Approximately 3% of these lesions progress to carcinoma if left untreated.
3. **Atypical simple hyperplasia** involves cellular atypia and mitotic figures in addition to glandular crowding and complexity. These lesions progress to carcinoma in about 10% of cases if untreated.
4. **Atypical complex hyperplasia** is the most severe form of endometrial hyperplasia. It progresses to carcinoma in approximately 30% of untreated cases.

EPIDEMIOLOGY

Endometrial hyperplasia typically occurs in the menopausal or perimenopausal woman, but may also occur in premenopausal women who have prolonged **oligomenorrhea and/or obesity** such as those with polycystic ovarian syndrome (PCOS).

RISK FACTORS

Patients at risk for endometrial hyperplasia, like those at risk for endometrial carcinoma, are at risk due to **unopposed estrogen exposure** (Table 14-7). This includes women with obesity, nulliparity, late menopause, and exogenous estrogen use without progesterone. Chronic anovulation, polycystic ovarian syndrome, and estrogen-producing tumors such as granulosa-theca cell tumors also put women at increased risk for endometrial hyperplasia. Because it has weak estrogenic agonist activity, tamoxifen use increases the risk of endometrial hyperplasia by stimulating the endometrial lining. Both **hypertension** and **diabetes mellitus** are independent risk factors for endometrial hyperplasia. Women with Lynch II syndrome (hereditary nonpolyposis colorectal cancer) have more than a 10-fold increased lifetime risk of endometrial hyperplasia and cancer.

CLINICAL MANIFESTATIONS

History

Patients with endometrial hyperplasia typically present with long periods of **oligomenorrhea** or amenorrhea followed by

TABLE 14-7 Risk Factors for Endometrial Hyperplasia (Mnemonic: ENDOMETRIUM)

E: Excess exogenous estrogen use without progesterone
N: Nulliparity
D: Diabetes mellitus
O: Obesity
M: Menstrual irregularity
E: Elevated blood pressure
T: Tamoxifen use
R: Rectal cancer (personal history of hereditary nonpolyposis colorectal cancer)
I: Infertility history
U: Unopposed estrogen
M: Menopause late (> age 55)

irregular or excessive uterine bleeding. **Uterine bleeding** in a postmenopausal woman should raise suspicion of endometrial hyperplasia or carcinoma (Chapter 29) until proven otherwise.

Physical Examination

Occasionally, the uterus will be enlarged from endometrial hyperplasia. This is attributed to both the increase in the mass of the endometrium and to the growth of the myometrium in response to continuous estrogen stimulation. More commonly, the **pelvic examination is unremarkable.** Patients may also have stigmata associated with chronic anovulation such as abdominal **obesity**, **acanthosis**, **acne**, **or hirsutism**.

Diagnostic Evaluation

Pelvic ultrasound may reveal a thickened endometrial stripe that might be suggestive of endometrial hyperplasia. However, **tissue diagnosis is required** for the diagnosis of endometrial hyperplasia. Although dilation and curettage (D&C) was once the gold standard for sampling the endometrium, **endometrial biopsies** (EMBs) enjoy a 90% to 95% accuracy rate without the operative and anesthetic risks. This rate is lower in premenopausal and perimenopausal women. Focal endometrial lesions are more commonly missed with EMB, up to 18% of samples. Given this, EMBs have thus become the **method of choice** for evaluation of abnormal uterine bleeding including that from endometrial hyperplasia. However, when an office biopsy cannot be obtained due to insufficient tissue, patient discomfort, or cervical stenosis, then D&C in the operating room is required to rule out endometrial hyperplasia and carcinoma, for women ≥ 45 and for younger women with risk factors for hyperplasia and cancer. D&C is also recommended in patients who have atypical complex hyperplasia on biopsy because approximately 30% of those patients will have a coexistent endometrial carcinoma.

TREATMENT

The treatment of endometrial hyperplasia depends on the histologic variant of the disease and on the age of the patient. The goal of treatment is to prevent progression of disease and the control abnormal bleeding. Simple and complex hyperplasia without atypia can be treated medically with **progestin therapy**. Progestins reverse endometrial hyperplasia by activating progesterone receptors, resulting in stromal decidualization, and thinning of the endometrium. Side effects can include irregular bleeding, bloating, headaches, irritability, and depression. Typically, injectable (Depo-Provera) or oral (Provera) **medroxyprogesterone** or other oral progestins such as megestrol (Megace) or norethindrone (Aygestin) are used at doses that will inhibit and eventually reverse the endometrial hyperplasia. **Micronized vaginal progesterone** (Prometrium) and the **levonorgestrel intrauterine system** (Mirena) are alternative treatment modalities. The progestin is usually administered in cyclic or continuous fashion for 3 to 6 months and then a **repeat EMB** is performed to evaluate for regression of disease. The progestin therapy may be repeated at a higher dose or in concert with a levonorgestrel-containing IUD if residual disease is found on repeat biopsy. Once the hyperplasia has been treated, preventative therapy should be initiated with regular cyclic or continuous progestin to prevent recurrence.

Atypical hyperplasia on initial EMB is further evaluated with D&C in the operating room given the significant (30%) risk of having coexistent endometrial cancer or developing endometrial cancer. Hysterectomy is the treatment of choice for women with endometrial hyperplasia with atypia who do not desire future fertility. Most women with atypical complex hyperplasia are either perimenopausal or postmenopausal.

However, in younger patients with atypical complex hyperplasia and chronic anovulation who wish to preserve fertility or if the patient is a poor surgical candidate, longer-term progestin management and weight loss are recommended first. A repeat EMB is performed at 3 months. If persistence is noted, the progestin dose can be increased. Persistence after 9 months is predictive of failure and hysterectomy is recommended. Once EMB has demonstrated no evidence of hyperplasia, the patient should actively pursue fertility options.

OVARIAN CYSTS

PATHOGENESIS

In general, ovarian masses can be divided into functional cysts and neoplastic growths. Benign and malignant neoplasms of the ovary are discussed in detail in Chapter 30. **Functional cysts** of the ovaries result from normal physiologic functioning of the ovaries (Chapter 20) and are divided into follicular cysts and corpus luteum cysts.

Follicular cysts are the most common functional cysts. They arise after failure of a follicle to rupture during the follicular maturation phase of the menstrual cycle. Functional cysts may vary in size from 3 to 8 cm and are classically asymptomatic and usually unilateral (Color Plate 9). Large follicular cysts can cause a tender palpable ovarian mass and can lead to ovarian torsion when greater than 4 cm in size. Most follicular cysts resolve spontaneously in 60 to 90 days. Simple cysts smaller than 2.5 cm are physiologic.

Corpus luteum cysts are common functional cysts that occur during the luteal phase of the menstrual cycle. Most corpus luteum cysts are formed when the corpus luteum fails to regress after 14 days and becomes enlarged (>3 cm) or hemorrhagic (corpus hemorrhagicum). These cysts can cause a delay in menstruation and dull lower quadrant pain. Patients with a ruptured corpus luteum cyst can present with acute pain and signs of hemoperitoneum late in the luteal phase.

Theca lutein cysts are large bilateral cysts filled with clear, straw-colored fluid. These ovarian cysts result from stimulation by abnormally high ß-human chorionic gonadotropin (e.g., from a molar pregnancy, choriocarcinoma, or ovulation induction therapy).

Endometriomas arise from the growth of ectopic endometrial tissue within the ovary. These cysts are also called "chocolate cysts," which comes from the thick brown old blood contained in them. Patients can present with the symptoms of endometriosis such as pelvic pain, dysmenorrhea, dyspareunia, and infertility.

EPIDEMIOLOGY

More than 75% of ovarian masses in women of reproductive age are **functional cysts** and less than 25% are nonfunctional neoplasms. Although functional ovarian cysts can be found in females of any age, they most commonly occur between puberty and menopause. Women who smoke have a twofold increase for functional cysts.

CLINICAL MANIFESTATIONS

History

Patients with functional cysts present with a variety of symptoms depending on the type of cyst. Follicular cysts tend to be **asymptomatic** and only occasionally cause menstrual disturbances such as prolonged intermenstrual intervals or short cycles. Larger follicular cysts can cause achy **pelvic pain**, dyspareunia, and ovarian torsion. Corpus luteum cysts may cause local pelvic pain and either amenorrhea or delayed menses. Acute abdominal pain may result from a **hemorrhagic corpus luteum cyst**, a torsed ovary, or a ruptured follicular cyst.

Physical Examination

The findings on bimanual pelvic examination vary with the type of cyst. Follicular cysts tend to be less than 8 cm and simple or unilocular in structure. Lutein cysts are generally larger than follicular cysts and often feel firmer or more solid on palpation. A ruptured cyst can cause pain on palpation, acute abdominal pain, and rebound tenderness. When an ovarian cyst results in a torsed adnexa, the classic presentation is **waxing and waning pain, and nausea and vomiting**.

Diagnostic Evaluation

After a thorough history and physical, the primary diagnostic tool for the workup of ovarian cyst is the **pelvic ultrasound**. Ultrasonography allows for better characterization of the cyst that can guide the workup and treatment. Because most functional cysts will spontaneously resolve over 60 to 90 days, **serial ultrasounds** may be used to check for cyst resolution. A CA-125 level is often obtained from patients who are at high risk for ovarian cancer. This should be used solely as a means of evaluating the treatment response to chemotherapy and not as a diagnostic or screening test per the American College of Obstetrics and Gynecology (ACOG) guidelines (see Chapter 30).

The **differential diagnoses** for ovarian cysts include ectopic pregnancy, pelvic inflammatory disease, torsed adnexa, tubo-ovarian abscess, endometriosis, fibroids, and ovarian neoplasms.

Treatment

Treatment of ovarian cysts depends on the age of the patient and the characteristics of the cyst. Table 14-8 outlines

TABLE 14-8 Management of a Cystic Adnexal Mass

Age	Type	Size of Cyst (cm)	Management
Premenarchal	Any	>2 cm	Surgical evaluation
Reproductive	Simple	≤5	No follow-up necessary
		>5 and ≤7	Repeat ultrasound in 1 y
		>7	Further imaging or surgical evaluation
	Hemorrhagic	≤5	No follow-up necessary
		>5	Repeat ultrasound in 6–12 wk
	Endometrioma	Any	Repeat ultrasound in 6–12 wk. Then if not surgically removed, follow yearly
	Nodule without flow or multiple thin septations	Any	Surgical evaluation or MRI
Postmenopausal	Simple	<1	No follow-up necessary
		>1 and ≤7	Repeat ultrasound in 1 y
		>7	Further imaging or surgical evaluation
	Hemorrhagic		Early menopause: repeat ultrasound in 6–12 wk
Late menopause: surgical evaluation			
	Nodule without flow or multiple thin septations	Any	Surgical evaluation or MRI

Any cystic mass that contains thick septations, nodules/solid components with abnormal Doppler flow, and cyst wall thickening or has presence of ascites and of omental/peritoneal masses merits surgical evaluation due to increased suspicion for malignancy.

the management options using these criteria. In general, a palpable ovary or adnexal mass in a **premenarchal or postmenopausal** patient is suggestive of an ovarian neoplasm rather than a functional cyst and surgical exploration is in order. Likewise, reproductive-age women with cysts larger than 7 cm or that **persist** or that are solid or complex on ultrasound probably do not have a functional cyst. These lesions should be closely investigated with MRI or surgical exploration.

For patients of reproductive age with cysts less than 7 cm in size, **observation** with a **follow-up ultrasound** is the appropriate action. Most follicular cysts should resolve spontaneously within 60 to 90 days. During this observation period, patients are often started on **oral contraceptives**. This is not a treatment for existing cysts but rather to **suppress ovulation** in order to prevent the formation of future cysts. Cysts that do not resolve within 60 to 90 days require evaluation with **cystectomy** and (rarely) oophorectomy via laparoscopy or laparotomy.

KEY POINTS

- Anatomic anomalies of the uterus are extremely rare and result from problems in the fusion of the paramesonephric (müllerian) ducts. Therefore, they are often associated with urinary tract anomalies and inguinal hernias.
- If present, symptoms include amenorrhea, dysmenorrhea, cyclic pelvic pain, infertility, recurrent pregnancy loss, and premature labor.
- Anomalies are diagnosed by physical examination, pelvic ultrasound, CT, MRI, hysterosalpingogram, hysteroscopy, and laparoscopy.
- Both septated uteri and bicornuate uteri can be treated surgically if symptomatic.
- Fibroids are benign, estrogen-sensitive, smooth muscle tumors of unclear etiology found in 50% of reproductive-age women.
- Fibroid incidence is three to nine times higher in black women compared to white, Asian, and Hispanic women. Risk is also increased in obese, nonsmoking, and perimenopausal women.
- Fibroids may be submucosal, intramural, or subserosal and can grow to great size, especially during pregnancy. They are asymptomatic in 50% to 65% of patients; when symptomatic, they can cause heavy or prolonged bleeding (most common), pressure, pain, and infertility (rare).
- Fibroids are typically diagnosed by pelvic ultrasound. In most cases, no treatment is necessary. However, they can be treated temporarily with Provera, danazol, or GnRH analogs to decrease estrogen and shrink the tumors, or myomectomy to resect the tumors when future fertility is desired.
- Fibroids are treated definitively by hysterectomy in the case of severe pain, when large or multiple, when causing pressure symptoms, or when there is evidence of postmenopausal or rapid growth.
- Endometrial hyperplasia is classified as simple or complex if only architectural alterations (glandular crowding) exist or as atypical simple or atypical complex if cytologic (cellular) atypia is also present.
- It is caused by prolonged exposure to exogenous or endogenous estrogen in the absence of progesterone. Risk factors include chronic anovulation, obesity, nulliparity, late menopause, and unopposed estrogen use.
- Risk of malignant transformation is 1% in simple hyperplasia, 3% in complex hyperplasia, 10% in atypical simple hyperplasia, and 30% in atypical complex hyperplasia.
- Endometrial hyperplasia is diagnosed by EMB or D&C and if no atypia is present it is usually treated medically with progestin therapy for 3 to 6 months, followed by resampling of the endometrium.
- The risk of atypical complex hyperplasia progressing to endometrial cancer is 30%. Thus, the recommended treatment for atypical complex hyperplasia is hysterectomy.
- Follicular cysts result from unruptured follicles. These are usually asymptomatic unless torsion occurs. Management includes observation with or without oral contraceptives to suppress future cyst formation, followed by repeat pelvic ultrasound.
- Corpus luteum cysts result from an enlarged and/or hemorrhagic corpus luteum. These may cause a missed period or dull lower quadrant pain. When ruptured, these cysts can cause acute abdominal pain and intra-abdominal hemorrhage. Corpus luteum cysts should resolve spontaneously or may be suppressed with oral contraceptives if recurrent.
- The differential diagnoses for ovarian cysts include ectopic pregnancy, pelvic inflammatory disease, torsed adnexa, tubo-ovarian abscess, endometriosis, fibroids, and ovarian neoplasms.
- Any palpable ovarian or adnexal mass in a premenarchal or postmenopausal patient is suggestive of ovarian neoplasm and should be investigated with exploratory laparoscopy or laparotomy.
- Cysts that do not resolve spontaneously in 60 to 90 days require further evaluation and treatment with cystectomy or oophorectomy (rarely) via laparoscopy or laparotomy.

C Clinical Vignettes

Vignette 1

A mother brings her 13-year-old daughter in to see you because she is experiencing cyclic lower abdominal pain every month that lasts for about 4 days. She is also concerned that the patient has not started her period like most of her classmates, and wants to know if you think this is normal. Physical examination reveals Tanner stage 4 breast and pubic hair development. Vaginal examination shows an intact hymen and a small, nulliparous cervix without lesions.

1. All of the following are formed by the paramesonephric ducts *except*:
   a. superior vagina
   b. cervix
   c. ovaries
   d. uterus
   e. Fallopian tubes
2. In addition to a detailed evaluation of her uterus, you perform an additional workup knowing that all of the following are commonly associated with uterine anomalies *except*:
   a. Unilateral renal agenesis
   b. Pelvic or horseshoe kidney
   c. Inguinal hernia
   d. Imperforate anus
   e. Ureteral duplication
3. Which of the following is the most common mullerian anomaly?
   a. Bicornuate uterus
   b. Septate uterus
   c. Uterine didelphys
   d. Unicornuate uterus
   e. Arcuate uterus
4. You see another patient following the one previously described. She is a 22-year-old who has been diagnosed with a septate uterus. You counsel her that she is at highest risk for which of the following complications of pregnancy?
   a. Recurrent first-trimester pregnancy loss
   b. Placental abruption
   c. Fetal genitourinary anomalies
   d. Second-trimester fetal loss
   e. Premature rupture of membranes

Vignette 2

A 30-year-old African American G0 woman comes to your office for her annual examination. During the history assessment, she reports increased pelvic pressure, constipation, and worsening menorrhagia with menses. During menstrual cycles she is using about 10 large pads per day with her heaviest flow and passing "quarter sized" blood clots.

On physical examination, you palpate a nontender, irregularly enlarged uterus with a lumpy-bumpy, firm contour. Her cervix appears normal, and she has no evidence of ascites or other abnormal physical findings. You suspect that she has uterine fibroids.

1. Which of the following tests is most commonly used for diagnosis of uterine fibroids?
   a. CT scan
   b. Pelvic x-ray
   c. Pelvic ultrasound
   d. MRI
   e. Hysterosalpingogram
2. All of the following medical therapies can be used to treat menorrhagia in women with uterine fibroids *except*:
   a. combined oral contraceptive pills
   b. antifibrinolytic agent (tranexamic acid)
   c. nonsteroidal anti-inflammatory drugs
   d. progestin only pills
   e. opioid agonists
3. Which of the following fibroid locations is most commonly associated with abnormal vaginal bleeding?
   a. Submucosal
   b. Intramural
   c. Subserosal
   d. Pedunculated
   e. Parasitic
4. All of the following are risk factors for uterine fibroids *except*:
   a. African American heritage
   b. multiparity
   c. early menarche
   d. perimenopause
   e. hypertension

Vignette 3

A 53-year-old G0 woman comes to your office to report that her menses have returned. She underwent menopause 4 years ago, and had not experienced any bleeding until the past 3 months. She reports several episodes of bleeding. She has a normal Pap smear history and had a normal pap and negative high-risk HPV screen performed 2 years ago. She has been taking over-the-counter medications and supplements for hot flashes, but cannot recall the names of them. She is in a monogamous relationship with her husband of 20 years. Further history reveals that she has type 2 diabetes and has a lifelong history of oligomenorrhea with heavy or prolonged bleeds when she does have a cycle. She had a prior laparoscopic cholecystectomy 8 years ago as her only surgical history. Physical examination reveals the following: BP: 150/85 mm Hg; BMI: 48; general characteristics: obese female with moderate acanthosis over posterior neck, inner thighs and inguinal area, moderate hirsutism over chin/neck area; Abdomen: well-healed laparoscopic scars; GU: uterus mobile, 9 weeks' sized (mildly enlarged), limited palpation of adnexa due to habitus, overall nontender, without discrete masses.

1. In addition to a thorough physical examination, which of the following is the next best step in evaluation of this patient?
   a. Transvaginal ultrasound
   b. CT scan of pelvis
   c. Hysterosalpingogram
   d. Pelvic MRI
   e. Cervical bacterial culture
2. In addition to a complete examination and additional workup as chosen above, which of the following is the next best step in evaluation?
   a. Cystourethroscopy
   b. Endometrial biopsy
   c. Colonoscopy
   d. Diagnostic laparoscopy
   e. Serum FSH
3. You are concerned that she is at high risk for endometrial hyperplasia or carcinoma. You explain to her the risk factors for endometrial hyperplasia include all of the following *except*:
   a. chronic anovulation
   b. obesity
   c. multiparity
   d. late menopause
   e. unopposed estrogen exposure
4. Her pathology returns with evidence of endometrial hyperplasia. Which of the following histologic variations of hyperplasia you counsel her has the highest risk of progression to endometrial cancer as well as the highest rate of coexistent underlying cancer?
   a. Simple hyperplasia without atypia
   b. Simple hyperplasia with atypia
   c. Complex hyperplasia without atypia
   d. Complex hyperplasia with atypia
   e. Mixed endometrial hyperplasia

Vignette 4

An 18-year-old G0 young woman presents to your office for routine gynecologic examination. She reports that her last menstrual period began about 23 days ago. It was light in flow, and lasted 4 days in length. She has minimal dysmenorrhea. She denies any history of sexually transmitted infections, and has been sexually active with two male partners in the last 2 weeks. She was given a prescription for oral contraceptives 3 months ago; however, she has not started taking these. She has no other complaints or medical/surgical history.

During her pelvic examination, you obtain a wet prep, which has normal squamous cells, rare WBCs, and no yeast. On bimanual examination, you palpate a 6 cm nontender left adnexal mass that is mobile. She has no rebound tenderness or guarding.

1. You suspect that she has an ovarian cyst. Which of the following is the most common diagnosis in a patient with this presentation?
   a. Theca lutein cyst
   b. Functional ovarian cyst
   c. Ectopic pregnancy
   d. Tubo-ovarian abscess
   e. Endometrioma
2. You determine that she does indeed have an ovarian cyst on ultrasound. She calls your office 3 days later to report acute onset of sharp left abdominal pain with waxing and waning pain, nausea and vomiting. An ovarian cyst of which size is concerning for torsion?
   a. 2.5 cm
   b. >1 cm
   c. <4 cm
   d. >4 cm
   e. 3 cm
3. Repeat ultrasound reveals that there is excellent flow to and from the ovary. However, the ovary now has a small amount of free fluid surrounding it. Her pain subsides and her hematocrit is stable. You diagnose a ruptured hemorrhagic cyst. She and her mother ask about options for preventing further cysts from occurring. You advise:
   a. expectant management
   b. removal of the cyst
   c. removal of the ovary
   d. progesterone-containing IUD (Mirena)
   e. combination estrogen and progesterone contraceptive

A Answers

Vignette 1 Question 1
Answer C: All reproductive structures arise from the müllerian system except the ovaries (which arise from the genital ridge) and the lower one-third of the vagina (which arises from the urogenital diaphragm). Specifically, the superior vagina, cervix, uterus, and fallopian tubes are formed by fusion of the paramesonephric (müllerian) ducts (see Fig. 13-1). Uterine anomalies are generally a result of incomplete fusion of the ducts during embryologic development, incomplete development of one or both ducts, or degeneration of the ducts (müllerian agenesis).

Vignette 1 Question 2
Answer D: Imperforate anus is commonly associated with other birth defects such as vertebral, cardiovascular, tracheoesophageal fistulae, esophageal atresia, and renal or limb defects (VACTERL). Müllerian anomalies are commonly associated with inguinal hernias or urinary tract anomalies (unilateral renal agenesis, pelvic or horseshoe kidney, and irregularities in the collecting system).

Vignette 1 Question 3
Answer B: Septate uterus is the most common mullerian anomaly due to malfusion of the paramesonephric (müllerian) ducts, and is usually recognized in women presenting during routine evaluation for obstetric or gynecologic reasons. The others listed are less common than septate uterus. Many uterine anomalies require no treatment unless there is a concern for significant future pregnancy complication or if the patient is symptomatic, for example, from bleeding into a noncommunicating uterine horn or nonpatent vaginal septum.

Vignette 1 Question 4
Answer A: Uterine septa can vary in thickness and are composed of collagen fibers and often lack an adequate blood supply to facilitate and support placental growth. For this reason, recurrent pregnancy loss is the most common complication for these patients. Once a pregnancy is successful beyond the first trimester in these women, they usually do not have further complications. Placental abruption, second-trimester fetal loss and premature rupture of membranes occurs more often in patients with bicornuate or unicornuate uteri. Fetal genitourinary anomalies are not associated with isolated maternal müllerian anomalies.

Vignette 2 Question 1
Answer C: Pelvic ultrasound is relatively inexpensive and delineates female pelvic anatomy as well as an MRI. It is the first line imaging for evaluation of gynecologic conditions and does not require the use of contrast dye for enhanced imaging, such as CT scan. Pelvic X-ray is best used to differentiate calcified components and air fluid levels, but does not outline pelvic anatomy. Hysterosalpingogram is similar to a plain film X-ray with added used of intrauterine contrast and fluoroscopy to demonstrate uterine cavity shape and tubal patency (with spill into the peritoneum). This is usually only reserved for workup of infertility or to confirm tubal occlusion following permanent sterilization.

Vignette 2 Question 2
Answer E: Opioid agonists are narcotic medications used to treat pain. These have no role in the treatment of heavy bleeding in women with uterine fibroids. Combined oral contraceptive pills, antifibrinolytics, and progestin therapy (oral, injectable or IUD) help reduce the amount of menstrual bleeding, which can also aid in reduction of pain during menstruation. Nonsteroidal anti-inflammatory drugs reduce levels of prostaglandin, which are produced by the uterus during menses and cause uterine contractions that augment pain from the fibroids. These are commonly used to treat dysmenorrhea associated with menses in women with and without uterine fibroids.

Vignette 2 Question 3
Answer A: Several mechanisms of fibroid induced menorrhagia have been described. It is well-known that submucosal fibroids can mechanically distort the endometrial lining, prohibiting it from building an organized endometrial layer. Other effects could be related to altered vascular growth due to expression of angiogenic growth factors by the fibroids themselves. Intramural fibroids involve the myometrial layer of the uterus and the most common symptom is dysmenorrhea. Subserosal fibroids are on the surface of the uterus and typically are asymptomatic. Parasitic fibroids are pedunculated off of the uterine serosa and grow within the peritoneal cavity. They recruit additional blood supply from nearby organs, but do not directly affect endometrial blood flow. All of the different types of fibroids can cause pressure and pain symptoms if their sizes are significantly increased and result in mass effect in the pelvis.

Vignette 2 Question 4
Answer B: Uterine fibroids are more commonly associated with nulliparity. Other known risk factors include African American heritage, nonsmoking status, early menarche, increased alcohol use, and hypertension. Generally, low-dose oral contraceptive pills do not cause growth of fibroids and depot-medroxyprogesterone acetate (Depo-Provera) is protective against fibroid formation. The use of hormone replacement in postmenopausal women with fibroids can

be associated with fibroid growth but typically does not result in clinical symptoms.

Vignette 3 Question 1

Answer A: A transvaginal ultrasound is the initial best imaging test for postmenopausal bleeding. This will discern if there are any uterine leiomyomas, potential masses or polyps, and evaluate the thickness of the endometrium. This has lower specificity in regards to diagnosing polyps when compared to hysteroscopy (direct visualization of the endometrial cavity), but hysteroscopy is more invasive and may need to be performed in the operating room. CT scan and MRI of the pelvis are costly and not used in the initial workup of a postmenopausal female with vaginal bleeding. Hysterosalpingogram is used to assess the shape and contour of the endometrial cavity. Radiopaque contrast medium is injected through the cervical canal and fluoroscopy is used to image the uterine cavity and fallopian tubes. Tubal patency is determined by spillage into the peritoneal cavity. This test will not evaluate the myometrium or endometrial thickness, and is not used for postmenopausal vaginal bleeding. Cervical culture (i.e., gonorrhea, chlamydia testing) is indicated in high-risk populations; however, this patient is not involved in high-risk sexual behavior (as evident from her history) and so this testing is not indicated.

Vignette 3 Question 2

Answer B: It is prudent that you consider endometrial polyps, hyperplasia, and endometrial carcinoma in the differential diagnosis of patients presenting with abnormal menstrual bleeding, including those older than 45 years, but especially in postmenopausal women with any bleeding. Endometrial biopsy (EMB) is the first-line test for evaluating endometrial pathology. It is up to 95% accurate and should be performed in all postmenopausal women with a thickened endometrial stripe (>4 mm) or with persistent vaginal bleeding. It is performed in the office without the use of anesthesia. A cystourethroscopy will not aid in determination of the cause of her vaginal bleeding at this time because it evaluates the bladder and urethra. Given her age of greater than 50, she does need a colonoscopy for routine colo-rectal cancer screening however, this is not used in the initial gynecologic workup for postmenopausal bleeding. Diagnostic laparoscopy is an invasive test and will not help to determine the pathologic nature of her endometrial cavity, which is causing the heavy bleeding. Serum FSH would confirm that this patient is postmenopausal but would not give information about the endometrial lining.

Vignette 3 Question 3

Answer C: Nulliparity (instead of multiparity) is a known risk factor for endometrial hyperplasia. Chronic anovulation, which can be caused by PCOS and obesity, allows for unopposed estrogen that causes excess stimulation of the endometrial lining without shedding in a systematic fashion. This can lead to disordered endometrial glandular growth and subsequently endometrial hyperplasia or carcinoma. Late menopause also has the same effect as continued estrogen exposure to the endometrial lining. Unopposed estrogen exposure is the underlying cause in the majority of cases of hyperplasia and even most endometrial carcinomas. This is seen in various clinical situations, including peripheral conversion of androgens to estrogen by adipocytes in obese women or in women who are taking exogenous estrogen without progesterone to help stabilize the endometrium and prevent overgrowth. This patient has multiple risk factors in her history including chronic anovulation, obesity, and hirsutism—likely PCOS—and is taking an unknown over-the-counter hormone replacement supplement, which could simulate unopposed estrogens in some situations.

Vignette 3 Question 4

Answer D: Atypical complex hyperplasia is the most severe form of endometrial hyperplasia. It progresses to carcinoma in approximately 30% of untreated cases. The histologic variations of endometrial hyperplasia and their rates of progression to cancer are outlined in Table 14-6. Simple and complex refer to glandular crowding of cytologically normal cells, and atypia describes the cytologically abnormal cells in more severe endometrial hyperplasia. These cytologic changes include large nuclei with lost polarity, increased nuclear-to-cytoplasmic ratios, prominent nuclei, and irregular clumped chromatin. Simple hyperplasia without atypia is the simplest form of hyperplasia, less than 1% of these lesions progress to carcinoma. Complex hyperplasia without atypia consists of abnormal proliferation of the glandular endometrial elements without proliferation of the stromal elements. The glands are crowded in a back-to-back fashion and are of varying shapes and sizes. Approximately 3% of these lesions progress to carcinoma if left untreated. Simple hyperplasia with atypia involves cellular atypia and mitotic figures in addition to glandular crowding and complexity and progresses to carcinoma in about 10% of cases if untreated. As many as 17% to 52% of patients with complex hyperplasia with atypia have coexistent cancer at the time of diagnosis. Mixed endometrial hyperplasia is not a histologic diagnosis.

Vignette 4 Question 1

Answer B: This patient is asymptomatic. Functional ovarian cysts are classically asymptomatic, unilateral, and arise after failure of a follicle to rupture during the follicular maturation phase of the menstrual cycle. Theca lutein cysts are large bilateral cysts with clear fluid that result from stimulation by abnormally high ß-human chorionic gonadotropin. Ectopic pregnancies are often tender to palpation, and her menstrual history suggests that she may not be pregnant with the recent menstrual cycle; however, a pregnancy test is still indicated for this patient who is sexually active and not using any contraception. Implantation or first-trimester bleeding in pregnancy can sometimes be mistaken for a "light" menstrual cycle. Endometriomas are present in patients with endometriosis. Her asymptomatic menstrual history does not suggest endometriosis because she does not report dysmenorrhea. An ultrasound will aid in diagnosis of the cyst appearance and internal components. Tubo-ovarian abscess is present in patients with pelvic inflammatory disease. You would suspect this in someone with abundant WBCs on wet prep, tenderness on examination, or other systemic signs such as abdominal pain or fever.

Vignette 4 Question 2

Answer D: When cysts reach a size of greater than 4 cm, they are at risk for torsion. This is somewhat determined by the contents of the cyst, with mature teratomas having a slight higher risk of torsion if solid internal components are present to act as a leading edge of the fulcrum for torsion. Acute pain in a gynecologic situation could also be caused by ruptured hemorrhagic corpus luteum cyst, a torsed ovary, or a ruptured follicular cyst. Emergent evaluation of this patient is recommended as she is at risk for ovarian necrosis if torsion is present. It is also important to counsel your patients who have a large ovarian cysts of this risk and to encourage early evaluation if pain arises.

Vignette 4 Question 3

Answer E: Combination estrogen and progesterone contraceptives such as oral contraceptive pills (OCPs), the Nuvaring, and the Ortho Evra patch work to prevent formation of future cysts by suppressing ovulation. These medications provide steady estrogen levels (as opposed to the fluctuating levels in a patient who is not on these medications). Therefore, the immature follicles never develop, there is no ovulation and the probability of a functional cyst is decreased. Women with recurrent ovarian cysts are often placed on combination estrogen–progesterone contraceptives to prevent the formation of new cysts. Of note, these medications do not *treat* current cysts, they *prevent* future cysts by suppressing ovulation. In this clinical setting, expectant management is reasonable but will not help to prevent cyst formation. Surgical removal of the cyst and ovary are much too invasive and are not indicated for a benign functional cyst that is not torsed and is not bleeding. The progesterone-containing IUD (Mirena) has only results in a partial inhibition of follicular cyst formation and ovulation. Therefore, most women (75%) using this contraceptive method can still get functional cysts.

Chapter

15 Endometriosis and Adenomyosis

ENDOMETRIOSIS

PATHOGENESIS

Endometriosis is a chronic disease marked by the presence of endometrial tissue **(glands and stroma)** outside the endometrial cavity. Endometrial tissue can be found anywhere in the body, but the most common sites are the **ovary** and the **pelvic peritoneum** including the anterior and posterior cul de sacs. Endometriosis in the ovary appears as a cystic collection known as an **endometrioma**. Other common sites include the most dependent parts of the pelvis such as the posterior uterus and broad ligaments, the uterosacral ligaments, fallopian tubes, colon, and appendix (Fig. 15-1). Although not commonly found, endometriosis has been identified as far away as the breast, lung, and brain.

There are three main theories about the etiology of endometriosis. The Halban theory proposes that endometrial tissue is transported via the **lymphatic system** to various sites in the pelvis, where it grows ectopically. Meyer proposes that multipotential cells in peritoneal tissue undergo **metaplastic transformation** into functional endometrial tissue. Finally, Sampson suggests that endometrial tissue is transported through the fallopian tubes during **retrograde menstruation**, resulting in intra-abdominal pelvic implants.

A prevailing theory is that women who develop endometriosis may have an **altered immune system** that is less likely to recognize and attack ectopic endometrial implants. These women may even have an increased concentration of inflammatory cells in the peritoneum that contribute to the growth and stimulation of the endometrial implants. Endometrial implants cause symptoms by disrupting normal tissue, forming adhesions and fibrosis, and causing severe inflammation. Interestingly, the **severity of symptoms does not necessarily correlate with the amount of endometriosis**. Women with widely disseminated endometriosis or a large endometrioma may experience little pain, whereas women with minimal disease in the cul-de-sac may suffer severe chronic pain.

EPIDEMIOLOGY

The estimated prevalence of endometriosis is between 10% and 15%. Because **surgical confirmation** is necessary for the diagnosis of endometriosis, the true prevalence of the disease is unknown. It is found almost exclusively in women of reproductive age, and is the single most common reason for hospitalization of women in this age group. Approximately 20% of women with **chronic pelvic pain** and 30% to 40% of women **with infertility** have endometriosis.

RISK FACTORS

Nulliparity, early menarche, prolonged menses, and müllerian anomalies are associated with an increased risk of diagnosis with endometriosis. Women with **first-degree relatives** (mother or sisters) with endometriosis have a 7% chance of developing the disorder compared to 1% chance in women without a family history. A relationship has also been observed between endometriosis and increased rates of some **autoimmune inflammatory disorders** such as lupus, asthma, hypothyroidism, chronic fatigue syndrome, fibromyalgia, and allergies. For unclear reasons, endometriosis is identified less often in black and Asian women.

CLINICAL MANIFESTATIONS

History

The hallmark of endometriosis is **cyclic pelvic pain** beginning 1 or 2 weeks before menses, **peaking 1 to 2 days before the onset of menses**, and subsiding at the onset of menses or shortly thereafter. Women with chronic endometriosis and teenagers with endometriosis may not demonstrate this classic pain pattern. Other symptoms associated with endometriosis are **dysmenorrhea**, **dyspareunia**, **abnormal bleeding**, **bowel and bladder symptoms, and subfertility**. Endometriosis is one of the most common diagnoses in the evaluation of infertile couples.

Symptoms of endometriosis vary depending on the area involved. Over 75% of women with symptomatic endometriosis will have pelvic pain and/or dysmenorrhea. **Dysmenorrhea** usually begins in the third decade, worsens with age, and should raise concern for endometriosis in women who develop dysmenorrhea after years of pain-free cycles. **Dyspareunia** is usually associated with deep penetration that can aggravate endometrial lesions in the cul-de-sac or on the uterosacral ligaments.

Endometriosis is also a cause of **infertility**. Although the exact mechanism is unclear, moderate to severe endometriosis can cause **dense adhesions,** which can distort the pelvic architecture, interfere with tubal mobility, impair oocyte release, and cause tubal obstruction.

Physical Examination

The physical findings associated with early endometriosis may be **subtle or nonexistent**. To maximize the likelihood of physical findings, the physical examination should be performed during early menses when implants are likely to be largest and most tender. When more disseminated disease is present, the clinician may find **uterosacral nodularity** and tenderness on rectovaginal

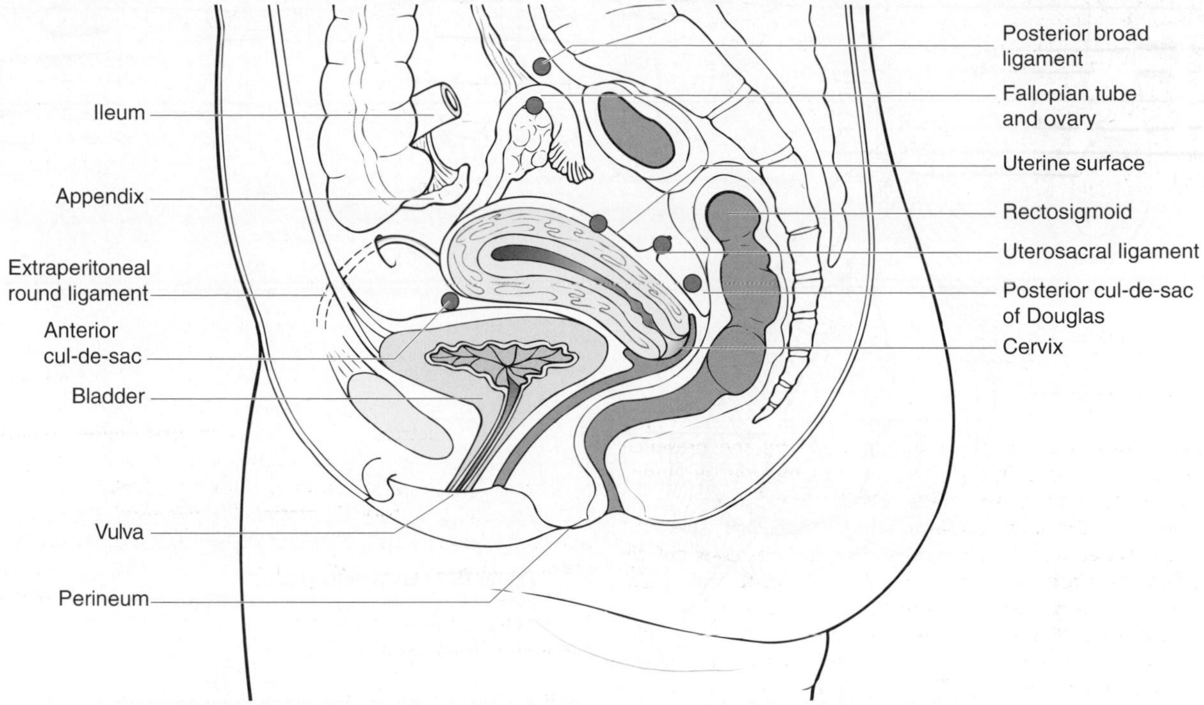

Figure 15-1 • Potential sites for endometriosis. The most common sites (indicated by blue dots) include the ovaries, the anterior and posterior cul de sacs, the uterosacral ligaments, and the posterior uterus and posterior broad ligaments.

examination or a **fixed retroverted uterus**. Pain with movement of the uterus can often be seen. When the ovary is involved, a tender, fixed **adnexal mass** may be palpable on bimanual examination or viewed on pelvic ultrasound (Fig. 15-2).

Diagnostic Evaluation

When the clinical impression and initial evaluation is consistent with endometriosis, **empiric medical therapy** is often favored over surgical intervention as a safe approach to management.

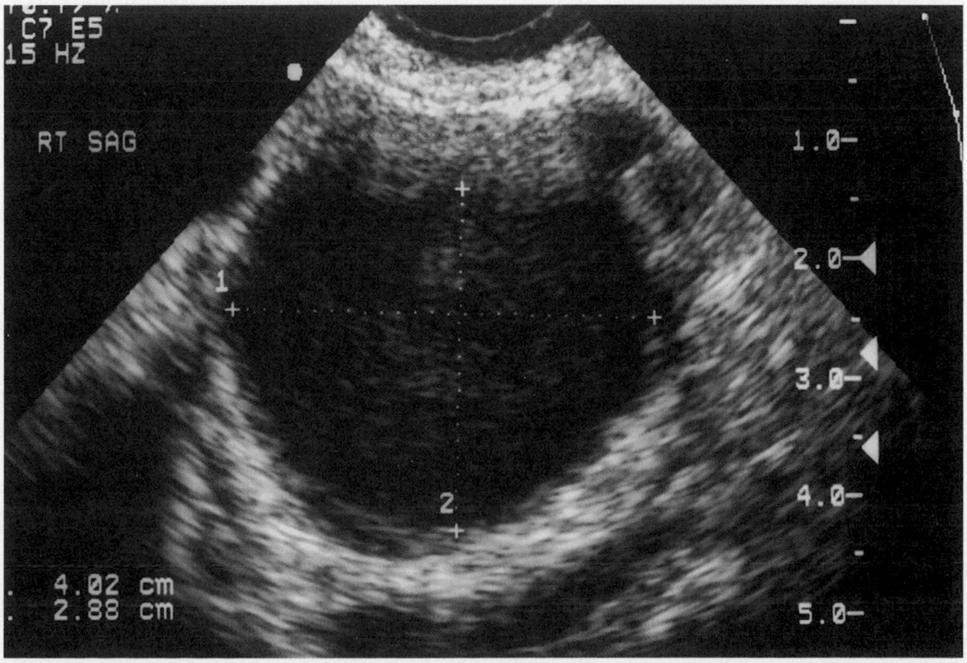

Figure 15-2 • Transvaginal ultrasound of an endometrioma of the ovary. Note the characteristic "ground glass" appearance of the endometrioma on ultrasound.

(From Berek JS. *Berek & Novak's Gynecology*, 14th ed. Philadelphia, PA: Lippincott Williams & Wilkins; 2006.)

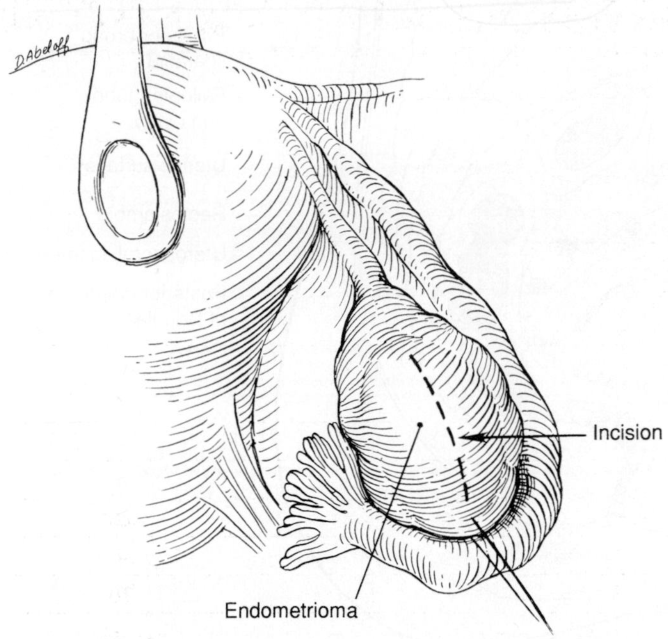

Figure 15-3 • Endometrioma.

However, the only way to definitively diagnose endometriosis is through **direct visualization** with laparoscopy or laparotomy. When surgical intervention is used, endometrial implants vary widely in terms of size, texture, and appearance. They may appear as rust-colored to dark brown powder burns or raised, blue-colored mulberry or raspberry lesions. The areas may be surrounded by reactive fibrosis that can lead to dense adhesions in extensive disease. The ovary itself can develop large cystic collections of endometriosis filled with thick, dark, old blood and debris known as **endometriomas or chocolate cysts** (Fig. 15-3). **Peritoneal biopsy** is not absolutely necessary but is recommended for histologic confirmation of the diagnosis of endometriosis.

Once the diagnosis of endometriosis is confirmed, the anatomic location and extent of the disease can be used to properly classify the operative findings. In general, endometriosis is categorized as minimal, mild, moderate, or severe. The American Fertility Society's revised classification schema is reproduced in Table 15-1. Although not commonly used, this classification method uses a point system to stage endometriosis based on the location, depth, and diameter of lesions and density of adhesions.

DIFFERENTIAL DIAGNOSIS

The differential diagnosis for endometriosis includes other chronic processes that result in recurring pelvic pain or an ovarian mass such as pelvic inflammatory disease, adenomyosis, irritable bowel syndrome, interstitial cystitis, pelvic adhesions, functional ovarian cysts, ectopic pregnancy, and ovarian neoplasms.

TREATMENT

The treatment choice for patients with endometriosis depends on the extent and location of disease, the severity of symptoms, and the patient's desire for future fertility. Treatment should be embarked upon with the mindset that the endometriosis is a chronic disease that may require long-term management and multiple interventions. **Expectant management** may be used in patients with minimal or nonexistent symptoms. For other patients, both surgical and medical options are available. In the case of severe or chronic endometriosis, a multidisciplinary approach incorporating medical and surgical management as well as pain center involvement and psychiatric support may provide the most comprehensive care.

Medical treatment for endometriosis is aimed at **suppression and atrophy of the endometrial tissue**. Although medical therapies can be quite effective, these are **temporizing measures** rather than definitive treatments. Endometrial implants and symptoms often recur following cessation of treatment. **There is no role for medical management in patients attempting to conceive**. Medical management does not improve conception rates and serves only to delay attempts at conception and/or employment of surgical treatments that have been shown to improve conception rates.

Current medical regimens for the treatment of endometriosis include **NSAIDs**, cyclic or continuous **estrogen–progestin contraceptives** (pills, patches, rings), and menstrual suppression with **progestins** (oral, injectable, or intrauterine). These treatments induce a state of " **pseudopregnancy**" by suppressing both ovulation and menstruation and by decidualizing the endometrial implants, thereby alleviating the cyclic pelvic pain and dysmenorrhea. These options are best for patients with mild endometriosis who are not currently seeking to conceive.

Patients with moderate to severe endometriosis can also be placed in a reversible state of **pseudomenopause** with the use of danazol (Danocrine), an androgen derivative, or gonadotropin-releasing hormone (GnRH) agonists such as leuprolide acetate (Lupron) and nafarelin (Synarel). Both classes of drugs suppress follicle-stimulating hormone (FSH) and luteinizing hormone (LH). As a result, the ovaries do not produce estrogen, resulting in decreased stimulation of endometrial implants. Subsequently, existing endometrial **implants atrophy**, and new implants are **prevented**. More recently, **aromatase inhibitors** such as anastrozole (Arimidex) and letrozole (Femara) have been used *off-label* to treat severe

TABLE 15-1 Classification of Endometriosis

Tube		**American Society for Reproductive Medicine Revised Classification of Endometriosis**			
		Patient's name______________ Date ______________			
		Stage I (minimal) 1–5			
		Stage II (mild) 6–15 Laparoscopy __________ Laparotomy __________			
		Photography______________			
		Stage III (moderate) 16–40 Recommend treatment ______________			
		Stage IV (severe) >40 ______________			
		Total______________ Prognosis ______________			
Ovary		**Endometriosis**	**<1 cm**	**1–3 cm**	**<3 cm**
		Superficial	1	2	4
		Deep	2	4	6
	R	Superficial	1	2	4
		Deep	4	16	20
	L	Superficial	1	2	4
		Deep	4	16	20
		Posterior	Partial		Complete
		Cul-de-sac			
		Obliteration	4		40
Ovary		**Adhesions**	**<1/3 Enclosure**	**1/3–2/3 Enclosure**	**>2/3 Enclosure**
	R	Filmy	1	2	4
		Dense	4	8	16
	L	Filmy	1	2	4
		Dense	4	8	16
	R	Filmy	1	2	4
		Dense	4[a]	8[a]	16
	L	Filmy	1	2	4
Peritoneum		Dense	4[a]	8[a]	16

Denote appearance of superficial implant types as red ([R], red, red-pink, flame-like, vesicular blobs, clear vesicles), white ([W], opacifications, peritoneal defects, yellow-brown), or black ([B] black, hemosiderin deposits, blue). Denote percent of total described as R__%, W__%, and B__%. Total should equal 100%.

[a]If the fimbriated end of the fallopian tube is completely enclosed, change the point assignment to 16.

endometriosis. These medications lower circulating estrogen levels by blocking conversion of androgens to estrogens in the ovary, brain, and periphery. These have not been approved for use in endometriosis, can cause bone loss, hot flashes, and nausea and vomiting, and must be used with combination OCPs or GnRH agonists to prevent development of follicular cysts.

Side effects associated with OCPs and progestin agents include irritability, depression, breakthrough bleeding, and bloating. The drawback to danazol is that patients may experience some **androgen-related, anabolic side effects** including acne, oily skin, weight gain, edema, hirsutism, and deepening of the voice. GnRH agonists such as Lupron result in **estrogen deficiency**. The side effects of these medications are similar to those seen during menopause including hot flashes, decreased bone density, headaches, and vaginal atrophy and dryness. Moreover, these treatments can be costly and often have limited insurance coverage. Therefore, the use of these medications is generally limited to 6 months.

Fortunately, newer treatment regimens known as **add-back therapy** have been designed for use in conjunction with GnRH agonists. These regimens add a small amount of progestin with or without estrogen to the GnRH agonist to minimize the symptoms caused by estrogen deficiency such as hot flashes and bone density loss. With add-back therapy, the patient receives the benefits of the GnRH agonist (endometriosis suppression and relief of pelvic pain and dysmenorrhea) while the small dose of progestin with or without estrogen minimizes the adverse effects of hypoestrogenation allowing the treatment to be continued up to 1 year.

Women with advanced endometriosis, endometriomas, and infertility may be best served by surgical management. Surgical treatment for endometriosis can be classified as either conservative or definitive. **Conservative surgical therapy** typically

TABLE 15-2 Conception Rates after Ablation of Endometrial Implants

Extent of Disease	Stage of Disease	Conception Rates (in %)
Mild	1 & 2	75
Moderate	3	50–60
Severe	4	30–40

involves laparoscopy and fulguration or excision of any visible endometrial implants. Endometriomas are best treated using laparoscopic cystectomy with removal of as much of the cyst wall as possible (Fig. 15-4). With conservative therapy, the uterus and ovaries are left in situ. For these women, the pregnancy rate after conservative surgical treatment depends on the extent of the disease at the time of surgery (Table 15-2). For patients with pain who do not desire immediate pregnancy, pain control can be optimized and recurrences delayed by starting or **restarting medical therapy** immediately after surgical treatment.

Definitive surgical therapy includes total hysterectomy and bilateral salpingo-oophorectomy (by abdominal or laparoscopic approach), lysis of adhesions, and removal of any visible endometriosis lesions. This therapy is reserved for cases in which childbearing is complete and for women with severe disease or symptoms that are refractory to conservative medical or surgical treatment. If postsurgical **hormone replacement therapy** is started after hysterectomy and oophorectomy, some providers will still employ combination hormone therapy due to the theoretical possibility of stimulating transformation of residual implants into an endometrial cancer by the use of estrogen-only replacement therapy.

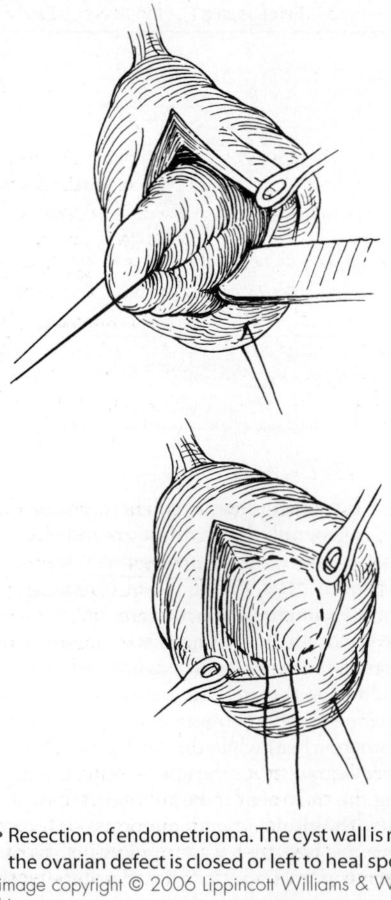

Figure 15-4 • Resection of endometrioma. The cyst wall is removed and the ovarian defect is closed or left to heal spontaneously.

ADENOMYOSIS

PATHOGENESIS

Adenomyosis is an **extension of endometrial tissue (glands and stroma) into the uterine myometrium** (Fig. 15-5). In the past, adenomyosis was referred to as *endometriosis interna*. This terminology is no longer used because adenomyosis and endometriosis are two distinct and different clinical entities (Table 15-3).

The cause of adenomyosis is not known. A current theory is that high levels of estrogen stimulate **hyperplasia of the basalis layer of the endometrium**. For unknown reasons, the barrier between the endometrium and myometrium is broken and the endometrial cells can then invade the myometrium. Because this disease occurs most frequently in parous women, it is thought that subclinical endomyometritis may be the first insult to the endometrial–myometrial barrier and eventually predisposes the myometrium to subsequent invasion. Another theory is that adenomyosis develops de novo from **metaplastic transformation** of müllerian rests cells located within the myometrium.

TABLE 15-3 Terminology of Aberrant Endometrial and Myometrial Tissue

Adenomyosis	An extension of endometrial tissue into the uterine myometrium leading to abnormal bleeding and pain. The uterus becomes soft, globular. Progestin-containing IUD and hysterectomy are the most effective means of treatment.
Adenomyoma	A well-circumscribed collection of endometrial tissue within the uterine wall. They may also contain smooth muscle cells and are not encapsulated. Adenomyomas can also prolapse into the endometrial cavity similar to a classic endometrial polyp.
Endometriosis	The presence of endometrial cells outside the uterine cavity. The hallmark of this chronic disease is cyclic pelvic pain. These estrogen-sensitive lesions can be treated with NSAIDs, OCPs, progestins, GnRH agonists, or surgery.
Endometrioma	A cystic collection of endometrial cells, old blood, and menstrual debris on the ovary; also known as "chocolate cysts."
Leiomyoma	Local proliferations of smooth muscle cells within the myometrium, often surrounded by a pseudocapsule. Also known as fibroids, these benign growths may be located on the intramural, subserosal, or submucosal portion of the uterus.

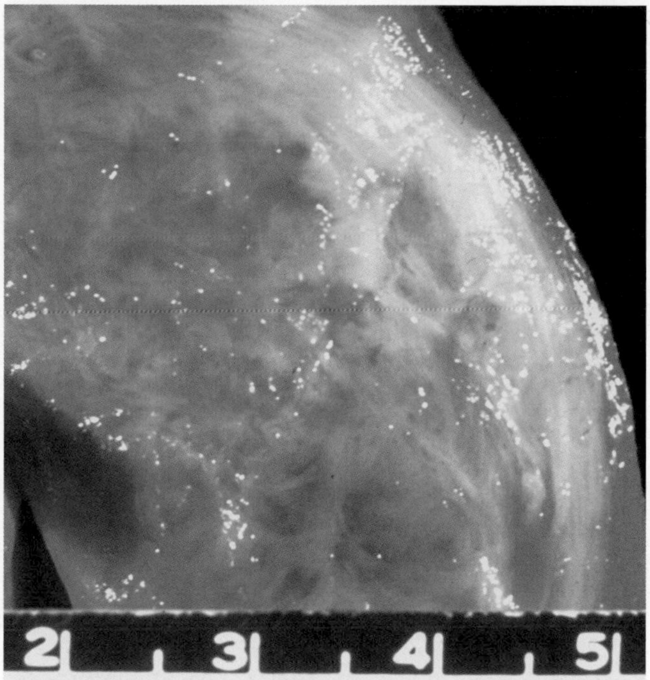

Figure 15-5 • Adenomyosis.
(From Rubin E, Farber JL. *Pathology*, 3rd ed. Philadelphia, PA: Lippincott Williams & Wilkins; 1999.)

Adenomyosis causes the uterus to become diffusely enlarged and globular due to **hypertrophy and hyperplasia** of the myometrium *adjacent to* the ectopic endometrial tissue. The disease is usually most extensive in the **fundus and posterior uterine wall**. Because the endometrial tissue in adenomyosis extends from the basalis layer of the endometrium, it does not undergo the proliferative and secretory changes traditionally seen in normally located endometrium or in endometriosis. Thus, unlike endometriosis, which contains both glandular and stromal endometrial tissue, adenomyosis is **less responsive to treatment with OCPs or other hormonal treatments**.

Adenomyosis may also present as a well-circumscribed, isolated region known as an **adenomyoma**. Adenomyomas contain smooth muscle cells as well as endometrial glands and stroma. These nodular growths may be located in the myometrium or extend into the endometrial cavity. Unlike uterine fibroids, which have a characteristic pseudocapsule, individual areas of adenomyosis are not encapsulated. Instead, adenomyosis can infiltrate throughout the myometrium giving the uterus a characteristic boggy feel on palpation.

EPIDEMIOLOGY

The incidence of adenomyosis is generally estimated to be about 20%. However, 40 - 65% of hysterectomy specimens contain some evidence of adenomyosis. Adenomyosis generally develops in parous women in their late 30s or early 40s. It occurs very infrequently in nulliparous women.

RISK FACTORS

Adenomyosis, endometriosis, and uterine fibroids frequently coexist. About 15% to 20% of patients with adenomyosis also have **endometriosis**, and 50% to 60% of patients with adenomyosis also have **uterine fibroids**. Patients with dyspareunia, dyschezia, and menorrhagia or menometrorrhagia have an increased probability of having adenomyosis.

CLINICAL MANIFESTATIONS

History

Thirty percent of patients with adenomyosis are **asymptomatic** or have symptoms minor enough that medical attention is not sought. Symptomatic adenomyosis occurs most often in parous women between age 35 and 50. When symptoms do occur, the most common are **secondary dysmenorrhea** (30%), **menorrhagia** (50%), or both (20%). Patients typically present with increasingly heavy or prolonged menstrual bleeding (menorrhagia). They may also complain of increasingly severe dysmenorrhea that may begin up to 1 week before menses and last until cessation of bleeding. Other patients may only experience pressure on the bladder or rectum due to an enlarged uterus.

Physical Examination

The pelvic examination of a patient with adenomyosis may reveal a **diffusely enlarged globular uterus**. The uterus is usually less than 14 cm. The consistency of the uterus is typically softer and boggier than the firmer, rubbery uterus containing fibroids. The adenomyomatous uterus may be mildly tender just before or during menses but should have normal mobility and no associated adnexal pathology.

DIAGNOSTIC EVALUATION

Prior to treating adenomyosis, any patient age 45 or older with change in menstrual quantity or pattern should have a TSH, pelvic ultrasound, and an endometrial biopsy to rule out other causes of abnormal uterine bleeding. **MRI is the most accurate imaging tool** for identifying adenomyosis. However, because the cost of MRI can be prohibitive, pelvic ultrasound is the most common imaging modality. MRI is then used if adenomyosis is suggested by **pelvic ultrasound** by an indistinct endometrial-myometrial junction or glandular tissue within the myometrium. This is usually reserved for situations where myomectomy is being planned and it is important to distinguish adenomyosis from uterine fibroids. Ultimately, hysterectomy is the only definitive means of diagnosing adenomyosis.

DIFFERENTIAL DIAGNOSIS

The differential diagnosis for adenomyosis includes disease processes resulting in uterine enlargement, menorrhagia, and/or dysmenorrhea including uterine fibroids, polyps, menstrual disorders, endometrial hyperplasia, endometrial cancer, pregnancy, and adnexal masses.

TREATMENT

The treatment for adenomyosis depends on the severity of the dysmenorrhea and menorrhagia. Women with minimal symptoms or those near menopause may be expectantly managed or managed with analgesics alone. Nonsteroidal anti-inflammatory drugs (**NSAIDs**), cyclic or continuous **estrogen–progestin contraceptives** (pills, patches, rings) and menstrual suppression with **progestins** (oral, injectable, or intrauterine) have also been found to be temporarily helpful. Short-term relief has also been achieved using **endometrial ablation;** however, pain and bleeding recur more frequently when adenomyosis is involved. The **levonorgetrel-containing IUD** has been found to be the most effective temporary means of managing the symptoms of adenomyosis.

Hysterectomy is the only definitive treatment for adenomyosis. Endometrial biopsy should be performed to rule out concomitant endometrial hyperplasia and cancer in women >45 before a hysterectomy is performed for adenomyosis. Prior to the surgery, it also is particularly important to distinguish adenomyosis from uterine fibroids. If adenomyosis is mistaken for uterine fibroids, a surgeon attempting a myomectomy may find only diffuse adenomyosis and be forced to perform a hysterectomy instead.

KEY POINTS

- Endometriosis is the presence of endometrial tissue outside the endometrial cavity, most often in the ovary or pelvic peritoneum. It occurs in 10% to 15% of women of reproductive age.
- The hallmark of endometriosis is cyclic pelvic pain, which is at its worst 1 to 2 days before menses and subsides at the onset of flow or shortly thereafter.
- The severity of symptoms of (dysmenorrhea, dyspareunia, abnormal bleeding, and infertility) may not correlate with extent of disease.
- Complications of endometriosis include intra-abdominal inflammation and bleeding that can cause scarring, pain, and adhesion formation, which can lead to infertility and chronic pelvic pain.
- Direct visualization with diagnostic laparoscopy or laparotomy (preferably with histologic confirmation with biopsy) is the only way to definitively diagnose endometriosis.
- Endometriosis can be treated medically (NSAIDs, OCPs, progestins, danazol, GnRH agonists) to reduce pain, but these methods are used mainly as temporizing agents.
- There is no role for the use of medical management in patients trying to conceive or those diagnosed with infertility.
- Endometriosis can be treated surgically with conservative therapy to ablate implants and lyse adhesions while preserving the uterus and ovaries. Surgery should be followed immediately by medical therapy to delay the recurrence of endometrial implants and pain.
- Endometriosis can be treated definitively with surgery, including total hysterectomy (often with bilateral salpingo-oophorectomy) lysis of adhesions, and removal of endometriosis lesions.
- Adenomyosis is the extension of endometrial tissue into the myometrium making the uterus diffusely enlarged, boggy, and globular. It occurs in 20% of women, most of whom are parous and in their late 30s or early 40s.
- Patients typically present with increasing secondary dysmenorrhea and/or menorrhagia; 30% of patients are asymptomatic.
- Adenomyosis may be suggested on pelvic ultrasound. MRI can best distinguish between adenomyosis and fibroids. Patients age 45 and older with abnormal uterine bleeding should also have an endometrial biopsy to rule out hyperplasia and cancer.
- Minimal symptoms may be treated with analgesics, NSAIDs, OCPs, or progestins, although adenomyosis is less responsive to hormonal management than endometriosis.
- The levonorgestrel-containing IUD is the most effective temporary means of treating the symptoms of adenomyosis.
- Hysterectomy is the only definitive means of definitively diagnosing and treating adenomyosis.

C Clinical Vignettes

Vignette 1

A 23-year-old G0 woman presents complaining of increasing pelvic pain with her menses over the last year since she stopped her OCPs. In particular, she has noticed more pain on her left side in the last couple of months. She denies any changes in her bladder or bowel habits but reports that she has begun to have pain with deep penetration during intercourse. She started OCPs when she was 17 for painful irregular cycles but stopped them a year ago when her insurance changed. She has had only one lifetime sexual partner and no history of sexually transmitted infections. She would like to preserve fertility. On examination, she has no abnormal discharge but her uterus is tender as well as her left adnexa. You appreciate a fullness that you suspect may be a mass. On pelvic ultrasound she has a 5 cm cystic ovarian mass thought to be an endometrioma. It persists in repeat ultrasound 8 weeks later and the patient is still symptomatic.

1. What would be the most appropriate next step in her care?
   a. Resume an oral contraceptive
   b. Schedule diagnostic laparoscopy with left ovarian cystectomy
   c. Prescribe an NSAID for her pain and repeat the ultrasound in 6 to 8 weeks
   d. Prescribe a GNRH agonist (i.e., Depo-Lupron)
   e. Refer her to a gynecologic oncologist

2. You perform a laparoscopic left ovarian cystectomy and note that the cyst is a "chocolate cyst." She also has other superficial implants of endometriosis on the uterosacral ligaments. The final pathology report is consistent with an endometrioma. At your patient's postoperative visit 2 weeks after surgery she tells you that her pain is resolved and she is feeling well. What do you recommend for the continued postoperative management of her endometriosis?
   a. Because endometriosis cannot be cured medically, she should undergo total hysterectomy with bilateral salpingo-oophorectomy
   b. You were able to completely remove the cyst, so she does not need any further therapy at this time
   c. Wait 6 months and then schedule a repeat laparoscopy to make sure there is no further endometriosis that needs to be treated
   d. Initiate therapy with a combined oral contraceptive or a progestin to delay the return of her previous symptoms
   e. Endometrial ablation because that will destroy her endometrium and decrease the risk of new implants developing from retrograde menstruation

3. Your patient would like to know more about the GnRH agonist, Lupron. You explain how it works and that the side effects include all of the following *except*:
   a. hot flashes
   b. headaches
   c. decreased bone density
   d. weight gain
   e. deepening of the voice

Vignette 2

A couple presents because they have been trying to conceive for 18 months. During the interview you learn that the man has fathered a child in a previous relationship and is in good health. The woman is 28 and reports that she has had painful menses for the past 5 or 6 years.

1. You begin to suspect that she may have endometriosis. All of information below would increase that suspicion *except*:
   a. she reports that a maternal cousin has a history of endometriosis
   b. she has experienced dyspareunia with deep penetration for several years
   c. her ethnicity is Caucasian
   d. she report the development of abnormal bleeding in the last year
   e. her menarche began at age 9

2. After completing your history you explain to your patient that you need to perform an examination before making any recommendations. You explain that women with endometriosis often have a normal examination but that there are certain findings that are associated with endometriosis. During your examination, which of the findings listed below would NOT increase your suspicion that she has endometriosis.
   a. A fixed deviated uterus
   b. Uterosacral nodularity on rectovaginal examination
   c. Tender adnexa
   d. An enlarged irregular uterus
   e. A fixed adnexal mass

3. After your examination where you did find uterosacral nodularity, you discuss with your patient your concern that she has endometriosis. You recommend that as part of her continued evaluation and treatment for infertility that she undergoes a diagnostic laparoscopy with ablation or excision of endometriosis if it is found. Your patient is very concerned about the diagnosis and wonders

what percent of women with infertility have endometriosis. You tell her:
a. 10%
b. 30%
c. 50%
d. 70%
e. 90%

Vignette 3

A 46-year-old G2P2 obese woman is referred from her primary care physician because of increasingly heavy and painful menses over the last 18 months. She has tried an oral contraceptive with some improvement of her bleeding but no improvement in her pain. She reports no other history of pelvic pain or abnormal bleeding in the past. She has never had an abnormal Pap smear and states she has never had any infections, "down there." Her only medical problems are her obesity, hypertension and gastroesophageal reflux disease. On examination, you note normal external genitalia, vagina, and cervix. However, her uterus is slightly enlarged, mildly tender, and softer than you expected. She has no adnexal mass or tenderness.

1. Which of these diagnoses is the least likely choice to keep in your differential?
a. Leiomyoma
b. Adenomyosis
c. Irritable bowel syndrome
d. Endometrial hyperplasia
e. Endometriosis

2. You explain to your patient that you think she may have adenomyosis and that it is most likely causing her symptoms. However, you would like to make sure whether or not she has fibroids as well. You explain that she will need an imaging study to help clarify this. Which study listed below would best differentiate between adenomyosis and uterine fibroids?
a. Pelvic ultrasound
b. Pelvic CT
c. Sonohysterogram
d. Pelvic MRI
e. Hysterosalpingogram

3. After further evaluation suggesting adenomyosis, your patient wants to proceed with hysterectomy because she is tired of bleeding and experiencing pain. You explain to her that she needs to undergo a test prior to scheduling her hysterectomy. What test does the patient need to undergo?
a. Wet prep
b. Endometrial biopsy
c. Mammogram
d. Colonoscopy
e. Chest X-ray

Vignette 4

A 38-year-old G3P3 woman with 12 months of increasingly heavy menses and worsening dysmenorrhea comes to you for a second opinion. She underwent a pelvic ultrasound that suggested adenomyosis and her gynecologist recommended a hysterectomy. She states that she does not trust the ultrasound results and wants to know if there is anything else that can be done to confirm the diagnosis.

1. What would be the most appropriate next step?
a. Review the ultrasound results and reassure her that her gynecologist is correct
b. Repeat the pelvic ultrasound
c. Tell her that hysterectomy is the only thing that will help to clarify her diagnosis
d. Suggest a 3-month trial of an oral contraceptive pill
e. Examine her and recommend obtaining a pelvic MRI

2. After you complete your evaluation, you agree that she likely has adenomyosis. She is very busy with work right now and wants to avoid surgery for several months. You recommend one or a combination of the options listed *except*:
a. Levonorgestrel-containing IUD
b. NSAID
c. oral contraceptive pill
d. progestin therapy
e. doxycycline for 14 days

3. When discussing hysterectomy and the timing for surgery, she tells you that she has a younger sister who is a 29-year-old G0. Your patient would like to know if her younger sister is likely to develop adenomyosis and subsequent menorrhagia and dysmenorrhea. You explain that all of the following may increase the risk for developing adenomyosis *except*:
a. parous women
b. fibroids
c. endometriosis
d. menopause
e. age 30 to 50

A Answers

Vignette 1 Question 1
Answer B: This patient's history, examination, and ultrasound findings are consistent with endometriosis. Because of her significant symptoms and the findings of a persistent endometrioma, laparoscopy with planned cystectomy is the best option for her. Large endometriomas are not likely to resolve on their own with time in contrast with functional ovarian cysts. They are also unlikely to respond to medical management with an oral contraceptive or GNRH agonist. In this young woman with findings consistent with an endometrioma, referral to an oncologist would not be necessary because of low risk of malignancy and because sensitivity with ultrasound to correctly diagnose endometriomas is high.

Vignette 1 Question 2
Answer D: For patients with pain who do not desire pregnancy, pain control can be optimized and recurrence delayed by starting medical therapy immediately after surgical treatment. For patients who desire fertility in the future, hysterectomy is not an appropriate option. Even though removal of the cyst significantly decreases the risk of endometrioma recurrence, the patient is at increased risk of developing the return of her symptoms and new implants with expectant management compared to medical therapy to suppress recurrent endometriosis and symptoms. Because of the risks of surgery and unlikely return of symptoms within 6 months, medical therapy would be the most appropriate initial step. Endometrial ablation is not recommended for those desiring pregnancy in the future and has not been shown to decrease the risk of recurrent symptoms from endometriosis.

Vignette 1 Question 3
Answer E: Deepening of the voice occurs with an androgen derivative, danazol, which initiates a pseudomenopause state. However, this symptom is not associated with the GnRH agonists. Hot flashes, headaches, decreased bone density, and weight gain can all occur secondary to GnRH agonists such as Lupron that initiate a medical pseudomenopause and create a relatively estrogen deficient state, which helps to prevent the development of new foci of endometriosis.

Vignette 2 Question 1
Answer A: Genetic factors probably are associated with the risk of developing endometriosis and an increased risk of developing endometriosis has been observed in first-degree relatives. However, this association has not been observed in third-degree relatives. Other risk factors include Caucasian ethnicity as compared to black or Asian ethnicity and early menarche. The report of deep dyspareunia, dysmenorrhea, and abnormal menstrual bleeding are all symptoms that are associated with endometriosis.

Vignette 2 Question 2
Answer D: An enlarged irregular uterus is typically associated with leiomyomas and not necessarily with endometriosis, although the two can be found concomitantly. Physical findings with early stage endometriosis can be subtle or nonexistent. However, with more disseminated disease a clinician may find uterosacral nodularity on rectovaginal examination, a fixed often retroverted uterus, tender adnexa, and/or a fixed adnexal mass when a large endometrioma is present.

Vignette 2 Question 3
Answer B: Approximately 30% to 40% of women who have infertility also have the diagnosis of endometriosis. The overall incidence of endometriosis in the US population is thought to be approximately 10% to 15%.

Vignette 3 Question 1
Answer C: Although irritable bowel syndrome is associated with pelvic pain and is likely underdiagnosed, it is not associated with menorrhagia or dysmenorrhea in particular. Leiomyomas are commonly associated with menorrhagia and sometimes dysmenorrhea. Two of the hallmarks for adenomyosis are menorrhagia and dysmenorrhea especially when it develops in women who are 30 to 50 years of age. Endometrial hyperplasia must be considered in an obese woman with hypertension and abnormal bleeding, especially if she is older than 45 years. Endometriosis would be less likely due to the age at which the onset of symptoms of abnormal bleeding and dysmenorrhea started. Typically these begin to present in the second and third decade. However, adenomyosis, endometriosis, and leiomyomas often coexist.

Vignette 3 Question 2
Answer D: Pelvic MRI is the most accurate imaging tool for identifying adenomyosis. Because the cost of MRI can be prohibitive, ultrasound is the most common means of diagnosis. If there is difficulty in differentiating between uterine fibroids and adenomyosis, then MRI is used. CT imaging is not a helpful tool in evaluating for adenomyosis. Sonohysterography is typically used to screen for intracavitary lesions such as endometrial polyps or submucosal fibroids. Hysterosalpingography is typically used to evaluate the uterine cavity and the patency of the fallopian tubes.

Vignette 3 Question 3

Answer B: Because of her abnormal bleeding and age older than 45 and obesity, endometrial biopsy should be performed prior to scheduling hysterectomy to rule out concomitant endometrial hyperplasia or carcinoma. A screening wet prep is not necessary prior to hysterectomy and only needs to be performed if the patient is complaining of symptoms consistent with bacterial vaginosis. Mammography is suggested every 1 to 2 years for women in their 40s but is not required prior to scheduling a hysterectomy. Routine colo-rectal cancer screening with colonoscopy begins at age 50. The patient is not having other symptoms that would require a colonoscopy. Routine chest X-rays are not necessary prior to a major gynecologic procedure and should be reserved for those where there is concern for cardiopulmonary disease.

Vignette 4 Question 1

Answer E: Both the examination and the pelvic MRI can increase or decrease the likelihood of adenomyosis and would be the most appropriate next step. Repeat ultrasound is unlikely to add new information to the initial ultrasound. Although hysterectomy may be eventually necessary and ultimately provides tissue to make the definitive diagnosis, MRI is a noninvasive method that is fairly sensitive in this patient looking for a second opinion. An oral contraceptive is used for a number of conditions including adenomyosis. A response or lack of response to it would not necessarily help clarify the diagnosis of adenomyosis.

Vignette 4 Question 2

Answer E: If you suspected an underlying chronic endometritis or if endometritis was found on endometrial biopsy, then doxycycline may be appropriate. It would not typically be effective for management of her menorrhagia and dysmenorrhea for NSAIDs can be used alone with mild symptoms or in combination with either an oral contraceptive or a progestin. Other than hysterectomy, the levonorgestrel-containing IUD is the most effective treatments for treating the symptoms of adenomyosis.

Vignette 4 Question 3

Answer D: Menopause is not associated with the development of adenomyosis and often symptoms related to adenomyosis will resolve at menopause. Women in their late reproductive years who are parous have an increased risk compared with younger nulliparous women. Endometriosis and fibroids have also been associated with adenomyosis.

Chapter 16 Infections of the Lower Female Reproductive Tract

URINARY TRACT INFECTIONS

Urinary tract infections (UTIs) are one of the most common infections of the lower genitourinary tract treated by clinicians. Approximately 50% of women will be diagnosed with a UTI during their lives and at an incidence of approximately 1% per year in adult women; 5% will have recurrent episodes. Women commonly present with symptoms of urethritis (discomfort or pain at the urethral meatus or a burning sensation throughout the urethra with micturition) or cystitis (pain in the midline suprapubic region and/or frequent urination). UTIs are most common in sexually active women, and increased in women with obesity, increasing age, anatomic or neurologic abnormalities, diabetes mellitus, and sickle cell disease. The rates are higher in women than men secondary to the shorter length of the urethra and its proximity to the vagina and rectum.

DIAGNOSIS

When a woman presents with dysuria, urinary urgency, and frequency, the diagnosis of UTI should lead the differential. A clean voided midstream urine sample can be sent for urinalysis and microscopic examination. Hematuria, leukocytes, leukocyte esterase, or nitrates in the absence of a vaginal infection are indicative of a UTI. Microscopic bacteruria without the presence of inflammatory cells or in the presence of squamous epithelial cell is most likely contamination. To distinguish contamination from true infection, the urinalysis and microscopic examination can be repeated with urine collected via catheterization. Patients are often diagnosed and treated for UTI in the setting of a positive urinalysis with concomitant symptoms of dysuria and urinary frequency once **pyelonephritis** is ruled out with evaluation for fevers and costovertebral angle tenderness (CVAT). The diagnosis of a UTI can be confirmed with a urine culture, but is not required in uncomplicated cases. Approximately 80% to 85% of UTIs are caused by *Escherichia coli* and other organisms that colonize the GI tract. Other common organisms that cause UTIs are *Staphylococcus saprophyticus*, *Proteus mirabilis*, *Klebsiella pneumoniae*, and *Enterococcus*. If the urine culture is negative, the diagnosis should be reconsidered. In patients with symptoms consistent with urethritis, organisms such as *Chlamydia trachomatis* and *Neisseria gonorrhoeae* should be considered and screened for using a midstream collection. Another etiology of urethritis is herpes simplex virus (HSV) infection. In patients with symptoms of cystitis, but a negative culture, the diagnosis of overactive bladder or painful bladder syndrome (interstitial cystitis) should be entertained.

TREATMENT

Most uncomplicated UTIs can be treated with oral antibiotics. It is important to both begin treatment on initial diagnosis as well as follow-up culture sensitivities to be certain that the pathologic organisms are treated adequately. Initial treatment is often begun with trimethoprim-sulfamethoxazole, nitrofurantoin, or a fluoroquinolone for 3 to 7 days. Ampicillin or cephalexin has also been used; however, more recently, beta-lactams have become less effective in the treatment of uncomplicated UTIs. The local sensitivities of common organisms should be known. For example, the rates of ampicillin-resistant *E. coli* can range from 5% to 35% in different hospitals. Patients with symptoms consistent with pyelonephritis are usually treated as an inpatient with IV antibiotics. Outpatient management has been studied and is used increasingly in reliable patients without other medical issues. A 14-day antimicrobial therapy should be completed.

THE EXTERNAL ANOGENITAL REGION

Various infectious diseases affect the external genitalia. In the female patient, the entire perianal area and mons should be considered in addition to the vulva. The skin overlying these areas is subject to the same infections that can occur anywhere on the epidermis, but the exposure and environment differ and must be considered when discussing these infections. There are also a variety of focal and systemic processes that can cause lesions or symptoms in this region. Anogenital lesions are usually categorized as ulcerative or nonulcerative and common symptoms include pain and itching.

VULVITIS

The most common cause of vulvitis, and usually of vulvar pruritus, is **candidiasis**. It is also a common cause of vaginitis and is discussed in greater detail later in this chapter. A candidal vulvitis usually presents with vulvar erythema, pruritus, and small satellite lesions. If the vulvitis does not respond to the usual treatment with topical or systemic antifungals, symptoms may be due to other causes such as allergic reaction, chemical or fabric irritants, and vulvar dystrophies. Malignancy should always be ruled out in the setting of chronic vulvar irritation.

ULCERATED LESIONS

Many primary vulvar ulcers are caused by sexually transmitted infections (STIs) (Table 16-1) such as **herpes**, **syphilis**, **chancroid**, and **lymphogranuloma venereum**. However, even with a diagnosis of an infectious process, these lesions can be

TABLE 16-1 Infectious Causes of Ulcerated Lesions

	Syphilis	Herpes	Chancroid	LGV
Incubation period (days)	7–14	2–10	4–7	3–12
Primary lesion	Papule	Vesicle	Papule/pustule	Papule/vesicle
Number of lesions	Single	Multiple	1–3, occasionally more	Single
Size (mm)	5–15	1–3	2–20	2–10
Painful	No	Yes	Yes	No
Diagnostic test	Dark-field microscopy RPR/MHA-TP/ FTA-ABS	Viral culture	Gram stain with "school of fish" appearance	Complement fixation
Treatment	Penicillin	Acyclovir	Ceftriaxone or azithromycin	Doxycycline

associated with malignant processes as well. Up to 25% of patients with genital ulcers will not have a laboratory-confirmed diagnosis. Treatment should be based on presentation and clinical findings.

There are conditions other than infections that can lead to vulvar ulcerations. Crohn's disease can have linear "knife cut" vulvar ulcers as its first manifestation, preceding gastrointestinal or other systemic manifestations by months to years. Behçet disease leads to tender and highly destructive vulvar lesions that often cause fenestrations in the labia and extensive scarring.

SYPHILIS

Syphilis is a chronic systemic infection caused by the spirochete ***Treponema pallidum***. It is transmitted primarily through direct sexual contact; however, infections can also occur transplacentally during pregnancy. The incidence of primary and secondary syphilis in the United States increased through the 1980s until 1990, when the CDC noted a peak of 50,578 reported cases followed by an almost 90% decrease between 1990 and 2000 to 5,979 reported cases. Unfortunately, between 2001 and 2009 there has been a steady increase in reported cases of primary and secondary syphilis with 15,997 cases reported in 2009. However, 2009 also marked the first time in 5 years that the rate of primary and secondary syphilis decreased in women. Cases of congential syphilis also declined in 2009 (427 cases reported).

Syphilis is divided into different stages of disease to help guide treatment and follow up. *T. pallidum* most likely enters the body through minute abrasions in the skin or mucosal surface and replicates locally. Initial lesions therefore commonly occur on the vulva, vagina, cervix, anus, nipples, or lips. The initial lesion that characterizes primary syphilis is a painless, red, round, firm ulcer approximately 1 cm in size with raised edges known as a **chancre** (Fig. 16-1). It develops approximately 3 weeks after inoculation and is usually associated with concomitant regional adenopathy. The lesions develop primarily from the patient's immune response and will heal without therapy. Material expressed from the chancre usually reveals motile spirochetes under dark-field microscopy.

Secondary syphilis is a systemic disease that occurs as *T. pallidum* disseminates and begins around 1 to 3 months after the primary stage resolves. Patients typically develop flu-like symptoms with fever and myalgias. Classically, a maculopapular rash may appear on the palms of the hands or soles of the feet. Moist papules and mucous patches can also occur. The dermatologic manifestations of secondary syphilis are why syphilis is known as the "great imitator." There may be other organ system involvement with meningitis, osteitis, nephritis, or hepatitis. All lesions resolve spontaneously, and this stage can be entirely asymptomatic. After resolution of this stage, the infection enters a latent phase that can last for years. Latent syphilis is further divided as early (acquired <1 year) or late (acquired >1 year) based on the time of initial symptoms.

Tertiary syphilis is quite uncommon today but is characterized by granulomas (gummas) of the skin and bones; cardiovascular syphilis with aortitis; and neurosyphilis with meningovascular disease, paresis, and tabes dorsalis.

Diagnosis

Screening for *T. pallidum* may be performed with nontreponemal anticardiolipin antibodies. Two types of nontreponemal serologic tests for syphilis are available: the Venereal Disease Research Laboratory (VDRL) test and the rapid plasma reagin (RPR) test. These tests remain positive for 6 to 12 months after treatment of primary syphilis, usually with progressively decreasing antibody titers. In primary syphilis, serologic assays may be negative during early infection, resulting in a lower sensitivity. These tests will become positive several weeks after the initial visit, and should therefore be repeated 1 and 3 months after appearance of the ulcer in the compliant patient in whom the diagnosis cannot be made at first presentation. False-positive nontreponemal tests can occur with various autoimmune conditions, other infections, malignancy, pregnancy, and IV drug use. Therefore, a positive result must be confirmed with specific treponemal antibody studies, such as the fluorescent treponemal antibody absorption (FTA-ABS) test and the *Treponema pallidum* particle agglutination assay (TPPA). The microhemagglutination test for antibodies to *Treponema pallidum* (MHA-TP) is no longer available in the United States. False-positive results in confirmatory testing occur less than 1% of the time. Primary, secondary, tertiary, and neurosyphilis can be diagnosed by the presenting signs and symptoms described above. However, patients who are asymptomatic with a positive titer are considered to be in early latent (acquired <1 year) or late latent (acquired >1 year) syphilis.

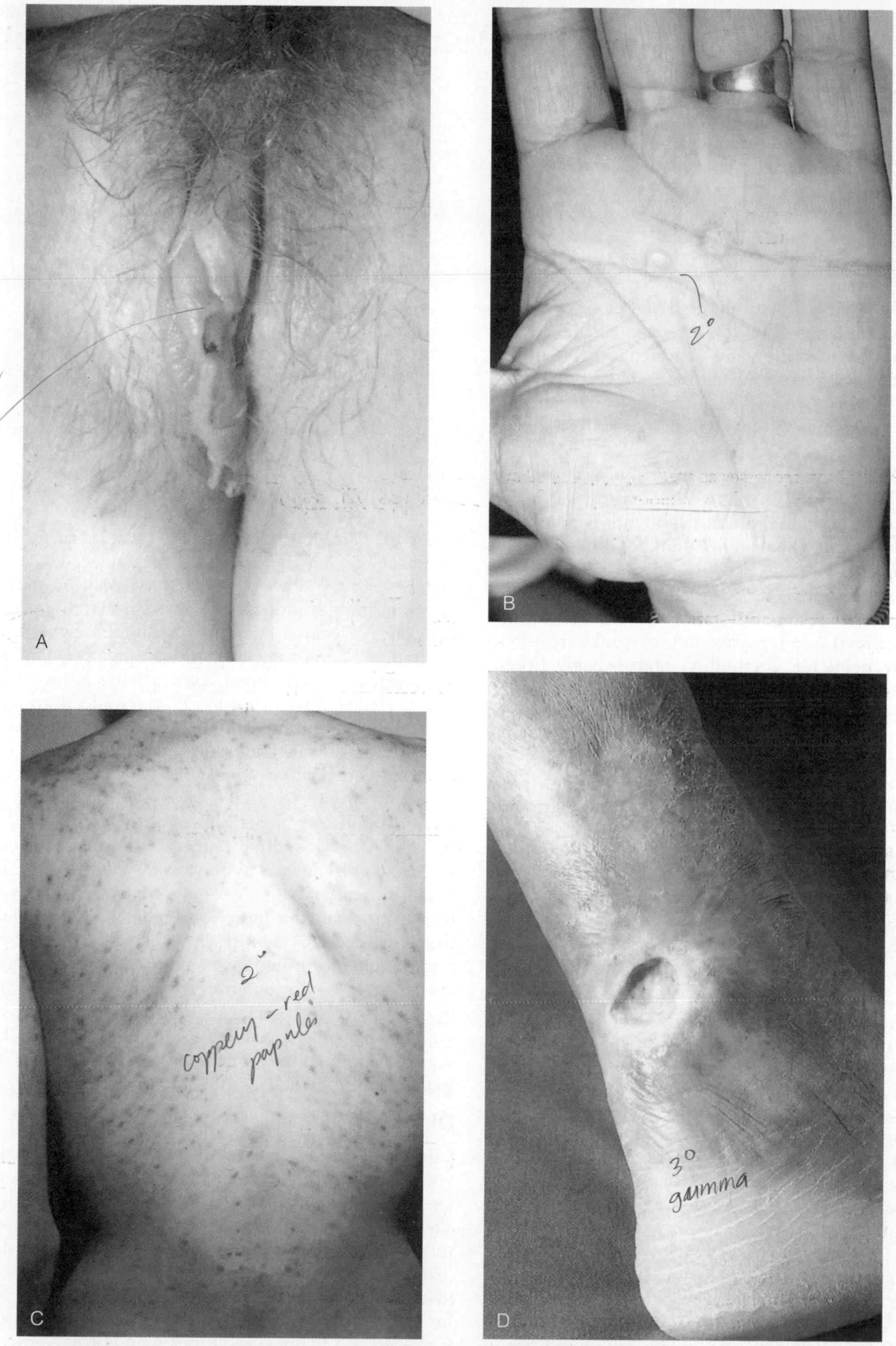

Figure 16-1 • (A) Slightly indurated primary chancre of 2 days' duration that was neither painful nor tender. It points to the need for a high index of suspicion concerning all genital lesions. Dark-filled microscopy prevents diagnostic error and embarrassment. (B) Papulosquamous secondary syphilis involving the palm. (C) Typical coppery-red papules in secondary syphilis. (D) Healing gumma. Delay in diagnosis is suggested by widespread pigmentation and scarring. Response to treatment was slow and the final scarring led to permanent edema of the foot, sometimes called paradoxical healing.
(Reproduced with permission from Champion RH. *Textbook of Dermatology*, 5th ed. Oxford: Blackwell Science; 1992:2852.)

Treatment

Penicillin remains the drug of choice for treatment of syphilis. Primary, secondary, or early latent syphilis can be treated with benzathine penicillin G, 2.4 million units IM one time. For late latent or latent of unknown duration syphilis, treatment consists of penicillin G 2.4 million units IM weekly for 3 weeks. For penicillin-allergic, nonpregnant patients with primary or secondary syphilis, several alternative regimens might be effective including doxycycline 100 mg orally twice a day for 14 days, tetracycline 500 mg orally four times a day for 14 days, ceftriaxone 1 g IM or IV daily for 10 to 14 days, or azithromycin 2 g single oral dose. However, data to support use of alternative regimens is still limited and close follow up is essential. If compliance is of concern in penicillin-allergic individuals, then desensitization and treatment with penicillin are recommended. Penicillin remains the only recommended treatment in pregnancy, with sufficient evidence demonstrating efficacy for preventing maternal syphilis transmission to the fetus and for treating fetal infection.

Neurosyphilis is a more serious infection and requires aqueous crystalline penicillin G, 3 to 4 million units IV every 4 hours for 10 to 14 days. In individuals in whom compliance may be ensured, procaine penicillin 2.4 million units IM once daily plus probenecid 500 mg orally four times a day both for 10 to 14 days is recommended as a treatment alternative for neurosyphilis. Some authorities further recommend following the recommended or alternative neurosyphilis treatment with benzathine penicillin 2.4 million units weekly IM for 3 weeks after completion of either regimen. Patients with a penicillin allergy in whom compliance issues are of concern will therefore require desensitization. Treatment success can be verified by following RPR or VDRL titers at 6, 12, and 24 months. Titers should decrease fourfold by 6 months and become nonreactive by 12 to 24 months after completion of treatment.

The Jarisch-Herxheimer reaction is an acute febrile reaction frequently accompanied by fever, chills, headache, myalgia, malaise, pharyngitis, rash, and other symptoms that usually occur within the first 24 hours (generally within the first 8 hours) after any therapy for syphilis. This reaction was initially recognized in the treatment of neurosyphilis, but can be seen with any syphilitic treatment, most commonly with early syphilis (up to 90% of patients with secondary syphilis). Antipyretics may be used, but they have not been proven to prevent this reaction. The Jarisch-Herxheimer reaction might induce preterm contractions or cause fetal distress in pregnant women, but this should not prevent or delay therapy. This transient inflammatory reaction is not considered a drug reaction, but is related to the treatment of syphilis, and can be seen with the treatment of other spirochetes as well, such as Lyme disease, when injured or dead organisms release endotoxins into the circulation marked by systemic release of cytokines.

GENITAL HERPES

Herpes simplex virus (HSV) infections are quite common in the perioral and genital regions. Although only about 5% of women report a history of genital herpes infection, as many as 25% to 30% have antibodies on serologic testing. Although some women have the classic severe presentation of genital herpes with painful genital ulcers, many women have a mild initial presentation or are entirely asymptomatic. Because of the asymptomatic nature of many initial presentations, it is difficult to get an estimate on the true incidence of disease; however, there has been a steady increase in patient visits to a clinician for herpes over the past two decades, with approximately 270,000 office visits in 2004. Although the majority of genital herpes lesions are caused by HSV-2, up to 80% of new cases of genital HSV are attributable to HSV-1, particularly among adolescent and young adult populations. HSV is transmitted through direct contact with an incubation period of 2 to 10 days after exposure. Primary infections usually begin with flulike symptoms including malaise, myalgias, nausea, diarrhea, and fever. Vulvar burning and pruritus precede the multiple vesicles that appear next and usually remain intact for 24 to 36 hours before evolving into painful genital ulcers (Fig. 16-2). These ulcers can require a mean of 10 to 22 days to heal. After this initial herpes outbreak, recurrent episodes can occur as frequently as one to six times per year. Recurrence is more frequent in HSV-2 infections. Symptoms tend to be less severe than the initial outbreak. It is important to note that subclinical or asymptomatic shedding can occur and is more frequent during the first 6 months after acquisition and immediately before or after recurrent outbreaks. Because of the possibility of frequent recurrence and the devastating consequences of neonatal herpes, pregnant women should have vaginal examinations around the time of delivery. Those with lesions should be delivered by cesarean delivery.

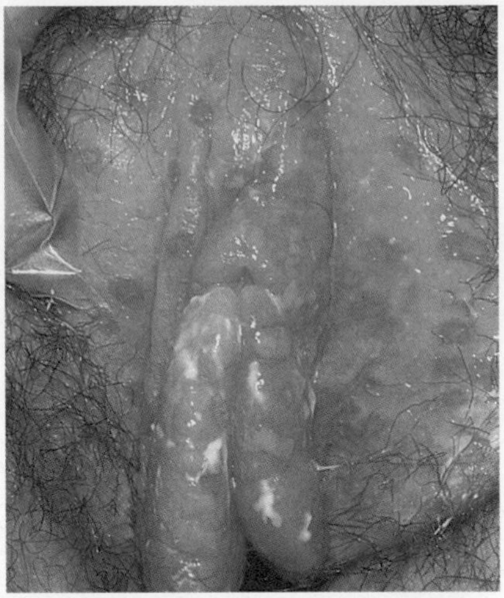

Figure 16-2 • Genital herpes.

HSV I now?

Diagnosis

Clinical diagnosis is often made with an examination of the vesicles and ulcers in conjunction with a sexual history. However, this modality has suboptimal sensitivity and specificity. Therefore, clinical diagnosis should be confirmed with laboratory testing. Viral cultures are used as the gold standard for diagnosis; however, sensitivity of culture is low, especially in recurrent or healing lesions. Although DNA PCR assays for HSV are more sensitive than culture, they are not FDA approved and many laboratories may not have this testing capacity. A **Tzanck smear** prepared of the lesions and examined for multinucleated giant cells with a characteristic appearance may reveal typical cytologic changes, but this study is also neither sensitive nor specific. Alternatively, type-specific antibodies for HSV-1 and HSV-2 IgG may be used to determine whether the patient has a primary infection as well as the serotype of the causative organism.

Treatment

Although many palliative treatments have evolved over the years such as sitz baths for comfort and analgesics to reduce the pain, there is no cure for herpes. For a **primary infection**, acyclovir 200 mg five times per day, acyclovir 400 mg three times per day, famciclovir 250 mg three times per day, or valacyclovir 1 g twice per day orally for 7 to 10 days are recommended therapies in treatment of first clinical outbreak reducing the length of infection and the length of time a patient has viral shedding. With severe HSV infections, such as those that occur in immunocompromised patients, IV acyclovir should be used at a dose of 5 to 10 mg/kg every 8 hours. Oral acyclovir 400 mg three times daily or 800 mg twice daily for 5 days may be used for treatment of recurrent lesions. For individuals with frequent recurrences, prophylactic or suppression therapy of 400 mg orally twice daily is recommended and can reduce recurrences by 80%. Alternatively, more costly antiviral medications may also be used, such as valacyclovir, particularly for easier dosing regimens. Additionally, daily treatment with valacyclovir 500 mg daily in the infected partner has been demonstrated to decrease the rate of HSV-2 transmission in discordant, heterosexual couples in which the source partner has a history of genital HSV-2 infection.

CHANCROID

Chancroid is caused by ***Haemophilus ducreyi***. Globally, it is a common STI, although the incidence in North America has declined steadily since 1987, with just 28 reported cases in 2009. Reported cases are likely to grossly underestimate true incidence because *H. ducreyi* is difficult to culture. Males are affected more than females by ratios of 3:1 to 25:1. Chancroid is a cofactor for HIV transmission; high rates of HIV infection among patients who have chancroid occur in the United States and other countries. Additionally, approximately 10% of persons who have chancroid that was acquired in the United States are coinfected with *T. pallidum* or HSV.

Chancroid appears as a painful, demarcated, nonindurated ulcer located anywhere in the anogenital region. There is often concomitant painful suppurative inguinal lymphadenopathy. Usually, just a single ulcer is present, but multiple ulcers and occasionally extragenital infections have been known to occur.

Diagnosis

Diagnosis is a challenge because *H. ducreyi* is difficult to culture. A definitive diagnosis of chancroid requires the identification of *H. ducreyi* on special culture media that are not widely available from commercial sources; even when these media are used, sensitivity is less than 80%. Often, transporting the culture swab in Amies or Stuart transport media or chocolate agar can aid in the culture. Direct Gram stains have not been a consistent method of diagnosis, and FDA-approved PCR test for *H. ducreyi* is also not available in the United States. The diagnosis is therefore often made clinically by ruling out other sources of infection, such as HSV and syphilis.

Treatment

Treatment regimens include ceftriaxone 250 mg IM once, azithromycin 1 g orally once, ciprofloxacin 500 mg orally twice a day for 3 days, or erythromycin 500 mg four times a day for 7 days. As with most other STIs, sexual partners should be treated as well.

LYMPHOGRANULOMA VENEREUM

The C. *trachomatis* L-serotypes (L1, L2, or L3) cause the systemic disease **lymphogranuloma venereum** (LGV). The primary stage of this illness is often a local lesion that may be either a papule or a shallow ulcer, and is often painless, transient, and can go unnoticed. The secondary stage (inguinal syndrome) occurs 2 to 6 weeks after the primary lesion and is characterized by painful inflammation and enlargement of the inguinal nodes (typically unilateral). Systemic manifestations include fever, headaches, malaise, and anorexia. Rectal exposure can result in the tertiary stage (anogenital syndrome), which is characterized by proctocolitis, rectal stricture, rectovaginal fistula, and elephantiasis (lymphatic filariasis). Initially, an anal pruritus will develop with a concomitant mucous rectal discharge. Although diagnosis is generally made per clinical suspicion, genital and lymph node specimens may be tested for C. *trachomatis* by culture, direct immunofluorescence, or nucleic acid detection.

Treatment

Treatment of LGV includes doxycycline 100 mg orally twice a day or erythromycin 500 mg orally four times a day for 21 days. With persistent illness, the antibiotic regimen can be repeated. If the external genitalia and rectum are disfigured and scarred, surgical measures may be required.

NONULCERATIVE LESIONS

One of the most common nonulcerative lesions is the condyloma (Fig. 16-3). **Condyloma acuminata** are warty lesions that occur anywhere in the anogenital region and are considered an STI. Other nonulcerative lesions include **molluscum contagiosum**, caused by a pox virus, and lesions caused by ***Phthirus pubis***, the crab louse, and ***Sarcoptes scabiei***, the itch mite.

Finally, when considering nonulcerative lesions, folliculitis should always be included in the differential diagnosis because

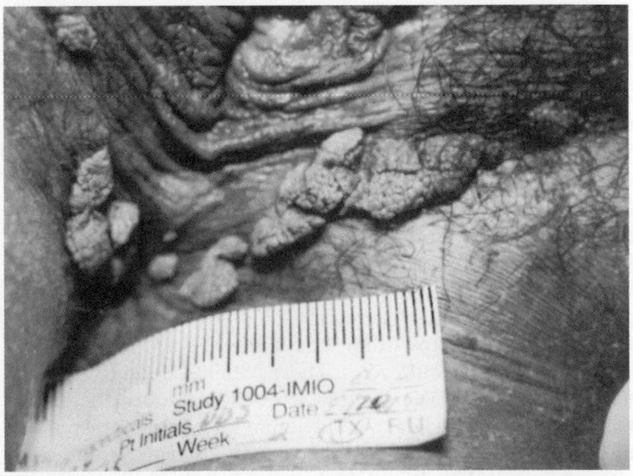

Figure 16-3 • Extensive external condylomata acuminata. These fleshy, exophytic growths are covered with small, papillary surface projections. Some of the lesions are pedunculated; others are sessile.

(Reproduced with permission from Blackwell RE. *Women's Medicine*. Cambridge, MA: Blackwell Science; 1996:317.)

the skin in the pubic region has hair follicles. In rare cases, folliculitis can lead to larger lesions such as boils, carbuncles, and abscesses. The usual source of these infections is skin flora, primarily *Staphylococcus aureus*. Factors contributing to these lesions in the anogenital region include tight undergarments, sanitary pads, poor hygiene, diabetes, and immunosuppression.

HUMAN PAPILLOMAVIRUS

The most clinically evident results of infection with human papillomavirus (HPV) are **condyloma acuminata** or **genital warts**. Approximately 5.6% of sexually active adults aged 18 to 59 self-reported a history of genital warts. However, of more significance in terms of morbidity and mortality, HPV is associated with cervical cancer and other squamous cell malignancies of the female and male reproductive tracts. It is estimated that the incidence of HPV has been increasing in the United States, with an estimated prevalence between 20% and 45%. It is clearly an STI with 60% to 80% of partners being affected.

Although genital warts often occur throughout the lower reproductive tract, patients usually present with anogenital lesions that they have identified or that have become pruritic or caused bleeding. An estimated 90% of genital warts are caused by serotypes 6 and 11, whereas cervical cancer is more often associated with serotypes 16, 18, and 31. HPV testing is not indicated for patients with genital warts.

Diagnosis

Genital warts are typically asymptomatic but can be painful or pruritic. The diagnosis is usually made via clinical examination. The wart has a raised papillomatous or spiked surface. Initially, the lesions are small, 1 to 5 mm diameter lesions, but these can evolve into larger pedunculated lesions and eventually into cauliflower-like growths, particularly in immunocompromised patients. In addition to the vulva, perineal body, and anogenital region, these lesions can also arise in the anal canal, on the walls of the vagina, and on the cervix. When uncertain of diagnosis or for lesions that are unresponsive to therapy, a biopsy of the lesion can be made for definitive diagnosis.

Treatment

Treatment of the lesions includes local excision, cryotherapy, topical trichloroacetic acid, topical 25% podophyllin, and 5-fluorouracil cream (Efudex 5%). The medical treatments are usually repeated weekly by the clinician until all lesions are gone. For motivated patients with uncomplicated condyloma that can be reached, both imiquimod (Aldara) and podofilox (Condylox) can be used. Imiquimod is used three times per week and needs to be washed off after 6 to 10 hours, whereas podofilox is applied twice a day for 3 days and left in place followed by no treatment for 4 days; this therapy regimen may be repeated up to four cycles. These patients can self-treat and follow up with clinicians every 3 to 4 weeks until the lesions have resolved. For larger condylomas or those unresponsive to medical treatment, CO_2 laser may be used to vaporize the lesion or surgical excision may be required. Regardless of treatment modality, a recurrence rate of approximately 20% is seen in all patients.

For prevention of HPV, two vaccines are available in the United States. The bivalent vaccine (Cervarix) protects against serotypes 16 and 18 and is FDA approved for girls and women aged 10 to 25. The quadravalent vaccine (Gardasil) protects against serotypes 6, 11, 16 and 18 and is FDA approved for girls and women as well as boys and men aged 9 to 26.

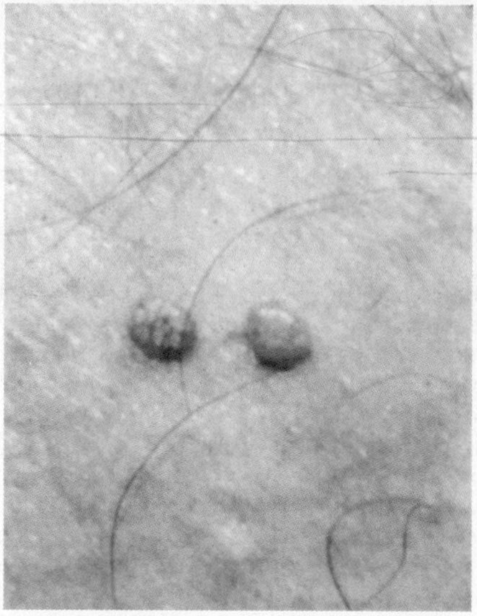

Figure 16-4 • Two typical molluscum lesions, one of which shows a mosaic appearance.

MOLLUSCUM CONTAGIOSUM

Molluscum contagiosum is caused by a pox virus that is spread via close contact with an infected person or via autoinoculation. The lesion is a small, 1 to 5 mm, domed papule with an umbilicated center (Fig. 16-4). Also known as *water warts*, these lesions contain a waxy material that reveals intracytoplasmic molluscum bodies under microscopic examination when stained with Wright stain or Giemsa stain. Molluscum lesions can occur anywhere on the skin except on the palms of the hands and soles of the feet. These lesions are often asymptomatic and generally resolve on their own. Diagnosis is generally made clinically; however, diagnosis may be confirmed with lesion biopsy for histologic or electron microscopic examination. These can be removed via local excision and/or treatment of the nodule base with trichloroacetic acid or cryotherapy.

PHTHIRUS PUBIS AND SARCOPTES SCABIEI

The nonulcerative lesions caused by ***Phthirus pubis***, the crab louse, and ***Sarcoptes scabiei***, the itch mite, are similar. Signs and symptoms of these two infections include pruritus, irritated skin, vesicles, and burrows. The primary difference is that lesions from *P. pubis*, or **pediculosis**, are usually confined to the pubic hair, whereas **scabies** may spread throughout the body. Thus, treatment is site specific: pediculosis can be cured with therapy application to specific areas, whereas it is more effective to treat scabies by applying treatment over the entire body. Pediculosis pubis is generally sexually transmitted. Treatment includes permethrin 1% cream rinse applied to affected areas and washed off after 10 minutes or pyrethrins with piperonyl butoxide applied to the affected area and washed off after 10 minutes. Scabies is commonly sexually transmitted in adults and transmitted by direct contact in children. Treatment for scabies includes permethrin cream

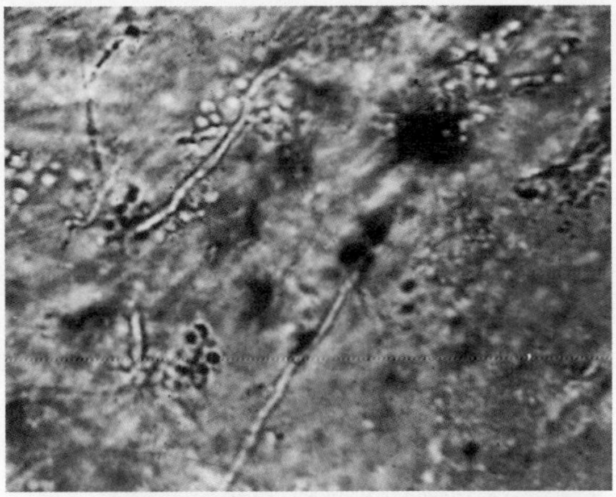

Figure 16-5 • *Candida albicans*, KOH mount of skin scraping. (Reproduced with permission from Crissey JT. *Manual of Medical Mycology*. Boston, MA: Blackwell Science; 1995:90.)

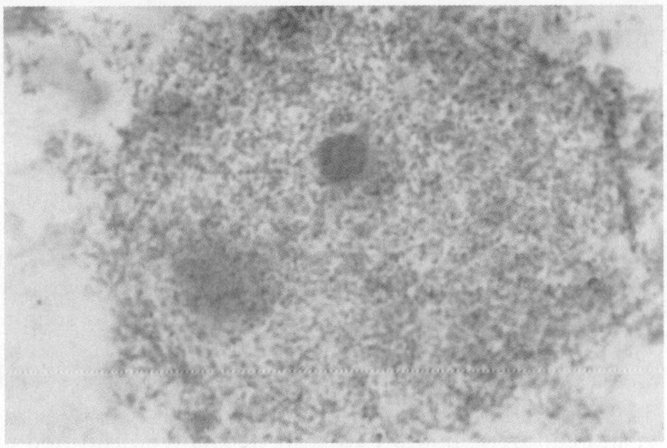

Figure 16-6 • Bacterial vaginosis.

(5%) applied to all areas of the body from the neck down and washed off after 8 to 14 hours or ivermectin 200 μg/kg orally, repeated in 2 weeks.

VAGINAL INFECTIONS

Symptoms related to vaginal infections are the leading cause of visits to a gynecologist. The vagina provides a warm, moist environment that can be colonized by various organisms. Imbalance of microflora in the vagina caused by antibiotics, diet, systemic illness; the introduction of a pathogen; or the overgrowth of one variety of organism can lead to symptoms including itching, pain, discharge, burning, and odor. Common organisms that cause symptoms with overgrowth include *Candida* (Fig. 16-5) and *Gardnerella*; the most common pathogenic protozoan is *Trichomonas*. These can each be easily diagnosed and treated quite effectively with antimicrobials. However, any chronic vaginitis with pruritus, pain, bleeding, and/or ulcerated lesions that do not respond to drug therapy should be investigated to rule out malignancy.

BACTERIAL VAGINOSIS

The vagina is commonly colonized with multiple bacteria, predominantly *Lactobacillus* sp. that generally maintain the vaginal pH below 4. **Bacterial vaginosis** (BV) can develop when there is a shift in the predominant bacterial species in the vagina (Fig. 16-6). Although BV is likely to be polymicrobial, one of the most common organisms present in culture is *Gardnerella vaginalis*. BV is quite common and is the leading cause of vaginitis, with prevalence rates of 5% of college populations and as high as 60% in STI clinics. Risk factors include new or multiple sexual partners, douching, lack of vaginal lactobacilli, female sexual partners, and cigarette smoking. BV is associated with acquisition of some STIs, complications after gynecologic surgery, complications of pregnancy (preterm birth), and recurrence of BV.

Diagnosis

Many patients with BV may be asymptomatic or have an isolated increase in vaginal discharge. However, symptomatic patients complain of a profuse nonirritating discharge, often with a malodorous fishy amine odor. Diagnosis can be made with three of the following findings: presence of thin, white, homogeneous discharge coating the vaginal walls; an amine odor noted with addition of 10% KOH ("whiff" test); pH greater than 4.5; or presence of clue cells (vaginal epithelial cells that are diffusely covered with bacteria) on microscopic examination. Gram stain with examination of bacteria in the vaginal discharge is considered the gold standard diagnostic test for BV.

Performance of vaginal culture for *G. vaginalis*, *Bacteroides*, and other anaerobes is generally not recommended as this is not a specific diagnostic method. Therefore, the clinical diagnosis is usually made from vaginal preps.

Treatment

Treatment of BV is recommended for symptomatic women and include either metronidazole 500 mg orally twice a day for 7 days or clindamycin 300 mg orally twice a day for 7 days. Both antibiotics are also available in gel or cream and can be used topically (metronidazole gel 0.75% one applicator intravaginally daily for 5 days or clindamycin cream 2% one applicator intravaginally daily for 7 days). A metronidazole 2 g single-dose therapy has been studied. However, it is less than 75% effective in BV when compared to 85% to 90% cure rates for the week-long treatment. Patients should be advised to avoid alcohol consumption during metronidazole treatment due to its antabuse effect. Up to 30% of women will have recurrence of BV within 3 months.

YEAST INFECTIONS

Candidiasis probably causes 30% of the vaginitis that leads women to be seen by a gynecologist. Many more of these infections are treated by women using over-the-counter (OTC) preparations. Candidiasis is caused by *Candida albicans* in 80% to 90% of all cases, with the remaining cases caused by other candidal species. Predisposing factors for candidal overgrowth include the use of broad-spectrum antibiotics, diabetes mellitus, and decreased cellular immunity as seen in AIDS patients or those on immunosuppressive therapies. Yeast infections are also associated with intercourse and may increase during the late luteal phase of the menstrual cycle.

Diagnosis

Typical symptoms of genital candidiasis include vulvar and vaginal pruritus, burning, dysuria, dyspareunia, and vaginal discharge. On physical examination, there is vulvar edema and erythema with a scant vaginal discharge. Only approximately 20% of patients display the characteristic white plaques adherent to the vaginal mucosa or thick curdy vaginal discharge. Diagnosis is usually made by microscopic examination of a 10% KOH preparation of the vaginal discharge, which improves visualization of characteristic branching hyphae and spores compared to saline preparation alone. However, the KOH preparation is estimated to have a sensitivity of 25% to 80%. Other diagnostic options include Gram stain and culture. Clinically, treatment is often instituted on the basis of clinical signs and symptoms. In recurrent vaginal yeast infection cases (more than four symptomatic episodes in 1 year), vaginal culture should be obtained to identify non-*albicans* species such as C. *glabrata* that may be less responsive to azole therapy.

Treatment

Treatment includes a short course (1 to 3 days) of any of the azole agents via topical applications or vaginal suppository, including miconazole as an OTC preparation or terconazole by prescription. Nystatin suppositories are less effective. Oral therapy includes fluconazole (Diflucan) 150 mg orally once, which has been shown to be as effective as any of the local treatments. Longer duration of therapy, such as 7 to 14 days of topical regimen or two to three doses of fluconazole oral therapy every 72 hours, is recommended for treatment for recurrent cases or complicated infections (women who are immunosuppressed, diabetic patients, pregnant, or have severe symptoms). First-line maintenance therapy for recurrent cases consists of oral fluconazole weekly for 6 months. In non-albicans candidiasis, treatment with 600 mg vaginal boric acid capsules daily for 14 days is 70% effective.

TRICHOMONAS VAGINALIS

Trichomonas vaginalis is a unicellular, anaerobic flagellated protozoan that can cause vaginitis. It inhabits the lower genitourinary tracts of women and men, and there are approximately 8 million cases diagnosed annually in the United States. The disease is sexually transmitted, with 75% of sexual partners possessing positive cultures.

Diagnosis

The signs and symptoms of *T. vaginalis* include a profuse discharge with an unpleasant odor. The discharge may be yellow, gray, or green in color and may be frothy in appearance. Vaginal pH is in the 6 to 7 range. Vulvar erythema, edema, and pruritus can also be noted. The characteristic erythematous, punctate epithelial papillae, or "strawberry" appearance of the cervix is apparent in only 10% of cases. Symptoms are usually worse immediately after menses because of the transient increase in vaginal pH at that time.

Diagnosis of *Trichomonas* is made via wet prep microscopic examination of vaginal swabs. The protozoan is slightly larger than a WBC with three to five flagella. Often, active movement of the flagella and propulsion of the organism can be seen (Fig. 16-7). However, microscopy has only 60% to 70% sensitivity. Other more sensitive tests are available, including nucleic acid probe study and immunochromatographic capillary flow dipstick technology. The diagnosis can be confirmed when necessary with culture, which is the most sensitive and specific study.

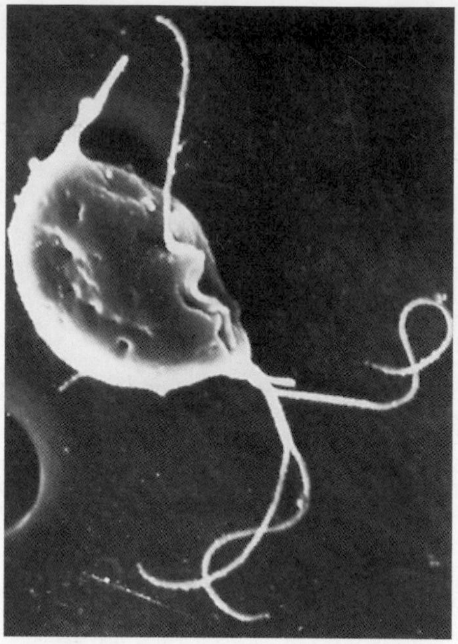

Figure 16-7 • Scanning electron micrograph of *Trichomonas vaginalis*. The undulating membrane and flagella of *Trichomonas* are its characteristic features.
(Reproduced with permission from Cox FEG, ed. *Modern Parasitology: A Textbook of Parasitology*, 2nd ed. Oxford: Blackwell Science; 1993:9.)

Treatment

The mainstay of treatment for *T. vaginalis* infections is metronidazole (Flagyl) 2 g orally or tinidazole 2 g orally in a single dose. As opposed to BV management, this regimen has been found to be as effective as the more traditional 500 mg orally twice a day for 7 days. However, metronidazole resistance may be present in 2% to 5% of vaginal trichomoniasis cases. In cases of metronidazole single-dose treatment failure, metronidazole 500 mg orally twice a day for 7 days is prescribed. If this treatment is unsuccessful, then tinidazole or metronidazole 2 g orally daily for 5 days, consultation with specialist, and *T. vaginalis* susceptibility through the CDC should be considered. Because of the high rate of concomitant infections in sexual partners, both partners should be treated to prevent reinfection.

INFECTIONS OF THE CERVIX

The organisms that most commonly cause cervicitis and infections of the upper reproductive tract differ from those that most commonly cause infections of the lower reproductive tract. ***N. gonorrhoeae*** and C. ***trachomatis*** are the two most common organisms that cause cervicitis and the only organisms shown to cause mucopurulent cervicitis. Clinically, cervicitis is diagnosed as cervical motion tenderness in the absence of other signs of pelvic inflammatory disease (PID).

Other organisms can also cause infections of the cervix, including HSV, HPV, and *Mycoplasma genitalium* as well as organisms causing BV. HSV causes either herpes lesions or a white plaque that resembles cervical cancer. Infection with HPV leads to condyloma and, depending on the subtype, is also an etiology of cervical cancer. Additionally, frequent douching may also cause cervicitis.

NEISSERIA GONORRHOEAE

Despite a 50% decrease in incidence in the 1990s, **gonococcal** infections remain the second leading reported STIs in the United States, with an estimated 700,000 infections occurring each year. Most cases occur in the 15- to 24-year-old age group. Among sexually active women, 15- to 19-year-olds have two times the incidence of 20- to 24-year-olds.

Multiple risk factors have been associated with gonococcal infections, including low socioeconomic status, urban residence, nonwhite and non-Asian ethnicity, early age of first sexual activity, illicit drug use, being unmarried, and history of STIs. Condoms, diaphragms, and spermicides decrease the risk of transmission. There are also seasonal variations in the incidence of gonorrhea in the United States with a peak observed in late summer.

Transmission between the sexes is unequal, with male-to-female transmission estimated at 80% to 90% compared to an estimated 20% to 25% female-to-male transmission rate after a single sexual encounter. This difference in transmission is most likely related to the type of epithelium exposed in the different sexes. In males, the external surface of the penis is primarily keratinized epithelium, whereas females receive primary contact with mucosa of the vagina and the nonkeratinized epithelium of the cervix. Further, male ejaculation increases the amount of exposure time in women, which supports the use of condoms as an exceptional prophylactic measure against gonococcal transmission.

Gonococcus can infect the anal canal, the urethra, the oropharynx, and Bartholin glands, in addition to the more commonly reported cervicitis, PID, or tubo-ovarian abscess (TOA). Up to 50% of women with gonorrhea are asymptomatic. Gonococcal exposure in neonates can cause conjunctivitis. As many as 1% of recognized gonococcal infections may proceed to a disseminated infection. This infection begins with fevers and erythematous macular skin lesions and proceeds to a tenosynovitis and septic arthritis.

Diagnosis

Identification of the causative organism, *N. gonorrhoeae*, a gram-negative diplococcus resembling paired kidney beans, is necessary for definitive diagnosis. Isolation using the modified Thayer-Martin chocolate agar has a sensitivity of 96% in endocervical cultures and provides the option of antimicrobial susceptibility identification. However, specific nucleic acid amplification tests (NAAT) for both gonorrhea and chlamydial infection have largely supplanted the use of culture. NAAT yield high sensitivity and specificity and provide increased female specimen testing options, including urine, endocervical swabs, and vaginal swabs.

Treatment

The recommended treatment for uncomplicated gonococcal infection is ceftriaxone 125 mg IM once or cefixime 400 mg orally once. Because of increasing resistance, fluoroquinolones are no longer recommended in the United States for the treatment of gonorrhea infections. Additionally, because patients infected with *N. gonorrhoeae* frequently are coinfected with *C. trachomatis*, it is recommended that patients diagnosed with gonorrhea infection should also be treated for chlamydial infection with azithromycin 1 g orally once or doxycycline 100 mg twice daily for 7 days, unless chlamydial coinfection has been ruled out by NAAT.

CHLAMYDIA TRACHOMATIS

C. trachomatis is a pathogen that causes ocular, respiratory, and reproductive tract infections. In the United States, its transmission is primarily via sexual contact, although vertical transmission from a mother to a newborn is also seen. Chlamydial infection is the most prevalent bacterial STI with an estimated 2.8 million infections occurring annually. There has been a steady increase in chlamydial infections, which is most likely secondary to the advent of NAATs for *C. trachomatis* (traditionally difficult to diagnose because they are obligate intracellular organisms and culture poorly) and aggressive screening programs of sexually active women. Prevalence is estimated at 3% to 5% in asymptomatic women, and 5% to 7% of pregnant women have had positive *Chlamydia* tests. Epidemiologically, *C. trachomatis* infections are parallel to those of *N. gonorrhoeae*, with higher rates seen among women 15- to 24-year-old, with earlier age of first coitus, and greater number of sexual partners.

Another reason for the higher prevalence of chlamydial infections is that carriers of both sexes are often entirely asymptomatic. Up to 70% of women are asymptomatic. If left untreated, approximately 10% to 15% of women will develop PID that may result in infertility or increased risk of ectopic pregnancies. Because of these devastating effects, the CDC recommends annual *Chlamydia* screening for sexually active women age 25 or younger, older women with risk factors for chlamydial infections (those with new sexual parters or multiple sexual partners), and all pregnant women. Common sites of infection include the endocervix, urethra, and rectum. Clinical manifestations of symptomatic chlamydial infections are often quite similar to those of *N. gonorrhoeae* and include symptoms of cervicitis, urethritis, and PID. As previously discussed, the L-serotypes of *C. trachomatis* can cause the systemic disease LGV.

Treatment

Treatment of choice for chlamydial infections is azithromycin 1 g orally single dose or doxycycline 100 mg orally twice a day for 7 days. Alternative regimens include erythromycin 500 mg orally four times a day for 7 days. For LGV, the treatment regimen consists of doxycycline 100 mg orally twice a day for 3 weeks.

KEY POINTS

- Syphilis is screened for with the RPR and VDRL tests and confirmed with either the TPPA or FTA-ABS.
- Benzathine penicillin is the drug of choice for treating syphilis. Neurosyphilis requires IV penicillin.
- Patients being treated for syphilis may experience the Jarisch-Herxheimer reaction, seen most commonly in the treatment of secondary syphilis.
- Up to 80% of newly acquired genital herpes infections are caused by HSV-1.
- Primary herpes infection classically appears as multiple vesicles that develop into painful ulcers.
- Treatment of genital herpes is usually palliative, although acyclovir can reduce the length of primary infection and suppressive therapy may decrease the number of recurrences.
- Chancroid manifests as a painful genital ulcer and usually concomitant lymphadenopathy, but can be difficult to diagnose as neither cultures nor Gram stain have been particularly consistent.
- Treatment of chancroid can include a variety of antibiotics; the simplest are single doses of PO azithromycin or IM ceftriaxone.
- Low-risk serotypes of HPV causes condylomata while high-risk serotypes are associated with cervical cancer.
- Bacterial vaginosis is polymicrobial but usually attributed to *Gardnerella,* and the first-line treatment is metronidazole (Flagyl) for a 7-day course.
- Seventy-five percent of sexual partners of those with *Trichomonas* will also be colonized and should be presumptively treated with first-line treatment of metronidazole 2 g orally single dose.
- *N. gonorrhoeae* causes an estimated 700,000 infections per year with common sequelae including cervicitis, PID, TOA, and Bartholin abscess.
- Treatment for uncomplicated gonorrhea infections is ceftriaxone 125 mg IM or cefixime 400 mg orally single dose. Treatment for gonorrhea infections should also include azithromycin 1 g orally once to treat likely concomitant chlamydial infections.
- Chlamydial infections tend to coincide with gonococcal infections. However, the incidence of gonococcal infections has remained stable, whereas the incidence of chlamydial infections has increased.
- Up to 70% of chlamydial infections are entirely asymptomatic.
- Treatment of chlamydial infections is a one-time 1 g oral dose of azithromycin.

C Clinical Vignettes

Vignette 1

An 18-year-old nulligravid woman presents to the student health clinic with a 4-week history of yellow vaginal discharge. She also reports vulvar itching and irritation. She is sexually active and monogamous with her boyfriend. They use condoms inconsistently. On physical examination, she is found to be nontoxic and afebrile. On genitourinary examination, vulvar and vaginal erythema is noted along with a yellow, frothy, malodorous discharge with a pH of 6.5. The cervix appears to have erythematous punctuations. There is no cervical, uterine, or adnexal tenderness. The addition of 10% KOH to the vaginal discharge does not produce an amine odor. Wet prep microscopic examination of the vaginal swabs is performed.

1. What would you expect to see under microscopy?
   a. Branching hyphae
   b. Multinucleated giant cells
   c. Scant WBC
   d. Flagellated, motile organisms
   e. Epithelial cells covered with bacteria

2. Which of the following is the most likely causal organism?
   a. Treponema pallidum
   b. Neisseria gonorrhoeae
   c. Trichomonas vaginalis
   d. Gardnerella vaginalis
   e. Haemophilus ducreyi

3. What is the best initial treatment for this patient?
   a. Metronidazole 2 g orally once
   b. Doxycycline 100 mg orally twice daily for 7 days
   c. Azithromycin 1 g orally once
   d. Clindamycin 300 mg orally twice daily for 7 days
   e. Metronidazole gel 0.75% one applicator intravaginally for 5 days

4. What is another important component of the treatment plan?
   a. Performing a test of cure in 3 months
   b. *T. vaginalis* susceptibility testing
   c. Treatment of sexual partner(s)
   d. Empiric treatment for chlamydial infection
   e. No further action is needed

5. The patient returns in 3 weeks with continued symptoms. She reports compliance with her initial treatment. Infection recurrence is confirmed on microscopy. Which of the following is the most appropriate treatment option?
   a. Tinidazole 2 g orally daily for 5 days
   b. Metronidazole 500 mg orally twice daily for 7 days
   c. Consultation with infectious disease specialist
   d. *T. vaginalis* susceptibility testing
   e. Clindamycin 300 mg orally twice times daily for 7 days

Vignette 2

A 16-year-old girl presents to the physician for annual examination. She denies any current symptoms or concerns. She has been sexually active for 1 year and is using Depo-Provera for contraception. She does not use condoms. On urogenital examination, she has a moderate amount of yellow mucopurulent discharge from the endocervix. There is no cervical motion, adnexal, or uterine tenderness. Microscopy of the vaginal discharge was normal except greater than 10 WBCs per high power field. Vaginal pH is normal.

1. What is the most appropriate next step in the management?
   a. Perform a Pap smear with reflex HPV testing
   b. Order a pelvic ultrasound
   c. Treat for presumptive chlamydial infection and gonorrhea
   d. Send vaginal discharge for culture and Gram stain
   e. Perform nucleic acid amplification test (NAAT) for chlamydial infection and gonorrhea

2. Test results confirm the diagnosis of gonorrhea. What is the best initial treatment for this patient?
   a. Ceftriaxone 125 mg IM once
   b. Ceftriaxone 125 mg IM once plus azithromycin 1 g orally once
   c. Doxycycline 100 mg orally twice daily for 7 days
   d. Ciprofloxacin 500 mg orally once
   e. Clindamycin 300 mg orally twice times daily for 7 days

3. If left untreated, this patient would be at risk for developing?
   a. Cervicitis
   b. Pelvic inflammatory disease
   c. Tubo-ovarian abscess
   d. Disseminated gonorrhea
   e. All of the above

Vignette 3

A 21-year-old nulligravid woman presents to her gynecologist with a 3-day history of painful genital ulcer. Last week she had a low-grade fever and generalized malaise, which has since resolved. She denies any history of genital ulcers. She has had four new sexual partners in the last year and uses oral contraceptives. She reports using condoms inconsistently. On genitourinary examination, several 1 to 2 mm painful vesicles are noted on the left labia minora. There is no inguinal lymphadenopathy.

1. Which of the following is the most likely causal organism?
   a. Treponema pallidum
   b. Herpes simplex virus
   c. Trichomonas vaginalis
   d. Chlamydia trachomatis L1, L2, or L3
   e. Haemophilus ducreyi

2. Assuming that additional testing was performed, which of the following results would you most likely expect to find?
   a. *T. pallidum* particle agglutination assay (TPPA), positive
   b. *H. ducreyi* culture, positive
   c. HSV-2 IgG, positive
   d. HSV-1 IgG, positive
   e. None of the above. Diagnostic testing is not reliable and treatment should be based on clinical suspicion

3. What is the best initial treatment for this patient?
   a. Ceftriaxone 250 mg IM once
   b. Imiquimod (Aldara) applied to affected area three times per week
   c. Acyclovir 200 mg orally five times daily for 7 days
   d. Benzathine penicillin G 2.4 million units IM once
   e. Doxycycline 100 mg orally twice daily for 21 days

4. The patient returns to clinic 3 months later for an annual examination. She is wondering how her diagnosis might impact her future health. You counsel her that:
   a. condom use will prevent sexual transmission
   b. there is no way to reduce recurrent outbreaks
   c. recurrence is more frequent with HSV-1
   d. asymptomatic viral shedding is an important mode of transmission
   e. she will need a cesarean section for future pregnancies

Vignette 4

A 36-year-old G2P2 woman presents to her gynecologist with a 3-week history of vaginal irritation and fish-smelling vaginal discharge. She recently tried an over-the-counter antifungal treatment without any improvement in her symptoms. She is sexually active in a monogamous relationship with a male partner of 5 years and she uses a contraceptive ring (NuvaRing). Genitourinary examination shows a thick white discharge. The remainder of her examination is normal. Microscopic evaluation of a saline "wet prep" of the vaginal secretions reveals decreased lactobacilli, a few WBCs, and vaginal epithelial cells with a stippled appearance.

1. Which of the following additional test(s) would support the diagnosis?
   a. Branching hyphae on 10% KOH prepared microscopic examination
   b. Positive NAAT for *Chlamydia*
   c. Vaginal pH less than 4.5
   d. Amine odor noted with the addition of 10% KOH
   e. None of the above

2. What is the best initial treatment for this patient?
   a. Metronidazole 2 g orally once
   b. Doxycycline 100 mg orally twice daily for 7 days
   c. Azithromycin 1 g orally once
   d. Metronidazole 500 mg orally twice daily for 7 days
   e. Fluconazole 150 mg orally once

3. Women diagnosed with this condition should be counseled regarding which of the following?
   a. There is a 30% risk of recurrence
   b. It is a sexually transmitted infection (STI)
   c. Sexual partner(s) should be treated
   d. Treatment should include empiric treatment for chlamydial infection
   e. Treatment should be initiated for both symptomatic and asymptomatic women

4. Risk factors for developing this condition include all of the following *except*:
   a. multiple sexual partners
   b. cigarette smoking
   c. douching
   d. contraceptive ring (NuvaRing)
   e. lack of vaginal lactobacilli

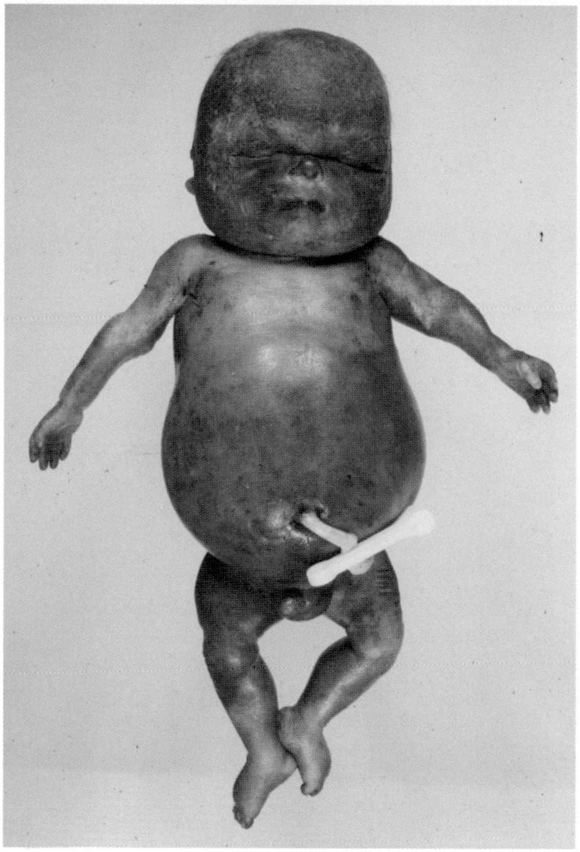

Color Plate 1 • Fetal hydrops caused by the accumulation of fluid in fetal tissues.

(From Sadler TW. *Langman's Medical Embryology*, 10th ed. Philadelphia, PA: Lippincott Williams & Wilkins; 2006.)

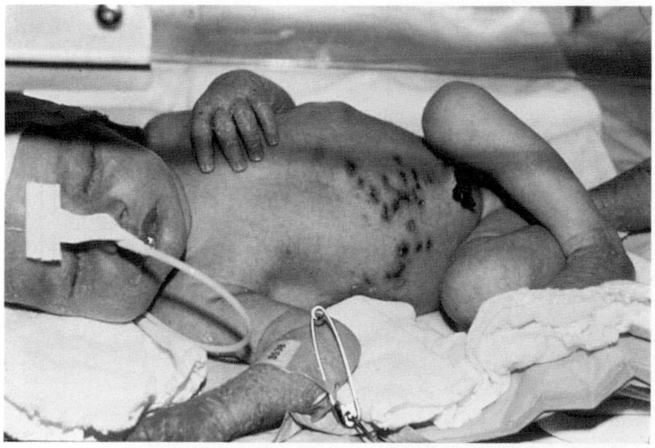

Color Plate 2 • Newborn with disseminated herpes simplex virus (HSV) infection. Note the healing ulcerations on the abdomen of the infant.

(From Sweet R, Gibbs R. *Atlas of Infectious Diseases of the Female Genital Tract.* Philadelphia, PA: Lippincott Williams & Wilkins; 2005.)

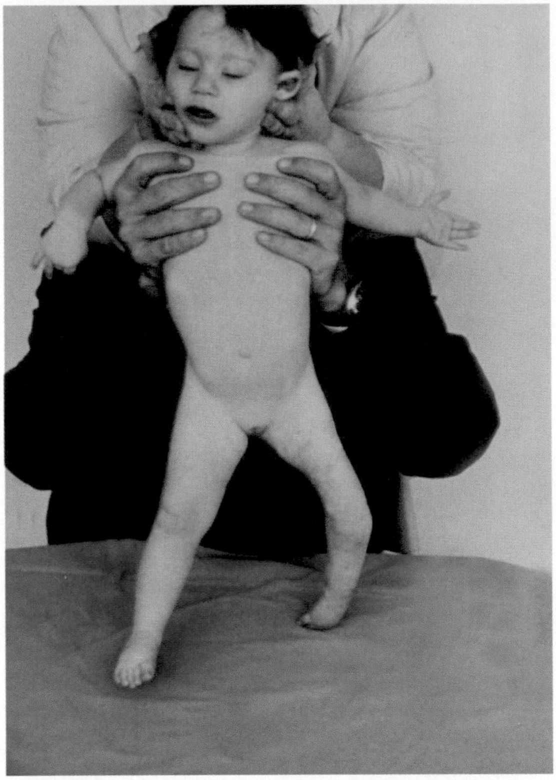

Color Plate 3 • Congenital varicella syndrome characterized by longbone defects, chorioretinitis, and cerebral cortical atrophy.
(From Sweet R, Gibbs R. *Atlas of Infectious Diseases of the Female Genital Tract*. Philadelphia, PA: Lippincott Williams & Wilkins; 2005.)

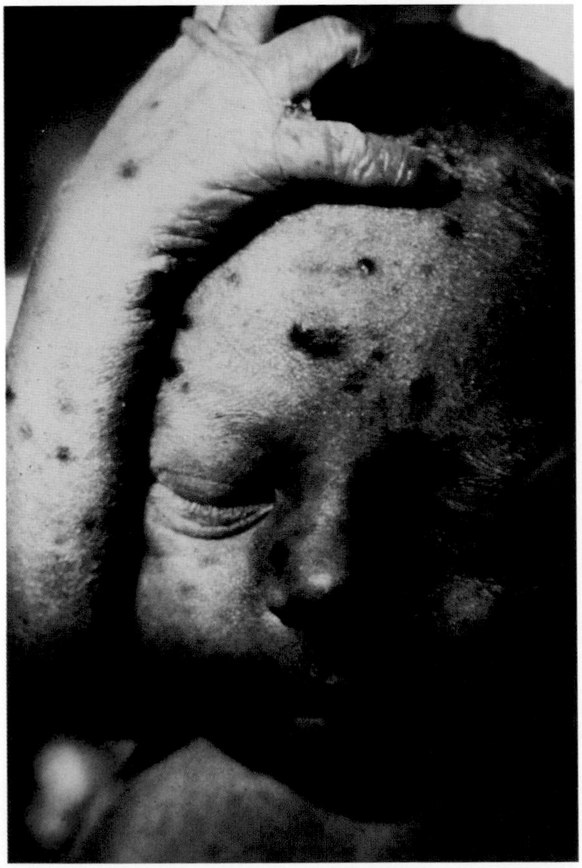

Color Plate 4 • Congenital CMV "blueberry muffin" baby with jaundice and thrombocytopenia purpura.
(From Sweet R, Gibbs R. *Atlas of Infectious Diseases of the Female Genital Tract*. Philadelphia, PA: Lippincott Williams & Wilkins; 2005.)

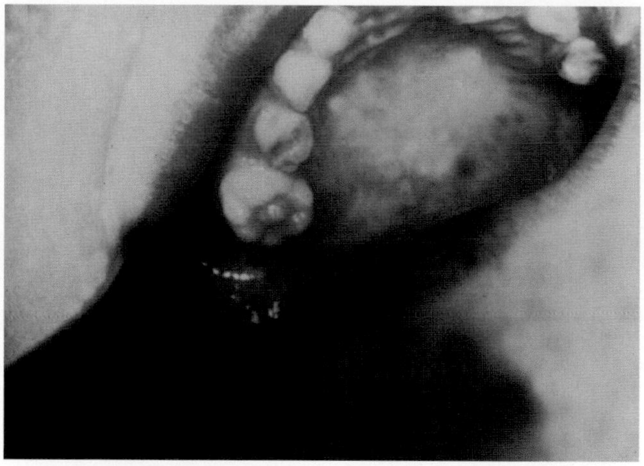

Color Plate 5 • Congenital syphilis—mulberry molar.
(From Sweet R, Gibbs R. *Atlas of Infectious Diseases of the Female Genital Tract*. Philadelphia, PA: Lippincott Williams & Wilkins; 2005.)

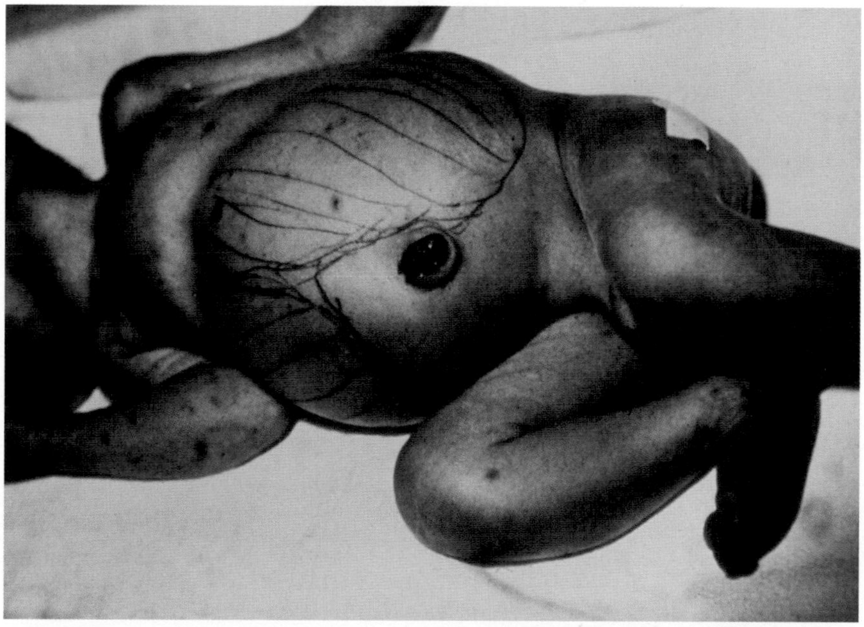

Color Plate 6 • Congenital toxoplasmosis with hepatosplenomegaly, jaundice, and thrombocytopenia purpura.
(From Sweet R, Gibbs R. *Atlas of Infectious Diseases of the Female Genital Tract*. Philadelphia, PA: Lippincott Williams & Wilkins; 2005.)

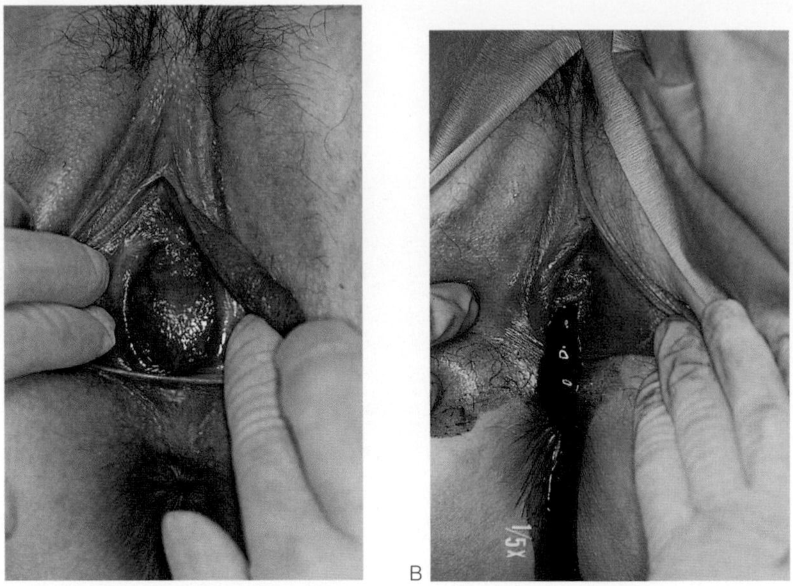

Color Plate 7 • Imperforate hymen. Note bulging hymen (A) and subsequent drainage of obstructed material once the hymenal tissue is excised (B)
(From Rock J, Johns H. *TeLinde's Operative Gynecology*, 9th ed. Philadelphia, PA: Lippincott Williams & Wilkins; 2003.)

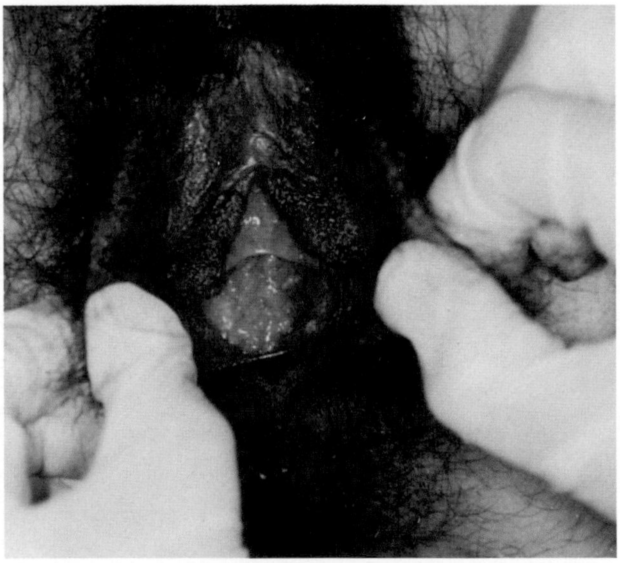

Color Plate 8 • Vaginal agenesis also known as Mayer-Rokinsky-Kuster-Hauser syndrome. Notable for congnital absence of the vagina with variable uterine development.
(From Emans J, Laufer M, Goldstein DP. *Pediatric and Adolescent Gynecology*, 5th ed. Philadelphia, PA: Lippincott Williams & Wilkins; 2005.)

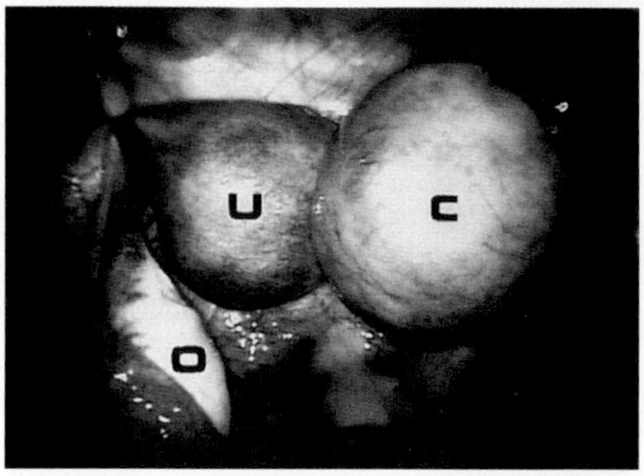

Color Plate 9 • Laparoscopic view of a large ovarian cyst.
C = ovary with cyst
U = uterus
O = normal ovary

(From Emans J, Laufer M, Goldstein DP. *Pediatric and Adolescent Gynecology*, 5th ed. Philadelphia, PA: Lippincott Williams & Wilkins; 2005.)

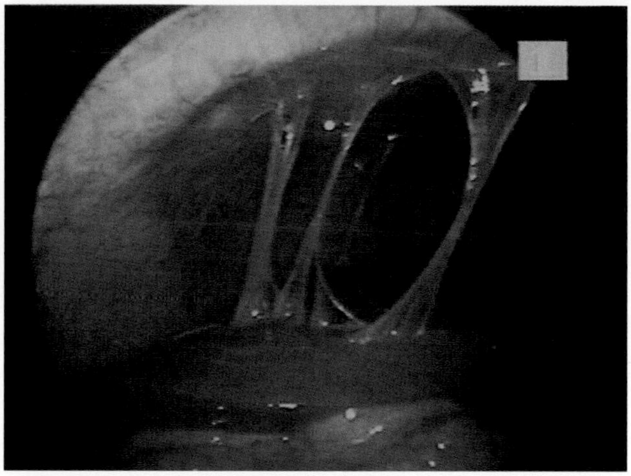

Color Plate 10 • Fitzhugh-Curtis syndrome.

(From Sweet R, Gibbs R. *Atlas of Infectious Diseases of the Female Genital Tract*. Philadelphia, PA: Lippincott Williams & Wilkins; 2005.)

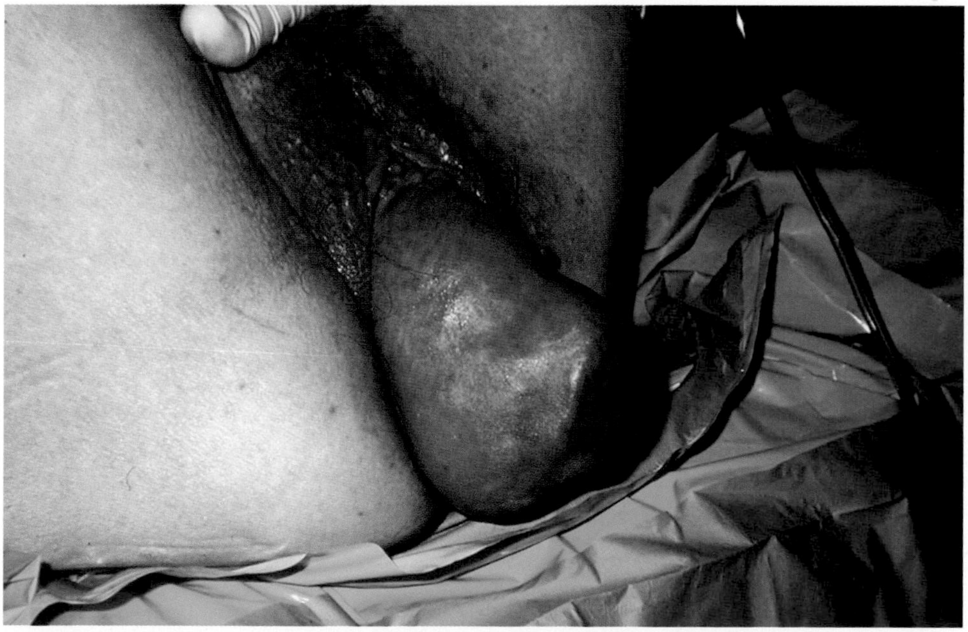

Color Plate 11 • Complete procidentia (prolapse) of the uterus and vagina.

(From Berek, JS. *Berek & Novak's Gynecology*, 14th ed. Philadelphia, PA: Lippincott Williams & Wilkins; 2006.)

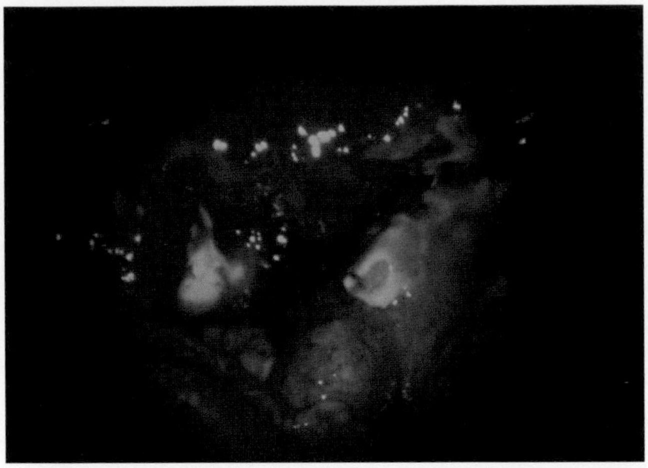

Color Plate 12 • Laparoscopic view of adult pelvic inflammatory disease.
(From Sweet R, Gibbs R. *Atlas of Infectious Diseases of the Female Genital Tract.* Philadelphia, PA: Lippincott Williams & Wilkins; 2005.)

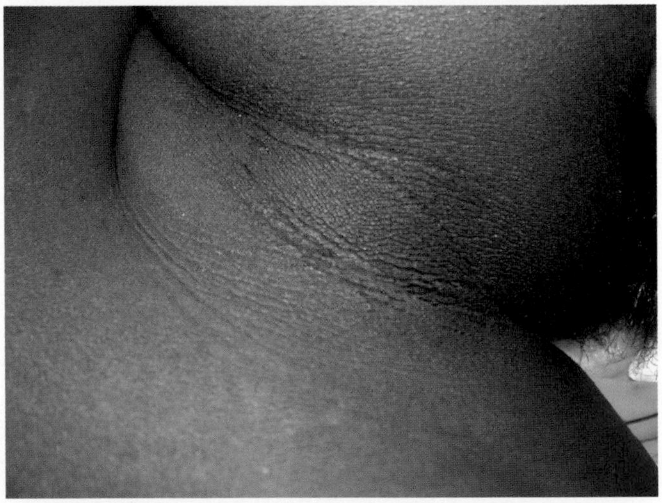

Color Plate 13 • Acanthosis nigricans associated with insulin resistance.
(From Berek JS. *Berek & Novak's Gynecology,* 14th ed. Philadelphia, PA: Lippincott Williams & Wilkins; 2006.)

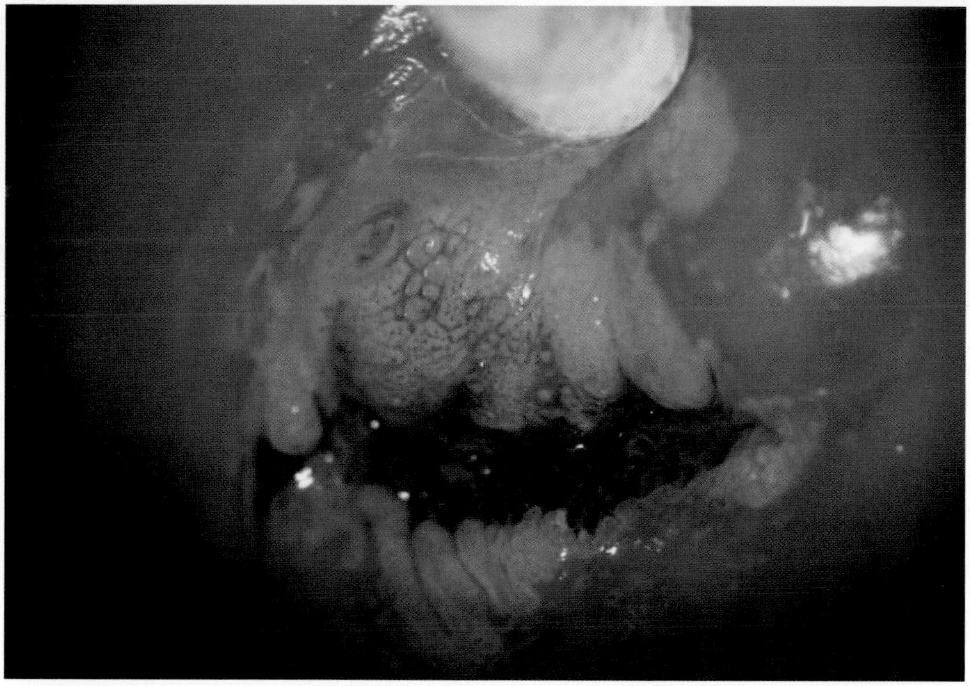

Color Plate 14 • Colposcopic view of cervix with CIN III showing mosaicism and punctations.
(From Berek JS. *Berek & Novak's Gynecology*, 14th ed. Philadelphia, PA: Lippincott Williams & Wilkins; 2006.)

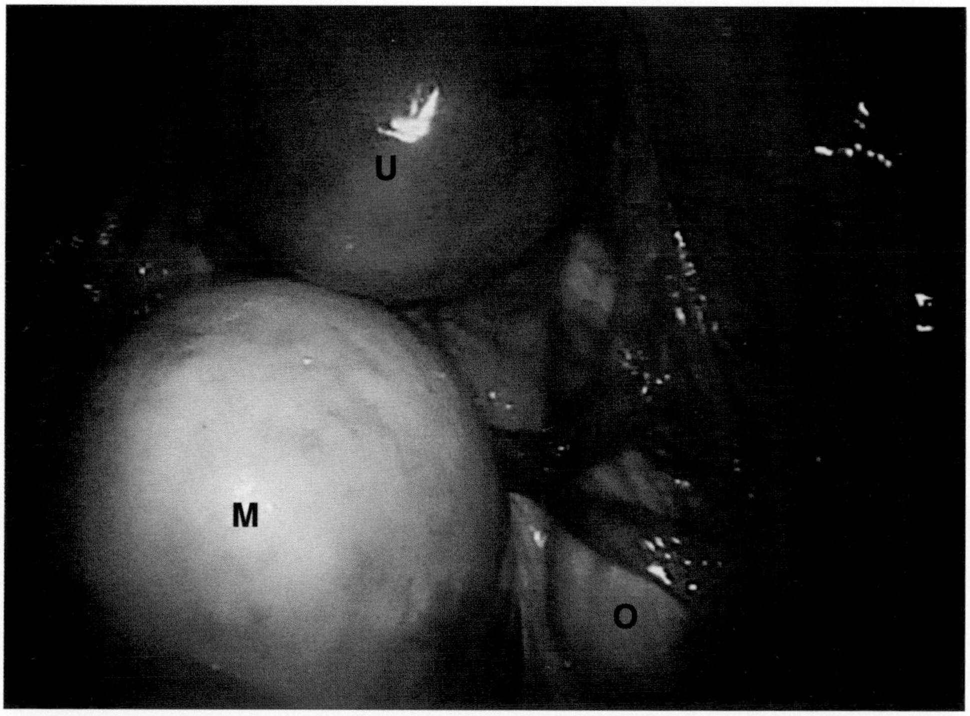

Color Plate 15 • Laparoscopic view of large ovarian mass (M) and normal uterus (U) and ovary (O).
(From Berek JS. *Berek & Novak's Gynecology*, 14th ed. Philadelphia, PA: Lippincott Williams & Wilkins; 2006.)

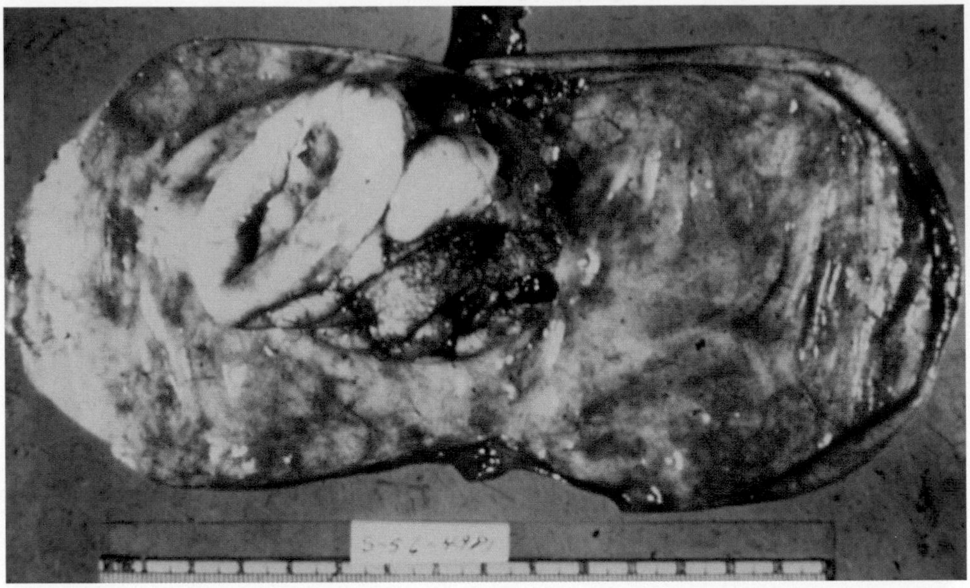

Color Plate 16 • Mature cystic teratoma (dermoid cyst).
(From Berek JS. *Berek & Novak's Gynecology*, 14th ed. Philadelphia, PA: Lippincott Williams & Wilkins; 2006.)

A Answers

Vignette 1 Question 1

Answer D: The symptoms and findings are most consistent with *Trichomonas*. Symptomatic patients report a frothy vaginal discharge that may be yellow, gray, or green. Vaginal pH is typically 6 to 7 and vulvar or vaginal mucosa is erythematous. The classical cervical findings include erythematous, punctate epithelial papillae, or "strawberry" appearance. Motile, flagellated protozoans are visible on wet prep microscopic examination.

Branching hyphae is seen with yeast infections. Symptoms include vaginal burning, pruritus, and increased thick, white, curdy vaginal discharge. Multinucleated giant cells can be seen on Tzanck smear preparation of herpetic lesions. Genital herpes is typically described as multiple 1 to 3 mm painful vesicles. You would expect to see increased WBCs with *Trichomonas*. Epithelial cells covered with bacteria, also known as clue cells, are seen with bacterial vaginosis (BV). Typical findings of BV include pH greater than 4.5 as well as an increase thin, white, malodorous, fishy vaginal discharge coating the vaginal walls. The addition of 10% KOH to the vaginal discharge typically produces a fishy amine odor. BV does not usually cause vaginal inflammation.

Vignette 1 Question 2

Answer C: Trichomoniasis is caused by *Trichomonas vaginalis*. Syphilis is caused by *Treponema pallidum*. Syphilis is divided into different stages. Primary syphilis is characterized by a nontender, red, round, firm ulcer approximately 1 cm in size with raised edges, known as a chancre. None of these findings were presents in this patient. *Neisseria gonorrhoeae* causes gonorrhea. Approximately 50% of women with gonorrhea are asymptomatic. *N. gonorrhoeae* is a common cause of mucopurulent cervicitis and pelvic inflammatory disease. This patient does not have clinical findings of either of these conditions. Bacterial vaginosis is typically caused by *Gardnerella vaginalis*. *Haemophilus ducreyi* causes chancroid, which is an ulcerated genital lesion. This patient did not present with an ulcerated lesion.

Vignette 1 Question 3

Answer A: A single-dose regimen with metronidazole or tinidazole is the mainstay treatment of trichomoniasis. An alternative multidose regimen is metronidazole 500 mg orally twice daily for 7 days. Compliance may be improved with the single-dose therapy. Doxycycline can be used to treat chlamydial infections. Azithromycin can be used to treat chlamydial infections and chancroid. Clindamycin can be used as an alternative regimen for the treatment of bacterial vaginosis. Metronidazole gel is considerable less efficacious for the treatment of trichomoniasis. The use of topical antimicrobial preparation is unlikely to achieve therapeutic levels in the perivaginal glands and is not recommended.

Vignette 1 Question 4

Answer C: Because of the high rate of concomitant *Trichomonas* infections in sexual partners, all partners should be treated to prevent reinfection. No data supports the rescreening for *T. vaginalis* at 3 months following initial infection. This is likely due to the high efficacy of nitroimidazole drugs, with a 90% to 95% cure rate. *T. vaginalis* susceptibility testing is available through the CDC. It is only recommended for refractory cases after multiple treatment failures. Reinfection and noncompliance should be ruled out. Empiric treatment for chlamydial infection is not recommended with the diagnosis of *Trichomonas* infections. On the other hand, empiric treatment of chlamydial infection is recommended in patients infected with *N. gonorrhoeae* due to the high frequency of coinfection (unless chlamydial coinfection has been ruled out by nucleic acid amplification testing). Sexual partners should receive treatment.

Vignette 1 Question 5

Answer B: Metronidazole 500 mg orally twice a day for 7 days is recommended for cases of metronidazole single-dose treatment failure. Treatment with tinidazole 2 g orally daily for 5 days is recommended after treatment failure with both the single-dose and the multidose metronidazole regimens. Consultation with infectious disease specialist is recommended only for refractory cases after multiple treatment failures. Reinfection and noncompliance should be ruled out. *T. vaginalis* susceptibility testing is available through the CDC. It is recommended only for refractory cases after multiple treatment failures. Reinfection and noncompliance should be ruled out. Clindamycin can be used as an alternative regimen for the treatment of bacterial vaginosis. Nitroimidazoles are the only class of drugs useful for the treatment of *Trichomonas* infections.

Vignette 2 Question 1

Answer E: In patients with mucopurulent discharge, an NAAT for chlamydial infection and gonorrhea should be performed. In addition, the CDC recommends annual screening of all sexually active women aged 25 years and less. Screening for cervical cancer is not indicated in this patient. Pap smears should begin at 21 years of age regardless of age at first intercourse. A pelvic ultrasound is not indicated based on lack of current symptoms and physical examination findings. A diagnosis of chlamydial infection or gonorrhea should be made prior to treatment. Vaginal cultures are typically not a useful diagnostic tool because they are nonspecific. Vaginal cultures can be useful if yeast or trichomoniasis is suspected and microscopy is normal. Gram stain can be useful in diagnosing bacterial vaginosis. The sensitivity of Gram stain to the diagnosis of chlamydial infection or gonorrhea is low. In addition, the patient has no findings consistent with BV, yeast, or trichomoniasis. Performing NAAT for chlamydial infection and gonorrhea is the most appropriate next step.

Vignette 2 Question 2

Answer A: In patients with a confirmed diagnosis of gonorrhea without a chlamydial coinfection, the correct treatment is ceftriaxone 125 mg IM once. Unless chlamydial co-infection has been ruled out, patients diagnosed with gonorrhea should be empirically treated for chlamydial infection with ceftriaxone and azithromycin. In this case, a chlamydial coinfection has already been excluded through NAAT and treatment should only include ceftriaxone. Doxycycline 100 mg orally twice daily for 7 days is the correct treatment for chlamydial infection. Because of increasing resistance, fluoroquinolones are no longer recommended in the United States for the treatment of gonorrhea. Clindamycin can be used as an alternative regimen for the treatment of bacterial vaginosis.

Vignette 2 Question 3

Answer E: If left untreated, this patient would be at risk for developing cervicitis, pelvic inflammatory disease (PID), tubo-ovarian abscess (TOA), or disseminated gonorrhea. Cervicitis is most commonly caused by chlamydial infection and gonorrhea. PID occurs in approximately 10% to 40% of women with cervical gonorrhea. Estimates of the progression to TOA occur in approximately 3% to 16% with PID. Disseminated gonorrhea occurs in 0.5% to 3% of *Neisseria gonorrhoeae* infections.

Vignette 3 Question 1

Answer B: Genital herpes classically presents with painful clusters of small vesicles and ulcers. Moreover, primary infections usually begin with flulike symptoms including malaise, myalgias, nausea, diarrhea, and fever. *Treponema pallidum* causes syphilis. Syphilis is divided into different stages. Primary syphilis is characterized by a nontender, red, round, firm ulcer approximately 1 cm in size with raised edges, known as a chancre. The vesicles described in this case are different than that typically seen in primary syphilis. *Trichomonas vaginalis* typically causes vaginitis, not genital ulcers. Symptomatic patients report a frothy vaginal discharge that may be yellow, gray, or green. Vaginal pH is typically elevated and vulvar or vaginal mucosa is erythematous. The classical cervical findings include erythematous, punctate epithelial papillae, or "strawberry" appearance. Motile, flagellated protozoans are visible on wet prep microscopic examination. *C. trachomatis* L-serotypes (L1, L2, or L3) cause lymphogranuloma venereum (LGV). The primary stage of LGV is characterized by nontender papules or shallow ulcers, which heal quickly and often go unnoticed. Painful inguinal lymphadenopathy typically occurs 2 to 6 weeks after the primary lesion. The vesicles described in this case are different than that typically seen in primary LGV. *Haemophilus ducreyi* causes chancroid. The lesion presents initially as an erythematous papule, which evolves to a pustule and ulcer. The ulcer is painful with an erythematous base and irregular, well-demarcated borders.

Vignette 3 Question 2

Answer D: A definitive diagnosis of genital herpes should be made through viral or serology testing. Many patients present with atypical lesions such as fissures or abrasions. It is estimated that up to 80% of new cases of genital herpes are attributable to HSV-1, particularly among adolescent and young adult populations. Thus, with a primary infection, you would expect to find HSV-1 IgG, positive. An HSV viral culture can be used to diagnose genital herpes; however, the culture has poor sensitivity. A positive *T. pallidum* particle agglutination assay (TPPA) would be diagnostic for syphilis. A positive *H. ducreyi* culture would be diagnostic for chancroid. This patient has a primary genital herpes infection. The majority of these infections are attributed to HSV-1, not HSV-2. Thus, the most likely finding would be HSV-1 IgG, positive. Finally, the diagnosis of genital herpes should not be based on clinical suspicion. Up to 20% of at-risk women with findings compatible with herpetic lesions will not have genital herpes. Thus, a definitive diagnosis should be made through viral or serology testing.

Vignette 3 Question 3

Answer C: For primary genital herpes infections, acyclovir 200 mg orally five times daily for 7 to 10 days is recommended to reduce the length of infection and the length of time a patient has viral shedding. Other options include a 7 to 10 day oral treatment with acyclovir 400 mg three times per day, famciclovir 250 mg three times per day, or valacyclovir 1 g twice per day. Ceftriaxone is used to treat chancroid and gonorrhea. Imiquimod (Aldara) is used to treat genital warts. Benzathine penicillin G is used to treat primary, secondary, or early latent syphilis. Extended regimens of doxycycline can be used to treat lymphogranuloma venereum caused by *C. trachomatis* L-serotypes (L1, L2, or L3).

Vignette 3 Question 4

Answer D: Viral shedding can occur both with and without genital herpes symptoms. It is important to counsel patients that they can transmit the virus even if they are asymptomatic. Subclinical viral shedding appears to be highest in the first 6 months following acquisition and is more common immediately before and after a clinical outbreak. Condom use can reduce the risk of transmission of genital herpes, but will not prevent the transmission. Both symptomatic and asymptomatic viral shedding can occur in genital areas not covered or protected by a condom. Recurrent outbreaks can be reduced through the use of daily suppressive antiviral drugs. Suppressive therapy prevents approximately 80% of recurrences. Recurrence is more frequent with HSV-2. Cesarean delivery is recommended only for those pregnant patients with active genital lesions or prodromal symptoms.

Vignette 4 Question 1

Answer D: This patient most likely has bacterial vaginosis (BV). BV is caused by an overgrowth of anaerobic bacteria (*Prevotella* sp. and *Mobiluncus* sp.), *Gardnerella vaginalis*, *Ureaplasma*, *Mycoplasma*, and numerous fastidious or uncultivated anaerobes. With this shift in vaginal flora, there is an accompanied decrease in lactobacilli. Patients usually complain of an increased vaginal discharge that often has a malodorous fishy amine odor. Diagnosis of BV can be made with three of the following findings: presence of thin, white, homogeneous discharge coating the vaginal walls; an amine odor noted with addition of 10% KOH ("whiff" test); pH of greater than 4.5; or presence of clue cells (vaginal epithelial cells that are diffusely covered with bacteria) on microscopic examination.

Branching hyphae on 10% KOH prepared microscopic examination would support the diagnosis of candidiasis. This patient does not have any major risk factor for chlamydial infection. Her examination findings do not reveal a mucopurulent discharge or any signs of cervicitis or PID. A vaginal pH greater than 4.5 would support the diagnosis of BV.

Vignette 4 Question 2

Answer D: Metronidazole 500 mg orally twice daily for 7 days is the correct treatment for BV. Alternatives include clindamycin 300 mg twice a day for 7 days or topical formulations of these antibiotics. Metronidazole 2 g orally once is only 75% effective in treating BV. However, it is the correct treatment for *Trichomonas vaginalis*. Doxycycline 100 mg orally twice daily for 7 days is the correct treatment for chlamydial infection. Azithromycin 1 g orally once is also the correct treatment option for chlamydial infection. Fluconazole 150 mg orally once is the treatment for candidiasis.

Vignette 4 Question 3

Answer A: There is a high risk of BV recurrence after treatment, reported up to 30%. Women should be advised to return for evaluation if symptoms recur. BV is not an STI. It is associated with the acquisition of other STIs as well as multiple sexual partners. However, women who have never been sexually active can also be affected. Treatment of sexual partners is not recommended with BV. Clinical trials indicate that treatment of sexual partners has not been beneficial in preventing BV recurrence. Although BV is associated with acquisition of some STIs, empiric treatment for chlamydial infection is not recommended. On the other hand, empiric treatment of chlamydial infection is recommended in patients infected with *N. gonorrhoeae* due to the high frequency of coinfection (unless chlamydial coinfection has been ruled out by NAAT). Treatment for BV is recommended only for symptomatic women.

Vignette 4 Question 4

Answer D: Risk factors for BV include new or multiple sexual partners, douching, lack of vaginal lactobacilli, female sexual partners, and cigarette smoking. The use of the contraceptive ring (NuvaRing) has not been associated with an increased risk of BV. On the other hand, the NuvaRing is more likely to promote lactobacilli and may be protective against developing BV.

Chapter 17 Upper Female Reproductive Tract and Systemic Infections

THE UPPER FEMALE REPRODUCTIVE TRACT

Women experience more upper reproductive tract, pelvic, and abdominal infections compared to men because of the absence of a mucosal lining or epithelium between these spaces and the external body in the female patient. Although defenses such as ciliary movement creating flow and cervical mucus exist, there is essentially an open tract between the vagina, the pelvis, and abdomen. This can lead to ascending infections of the uterus, fallopian tubes, adnexa, pelvis, and abdomen. This open ascending tract may also lead to the acquisition of toxic shock syndrome (TSS). Further, because the vaginal epithelium is easily abraded during intercourse, transmission of systemic infections such as HIV and hepatitis B and C is more common from men to women than the converse.

ENDOMETRITIS

Pathogenesis

Endometritis is an infection of the uterine endometrium; if the infection invades into the myometrium, it is known as **endomyometritis**. Endometritis and endomyometritis are included in a spectrum of inflammatory disorders of the upper female genital tract that comprises pelvic inflammatory disease (PID). Risk factors include retained products of conception, sexually transmitted infections (STIs), intrauterine foreign bodies or growths, and instrumentation of the intrauterine cavity. It is seen most commonly after cesarean delivery, but also after vaginal deliveries and surgical pregnancy terminations. Endometritis is an uncommon complication of minimally invasive transcervical gynecologic procedures such as hysteroscopy, endometrial ablation, endometrial biopsy, and intrauterine device (IUD) placement. In such cases, routine use of antibiotic prophylaxis is not recommended. However, antibiotic prophylaxis is recommended for cesarean sections, surgical terminations of pregnancy, and hysterosalpingography or sonohysterography in women with a history of pelvic infection or if dilated tubes are demonstrated. Nonpuerperal endometritis is not commonly recognized but is probably coexistent with 70% to 80% of PID. Its etiology is related to ascent of infection from the cervix, which then proceeds to the fallopian tubes to cause acute salpingitis and, eventually, widespread PID. Diagnosis of endomyometritis is made in the clinical settings described above with a bimanual examination revealing uterine tenderness, as well as fever and elevated WBC count.

Chronic endometritis is often asymptomatic but is clinically significant because it leads to other pelvic infections and, uncommonly, endomyometritis. It is often a polymicrobial infection with a variety of pathogens, including skin and gastrointestinal flora in addition to the usual flora colonizing the lower reproductive tract. Mycobacterium tuberculosis is a rare cause of chronic endometritis in developed countries but is a leading cause of infertility in endemic countries. Chronic endometritis can be suspected in patients with chronic irregular bleeding, discharge, and pelvic pain. The diagnosis can be made in a nonpuerperal patient with endometrial biopsy showing plasma cells.

Treatment

Treatment of severe endomyometritis unrelated to pregnancy is the same as treatment for PID. For postpartum endomyometritis, treatment consists of clindamycin 900 mg IV every 8 hours and gentamicin loaded with 2 mg/kg IV and then maintained with 1.5 mg/kg IV every 8 hours. Single daily IV dosing of gentamicin (5 mg/kg every 24 hours) may be substituted for 8-hour dosing. Single antibiotic agent treatment of endometritis may also be considered, including cephalosporins such as cefoxitin 2 g IV every 6 hours. Treatment course continues until clinical improvement and afebrile status for 24 to 48 hours. Oral antibiotic therapy is not required following successful parenteral treatment. In nonpuerperal infections where chlamydial infection may be the suspected cause, doxycycline should be added to the regimen for a total of 14 days. Chronic endometritis, on the other hand, is treated with a 10- to 14-day course of doxycycline 100 mg PO BID.

PELVIC INFLAMMATORY DISEASE

Pelvic inflammatory disease (PID) is an infection of the upper female genital tract including any combination of endometritis, salpingitis, tubo-ovarian abscess, and pelvic peritonitis. It is the most common serious complication of STIs. An estimated 750,000 to 1 million cases occur annually in the United States. The annual expense of initial treatment is estimated at $3.5 to $5 billion, which does not account for possible future treatment for the principal sequelae, including infertility and increased ectopic pregnancies. PID is strongly associated with infertility. Specifically, infertility risk increases with the number of PID episodes: 12% with one episode, approximately 20% with two episodes, and 40% with three or more episodes. Additionally, the risk of ectopic pregnancy is increased as much as 7- to 10-fold and approximately 20% of women develop chronic pelvic pain during their lifetime. Sequelae, including chronic pelvic pain, dyspareunia, and pelvic adhesions, may also require surgical therapy, contributing to the economic costs and morbidity of this disease.

Among sexually active women, the incidence of this disease is highest in the 15- to 25-year-old age group (at least three times greater than in the 25- to 29-year-old age group). This may be attributed to higher-risk behavior of this age group. It may also be related to decreased immunity to STI agents in younger women, although the pathophysiology is unclear. Finally, the younger age group is less likely to have regular gynecological care or to seek medical attention until bacterial vaginosis or cervicitis has progressed to the more symptomatic PID (Fig. 17-1).

Other risk factors for PID include nonwhite and non-Asian ethnicity, multiple partners, recent history of douching, prior history of PID, and cigarette smoking. IUDs are considered a risk factor for PID when insertion occurs in the setting of concurrent chlamydial infection or gonorrhea, where the prevalence of STIs is high, and when aseptic conditions cannot be assured. In contrast, barrier contraceptives have been shown to decrease the incidence of PID, and use of oral contraceptives appears to diminish the severity of PID.

Clinical Manifestations

The principal symptom of acute salpingitis is abdominal or pelvic/adnexal pain. The character of the pain can range (burning, cramping, stabbing) and can be unilateral or bilateral. Pain may also be absent in what has been deemed "silent" PID. Other associated symptoms include increased vaginal discharge, abnormal odor, abnormal bleeding, gastrointestinal disturbances, and urinary tract symptoms. Fever is a less common symptom, seen in only 20% of women with PID.

Diagnosis

Because untreated PID can lead to serious sequelae (e.g., infertility), a low threshold for diagnosis and treatment should be maintained. Minimum criteria for empiric treatment include pelvic or lower abdominal pain in sexually active young women or women at risk for STIs, and one or more of the following: cervical motion tenderness, uterine tenderness, or adnexal tenderness. Additional diagnostic criteria that supports the diagnosis of PID include fever (>38.3°C), abnormal cervical or vaginal mucopurulent discharge, abundant WBC on saline microscopy of vaginal secretions, elevated erythrocyte sedimentation rate, elevated C-reactive protein, and cervical *Neisseria gonorrhoeae* or *Chlamydia trachomatis* infections. Cervical cultures are performed to find a causative organism but, because of the disease's polymicrobial nature, should not dictate the treatment regimen. The definitive diagnosis is made via laparoscopy, endometrial biopsy, or pelvic imaging with PID findings. In practice, a more invasive diagnostic laparoscopic surgical procedure is usually performed only when appendicitis cannot be ruled out by clinical examination or when there is a poor response to treatment with antibiotics. Occasionally, PID is complicated by **Fitzhugh-Curtis syndrome** (Color Plate 10). This is a perihepatitis from the ascending infection resulting in right upper quadrant pain and tenderness and liver function test (LFT) elevations.

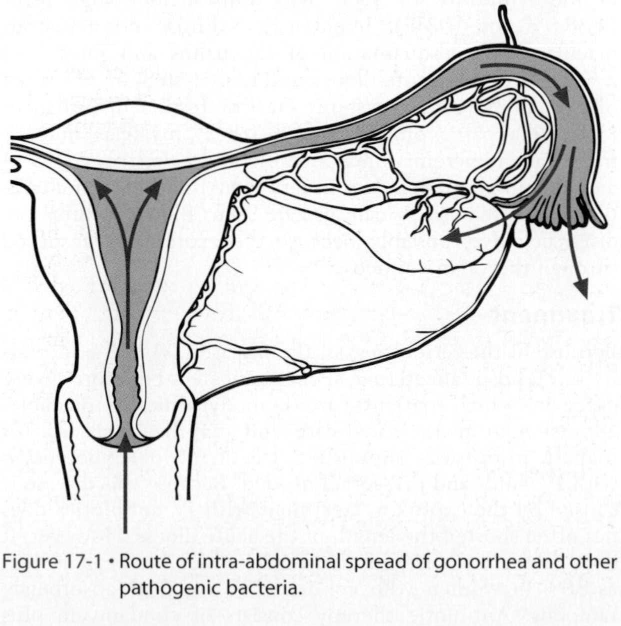

Figure 17-1 • Route of intra-abdominal spread of gonorrhea and other pathogenic bacteria.

The principal organisms suspected of causing PID are *N. gonorrhoeae* and *C. trachomatis*; these two organisms together account for approximately 40% of all PID cases. However, cultures from the upper reproductive tract have shown that most PID is likely to be polymicrobial, including anaerobic organisms such as *Bacteroides* species and facultative bacteria such as *Gardnerella*, *Escherichia coli*, *Haemophilus influenzae*, and streptococci.

Treatment

Because of the high rate of ambulatory treatment failures and the seriousness of sequelae, patients are often hospitalized for treatment of PID, particularly those who are teenagers, unable to tolerate POs, pregnant, noncompliant, febrile, or who have been refractory to outpatient therapy. PID is usually treated with a broad-spectrum cephalosporin, such as cefoxitin 2 g IV every 6 hours or cefotetan 2 g IV every 12 hours plus doxycycline 100 mg IV or orally every 12 hours because of its polymicrobial nature. The IV antibiotic regimen is continued until the patient demonstrates clinical improvement for 24 hours, and doxycycline 100 mg orally twice a day is continued for a total 14-day course. In patients allergic to cephalosporins, IV clindamycin and gentamicin can be used. On an outpatient basis, a single dose of ceftriaxone 250 mg IM or cefoxitin 2 g IM plus 1 g of probenecid orally along with oral doxycycline 100 mg orally twice a day for 14 days is used with close follow-up for resolution of symptoms. If patients have BV or *Trichomonas*, then metronidazole 500 mg orally twice a day for 14 days must be added. PID is rare in pregnant patients; because tetracyclines and fluoroquinolones are avoided in pregnancy, clindamycin and gentamicin is the treatment of choice during pregnancy. Additionally, because of the emergence of fluoroquinolone-resistant *N. gonorrhoeae* in the United States, fluoroquinolones are no longer recommended by the CDC for treatment of gonorrhea or of PID cases in which *N. gonorrhoeae* may be a causative agent.

TUBO-OVARIAN ABSCESS

Persistent PID can lead to the development of tubo-ovarian abscess (TOA) (Fig. 17-2). Most so-called TOAs are actually tubo-ovarian complexes (TOC), the difference being that complexes are not walled off like the true abscess and are thus more responsive to antimicrobial therapy. Estimates of the progression from PID to TOA range from 3% to 16%; thus, any PID not responsive to therapy should

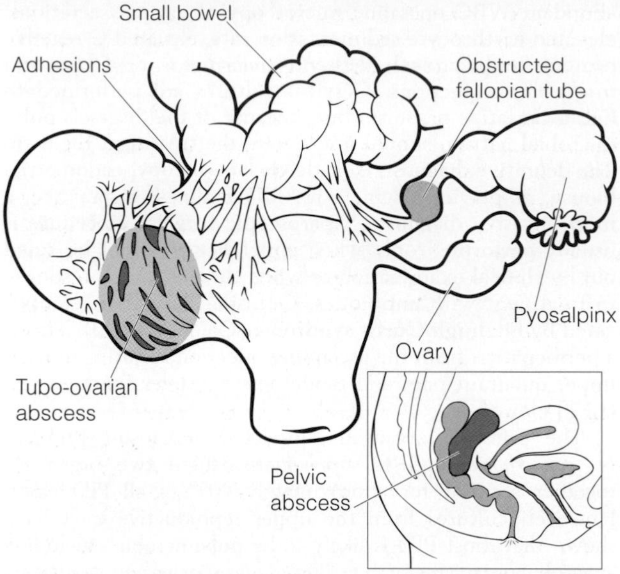

Figure 17-2 • Findings associated with chronic pelvic inflammatory disease, including tubo-ovarian abscess, adhesions, pyosalpinx, and an abscess located in the posterior cul-de-sac.

be investigated further to rule out TOA. Furthermore, HIV-infected women with PID are at increased risk of development of TOA.

Diagnosis

The diagnosis of TOA can be made clinically in the setting of PID and the appreciation of an adnexal or posterior cul-de-sac mass or fullness. Most patients will endorse abdominal and/or pelvic pain (90%) and demonstrate fever and leukocytosis (60% to 80%). WBC count is usually elevated with a left shift and the erythrocyte sedimentation rate (ESR) is often elevated as well. Cultures should include endocervical swabs and blood cultures to rule out sepsis. Culdocentesis that reveals gross pus is diagnostic but has been used less as advances in imaging studies have been made. Although most TOA are appreciated by clinical examination, a negative examination does not rule out a TOA. Ultrasound is the imaging study of choice to diagnose TOAs and is able to distinguish between TOAs and TOCs. However, pelvic CT may be required, particularly in obese patients for whom ultrasound use is limited. Finally, laparoscopy can lead to a definitive diagnosis but is usually used only when the clinical picture is unclear.

Treatment

While treatment of TOAs can be medical or surgical, a trial of medical management with broad-spectrum antibiotics in an inpatient setting is frequently the first step. Unless the abscess is ruptured and causing peritoneal signs or is impenetrable by antibiotics, surgical treatment can often be avoided. Treatment is the same as that for the parenteral treatment for PID and include broad-spectrum cephalosporin (cefotetan 2 g IV every 12 hours or cefoxitin 2 g IV every 6 hours) plus doxycycline (100 mg PO or IV every 12 hours). Clindamycin (900 mg every 8 hours) plus gentamicin (loading dose of 2 mg/kg, followed by 1.5 mg/kg IV every 8 hours or 5 mg/kg IV every 24 hours) with or without ampicillin (3 g IV every 6 hours) is another recommended regimen. The course of this disease can be monitored by symptoms, clinical examination, temperature, WBC count, and, if these are equivocal, imaging studies. Typically, a repeat pelvic examination is performed after the patient has been afebrile for 24 to 48 hours to monitor for improvement and eventual resolution of tenderness. If responsive to medical management, the patient can be converted to oral antibiotics to complete a 10- to 14-day course with doxycycline plus clindamycin or metronidazole.

For more serious TOAs, either unresponsive to antibiotic therapy or with gross rupture, surgical intervention is necessary. Drainage of TOA using ultrasound guidance or laparoscopy may be considered in patients who do not respond to 48 hours of medical therapy. Unilateral salpingo-oophorectomy is considered as a curative therapy for the unilateral TOA by some authorities. For bilateral TOAs, often a total abdominal hysterectomy and bilateral salpingo-oophorectomy (TAHBSO) may be necessary.

TOXIC SHOCK SYNDROME

Toxic shock syndrome (TSS) reached its peak in the United States in 1980 when the rate was 6 to 12:100,000 menstruating women. Since 1984, the incidence has decreased dramatically and the current annual incidence is estimated at 1 to 2:100,000 women. Initially, TSS was correlated with high-absorbency tampons and menstruation in approximately 50% to 70% of cases over the past two decades. Of note, the proportion of menstrual-related TSS has been decreasing over time. Nonmenstrual-related TSS has been associated with vaginal infections, vaginal delivery, cesarean section, postpartum endometritis, miscarriage, and laser treatment of condylomata.

Diagnosis

TSS is caused by colonization or infection with specific strains of *Staphylococcus aureus* that produce an epidermal toxin—toxic shock syndrome toxin-1 (TSST-1). This toxin and other staphylococcal toxins are likely to cause most of the symptoms of TSS. Symptoms include high fever (>38.9°C or 102°F), hypotension, diffuse erythematous macular rash, desquamation of the palms and soles 1 to 2 weeks after the acute illness, and multisystem involvement of three or more organ systems. Gastrointestinal disturbances (abdominal pain, vomiting, and diarrhea), myalgias, mucous membrane hyperemia, increased blood urea nitrogen (BUN) and creatinine, platelet count less than 100,000, and alteration in consciousness can also be seen. Blood cultures are often negative, possibly because the exotoxin is absorbed through the vaginal mucosa.

Treatment

Because of the seriousness of the disease (2% to 8% mortality rate), hospitalization is always indicated. For more severe cases in which patients are hemodynamically unstable, admission to an intensive care unit may be necessary. Of highest priority is supportive treatment of hypotension with IV fluids and pressors if needed. Because this disease is caused by the exotoxin, treatment with IV antibiotics does not often shorten the length of the acute illness. However, it does decrease the risk of recurrence, which has been as high as 30% in women who continued to use high-absorbency tampons. Antibiotic therapy consists of clindamycin plus vancomycin for empiric treatment when specific *S. aureus* isolate sensitivity is unknown, clindamycin plus vancomycin or linezolid in MRSA TSS cases, and clindamycin plus nafcillin or oxacillin in MSSA TSS cases. Treatment duration is generally 10 to 14 days. Currently, there is a lack of controlled studies to support the use of IV immune globulin or corticosteroid therapy.

HUMAN IMMUNODEFICIENCY VIRUS

HIV is the causative agent of AIDS. HIV is transmitted via sexual contact, via parenteral inoculation, and vertically from mothers to infants via a transplacental route, during birth from direct exposure, and via breast milk. There were an estimated 11,200 new HIV infections among women in the United States in 2009, comprising 23% of all new HIV infections. Women of color are disproportionally affected at all stages of HIV infection. In 2009, African American women made up 14% of the female population but accounted for approximately 66% of HIV infections among female patients. Similarly, Latina women made up 11% of the female population but accounted for 14% of HIV infections among female patients. The proportion of AIDS cases among adult and adolescent females (age ≥13 years) in the United States increased from 7% in 1985 to 25% in 2008. However, between 2006 and 2009, the number of diagnoses of HIV infection and AIDS has decreased among women. Worldwide, women represent a far more substantial proportion of those affected with HIV. According to the Joint United Nations Program on HIV/AIDS, in 2009, nearly 52% of adults living with HIV worldwide were women. In 2009, there were approximately 33.3 million people living with HIV and 1.8 million AIDS-related deaths. Worldwide, the number of new HIV infections, mother-to-child transmission of HIV, and AIDS-related deaths are decreasing. The effects of antiretrovirals are especially evident in sub-Saharan Africa since 2004 with the expansion of antiretroviral therapy (ART).

Infection with HIV—a retrovirus—leads to decreased cellular immunity because various cells carrying the CD4 antigen become infected, including helper T cells, B cells, monocytes, and macrophages. Initially, the infection is entirely asymptomatic, although the individual is a carrier of the disease; this stage can last from 5 to 7 years. This disease may appear initially with the AIDS-related complex, which includes lymphadenopathy, night sweats, malaise, diarrhea, weight loss, and unusual recurrent infections such as oral candidiasis, varicella zoster, or herpes simplex. As the infection further decreases cellular immunity, full-blown AIDS develops with opportunistic infections such as *Pneumocystis carinii* pneumonia, toxoplasmosis, *Mycobacterium avium-intracellulare*, cytomegalovirus, and various malignancies such as Kaposi sarcoma and non-Hodgkin lymphoma.

Diagnosis

The diagnosis of HIV infection is made initially via a screening test. Most commonly, the test is an enzyme-linked immunosorbent assay (ELISA), using HIV antigens, to which patient serum is added. A positive test results when antigen–antibody complexes form. This test does have false-positive results, which, in low-risk populations, may occur more often than true positive results. Positive tests are therefore confirmed by a Western blot. Another level of confirmation may be obtained if a viral load is sent and is positive. Viral loads and CD4 cell counts are used to follow the progression of disease. The CDC currently recommends routine HIV screening as a normal part of medical practice for nonpregnant patients and as a normal part of prenatal screening for pregnant women.

Treatment

There is no known cure for HIV or AIDS. The approach to this disease is prevention of transmission, prophylaxis of opportunistic infections, and prolonging the lives of infected patients by slowing progression of disease with antiretroviral agents. Great efforts are being directed toward prevention of HIV transmission by encouraging modification of risky behavior. In addition, in 2012, the FDA approved of the combination medication, tenofovir disoproxil fumarate plus emtricitabine (TDF/FTC), for use as "pre-exposure prophylaxis" among sexually active adults without HIV to reduce their risk of becoming infected. Condoms are recommended for sexually active patients. IV drug users should avoid sharing needles and use clean needles. With improved screening methods, the risk of HIV infection from blood transfusion is currently estimated at less than 1:1,000,000.

Prophylaxis and treatment of the opportunistic infections in HIV-positive patients are discussed in *Blueprints Medicine*. Delaying the progress of the disease is accomplished primarily with nucleoside analogs and protease inhibitors. The nucleoside analogs—zidovudine (AZT), lamivudine (3TC), abacavir, didanosine, and stavudine—act to inhibit reverse transcriptase and interfere with viral replication. Protease inhibitors (lopinavir, atazanavir, indinavir, saquinavir, ritonavir) interfere with the synthesis of viral particles and have been effective in increasing CD4 counts and decreasing viral load. Because the action mechanisms of these two groups differ, a synergistic effect is seen with combination therapy known as highly active antiretroviral therapy (HAART). Multiagent therapy also decreases drug resistance. Other antiretroviral drug classes include nonnucleoside reverse transcriptase inhibitors, and newer drug classes including entry inhibitors, CCR5 receptor antagonists, and integrase inhibitors.

Beyond this simple review of HIV management, there are issues regarding HIV infection in women that deserve special emphasis. First, obstetric care of the HIV patient demands attention to both the ongoing care of the patient as well as the prevention of vertical transmission to the fetus. Second, the high incidence of invasive cervical cancer in this population requires more aggressive screening than in the general population.

In the United States, approximately 7,000 infants are born annually to mothers who are infected with HIV. With no treatment, approximately 25% of infants born to HIV-infected mothers will become infected with HIV. Increased transmission can be seen with higher viral burden or advanced disease in the mother, rupture of the membranes, and invasive procedures during labor and delivery that increase neonatal exposure to maternal blood. Vertical transmission can occur intrauterine (20% to 50%), intrapartum (50% to 80%), or postpartum (15%). In 1994, Pediatric AIDS Clinical Trials Group (PACTG) protocol 076 demonstrated that a three-part regimen of **zidovudine** (ZDV) administered during pregnancy and labor and to the newborn could reduce the risk of perinatal transmission by two-thirds in women. Additionally, with the use of HAART to further decrease viral load with potent regimens, the rate of transmission can be further decreased to less than 1% to 2% with an undetectable viral load. Currently, ART in pregnancy includes a three-drug regimen generally started in the second trimester with a goal for viral suppression by the third trimester, regardless of need for antiretrovirals for maternal health indication. Cesarean delivery has been shown to lower transmission rates by roughly two-thirds compared to vaginal delivery in patients on no therapy and particularly without onset of labor or rupture of membranes or in the setting of high viral load. However, in women with viral loads less than 1,000 copies/mL, there is no additional benefit of cesarean delivery versus vaginal delivery in HIV perinatal transmission. Therefore, cesarean delivery should be considered in HIV-infected pregnant women with viral loads greater than 1,000 copies/mL and without longstanding onset of labor or rupture of membranes. Because of the effective interventions in HIV-positive women to decrease vertical transmission, it is recommended that HIV screening be offered to all pregnant women at their first prenatal visit and again in the third trimester if the woman has specified risk factors for HIV infection. Furthermore, in resource-rich nations where safe bottle feeding alternatives are available, breastfeeding is contraindicated in HIV-infected woman as virus is found in breast milk and is responsible for HIV transmission to the infant. Postnatal HIV transmission from breast milk at 2 years may be as high as 15%. Furthermore, studies are lacking regarding the efficacy of maternal ART for prevention of transmission of HIV through breast milk and the toxicity of antiretroviral exposure of the infant via breast milk.

The high incidence of invasive cervical cancer in HIV-infected women is an important issue in gynecologic outpatient management. Studies confirm the synergistic association of HIV and human papillomavirus (HPV), the causative agent in squamous cell carcinoma of the cervix. The Centers for Disease Control and Prevention currently recommends routine Pap smears at initial evaluation and 6 months later. Thereafter, yearly evaluations are sufficient if results are negative unless there is documentation of previous HPV infection, squamous intraepithelial lesion, or symptomatic HIV disease, in which case the Pap smear should be repeated at 6-month intervals.

KEY POINTS

- Endomyometritis occurs most commonly after a delivery or instrumentation of the endometrial cavity.
- Diagnosis of endomyometritis is made clinically with findings of uterine tenderness, fever, and elevated WBC count.
- Endomyometritis unrelated to pregnancy is treated the same as PID. Endomyometritis related to pregnancy is treated with broad-spectrum antibiotics such as IV clindamycin and gentamicin or IV cephalosporins.
- There may be as many as one million cases of PID reported annually.
- Twelve percent of patients with one episode of PID will become infertile.
- Minimal diagnosis criteria for PID consists of pelvic or lower abdominal pain, plus uterine, adnexal, or cervical motion tenderness.
- Because of the seriousness of this disease and its sequelae, patients are often hospitalized and treated with IV antibiotics.
- Chronic or acute PID can lead to TOAs or TOCs.
- Diagnosis of TOA or TOC is most likely when there is an adnexal mass in the setting of PID symptoms. Confirmation is usually achieved with an imaging study such as pelvic ultrasound or CT.
- TOA treatment includes hospitalization and broad-spectrum IV antibiotics. For TOAs not responsive to antibiotics, surgical drainage of TOA is recommended.
- TSS peaked in 1984; since then the incidence has decreased dramatically and the current annual incidence is 1 to 2:100,000 women.
- TSS symptoms, which include fever, rash, and desquamation of palms and soles, are most likely caused by an *S. aureus* toxin, TSST-1.
- Because of the seriousness of TSS, patients are hospitalized and treated with IV antibiotics and, if necessary, hemodynamic support.
- HIV is transmitted via sexual contact, shared IV needles, and any activity where infected blood is introduced to a noninfected host.
- HIV infection is screened for with the ELISA test and confirmed with a Western blot.
- There is currently no cure for HIV infection, so treatment focuses on antiretroviral agents such as nucleoside analogs and protease inhibitors and treatment of the multiple opportunistic infections.
- Vertical transmission rates during pregnancy have been shown to decrease with antiretroviral treatment and are positively associated with viral load.

C Clinical Vignettes

Vignette 1

A 28-year-old G1P1 presents to the emergency department 4 days after primary cesarean section with complaints of fever, malaise, and increased lower abdominal pain for the past 6 hours. Her labor course was complicated by prolonged rupture of membranes and stage 2 arrest due to cephalopelvic disproportion resulting in a cesarean delivery. Her postoperative course was uncomplicated and she had been discharged home stable the day prior to presentation. Her temperature is 38.1°C (100.6°F), pulse rate is 102/min, respirations are 20/min, and BP is 110/70 mm Hg. Abdominal examination shows fundal tenderness. The incision is intact without erythema, warmth, or discharge. On pelvic examination, there is foul-smelling lochia. Her WBC count is elevated and there is moderate blood on urine analysis.

1. Which of the following is the leading differential diagnosis?
   a. Pyelonephritis
   b. Endomyometritis
   c. Chorioamnionitis
   d. Septic pelvic thrombophlebitis
   e. Cellulitis
2. Which of the following is the most appropriate next step in management?
   a. Dilation and curettage
   b. Discharge home with oral doxycycline
   c. Exploratory laparotomy
   d. CT scan of abdomen and pelvis
   e. Administer IV clindamycin and gentamicin
3. What is the most important risk factor for developing postpartum endomyometritis?
   a. Route of delivery
   b. Multiple vaginal examinations
   c. Prolonged rupture of membranes
   d. Internal fetal monitoring
   e. Low socioeconomic status

Vignette 2

A 20-year-old nulligravid young woman presents to the emergency department 4 hours after the onset of nausea, vomiting, and moderate lower abdominal pain. Her last menstrual period was 2 weeks ago. She reports three new sexual partners in the last 6 months and uses condoms intermittently. She denies any history of sexually transmitted infections. Her temperature is 38.0°C (100.4°F), pulse rate is 96/min, respirations are 20/min, and BP is 110/60 mm Hg. Examination shows a soft abdomen and lower quadrant tenderness without guarding or rebound. On pelvic examination, there is a mucopurulent cervical discharge, moderate cervical motion tenderness, and uterine tenderness. Bilateral adnexa are nontender and without enlargement.

1. What is the most likely diagnosis?
   a. Ectopic pregnancy
   b. Pelvic inflammatory disease
   c. Ovarian torsion
   d. Pyelonephritis
   e. Cervicitis
2. All of the following support the patient's diagnosis *except:*
   a. cervical motion tenderness and uterine tenderness
   b. mucopurulent cervical discharge
   c. abundant lactobacilli on saline prepared microscopy
   d. elevated C-reactive protein
   e. elevated erythrocyte sedimentation rate
3. What is the best initial treatment for this patient?
   a. Ceftriaxone 250 mg IM once plus doxycycline 100 mg orally twice daily for 14 days
   b. Ceftriaxone 250 mg IM once plus doxycycline 100 mg orally twice daily for 14 days plus metronidazole 500 mg orally twice daily for 14 days
   c. Doxycycline 100 mg orally twice daily for 14 days
   d. Cefoxitin 2 g IV every 6 hours plus doxycycline 100 mg IV every 12 hours
   e. Clindamycin 900 mg IV every 8 hours
4. What is this patient's future risk of infertility?
   a. 1%
   b. 12%
   c. 20%
   d. 40%
   e. 60%
5. Which of the following has been demonstrated to be protective against PID?
   a. Condoms
   b. Diaphragm with spermicide
   c. Oral contraceptive pill
   d. All of the above
   e. None of the above

Vignette 3

A 32-year-old primigravid woman at 8 weeks' gestation presents to establish prenatal care. She was diagnosed with HIV 6 years ago and is not currently on antiretroviral therapy (ART). Four months ago, her HIV viral load was 7,000 copies/mL and her CD4 count was 850 cells/mm^3. This is a planned and desired pregnancy.

1. What is the best initial treatment for this patient?
   a. Follow viral load and start ART only if viral load is greater than 100,000 copies/mL
   b. Start ART immediately
   c. Follow CD4 count and start ART only if viral load is less than 500 cells/mm^3
   d. Start ART at 36 weeks regardless of viral load
   e. Start ART in second trimester regardless of viral load

2. During what time period is vertical transmission of HIV most likely to occur?
   a. Early antepartum
   b. Late antepartum
   c. Intrapartum/labor and delivery
   d. Postpartum
   e. All of the above confer equal risk of vertical transmission

3. The patient presents to triage with painful contractions. On vaginal examination, her cervix is dilated to 6 cm with a bulging bag of water. She is admitted to labor and delivery triage. Last week, her viral load was found to be 450 copies/mL. Which of the following is the most appropriate next step?
   a. Start zidovudine IV and expectantly manage labor
   b. Perform an urgent cesarean section
   c. Continue her antenatal ART and expectantly manage labor
   d. Check CD4 count
   e. Start zidovudine IV and then artificially rupture membranes to expedite labor

4. The patient is wondering if it safe for her to breastfeed. Which of the following is the most appropriate recommendation?
   a. Breast and bottle feed
   b. Breastfeed as long as she remains on ART
   c. Bottle feed only
   d. Breast feed as long as her viral load is low
   e. None of the above

Vignette 4

A 34-year-old G2P2 woman comes to the emergency department with 8 hours of increasing right lower quadrant pain, inability to tolerate orals, and nausea. She is sexually active and uses Depo-Provera for contraception. She was treated for gonorrhea and reports compliance with treatment. Her temperature is 38.5°C (101.3°F), pulse rate is 114/min, respirations are 22/min, and BP is 110/70 mm Hg. On examination, her abdomen is soft with right lower quadrant tenderness. Voluntary guarding is present without rebound. Pelvic examination shows no cervical motion tenderness or uterine tenderness. The right adnexa is exquisitely tender and fullness is appreciated. Her WBC count is 17,000 cells/μL and there are 15% bands. Urine HCG is negative.

1. What is the most likely diagnosis?
   a. Ovarian torsion
   b. Appendicitis
   c. Tubo-ovarian abscess
   d. Cervicitis
   e. Ectopic pregnancy

2. Which of the following is the most appropriate next step in management?
   a. Pelvic ultrasound
   b. Abdominal X-ray
   c. Measurement of serum β-hCG concentration
   d. Dilation and curettage
   e. Discharge home on oral antibiotics

3. What is the best initial treatment for this patient?
   a. Ceftriaxone 250 mg IM once plus doxycycline 100 mg orally twice daily for 14 days
   b. Gentamicin 5 mg/kg IV every 24 hours
   c. Doxycycline 100 mg orally twice daily for 14 days
   d. Cefoxitin 2 g IV every 6 hours plus doxycycline 100 mg IV every 12 hours
   e. Clindamycin 900 mg IV every 8 hours

4. After 48 hours the patient is found to be in moderate distress. Her temperature is 39.1°C (102.4°F), pulse rate is 130/min, respirations are 26/min, and BP is 105/55 mm Hg. On examination, her abdomen is diffusely tender with guarding and rebound present. Which of the following is the most appropriate next step in management?
   a. Exploratory laparotomy
   b. Repeat pelvic ultrasound
   c. Add metronidazole 500 mg IV twice daily
   d. Consult infectious disease specialist
   e. Perform a CT scan of abdomen and pelvis

A Answers

Vignette 1 Question 1

Answer B: One of the most common causes of postpartum fever is endomyometritis. The diagnosis is largely made clinically with findings of fever and uterine tenderness in a postpartum woman. Other findings that support the diagnosis are foul-smelling lochia, lower abdominal pain and elevated WBC count.

Pyelonephritis should be suspected in a patient with fever, flank pain, and costovertebral angle tenderness. Urinalysis should reveal pyuria and bacteruria. The hematuria in this patient is likely due to contamination from the lochia postpartum. Chorioamnionitis or intra-amniotic infection is a maternal febrile morbidity exclusive to the intrapartum period. Septic pelvic thrombophlebitis is often a diagnosis of exclusion and should be considered in the setting of persistent unexplained fever in the postpartum period. This patient has a normal appearing incision making wound cellulitis very unlikely.

Vignette 1 Question 2

Answer E: Postpartum endomyometritis is typically a polymicrobial infection involving both aerobes and anaerobes from the genital tract. After diagnosing endomyometritis, treatment should be initiated with broad-spectrum parenteral antibiotics such as IV clindamycin plus gentamicin or cephalosporins. Treatment course continues until clinical improvement and afebrile status for 24 to 48 hours. Oral antibiotic therapy is not required following successful parenteral treatment.

Although retained products of conception can cause endomyometritis, performing a dilation and curettage is not the most appropriate next step. In patients refractory to broad-spectrum parenteral antibiotics, additional imaging should be performed to look for other causes of fever. If retained tissue is found, a dilation and curettage may be necessary to remove the necrotic material. Patients with postpartum endomyometritis should be treated with broad-spectrum parenteral antibiotics. Oral doxycycline is typically used to treat chronic endometritis and chlamydial infections. Exploratory laparotomy is not indicated in a patient with postpartum endomyometritis. The diagnosis of postpartum endomyometritis is largely based on clinical findings. Imaging studies can be helpful in patient refractory to broad-spectrum parenteral antibiotics to look for an abscess, retained products, or septic pelvic thrombophlebitis.

Vignette 1 Question 3

Answer A: Cesarean delivery is the most important risk factor for developing postpartum endomyometritis. In the absence of prophylactic antibiotics, there is a 30% rate of developing postpartum endomyometritis after a nonelective cesarean delivery versus 3% for a vaginal delivery. Additional risk factors may include multiple vaginal examinations, prolonged rupture of membranes, internal fetal monitoring, low socioeconomic status, manual removal of the placenta, and prolonged labor.

Vignette 2 Question 1

Answer B: Pelvic inflammatory disease (PID) should be suspected in sexually active young women or women at risk for STIs who have pelvic or lower abdominal pain and one or more of the following: cervical motion tenderness, uterine tenderness, or adnexal tenderness. By using condoms intermittently, this patient is at risk for pregnancy. However, clinical manifestations of ectopic pregnancies typically appear 6 to 7 weeks after the last normal menstrual period. Women also typically have vaginal bleeding, pain, and symptoms of early pregnancy. Women with ovarian torsion typically complain of a sudden onset sharp lower abdominal pain. Intermittent nausea and vomiting are often present. Fever and mucopurulent discharge are unlikely findings. Pyelonephritis should be suspected in a patient with fever, flank pain, and costovertebral angle tenderness. Cervicitis should be suspected in women with mucopurulent discharge and cervical motion tenderness in the absence of other signs of PID. In this case, the patient is febrile and with concurrent uterine tenderness.

Vignette 2 Question 2

Answer C: Lactobacilli are part of the normal flora of the female genital tract and are not indicative of an infection. Minimal criteria are used to diagnose PID. The CDC recommends that empiric treatment for PID be initiated in sexually active young women or women at risk for STIs who have pelvic or lower abdominal pain and one or more of the following: cervical motion tenderness, uterine tenderness, or adnexal tenderness. Additional diagnostic criteria that supports the diagnosis of PID include fever (>38.3°C), abnormal cervical or vaginal mucopurulent discharge, abundant WBC on saline microscopy of vaginal secretions, elevated erythrocyte sedimentation rate, elevated C-reactive protein, and cervical *Neisseria gonorrhoeae* or *Chlamydia trachomatis* infection.

Vignette 2 Question 3

Answer D: This patient should be admitted for treatment of PID with parenteral antibiotics due to her inability to tolerate PO. PID is usually treated with a broad-spectrum cephalosporin, such as cefoxitin 2 g IV every 6 hours or cefotetan 2 g IV every 12 hours plus doxycycline 100 mg IV or orally every 12 hours because of its polymicrobial nature.
For those patients who are candidates for outpatient treatment of PID, the recommended treatment is ceftriaxone 250 mg IM once plus doxycycline 100 mg orally twice daily for 14 days. For those patients who are candidates for outpatient treatment of PID and who have

been diagnosed with BV or *Trichomonas*, the recommended treatment is ceftriaxone 250 mg IM once plus doxycycline 100 mg orally twice daily for 14 days plus metronidazole 500 mg orally twice daily for 14 days. Doxycycline 100 mg orally twice daily for 14 days is the treatment regimen for chronic endometritis. For those patients with a cephalosporin allergy, clindamycin can be used with gentamicin. Using clindamycin as a single agent to treat PID is not recommended.

Vignette 2 Question 4
Answer B: PID is strongly associated with infertility. Specifically, infertility risk increases with the number of PID episodes: 12% with one episode, approximately 20% with two episodes, and 40% with three or more episodes.

Vignette 2 Question 5
Answer D: Barrier contraceptives, such as the condom or diaphragm, have been shown to reduce the risk of sexually transmitted infections and PID. The use of oral contraceptives appears to diminish the severity of PID.

Vignette 3 Question 1
Answer E: ART in pregnancy is generally started in the second trimester with a goal for viral suppression by the third trimester. ART is generally avoided in the first trimester for fear of potential teratogenic side effects. However, ART should be initiated immediately for women who require treatment for her own health, regardless of gestational age.

Vignette 3 Question 2
Answer C: Approximately 50% to 80% of vertical transmission of HIV occurs intrapartum. Twenty percent to 50% of transmissions occur during the antepartum period, as early as 8 to 15 weeks' gestation. Fifteen percent of transmissions occur postpartum through breastfeeding.

Vignette 3 Question 3
Answer A: In women with viral loads less than 1,000 copies/mL, there is no additional benefit of cesarean delivery versus vaginal delivery in HIV perinatal transmission. This patient is a candidate for a trial of labor. Use of zidovudine IV during labor and delivery has been proven to reduce the risk of perinatal transmission. Invasive procedures including artificial rupture of membranes and use of fetal scalp electrodes should be avoided.

Women with a viral load greater than 1,000 copies/mL should be offered and recommended a cesarean section. These women are at increased risk of vertical transmission of HIV. Women should continue on their antepartum combination ART during labor. However, intrapartum zidovudine IV should also be added as it has been proven to reduce the risk of perinatal transmission. The CD4 count was recently checked and repeating this test is not needed in managing this patient.

Vignette 3 Question 4
Answer C: In resource-rich nations, breastfeeding is contraindicated in HIV-infected woman, regardless of viral load or use of ART. Postnatal HIV transmission from breast milk at 2 years may be as high as 15%. Use of concurrent breast and bottle feeding is not recommended as it has been shown to have higher rates of postnatal HIV transmission from breast milk.

Vignette 4 Question 1
Answer C: This patient most likely has a tubo-ovarian abscess (TOA). The diagnosis of TOA can be made clinically in the setting of PID and the appreciation of an adnexal or posterior cul-de-sac mass or fullness. The diagnosis is further supported by a fever, leukocytosis, and bandemia.

Women with ovarian torsion typically complain of a sudden onset sharp lower abdominal pain. Intermittent nausea and vomiting are often present. Fever, adnexal tenderness, and fullness are unlikely findings. Appendicitis should be suspected in any patient with right lower quadrant pain. However, this patient has a recent gonorrhea infection and has adnexal tenderness and fullness on examination that supports the diagnosis of TOA. Cervicitis should be suspected in women with mucopurulent discharge and cervical motion tenderness in the absence of other signs of PID. In this case, the patient is febrile with adnexal tenderness and fullness. An ectopic pregnancy is essentially ruled out with a negative urine HCG.

Vignette 4 Question 2
Answer A: Pelvic ultrasound is the imaging study of choice to diagnose TOAs. In addition, it is able to distinguish between TOAs and tubo-ovarian complexes (TOC). TOCs are not walled off like the true abscess and are thus more responsive to antimicrobial therapy. An abdominal X-ray is a poor imaging technique for female reproductive organs. A negative urine HCG is very accurate and sufficient to rule out pregnancy. Performing a dilation and curettage will provide no therapeutic or diagnostic utility for TOAs. This patient needs to be treated with broad-spectrum parenteral antibiotics due to her inability to tolerate PO.

Vignette 4 Question 3
Answer D: A trial of medical management with broad-spectrum antibiotics in an inpatient setting is frequently the first step in the treatment of TOAs. Treatment options include a broad-spectrum cephalosporin like cefoxitin 2 g IV every 6 hours plus doxycycline 100 mg IV every 12 hours. Other options include clindamycin plus gentamicin with or without ampicillin. The patient should be monitored with a repeat pelvic examination after the patient has been afebrile for 24 to 48 hours. If the patient is responsive to medical management, the patient can be converted to oral antibiotics with doxycycline plus clindamycin or metronidazole for 10 to 14 days.

Ceftriaxone 250 mg IM once plus doxycycline 100 mg orally twice daily for 14 days is the outpatient treatment for PID. Gentamicin can be used for the treatment of TOAs but only in conjunction with clindamycin to provide coverage for anaerobic bacteria. Ampicillin can also be added to this regimen to increase coverage for gram-positive bacteria. Doxycycline 100 mg orally twice daily for 14 days is the treatment regimen for chronic endometritis. Clindamycin can be used for the treatment of TOAs but only in conjunction with gentamicin to provide coverage for gram-negative bacteria. Ampicillin can also be added to this regimen to increase coverage for gram-positive bacteria.

Vignette 4 Question 4
Answer A: This patient has a clinical picture concerning for a ruptured tubo-ovarian abscess. Surgical management is necessary at this time. A delaying surgery will lead to further deterioration and septic shock. Repeat imaging would delay surgical management. Change in antibiotic regimen is not indicated. Consulting infectious disease specialist is not appropriate in a potentially unstable patient. Repeat imaging would delay surgical management.

Chapter 18 Pelvic Organ Prolapse

PELVIC ORGAN PROLAPSE

PATHOGENESIS

As shown in Figure 18-1, normal structural support of the pelvic organs is provided by a complex interaction between the muscles of the pelvic floor and connective tissue attachments to the bony pelvis. This network of **muscles** (e.g., levator ani muscles), **fascia** (e.g., urogenital diaphragm, endopelvic fascia including the pubocervical and rectovaginal), **nerves**, and **ligaments** (e.g., uterosacral and cardinal ligaments) provides support on which the pelvic organs rest. Damage to any one of these structures can potentially result in a weakening or loss of support to the pelvic organs (Fig. 18-2). Damage to the anterior vaginal wall pubocervical fascia can result in herniation of the bladder (**cystocele**) and/or urethra (**urethrocele**) into the vaginal lumen. Injuries to the endopelvic fascia of the rectovaginal septum in the posterior vaginal wall can result in herniation of the rectum (**rectocele**) into the vaginal lumen. Injury or stretching of the uterosacral and cardinal ligaments can result in descensus, or prolapse, of the uterus (**uterine prolapse**). After hysterectomy, some women may experience

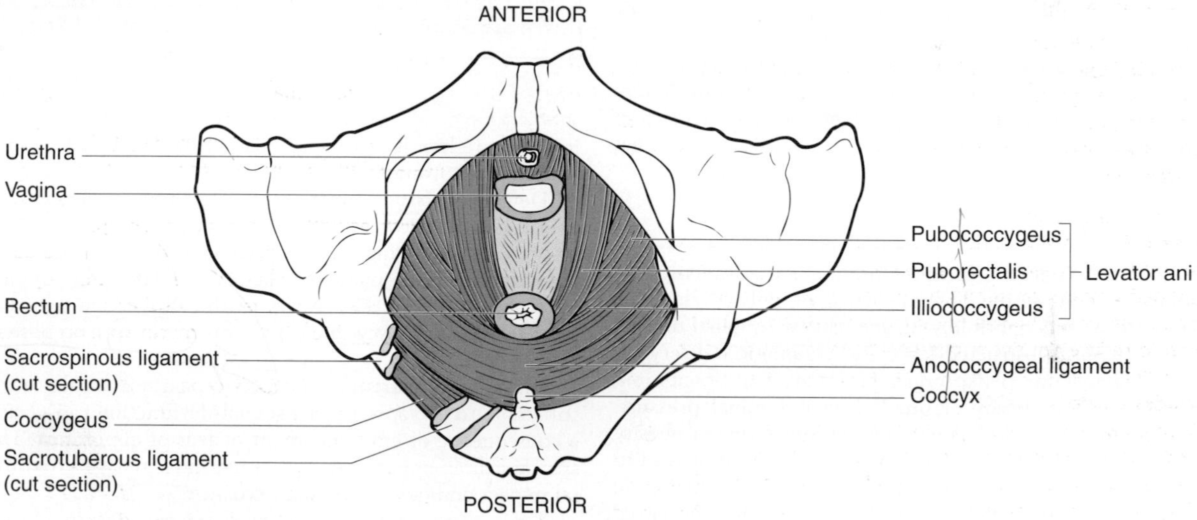

Figure 18-1 • Normal structural support of the pelvic floor as seen from above.

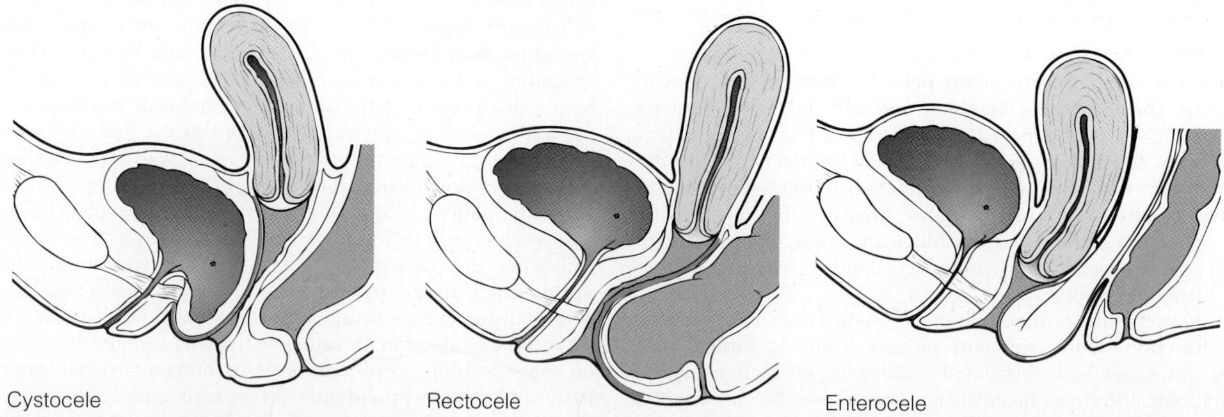

Figure 18-2 • Anatomic defects in pelvic relaxation.

prolapse of the small intestine (**enterocele**) or the apex of the vagina (**vaginal vault prolapse**) secondary to loss of the support structures upon removal of the uterus and cervix.

Pelvic organ prolapse presents with a variety of symptoms including **pelvic pressure** and discomfort, **dyspareunia**, difficulty evacuating the bowels and bladder, and low back discomfort. These clinical symptoms are often associated with a visible or **palpable bulge in the vagina**. Pelvic support is most commonly compromised by pregnancy and subsequent delivery; chronic increases in intra-abdominal pressure from obesity, chronic cough (COPD and emphysema), or chronic heavy lifting; connective tissue disorders; and atrophic changes due to aging or estrogen deficiency.

EPIDEMIOLOGY

Pelvic relaxation is especially apparent in the **postmenopausal** population. This increase is attributed to **decreased endogenous estrogen**, the effects of gravity over time, and normal aging in the setting of previous pregnancy and vaginal delivery. **Atrophy** is associated with compromised elasticity, diminished vascular support, and laxity in structural elements. Tissues become less resilient to forces of gravity and increased intra-abdominal pressure, and accumulative stresses on the pelvic support system take effect. The **reported prevalence** of pelvic organ prolapse in population-based surveys ranges from 2.9% to 9%. Population-based surgical intervention studies report a higher prevalence of symptomatic prolapse quoting an 11% to 19% lifetime risk for undergoing surgery. Previous studies have asserted that lower rates of prolapse are seen in African American women compared to Caucasian women, but this has not been consistently demonstrated in the literature.

RISK FACTORS

Risk factors for pelvic organ prolapse include **advancing age, menopause, and parity.** The incidence of pelvic relaxation increases four- and eightfold with the first two **vaginal deliveries**, respectively. Obstructed labor and **traumatic delivery** are also risk factors for pelvic organ prolapse as are conditions that result in chronically **elevated intra-abdominal pressure**. This pressure differential can be seen in the setting of obesity, chronic cough, COPD, chronic constipation, repeat heavy lifting, and large pelvic tumors. Additionally, a surgical history of **hysterectomy** is associated with an increase in apical prolapse.

CLINICAL MANIFESTATIONS

History

The symptoms reported with pelvic relaxation vary depending on the structures involved and the degree of prolapse (Table 18-1). With small degrees of pelvic relaxation, patients are often asymptomatic; however, prolapse severity and symptoms are not always well-correlated. When symptomatic, patients often complain of **pelvic pressure**, heaviness in the lower abdomen, or a **vaginal bulge** that may worsen at night or become aggravated by prolonged standing, vigorous activity, or lifting heavy objects.

Women with prolapse often experience concurrent **urinary dysfunction** with complaints ranging from incomplete bladder emptying and obstructed voiding to overactive bladder. Paradoxically, stress incontinence can appear to "improve" as the prolapse worsens. As the support for the anterior vaginal wall weakens and the bladder descends, a kink is introduced into the urethra. It is a mechanical obstruction that masquerades as "improvement."

TABLE 18-1 Symptoms That May Be Manifested in Pelvic Organ Prolapse

Vaginal/sexual symptoms
Pelvic pressure and/or heaviness
Palpable or visible vaginal bulging
Backache
Urinary symptoms
Urinary frequency
Urinary urgency
Incomplete/interrupted voiding
Difficulty starting urinary stream
Urinary incontinence
Bowel symptoms
Obstructed defecation
Constipation
Painful defecation
Incomplete defecation
Splinting[a]

[a]Placing fingers in or around the vagina/perineum to aid in defecation.

Defecatory issues can be associated with prolapse of the apical and posterior aspects of the vaginal wall and include incomplete emptying, fecal urgency, or constipation. Some patients perform a maneuver known as **"splinting"** to aid in evacuation of stool. This refers to the application of manual pressure (usually by a finger) to the perineum or posterior vaginal wall.

Although dyspareunia and pelvic pain are usually not attributable to prolapse per se, **sexual dysfunction** can occur as a consequence of embarrassment or fear of discomfort. These symptoms can impact daily activities, and can have a detrimental impact on body image and sexuality.

Physical Examination

Pelvic relaxation is best observed by separating the labia and viewing the vagina while the patient strains or coughs. A **split-speculum examination** should be performed by using a Sims speculum or the lower half of a Grave speculum to provide better visualization of the anterior vaginal wall, posterior vaginal wall, and apex individually. Using this method, the speculum is used to retract the posterior vaginal wall and a **cystocele** may cause a downward movement of the anterior vaginal wall when the patient strains (Fig. 18-3). Similarly, **rectoceles and enteroceles** result in an upward bulging of the posterior vaginal wall when the patient strains with the split speculum placed upside down retracting the anterior vaginal wall (Fig. 18-4). This laxity in the rectovaginal wall can also be demonstrated on **rectal examination**. A **prolapsed uterus** can also be viewed on split-speculum examination or by bimanual pelvic examination. **Complete procidentia** refers to complete eversion of the vagina with the entire uterus prolapsing outside the vagina (Color Plate 11).

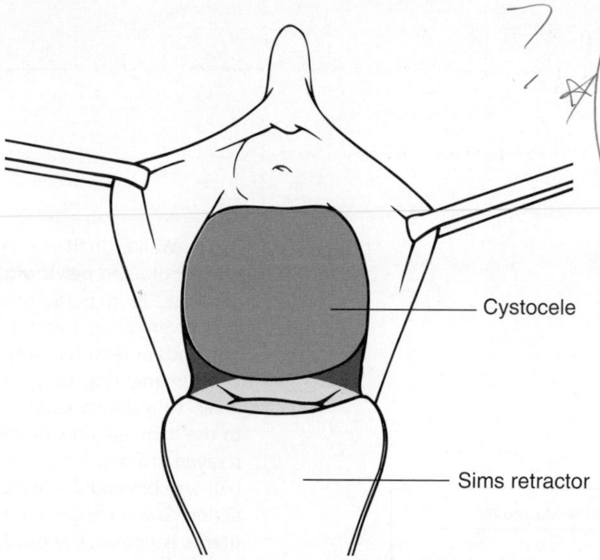

Figure 18-3 • A cystocele (*seen here via split-speculum examination*) is the bulging of the bladder into the anterior vaginal wall. It is usually caused by an acquired defect in the anterior endopelvic fascial anatomy. It can be repaired with an anterior colporrhaphy.

Many clinicians formerly use the **Baden-Walker Halfway Scoring System** for quantifying pelvic organ prolapse. It records the amount of descent of the structure (bladder, rectum, etc.) using a four-point system with the hymen as a fixed point of reference (Fig. 18-5). Zero represents normal anatomic position (i.e., no descensus), 1 represents descensus halfway to the hymen, 2 represents descensus to the hymen, 3 represents descensus halfway past the hymen, and 4 represents maximum descent. The examination is conducted with the patient straining in order to record maximum descent.

More commonly, however, the **Pelvic Organ Prolapse Quantitative scale** (POP-Q) is used as an objective, site-specific system for describing, quantifying, and staging pelvic support in women. It provides a standardized means for documenting, comparing, and communicating clinical findings of pelvic organ prolapse that **focuses on the physical extent of the vaginal wall prolapse,** and not on which organ is presumed to be prolapsing within that defect (Fig. 18-6). In order to quantitatively assess the degree of prolapse involved, the POP-Q uses six points within the vagina that are measured relative to a **fixed point of reference: the hymen**. POP-Q is particularly helpful in both the clinical and research settings for comparing patients' examinations over time and among different examiners.

DIAGNOSTIC EVALUATION

The diagnosis of pelvic organ prolapse depends primarily on an accurate history and thorough physical examination. Other tools that may be useful in the diagnosis and preoperative evaluation of cystoceles and urethroceles include urine cultures, cystoscopy, urethroscopy, and urodynamic studies, if indicated. When a rectocele is suspected from a history of chronic constipation and difficulty passing stool, obstructive lesions should be ruled out using anoscopy or sigmoidoscopy. A defecography study (similar to a barium enema) may also help to show a rectocele or enterocele but is not essential to diagnosis.

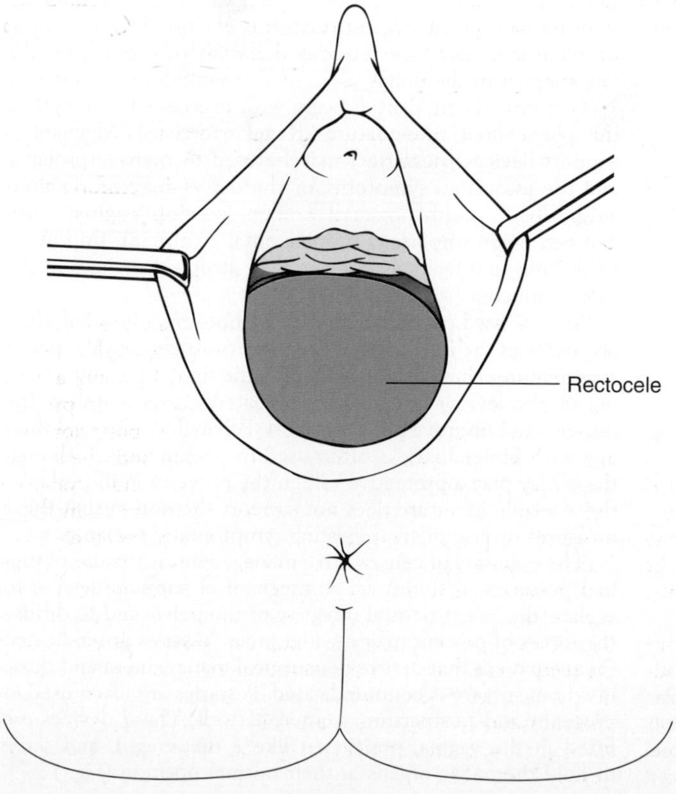

Figure 18-4 • A rectocele is the bulging of the rectum into the posterior vaginal wall.It is usually caused by an acquired defect in the posterior endopelvic fascial anatomy. It can be repaired with a posterior colporrhaphy.

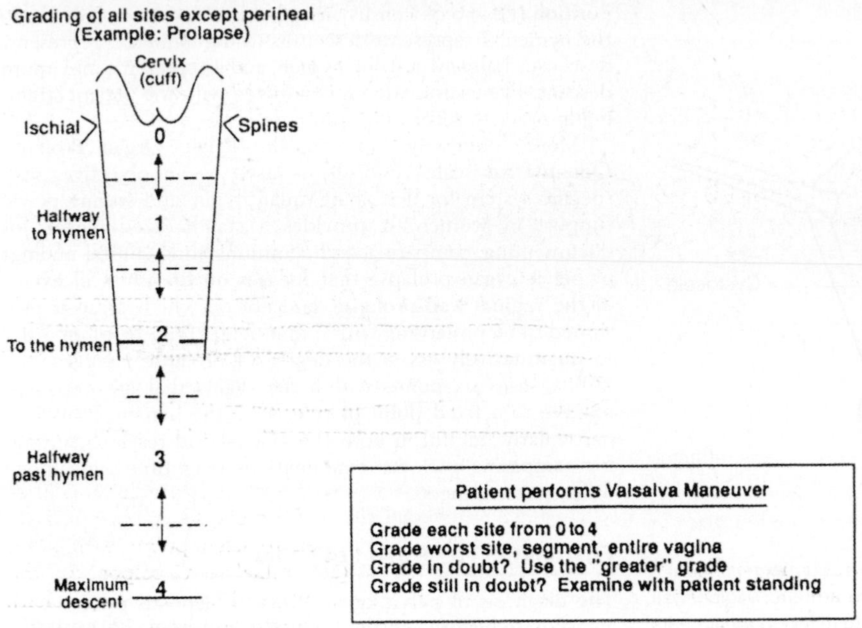

Figure 18-5 • Baden-Walker halfway system for grading pelvic organ prolapse. In general, grade 1 is given to a defect that descends at least half-way to the hymenal ring. Grade 2 is given to a defect extending to the hymenal ring. Grade 3 is given to a defect extending half-way beyond the hymenal ring. Grade 4 is given if the uterus is completely outside of the vagina.
(Image from Rock J, Jones H. *TeLinde's Operative Gynecology*, 10th ed. Philadelphia, PA: Lippincott Williams & Wilkins; 2008.)

DIFFERENTIAL DIAGNOSIS

Although rare in comparison, the differential diagnosis for cystocele and urethrocele includes urethral diverticula, Gartner cysts, Skene gland cysts, and tumors of the urethra and bladder. When a rectocele is suspected, obstructive lesions of the colon and rectum (lipomas, fibromas, sarcomas) should be investigated. Cervical elongation, prolapsed cervical polyp, prolapsed uterine fibroid, and prolapsed cervical and endometrial tumors may be mistaken for uterine prolapse as can lower uterine segment fibroids.

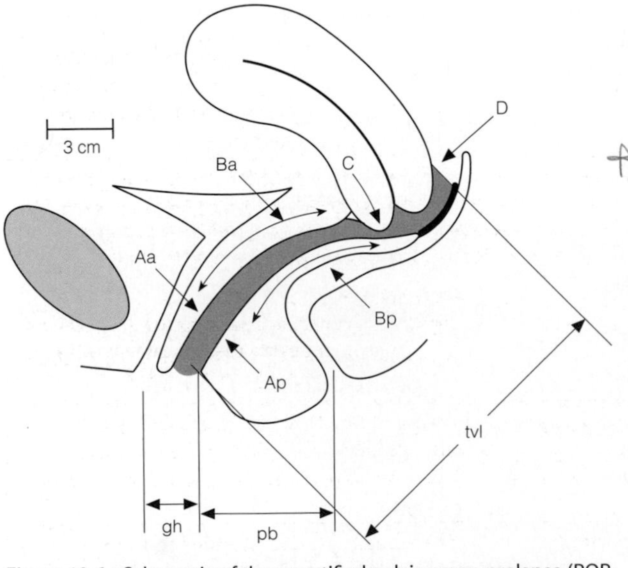

Figure 18-6 • Schematic of the quantified pelvic organ prolapse (POP-Q) system. Six sites (*points Aa, Ba, C, D, Bp, Ap*), genital hiatus (gh), perineal body (pb), and total vaginal length (tvl) are used to quantify the degree of pelvic organ prolapse. The vagina and hymenal ring are shown in blue.

TREATMENT

Prolapse is generally a benign condition and further evaluation and treatment is guided by the patient's goals for improvement in her quality of life. Thus, asymptomatic prolapse can be monitored but does not require any further treatment and **expectant management** is acceptable. For those patients who have significant bother from her prolapse symptoms, intervention is appropriate. Regardless of the etiology, symptomatic pelvic organ prolapse is essentially **a structural problem** and therefore requires therapies that reinforce the lost support to the pelvis.

Conservative modalities begin with exercises to strengthen the pelvic floor musculature (**Kegel exercises**). Mechanical support devices (**pessaries**) may be used to manage prolapse and the associated symptoms, or the defect **may be repaired surgically**. In postmenopausal women, **low-dose vaginal estrogen** can be an important supplemental treatment, improving tissue tone and facilitating reversal of atrophic changes in the vaginal mucosa.

In motivated patients with mild symptoms, a first-line therapy involves the use of **Kegel exercises** to strengthen the pelvic musculature. These exercises involve the tightening and releasing of the levator ani muscles repeatedly to strengthen the muscles and improve pelvic support. Pelvic floor **physical therapy** with **biofeedback** is often used in conjunction. Although these may play a protective role in the prevention of prolapse, the available literature does not support the notion that these measures reverse or treat existing symptomatic prolapse.

The mainstay of conservative management is the use of **vaginal pessaries**. Pessaries act as mechanical support devices to replace the lost structural integrity of the pelvis and to diffuse the forces of descent over a wider area. Pessaries are indicated for any patient that desires **nonsurgical management** and those in whom surgery is contraindicated. Pessaries are often used in pregnant and postpartum women as well. These devices are fitted in the vagina, positioned like a diaphragm, and serve to hold the pelvic organs in their normal position (Fig. 18-7).

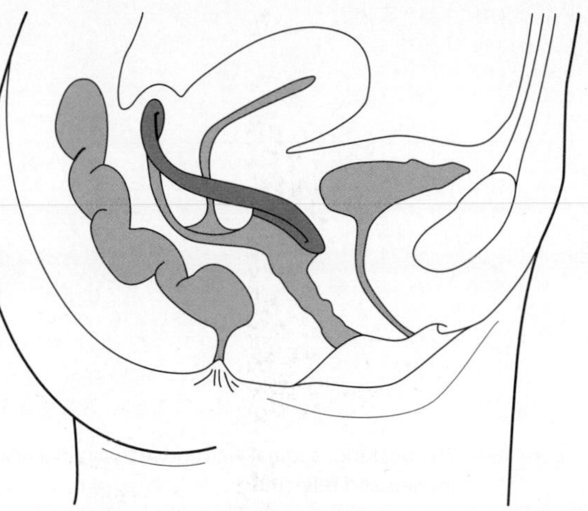

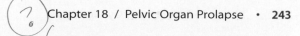

Figure 18-7 • Placement of a vaginal pessary to treat pelvic organ prolapse.

Studies suggest that certain physical characteristics like longer vagina, smaller introitus, and lower weight are associated with more successful pessary placement. The use of vaginal pessaries requires a highly motivated patient who is willing to accept an intravaginal device and the small risks of pain, ulcerations, bleeding, leukorrhea, and infection. Pessaries may be used intermittently (interval removal and self-replacement) or may remain inside the vagina for up to 3 to 6 months at a time. Close follow-up with removal, vaginal examination, cleaning, and replacement ensures proper placement and hygiene and minimizes the small associated risks.

Symptomatic patients who are not happy with nonoperative approaches may require **surgical correction**. In general, surgical repair for pelvic relaxation produces good results although the recurrence rate over time may be as high as 30%. As outlined in Table 18-2, correction of cystoceles and rectoceles can be accomplished by **anterior and posterior colporrhaphy**, respectively. These procedures repair the **fascial defect** through which the herniation occurred (see Figs. 18-8 to 18-10). **Enteroceles**, which represent the herniation of small bowel into the vaginal canal, can be repaired along with the reinforcement of the rectovaginal fascia and the posterior vaginal wall. The key to the repair of any and all compartments is the re-establishment of the normal connection of the respective fascial layers to each other and the support ligaments. With significant uterine prolapse, abdominal or vaginal **hysterectomy** may be indicated although the removal of the uterus in and of itself is not curative for descent. In addition to the hysterectomy, an **apical suspension procedure** is often performed to prevent later prolapse of the vaginal vault.

In women who have prolapse of the vaginal vault after hysterectomy, the **vaginal vault prolapse** is corrected by suspension of the vaginal apex to fixed points within the pelvis such as the sacrum (abdominal sacral colpopexy), the uterosacral ligaments (high uterosacral ligament suspension), or sacrospinous ligaments (sacrospinous ligament fixation). The degree of success depends on the skill of the surgeon, the degree of pelvic relaxation, and the age, weight, and lifestyle of the patient.

Women who are poor surgical candidates and who no longer plan vaginal intercourse may be offered a colpocleisis. This is a vaginal obliterative procedure closes off the vaginal canal as a means of treating symptomatic pelvic organ prolapse. These procedures are less invasive with a shorter operative time, fewer complications and recurrences and a high patient satisfaction rate.

TABLE 18-2 Surgical Treatment of Pelvic Organ Prolapse

Anatomical Defect	Repair Procedure	Details of Repair
Cystocele	Anterior colporrhaphy	Plication (reinforcement) of the endopelvic fascia and reattachment to the apex or uterine cervix (if present) to resuspend the anterior vaginal wall and bladder
Rectocele	Posterior colporrhaphy	Similar to anterior colporrhaphy, except the posterior endopelvic fascia is identified and reattached to the apical support or uterine cervix (if present) and distally to the perineal body
Enterocele	Vaginal enterocele repair	The enterocele is repaired along with the reattachment of the rectovaginal fascia to the apex or uterine cervix (if present)
Uterine prolapse	Hysterectomy (abdominal or vaginal) and McCall culdoplasty	Hysterectomy followed by attachment of the resulting vaginal cuff to the uterosacral ligaments to decrease the risk of future vault prolapse
Vaginal vault prolapse (after hysterectomy)	Sacrospinous ligament fixation Or Abdominal sacral colpopexy	The vaginal apex is suspended to the sacrospinous ligaments via a vaginal approach Uses mesh to attach the vaginal apex to the sacrum via an abdominal, laparoscopic, or robotic approach

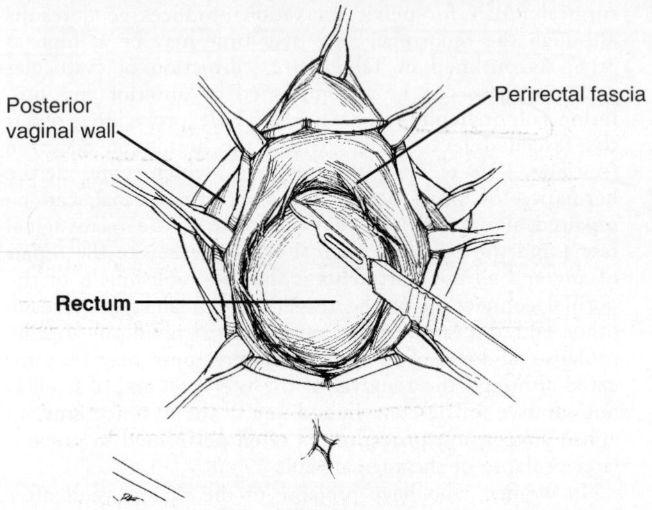

Figure 18-8 • The posterior vaginal wall and rectovaginal fascia are incised and reflected.
(From Bourgeois FJ. *Obstetrics & Gynecology Recall*, 3rd ed. Philadelphia, PA: Lippincott Williams & Wilkins; 2008.)

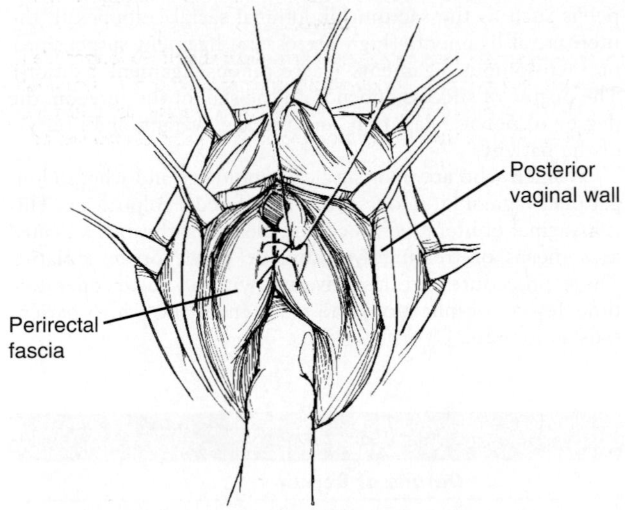

Figure 18-9 • The rectocele is reduced by plicating (reinforcing) the perirectal fascia to the midline.
(From Bourgeois FJ. *Obstetrics & Gynecology Recall*, 3rd ed. Philadelphia, PA: Lippincott Williams & Wilkins; 2008.)

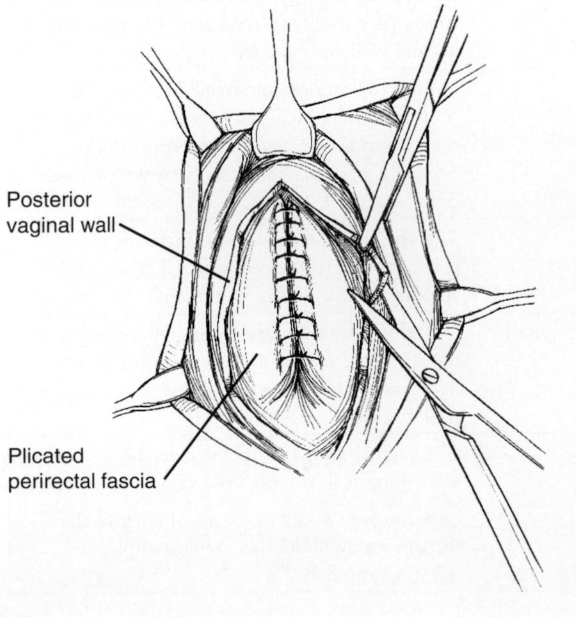

Figure 18-10 • The excess vaginal mucosa is trimmed from the posterior vaginal wall, and the vaginal incision is closed in the midline.
(From Bourgeois FJ. *Obstetrics & Gynecology Recall*, 3rd ed. Philadelphia, PA: Lippincott Williams & Wilkins; 2008.)

KEY POINTS

- Pelvic organ prolapse is a general term used to denote a herniation of the anterior, apical, or posterior vaginal walls into the vaginal lumen. Traditionally, these were named by the organ presumed to be behind the prolapse including bladder (cystocele), urethra (urethrocele), rectum (rectocele), small bowel (enterocele), and/or uterus (uterine prolapse).
- Vaginal vault prolapse occurs most commonly in patients who have undergone hysterectomy but may occur in conjunction with weakness or laxity of the cardinal/uterosacral ligaments as seen with uterine prolapse. The vagina can then invert into the vaginal canal and potentially prolapse outside the body in its most severe form.
- Debate exists as to the exact contribution of individual risk factors for prolapse but include obstetric trauma, chronic elevations in intra-abdominal pressure, hypoestrogenic state, and inherent poor tissue quality, such as associated with musculoskeletal syndromes.
- Pelvic organ prolapse primarily manifests as pelvic pressure and vaginal bulging although urinary, defecatory, and sexual dysfunction can be present.
- Pelvic organ prolapse is diagnosed primarily by history and physical examination, but may also require urine cultures, cystoscopy, urethroscopy, urinary dynamic studies, anoscopy, sigmoidoscopy, and defecography as indicated.
- Both the POP-Q and the Baden-Walker systems are used for the quantification of pelvic organ prolapse. POP-Q is used more in research, whereas Baden-Walker halfway system is used more clinically to quantify the degree of pelvic organ prolapse.
- Treatment of pelvic organ prolapse is guided by the severity of symptom. Pelvic organ prolapse can be treated nonsurgically with Kegel exercises, pelvic floor physical therapy, and biofeedback. Vaginal pessary use is the mainstay of nonsurgical management of pelvic organ prolapse.
- Surgical treatment options for pelvic organ prolapse include anterior and posterior colporrhaphy for cystoceles and rectoceles, respectively. These procedures repair the fascial defect and strengthen the existing vaginal wall support.
- Uterine prolapse is most commonly treated with abdominal or vaginal hysterectomy with apical suspension of the vault. Vaginal vault prolapse is repaired by resuspending the vaginal vault to a fixed structure in the pelvis.
- women who are poor surgical candidates and no longer plan vaginal intercourse may be offered a colpocleisis. This vaginal obliterative procedure is less invasive with a shorter operative time, fewer complications and recurrences and a high patient satisfaction rate.

C Clinical Vignettes

Vignette 1

A 69-year-old woman with pelvic pressure and palpable bulge presents for evaluation. She recalls some mention of a cystocele diagnosis, given by her primary care provider. Today, she requests formal evaluation by a gynecologist.

1. When performing the physical examination, what is one type of staging system to describe prolapse?
   a. Pelvic organ prolapse quantification scale (POP-Q)
   b. Gray scale
   c. Visual analog scale
   d. Breslow scale
   e. Clark scale

2. In discussing her symptoms, the patient points out that her voiding function has changed as the prolapse has grown in severity. Initially, the patient reported stress urinary incontinence, but as the prolapse worsened, the incontinence improved. While she is happy with the resolution of her incontinence, she currently experiences some incomplete bladder emptying, which is improved upon manual reduction of the prolapse. How do you counsel her about her risk of incontinence after an isolated anterior wall repair (with no other concomitant surgery)?
   a. High likelihood of de novo urgency and urge urinary incontinence
   b. High likelihood of urinary frequency
   c. High likelihood that her stress incontinence will be cured by anterior repair
   d. High likelihood that an anterior repair will unmask and potentially "worsen" her stress urinary incontinence symptoms
   e. High likelihood of de novo fecal incontinence

3. In assessing the above patient, you also find a posterior vaginal wall defect. What is a common symptom that is associated with rectoceles?
   a. Urinary urgency
   b. Hematuria
   c. Incomplete evacuation of stool that may require splinting
   d. Vaginal bleeding
   e. Vaginal wall erosion

Vignette 2

A 53-year-old woman presents for counseling and management of her low-grade anterior wall prolapse. She is only symptomatic on days when she has engaged in heavy lifting or particularly strenuous activity. She is morbidly obese and would like to begin a formal weight loss program. She is curious about management options.

1. Of the following, which do you recommend?
   a. Conservative management (may include pelvic floor exercises, weight loss, or pessary)
   b. Colpocleisis obliterative procedure
   c. Gellhorn space occupying pessary
   d. Round ligament suspension
   e. Hysterectomy

2. She agrees to a trial with a pessary. You choose a supportive pessary and counsel her regarding pessary insertion, removal, cleaning, etc. Which of the following are factors associated with a successful pessary fitting?
   a. Short vaginal length
   b. Long vaginal length
   c. Obesity
   d. History of traumatic vaginal deliveries
   e. Menopausal state

Vignette 3

An 89-year-old female patient with multiple, serious medical comorbidities presents to discuss options for treatment of her high-grade prolapse. The prolapse is externalized and becoming ulcerated from friction against her undergarments. She cannot tolerate a pessary. Her main priority is to "fix or get rid of this thing," but her primary care provider has cautioned against a lengthy or open abdominal procedure. She is not interested in future intercourse.

1. What can you offer this patient?
   a. Nothing can be done
   b. Open abdominal sacral colpopexy
   c. Robot-assisted laparoscopic sacral colpopexy
   d. Hysterectomy with anterior and posterior colporrhaphy, vault suspension
   e. Colpocleisis

2. After counseling the patient about colpocleisis, she expresses concern about losing her potential for future intercourse. She is not ready to proceed with any surgical repairs. She asks about the use of topical estrogen cream. Which of the following is NOT a contraindication to estrogen administration?
   a. Endometrial cancer
   b. Stroke
   c. Active arterial thromboembolic disease (i.e., myocardial infarction)

d. Administration of progestin
e. Hormone receptor positive breast cancer

Vignette 4

A 29-year-old G2P1 woman is 22 weeks' pregnant with reports of pelvic bulge and bothersome pressure. Physical examination reveals cervical prolapse, approaching the opening of the vaginal introitus. She is worried that the prolapse will worsen as the pregnancy progresses.

1. What can you offer this patient for her symptomatic prolapse?
   a. Pessary trial
   b. Reassessment after delivery but nothing during the pregnancy
   c. Cerclage
   d. Hysteropexy
   e. Uterosacral ligament fixation
2. The patient also complains of occasional small volume stress incontinence with coughing or sneezing, only during her pregnancy. How would you counsel this patient on incontinence treatment during pregnancy?
   a. Offer trial of anti-cholinergic medication
   b. Offer sling procedure
   c. Offer bulking injections
   d. Offer reassurance, encourage expectant management
   e. Offer Burch procedure

A Answers

Vignette 1 Question 1
Answer A: Both the Baden-Walker system and the pelvic organ prolapse quantification scale (POP-Q) are used to describe prolapse and quantify the degree of descent. In the past, the Baden-Walker Halfway Scoring System was in wide use among gynecologic providers. Conversely, initially the POP-Q system was regarded as being useful for research purposes, but with the documentation of nine separate points, it has become one of the most clinical used systems for grading POP. The gray scale simply refers to non–color-Doppler sonographic images. The Breslow and Clark classifications refer to staging for melanoma.

Vignette 1 Question 2
Answer D: Typically, symptoms of urgency and frequency are not related to prolapse. However, with the spectrum of pelvic floor relaxation and its associated disease processes, it is not uncommon to diagnose patients with both prolapse and stress urinary incontinence. With advanced anterior wall prolapse, the urethra may be kinked upon itself, thus introducing a dynamic barrier to the frank leakage of urine. These patients may relay a history of stress incontinence that improved as the prolapse worsened. With reconstruction of the anterior vaginal wall and restoration of normal anatomy, this mechanical obstruction is removed and the outflow tract is restored. In other words, once the kink is removed—it may be easier for the urine to pass freely, thus exacerbating the symptoms of stress urinary incontinence.

Vignette 1 Question 3
Answer C: Prolapse can be a dynamic entity with symptoms waxing and waning with level of activity, time of day, etc. Also, severity of symptoms may not necessarily correlate with the extent of prolapse. Further compounding the issue of obtaining an accurate patient history is the sensitive nature of the involved anatomy and patients may not always readily offer a full account of symptoms. In consideration of the above, the provider should make specific inquiries about voiding, defecatory, and sexual function. With a posterior vaginal defect, incomplete or difficulty with evacuation of the bowels is a common finding and some patients manually apply pressure (i.e.,"splint") to aid in defecation. Rectoceles are not routinely associated with any of the other answer choices.

Vignette 2 Question 1
Answer A: Treatment for pelvic organ prolapse is guided by patient's request and desire for symptom control. As with many other areas of medicine, the least invasive modality is recommended with escalation to more invasive methods if resultant improvement is not achieved. Although there is no strong data to support the role of pelvic floor muscle exercises in preventing progression of prolapse, there is evidence that it may improve concurrent issues such as stress urinary incontinence. Additionally, weight loss has been shown to improve pelvic floor pathology. Colpocleisis is generally not considered a first-line option, as this obliterative procedure closes off the vaginal introitus and permanently removes the potential for vaginal intercourse. Round ligament suspensions are not effective. A Gellhorn pessary is a space occupying device and is usually used in high-grade prolapse. With low-grade prolapse, a smaller, supportive pessary might be a better option. A hysterectomy, in and of itself, will not correct the prolapse.

Vignette 2 Question 2
Answer B: There is some data to suggest that a longer vaginal length (>7 cm) and a narrower introitus (<4 finger breadths) may influence the success of pessary fitting. None of the other answer choices seem to benefit pessary fitting or positively impact continuation rates in the short term. Pessaries are offered as first-line therapy for all types of prolapse and can be fitted regardless of stage or dominant compartment (cystocele vs. rectocele). Pessaries are available in many shapes and sizes and many patients will maintain use after a successful fitting (41% to 67%).

Vignette 3 Question 1
Answer E: Because reconstructive surgery for pelvic organ prolapse is considered an elective procedure (as opposed to surgeries that are vital to survival), the severity of a patient's medical co-morbidities may preclude a surgical approach, especially one that requires an open abdominal incision, insufflation of the abdomen, or steep Trendelenburg. In poor surgical candidates, first-line therapy will entail noninvasive modalities such as pessaries or expectant management. However, if conservative management has been exhausted and the patient desires to proceed with surgery, a colpocleisis is one procedure that may be offered. Appropriate candidates are those who no longer desire the potential for vaginal intercourse and understand the anatomical consequences of an obliterative procedure. This procedure essentially closes off the vaginal opening by approximating the anterior and posterior walls, thereby reducing the prolapse in the process. The peritoneal cavity is never entered, operative time is short, and recovery is rapid. Generally, satisfaction rates are very high and recurrence rates exceedingly low.

Vignette 3 Question 2
Answer D: Either a strict contraindication or "warning" has been issued against all of the above answer options except for D (i.e.,

progestin use). In fact, unopposed estrogen can be dangerous in women who have not undergone hysterectomy; progesterone is *recommended* to offset the hyperplastic potential of unopposed systemic estrogen. Although very low systemic levels of estrogen can be detected in women using low-dose vaginal estrogen for treatment of atrophy, use of *low-dose vaginal estrogen* does not require similar concomitant use of a progestin.

Vignette 4 Question 1

Answer A: If the patient is asymptomatic, evaluation and management can be deferred until after the delivery, but this patient reports discomfort. A pessary can be used during pregnancy for symptomatic prolapse. Similar to nongravid patients, women should be counseled regarding removal, cleaning, and maintenance. This patient should be followed to monitor for vaginal erosions, lesions, or ulcerations. A cerclage is indicated for cervical insufficiency and will not address pelvic floor relaxation or descent. A hysteropexy is not an effective procedure for prolapse; furthermore, operative manipulation of the uterus during the pregnant state is not recommended, especially for an elective procedure. A uterosacral ligament fixation during pregnancy is not recommended for several reasons, including laxity of these ligaments during pregnancy and because the enlarged uterus will interfere with access to these structures. Lastly, elective procedures should be deferred until completion of the pregnancy and postpartum recovery for both maternal and fetal safety.

Vignette 4 Question 2

Answer D: Secondary to the anatomic changes of an expanding uterus in pregnancy, the incidence of stress incontinence can be quite high. In many cases, incontinence resolves after recovery from the peripartum period. If the patient has incontinence that is both persistent and bothersome after delivery, formal evaluation can be undertaken after healing is complete. No elective invasive procedures are recommended during the pregnancy itself, especially with the risk of blood loss associated with the engorged pelvic vasculature. Anti-cholinergic medication is indicated for urge incontinence.

Chapter

19 Urinary Incontinence

URINARY INCONTINENCE

EPIDEMIOLOGY

The involuntary loss of urine is common, affecting an estimated 18.3 million American women in 2010, with an expected 55% increase to 28.4 million in 2050. Nearly 50% of all women experience occasional urinary incontinence, and 20% of women older than 75 years are affected daily. Urinary incontinence is often a major reason for placing individuals in nursing homes, with some 30% of nursing home residents suffering from urinary incontinence. In a large survey study of noninstitutionalized US women, 49.6% reported incontinence symptoms, of which 49.8% reported stress incontinence, 34.3% reported mixed incontinence, and 15.9% reported pure urge incontinence. It is estimated that more than $12 billion are spent annually on the treatment of stress incontinence.

Urinary incontinence is failure of the bladder to store urine appropriately (Table 19-1). The most common urine storage disorder is **stress (urinary) incontinence,** which is characterized by involuntary urine loss on effort or physical exertion (e.g., sporting activities), or on sneezing or coughing. The annual incidence of stress incontinence is estimated to be 4% to 11% and the annual remission rates have been reported as 4% to 5%. **Urgency (urinary) incontinence**, the complaint of involuntary loss of urine associated with urgency, that may be associated with detrusor overactivity, occurs in 5% to 10% of women at least monthly. Many women will suffer from a combination of urgency and stress incontinence; this is known as **mixed (urinary) incontinence.**

There are several other conditions that lead to involuntary loss of urine (Table 19-1). **Urinary retention** secondary to detrusor underactivity, an acontractile detrusor, or bladder outlet obstruction can result in urinary incontinence; this is often referred to as **overflow (urinary) incontinence**. Conditions that may be associated with this type of incontinence include diabetes, neurologic diseases, severe genital prolapse, and postsurgical obstruction from urinary continence procedures. **Bypass (urinary) incontinence** or continuous (urinary) incontinence is typically the result of a **urinary fistula** formed between the urinary tract and the vagina. In the United States, almost all cases of urinary fistula result from pelvic surgery or pelvic radiation; whereas in developing countries the etiology is usually obstetric birth trauma and obstructed labor. **Functional (urinary) incontinence** can result when a woman has any condition that interferes with her ability to reach a toilet in a timely fashion or attend to her toileting needs; this includes cognitive, psychological, or physical impairments. This type of incontinence is often seen in the elderly with limited mobility and those with dementia.

RISK FACTORS

Age is an important risk factor for all types of urinary incontinence. The prevalence of urinary incontinence rises from 15% in the second decade of life to 30% in the fifth decade, at which time it plateaus, then rises again in the seventh decade. Stress incontinence is more predominant in younger and middle-aged women, whereas urgency incontinence and mixed incontinence are more predominant in older women. The effect of **menopause and hormonal status** on urinary incontinence has been investigated in several studies with conflicting results. In postmenopausal women, low estrogen levels may contribute to urinary incontinence. Treatment with local (vaginal) estrogen was shown to improve symptoms, whereas oral hormone replacement therapy worsened symptoms. **Obesity** has been shown to be a significant risk factor for urinary incontinence in multiple large-scale studies, with a greater impact on stress incontinence compared with urgency and mixed incontinence. **Type 2 diabetes mellitus** is a strong independent risk factor for urinary incontinence, particularly urgency incontinence. Pregnancy, vaginal delivery, pelvic surgery, medication (e.g., alpha-blockers), smoking, and genetic factors have also all been implicated as risk factors for urinary incontinence. Table 19-2 delineates the risk factors specific to stress urinary incontinence.

PATHOPHYSIOLOGY

Understanding the anatomy and physiology of the lower urinary tract and pelvic floor is crucial to understanding the mechanism behind each type of urinary incontinence. The bladder, or detrusor muscle, is a meshwork of smooth muscle layers ending in the trigone area at its base (Fig. 19-1). The **internal sphincter** is at the junction of the bladder and the urethra. This is also known as the **urethrovesical junction (UVJ)**. The urethra is also made of smooth muscle. It is suspended by the pubourethral ligaments that originate at the lower pubic bone and extend to the middle third of the urethra to form the **external sphincter**.

Urinary continence at rest is possible because the **intraurethral pressure** exceeds the **intravesical pressure**. Continuous contraction of the **internal sphincter** is one of the primary mechanisms for maintaining continence at rest. The **external sphincter** provides about 50% of urethral resistance and is the second line of defense against incontinence. When the urethrovesical junction is in its proper position, any sudden increase in intra-abdominal pressure is **transmitted equally to the bladder and proximal third of the urethra**. Therefore, as long as

TABLE 19-1 Types of Urinary Incontinence

Stress (urinary) incontinence
Involuntary loss of urine on effort or physical exertion, or on sneezing or coughing
Urgency (urinary) incontinence
Involuntary loss of urine associated with urgency
Mixed (urinary) incontinence
Involuntary loss of urine associated with urgency and also with effort or physical exertion or on sneezing or coughing
Overflow (urinary) incontinence
Loss of urine due to poor or absent bladder contractions or bladder outlet obstruction that leads to urinary retention with overdistention of the bladder and overflow incontinence
Continuous (urinary) incontinence secondary to urinary fistula
Loss of urine through a urinary fistula secondary to surgery, radiation, or obstructed labor
Functional (urinary) incontinence
Loss of urine due to a physical or psychological (e.g., dementia) inability to respond to voiding cues. Often seen in nursing home patients and geriatric patients

the intraurethral pressure exceeds the intravesical pressure, continence is preserved.

In addition to the internal and external sphincters, continence is also maintained via the action of the **submucosal vasculature** of the urethra. When this vasculature complex fills with blood, the intraurethral pressure is increased, thus preventing involuntary loss of urine (Fig. 19-2). Neurologic control of the bladder and urethra is provided by both the **autonomic** (sympathetic and parasympathetic)

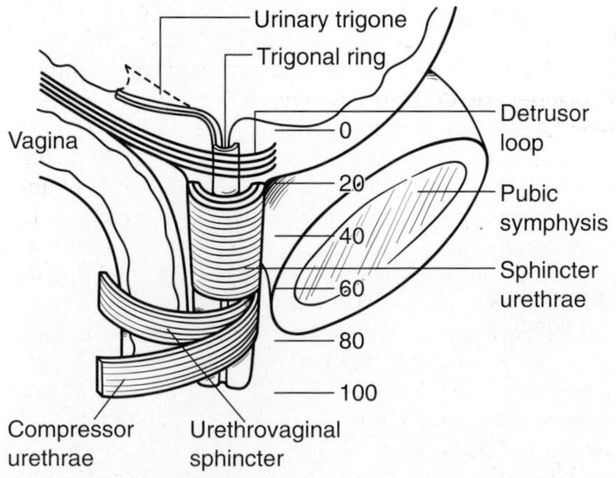

Figure 19-1 • Location of various structures along the urethra. (From Kursh ED, McGuire EJ. *Female Urology.* Philadelphia, PA: J. B. Lippincott Company; 1994.)

TABLE 19-2 Risk Factors for Urinary Stress Incontinence

Age
Obesity
Diabetes mellitus
Pregnancy and vaginal delivery
Genetics
Hormonal status
Pelvic surgery
Smoking
Chronic cough
Medications

and **somatic nervous systems** (Fig. 19-3). The **sympathetic nervous system** provides continence and prevents micturition by contracting the bladder neck and internal sphincter. Sympathetic control of the bladder is achieved via the **hypogastric nerve** originating from T10 to L2 of the spinal cord. The **parasympathetic nervous system** allows micturition to occur. Parasympathetic control of the bladder is supplied by the **pelvic nerve** derived from S2, S3, and S4 of the spinal cord. Finally, the somatic nervous system aids in voluntary prevention of micturition by innervating the striated muscle of the external sphincter and pelvic floor through the **pudendal nerve**.

During micturition, the bladder releases its contents under voluntary control through a series of coordinated activities, resulting in urethral relaxation and bladder contraction. Stretch receptors in the bladder wall send a signal to the CNS to begin voluntary voiding. This triggers inhibition of the sympathetic sacral and pudendal nerves, thereby causing relaxation of the urethra, external sphincter, and levator ani muscles. This is closely followed by activation of the parasympathetic pelvic nerve, resulting in contraction of the detrusor muscle, and micturition begins.

HISTORY

Care of all patients with urinary incontinence should begin with obtaining a thorough medical and surgical history. Terminology developed by the International Continence Society (ICS) and International Urogynecological Association (IUGA) can be helpful in obtaining and documenting the patients symptoms. These include symptoms discreetly categorized into a comprehensive, user-friendly, female-specific, clinically based system (Table 19-3).

PHYSICAL EXAMINATION

The **physical examination** should include both internal and external pelvic examinations. Pelvic organ prolapse is often found in patients with urinary incontinence and should be evaluated and documented. Because the innervation of the lower urinary tract is closely associated with the innervation of the lower extremities and rectum, patients should receive a thorough

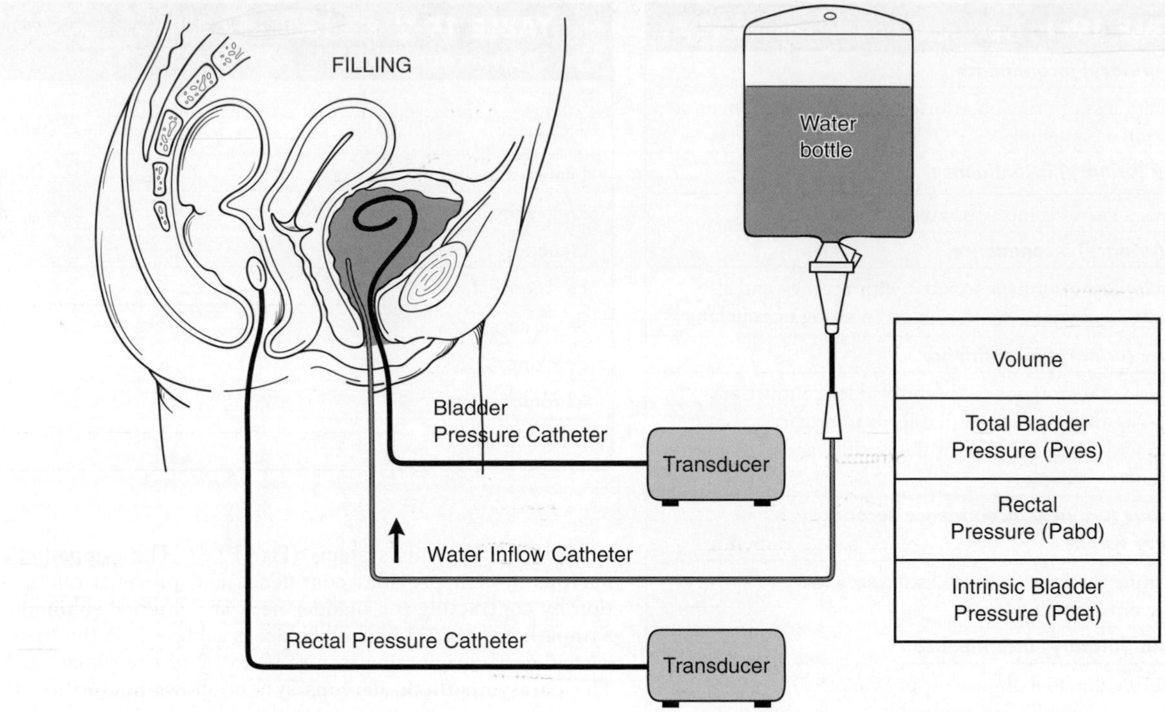

Figure 19-2 • Complex cystometry.
(From Wall LL, Norton PA, DeLancy JOL. *Practical Urogynecology*. Baltimore, MD: Williams & Wilkins; 2003.)

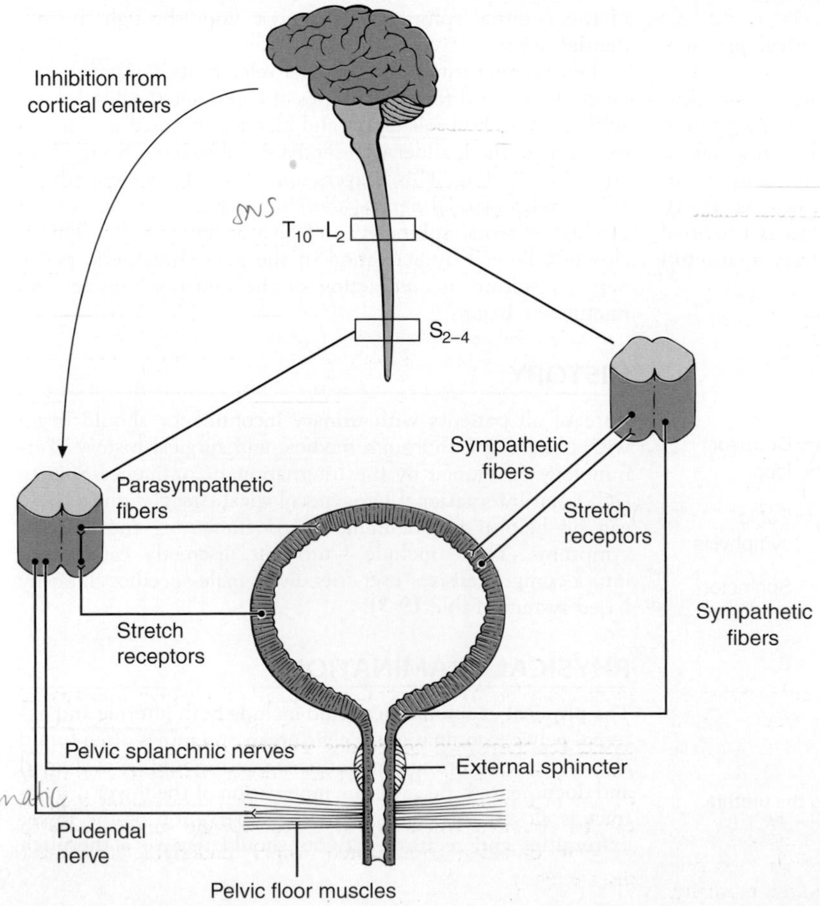

Figure 19-3 • Innervation of the lower urinary tract.

TABLE 19-3 IUGA/ICS Terminology for Symptoms of Pelvic Floor Dysfunction

Urinary incontinence symptoms		
Incontinence	Positional	Insensible (unaware)
Stress incontinence	Nocturnal	Coital incontinence
Urge incontinence	Continuous	Mixed symptomatology
Bladder storage symptoms		
Daytime frequency	Urgency	Nocturia
Sensory symptoms		
Increased bladder sensation	Reduced bladder sensation	Absent bladder sensation
Voiding symptoms		
Hesitancy	Straining	Immediate revoiding
Slow stream	Spraying	Postvoid leakage
Intermittency	Incomplete emptying	Position-dependent voiding
Dysuria	Retention	
Prolapse symptoms		
Vaginal bulging	Bleeding, discharge, infection	Low back pain
Pelvic pressure	Splinting/digitation	
Sexual dysfunction		
Dyspareunia	Deep dyspareunia	Vaginal laxity
Introital dyspareunia	Obstructed intercourse	Other symptoms
Anorectal dysfunction		
Anal incontinence	Straining	Rectal prolapse
Fecal incontinence	Incomplete evacuation	Rectal bleeding/mucus
Fecal urgency	Diminished rectal sensation	Coital fecal incontinence
Fecal urgency	Constipation	Passive fecal incontinence
Lower urinary tract pain/pelvic pain		
Bladder pain	Vulvar pain	Perineal pain
Urethral pain	Vaginal pain	Pelvic pain
Lower urinary tract infection		
Urinary tract infection	Recurrent UTI	Hematuria

From Haylen BT, de Ridder D, Freeman RM, et al. An International Urogynecological Association (IUGA)/International Continence Society (ICS) joint report on the terminology for female pelvic floor dysfunction. *Int Urogynecol J.* 2010;21:5–26.

neurologic examination. In particular, deep tendon reflexes, anal reflex, pelvic floor contractions, and the bulbocavernosus reflex should be elicited.

DIAGNOSTIC EVALUATION

Fortunately, a variety of diagnostic tests are available for the evaluation of urinary incontinence. The scope of this text precludes an exhaustive compilation of every diagnostic modality. In general, the goal of diagnostic testing is to distinguish between **stress incontinence** and **urgency incontinence** since the treatments for these two conditions are very different. Initial tests typically include the stress test, the cotton swab test, cystometrogram, and uroflowmetry. More complex urodynamic studies can be obtained when indicated (considering surgery, patient 65 years or older, complicated history, underlying neurologic disease, etc.).

A voiding diary or bladder chart (Fig. 19-4) can be used to document the specific circumstances of the patient's voiding habits (e.g., intake, amount voided, leak volume, associated activity, urgency presence). A **urinalysis** and **urine culture** should be obtained to rule out infection as a cause of incontinence.

A **stress test** is performed by filling the bladder with up to 300 mL of normal saline or sterile water through a catheter. The patient is asked to cough, and the clinician observes to verify the loss of urine. This can be done standing or in the lithotomy position. If urine leakage is witnessed by the clinician, the patient is then said to have genuine **stress incontinence**. A **postvoid residual** (PVR) is obtained by catheterization of the bladder after voiding. This specimen can then be used to rule out urinary retention and infection. An alternative is to measure the postvoid residual with an ultrasound bladder scanner. The upper limits of a normal postvoid residual have been reported as 50 to 100 mL.

The purpose of the **cotton swab test** is to diagnose a hypermobile urethra associated with stress incontinence. The clinician inserts a lubricated cotton swab into the urethra to the angle of the urethrovesical junction (Fig. 19-5). When the patient strains as if urinating, the urethrovesical junction descends and the cotton swab moves upward. The change in cotton swab angle is normally less than 30 degrees (Fig. 19-5A), and a value of greater than 30 degrees is consistent with a hypermobile urethra (Fig. 19-5B).

Urodynamics, the functional study of the lower urinary tract, are usually reserved for patients contemplating surgery and for those in whom a clear diagnosis cannot be made on preliminary tests. The three major components of urodynamic studies include evaluation of urethral function (urethrocystometry, urethral pressure profilometry), bladder filling (cystometry), and bladder emptying (uroflowmetry and voiding cystometry or pressure flow studies).

As part of urodynamic testing, **cystometry** measures the pressure and volume relationship of the bladder during filling and/or pressure flow study during voiding. To achieve this, pressure sensors are placed into the bladder to measure intravesical pressure and into either the vagina or rectum to measure abdominal pressure as the bladder is filled with fluid in a retrograde fashion. Cystometry assesses bladder sensation, bladder capacity, detrusor activity, and bladder compliance. The sensation to void typically occurs after the bladder is instilled with 150 mL of fluid. Normal bladder capacity is 400 to 600 mL.

Urodynamic measurements may also include **uroflowmetry**, which measures the rate of urine flow and flow time through the urethra when a patient is asked to spontaneously void while sitting on an uroflow chair. Uroflowmetry is useful in diagnosing outflow obstruction and abnormal bladder reflexes, especially in patients complaining of hesitancy, incomplete bladder emptying, poor stream, and urinary retention.

Number of pads changed today 1
Type of pad used Maxi pad

	Urinate in toilet (time and amount)	Accident (time)	Activity during accident	Fluid intake (time, type, amount)
To Bed →	2200 240 cc			1 glass water
	0300 660 cc	0300	Leak on way to bathroom	
	0500 540 cc	0500	Preparing to urinate	
Up For Day →	0700 150 cc			16 oz coffee 1 cup water
	0845 35 cc			
	1145 160 cc			
	1200			16 oz lemonade
	1540 60 cc			
	1800 100 cc			2 glasses wine 2 cups water
	1940 60 cc			16 oz diet coke 1 glass water

Figure 19-4 • Voiding diary (also called bladder chart). This patient's diary demonstrates urinary frequency, nocturia, urge incontinence, and greater consumption of fluid, caffeine, and alcohol in the evening.
(From Berek JS. *Berek & Novak's Gynecology*, 14th ed. Philadelphia, PA: Lippincott Williams & Wilkins; 2006.)

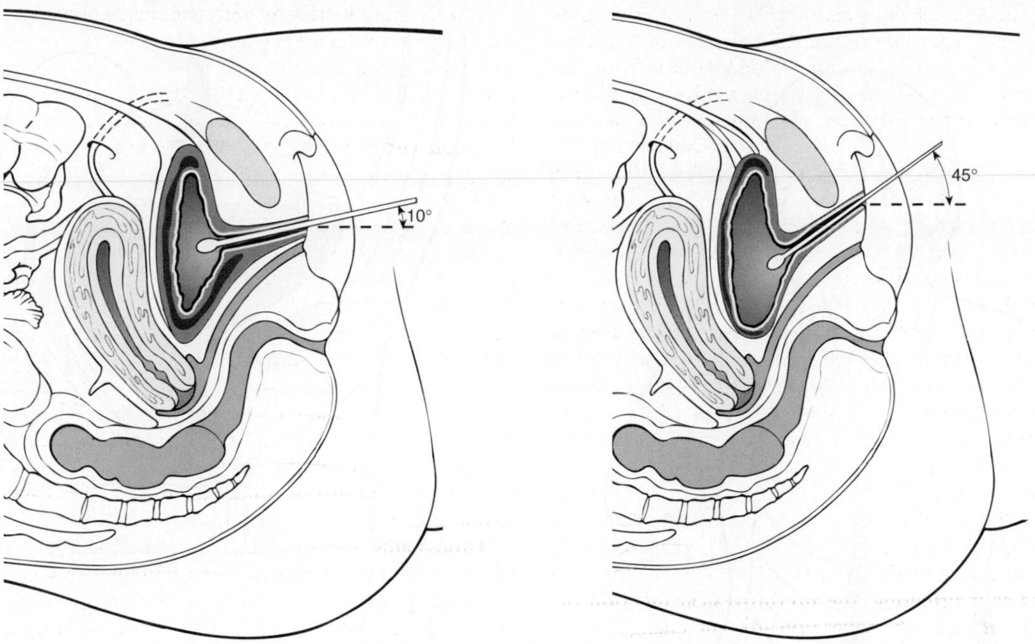

A: During the cotton swab test, a swab is placed in the urethra to the bladder neck. Normal movement of the UVJ with Valsalva (straining) should be less than 30°.

B: When pelvic relaxation results in hypermobility of the bladder neck, there is a large change (30° to 60°) of the UVJ with Valsalva (straining).

Figure 19-5 • (A, B) Cotton swab test.

STRESS INCONTINENCE

PATHOGENESIS

Stress incontinence is the involuntary loss of urine through the intact urethra in response to an increase in **intra-abdominal pressure** such as coughing, sneezing, or exercise. In many cases patients with stress incontinence will have a **hypermobile urethra**. As a result, increases in intra-abdominal pressure are no longer transmitted equally to the bladder and urethra. Instead, increases in intra-abdominal pressure are transmitted primarily to the bladder. Therefore, as **intravesical pressures exceed intraurethral pressure**, urinary stress incontinence occurs (Fig. 19-6). In 1990, the **integral theory** was introduced by Petros and Umsten. This landmark theory proposes that the control of urethral closure is mainly the interplay of the pubourethral ligaments, suburethral vaginal hammock, and pubococcygeus muscles. This theory led to the development of midurethral slings. DeLancey introduced the **hammock theory** in 1994 which states that the urethra lies on the supportive layer of the endopelvic fascia and anterior vaginal wall. This supportive layer gains structural support through its lateral attachments to the arcus tendineus fascia and levator ani muscles. During a cough the urethra is compressed against this hammock-like supportive layer with a resultant increase in urethral closure pressure. In a smaller percentage of women, stress urinary incontinence may be due to weakness in the internal urethral sphincter known as **intrinsic sphincter deficiency**.

HISTORY

Patients with stress incontinence may present with a complaint of involuntary loss of urine with coughing, laughing, sneezing, and straining. With more severe stress incontinence, urine leakage may occur with activities that cause even small increases in intra-abdominal pressure, such as walking standing, or changing positions.

DIAGNOSTIC EVALUATION

Leakage of urine with an increase in intra-abdominal pressure (coughing, jumping, Valsalva effort) during either a simple stress test or during more complex urodynamics can be used to make the diagnosis of stress incontinence. Urodynamics should be reserved for elucidating more complex presentations of incontinence.

TREATMENT

Treatment of stress incontinence includes a multifaceted approach including lifestyle and behavioral modification and medical and surgical management.

Lifestyle and behavioral modifications include weight loss, caffeine restriction, fluid management, bladder training, pelvic floor muscle exercises (Kegel exercises), and physical therapy (biofeedback, magnetic therapy, and electrical stimulation). Pelvic floor muscle exercises (**Kegel exercises**) result in an increase in resting and active muscle tone and thereby increase

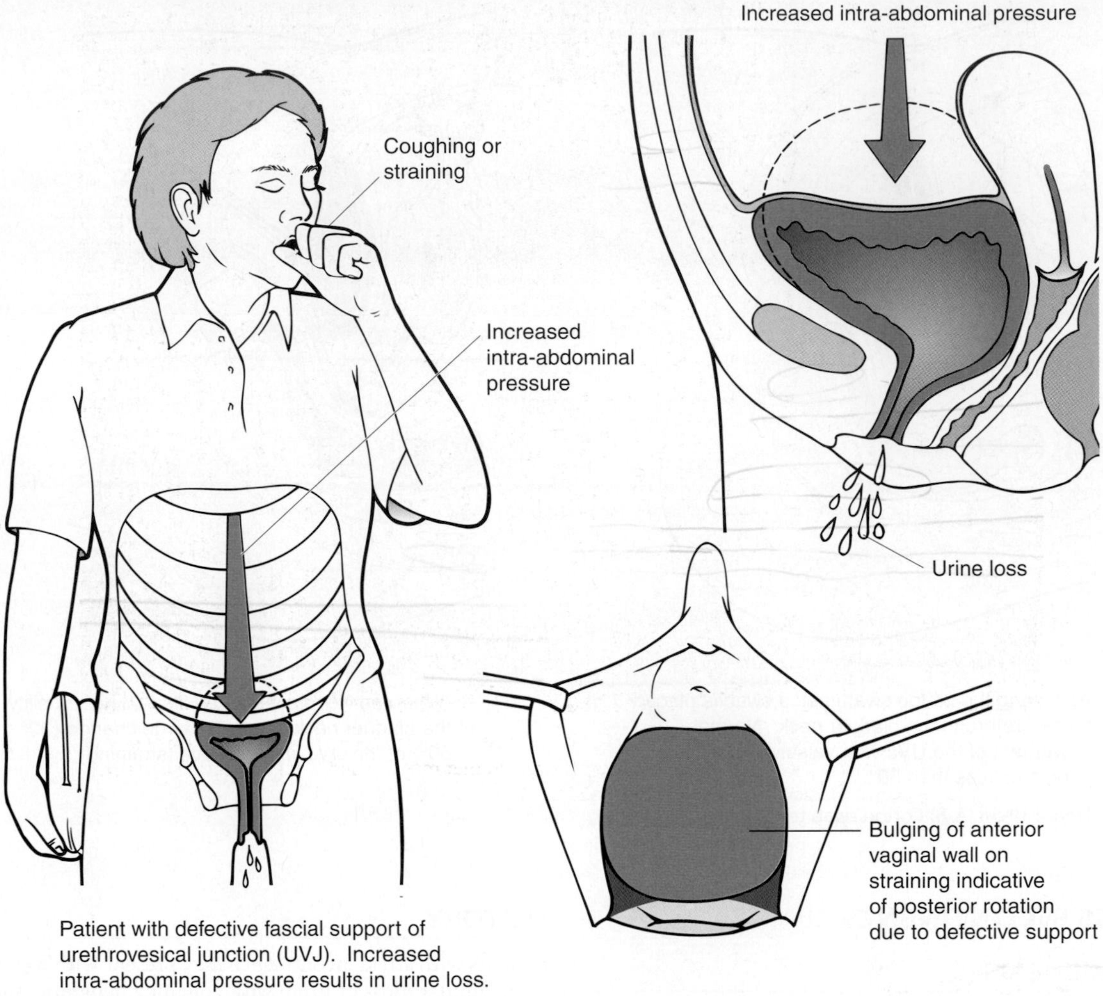
Increased intra-abdominal pressure
Coughing or straining
Increased intra-abdominal pressure
Urine loss
Bulging of anterior vaginal wall on straining indicative of posterior rotation due to defective support
Patient with defective fascial support of urethrovesical junction (UVJ). Increased intra-abdominal pressure results in urine loss.

Figure 19-6 • Patient with urinary stress incontinence.

urethral closing pressure. These can be done with or without biofeedback and/or electrical stimulation.

Medical therapy for the treatment of stress incontinence is limited and no mediations are FDA approved for this purpose. Alpha-adrenergic agonists (midodrine, pseudoephedrine), beta-adrenergic receptor antagonists and agonists (clenbuterol, propranolol), tricyclic antidepressants (imipramine), and serotonergic/noradrenergic reuptake inhibitors (duloxetine) have been tried, but limited data exists for their use. The side effects from these various medications must be weighed against the benefit. The use of systemic estrogen to treat stress incontinence has been controversial, and in recent publications, it has not been shown to improve the symptoms and may worsen or lead to the development of stress incontinence in some women.

Incontinence pessaries and other intravaginal devices are used to physically elevate and support the urethra, which restores normal anatomic relationships. As a result, increases in intra-abdominal pressures are transmitted equally to the bladder and urethra and continence is maintained. Incontinence pessaries differ from pessaries for pelvic relaxation in that incontinence pessaries have added features to specifically support the urethra (Fig. 19-7). Because pessaries are non-invasive, they are useful in patients for whom surgery is contraindicated (elderly, ill, or pregnant women). These devices require close medical supervision to avoid infection of the vaginal epithelium or damage to the vaginal tissues. Patients are often given vaginal estrogen to decrease the risk of vaginal trauma and ulceration.

Surgery is frequently the treatment of choice for stress incontinence. Several approaches have been employed with roughly equal success. These include the abdominal retropubic urethropexies (Burch procedures), bladder neck slings, and tension-free midurethral slings (tension-free vaginal tape, transobturator tape). Most of the abdominal procedures and bladder neck slings aim to **resuspend the hypermobile urethra** to its normal anatomic position (Fig. 19-8), whereas the aim of the **tension-free midurethral sling** is to provide reinforcement at the midurethra to the pubic bone, suburethral vaginal hammock, and pubococcygeus muscles. Disadvantages of surgery include the risks of an invasive procedure and the risk of failure with resumption of symptoms over time. Patients with **intrinsic sphincter deficiency** may benefit from periurethral or transurethral placement of bulking agents to improve sphincter tone (Fig. 19-9).

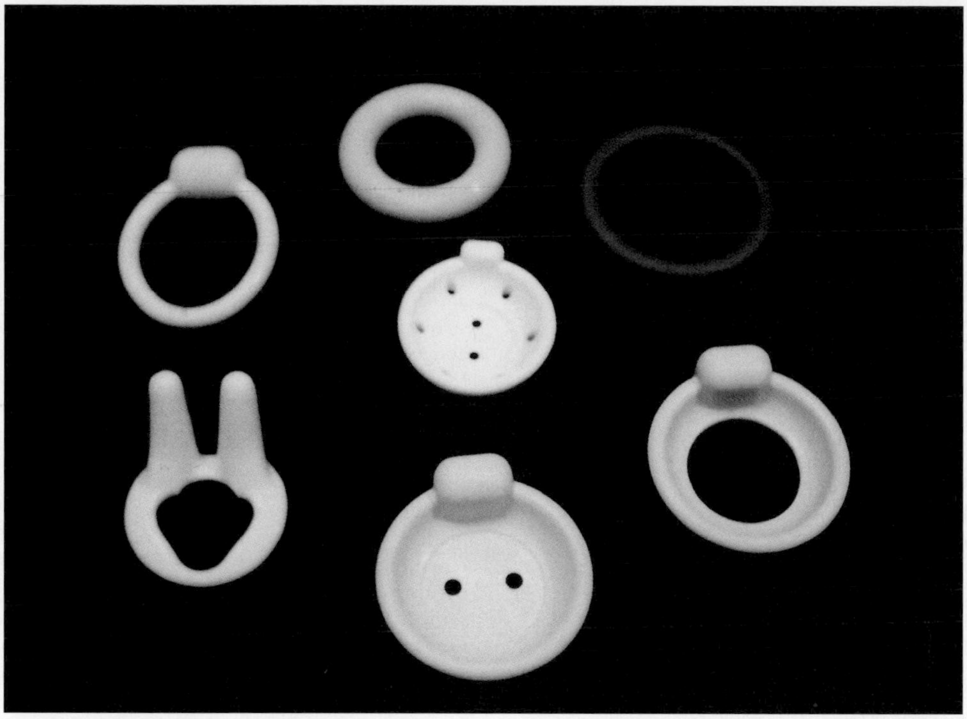

Figure 19-7 • Vaginal incontinence pessaries for treating stress urinary incontinence. Incontinence pessaries differ from more common prolapse pessaries in that most incontinence pessaries have a portion of the device specifically designed to support the bladder neck.
(From Berek JS. *Berek & Novak's Gynecology*, 14th ed. Philadelphia, PA: Lippincott Williams & Wilkins; 2006.)

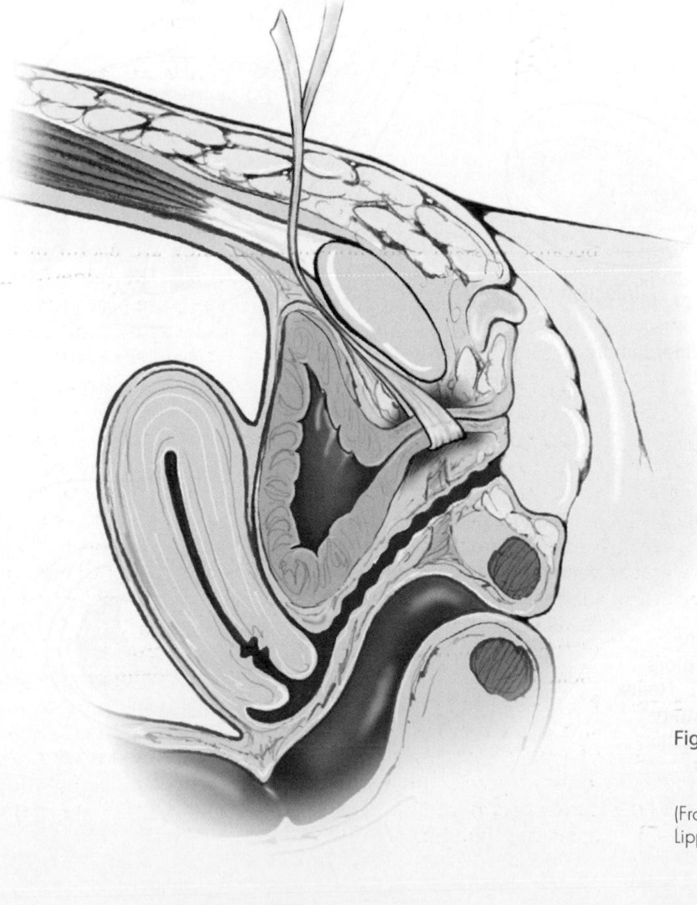

Figure 19-8 • Suburethral sling. The sling is supporting the urethra and bladder neck and the ends are anchored to or above the rectus fascia.
(From Berek JS. *Berek & Novak's Gynecology*, 14th ed. Philadelphia, PA: Lippincott Williams & Wilkins; 2006.)

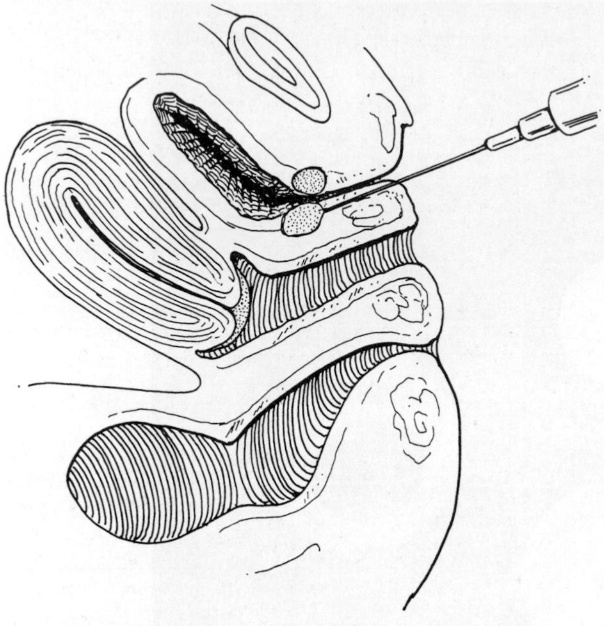

Figure 19-9 • Periurethral injection of collagen around the bladder neck.
(Image from Rock J, Jones H. *TeLinde's Operative Gynecology*, 10th ed. Philadelphia, PA: Lippincott Williams & Wilkins; 2008.)

URGENCY INCONTINENCE

PATHOGENESIS

Urgency incontinence is the involuntary loss of urine associated with urgency and has traditionally been associated with detrusor overactivity; however, a patient may have urgency incontinence without discernible detrusor overactivity. Most detrusor overactivity is **idiopathic**. Some conditions known to cause involuntary bladder contractions include urinary tract infections (UTIs), bladder stones, bladder cancer, urethral diverticula, and foreign bodies (Fig. 19-10). Neurologic disorders such as stroke, spinal cord injury, Parkinson disease, multiple sclerosis, and diabetes mellitus can also cause detrusor overactivity (Table 19-4).

CLINICAL MANIFESTATIONS

Patients with urgency incontinence usually present with a history of involuntary urine loss and urgency whether or not the bladder is full. Many women complain of not being able to reach the bathroom in time or of dribbling or leaking triggered by just seeing a bathroom. Detrusor overactivity presents with symptoms including urinary urgency, frequency, and nocturia. Given the wide differential for detrusor overactivity, patients should also be asked about neurologic symptoms, history of previous anti-incontinence surgery, and hematuria (suggestive of cancer, stones, or infection).

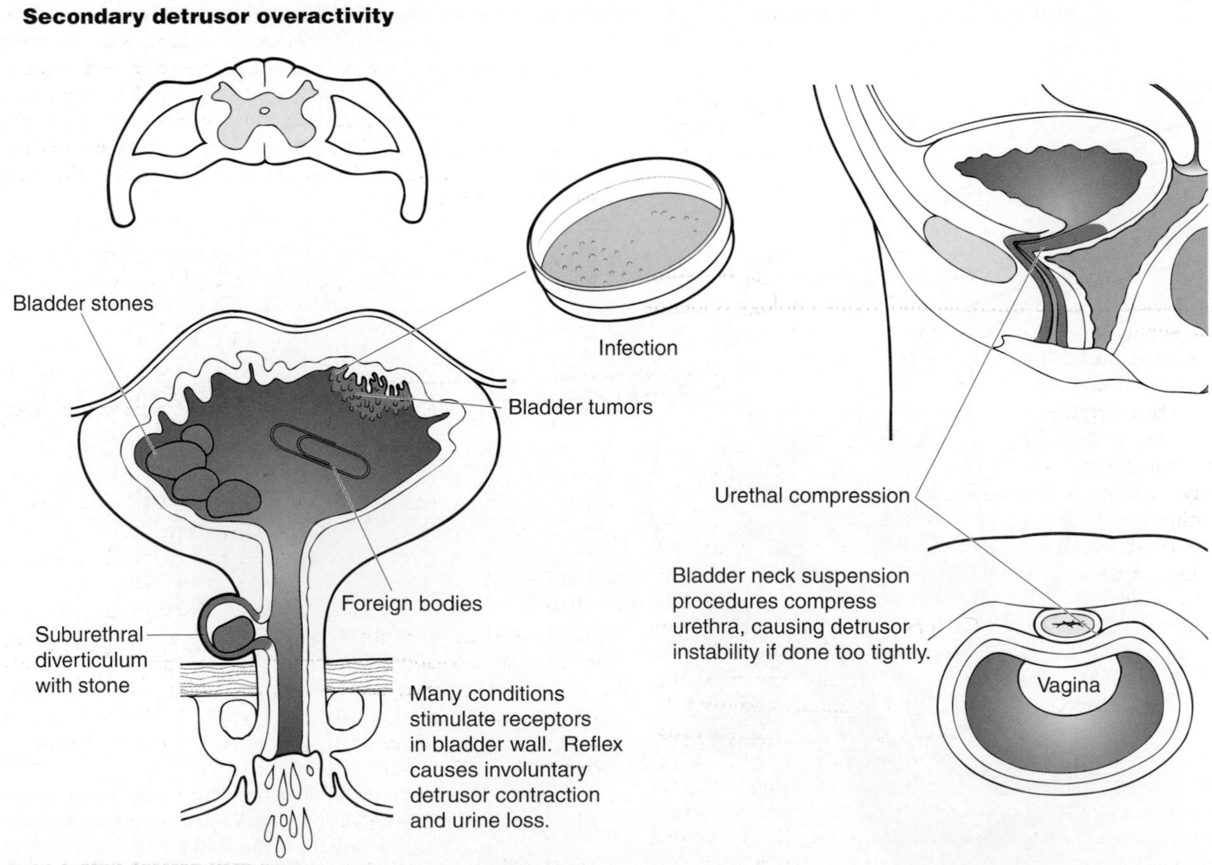

Figure 19-10 • Causes of detrusor overactivity.

TABLE 19-4 Common Causes of Detrusor Overactivity

Nonneurologic causes
UTIs
Urethral obstruction
Urethral obstruction (previous surgery)
Bladder stones
Bladder cancer
Suburethral diverticula
Foreign bodies
Neurologic causes
Cerebrovascular accident
Alzheimer disease
Parkinsonism
Multiple sclerosis
Diabetes
Peripheral neuropathies
Autonomic neuropathies
Cauda equine lesions

DIAGNOSTIC EVALUATION

The diagnosis of urgency incontinence is clinical and does not require specialized testing. Urodynamic studies should be reserved for cases resistant to initial treatment, complex cases, or if surgery is planned.

TREATMENT

The treatment of urge incontinence will depend on the etiology of disease. In cases where an underlying etiology is identified, it should be treated appropriately. **Idiopathic urgency incontinence**, the most common type, is managed with a combination of lifestyle and behavior modifications, medication, and sometimes surgery. **Lifestyle and behavioral modifications** include weight loss, caffeine restriction, fluid management, bladder training, pelvic floor muscle exercises (Kegel exercises), and physical therapy (biofeedback, magnetic therapy, and electrical stimulation).

The most common medications used to treat urgency incontinence are **anticholinergic drugs** with antimuscarinic effects (Table 19-5). Anticholinergic drugs act by increasing bladder capacity and decreasing urgency resulting in decreased incidences of incontinence and decreased voids overall. The effect may take up to 4 weeks, and therefore, premature discontinuation and dose changes should be avoided before this time. Side effects of anticholinergic drugs include dry mouth, blurred near vision, tachycardia, drowsiness, decreased cognitive function and constipation. They are contraindicated in patients with gastric retention and angle closure glaucoma. Anticholinergic drugs should be avoided or used with caution in patients with dementia, as they may worsen this condition.

TABLE 19-5 Medications Indicated for Urgency Incontinence

Oxybutynin (Ditropan) 5 mg PO TID to QID
Oxybutynin extended release (Ditropan XL) 5, 10, 15 mg PO QD
Oxybutynin transdermal patch (Oxytrol) one patch twice weekly
Oxybutynin gel 10% (Gelnique) one sachet QD
Tolterodine (Detrol) 2 mg PO BID
Tolterodine extended release (Detrol LA) 4 mg PO QD
Fesoterodine (Toviaz) 4, 8 mg PO QD
Solifenacin (Vesicare) 5, 10 mg PO QD
Trospium (Sanctura) 20 mg PO BID
Trospium extended release (Sanctura XR) 60 mg PO QD
Darifenacin (Enablex) 7.5, 15 mg PO QD

Surgical treatments for urgency incontinence include sacral and peripheral neuromodulation, bladder injections, and augmentation cystoplasty. The Food and Drug Administration (FDA) has approved **sacral neuromodulation** for the treatment of urinary retention and the symptoms of overactive bladder, including urinary urge incontinence and significant symptoms of urgency frequency alone or in combination, in patients who have failed or could not tolerate more conservative treatments. **Posterior tibial nerve stimulation** has been approved for urinary frequency, urinary urgency, and urgency incontinence. **Botulinum toxin**, although not FDA approved for this purpose, is injected into the detrusor muscle for the treatment of urgency incontinence. Rarely, **augmentation cystoplasty** is required in patients with severe refractory urgency incontinence.

OVERFLOW INCONTINENCE

PATHOGENESIS

Overflow incontinence in women is usually due to **an underactive or acontractile detrusor muscle**. As a result, bladder contractions are weak or nonexistent, causing incomplete voiding, urinary retention, and overdistension of the bladder (Fig. 19-11). The causes of overflow incontinence due to detrusor underactivity vary widely from fecal compaction, to use of certain medications, to neurologic diseases such as spinal cord injuries and multiple sclerosis (Table 19-6).

Bladder outlet obstruction, typically due to surgical procedures that result in urethral kinking, stenosis, or obstruction, can also cause bladder overdistension and overflow incontinence, but it is rarely seen in women. **Postoperative overdistension** of the bladder due to unrecognized urinary retention and the use of epidural anesthesia are common causes of overflow incontinence.

CLINICAL MANIFESTATIONS

Patients with overflow incontinence may present with a wide variety of symptoms including frequent or **constant urinary**

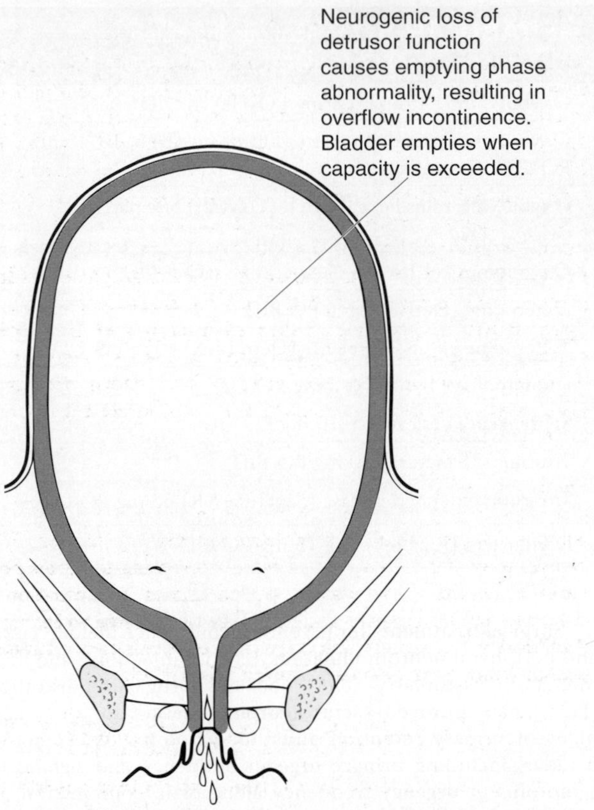

Neurogenic loss of detrusor function causes emptying phase abnormality, resulting in overflow incontinence. Bladder empties when capacity is exceeded.

Figure 19-11 • Overdistended bladder with overflow incontinence.

■ TABLE 19-6 Causes of Overflow Incontinence
Neurogenic causes
Lower motor neuron disease
Spinal cord injuries
Diabetes mellitus (autonomic neuropathy)
Multiple sclerosis
Obstructive causes
Postsurgical urethral obstruction
Postoperative overdistention
Pelvic masses
Fecal impaction
Pharmacologic causes
Anticholinergic drugs
Alpha-adrenergic agonists
Epidural and spinal anesthesia
Other causes
Cystitis and urethritis
Psychogenic (psychosis or severe depression)
Idiopathic

dribbling, along with the symptoms of stress incontinence and urge incontinence. Outflow obstruction (rare) involves a history of urinary retention, straining to void, poor stream, and incomplete emptying. Bladder outlet obstruction may occur following continence procedures such as bladder neck and midurethral slings.

TREATMENT

Treatment strategy in overflow incontinence is geared toward relieving urinary retention, increasing bladder contractility, and decreasing urethral obstruction. **Medical management** of overflow incontinence includes the use of various agents to reduce urethral closing pressure (prazosin, terazosin, phenoxybenzamine) and **striated muscle relaxants** (diazepam, dantrolene) to reduce bladder outlet resistance. **Cholinergic agents** (bethanechol) are used to increase bladder contractility. Intermittent **self-catheterization** may also be used in overflow incontinence to avoid chronic urinary retention and infection.

Patients with overflow incontinence due to **bladder outlet obstruction** caused by a continence procedure benefit from surgical correction of the obstruction. Postoperative overdistension of the bladder is typically temporary and may be managed by continuous bladder drainage for 24 to 48 hours.

BYPASS INCONTINENCE (URINARY FISTULA)

PATHOGENESIS

Bypass incontinence (continuous urinary incontinence) is typically the result of a **urinary fistula** formed between the bladder and the vagina (vesicovaginal fistula), as shown in Figure 19-12, or between the urethra and the vagina (urethrovaginal fistula) or the ureter and the vagina (ureterovaginal fistula).

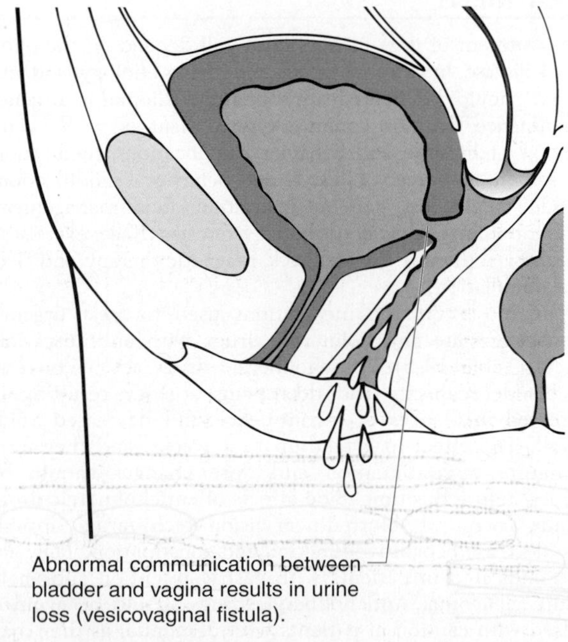

Abnormal communication between bladder and vagina results in urine loss (vesicovaginal fistula).

Figure 19-12 • Vesicovaginal fistula.

A urinary fistula will result in extra urethral leakage of urine, which is usually reported by the patient as **continuous incontinence.** Pelvic radiation and pelvic surgery account for more than 95% of urinary fistula incontinence cases in the United States. In particular, simple abdominal hysterectomy and vaginal hysterectomy alone account for more than 50% of **vesicovaginal fistulas**. **Urethrovaginal fistulas** may also occur as complications of surgery for urethral diverticula, anterior vaginal wall prolapse, or stress urinary incontinence. **Ureterovaginal fistulas**, as seen after 1% to 2% of radical hysterectomies, are usually due to devascularization rather than direct injury. Obstetric injuries associated with operative vaginal deliveries (forceps, vacuum) were once the leading cause of urinary fistulas but are now rare causes of urinary fistula in the United States, Canada, and western Europe. In many developing nations, urinary fistula often results from birth trauma and obstructed labor. Ectopic ureters and urethral diverticula may also produce total incontinence.

RISK FACTORS

The incidence of fistula formation after surgery is higher if the patient has a history of preoperative radiation, endometriosis, pelvic inflammatory disease (PID), or previous pelvic surgery. In developing countries, risks for urinary fistula are linked to obstructed labor and may include absent or untrained birth attendants, inadequate pelvic dimensions (secondary to early childbearing, chronic disease, and malnutrition), inadequate labor, malpresentations, hydrocephalus, and introital stenosis secondary to tribal circumcision.

HISTORY

Patients with a urinary fistula usually present with a history of painless and continuous loss of urine, usually after pelvic surgery, pelvic radiation, or obstetric trauma. Fistulas due to surgery usually become clinically apparent within 14 postoperative days.

DIAGNOSTIC EVALUATION

Methylene blue or indigo carmine instilled **into the bladder** in a retrograde fashion can be visualized leaking through the fistula into the vagina. If the fistula is very small and difficult to visualize, a tampon can be placed in the vagina following the instillation of dye; the blue dye will stain the tampon if a vesicovaginal fistula is present. To diagnose a ureterovaginal fistula, **indigo carmine** is given intravenously. As the compound is filtered through the kidneys and passes through the ureters, it will stain the tampon. If a ureterovaginal fistula is present, the retrograde dye test will be negative and the IV dye test will be positive. **Cystourethroscopy** and the **voiding cystourethrogram** (VCUG) can then be used to identify the number and location of the fistulas. Intravenous pyelogram (IVP) and retrograde pyelogram may also be used to localize urinary fistulas as well.

TREATMENT

Surgery is the primary treatment for urinary fistulas. It is typical to wait 3 to 6 months before attempting to repair **post-surgical fistulas**. This waiting period allows inflammation to decrease and vascularity and pliability of the area to increase. **Antibiotics** for urinary infection and **estrogen** for postmenopausal women are also used during this period.

FUNCTIONAL INCONTINENCE

Functional incontinence is attributed to factors outside the lower urinary tract. These might include **physical or mental impairments** that prevent the patient from being able to respond normally to cues to void. These are particularly common in nursing home residents and in geriatric patients in general. Factors such as physical immobility, dementia, delirium, medications, and systemic illness can all contribute to functional incontinence. Once an etiologic agent is identified, treatment should be aimed at addressing the root cause.

KEY POINTS

- Under normal circumstances, urinary incontinence is avoided due to the complex system of muscles, ligaments, sphincters, and nerves that keep the intraurethral pressure greater than the intravesical pressure.
- Diagnostic evaluation includes a thorough history and physical examination, urine analysis and culture, stress test, cotton-swab test, and use of a voiding diary. Urodynamics (cystometrogram, uroflowmetry) can be used as indicated.
- Risk factors for urinary incontinence include age, hormonal status, obesity, diabetes, impaired functional status, and some neurologic disorders.
- Stress incontinence is characterized by leaking with physical activity such as coughing, sneezing, lifting, or exercising.
- Stress incontinence can be treated with lifestyle and behavioral modification, incontinence pessaries, and surgical management. Common surgical treatments include supportive slings for the urethra and bladder neck.
- Urgency incontinence is characterized by leaking associated with urgency and may exhibit detrusor overactivity. Most cases of detrusor overactivity are idiopathic. Other cases are caused by UTI, bladder stones, cancer, diverticula, and neurologic disorders (stroke, multiple sclerosis, Alzheimer disease).
- The goal of treatment is to relax the bladder, suppress involuntary bladder contractions, and enhance urine storage. This can be achieved with lifestyle and behavioral modification as well as anticholinergic medication. Surgical procedures include sacral and peripheral nerve stimulation, bladder injections, and augmentation cystoplasty.
- When neurologic etiologies exist, treatment of the disorder may result in improved detrusor stability.

- Overflow incontinence is most commonly due to decreased detrusor contractions caused by medications or neurologic disease; obstruction and postoperative overdistension occur less frequently in women.
- The primary symptom of overflow incontinence is urinary retention with continuous dribbling. It is usually treated with self-catheterization and/or medications to increase bladder contractility (cholinergic agents) and lower urethral resistance (alpha-adrenergic agents).
- Bypass incontinence is painless, continuous urine leakage usually due to vesicovaginal, urethrovaginal, or ureterovaginal fistulas. Bypass incontinence is treated surgically with repair of the urinary fistula.
- The most common causes of urinary fistulas in the United States are pelvic radiation and pelvic surgery. In developing countries, total incontinence is attributable to obstetric trauma, often leading to urinary fistula.
- Functional incontinence is urinary loss due to the physical and/or mental inability to attend to voiding cues. Causes include physical impairment, dementia and delirium, and medications.
- Functional incontinence occurs most commonly in nursing homes and in geriatric and psychiatric patients.

C Clinical Vignettes

Vignette 1

A 56-year-old G3P3 woman is referred to the urogynecology clinic for urinary leakage by her PCP. She has leaked urine when coughing, sneezing, and jogging for the past 3 years. She denies leakage of urine with urgency. Her BMI is 33. She uses three pads per day for urinary leakage. Urinalysis and urine cultures done in her PCP's office 1 week ago were negative.

1. Which of the following is NOT a first-line treatment for this patient?
   a. Pelvic floor muscle exercises (Kegel exercises)
   b. Caffeine restriction
   c. Oxybutynin (anticholinergic medication)
   d. Bladder training
   e. Weight loss

2. After trying behavioral and lifestyle modifications, the patient continues to be symptomatic. Urodynamic studies are done to further evaluate the incontinence. Cystometry reveals leakage of urine with increases in intra-abdominal pressure during Valsalva effort and coughing. No involuntary detrusor contractions are seen. Bladder compliance is normal. The pressure flow pattern is continuous and normal with a void initiated by urethral relaxation and a normal detrusor contraction. What type of urinary incontinence does this patient most likely have?
   a. Stress incontinence
   b. Urgency incontinence
   c. Overflow incontinence
   d. Mixed incontinence
   e. Functional incontinence

3. After trying conservative management with behavioral and lifestyle modifications, the patient has not had complete resolution of her symptoms and is still bothered by the loss of urine with coughing, sneezing, and exercise. After appropriate counseling she opts to proceed with surgery. Which of the following is an appropriate surgical choice for her?
   a. Vaginal hysterectomy
   b. Midurethral sling
   c. Cystourethroscopy
   d. Sacral neuromodulation (InterStim)
   e. colpocleisis

4. Following surgery for urinary incontinence, the patient complains of difficulty starting a stream of urine, a weak and interrupted stream, and feeling as if she is not completely empty. She is also experiencing urinary leakage. A postvoid residual measured with a catheter is 250 mL. What is the most likely diagnosis?
   a. Urgency incontinence
   b. Continuous incontinence
   c. Stress incontinence
   d. Bladder outlet obstruction with overflow urinary incontinence
   e. Functional incontinence

Vignette 2

A 45-year-old G5P5 woman who had three vaginal deliveries and two caesarian sections underwent an abdominal hysterectomy for large symptomatic fibroids 3 months ago. On postoperative day 10, she began leaking urine continuously, even at night. She is wearing adult diapers (Depends) and protective pads all of the time and sleeps with an additional pad under her at night. Urinalysis and urine cultures are negative.

1. From this history, you are suspicious that this patient may have:
   a. Overflow incontinence
   b. Stress incontinence
   c. Continuous incontinence secondary to a urinary fistula
   d. Urgency incontinence
   e. Functional incontinence

2. On pelvic examination the vagina is well-healed, and you do not see any lesions or active leaking of urine into the vagina. Further testing at this time may include:
   a. Cystourethroscopy
   b. Dye testing with retrograde filling of the bladder with methylene blue or indigo carmine
   c. IV dye testing with indigo carmine
   d. All of the above
   e. None of the above

3. You fill the bladder with methylene blue dye in a retrograde fashion and still cannot see any dye leaking into the vagina. A tampon is placed for 1 hour and it is also negative when removed. Indigo carmine is given intravenously and a tampon placed in the vagina for an hour, when the tampon is removed, it is stained with blue dye. What type of defect does this patient have?
   a. Vesicovaginal fistula
   b. Urethrovaginal fistula
   c. Ureterovaginal fistula
   d. Vesicouterine fistula
   e. Rectovaginal fistula

Vignette 3

An 82-year-old G3P2 woman is brought to your office by her caregiver from a local retirement home. She has a diagnosis of dementia that has been worsening over the past year. She is followed closely by her PCP and saw him recently for her general conditions. She is communicative but has a poor memory. Her history is obtained from her caregiver. She is ambulatory with minimal assistance and is able to follow commands. Her BMI is 23.5. Her caregiver tells you that over the past year she has had an increase in the number of urinary leakage episodes. She wears adult diapers (Depends), which have to be changed at least two times per day due to leakage. In the morning she wakes up with a wet pad. Her pelvic examination is normal except for atrophic vaginitis (consistent with menopause).

1. Which of the following laboratory tests would you order on this patient?
   a. Urinalysis with culture and sensitivity
   b. Urine microscopy
   c. Urine cytology
   d. Serum creatinine
   e. All of the above
2. Your test results are negative. What is the most likely diagnosis for this patient?
   a. Stress incontinence
   b. Urgency incontinence
   c. Functional incontinence
   d. Overflow incontinence
   e. Continuous incontinence secondary to fistula
3. What is the initial management of this patient?
   a. Pelvic floor muscle exercises, 3 sets of 10 per day
   b. Bladder training, she should be instructed to empty her bladder every 2 to 3 hours
   c. Weight loss
   d. Incontinence pessary
   e. Expectant management
4. Upon physical examination this patient was noted to have atrophic vaginitis. What is your treatment of choice for this?
   a. Hormone replacement therapy (systemic estrogen/progesterone)
   b. Detrol LA (anticholinergic medication)
   c. Low-dose vaginal estrogen
   d. Midodrine (alpha-adrenergic agonists)
   e. Oxybutinin (anticholinergic)

Vignette 4

A 63-year-old G3P2 woman is referred to the urogynecology clinic for evaluation of urinary incontinence. Urinalysis and urine culture done by her PCP 1 week earlier were negative. Her medical history is positive for hypertension and osteoarthritis. She is complaining of leakage of urine following an overwhelming need to void. She runs to the bathroom, but leaks a large amount before she makes it to the toilet. She also has urinary frequency and empties her bladder every 1 to 1.5 hours during the day and gets up four times at night to void. She denies loss of urine with cough, sneeze, and exercise.

1. From this patient's history, what is your initial diagnosis?
   a. Urgency incontinence
   b. Overflow incontinence
   c. Stress incontinence
   d. Mixed incontinence
   e. Continuous incontinence secondary to a urinary fistula
2. What is the most likely cause of this patient's urinary incontinence?
   a. Neurogenic bladder
   b. Bladder outlet obstruction
   c. Idiopathic urgency incontinence
   d. Urinary fistula
   e. Pelvic mass
3. On physical examination she has mild pelvic organ prolapse that is not bothersome, vaginal atrophy, and her BMI is 32. Which of the following would you recommend for this patient as initial management for her condition?
   a. Midurethral sling
   b. Sacral neuromodulation
   c. Lifestyle and behavioral modifications including, weight loss, caffeine restriction, fluid management, bladder training, pelvic floor muscle exercises, and physical therapy
   d. Botulinum toxin A
   e. Vaginal hysterectomy
4. The patient returns for a follow-up appointment, she has implemented your suggestions and has noticed a moderate improvement in her urinary incontinence, urgency and frequency. You suggest that she begin which treatment?
   a. Sacral neuromodulation
   b. Botulinum toxin A injections
   c. Detrol LA (anticholinergic medication)
   d. Posterior tibial nerve stimulation
   e. Midurethral sling

A Answers

Vignette 1 Question 1

Answer C: This patient has a history consistent with stress incontinence, her initial treatment should include behavioral and lifestyle modifications such as weight loss, caffeine restriction, fluid management, bladder training, and pelvic floor muscle exercises (Kegel exercises). Oxybutynin is an anticholinergic medication used to treat urgency incontinence; this patient does not give a history of urgency incontinence.

Vignette 1 Question 2

Answer A: Urodynamic studies support the history of stress incontinence given by this patient. The loss of urine with increases in abdominal pressure and no increase in detrusor pressure during cystometry are consistent with the diagnosis of stress (urinary) incontinence. Urgency incontinence is usually a clinical diagnosis, but can be associated with detrusor overactivity on urodynamics; this patient does not give a history of or demonstrate urgency incontinence. Overflow incontinence is associated with either an underactive/acontractile detrusor or outlet obstruction; this patient has a normal detrusor contraction when voiding and a normal urine flow pattern. Mixed incontinence is a combination of urgency and stress incontinence. Functional incontinence is attributed to factors outside the lower urinary tract including physical or mental impairments that prevent the patient from being able to response normally to cues to void.

Vignette 1 Question 3

Answer B: A midurethral sling such as a TVT (tension-free transvaginal sling) or TOT (transobturator approach midurethral sling) would be the treatment of choice for stress incontinence in this patient. Vaginal hysterectomy is not a procedure for stress incontinence. Cystourethroscopy is an endoscopic procedure used to evaluate the interior of the bladder and urethra and is not a procedure for the treatment of urinary incontinence. Sacral neuromodulation (InterStim) is used for the treatment of urgency incontinence, not stress incontinence. Colpocleisis is a vaginal obliteration procedure used to treat pelvic organ prolapse in patients who are poor surgical candidates and no longer plan on vaginal intercourse.

Vignette 1 Question 4

Answer D: Bladder outlet obstruction with overflow urinary incontinence is the most likely diagnosis, and urodynamics with pressure flow studies can help to better evaluate her problem. The treatment for bladder outlet obstruction from a midurethral sling would be surgical release/revision of the sling.

Vignette 2 Question 1

Answer C: This patient's history of continuous urinary incontinence following an abdominal hysterectomy is consistent with a urinary fistula. She has risk factors for fistula, including prior pelvic surgery and large uterine fibroids. She has no history of surgery for urinary stress incontinence or of an underactive bladder, making overflow incontinence unlikely. Stress incontinence is characterized as involuntary urine loss on effort or physical exertion (e.g., sporting activities) or on sneezing or coughing. She also does not have the complaint of involuntary loss of urine associated with urgency. Functional incontinence is due to physical or mental impairments that prevent the patient from being able to response normally to cues to void.

Vignette 2 Question 2

Answer D: Methylene blue or indigo carmine instilled into the bladder in a retrograde fashion can be visualized leaking through the fistula into the vagina. If the fistula is very small and difficult to visualize, a tampon can be placed in the vagina following the instillation of dye; the blue dye will stain the tampon if a vesicovaginal fistula is present. To diagnose a ureterovaginal fistula, indigo carmine is given intravenously. As the compound is filtered through the kidneys and passes through the ureters, it will stain the tampon. If a ureterovaginal fistula is present, the retrograde dye test will be negative and the IV dye test will be positive. Cystourethroscopy and the voiding cystourethrogram (VCUG) can then be used to identify the number and location of the fistulas.

Vignette 2 Question 3

Answer C: This patient has continuous (urinary) incontinence following an abdominal hysterectomy. She has several risk factors for complications such as urinary tract fistula. A retrograde dye test with methylene blue dye is negative; however, an IV indigo carmine dye test is positive. This would indicate a communication between a ureter and the vagina, or a ureterovaginal fistula. A vesicovaginal fistula would allow leakage of urine between the bladder and vagina and would have had a positive retrograde methylene blue test. A urethrovaginal fistula between the urethra and vagina may be visualized on urethroscopy or require imaging to identify and would not be expected to result from a hysterectomy. A vesicouterine fistula is a communication between the bladder and uterus; this patient had a hysterectomy and does not have a uterus. A rectovaginal fistula is a communication between the rectum and vagina that can occur following hysterectomy, but is more likely to occur following a traumatic vaginal delivery. A rectovaginal fistula results in stool or gas passing through the vagina.

Vignette 3 Question 1

Answer A: Urinary tract infection is a reversible cause of urinary incontinence and should always be ruled out in a patient with urinary incontinence. Urine microscopy is used to evaluate abnormalities of the urine such as hematuria. Urine cytology looks at cells is the urine to rule out evidence of malignancy. Serum creatinine is a blood test used to assess kidney function.

Vignette 3 Question 2

Answer C: Functional incontinence is attributed to factors outside the lower urinary tract including physical or mental impairments that prevent the patient from being able to response normally to cues to void. These are particularly common in nursing home residents and in geriatric patients in general. Factors such as physical immobility, dementia, delirium, medications, and systemic illness can all contribute to functional incontinence. To make the diagnosis of functional incontinence, a history of the other types of urinary incontinence such as stress or urgency incontinence should be ruled out. It is possible that this patient is also experiencing other types of incontinence; however, with the information given, functional incontinence is the most likely diagnosis at this time.

Vignette 3 Question 3

Answer B: Instructing the patient to void on a schedule every 2 to 3 hours is one of the first interventions to recommend in this patient. Management of her fluid and caffeine intake should also be encouraged. This patient is probably not capable of performing pelvic floor muscle exercises. She does not need to lose weight; her BMI is in the normal range. A pessary is used to treat stress incontinence and will not benefit a patient with functional incontinence. Expectant management is insufficient since she is symptomatic and capable of following instructions.

Vignette 3 Question 4

Answer C: Vaginal estrogen is used to treat atrophic vaginitis secondary to menopausal estrogen deficiency. Treatment with topical estrogen may relieve this patient of her urinary symptoms. Hormone replacement therapy is not indicated and may cause or worsen urinary incontinence. Detrol LA and oxybutinin are anticholinergic medications used to treat urgency incontinence. Midodrine, an alpha-adrenergic agonist, has been used "off-label" in the treatment of stress incontinence, although there is little evidence to support its use for this indication. It does not play a role in the treatment of atrophic vaginitis.

Vignette 4 Question 1

Answer A: This patient meets the definition of urgency incontinence—involuntary urine loss and urgency whether or not the bladder is full. Many women complain of not being able to reach the bathroom in time or of dribbling or leaking triggered by just seeing a bathroom.

Vignette 4 Question 2

Answer C: Idiopathic urgency incontinence is the most common cause of urgency incontinence, there is no reason to believe that this patient is experiencing neurogenic bladder, bladder outlet obstruction, urinary fistula, or a pelvic mass.

Vignette 4 Question 3

Answer C: The initial first-line therapy in a patient with urgency incontinence should include lifestyle and behavioral modifications. Midurethral sling is a surgical treatment for stress incontinence. Sacral neuromodulation and botulinum toxin A are treatments for medication refractory urgency incontinence. There are no indications for hysterectomy described here.

Vignette 4 Question 4

Answer C: An anticholinergic medication such as Detrol LA would be the next most logical treatment to try in this patient for the treatment of urgency incontinence, frequency, and nocturia. Sacral neuromodulation, botulinum toxin A injections, and posterior tibial nerve stimulation are reserved for patients refractory to medications. A midurethral sling is one treatment for stress incontinence.

Chapter

20 Puberty, the Menstrual Cycle, and Menopause

PUBERTY

Puberty describes the series of events in which a child matures into a young adult. It encompasses a series of neuroendocrine and physiologic changes, which result in the ability to ovulate and menstruate. These changes include the development of secondary sex characteristics, the growth spurt, and achievement of fertility. Before any perceived phenotypic change, **adrenarche** occurs with regeneration of the zona reticularis in the adrenal cortex and production of androgens, and ultimately stimulates the appearance of pubic hair. **Gonadarche** describes the activation of the hypothalamic-pituitary-gonadal axis, which involves pulsatile gonadotropin-releasing hormone (GnRH) secretion stimulating the anterior pituitary to produce luteinizing hormone (LH) and follicle-stimulating hormone (FSH). These in turn trigger the ovary to produce estrogens (Fig. 20.1).

The pubertal sequence includes accelerated growth, breast development (**thelarche**), development of pubic and axillary hair (**pubarche**), and onset of menstruation (**menarche**). These stages usually occur in that order (Fig. 20-2). Concerned parents can be reassured by knowing that, on average, the length of time from breast bud development to menstruation is typically 2.5 years.

ADRENARCHE AND GONADARCHE

Adrenarche occurs between ages 6 and 8 when the adrenal gland begins regeneration of the zona reticularis. This inner layer of the adrenal cortex is responsible for the **secretion of sex steroid hormones**. As a result of the regeneration, the adrenal gland produces increased quantities of the androgens dehydroepiandrosterone sulfate (DHEAS), dehydroepiandrosterone (DHEA), and androstenedione. Production of these androgenic steroid hormones increases from age 6 to 8 up until age 13 to 15. The primary stimulus of adrenarche is unknown.

Gonadarche is independent of adrenarche and begins around age 8, when pulsatile GnRH secretion from the hypothalamus is increased. There is also changing sensitivity of the neuroendocrine system to negative feedback by gonadal hormones. This leads to subsequent pulsatile secretion of LH and FSH from the anterior pituitary. Initially, these increases occur mostly during sleep and fail to lead to any phenotypic changes. As a girl enters early puberty, the LH and FSH pulsatility lasts throughout the day, eventually leading to stimulation of the ovary and subsequent estrogen release. This, in turn, triggers the characteristic breast bud development associated with puberty. The positive feedback of estradiol also results in the initiation of the LH surge and the ability to ovulate.

ACCELERATED GROWTH

The growth spurt is characterized by an acceleration in the growth rate around age 9 to 10, leading to a mean peak growth velocity around age 12 of about 9 cm per year. The increased rate of growth is due to the direct effect of **sex steroids** on epiphyseal growth and due to the increased pituitary **growth hormone** secretion in response to sex steroids (Fig. 20-2).

THELARCHE

The first stage of **thelarche**, the development of breast buds, usually occurs around age 10. Thelarche is usually the **first phenotypic sign of puberty** and occurs in response to the increase in levels of circulating estrogen. Concomitantly, there is estrogenation of the vaginal mucosa and growth of the vagina and uterus. Further development of the breast will continue throughout puberty and adolescence, as described by Marshall and Tanner (Table 20-1 and Fig. 20-3).

PUBARCHE

The onset of **growth of pubic hair** (Fig. 20-3) usually occurs around age 11 and is often accompanied by growth of **axillary hair**. Pubarche usually follows thelarche, but a normal variant may occur with pubarche preceding thelarche, particularly in African American girls. The growth of pubic and axillary hair is likely secondary to the increase in **circulating androgens**.

MENARCHE

The average age at onset of menstruation is between 12 and 13 or **2.5 years after the development of breast buds**. As gondal estrogen production increases during puberty, it increases enough to stimulate endometrial proliferation, ultimately resulting in the start of menses. The adolescent menstrual cycle is usually **irregular for the first 1 to 2 years** after menarche, reflecting anovulatory cycles. On average, it takes about 2 years after menarche before regular ovulatory cycles are achieved. Failure to achieve a regular menstrual cycle after this point may represent a reproductive disorder. Menarche is often delayed in gymnasts, distance runners, and ballet dancers. Some theories propose that this is due to an **insufficient percentage of body fat** that may result in hypothalamic anovulation and amenorrhea. Others postulate that the **exercise and stress** on the body may inhibit ovulation through positive effects on norepinephrine and GnRH, thus interfering with menarche.

ABNORMAL PUBERTY

Precocious puberty is defined as pubarche or thelarche before 7 years of age in Caucasian girls and before 6 years of age in

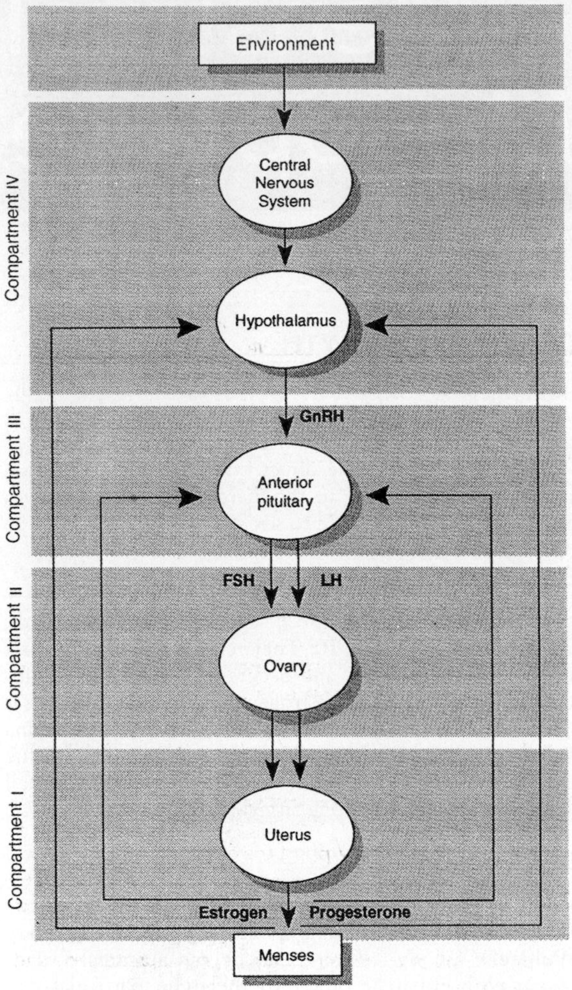

Figure 20-1 • Basic principles of menstrual function. The hypothalamic-pituitary-ovarian axis can be segmented into distinct compartments; each is necessary for normal menstrual function.
(From Bourgeois FJ. *Obstetrics & Gynecology Recall*, 3rd ed. Philadelphia, PA: Lippincott Williams & Wilkins; 2008.)

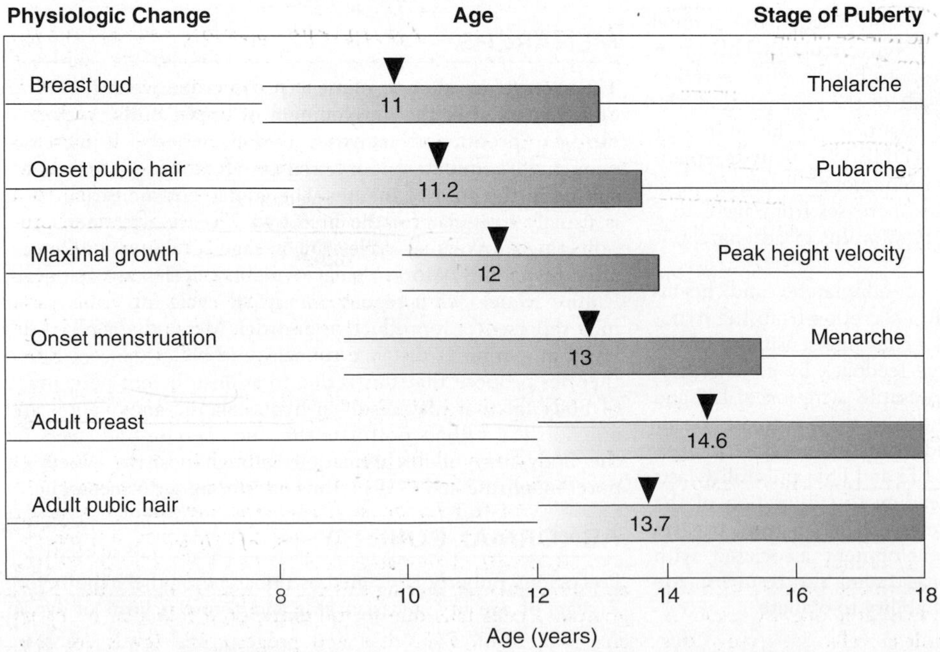

Figure 20-2 • Average age and age range for onset of the major physical changes associated with puberty.

TABLE 20-1 The Tanner Stages of Breast Development

Stage 1	Preadolescent: elevation of papilla only
Stage 2	Breast bud stage: elevation of breast and papilla, areolar enlargement
Stage 3	Further enlargement of breast and areola without separation of contours
Stage 4	Projection of areola and papilla to form a secondary mound
Stage 5	Mature stage: projection of papilla only as areola recesses to breast contour

Adapted from Speroff L, Glass RH, Kase NG. *Clinical Gynecologic Endocrinology and Infertility*, 5th ed. Baltimore, MD: Williams & Wilkins; 1994:377.

African American girls. Absent or incomplete breast development by the age of 12 years is defined as **delayed puberty** and also needs further workup. The initial workup for both includes a careful history, physical examination, hormone assessment and bone age determination.

THE MENSTRUAL CYCLE

The hypothalamus, pituitary, ovaries, and uterus are all involved in maintaining the menstrual cycle (Fig. 20-1). The menstrual cycle is divided into two 14-day phases, **the follicular and luteal phases**, which describe changes in the ovary over the length of the cycle, and the **proliferative and secretory phases**, which describe concurrent changes in the endometrium over the same period of time (Fig. 20-4).

During the **follicular phase,** the release of **FSH** from the pituitary gland results in development of a primary ovarian follicle. The ovarian **follicle produces estrogen**, which causes the uterine lining to proliferate. At midcycle—approximately day 14-there is an LH spike in response to a preceding estrogen surge, which stimulates ovulation, the release of the ovum from the follicle (Fig. 20-4). After ovulation the **luteal phase** begins. The remnants of the follicle left behind in the ovary develop into the corpus luteum. This corpus luteum is responsible for the **secretion of progesterone**, which maintains the endometrial lining in preparation to receive a fertilized ovum. If fertilization does not occur, the corpus luteum degenerates and progesterone levels fall. Without progesterone, the endometrial lining is sloughed off, which is known as *menstruation* (Fig. 20-4).

FOLLICULAR PHASE

The withdrawal of estrogen and progesterone during the luteal phase of the prior cycle causes a gradual increase in FSH. In turn, FSH stimulates the growth of approximately 5 to 15 **primordial ovarian follicles**, initiating the **follicular phase again.** Of these primordial follicles, one becomes the **dominant follicle** and develops and matures until ovulation. The developing dominant follicle, destined to ovulate, produces estrogen that enhances follicular maturation and increases the production of FSH and LH receptors in an autocrine fashion.

The estrogens are produced in a two-cell process with the **theca interna cells** producing **androstenedione** in response to LH stimulation and the **granulosa cells** converting this **androstenedione to estradiol** when stimulated by FSH. LH also rises and stimulates the synthesis of androgens, which are converted to estrogen. As rising estrogen levels negatively feed back on pituitary FSH secretion, the dominant follicle is protected from the decrease in FSH by its increased number of FSH receptors (Fig. 20-5).

OVULATION

Toward the end of the follicular phase, estrogen levels eventually surge to reach a critical level that triggers the anterior pituitary to release an LH spike. The LH surge triggers the resumption of meiosis in the oocyte and induces production of progesterone and prostaglandins within the follicle. The progesterone and prostaglandins in turn are responsible for the rupture of the follicular wall with release of the mature ovum or ovulation (Fig. 20-5). The ovum usually passes into the adjoining fallopian tube and is swept down to the uterus by the cilia lining the tube. This process takes 3 to 4 days. **Fertilization of the ovum must occur within 24 hours of ovulation** or it degenerates.

LUTEAL PHASE

After ovulation, the luteal phase ensues. The **granulosa and theca interna cells** lining the wall of the follicle form the corpus luteum under stimulation by LH. The corpus luteum synthesizes estrogen and significant quantities of progesterone, which cause the endometrium to become more glandular and secretory in preparation for implantation of a fertilized ovum (Fig. 20-5). If fertilization occurs, the developing **trophoblast synthesizes human chorionic gonadotropin (hCG)**—a glycoprotein very similar to LH—which maintains the corpus luteum so that it can continue production of estrogen and progesterone to support the endometrium. This continues until **the placenta develops its own synthetic function at 8 to 10 weeks' gestation**. If fertilization, with its concomitant rise in hCG, does not occur, the corpus luteum degenerates, progesterone levels fall, the endometrium is not maintained, and menstruation occurs.

MENSTRUATION

The endometrium of the uterus undergoes cyclical changes during the menstrual cycle (Fig. 20-4). During the follicular phase, the endometrium is in the **proliferative phase**, growing in response to estrogen. During the luteal phase, the endometrium enters the **secretory phase** as it matures and is prepared to support implantation. If the ovum is not fertilized, the corpus luteum degenerates after approximately 14 days, leading to a fall in estrogen and progesterone levels. The withdrawal of progesterone causes the endometrium to slough, initiating the **menstrual phase.** At the same time, FSH levels begin to slowly rise in the absence of negative feedback and the follicular phase starts again. A menstrual cycle less than 24 days or longer than 35 days or a menses that lasts more than 7 days merit further evaluation.

PERIMENOPAUSE

The menopausal transition, or perimenopause is the transition from **normal ovulatory cycles to menopause**. It can begin 2 to 8 years prior to menopause. These years are characterized by **irregular menstrual cycles** and some of the symptoms that are associated with menopause, such as hot flashes, night sweats, and mood swings. During this period, inhibin B secretion from granulosa cells falls due to the diminished follicular numbers and as a result FSH rises and progesterone levels are low.

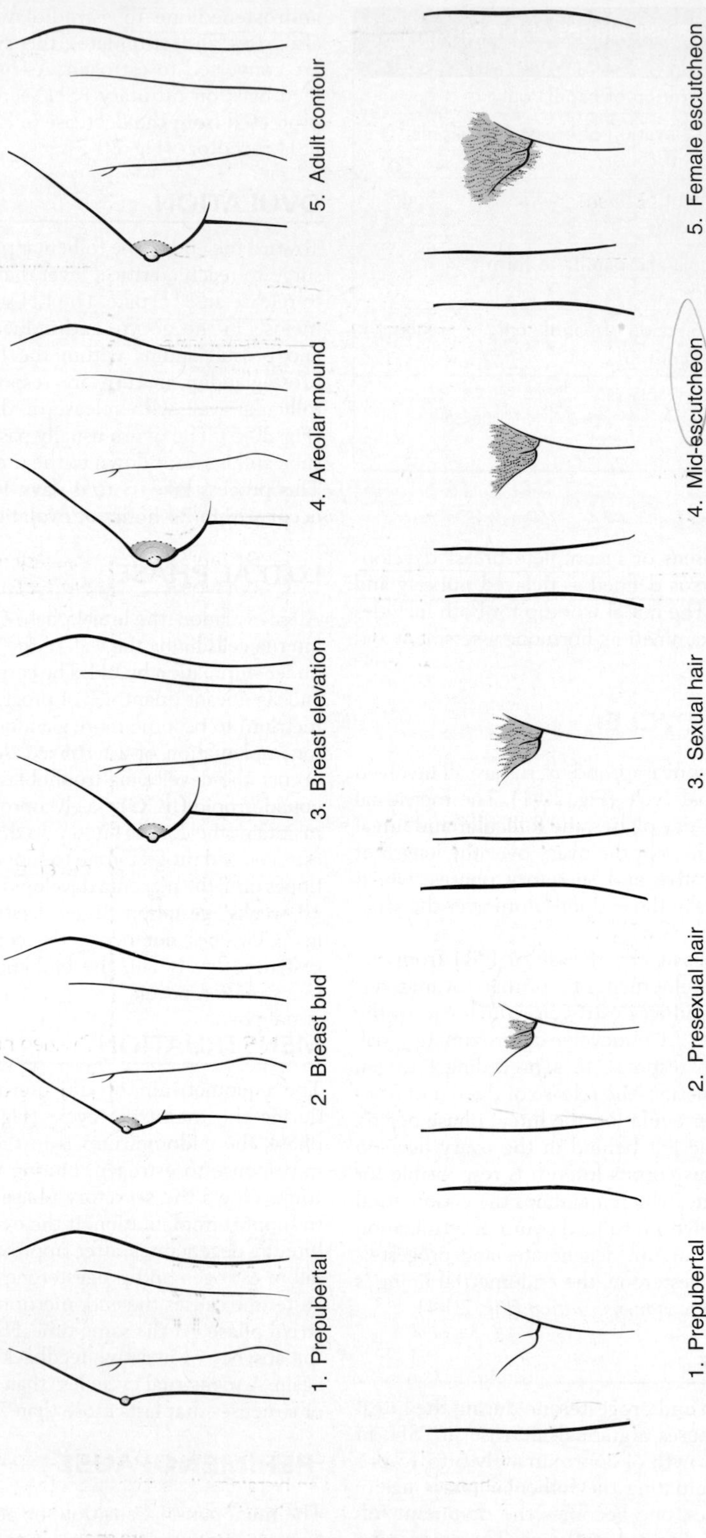

Figure 20-3 • Tanner stages of thelarche (breast development) and of pubarche (onset of pubic hair growth).

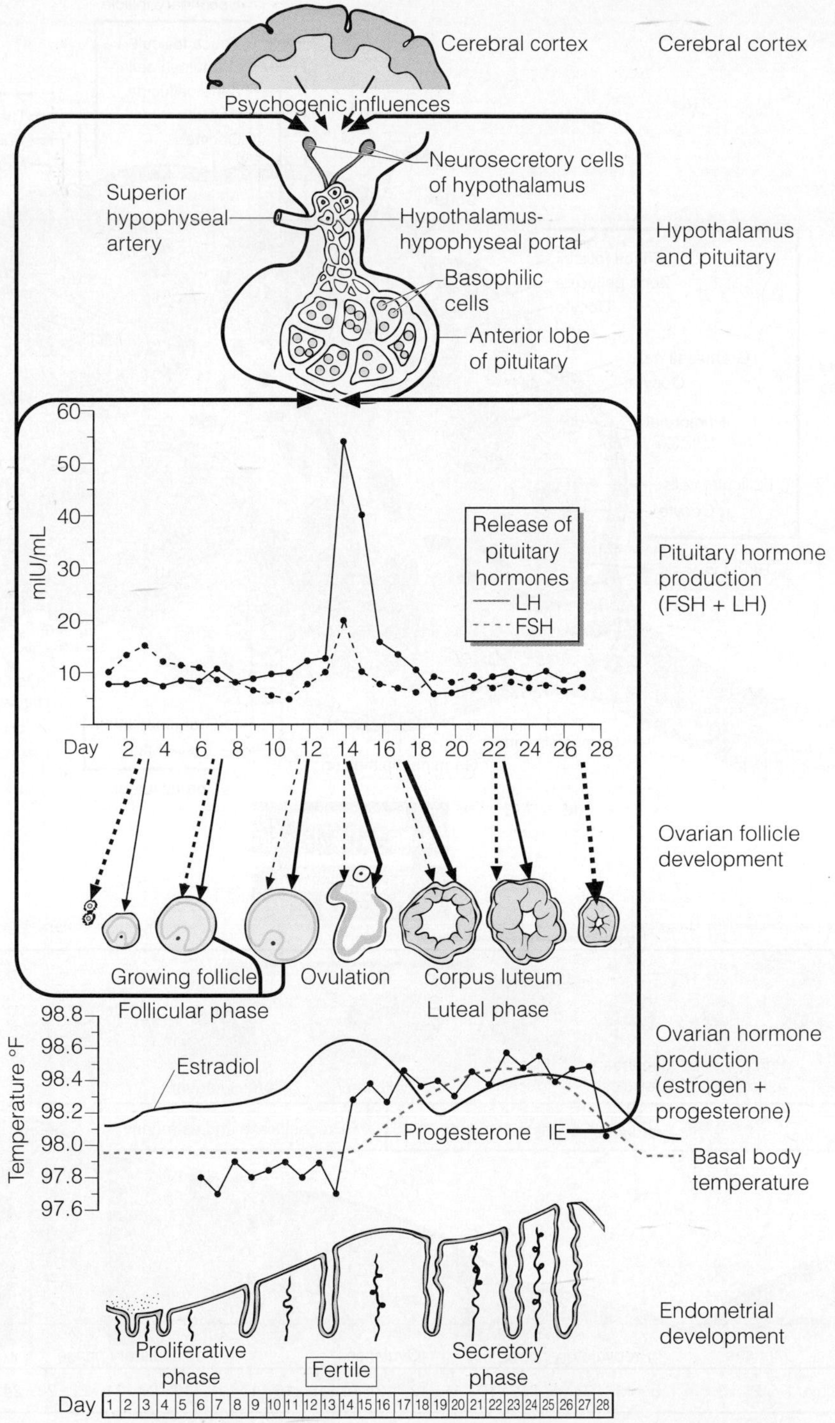

Figure 20-4 • Normal menstrual cycle, day 1 to day 28. The cyclic changes of FSH and LH and the resultant changes in the ovarian histology (follicular and luteal phases) in estrogen and progesterone levels, in basal body temperature, and the endometrial histology (proliferative and secretory phases) are shown. Note how the LH surge near day 14 of a 28-day cycle triggers ovulation and a rise in basal body temperature, signifying the time of maximum fertility during the cycle.

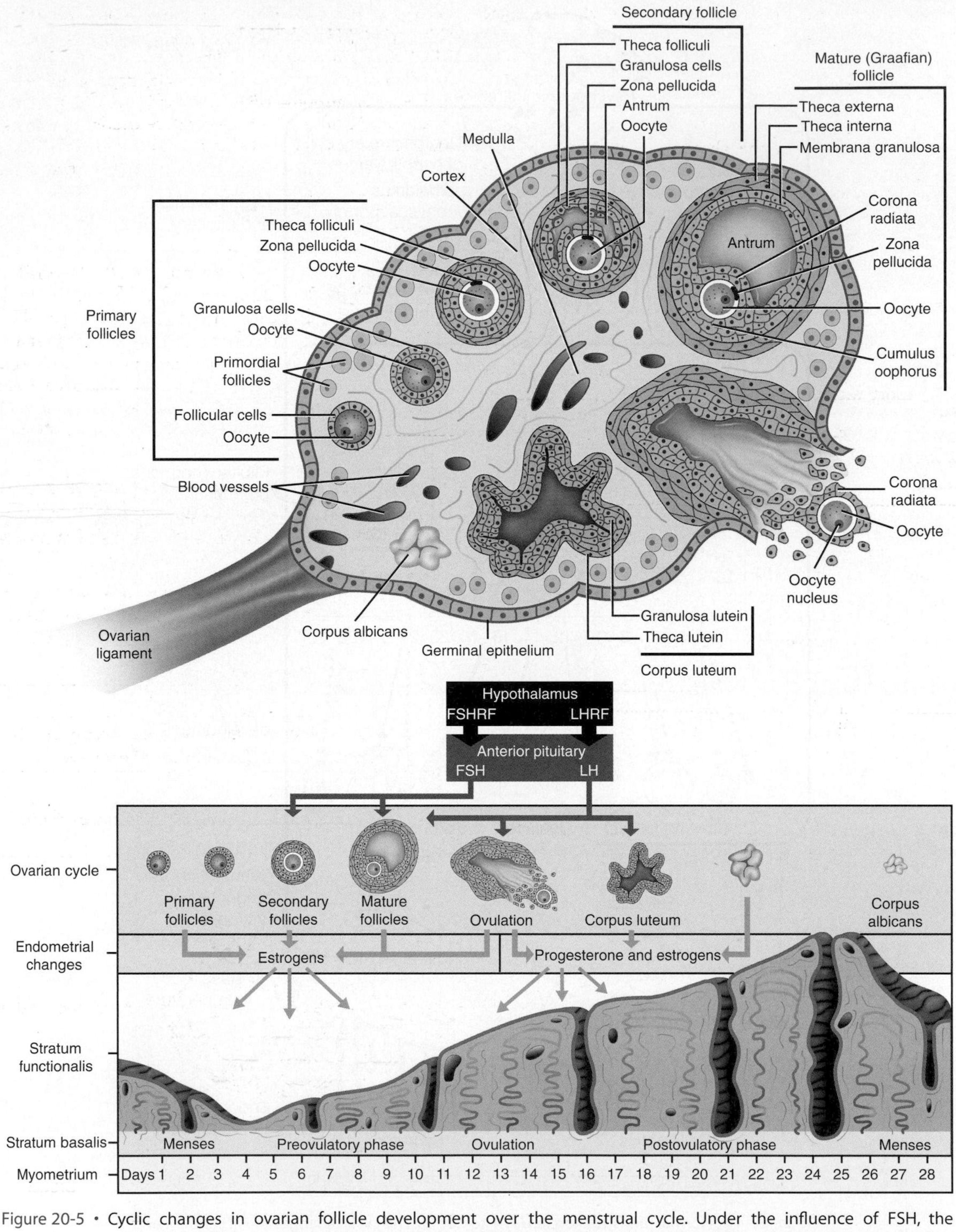

Figure 20-5 • Cyclic changes in ovarian follicle development over the menstrual cycle. Under the influence of FSH, the primordial follicle matures into the preantral follicle and then into the graafian follicle. During the last few days of the growing period, the estrogen produced by the follicular and theca cells stimulate the formation of LH in the pituitary. The LH surge triggers ovulation and the oocyte is discharged from the ovary together. During the luteal phase of the cycle, the follicular cells remaining inside the collapsed follicle differentiate into luteal cells. The corpus luteum is formed by hypertrophy and accumulation of lipid in the granulose and theca interna cells. The remaining cavity of the follicle is filled with fibrin. If pregnancy does not occur, the corpus luteum then degenerates into the corpus albicans and menstruation begins.

(From Eroschenko VP. *Di Fiore's Atlas of Histology, with Functional Correlations*, 9th ed. Baltimore, MD: Lippincott Williams & Wilkins; 2000.)

Estradiol is preserved until late perimenopause when FSH and estradiol both fluctuate.

MENOPAUSE AND POSTMENOPAUSE

Menopause is defined by **12 months of amenorrhea after the final menstrual period** in the absence of any other pathological or physiological causes. At this point, nearly all the oocytes have undergone atresia, although a few remain and can be found on histologic examination. It is characterized by complete, or near complete, ovarian follicular depletion and absence of ovarian estrogen secretion.

The average age at menopause in the United States is 51 years. Five percent of women will have late menopause (occurring after age 55) and another 5% of women have early menopause (occurring between ages 40 and 45). Early menopause is more common in women with a history of cigarette smoking, short menstrual cycles, nulliparity, type 1 diabetes, and family history of early menopause. Primary ovarian insufficiency (PMOI), formerly premature ovarian failure (PMOF) is the onset of spontaneous menopause before the age of 40 and requires further testing.

Various physiologic and hormonal changes occur during this period, including a decrease in estrogen, increase in FSH, and classic symptoms such as hot flashes, night sweats, mood swings, and vaginal dryness. Forty to eighty percent of women will begin having mild symptoms during perimenopause and 50% will experience an increase in frequency and intensity of symptoms during menopause. For most women, symptoms may last during the first year or two of menopause before gradually decreasing and stopping. Even though a quarter of women have hot flashes and/or night sweats that do extend beyond the first 5 years of menopause, it is important to look for other causes for the symptoms when this does occur.

ETIOLOGY

Menopause is generally heralded by menstrual irregularity as the number of oocytes capable of responding to FSH and LH decreases and **anovulation** becomes more frequent. During this period, LH and FSH levels gradually rise because of **diminished estrogen production**. The fall in estradiol levels leads to hot flashes, mood changes, insomnia, depression, osteoporosis, and vaginal atrophy (Fig. 20-6 and Table 20-2). Premature menopause resulting from premature ovarian failure is usually idiopathic or autoimmune. If it occurs before age 30, chromosomal studies can be ordered to rule out a genetic basis (e.g., mosaicism).

DIAGNOSIS

The diagnosis of menopause can usually be made by history and physical examination and confirmed by testing FSH levels. Patients classically present between ages 48 and 52 (average age is 51) complaining of amenorrhea, and vasomotor instability, sweats, mood changes, depression, dyspareunia, and dysuria. These symptoms generally **disappear within first 1 to 2 years**, although a substantial proportion of women can remain symptomatic beyond the first 5 years of menopause.

TABLE 20-2 Menopausal Symptoms and Long-Term Effects (Mnemonic: FSH > 40 IU/L)

F	Flushes, forgetful (Alzheimer disease)
S	Sweats at night, sad (depression) stroke, skeletal changes (accelerated bone loss leading to osteoporosis), skin changes, sexual dysfunction
H	Headaches, heart disease
I	Insomnia
U	Urinary symptoms (stress and urge incontinence), urogenital atrophy (loss of pelvic floor muscles)
L	Libido decreases

Remember that an FSH level >40 IU/L is the blood test to confirm menopause.

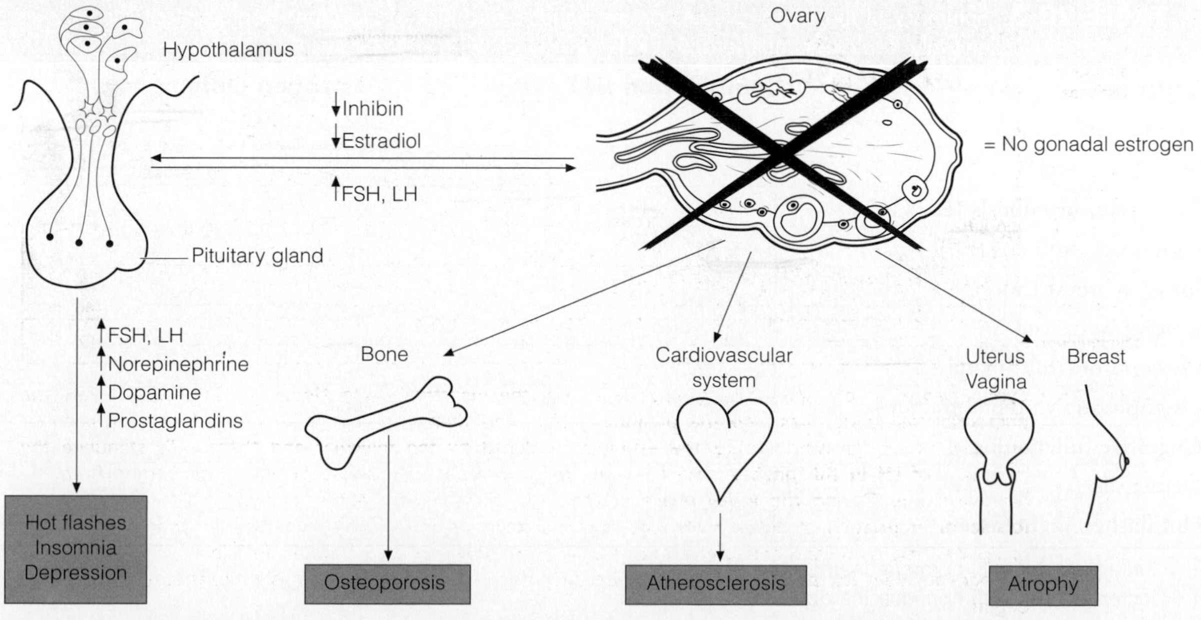

Figure 20-6 • Changes in both the ovary and the hypothalamus contribute to the physiologic changes of menopause.

On physical examination, there may be a decrease in breast size and change in texture. Vaginal, urethral, and cervical **atrophy** may be seen, which is consistent with **decreased estrogen levels**. If there is any question about the diagnosis, an **elevated FSH** greater than 40 IU/L is diagnostic of menopause. During the perimenopausal period, the FSH level may be increased or decreased. Therefore, as a diagnostic test, FSH is best reserved for patients with a combination of amenorrhea or oligomenorrhea and menopausal symptoms.

PATHOGENESIS

Although menopause is a naturally occurring event, there are two important long-term consequences of the estrogen decrease (Fig. 20-6). First, from a cardiovascular standpoint, the protective benefits of estrogen on the lipid profile (increased high-density lipoprotein [HDL] and decreased low-density lipoprotein [LDL]) and on the vascular endothelium (prevents atherogenesis, increases vasodilatation, and inhibits platelet adherence) are lost, and women are at **increased risk for coronary artery disease**. Secondly, with menopause, **bone resorption accelerates** because estrogen plays an important role in regulating osteoclast activity. The increased bone resorption can lead to osteopenia and potentially osteoporosis, particularly in thin (weight <127 lbs.), Caucasian and Asian background, and those with a family history of osteoporosis. This is a particularly important since 15% of women older than 50 years will be diagnosed with osteoporosis and 50% with osteopenia. In fact, a woman can lose 20% of her original bone density in the first 5 to 7 years after menopause. Subsequently, menopausal patients are at risk of hip and vertebral fractures, pain, loss of height, and immobility.

HORMONE-REPLACEMENT THERAPY AND ESTROGEN-REPLACEMENT THERAPY

Hormone-replacement therapy (HRT) refers to the use of a **combination of estrogen and progesterone** to treat menopausal-related symptoms in women who still have their uterus in situ. Menopausal symptoms are due to decreased estrogen levels. The estrogen component on HRT supplies the patient with an exogenous source of estrogen and thereby treats the symptoms of menopause. However, **unopposed estrogen exposure**, whether endogenous or exogenous, can result in endometrial hyperplasia and/or endometrial cancer. Therefore, when estrogens are being used to treat menopausal symptoms in women who still have their uterus in situ, **progestins must be used to decrease the risk of endometrial hyperplasia and cancer**. In menopausal patients who have undergone a hysterectomy, there is no risk of endometrial hyperplasia or endometrial cancer from unopposed estrogen exposure. Thus, these women can use **estrogen-replacement therapy** (ERT) for the treatment of their menopausal symptoms. This therapy uses estrogen only and does not require complementary progesterone use.

The risks and benefits of HRT and ERT have been the subject of numerous studies over the past 30 years. These trials have been designed to evaluate the most common causes of death, disability, and poor quality of life in postmenopausal women including cardiovascular disease, venous thromboembolism, cancer, osteoporosis, and loss of cognitive function. Among the studies contributing to our knowledge of the safety and efficacy of HRT and ERT were the Heart and Estrogen/Progestin Replacement Studies (HERS I and II), Postmenopausal Estrogen/Progestin Interventions (PEPI) Trial, the WHI Memory Study (WHIMS), and the Women's Health Initiative (WHI). Although initially some epidemiologic studies suggested a cardioprotective effect or HRT with preservation of cognitive function and prevention of dementia, later data from WHI, HERS I and II, and others did not support these conclusions. The collective findings from the major studies are summarized in Table 20-3.

TABLE 20-3 Summary of the Major Studies on the Benefits and Risk of Hormone-Replacement Therapy (HRT) and Estrogen-Only Replacement Therapy (ERT)

Outcome	Combination HRT	Estrogen Only
Heart attack	↑	↔
Stroke (ischemic)	↑	↑
Deep vein thrombosis (DVT)	↑	↑
Pulmonary embolus (PE)	↑	↔
Invasive breast cancer	↑	↔
Colorectal cancer	↓	↑
Osteoporotic hip fracture	↓	↓
Osteoporotic vertebral fracture	↓	↓
Cognitive functioning	↔	↔
Dementia	↑	↑
Hot flashes, night sweats	↓	↓

↑ = increased risk with hormone therapy use.
↑ = increased risk with hormone therapy use.
↔ = no change risk with hormone therapy use.

Benefits of HRT and ERT

In general, both HRT and ERT use result in excellent control of menopausal symptoms including reduction of vasomotor flushing, improvement in mood and sleep dysfunction, prevention of urogenital and vaginal atrophy, and improvement in skin and muscle tone. HRT also resulted in decreased risk of colorectal cancer, and both HRT and ERT provided protection from osteoporotic fractures in the hip and the vertebra.

Risks of HRT and ERT

Conversely, combination HRT use resulted in increased coronary artery events, increased DVTs and PEs, and an increased risk of invasive breast cancer in women who used HRT for a prolonged period of time (i.e., >5 years' duration). Estrogen-only replacement therapy was associated with an increased risk of stroke (age independent) and DVTs. It did NOT impact heart attacks (age dependent) or the risk of colorectal cancer. While the risk of PEs and invasive breast cancer were not statistically significant, ERT use was associated with a trend toward more PEs and fewer invasive breast cancers. While statistically significant, the absolute risk of most of these outcomes was very small.

The major limitation of the WHI trials is that the participants were much older (average age of 63) and had higher BMIs (average BMI of 34), and the sample had a higher percentage of smokers than subjects in most epidemiologic studies. This makes it more difficult to generalize the findings to healthy, younger, newly menopausal women with symptoms for whom the benefits of short-term use often far outweigh the risks.

Recommendations and Contraindications

As a result of cumulative studies, the current national recommendation is that HRT and ERT be used only for the **treatment of menopausal symptoms** and at **the lowest effective dose** for the **shortest period of time** needed **(generally 1 to 5 years)**. HRT should not be started for the prevention of health conditions such as cardiovascular disease, osteoporosis, or dementia. Treatment must be considered carefully, however, and each patient's symptoms, risk factors, and relative risks and benefits should be individually evaluated. **Contraindications to HRT** include chronic liver impairment, pregnancy, known estrogen-dependent neoplasm (breast, ovary, uterus), history of thromboembolic disease (DVT, PE, CVA), and undiagnosed vaginal bleeding.

Nonhormonal Treatment of Menopausal Symptoms

Alternative regimens for postmenopausal women who are unable or unwilling to take HRT or who have completed short-term HRT or ERT should be targeted toward the individual's symptoms and treatment goals (Table 20-4).

Vasomotor symptoms (hot flashes and night sweats) can be managed with clonidine (Catapres), selective serotonin reuptake inhibitors (SSRIs) such as paroxetine (Paxil) and serotonin and norepinephrine reuptake inhibitors (SNRIs) such as venlafaxine (Effexor). Low-dose gabapentin (Neurontin) has been found to provide effective relief of night sweats and sleep disturbances resulting from vasomotor symptoms. Where indicated, other causes for hot flashes such as thyroid disease, autoimmune disorders, carcinoid and pheochromocytoma tumors, and selective estrogen receptor modulator (SERMs; tamoxifen/raloxifene) use should be ruled out. Complementary and alternative therapies (soy, black cohosh, phytoestrogens, dong quai, evening primrose oil) have not been found to be more effective than placebos in the treatment of vasomotor symptoms.

Vaginal and urogenital atrophy can be managed locally with lubricants and moisturizers. Low-dose vaginal estrogen can have excellent local effects on vaginal and urethral atrophy, with only minimal systemic absorption. When used at low vaginal dosing, these estrogen sources do not require opposing progestin use in women with an intact uterus.

The **prevention and treatment for osteoporosis** has been refined over the past few years and includes calcium and vitamin D supplementation; bisphosphonates (etidronate, alendronate, risedronate); calcitonin, raloxifene, and tamoxifen (SERMs); and weight-bearing exercise such as walking, hiking, and stair climbing. Reduction in smoking and in caffeine and alcohol intake has also been shown to lower the rate of bone loss. A bone-density measurement may be determined to follow bone mass in postmenopausal women. It is recommended that all postmenopausal women receive

TABLE 20-4 Treatment Options to Address the Various Symptoms/Conditions of Menopause

Menopausal Symptom	Treatment Option
Cardiovascular changes	BP and lipid control medications, smoking cessation, weight loss, exercise
Osteoporosis risk	HRT/ERT, calcium, Vitamin D, bisphosphonates, raloxifene, weight-bearing exercise
Vasomotor Symptoms (Hot flashes, night sweats)	HRT/ERT, clonidine, SSRIs SNRIs, gabapentin
Vaginal dryness/dyspareunia	Low-dose vaginal estrogen, water-based lubricant, vaginal moisturizers
Mood disturbances	HRT/ERT, SSRIs,

HRT, hormone replacement therapy; ERT, estrogen replacement therapy; SSRIs, selective serotonin reuptake inhibitors.

a bone-density measurement at age 65. Women who are at higher risk of osteoporosis (thin, Caucasian, Asian, smoker, family history, fracture history) or those using medications that predispose to bone loss (levothyroxine, steroids, heparin) should be scanned earlier, perhaps at the time of menopause or by age 60. Repeat bone-density measurements are done no more frequently than every 2 to 3 years.

With respect to **cardiovascular risks**, improvement in lifestyle and diet are key factors, as well as optimal blood pressure and weight control to decrease morbidity and mortality.

KEY POINTS

- The typical order of the events in puberty is accelerated growth, thelarche (breast development), pubarche (pubic hair development), and menarche (onset of menstruation).
- During the normal menstrual cycle, the ovary goes through a follicular and luteal phase at the same time that the endometrium goes through the proliferative and secretory phases.
- Ovulation occurs in response to the LH surge signaling the cascade for the mature follicle to break open and release the mature oocyte. Fertilization of the ovum must occur within 24 hours of ovulation.
- Menstruation occurs as the result of decreasing progestin levels resulting in the sloughing of the endometrium.
- Menopause marks the termination of the reproductive phase of a woman's life. It is characterized by the cessation of menses and the onset of an estrogen-deficient state.
- Perimenopause can begin 2 to 8 years prior to menopause. It is characterized by irregular menstrual cycles and milder, less frequent symptoms that are associated with menopause, such as hot flashes, night sweats, and mood swings.
- The average age of menopause is 51. Menopausal patients present with amenorrhea, hot flashes, vaginal atrophy, and mood and sleep changes, all consistent with decreased levels of estrogen.
- Menopause can be diagnosed with after 12 months of amenorrhea and the presence of menopausal symptoms, which may include hot flashes, night sweats, mood and sleep disturbances, and vaginal dryness. It can be confirmed by elevated levels of FSH.
- Women who wish to use hormone replacement for menopausal symptoms and who still have a uterus in place should use both estrogen and progesterone therapy (HRT). This decreases the risk of endometrial hyperplasia and endometrial cancer from unopposed estrogen exposure.
- Two major benefits of HRT and ERT are the prevention of bone loss and osteoporosis and the relief of symptoms associated with menopause.
- Combination hormone therapy (HRT) has been associated with an increased of heart attacks,strokes, DVTs, PEs, and invasive breast cancer.
- When used alone, estrogen replacement therapy (ERT) has been associated with an increased risk of strokes and DVTs.
- When used, HRT and ERT should be reserved for the treatment of vasomotor symptoms. In general, HRT/ERT use should be used for the shortest period of time needed-usually 1-5 years at the lowest effective dose to treat symptoms.
- If HRT is completed, not tolerated, or not desired, alternative therapies are available to address each of the symptoms and side effects of menopause.

C Clinical Vignettes

Vignette 1

An 8-year-old African American girl is brought to your office by her parents concerned that she has started developing breasts too soon. Physical examination reveals a Tanner stage II breast and pubic hair growth.

1. Breast bud development is the beginning of what stage of puberty?
   a. Thelarche
   b. Adrenarche
   c. Pubarche
   d. Menarche
   e. Accelerated growth

2. You reassure the parents that this is normal. What is typical pubertal sequence?
   a. Menarche, pubarche, thelarche, accelerated growth
   b. Pubarche, thelarche, accelerated growth, menarche
   c. Thelarche, pubarche, accelerated growth, menarche
   d. Accelerated growth, thelarche, pubarche, menarche
   e. Pubarche, accelerated growth, thelarche, menarche

3. When can the patient expect her first menses?
   a. At 14 years of age
   b. At 12 years of age
   c. At 11 years of age
   d. At 13 years of age
   e. It's impossible to tell from the data provided

Vignette 2

A 28-year-old patient is in your office to discuss the possibility of getting pregnant. As part of her history you take thorough menstrual history. She states that she had menarche at age 12. Initially her menses was irregular, but since she was 16 her menses has been every 30 days and last for 5 days. She uses four to five tampons a day and denies dysmenorrhea.

1. The menstrual cycle is divided into which two phases when describing the endometrium?
   a. Follicular and secretory phases
   b. Follicular and luteal phases
   c. Proliferative and luteal phases
   d. Proliferative and secretory phases
   e. Atrophic and menstrual

2. Which of these structures does NOT produce progesterone?
   a. Placenta
   b. Endometrium
   c. Corpus luteum
   d. Follicle
   e. Adrenal cortex

3. The patient comes back to your office and she is pregnant. What hormone does the developing trophoblast produce?
   a. Human chorionic gonadotropin (hCG)
   b. Progesterone
   c. Androstenedione
   d. LH
   e. Estrogen

Vignette 3

A 51-year-old woman presents to your office amenorrhea for the past year. Since she has not had any hot flashes, she is wondering if she is menopausal.

1. What blood test would confirm the diagnosis of menopause?
   a. FSH
   b. Estrogen
   c. Testosterone
   d. Human chorionic gonadotropin (hCG)
   e. Prolactin

2. Early menopause is more common in all of the following except:
   a. in nulliparous women
   b. women with hypertension
   c. women who smoke
   d. women with type 1 diabetes
   e. women with family history of early menopause

3. Which of the following is NOT a symptom of menopause?
   a. Hot flashes
   b. Insomnia
   c. Visual changes
   d. Vaginal atrophy
   e. Night sweats

Vignette 4

A 51-year-old woman presents to your office to discuss hormone replacement therapy (HRT). She has been amenorrheic for more than a year. She reports hot flashes multiple times a day and daily night sweats. These symptoms are interfering with her concentration and sleep.

1. Which of the following is NOT a contraindication to HRT?
   a. History of a deep vein thrombosis
   b. History of breast cancer
   c. Cirrhosis
   d. Smoking
   e. History of pulmonary emboli

2. What is the ONLY indication for HRT?
   a. Osteoporosis prevention
   b. Vaginal dryness treatment
   c. Hot flashes and night sweats interfering with quality of life
   d. Cardiovascular disease prevention
   e. Dementia prevention

3. The patient has not had a hysterectomy. If the patient is started on estrogen replacement, what other hormone also needs to be prescribed?
   a. Progesterone
   b. FSH
   c. Human chorionic gonadotropin (hCG)
   d. Testosterone
   e. Vaginal estrogen cream

A Answers

Vignette 1 Question 1
Answer A: The first stage of STET thelarche is breast bud development and is the first phenotypic sign of puberty. Adrenarche is when the adrenal gland begins regeneration of the zona reticularis, which is responsible for the secretion of sex steroid hormones. Pubarche is the onset of pubic hair growth. Menarche is the first menses.

Vignette 1 Question 2
Answer D: The normal pubertal sequence is initiated with accelerated growth. Breast development (thelarche) is next, followed by appearance of pubic hair (pubarche). Onset of menstruation (menarche) is at the end. A normal variant seen most commonly with African American girls is that pubarche precedes thelarche.

Vignette 1 Question 3
Answer C: Average length of time from breast bud development to menstruation in typically 2.5 years and so you would expect her to have her menses between 10 and 11 years of age. The other ages are all later than you would expect.

Vignette 2 Question 1
Answer D: The menstrual cycle is divided into the follicular and luteal phases in respect to changes in the ovary over the length of the cycle. The proliferative and secretory phases describe the concurrent changes in the endometrium. Options A and C are both wrong because these describe a phase in respect to both the ovary and endometrium. Atrophic and menstrual are terms used to describe the status of the endometrium but this terminology is not used for phases of the menstrual cycle.

Vignette 2 Question 2
Answer B: The endometrium does not produce progesterone. The corpus luteum produces progesterone to maintain the endometrium until the placenta takes over at 8 to 10 weeks gestation. In the absence of fertilization, the corpus luteum degenerates and the progesterone levels fall, so the endometrium is unable to be maintained resulting in a menstruation. The follicle produces progesterone in response to the LH surge and results in ovulation. This follicle then becomes the corpus luteum after ovulation.

Vignette 2 Question 3
Answer A: The trophoblast produces hCG to maintain the corpus luteum. Without this rise in hCG it signals to the corpus luteum that fertilization has not occurred and triggers the cascade that results in menstruation. The follicle produces progesterone in response to the LH surge and results in ovulation. This follicle then becomes the corpus luteum after ovulation. The corpus luteum produces progesterone to maintain the endometrium until the placenta takes over at 8 to 10 weeks gestation. Androstenedione is produced by the theca interna cells. LH is produced by the anterior pituitary gland.

Vignette 3 Question 1
Answer A: An FSH level greater than 40 IU/L is diagnostic of menopause. Estrogen levels do not consistently predict menopause, especially if there is peripheral conversion of estrogen in the morbidly obese patient. Testosterone has no role in predicting menopause. If there is a presence of hCG at this age, pregnancy (though unlikely) and gestational trophoblastic disease must be ruled out. Prolactin is produced in the anterior pituitary and causes milk secretion from the breast and preventing ovulation in lactating women. High prolactin levels (hyperprolactinemia) may result in galactorrhea and/or amenorrhea. It is not diagnostic of menopause.

Vignette 3 Question 2
Answer B: The average age of menopause is 51, with 90% of women experiencing this change between ages 47 and 55. Hysterectomy and tubal ligation are associated with a slightly earlier menopause (1-2 years). Early menopause is defined as occurring between ages 40 and 45. Early menopause is more common in women with a history of cigarette smoking, short cycles, nulliparity, type 1 diabetes, in utero exposure to diethylstilbestrol (DES), and family history of early menopause. Hypertension has not been shown to increase the risk of early menopause. Menopause occurring before age 40 is considered premature ovarian insufficiency (previously termed premature ovarian failure).

Vignette 3 Question 3
Answer C: Hot flashes, insomnia, and vaginal atrophy are all common symptoms of menopause and are a result of the diminished estrogen production. Visual changes are age related and not a direct effect of menopause.

Vignette 4 Question 1
Answer D: Contraindications to HRT include chronic liver impairment, pregnancy, known estrogen-dependent neoplasm (breast, ovary, uterus), history of thromboembolic disease (DVT, PE, CVA), and unevaluated vaginal bleeding. Oral contraceptives, but not HRT, are contraindicated in elderly smokers. However, the principal conclusion of the Women's Health Initiative (WHI) study was that the lowest dose possible should be chosen, especially in patients with an increased cardiovascular risk, as is the case in smokers.

Vignette 4 Question 2
Answer C: Currently, the only clinical indication for HRT is moderate to severe vasomotor symptoms including hot flashes and night

sweats. An added benefit of HRT is the prevention and treatment of osteoporosis, however, HRT should not be a first-line therapy for the prevention or treatment of osteoporosis HRT use should be limited to the lowest dose necessary to control vasomotor symptoms and for the shortest period of time needed. If vaginal dryness is the primary symptom, this patient would best be treated with lubricants and moisturizers first, followed by low-dose vaginal estrogen so that there is minimal systemic absorption. HRT should not be used to treat or prevent cardiovascular disease or dementia.

Vignette 4 Question 3

Answer A: When estrogens are being used to treat menopausal symptoms in women who still have uterus in situ, progestins must be used to decrease the risk of endometrial hyperplasia and cancer. None of the other options would be protective of the endometrium.

Chapter

21 Amenorrhea

1°: no menstruation by age 16 or 4 y after thelarche.
2°: absence for 3 cycles or 6 mo total

Amenorrhea—the absence of menses—is classified as either primary or secondary. **Primary** amenorrhea is the absence of menarche (first menses) by age 16 or no menstruation by 4 years after thelarche (the onset of breast development). **Secondary** amenorrhea is the absence of menses for three menstrual cycles or a total of 6 months in women who have previously had normal menstruation. The pathophysiology underlying these two processes differs greatly, as do the differential diagnoses.

PRIMARY AMENORRHEA

The diagnosis of primary amenorrhea is made if menses has not occurred by age 16 or within 4 years of thelarche. In the United States, the prevalence of primary amenorrhea is 1% to 2%. The causes of primary amenorrhea include congenital and chromosomal abnormalities, hormonal aberrations, hypothalamic–pituitary disorders, and the variety of causes of secondary amenorrhea that may present before menarche. Primary amenorrhea can be divided into three categories: outflow tract obstruction, end-organ disorders, and central regulatory disorders (Table 21-1).

OUTFLOW TRACT ANOMALIES

Imperforate Hymen

During fetal development, the hymen may fail to canalize, remaining a solid membrane across the vaginal introitus. If the hymen is imperforate, it will not allow egress of menstrual blood or menses. Thus, despite having begun to menstruate, patients appear to have primary amenorrhea. After a time, patients present with pelvic or abdominal pain from the accumulation and subsequent dilation of the vaginal vault and uterus by menses. On physical examination these patients have a bulging membrane just inside the introitus, often with purple-red discoloration behind it consistent with hematocolpos. The treatment of imperforate hymen is surgical; usually a cruciate incision is made and the hymen is sewn open to allow the passage of menstrual flow.

Transverse Vaginal Septum

A transverse vaginal septum may result from failure of the Müllerian-derived upper vagina to fuse with the urogenital sinus–derived lower vagina. The result of this failed fusion, an imperforate transverse vaginal septum, is commonly found at the level of the midvagina and its persistence may lead to primary amenorrhea by obstruction. The clinical history may include a young woman who presents with primary amenorrhea with cyclic pelvic pain. Diagnosis is made on careful examination of the female genital tract, examining for a bulging septum consistent with hematocolpos. The diagnosis is commonly mistaken as imperforate hymen, and can be differentiated by the presence of a hymeneal ring below the septum. Surgical correction involves resection of the septum.

Vaginal Agenesis

MRKH = agenesis

Patients with **Mayer-Rokitansky-Kuster-Hauser** (MRKH) syndrome have Müllerian agenesis or dysgenesis. They may have complete vaginal agenesis and absence of a uterus or partial vaginal agenesis with a rudimentary uterus and distal vagina. This differs from **vaginal atresia** where the Müllerian system is developed but the distal vagina is composed of fibrosed tissue. Diagnosis is made with physical examination that reveals no patent vagina, chromosomes that are 46,XX, and ovaries visualized on ultrasound. With partial vaginal agenesis or vaginal atresia, a rectal examination may reveal a pelvic mass consistent with a uterus. The uterus can be visualized with ultrasound, CT, or MRI. A neovagina can be created either by serial dilation of the perineal body by the patient over an extended period of time or by reconstructive surgery. In true vaginal atresia, the neovagina created may be connected with the upper genital tract.

Testicular Feminization

Testicular feminization, also known as androgen insensitivity syndrome (AIS), results from a dysfunction or absence of the testosterone receptor that leads to a phenotypical female with 46,XY chromosomes. This syndrome occurs in 1 in 50,000 women. Because these patients have testes, **Müllerian inhibiting factor** (MIF) is secreted early in development, and these patients therefore have an absence of all Müllerian-derived structures. Of note, the testes may be undescended or may have migrated down to the labia majora. The diminished testosterone sensitivity commonly leads to an absence of pubic and axillary hair. Usually estrogen is produced, and these patients develop breasts but present with primary amenorrhea because they have no uterus. Patients commonly have a vagina that ends as a blind pouch. For those patients with the absence of or a foreshortened vagina, therapy involves creating a neovagina for sexual function; however, these patients are unable to reproduce. Additional health consequences may include testicular cancer and complex psychosocial issues.

END-ORGAN DISORDERS

Ovarian Failure

Primary ovarian failure results in low levels of estradiol but elevated levels of gonadotropins termed **hypergonadotropic hypogonadism**. There are a variety of causes of primary ovarian failure (Table 21-2). **Savage syndrome** is characterized by failure of the ovaries to respond to follicle-stimulating hormone (FSH) and luteinizing hormone (LH) secondary to

TABLE 21-1 Etiologies of Primary Amenorrhea

Outflow tract abnormalities
Imperforate hymen
Transverse vaginal septum
Vaginal agenesis
Vaginal atresia
Testicular feminization
Uterine agenesis with vaginal dysgenesis
MRKH syndrome
End-organ disorders
Ovarian agenesis
Gonadal agenesis 46,XX
Swyer syndrome/gonadal agenesis 46,XY
Ovarian failure
Enzymatic defects leading to decreased steroid biosynthesis
Savage syndrome—ovary fails to respond to FSH and LH
Turner syndrome
Central disorders
Hypothalamic
Local tumor compression
Trauma
Tuberculosis
Sarcoidosis
Irradiation
Kallmann syndrome—congenital absence of GnRH
Pituitary
Damage from surgery or radiation therapy
Hemosiderosis deposition of iron in pituitary

TABLE 21-2 Causes of Primary Gonadal Failure (Hypergonadotropic Hypogonadism)

Idiopathic premature ovarian failure
Steroidogenic enzyme defects (primary amenorrhea)
Cholesterol side-chain cleavage
3β-ol-dehydrogenase
17-hydroxylase
17-desmolase
17-ketoreductase
Testicular regression syndrome
True hermaphroditism
Gonadal dysgenesis
Pure gonadal dysgenesis (Swyer syndrome) (46,XX and 46,XY)
Turner syndrome (45,XO)
Turner variants
Ovarian resistance syndrome (Savage syndrome)
Autoimmune oophoritis
Postinfection (e.g., mumps)
Postoophorectomy (also wedge resections)
Postirradiation
Postchemotherapy

Adapted from DeCherney A, Pernoll M. *Current Obstetric and Gynecologic Diagnosis and Treatment.* Norwalk, CT: Appleton & Lange; 1994:1009.

a receptor defect. In **Turner syndrome** (45,XO), the ovaries undergo such rapid atresia that by puberty there are usually no primordial oocytes. Defects in the enzymes involved in steroid biosynthesis, particularly 17-hydroxylase, can result in amenorrhea and absence of breast development given the lack of estradiol.

Gonadal Agenesis with 46,XY Chromosomes

If there is a defect in the enzymes that are involved in testicular steroid production—**17-α-hydroxylase** or **17,20 desmolase**—testosterone production will be absent. However, MIF will still be produced; hence, there will be no female internal reproductive organs. These patients will otherwise be phenotypically female, usually without breast development. Patients with an absence of or defect in the testosterone receptor develop testicular feminization syndrome.

While testicular feminization results from peripheral effects of diminished or absent sensitivity of testosterone receptors, another situation in which the patient is genetically male but phenotypically female is gonadal agenesis. The congenital absence of the testes in a genotypical male, **Swyer syndrome**, results in a phenotypical picture similar to that of ovarian agenesis. Because the testes never develop, MIF is not released and these patients have both internal and external female genitalia. However, without estrogen they will not develop breasts.

CENTRAL DISORDERS

Hypothalamic Disorders

The pituitary will not release FSH and LH if the hypothalamus is unable to produce gonadotropin-releasing hormone (GnRH), transport it to the pituitary, or release it in a pulsatile fashion. Anovulation and amenorrhea result from this hypogonadotropic hypogonadism. **Kallmann syndrome** is one form of hypogonadotropic hypogonadism, which involves the congenital absence of GnRH and is commonly associated with anosmia. In Kallmann syndrome, the normal migration of the GnRH neurons are disrupted in their travel from the olfactory placode to the hypothalamus, and the olfactory bulbs also do not form, leading to this combination of hypogonadotropic hypogonadism and anosmia. Other ways that GnRH transport may be disrupted includes compression or destruction of the pituitary stalk or arcuate nucleus. This can result from tumor mass effect, trauma, sarcoidosis, tuberculosis, irradiation, or Hand-Schuller-Christian disease. Finally, there may be defects in GnRH pulsatility in cases of anorexia nervosa, extreme stress, athletics, hyperprolactinemia, hypothyroidism, rapid or severe weight loss, and constitutionally delayed puberty.

Pituitary Disorders

Primary defects of the pituitary are a rare cause of primary amenorrhea. Pituitary dysfunction is usually secondary to hypothalamic dysfunction. It may be caused by tumors, infiltration of the pituitary gland, or infarcts of the pituitary. Surgery or irradiation of pituitary tumors may lead to decreases in or absence of LH and FSH. Hemosiderosis can result in iron deposition in the pituitary, leading to destruction of the gonadotrophs that produce FSH and LH.

DIAGNOSIS

A patient who presents with primary amenorrhea can be worked up based on the phenotypic picture (Table 21-3, Fig. 21-1). Lack of a uterus is seen in males because of the

TABLE 21-3 Diagnosis of Etiology of Primary Amenorrhea

	Uterus Absent	Uterus Present
Breasts absent	Gonadal agenesis in 46,XY	Gonadal failure/agenesis in 46,XX
Breasts present	Enzyme deficiencies in testosterone synthesis	Disruption of hypothalamic–pituitary axis
	Testicular feminization	Hypothalamic, pituitary, or ovarian pathogenesis similar to that of secondary amenorrhea
	Müllerian agenesis or MRKH	Congenital abnormalities of the genital tract

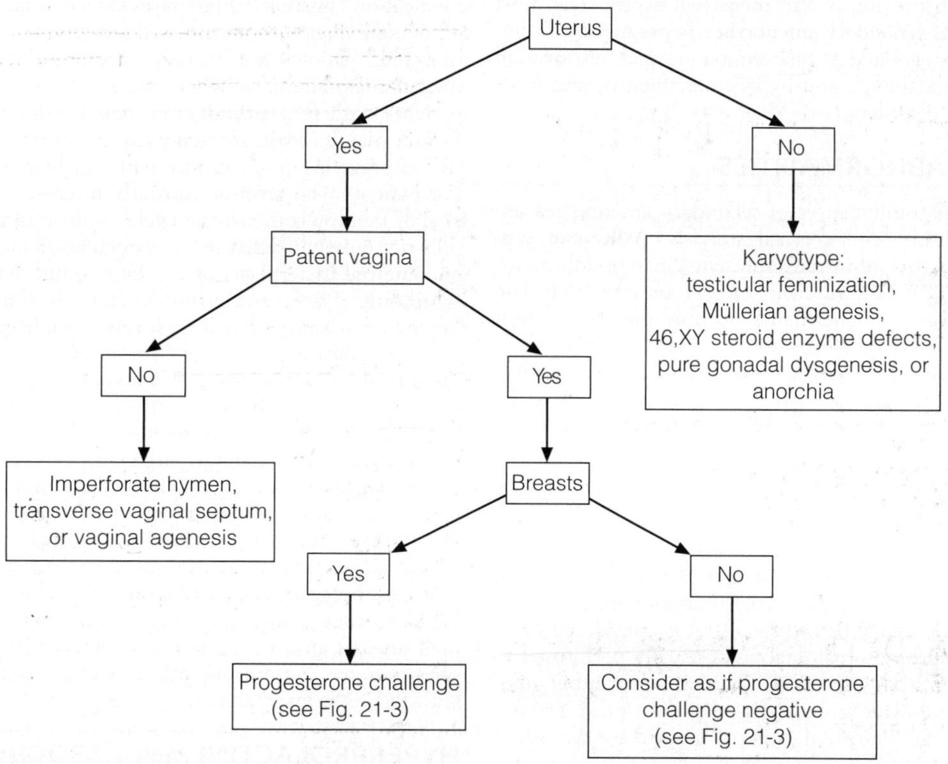

Figure 21-1 • Diagnostic flowchart for patients with primary amenorrhea.

release of MIF by the testes and in females with Müllerian agenesis. Breast development is dependent on estradiol secretion by the ovaries. Patients who have neither a uterus nor breasts are generally 46,XY males with steroid synthesis defects or varying degrees of gonadal dysgenesis, in which adequate MIF is produced by gonadal tissue but androgen synthesis is insufficient.

If breasts are present but no uterus, the etiologies can include congenital absence of the uterus (Müllerian agenesis) in the female or testicular feminization in the male. In the latter case, estradiol from direct testicular secretion as well as peripheral conversion of testosterone and androstenedione leads to breast development. The presence of a normal amount and distribution of pubic hair supports Müllerian agenesis, whereas absent or scant pubic hair indicate androgen insensitivity.

For patients who have a uterus but breast development is absent, the differential includes hypergonadotropic hypogonadism, as seen in gonadal dysgenesis in both sexes, and with defects in steroid pathways in 46,XX patients and hypogonadotropic hypogonadism, which is seen in CNS, hypothalamic, and pituitary dysfunction. A serum FSH level differentiates between these two, with elevation seen in hypergonadotropic hypogonadism.

The workup for amenorrhea in phenotypic females with the absence of either a uterus or breasts should include a karyotype analysis, followed by testosterone and FSH assays. Further biochemical and hormonal assays may be performed to elucidate specific enzyme defects. Patients with both a uterus and breast development should be evaluated to determine whether there is a patent outflow tract from the uterus. If the vagina, cervix, and uterus are continuous, these can be evaluated as if the patient were presenting with secondary amenorrhea.

TREATMENT

Patients with congenital abnormalities may be treated surgically with reconstructive procedures to allow egress of menses in those with a functional uterus or to create a functional vagina. Patients with an absent uterus and breasts can be treated with estrogen replacement to effect breast development and prevent osteoporosis. Patients who have breast development but an absent uterus may not require medical intervention.

Patients with a uterus but without breast development and with hypergonadotropic hypogonadism often have irreversible ovarian failure and will require estrogen replacement therapy. Patients with hypogonadotropic hypogonadism require further workup as patients with secondary amenorrhea.

SECONDARY AMENORRHEA

Secondary amenorrhea is the absence of menses for more than 6 months or for the equivalent of three menstrual cycles in a woman who previously had menstrual cycles. **The most common cause of secondary amenorrhea is pregnancy**. Other causes can be categorized as anatomic abnormalities, ovarian dysfunction, prolactinoma and hyperprolactinemia, and CNS or hypothalamic disorders.

ANATOMIC ABNORMALITIES

The common anatomic causes of secondary amenorrhea are Asherman syndrome and cervical stenosis. **Asherman syndrome** is the presence of intrauterine synechiae or adhesions, usually secondary to intrauterine surgery or infection. The potential etiologies of Asherman syndrome include dilation and curettage (D&C), myomectomy, cesarean delivery, or endometritis. **Cervical stenosis** can manifest as secondary amenorrhea and dysmenorrhea. It is usually caused by scarring of the cervical os secondary to surgical or obstetric trauma.

OVARIAN FAILURE

Ovarian failure may result from ovarian torsion, surgery, infection, radiation, or chemotherapy. **Premature ovarian failure** (POF) is often idiopathic. Any time menopause occurs without another etiology before age 40, it is considered POF. Before age 35, chromosomal analysis is usually performed to diagnose a genetic basis for POF. Patients with either idiopathic POF or a known cause of early ovarian failure are generally treated with supplemental estrogen to decrease the risk of cardiovascular disease and osteoporosis.

POLYCYSTIC OVARY SYNDROME

Polycystic ovary syndrome (PCOS), also known as Stein-Leventhal syndrome, was first described in 1935. However, it is now known as one of the most common hormonal disorders in women, and has a prevalence of 5% to 10% in the United States and developed world. Diagnosis is made when women meet two of three of the following: oligo or anovulation, clinical or laboratory evidence of hyperandrogenism, and polycystic ovaries on ultrasound. Clinical evidence of hyperandrogenism may include excessive hair growth (hirsutism) and male pattern hair loss as well as acne. It is not entirely clear what precipitates the disease, but once it begins, a self-perpetuating cycle occurs.

In the case of PCOS, chronic anovulation leads to elevated levels of estrogen and androgen. The increased androgen released from the ovaries and the adrenal cortex is converted peripherally in the adipose tissue into estrone. Further, the elevated androgens lead to a decrease in the production of sex hormone binding globulin (SHBG), resulting in even higher levels of free estrogens and androgens. This hyperestrogenic state leads to an increased LH:FSH ratio, atypical follicular development, anovulation, and increased androgen production. Once again, the androgens are peripherally converted to estrogens, leading to a cyclical propagation of the disease. Many patients with PCOS who are hyperandrogenic and obese also develop insulin resistance and hyperinsulinemia. Not surprisingly, the incidence of type 2 diabetes mellitus is increased in these patients.

Treatment of these patients depends on the particular symptoms and the desires of the patient. For patients desiring pregnancy, ovulation induction may be performed using clomiphene citrate (Clomid). Patients with PCOS may be particularly resistant to ovulation induction, even with medication. Further, there is evidence that the probability of ovulation can be significantly increased by weight loss; therefore, patients are strongly encouraged to take an active role in maintaining or losing weight prior to pregnancy. In patients with hyperinsulinemia and insulin resistance, metformin may increase spontaneous ovulation, and in the least will improve insulin resistance and may help with weight loss. For patients who are not currently interested in fertility, the goal of therapy is menstrual cycle control. Oral contraceptive pills not only will assist in cycle regulation and reduce risk of endometrial hyperplasia or carcinoma, but also may improve symptoms of acne and arrest further development of hirsutism by decreasing circulating levels of androgens. If estrogen is contraindicated, or patient preference indicates, progestin therapy alone in the form of a levonorgestrel IUD, oral pills (Provera), or injectable medications (Depo-Provera) will similarly decrease their risk of endometrial disease. Again, obese patients should be strongly urged to lose weight. Similar to the metabolic syndrome (also known as syndrome X), patients with PCOS have increased risk of hypertension, obstructive sleep apnea, coronary artery disease, insulin resistance, and type 2 diabetes. Weight loss can decrease these risks as well as break the cycle of anovulation. Most clinicians would recommend that patients undergo a screen for type 2 diabetes mellitus and ensure they are connected with a primary care physician for monitoring other health disorders associated with PCOS as listed above.

HYPERPROLACTINEMIA-ASSOCIATED AMENORRHEA

Excess prolactin leads to amenorrhea and galactorrhea. Menstrual irregularities often result from abnormal gonadotropin (FSH and LH) secretion due to alterations in dopamine levels typically seen in hyperprolactinemia. The etiologies and consequences of excess prolactin are numerous. Prolactin release is inhibited by dopamine and stimulated by serotonin and thyrotropin-releasing hormone (TRH). Because of the constant suppression of prolactin release by hypothalamic release of dopamine, any disturbance in this process by a hypothalamic or pituitary lesion can lead to disinhibition of prolactin secretion.

Hyperprolactinemia has several possible etiologies (Table 21-4). Primary hypothyroidism that leads to elevated thyroid-stimulating hormone (TSH) and TRH can cause hyperprolactinemia. Medications that increase prolactin levels (by a hypothalamic–pituitary effect) include dopamine antagonists (Haldol, Reglan, phenothiazine), tricyclic antidepressants, estrogen, monoamine oxidase (MAO) inhibitors, and opiates. A prolactin-secreting pituitary adenoma leads to elevated prolactin levels. The empty sella syndrome, in which the subarachnoid membrane herniates into the sella turcica, causing it to enlarge and flatten, is another cause of

TABLE 21-4 Differential Diagnosis of Galactorrhea-Hyperprolactinemia

Pituitary tumors secreting prolactin
Macroadenomas (>10 mm) Microadenomas (<10 mm)
Hypothyroidism
Idiopathic hyperprolactinemia
Drug-induced hyperprolactinemia
Dopamine antagonists Phenothiazines Thioxanthenes Butyrophenone Diphenylbutylpiperidine Dibenzoxazepine Dihydroindolone Procainamide derivatives Catecholamine-depleting agents False transmitters (α-methyldopa)
Interruption of normal hypothalamic–pituitary relationship
Pituitary stalk section
Peripheral neural stimulation
Chest wall stimulation Surgery (e.g., mastectomy) Burns Herpes zoster Bronchogenic tumors Bronchiectasis/chronic bronchitis
Nipple stimulation
Stimulation of nipples Chronic nipple irritation
Spinal cord lesion
Tabes dorsalis Syringomyelia
CNS disease
Encephalitis Craniopharyngioma Pineal and hypothalamic tumors Hypothalamic tumors Pseudotumor cerebri

hyperprolactinemia. Other conditions associated with high prolactin include pregnancy and breastfeeding. Any patient with an elevated prolactin level should have an imaging study to rule out prolactinoma.

DISRUPTION OF THE HYPOTHALAMIC–PITUITARY AXIS

As in the hypothalamic and pituitary causes of primary amenorrhea, disruption in the secretion and transport of GnRH, absence of pulsatility of GnRH, or acquired pituitary lesions will all cause hypogonadotropic hypogonadism (Table 21-5). Common causes of hypothalamic dysfunction include stress, exercise, anorexia nervosa, and weight loss.

TABLE 21-5 Differential Diagnosis of Hypoestrogenic Amenorrhea (Hypogonadotropic Hypogonadism)

Hypothalamic dysfunction
Kallmann syndrome Tumors of hypothalamus (craniopharyngioma) Constitutional delay of puberty Severe hypothalamic dysfunction Anorexia nervosa Severe weight loss Severe stress Exercise ***Pituitary disorder***
Sheehan syndrome Panhypopituitarism Isolated gonadotropin deficiency Hemosiderosis (primarily from thalassemia major)
Adapted from DeCherney A, Pernoll M. *Current Obstetric and Gynecologic Diagnosis and Treatment.* Norwalk, CT: Appleton & Lange; 1994:1013.

Diagnosis

The approach to secondary amenorrhea always begins with a beta human chorionic gonadotropin (β-hCG) assay to **rule out pregnancy** often before a formal history is taken. If this is negative, the standard history should include focused questions toward hypothyroidism (e.g., lethargy, weight gain, cold intolerance), hyperprolactinemia (e.g., nipple discharge, usually bilateral), and hyperandrogenism (e.g., recent changes in hirsutism, acne, or virilism; see Chapter 23). **TSH** and **prolactin** levels should then be checked to rule out hypothyroidism and hyperprolactinemia, both of which can cause amenorrhea. If both are elevated, the hypothyroidism should be treated and the prolactin level can be checked after thyroid studies have normalized to verify resolution.

If the prolactin level is elevated and TSH is normal, a workup for the other causes of prolactinemia should ensue (Fig. 21-2). In the diagnostic evaluation of the patient, a careful history should be taken, including a complete list of medications and clear documentation of the onset of symptoms. A thorough physical examination should include visual fields, cranial nerves, breast examination, and an attempt to express milk from the nipple. An MRI can rule out a hypothalamic or pituitary lesion.

If the prolactin level is normal, a **progesterone challenge test** (10 mg orally for 7 to 10 days to mimic progesterone withdrawal) can be performed to assess the adequacy of endogenous estrogen production and the outflow tract. Withdrawal bleeding occurring after the progesterone challenge indicates the presence of estrogen and an adequate outflow tract. In this case, amenorrhea is usually secondary to anovulation, which can be caused by a variety of endocrine disorders that alter pituitary/gonadal feedback such as polycystic ovaries, tumors of the ovary and adrenals, Cushing syndrome, thyroid disorders, and adult-onset adrenal hyperplasia (Table 21-6).

Absence of withdrawal bleeding in response to progesterone alone must then be evaluated with estrogen and progesterone administration. If there is still no menstrual bleeding, an outflow tract disorder such as Asherman syndrome or cervical stenosis is suspected. If menstrual bleeding does occur

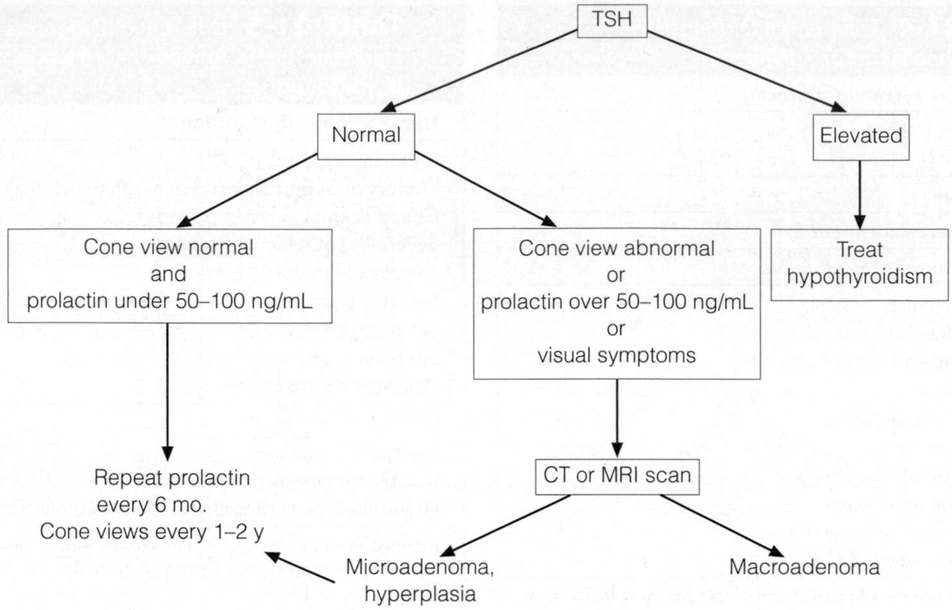

Figure 21-2 • Diagnostic flowchart for patients with amenorrhea-galactorrhea-hyperprolactinemia.

in response to estrogen and progesterone administration, this suggests an intact and functional uterus without adequate endogenous estrogen stimulation. Measurement of FSH and LH will help differentiate between a hypothalamic–pituitary disorder (low/normal FSH and LH levels) and ovarian failure (high FSH and LH levels) (Fig. 21-3).

TABLE 21-6 Differential Diagnosis of Eugonadotropic Eugonadism (Progesterone Challenge Positive)

Mild hypothalamic dysfunction
Emotional strdess
Psychologic disorder
Weight loss
Obesity
Exercise-induced
Idiopathic
Hirsutism-virilism
Polycystic ovary syndrome
Ovarian tumor
Adrenal tumor
Cushing syndrome
Congenital and adult-onset adrenal hyperplasia
Systemic disease
Hypothyroidism
Hyperthyroidism
Addison disease
Chronic renal failure
Many others seen in other chronic diseases

Adapted from DeCherney A, Pernoll M. *Current Obstetric and Gynecologic Diagnosis and Treatment.* Norwalk, CT: Appleton & Lange; 1994:1013.

Treatment

Patients with hypothyroidism are treated with thyroid hormone replacement. Those with pituitary macroadenomas are treated with surgical resection. Some patients with macroadenomas and most with microadenomas are treated with bromocriptine, a dopamine agonist that often causes tumor regression and the resumption of ovulation. Other hyperprolactinemic patients can also be treated with bromocriptine in order to resume ovulation. Further, this treatment should be followed with serial prolactin levels and cone view radiographs to diagnose development of a macroadenoma.

Patients who respond to a progesterone challenge should be withdrawn with progesterone on a regular basis to prevent endometrial hyperplasia. Oral contraceptive pills (OCPs) are useful in this case and may be beneficial in the management of hirsutism. However, if the patient is a smoker and older than 35 years, progesterone alone is indicated because of the increased risk of cerebrovascular accidents and venous thromboembolism with estrogen usage in these patients.

For patients who are hypoestrogenic, consideration should be given to estrogen and progesterone replacement for the effects these have on bone density and genital atrophy. OCPs are often used for women younger than 35 years or nonsmokers older than 35 years. For other patients, a regimen of 0.625 mg of conjugated estrogen cycled with 5 to 10 mg of medroxyprogesterone acetate is suitable. These patients should also receive 1.2 g of elemental calcium supplementation per day.

Ovulation Induction

Ovulation induction with bromocriptine can be used in patients with hyperprolactinemia. If the cause of hyperprolactinemia is medication related, discontinue or decrease the medication if possible. Patients who respond to the progesterone challenge have evidence of estrogenation. Any specific cause of this amenorrheic state should be corrected. If menses do not resume, ovulation induction may be performed with clomiphene citrate (Clomid), which acts as an antiestrogen to

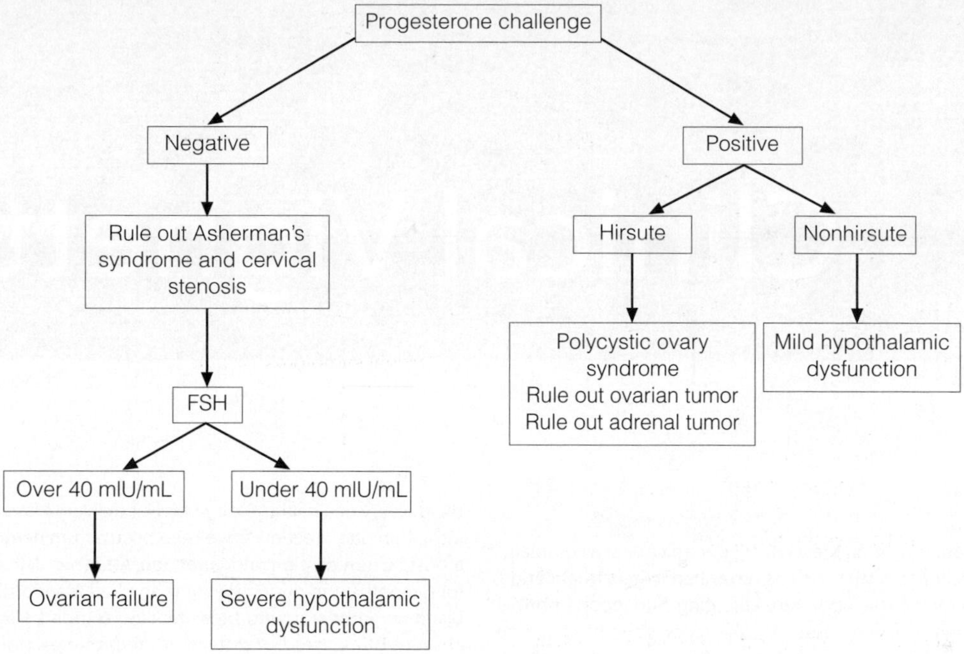

Figure 21-3 • Diagnostic flowchart for patients with secondary amenorrhea.

stimulate gonadotropin release. Patients with elevated androgens may need therapy with Clomid.

Patients who do not respond to progesterone alone are presumed to have low estrogen levels; however, these patients will occasionally respond to Clomid as well. For patients who do not respond to Clomid, human menopausal gonadotropin (hMG) or recombinant GnRH can be used to stimulate ovulation. Careful monitoring with ultrasound and estradiol levels should be done in the case of gonadotropin ovulation induction because of the risk of ovarian hyperstimulation.

KEY POINTS

- Primary amenorrhea is the absence of menarche by age 16 or 4 years after thelarche.
- Primary amenorrhea can be caused by congenital abnormalities of the genital tract, chromosomal abnormalities, enzyme or hormonal deficiencies, gonadal agenesis, ovarian failure, or disruption of the hypothalamic–pituitary axis.
- The workup of primary amenorrhea is usually organized into four categories based on the presence or absence of a uterus and the presence or absence of breast development.
- In the absence of both uterus and breasts, karyotype usually reveals 46,XY.
- In the absence of a uterus and presence of breasts, karyotype will differentiate between Müllerian agenesis and testicular feminization.
- In the absence of breasts and presence of a uterus, FSH will differentiate between hypergonadotropic and hypogonadotropic hypogonadism. Karyotype may be necessary to rule out gonadal agenesis in a 46,XY.
- Patients with both a uterus and breasts should be evaluated as if presenting with secondary amenorrhea.
- Anatomic abnormalities including Asherman syndrome and cervical stenosis may lead to secondary amenorrhea. These patients fail to respond to estrogen and progesterone withdrawal.
- Hyperprolactinemia is a common cause of secondary amenorrhea.
- Patients with normal prolactin levels may be given a progesterone challenge to investigate whether or not the endometrium is estrogenized.
- With progesterone challenge failure, the differential diagnosis becomes hypergonadotropic or hypogonadotropic hypogonadism that can be differentiated by an FSH measurement.
- For patients not seeking current fertility, it is important to treat the specific cause of amenorrhea and to consider hormone replacement in the hypoestrogenic patient.
- For patients who desire fertility, ovulation induction can usually be achieved. Patients with hyperprolactinemia require bromocriptine, whereas patients with other forms of hypogonadism may respond to clomiphene and gonadotropins.

C Clinical Vignettes

Vignette 1

An 18-year-old young woman presents to your office with a complaint of amenorrhea. She notes that she has never had a menstrual period, but that she has mild cyclic abdominal bloating. She reports normal breast development starting at age 12. She reports she has become sexually active, but she finds intercourse painful. Her past medical and surgical history is unremarkable. On physical examination, you note normal appearing axillary and pubic hair. Her breast development is normal. Pelvic examination reveals normal appearing external genitalia, and a shortened vagina ending in a blind pouch.

1. Which of the following tests would be your first step in determining the diagnosis?
   a. Karyotype
   b. Pelvic ultrasound
   c. Serum FSH
   d. Diagnostic laparoscopy

2. You perform a bedside ultrasound and find normal appearing bilateral ovaries as well as an absent uterus and fallopian tubes. What is your most likely diagnosis?
   a. Imperforate hymen
   b. Transverse vaginal septum
   c. Müllerian agenesis
   d. Androgen insensitivity syndrome

3. Which additional organ system should you be evaluating in a patient with this disorder?
   a. Pancreas and duodenum
   b. Cerebral circulation
   c. Olfactory system
   d. Renal and urinary collecting system

4. Your patient's concerned mother calls you later that afternoon. "How will my daughter be able to start a family?" You wisely counsel her about her options, which include:
   a. intrauterine insemination
   b. uterine transplant
   c. in vitro fertilization with gestational carrier
   d. the patient will not be able to reproduce using her genetic material

Vignette 2

A 32-year-old G1P1001 woman presents to your office with the chief complaint of amenorrhea since her most recent vaginal delivery 1 year ago. She notes that she had an uncomplicated pregnancy, followed by the delivery of a healthy baby boy. Her delivery was complicated by an intra-amniotic infection as well as a postpartum hemorrhage requiring a postpartum dilation and curettage. After her delivery, she breastfed for 6 months, and during this time she had scant and irregular vaginal bleeding. After stopping breastfeeding 6 months ago, she notes the absence of menses, but instead has monthly painful cramping, which seems to be getting worse. She remarks that prior to her pregnancy, she had normal, regular menses, which were not too heavy or painful. She and her husband would like to have another child, and have been having unprotected intercourse for the past 6 months without achieving a pregnancy. Your review of systems is otherwise negative. You perform a physical examination, which is normal other than a slightly enlarged, tender uterus. A urine pregnancy test in the office is negative.

1. What is the most likely diagnosis?
   a. Sheehan's syndrome
   b. Lactational amenorrhea
   c. Asherman's syndrome
   d. Premature ovarian failure

2. You suspect Asherman's syndrome, and perform a hysterosalpingogram, which reveals multiple synechiae within the uterus, confirming your suspicions. Your next step in therapy is which of the following?
   a. Diagnostic and operative hysteroscopy
   b. Provera 10 mg daily for 5 days in an attempt to achieve a withdrawal bleed
   c. In vitro fertilization
   d. Place an intrauterine device
   e. Inform your patient that unfortunately, she is "barren" and will not be able to carry a pregnancy again

3. What obstetrical complication might you be concerned about for your patient in her next pregnancy?
   a. Preterm labor
   b. Cervical insufficiency
   c. Preeclampsia
   d. Placenta accreta

Vignette 3

A 15-year-old female adolescent presents to your office with primary amenorrhea. She notably has short stature, a webbed neck, and widely spaced nipples. She has noticed that she has not developed breasts or pubic hair like her friends at school have, and this is frustrating to her. She is not sexually active. Physical examination confirms the absence of secondary sex characteristics, and auscultation of the chest reveals a harsh systolic murmur. Pelvic examination reveals normal appearing female external genitalia and a normal vagina, with a palpable uterus on bimanual examination.

1. To confirm your suspected diagnosis, which test would you first order?
   a. Pelvic ultrasound
   b. Serum FSH and LH
   c. Karyotype
   d. Serum estradiol
2. Suddenly you remember from medical school that there are other medical predispositions that Turner patients have, and you order all of the following tests except:
   a. thyroid function testing
   b. echocardiogram
   c. basic metabolic panel
   d. antiendomysial antibody test
   e. DEXA scan
3. The patient and her family are surprised about her diagnosis, but glad to have an explanation for her symptoms. The patient notes that what bothers her most is her lack of breasts and absent pubic hair. What therapy can you offer for her delayed puberty?
   a. Growth hormone therapy
   b. Gonadotropin therapy (FSH, LH)
   c. Estrogen plus progesterone
   d. Estrogen alone
4. Five years later, at age 20, your patient returns to your clinic for an infertility consultation. She has had surgical repair of her aortic coarctation, and has been on oral contraceptive pills for the last 2 years for hormone replacement. She is followed by an internist who reports that all other systems (hepatic, renal, etc.) have been stable. What advice might you give your patient about attempting pregnancy?
   a. None, she is not a good candidate for pregnancy
   b. Stop the birth control pills because they are preventing spontaneous conception
   c. Clomid ovulation induction
   d. In vitro fertilization

Vignette 4

A 19-year-old female college freshman presents with amenorrhea for the past 8 months. She states that she had normal menarche at age 12, and initially had irregular menses for the first few cycles, but they became regular quickly, and had been normal until 8 months ago. She denies sexual activity, has had no sexually transmitted infections, and is otherwise healthy with no past medical problems or surgeries. She reports that she eats a healthful diet and has been running approximately 15 miles per week with her cross-country team for the past year. She states that running is her "passion" and sometimes she puts in a few extra miles to blow off stress from her classes. Physical examination reveals a thin, athletic female with normal breast development and normal secondary sex characteristics. Pelvic examination reveals normal external genitalia and on bimanual examination, you palpate a small, anteverted uterus with no adnexal masses.

1. Which test would you first perform?
   a. Pelvic ultrasound
   b. Urinary LH test strips
   c. Serum FSH
   d. Serum β-hCG
   e. Prolactin
   f. TSH
2. You perform a serum β-hCG which is negative, and subsequently test FSH, prolactin, and TSH. Prolactin and TSH are within normal limits. FSH is low. What is your suspected diagnosis?
   a. Premature ovarian failure
   b. Exercise-induced amenorrhea
   c. Lactational amenorrhea
   d. Anorexia nervosa
   e. Bulimia nervosa
   f. Iatrogenic amenorrhea
3. What findings would you expect to see on laboratory testing in a patient with premature ovarian failure?
   a. Elevated TSH, normal FSH, low estradiol
   b. Normal TSH, elevated FSH, normal estradiol
   c. Normal TSH, elevated FSH, low estradiol
   d. Elevated TSH, elevated FSH, elevated estradiol
4. Another similar patient presents to your office with secondary amenorrhea, but she also reports galactorrhea and headache. Your laboratory findings include an elevated prolactin of 120 ng/mL, normal FSH, and normal TSH. What is your next step in diagnosis?
   a. MRI of the head
   b. Pelvic ultrasound
   c. Serum estradiol
   d. Serum testosterone
   e. No further testing is necessary
5. What therapy would you first initiate with this patient?
   a. Transsphenoidal resection
   b. Dopamine agonist
   c. Radiation
   d. Chemotherapy

A Answers

Vignette 1 Question 1
Answer B: A pelvic ultrasound should be the first step, aimed to determine the presence or absence of the uterus, tubes, and ovaries. Given the presence of normal telarche (breast development appears normal) and adrenarche (pubic hair is present), a random FSH would not be helpful. A karyotype and diagnostic laparoscopy may also be helpful in determining a final diagnosis, but an ultrasound should be the next step.

Vignette 1 Question 2
Answer C: Müllerian agenesis (also known as Mayer-Rokitansky-Kuster-Hauser syndrome) refers to the congenital absence of the uterus, tubes, and upper vagina. Variants of Müllerian agenesis may include rudimentary uterine horns with or without a functional endometrium, and may lead to cyclic abdominal pain.

Imperforate hymen and transverse vaginal septum typically would present with cyclic abdominal pain and evidence on examination of hematocolpos. Androgen insensitivity syndrome patients would have scant or absent pubic hair, but otherwise may present in a similar fashion—primary amenorrhea with normal appearing breast tissue in a young phenotypical female adult.

Vignette 1 Question 3
Answer D: Embryologically speaking, development of the uterus, cervix, and vagina is closely tied with the development of the urinary system. The Müllerian ducts (also known as the paramesonephric ducts) form bilaterally and fuse to form the uterus, tubes, cervix, and upper vagina in the female. Abnormalities in Müllerian duct fusion have been associated with renal agenesis or hypoplasia, ectopic kidney and horseshoe kidney.

Other systems that may be involved include skeletal, auditory, and cardiac systems. The gastrointestinal tract, cerebral circulation, and olfactory system have not been associated.

Vignette 1 Question 4
Answer C: Although this patient will not be able to reproduce spontaneously because of her absent uterus, tubes and cervix, she does have normal ovaries. With the addition of assisted reproductive technologies, she will be able to entertain the possibility of biological children. When she is interested in childbearing, she may opt to undergo stimulation of her ovaries with injectable gonadotropins followed by retrieval of her oocytes, fertilization with her partner's sperm, and embryo transfer to a gestational carrier.

Intrauterine insemination is not an option for her given her absent uterus. Uterine transplant has occurred only in rare circumstances, and subsequent pregnancy would be high risk (and likely contraindicated) given immunosuppressive medications needed for the success of the transplant; this is not currently an available therapy for women with Müllerian agenesis.

Vignette 2 Question 1
Answer C: This patient has secondary amenorrhea and the most likely cause given her clinical presentation is Asherman's syndrome. Intrauterine adhesions caused by prior obstetric procedures (typically dilation and curettage) obstruct the uterine cavity and cause cyclic pain and (in some cases) secondary amenorrhea. More commonly it presents as dysmenorrhea.

Lactational amenorrhea is unlikely given that she is no longer breastfeeding. Sheehan's syndrome is panhypopituitarism secondary to infarction of the pituitary gland caused by postpartum hemorrhage and relative hypotension: this is less likely given her ability to breastfeed without difficulty for 6 months after delivery. The patient's symptoms of cyclic pain make premature ovarian failure less likely given your suspicion that she is ovulatory (cyclic pain), although it is additionally a possibility.

Vignette 2 Question 2
Answer A: The correct answer is to offer surgical management with hysteroscopy to resect the scar tissue within her uterine cavity, which would allow the patient relief from her cyclic pain (by releasing the obstructed menstruation), and additionally would assist her in attaining a more hospitable uterine cavity for future pregnancy.

Inducing a withdrawal bleed with Provera would not improve her obstructed flow or increase her fertility. Although in vitro fertilization may be an option in her future should operative intervention fail, it is not the first step in management. Placement of an intrauterine device may prove challenging given her intrauterine scar tissue, and furthermore may cause increased pain and most importantly will not reduce her scar tissue. An intrauterine Foley catheter or IUD is frequently placed at the end of a hysteroscopic resection of scar to reduce re-formation of scar tissue, but the IUD should not be used as first line therapy.

Vignette 2 Question 3
Answer D: Because the endometrial surface is thought to be denuded in the setting of Asherman's syndrome, leading to the formation of scar tissue, patients are at risk for placenta accreta in a subsequent pregnancy. Placenta accreta is the abnormal implantation of the placenta past the decidual layer of the endometrium and into the myometrium. It leads to abnormal adherence of the placenta to the uterus, which in some cases can lead to placenta increta (deep invasion into the myometrium) and placenta percreta (invasion

through the uterine serosa and into other pelvic organs such as the bladder or rectum).

Preterm labor is unlikely to be increased in a subsequent pregnancy if the scar tissue is adequately resected and the uterine cavity is normal prior to pregnancy. Cervical insufficiency is the premature shortening and sometimes dilation of the cervix. A patient may be at risk for this secondary to prior cervical procedures (LEEPs, cold knife cones) as well as dilation and curettage, but in this setting of Asherman's the most correct answer is placenta accreta. There is no known association between Asherman's syndrome and preeclampsia.

Vignette 3 Question 1

Answer C: A karyotype in this case would confirm your suspected diagnosis of Turner syndrome, with a result of 46,X. Clues that led to this diagnosis include primary amenorrhea in the setting of absent secondary sex characteristics, physical examination findings of short stature, webbed neck, and widely spaced nipples (also known as "shield chest"). Additionally, her murmur is likely secondary to coarctation of the aorta, one of the more common cardiac anomalies patients with Turner syndrome may have. Other characteristic findings include "streak gonads," which are often nonfunctional and subsequent pregnancy is rare.

Pelvic ultrasound would likely reveal a normal appearing uterus, and may or may not identify streak gonads; it is less helpful in definitive diagnosis. Serum FSH and LH would likely be elevated and estradiol low for a patient with Turner syndrome, but this would be less helpful in confirming her diagnosis.

Vignette 3 Question 2

Answer E: Although patients with Turner syndrome commonly develop osteoporosis secondary to premature ovarian failure, at age 15 this is less likely, therefore you would not order a DEXA scan at this age.

It is reasonable to check a thyroid function panel, as patients are at increased risk of Hashimoto's thyroiditis. You heard a murmur on your physical examination, which prompts you to order an echocardiogram, especially in light of your knowledge that Turner syndrome carries an increased risk for aortic coarctation, bicuspid aortic valve, and aortic dissection. You look for hyperglycemia and abnormal renal function on your basic metabolic panel, given known increased risk of diabetes and renal disease in Turner syndrome. You ordered anti-endomysial antibodies to check for Celiac disease, which is also associated with this syndrome, although less commonly than the above disorders.

Vignette 3 Question 3

Answer C: The patient, now at age 15, is likely to have reached her full growth potential; therefore, initiation of estrogen therapy is indicated. Given the presence of a uterus (and risk for endometrial hyperplasia or carcinoma with unopposed estrogen), you would also administer a cyclic or daily progestin to protect her endometrium. Initially, estrogen is started at a low (prepubertal) dose and increased gradually over 3 to 4 years to physiologic adult levels. Estrogen and progesterone therapy should continue until she reaches the age of menopause.

Growth hormone therapy would be indicated if she had presented at an age prior to the fusion of her distal epiphyses, in order to maximize her height. In this setting, however, it would not be of assistance. Gonadotropin therapy would likely effect puberty as would estrogen and progesterone, but it should be given in a subcutaneous manner. The ease of oral estrogen and progestin with good effects make use of gonadotropins in this setting cumbersome and contraindicated.

Vignette 3 Question 4

Answer D: In vitro fertilization using donor eggs and most likely a gestational carrier are her options for conceiving a pregnancy. Given that most likely her gonads do not have functional tissue (from her presentation with absent breast development at age 15), most likely they also do not have functional follicles. Ovulation induction for in vitro fertilization therefore would likely fail and may put her health at risk. The patient's most safe route for pregnancy would be the use of donor eggs (with her partner's sperm) and a gestational carrier. The option for her to carry the pregnancy in her own uterus may be possible, but only after careful collaboration with a perinatologist and an infertility specialist.

In this case, birth control pills are functioning for hormone replacement rather than contraception. Clomid ovulation induction would also be contraindicated given her likely lack of functional ovarian follicles in her streak gonads.

Vignette 4 Question 1

Answer D: Although this patient reports no sexual activity, it is of utmost importance to rule out pregnancy in any case of secondary amenorrhea (and most cases of primary amenorrhea). A negative β-hCG test rules out the most common cause of secondary amenorrhea: pregnancy.

A pelvic ultrasound would not be useful in this setting, as the patient is without symptoms of pain (no concern for obstructive cause of amenorrhea). Urinary LH test strips are used for patients attempting to test for evidence of ovulation. Given that this patient is not menstruating, it follows that she is likely not ovulating, therefore urinary LH testing would not be helpful. Serum FSH, prolactin, and TSH would be helpful in your workup, but only after pregnancy has been ruled out.

Vignette 4 Question 2

Answer B: The most likely diagnosis is exercise-induced amenorrhea (hypogonadotropic hypogonadism), which would carry a normal prolactin and TSH, with a low FSH. Women who are involved in strenuous exercise commonly have menstrual irregularity and this may progress to amenorrhea as the intensity and/or duration of the exercise increases. Exercised-induced amenorrhea occurs when the reduction of weight below a threshold is achieved. It is hypothesized that when body weight is low and physical exertion is high for these extended periods, the pulsatile nature of GnRH is disturbed such that normal stimulation of the ovaries by FSH and LH is absent, and therefore anovulation and amenorrhea ensure. This process is reversible by decreasing exercise or increasing caloric intake.

The laboratory findings are not consistent with premature ovarian failure. The patient is not currently lactating; therefore she does not have lactational amenorrhea. Anorexia and bulimia nervosa may result in similar laboratory findings, but this patient gives no history of eating disorder. It is important, however, that during your evaluation you screen her for evidence of abnormal eating patterns and unusual weight control habits. Iatrogenic amenorrhea refers to medication-induced amenorrhea, as with Depo-Lupron or oral contraceptives. The patient gives no history of use of these medications.

Vignette 4 Question 3

Answer C: Premature ovarian failure is one type of hypergonadotropic hypogonadism, which presents as secondary amenorrhea at an age less than 40. Laboratory studies would show a markedly elevated FSH with low estradiol. TSH is not affected in this setting. Causes of premature ovarian failure may include chromosomal abnormalities and genetic disorders (Fragile X), although in most cases a definitive cause is not found. Young women with this diagnosis understandably may be devastated by these findings, particularly if they had planned childbearing. Fertility options include IVF with their own eggs, but most likely they will require egg donation, depending on the level of depletion of their own follicles. They will benefit from estrogen and progesterone replacement to reduce their risk of osteoporosis and improve their long-term cardiovascular health—this should be strongly recommended to them in your counseling. The three other combinations of laboratory tests above are not consistent with premature ovarian failure.

Vignette 4 Question 4

Answer A: Because of this patient's elevated prolactin, headache, and galactorrhea, you are most suspicious of a prolactinoma, therefore you order an MRI. Prolactinomas are the most common type of pituitary adenoma. Amenorrhea occurs secondary to inhibition of GnRH secretion, which causes decreased FSH and LH secretion leading to anovulation and another form of "hypogonadotropic hypogonadism."

A pelvic ultrasound would not be helpful in this case as it would likely be normal, with normal appearing ovaries and a thin endometrial stripe (secondary to lack of stimulation by ovulating ovaries). You more highly suspect a prolactinoma because of the serum prolactin. Estradiol and testosterone testing also would not be diagnostic in this case.

Vignette 4 Question 5

Answer B: You suspect this is a microadenoma given the PRL level is less than 200, so you opt to initiate therapy with a dopamine agonist. The two medications in use today include bromocriptine and cabergoline, both of which are highly effective in reducing the size of the adenoma. Many providers try bromocriptine before cabergoline because of the increased risk for valvular heart disease with cabergoline. Initiation of treatment with either drug should start at a low level, and slowly titrate up. You would follow serum prolactin levels to determine the final effective dose, and would additionally repeat the MRI in 3 to 6 months to evaluate for treatment effect.

Transsphenoidal resection is a treatment option for patients who do not respond to dopamine agonists or who cannot tolerate the treatment; however, this would not be your first line therapy given increased risk of surgery as well as risk of treatment failure (and persistently present prolactinoma cells). Radiation therapy is primarily used for women who fail resection or who have large adenomas refractory to other treatment. There is no role for chemotherapy in treating a prolactinoma.

Chapter 22 Abnormalities of the Menstrual Cycle

Characteristics of the menstrual cycle vary from woman to woman. Normal variances include a cycle length between 21 and 35 days, bleeding for up to 7 days, as well as mild to moderate cramping, often relieved with over-the-counter medications. Additionally, rare women also may have spotting to light bleeding at midcycle as a result of a slight decline in estrogen levels that precede ovulation. Bleeding that occurs outside of these parameters is defined as abnormal uterine bleeding and is a common reason to consult a gynecologist. This chapter will describe common abnormalities of the menstrual cycle, including appropriate diagnostic evaluation and treatment options.

DYSMENORRHEA

Dysmenorrhea is defined as **pain and cramping** during menstruation that **interferes with normal activities** and requires over-the-counter or prescription medication. Mild pain during menses is normal. Discomfort during menstruation ranges from mild discomfort to severe pain that causes some patients to be bedridden. Fifty percent of menstruating women suffer from dysmenorrhea and 10% of these are incapacitated for 1 to 3 days each month.

Dysmenorrhea is classified as primary or secondary. **Primary dysmenorrhea** is idiopathic menstrual pain without identifiable pathology; **secondary dysmenorrhea** is painful menses due to underlying pathology (endometriosis, fibroids, adenomyosis, PID, cervical stenosis).

PRIMARY DYSMENORRHEA

Primary dysmenorrhea usually occurs before age 20. Because primary dysmenorrhea is almost always associated with ovulatory cycles, it is usually diagnosed in late teens rather than at menarche when cycles are often anovulatory. Although there is no obvious organic cause, primary dysmenorrhea is thought to result from **increased levels of endometrial prostaglandin production** derived from the arachidonic acid pathway. Additionally, there may be a psychological component involved for some patients that depends on attitudes toward menstruation learned from mothers, sisters, and friends.

Diagnosis

The diagnosis of primary dysmenorrhea is made on the basis of history and the **absence of organic causes**. The most common misdiagnosis of primary dysmenorrhea is endometriosis. Often, the pain of dysmenorrhea occurs with ovulatory cycles on the first or second day of menstruation, whereas pain from endometriosis may begin 1 to 2 days to weeks before menstruation, worsens 1 to 2 days before menstruation, and is relieved at or right after the onset of menstrual flow (Chapter 15). Associated symptoms of primary dysmenorrhea include nausea, vomiting, and headache. On physical examination there are no obvious abnormalities except a generalized tenderness throughout the pelvis.

Treatment

The first-line medical treatment for primary dysmenorrhea is **nonsteroidal anti-inflammatory drugs** (NSAIDs). The most commonly used agents include aspirin, ibuprofen, ketoprofen, and naproxen. These drugs are all available without prescription; however, patients may need prescription-strength dosages to obtain adequate symptom relief. Because antiprostaglandins work by blocking prostaglandin synthesis and metabolism, these medications should be taken with the onset of menses, continued for 1 to 3 days, and then taken as needed. **COX-2 inhibitors** such as Celebrex (celecoxib) are another class of NSAIDs that have been shown to be effective in the treatment of primary dysmenorrhea. However, potential side effects have limited their use in the United States.

Oral contraceptive pills (OCPs) are the second line of treatment for women who do not get adequate pain relief from antiprostaglandin agents and NSAIDs alone or who cannot tolerate these drugs. More than 90% of women with primary dysmenorrhea find adequate pain relief with the use of oral contraceptives given in a continuous (preferred) or cyclic fashion. The same is true for other estrogen/progestin combination contraceptives such as the Ortho Evra patch and NuvaRing. The mechanism of relief is either secondary to the **cessation of ovulation** or due to the **decrease in endometrial proliferation** leading to **decreased prostaglandin production**. Most patients who have been cycled for 1 year on OCPs experience a reduction of symptoms even if the OCPs are discontinued. For women who cannot tolerate estrogens, several progestin-only contraceptives also provide relief, including Depo-Provera, Implanon, and the Mirena IUS.

Nonmedical options for the treatment of primary dysmenorrhea include the use of heating pads and patches to the lower abdomen, exercise, massage, acupuncture, and hypnosis. The use of transcutaneous electrical nerve stimulation (TENS) has been also shown to relieve or decrease pain in women suffering from primary dysmenorrhea.

Surgical therapies including cervical dilation, uterosacral ligament ligation, and presacral neurectomy have been used in the past but **have little use** in current management of true primary dysmenorrhea. Often, primary dysmenorrhea will decrease throughout a patient's 20s and early 30s. In addition, a pregnancy carried to viability will usually decrease the symptoms of primary dysmenorrhea. Very rarely, a patient with true primary dysmenorrhea may require hysterectomy to relieve her pain. Prior to this, a thorough evaluation, possibly including questioning about childhood molestation or sexual assault, pelvic ultrasound, MRI, and laparoscopy should be performed to look for secondary causes of dysmenorrhea.

SECONDARY DYSMENORRHEA

Secondary dysmenorrhea implies that the symptoms are secondary to an identifiable cause (Fig. 22-1) such as endometriosis and adenomyosis (Chapter 15), uterine fibroids (Chapter 14), cervical stenosis, or pelvic adhesions. Because the first three causes are discussed in other chapters, refer to those particular chapters for detailed management.

Cervical Stenosis

Cervical stenosis causes dysmenorrhea by obstructing blood flow during menstruation. The stenosis can be congenital or secondary to scarring from infection, trauma, or surgery. Patients often complain of scant or prolonged light menses associated with severe cramping pain that is relieved with increased menstrual flow. On physical examination there may be obvious scarring of the external os; often the clinician is unable to pass a uterine sound through the cervical canal.

Treatment

Cervical stenosis is treated by dilation of the cervix. Either a surgical dilation can be performed or laminaria tents can be used. Surgical dilation is usually performed in the operating room, but can be attempted in the office with a paracervical block. Progressively larger dilators are placed through the cervical canal until it becomes patent. Ultrasound guidance can be helpful in avoiding creation of a false passage or uterine perforation.

Laminaria may be placed in the cervix in the office setting. Made from seaweed, these dilate over a 24-hour period by absorbing water from the surrounding tissue. Slow dilation of the cervix results from expansion of the laminaria. Dilation will provide relief; however, symptoms often recur, requiring multiple dilations. Pregnancy with vaginal delivery often leads to a permanent cure.

Pelvic Adhesions

Patients with a history of **pelvic infections** including cervicitis, pelvic inflammatory disease (see Color Plate 12), or tubo-ovarian abscess may have symptoms of dysmenorrhea secondary to adhesion formation. Patients with other local **inflammatory diseases** (appendicitis, endometriosis, or Crohn's disease) or **prior pelvic surgery** (especially myomectomy) may also have adhesions leading to dysmenorrhea. If a patient has a history of any of these problems and reports pain associated with movement or activity, pelvic adhesions should be suspected. In some patients, pelvic adhesions can be so extensive as to "cement" the uterus into a fixed position, which may be noted on pelvic examination. Adhesions are **not visible on traditional imaging modalities** such as pelvic ultrasound, MRI, or CT.

Treatment

Patients with pelvic adhesions will occasionally respond to the antiprostaglandins prescribed for primary dysmenorrhea. When suspicions are high and the pain necessitates treatment, pelvic adhesions can be both **diagnosed and treated via laparoscopy**. Occasionally, the adhesions may be so dense as to necessitate laparotomy for safe lysis. However, the patient should be aware that surgery can lead to further adhesions and further problems with dysmenorrhea, infertility, and/or chronic pelvic pain.

PREMENSTRUAL SYNDROME AND PREMENSTRUAL DYSPHORIC DISORDER

Premenstrual syndrome (PMS) and its more severe variant, that is, premenstrual dysphoric disorder (PMDD) are characterized by a constellation of physical and/or behavioral changes that occur in the second half of the menstrual cycle. These changes might include headache, weight gain, bloating, breast tenderness, mood fluctuation, restlessness, irritability, anxiety,

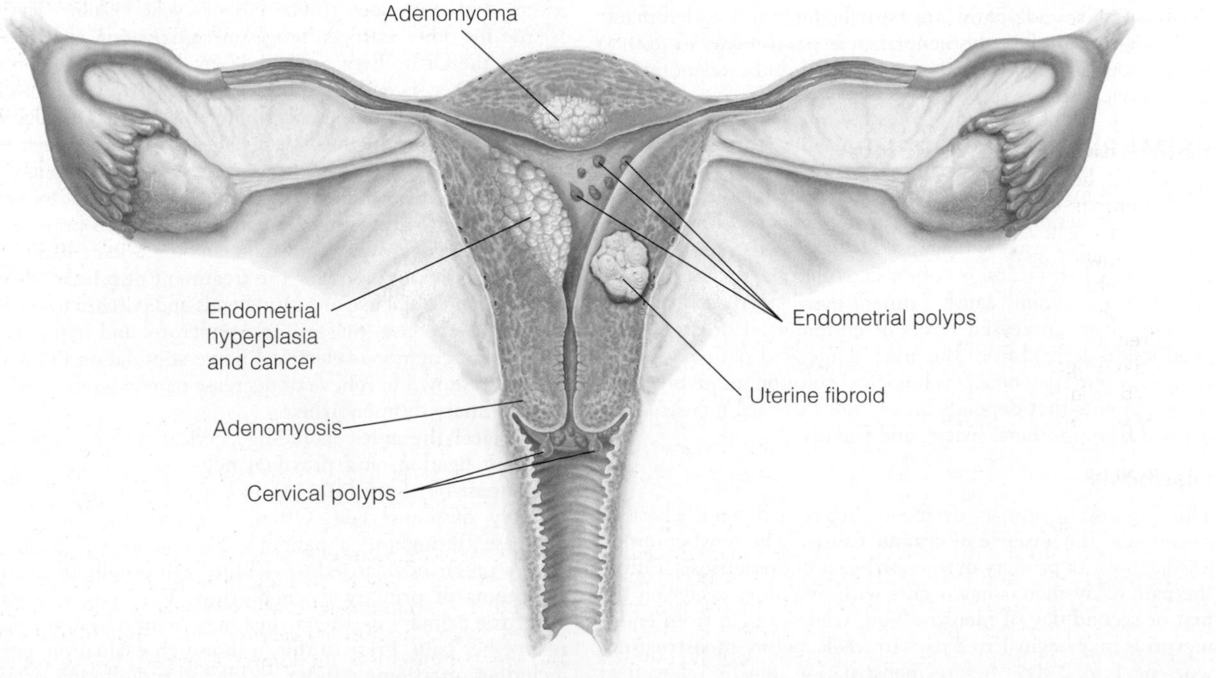

Figure 22-1 • Common causes of abnormal vaginal bleeding.
(From Anatomical Chart Co.)

depression, fatigue, and a feeling of being out of control. These symptoms must occur in the 2 weeks prior to menstruation and there must be at least a 7-day symptom-free interval in the first half of the menstrual cycle. Symptoms must occur in at least two consecutive cycles for the diagnosis to be made.

About 75% of women suffer from some recurrent PMS symptoms; of these, 30% report significant problems and 5% of women are incapacitated or severely distressed by PMDD at some point during their cycle. The highest incidence occurs among women in their late 20s to early 30s.

PATHOGENESIS

The exact etiology of PMS and PMDD is unknown but is likely **multifactorial** and includes both physiologic and psychological causes. Past hypotheses have included abnormalities in estrogen–progesterone balance, disturbance in the renin–angiotensin–aldosterone pathway, excess prostaglandin and prolactin production, and psychogenic factors. Recent studies also suggest that PMS and PMDD may be due to the interaction between the **neurotransmitter serotonin** and cyclic changes in the **ovarian steroids**. The serum concentrations of estrogen and progesterone are no different in patients with PMS/PMDD and those without. However, studies have suggested that although women with PMS and PMDD have normal levels of estrogen and progesterone, they may have **an abnormal response to normal hormonal changes**.

TREATMENT

Effective treatments for PMS and PMDD have been identified after systematic reviews. The **selective serotonin reuptake inhibitors** (SSRIs) have demonstrated clear efficacy in treating both the physical and mood symptoms of these disorders. **Prozac** (fluoxetine) has been approved by the U.S. FDA for the treatment of PMDD. Other drugs in this category, including Celexa (citalopram), Paxil (paroxetine), and Zoloft (sertraline), have also been shown to be effective.

The serotonin and norepinephrine reuptake inhibitor (SNRI) **Effexor** (venlafaxine) and the benzodiazepine **Xanax** (alprazolam) have also shown efficacy in treating these disorders. In small trials, both Lupron (leuprolide acetate) and Danocrine (danazol) have shown efficacy in treating PMS and PMDD. Their side effects, however, prevent widespread use of these options.

A number of additional medications may have possible efficacy in the treatment of PMS and PMDD. Several older studies showed oral contraceptives to have no greater efficacy than placebo in managing PMS and PMDD. A new OCP, **Yaz**, which is formulated with low-dose estrogen and uses **drospirenone** (a spironolactone with antimineralocorticoid and antiandrogenic activity) as its progestin, has been found to be effective in the treatment of PMS and has been approved for that use. Spironolactone itself has not consistently shown to be effective. There is some suggestion that **exercise** and **relaxation** techniques may improve the symptoms of PMS and PMDD.

Several studies have looked at **vitamin supplementation** as a treatment for PMS and PMDD. There appears to be some role for the use of calcium (600 mg BID), vitamin D (800 IU/day), vitamin B_6 ($\leq$100 mg/day), magnesium (200 to 360 mg/day), and chasteberry extract (one tablet/day) in the treatment of these disorders. Several studies have also showed that complex **carbohydrate-rich beverage** consumption improved both the psychological symptoms and appetite cravings. This is thought to work by modulating tryptophan and serotonin synthesis.

Other supplements such as evening primrose oil, essential fatty acids, and ginkgo biloba extract have not been found to be effective nor has the use of progesterone and progestins.

ABNORMAL UTERINE BLEEDING

The normal menstrual cycle consists of cyclic bleeding approximately **every 28 days** (normal range, 21 to 35 days), lasting **3 to 5 days** with about **30 to 50 mL** of blood loss per cycle. Abnormal uterine bleeding refers to any departure from the norm in the menstrual cycle. It can involve **too much bleeding** (heavy periods, frequent menses, or bleeding between periods) or **too little bleeding** (light periods, infrequent periods, or complete absence of periods). It may also refer to inappropriate unscheduled bleeding (postcoital spotting, postmenopausal bleeding). The most common causes of abnormal uterine bleeding are covered briefly in this chapter and in more detail in other chapters of this text (Fig. 22-1).

Dysfunctional uterine bleeding describes idiopathic heavy and/or irregular bleeding that **cannot be attributed to another cause** following a complete evaluation. DUB is most commonly due to anovulation or oligoovulation. The most common cause of anovulation in women of reproductive age is polycystic ovarian syndrome (PCOS). Amenorrhea—complete absence of periods for at least 6 consecutive months—is discussed in Chapter 21.

PATTERNS OF ABNORMAL UTERINE BLEEDING

The typical patterns of abnormal uterine bleeding are summarized in Table 22-1. It is generally agreed that these definitions to describe different types of abnormal uterine bleeding in non-pregnant reproductive aged women have been inconsistent and confusing. Efforts have been ongoing to simplify the terminology. This new classification system known by the acronym **PALM-COEIN** was introduced in 2011 by the International Federation of Gynecology and Obstetrics (FIGO) and is supported by the American College of OB/GYN (ACOG). This new nomenclature system classifies AUB by both the **pattern and the etiology** of the bleeding. PALM represents the structural causes of AUB including Polyps, Adenomyosis, Leiomyomas, and Malignancy and hyperplasia. **COEIN** delineates the nonstructural causes including Coagulopathy, Ovulatory dysfunction, Endometrial, Iatrogenic and those etiologies that are Not yet classified. Because the PALM-COEIN system has not yet been universally adopted, the traditional terminology is still described in this text.

MENORRHAGIA

Patients with menorrhagia have regularly timed menstrual cycles but the flow is either excessive in its duration (>7 days) or its volume (>80 mL/cycle). Patients with menorrhagia occasionally describe the blood as **flooding** or **gushing**, and may have blood clots along with their excessive flow. Most gynecologists use a history of greater than 24 menstrual pads in a day or soaking through a pad every hour as indicative of menorrhagia. Menorrhagia is most commonly caused by **uterine fibroids**, **adenomyosis**, **endometrial polyps**, and less commonly by endometrial hyperplasia or cancer or cervical polyps or cancer (Fig. 22-1). Teenagers with menorrhagia should be evaluated for **primary bleeding disorders** such as von Willebrand disease, idiopathic thrombocytopenic

TABLE 22-1 Patterns of Uterine Bleeding

Bleeding Pattern	Definition	Timing of Cycle	Flow Amount
Normal menses	Regular bleeding, average Q 28 d (range, 21–35), lasting 3–5 d, bleeding on average 30–50 mL/cycle	Regular	Normal
Menorrhagia (hypermenorrhea)	Heavy (>80 mL/cycle) or prolonged (>7 d) menstrual flow occurring at regular intervals	Regular	Heavy
Hypomenorrhea	Regularly timed menses but light flow	Regular	Light
Metrorrhagia (intermenstrual bleeding)	Any bleeding between normal menses, usually lighter than normal menstrual bleeding	Irregular	Normal–light
Menometrorrhagia	Excessive or prolonged bleeding at irregular intervals	Irregular	Heavy
Oligomenorrhea	Irregular cycles >35 d apart	Irregular	Varies
Polymenorrhea	Frequent regular cycles but <21 d apart	Regular	Normal
Amenorrhea, secondary	No menses for 6 or more consecutive months	N/A	N/A
Amenorrhea, primary	No menses by age 14 in the absence of secondary sexual characteristics *or* No menses by age 16 in the presence of secondary sexual characteristics	N/A	N/A
Dysfunctional uterine bleeding	Idiopathic heavy and/or irregular bleeding with no identifiable causes	Regular or irregular	Varies

purpura (ITP), platelet dysfunction, and thrombocytopenia from malignancy.

HYPOMENORRHEA

Patients with hypomenorrhea have **regularly timed menses** but an unusually **light amount of flow**. This is commonly caused by hypogonadotropic hypogonadism, which is seen most commonly in anorexic patients and athletes. Atrophic endometrium can also occur in the case of Asherman's syndrome (**intrauterine adhesions** or synechiae), congenital malformations, infection, and intrauterine trauma. Patients on **OCPs, Depo-Provera, and the progestin-containing IUDs** also have atrophic endometrium and often have light menses as do women who have undergone endometrial ablation. Outlet obstruction secondary to cervical stenosis or congenital abnormalities can also result in hypomenorrhea.

METRORRHAGIA AND MENOMETRORRHAGIA

Metrorrhagia is characterized by bleeding that occurs between regular menstrual periods. This bleeding is usually less than or equal to normal menstrual volume. Primary causes include cervical lesions (polyps, eversion, and carcinoma) and endometrial polyps and carcinoma. **Menometrorrhagia** is excessive (>80 mL) or prolonged bleeding at irregular intervals. The usual causes include uterine fibroids, adenomyosis, endometrial polyps, hyperplasia, and cancer (Fig. 22-1). Thyroid disorders can result in increased or decreased flow or no change in menstrual flow.

OLIGOMENORRHEA

Patients with periods **greater than 35 days apart** are described as having oligomenorrhea. The causes are similar to those for amenorrhea with disruption of the hypothalamic–pituitary–gonadal axis or systemic diseases such as hyperprolactinemia and thyroid disorders (Chapter 21). The most common causes of oligomenorrhea are PCOS, **chronic anovulation, and pregnancy. Thyroid disease** should also be considered. When a patient has no period for 6 consecutive months, secondary amenorrhea is diagnosed.

POLYMENORRHEA

Polymenorrhea, or **frequent periods**, describes regular periods that occur less than 21 days apart. Polymenorrhea can be confused with metrorrhagia (intermenstrual bleeding). However, if all of the bleeding episodes are similar in amount and fewer than 21 days apart, polymenorrhea should be considered. This is usually caused by **anovulation**.

EVALUATION OF ABNORMAL UTERINE BLEEDING

The workup for abnormal uterine bleeding includes a careful **history and physical** followed by diagnostic tests to determine the underlying etiology. The history should include timing of bleeding, quantity of bleeding, menstrual history with menarche and recent periods, and associated symptoms. It should also include a family history of bleeding disorders, particularly if menorrhagia appears at menarche.

On physical examination, **rectal, urethral, vaginal, and cervical causes of bleeding should be ruled out**. Care should be taken to look for sequelae of PCOS (hirsutism, acne, truncal obesity, acanthosis nigricans), thyroid disease (thyromegaly, skin changes, diaphoresis, increased pulse), and signs of bleeding disorder (bruising, petechiae). The bimanual examination may reveal uterine or adnexal masses consistent with fibroids, adenomyosis, pregnancy, or cancer. A **Pap smear** is used to screen for cervical dysplasia and cancer and **cervical cultures** should be taken to rule out infection.

Laboratory evaluation should be tailored to the type of menstrual irregularity. For light or skipped cycles, evaluation would include a **pregnancy test**, **TSH**, **PRL**, **and an FSH** if menopause or POI - primary ovarian insufficiency (formerly premature ovarian failure - PMOF) is suspected. The spectra of hormonal tests that can be performed are discussed with the workup of amenorrhea or PCOS, and PMOF are discussed elsewhere in the text.

For heavy, frequent, or prolonged cycles, appropriate laboratory tests would include a **pregnancy test**, **TSH**, **and CBC**. A primary bleeding disorder evaluation should be done when menorrhagia presents at menarche, in teenagers or in women with symptoms suggestive of a systemic or hematologic etiology such as easy bruising (>5 cm), frequent nosebleeds, bleeding gums, and excessive bleeding after surgery, dental extraction, or childbirth. Evaluation for these women might include a complete blood count **(CBC) including platelet count** and difference, **PT/PTT**, **factor VIII**, **and von Willebrand factor antigen and activity**.

Importantly, any woman age 45 or older with abnormal uterine bleeding (excessive or insufficient) should undergo an **endometrial biopsy** to rule out endometrial hyperplasia and cancer even if other testing reveals a potential explanation for the abnormal bleeding. **Obese patients with prolonged oligomenorrhea** should also undergo endometrial biopsy even if they are younger than 45 years. These women are at increased risk of endometrial hyperplasia and cancer due to the peripheral conversion of androgens into estrogens in their adipose cells.

A **pelvic ultrasound** can be used to identify endometrial polyps, fibroids, hyperplasia, cancers, and adnexal masses. If intrauterine pathology is suspected on pelvic ultrasound, a 3D ultrasound, **sonohysterogram,** or hysterosalpingogram can be performed to show intrauterine defects. **MRI** is expensive but useful in distinguishing adenomyosis from uterine fibroids. **Hysteroscopy** allows direct visualization of the intrauterine cavity. A dilation and curettage (D&C) provides tissue for diagnosis.

TREATMENT

The treatment of abnormal uterine bleeding **depends on the specific underlying etiology**. The most common causes and treatments are detailed in Table 22-2. Symptomatic fibroids and polyps can be treated by resection or removal (Chapter 14). **Adenomyosis** is occasionally responsive to hormonal regulation with combined estrogen/progesterone such as a combination OCP. The levonorgestrel-containing **IUD (Mirena)** has been found to substantially decrease the bleeding and pain associated with adenomyosis. Endometrial ablation or resection can be considered, although there is initial evidence suggesting an increased incidence of postablation pain and continued abnormal bleeding in women with adenomyosis. In patients with refractory pain and/or bleeding, hysterectomy may be required (Chapter 15). **Endometrial hyperplasia** is most commonly managed with **progestin therapy** if no cytologic atypia and occasionally with **D&C or hysterectomy** when atypia is present (Chapter 14). **Anovulation** is treated with menstrual regulation with estrogens and/or progestins and weight loss (Chapter 21). Treatment for POI/PMOF and menopause is directed toward relief of specific symptoms (Chapter 20). In cases where hyperplasia and cancer have been ruled out, tranexamic acid (Lysteda), which is a new antifibrinolytic agent, has been shown to decrease menstrual blood loss and is FDA approved for the treatment of menorrhagia.

TABLE 22-2 Common Causes and Treatments for Abnormal Uterine Bleeding

Bleeding Disorder	Bleeding Amount	Typical Treatment
Neoplasms		
Uterine fibroids	Heavy	Hormonal management, tranexamic acid, uterine artery embolization, myomectomy, endometrial ablation, hysterectomy
Adenomyosis	Heavy	Hormonal management, Mirena IUD, endometrial ablation hysterectomy
Cervical polyps	Light	Polypectomy
Endometrial polyps	Heavy	Hysteroscopy, polypectomy ± D&C, endometrial ablation, hysterectomy
Endometrial hyperplasia	Varies	Progestin therapy (if no atypia), D&C, hysterectomy if atypia is present
Endometrial cancer	Heavy	Hysterectomy, BSO, radiation
Pregnancy problems		
Pregnancy	Varies	Expectant management vs. delivery
Miscarriage	Heavy	Expectant management vs. D&C
Ectopic pregnancy	Varies	Methotrexate vs. surgical management
Hormonal problems		
Hypothyroidism	Varies	Thyroid hormone replacement
Hyperprolactinemia	None	Dopamine agonists
Anovulation	Varies	Combined estrogen/progestin pills, patch or ring, or cyclic progestin

In women who have completed childbearing, endometrial ablation can also be used to treat AUB by destroying the majority of the endometrium down to its basalis layer. A variety of ablation modalities are available including laser, roller bar/barrel, hydrothermal balloon, cryoablation, bipolar radiofrequency, microwave, and hydrothermal ablation (circulating hot water). Each of these carries an 85% to 97% success rate over 5 years. Success for the procedure is defined as reduction in uterine blood flow (NOT amenorrhea) and patient satisfaction. About 15% to 45% of patients will be amenorrheic after ablation and 10% to 30% will subsequently choose to have a hysterectomy for persistent bleeding or pain.

DYSFUNCTIONAL UTERINE BLEEDING

If **no pathologic cause** of abnormal uterine bleeding is identified, the diagnosis of dysfunctional uterine bleeding (DUB) is made. DUB is a **diagnosis of exclusion**. Most patients with DUB are **anovulatory**. In these instances, the ovary produces estrogen but no corpus luteum is formed, and thus no progesterone is produced. Subsequently, there is continuous estrogenic stimulation of the endometrium without the usual progesterone-induced bleeding. Instead, in DUB, the endometrium continues to proliferate until it outgrows its blood supply, breaks down, and sloughs off in an irregular fashion. DUB is most likely to occur with anovulatory cycles and thus is most common during times in a woman's life when she is most likely to be anovulatory such as adolescence, perimenopause, lactation, and pregnancy. Pathologic anovulation occurs in **hypothyroidism**, **hyperprolactinemia**, **hyperandrogenism**, **and POI/PMOF**.

DIAGNOSIS

The diagnosis of DUB is made by history, physical examination, laboratory tests, and imaging to **rule out other causes of abnormal bleeding** as described in the prior section. In **adolescence**, the risk of structural causes of abnormal bleeding is small. However, any congenital anomalies and bleeding disorders should be eliminated. In the **reproductive years**, there is an increased risk of structural and hormonal etiologies for abnormal bleeding. During **perimenopause**, the risk of DUB increases, but so does the risk of other causes of abnormal bleeding including fibroids, polyps, adenomyosis, and endometrial hyperplasia and cancer. A careful workup of abnormal uterine bleeding must therefore be performed before the diagnosis of DUB is given. Importantly, **any woman 45 years or older with abnormal uterine bleeding should undergo an endometrial biopsy to rule out endometrial hyperplasia and cancer**. The same is true for obese women younger than 45 years who have had extended periods of oligo.amenorrhea.

Because DUB is commonly associated with anovulation, efforts should be made to determine whether a patient is ovulating. A basal body temperature can be graphed daily to determine whether ovulation is occurring. This can also be accomplished with ovulation prediction kits, which are at-home tests for detecting the LH surge from urine samples. A midluteal, day 21 to 23 serum progesterone level may also indicate if a patient is ovulating. An endometrial biopsy, showing a decidualized or luteal phase endometrium, is evidence of ovulation and progesterone effect upon the endometrium.

TREATMENT

Once the diagnosis of DUB is made, treatment depends on the cause, the age of the patient, desire for fertility, and the acute versus chronic nature of the bleeding.

In the case of **acute hemorrhage**, therapy to stop the bleeding should be initiated immediately. **Intravenous estrogen** (25 mg conjugated estrogen every 4 hours up to 24 hours) provides a quick response but also carries an increased risk of venous thromboembolic events (DVT, PE). For patients with excessive blood loss who are hemodynamically stable, **high-dose oral estrogens** can control the bleeding within 24 to 48 hours. A typical dosing might be 2.5 mg every 4 hours for 14 to 21 days followed by medroxyprogesterone acetate 10 mg per day for 7 to 10 days. Instead of this sequential hormone therapy, an **OCP taper** can be used for endometrial stabilization. A typical taper would use a monophasic pill containing 35 mcg ethinyl estradiol given three times a day for 3 days, then two times a day for 2 days, and then daily for the remainder of the pack.

For chronic DUB, nonhormonal therapy with **NSAIDs** (e.g., 800 mg ibuprofen TID × 5 days) has been shown to decrease menstrual blood loss by 20% to 50%. This is typically reserved for ovulatory women with DUB. This therapy may be used alone or in conjunction with estrogen and progesterone therapy.

Menstrual regulation using hormonal therapy is the primary treatment for anovulatory DUB. This can include use of combination **estrogen and progesterone** in the form of oral contraceptive pills, Ortho Evra patch, or NuvaRing. These may be dosed in a continuous (preferred) or cyclic fashion depending on the patient's desire.

In patients in whom the use of estrogen is contraindicated (women with hypertension, thrombophilias, and history of DVT or PE and those 35 and older who smoke), or those who prefer an alternative to estrogen/progestin combination, similar cycle control can be achieved using **progestin-only options**. These include cyclic progestin administration (10 mg medroxyprogesterone acetate per day for 10 consecutive days each month), or progesterone in the form of Depo-Provera, levonorgestrel-releasing IUS (Mirena), or Implanon. These latter three are likely to result in light menses or amenorrhea over time. The Mirena IUD is particularly helpful in anovulatory and ovulatory patients with menorrhagia including those who are at increased risk for developing endometrial hyperplasia or cancer (obese, diabetic, hypertension, smoker, positive family history, or chronic anovulation due to polycystic ovary syndrome).

Surgical intervention may be required for patients with DUB who do not respond to medical therapy. **D&C** may be both diagnostic and therapeutic but the result is typically temporary.

Hysterectomy is the definitive surgery for DUB but should be reserved for those cases refractory to all other treatments or for women for whom childbearing is complete. Hysterectomy may be performed laparoscopically, vaginally, or abdominally. The patient's personal risk factors and age may be used to determine if the ovaries and/or cervix is left in situ or removed.

POSTMENOPAUSAL BLEEDING

Menopause is marked by 12 months of amenorrhea after the final menstrual period. Postmenopausal bleeding, then, is any vaginal bleeding that occurs more than 12 months after the last menstrual period. **Any postmenopausal bleeding is abnormal** and should be investigated given the increased

TABLE 22-3 Causes of Postmenopausal Bleeding

Etiology	Percentage
Vaginal/endometrial atrophy	30
Exogenous estrogens	30
Endometrial cancer	10
Endometrial polyps	10
Endometrial hyperplasia	10
Other	10

risk of reproductive cancers in women in this age group. The most common cause of postmenopausal bleeding, however, is **endometrial and/or vaginal atrophy**, not cancer (Table 22-3). Endometrial hyperplasia cancer in responsible for only 10% to 15% of all postmenopausal bleeding.

ETIOLOGIES

Bleeding in postmenopausal women can be due to nongynecologic etiologies, lower and upper genital tract sources, reproductive tumors, or exogenous hormonal stimulation. **Nongynecologic causes** include rectal bleeding from hemorrhoids, anal fissures, rectal prolapse, and lower gastrointestinal (GI) tumors. Urethral caruncles are another source of bleeding in the postmenopausal woman. These disorders can be identified by history and physical, anoscopy, fecal immunoassay test, barium enema, or colonoscopy.

Vaginal atrophy due to the lack of endogenous estrogen is the most common source of **lower genital tract** postmenopausal bleeding. The thin vaginal mucosa is easily traumatized and therefore likely to bleed. Other causes of lower genital tract bleeding are benign and malignant lesions of the vulva, vagina, or cervix.

Pathologic causes of postmenopausal bleeding from the **upper genital tract** include endometrial atrophy, endometrial polyps, endometrial hyperplasia, and endometrial cancer. Estrogen-secreting ovarian tumors can cause stimulation of the endometrium that presents as postmenopausal bleeding. Each of these disorders can be identified with a combination of Pap screen and high-risk HPV, endometrial biopsy, and pelvic ultrasound.

The use of **exogenous hormones** is another common cause of postmenopausal uterine bleeding. Despite the occurrence of bleeding with the use of hormone replacement therapy (50% in the first year of use), thorough evaluation of the postmenopausal patient with endometrial biopsy is still required to rule out endometrial hyperplasia and cancer.

DIAGNOSIS

A careful history is important. Physical examination should include a careful inspection of the external anogenital region, vulva, vagina, and cervix. A **Pap smear and high-risk HPV screen** should be performed as well as a digital rectal examination and fecal immunoassay test. Laboratory tests might include a **CBC, TSH, prolactin, and FSH levels.** If an ovarian mass is identified, tumor markers (Ca-125, LDH, hCG, AFP, CEA, inhibin, and estradiol) should also be considered.

A **pelvic ultrasound, sonohysterogram, and MRI** can be useful in the evaluation of the endometrial stripe and uterine cavity. In the postmenopausal woman, the endometrial stripe should be thin and less than or equal to 4 mm. **Endometrial biopsy** should be performed in a postmenopausal patient with an endometrial stripe greater than 4 mm or if the bleeding is persistent. This is done to rule out endometrial hyperplasia and cancer even if there is another identifiable source of postmenopausal bleeding. **Hysteroscopy**—either in the office or operating room—can further elucidate intrauterine abnormalities such as endometrial polyps and fibroids. **D&C** is both diagnostic and therapeutic for some lesions of the uterus and cervix.

TREATMENT

Treatment of postmenopausal bleeding should be directed at **treating the causal agent**. Lesions of the vulva and vagina should be biopsied and treated accordingly. Lacerations of the vaginal mucosa should be repaired. Vaginal atrophy can be treated with vaginal estrogen. Commonly, low-dose vaginal estrogen preparations (cream, pill, ring) are very effective. Systemic treatment can also be obtained with hormone replacement therapy (HRT) if the uterus is in situ or with estrogen replacement therapy (ERT) if the uterus has been removed.

Endometrial polyps may be removed by hysteroscopic resection or D&C. Endometrial hyperplasia (Chapter 14) can be treated with progestin therapy if no atypia is present or hysterectomy, when atypia is found. Endometrial cancer is usually treated by TAHBSO performed in conjunction with possible lymph node dissection, radiation, or chemotherapy therapy (less common).

KEY POINTS

- Primary dysmenorrhea is severe pain with menses that cannot be attributed to any identifiable cause. It is thought to be due to increased levels of prostaglandins.
- Most primary dysmenorrhea is managed with NSAIDs and/or contraceptive steroids in pill, patch, or ring form. TENS units, heating pads, exercise, massage, acupuncture, and hypnosis may also help. There is little role for surgery in the management of primary dysmenorrhea.
- Secondary dysmenorrhea is painful menses due to an identifiable cause such as adenomyosis, endometriosis, fibroids, cervical stenosis, or pelvic adhesions. The treatment should be tailored to the cause.
- PMS and PMDD represent a multifactorial disease spectrum with physiologic and psychological components including headache, weight gain, bloating, breast fluctuation, irritability, fatigue, and a feeling of being out of control.
- In order to make the diagnosis of dysmenorrhea, symptoms must be in the second half of the menstrual cycle with at least a 7-day symptom-free interval during the first half of the menstrual cycle. Symptoms must occur in at least two consecutive cycles.

- Although the cause of PMS/PMDD is unknown. A variety of treatments offer relief including SSRIs (Prozac, Zoloft), OCPs, as do diet modification, exercise, and vitamin supplementation (calcium, vitamin D, vitamin B_6, and magnesium).
- The normal menstrual cycle occurs, on average, every 28 days (range, 21 to 35 days) and lasts 3 to 5 days with 30 to 50 mL of blood loss per cycle.
- Menorrhagia is regular bleeding that is heavy or prolonged. Metrorrhagia is bleeding between periods and menometrorrhagia is heavy or prolonged irregular bleeding. The most common causes of heavy or prolonged bleeding include polyps, fibroids, adenomyosis, cancer, and pregnancy complications.
- The most common causes of oligomenorrhea (periods >35 days apart) include chronic ovulation, PCOS, and pregnancy.
- The initial evaluation of abnormal uterine bleeding should include a history and physical, laboratory tests (pregnancy test, TSH, prolactin, ± FSH), endometrial biopsy (for women 45 and older), and pelvic ultrasound. Treatment should be directed at the cause of the abnormal bleeding.
- DUB is a diagnosis of exclusion when no other source for abnormal bleeding can be identified. It is thought to be secondary to anovulation, and is therefore more prevalent in adolescents and perimenopausal woman.
- Most women with DUB can achieve menstrual regularity using a daily monophasic birth control pill, patch, ring, or by use of cyclic progestins when estrogens are contraindicated.
- In cases of acute hemorrhage, IV estrogens and high-dose oral estrogens can be used to stop acute bleeding. DUB that is not responsive to medical therapy may require surgical treatment with D&C, Mirena IUD, endometrial ablation, or, rarely, hysterectomy.
- The most common cause of postmenopausal bleeding is vaginal/endometrial atrophy. Other causes include cancer of the upper and lower genital tract, endometrial polyps, exogenous hormonal stimulation, and bleeding from nongynecologic sources.
- Postmenopausal bleeding should always be investigated to rule out endometrial hyperplasia and cancer. The evaluation of postmenopausal bleeding should include a thorough history and physical, TSH and other laboratory tests as indicated. A pelvic ultrasound should be performed to look for structural abnormalities.
- All postmenopausal women with an endometrial stripe <4mm or persistent bleeding should have an endometrial biopsy to rule out endometrial hyperplasia and cancer.

C Clinical Vignettes

Vignette 1

A 58-year-old G3P3003 Caucasian, postmenopausal woman comes to your office. She has been menopausal since age 50. She has a negative past medical and surgical history. She took hormone replacement for about 2 years but stopped due to concerns of an increased risk of cancer that she heard about from friends. Prior to the onset of menopause, she had a history of normal and regular menses. She has had annual GYN care with you, and has never been diagnosed with cervical dysplasia. Her last Pap smear with HPV was obtained last year and both were negative. She has recently become sexually active with a new partner and has noted some spotting with intercourse as well as intermittent spotting that she notices on wiping for the past 2 to 3 months associated with occasional mild lower abdominal cramping. She complains of a general feeling of vaginal dryness and does have pain and dryness with intercourse. She has no other complains what so ever.

1. Her most likely diagnosis is:
   a. endometrial cancer
   b. cervical cancer
   c. urogenital atrophy
   d. bleeding dyscrasia
   e. uterine fibroids
2. On examination, she has normal appearing external female genitalia. She has a normal appearing rectum and a fecal immunoassay test is negative for blood. On speculum examination, she has pale, thin vaginal epithelium without lesions, blood or discharge. Her cervix is pale and stenotic but without lesions. A bimanual examination reveals a small, non-tender mid-position uterus, with no adnexal masses. The most appropriate testing includes:
   a. endometrial biopsy
   b. transvaginal ultrasound
   c. STI testing (gonorrhea and chlamydia)
   d. all of the above
   e. none of the above
3. You perform an examination testing for gonorrhea and chlamydial infection as well as perform an endometrial biopsy. In addition, you order a pelvic ultrasound. STD testing is negative. Her endometrial biopsy returns with inactive, atrophic endometrium, negative for hyperplasia or malignancy. Her transvaginal ultrasound reveals a normal appearing uterus with evidence of a 2 cm intracavitary lesion consistent with an endometrial polyp. Ovaries are normal; there is no free fluid present in the peritoneal cavity. The next most appropriate step in the management of this patient is:
   a. reassurance and follow up in 1 year
   b. reassurance and follow up ultrasound in 1 year
   c. outpatient hysteroscopy D&C with polypectomy
   d. treat the urogenital atrophy with systemic or vaginal estrogens and follow up in 3 months

Vignette 2

An 18-year-old college student is referred to you due to worsening pain with her menses. She had onset of menses at age 14. She describes irregular periods until age 16 when her periods became more regular but also more painful. At this time, she is missing classes 1 or 2 days each month due to symptoms. She has tried OTC (over the counter) Midol and Tylenol without significant relief of her pain. She has a negative past medical and surgical history. She denies sexual activity, is on no medications, and has no allergies. Although she does not seem very clear about her family history, she is unaware of any significant medical conditions, heritable cancers or other conditions. She has never been pregnant and has never seen a gynecologist. She does not smoke, drink, or use alcohol or illicit drugs.

1. What is the best initial treatment for this patient?
   a. Trial of scheduled NSAIDs (nonsteroidal anti-inflammatory agents)
   b. Trial of oral contraceptive
   c. Diagnostic laparoscopy
   d. Transvaginal ultrasound
   e. endometrial ablation
2. You prescribe naproxen sodium 500 mg PO every 12 hours at onset of menses taken as a scheduled medication for the first 3 days of her period followed by prn administration. On follow up, she endorses partial relief of her symptoms. Although she is able to attend class, she continues to have significant pain for 3 to 4 days during her cycle. She also admits to being sexually active (she was afraid to discuss this at her first visits), and to using condoms infrequently. Her first sexual encounter occurred 2 months ago. At this point, what additional evaluation would you perform?
   a. Pap smear and HPV testing
   b. STI screening
   c. Transvaginal ultrasound
   d. Both options a and b
   e. Endometrial biopsy

3. The patient's screening returns as negative. An in-office pregnancy test is also negative. At this point, what would you offer to your patient for treatment of her dysmenorrhea?
   a. Continued use of NSAIDs
   b. Combination oral contraceptive pills
   c. Tranexamic acid
   d. Hydrocodone and acetaminophen
   e. Both options a and b

Vignette 3

A 35-year-old G1P0010 woman presents to your office with a concern that she has premenstrual syndrome (PMS). She states that she feels very "hormonal" most months in the week or so before her menses. She has been told that she is on edge and loses her temper easily with coworkers and at home with her family during these times. She does not feel like leaving the house or even getting dressed some days, has not been sleeping well, and is gaining weight due to overeating. Her menstrual cycles are regular; she is single and not sexually active. She has one child, born by SVD at term without complications. She recalls some depression following the delivery but was never treated and her symptoms resolved. Her past medical and surgical histories are negative. She wants to know what you can do to help her.

1. What diagnostic evaluation would you offer this patient at this visit?
   a. Reassurance and general stress reduction/healthy lifestyle tips
   b. Send her to see her PCP
   c. Ask her to fill out a symptom calendar for 2 months and return
   d. Send a CBC, TSH, and prolactin
   e. Start her on a selective serotonin reuptake inhibitor (SSRI)

2. The patient returns to your office in 2 months with a symptom calendar. Her calendar does show that her menstrual cycles are regular and occur every 30 days. She documented that her symptoms of emotional lability, sleep disturbances, "emotional eating," and decreased interest in activities are most prominent for about 10 days prior to the onset of a period, and last for 2 to 3 days into the start of period. She feels well in general for about 2 weeks although not completely symptom free on all days. Her severe symptoms begin to return 10 days prior to the next cycle. You diagnose PMS and outline her treatment options. These include:
   a. vitamin supplementation with calcium, vitamin E, vitamin B_6, and magnesium
   b. Prozac
   c. oral contraceptive Yaz
   d. exercise and relaxation techniques
   e. any of the above

3. The patient chooses to start vitamin supplements, and has taken calcium, vitamin E, vitamin B_6, and magnesium for the past 2 months, while continuing to keep a symptom calendar. You see her in follow up. She states that her symptoms prior to the onset of menses are somewhat improved but not sufficiently to allow her to feel like "herself" and to perform as she would like at work and in her home. You examine her calendar and note that she continues to have symptoms throughout the month, with rare isolated symptom-free days. At this point, what do you recommend?
   a. Stop the vitamin supplements and continue to keep a symptom calendar
   b. Continue the vitamin supplements and continue to keep a symptom calendar for 2 more months
   c. Start progesterone therapy
   d. Add an SSRI such as Prozac (dosed for PMS during the luteal phase only)
   e. Consider treatment for underlying depression

Vignette 4

A 27-year-old G0P0 woman presents to your office with a history of amenorrhea. She has a history of regular menstrual cycles in high school as well as while in college and medical school, when she began oral contraceptives for birth control. She stopped her birth control pills about 7 months ago and her period never resumed. She is sexually active with a male partner and uses condoms for contraception. She has a history of seasonal allergies, no prior surgeries, and no prior pregnancies. She has not has a Pap smear in 5 years, but has no history of dysplasia and no prior known STDs.

1. Additional significant history that you might want to ask about includes:
   a. the type/brand of oral contraception she was taking
   b. her typical diet and exercise pattern
   c. family history of amenorrhea
   d. the last time she had intercourse
   e. does she desire future fertility

2. When you question her about her general diet and activity, she states that she is a vegetarian. She is a resident, so often eats on the run or skips meals but does eat one to two meals per day and has no prior history of an eating disorder. She exercises when she can, about one to two times per week. She typically jogs or goes for a walk with her dog. Her BMI is elevated at 30. Which of the following tests are most appropriate to order at this visit?
   a. TSH, prolactin, and β-hCG
   b. 17-OH progesterone, DHEAS, and testosterone
   c. Transvaginal ultrasound
   d. Hysterosalpingogram to look for intrauterine adhesions
   e. All of the above

3. Her pregnancy tests as well as tests for thyroid and prolactin disorders are all negative. She has an elevated fasting insulin as well a high normal fasting glucose. Her androgens (testosterone and DHEAS) are elevated, but not in the range that you would be concerned for an androgen-producing tumor. You make a diagnosis of PCOS. You discuss the importance of a continued healthy balanced diet (and watching that she limits simple carbohydrate intake) as well as continued regular exercise. Additional appropriate treatment includes adding the following:
   a. Oral contraceptives
   b. Glucophage (Metformin)
   c. Mirena IUD
   d. Weight reduction
   e. Any of the above

A Answers

Vignette 1 Question 1

Answer C: Urogenital atrophy refers to changes in the epithelium of the lower urinary and genital tract as systemic levels of estrogen decline, as is seen in menopause. There is a thinning of the epithelium that can cause fragility, decreased compliance, and abrasions or tearing sufficient to cause clinically evident bleeding.

Endometrial cancer is the most common gynecological cancer in the United States. Although there are well-known associations and risk factors including anovulation, obesity, nulliparity, HTN and DM, a second subset of women with endometrial cancer lack these associated risks. This patient has no historical risks that place her at increased risk of endometrial cancer. Additionally, she does give symptoms that correlate with urogenital atrophy including general dryness and pain with intercourse.

Cervical cancer is similarly unlikely in a woman with a life-long history of normal findings on Pap smear (cervical cytology) and more recently, HPV testing. With a negative Pap smear and HPV test in the prior 12 months, the chance of a clinically relevant cervical lesion is so low, that our current screening guidelines do not recommend repeat testing for 5 years.

While it is possible for uterine fibroids to cause such symptoms, she has no history of fibroids and fibroids often shrink in response to decreased estrogen levels during menopause. Although hormonal replacement therapy can cause fibroids to grow, they typically do not cause clinical symptoms in menopause.

This patient has no prior past medical history of a bleeding disorder, and no additional history suggesting this diagnosis currently (frequent nose bleeds, bleeding gums, easy bruising). Although it is appropriate to consider in the differential diagnosis, it would be less likely that urogenital atrophy.

Vignette 1 Question 2

Answer D: In this case scenario, it is appropriate to consider all of the diagnostic tests listed. Postmenopausal bleeding is always pathological. Although not always neoplastic or cancerous, all occurrences of postmenopausal bleeding do need to be thoroughly evaluated.

Transvaginal ultrasound is appropriate to evaluate for structural lesions of the cervix, uterus, or adnexa including endometrial polyps, fibroids, and ovarian cysts or tumors. The endometrial thickness (EMS) can also be measured and reported. An EMS of less than or equal to 4 mm in a woman not taking hormone replacement is less likely to be associated with endometrial hyperplasia or malignancy, while an EMS of greater than 4 mm is associated with an increased risk of endometrial abnormalities. In women with an EMS greater than 4 mm and those with persistent postmenopausal bleeding, endometrial sampling with office-based endometrial biopsy or dilation and curettage is needed to rule out endometrial hyperplasia or cancer.

Any woman who is sexually active should undergo basic screening that includes a risk assessment for the acquisition of sexually transmitted infections including HIV on an annual basis. In this patient with a new sexual partner, STI testing is appropriate. Cervicitis from chlamydial infection or gonorrhea can cause irregular vaginal bleeding.

Vignette 1 Question 3

Answer C: Endometrial polyps are common, often benign neoplasms arising from the endometrial cavity. Although they are most commonly identified in women of reproductive age, they can present well into the menopausal years. While the clinical course of smaller polyps may include spontaneous regression in younger women, the finding of endometrial polyps in postmenopausal women is of sufficient concern and risk to recommend removal for patients who are candidates for an outpatient surgical procedure. It is possible to find endometrial hyperplasia or cancer in the base of an otherwise benign-appearing endometrial polyp.

Although this patient clearly has symptoms and physical findings associated with urogenital atrophy, the addition of exogenous estrogens is contraindicated in any woman with unexplained vaginal bleeding. Moreover, urogenital atrophy is not an indication for systemic HRT. Following polypectomy, she would likely benefit from low-dose vaginal estrogen to treat her atrophy.

Vignette 2 Question 1

Answer A: This patient's clinical presentation is classic for primary dysmenorrhea. Often, women begin to experience pain with menses in the late teens and early twenties as cycles become ovulatory. Nonsteroidal anti-inflammatory medications are considered first-line treatment for primary dysmenorrhea particularly in women who do not otherwise need contraception.

If the patient was at risk for pregnancy, or one whose pain is not controlled with NSAIDs, contraceptive steroids (pills, patch or ring) would also be a good choice. In addition to inhibiting ovulation, OCPs limit the growth of endometrial tissue and secondarily limit the production of prostaglandin in endometrial tissue. With such a straightforward history, neither pelvic ultrasound nor laparoscopy are warranted at this time. Endometrial ablation is used to treat menorrhagia in patients who have completed childbearing. It would be contraindicated in this case.

Vignette 2 Question 2

Answer B: Annual STI screening in indicated in all sexually active women <_ 24 years of age (<_ is for greater than equal to sign). Current recommendations for cervical screening with cytology include first Pap smear at age 21 regardless of the age of first intercourse. Previous recommendations to start at age 21 or 3 years from the first sexual intercourse have now been dropped. In this patient who is 18-year-old, a Pap smear is not indicated. Although she has only had a partial response to the trial of NSAIDs, as long as there are no obvious abnormalities on physical examination, it is not yet necessary to consider imaging. An endometrial biopsy (EMB) is generally reserved for ruling out endometrial hyperplasia and cancer in women 45 years or older and who have abnormal uterine bleeding. There is no indication for EMB in this patient. Most providers would consider an alternate first-line medication prior to conducting a more in-depth evaluation.

Vignette 2 Question 3

Answer E: Given that the patient is in need of contraception and needs additional management of her dysmenorrhea, a trial of oral contraceptives is an ideal option. This can be used alone or in combination with NSAIDs. Given that she has had only partial relief of her symptoms with a trial of NSAIDs, using both might provide her with greater relief. Hydrocodone (Lortab, Vicodin, Norco) is a potentially addictive opioid analgesic and is not indicated for the routine treatment of dysmenorrhea. These medications should be reserved for the short-term treatment of severe pain. Tranexamic acid is an antifibrinolytic agent used to treat menorrhagia. It is not indicated in the treatment of dysmenorrhea.

Vignette 3 Question 1

Answer C: This patient is presenting with symptoms that are interfering with her activities of daily living and appear to be affecting her overall quality of life, so evaluation and considering treatment options is appropriate for her. While general counseling regarding healthy lifestyle is important and may be helpful to women with a diagnosis of PMS, the severity of symptoms in this patient's presentation warrants a more assertive approach. This initial evaluation is within the scope of an OB/GYN provider.

Given the timing of symptoms relative to her menses, PMS is high on the differential. Diagnosis relies upon demonstrating that symptoms worsen in the luteal phase (1 to 2 weeks prior to the onset of menses), and resolve completely with the start or shortly following the onset of menses. This is the most common way that a provider can differentiate between PMS and an underlying mood disorder such as anxiety or depression.

PMS is a clinical diagnosis based upon analysis of a patient's symptoms and signs. There are no laboratory tests that support the diagnosis. While SSRIs have been very effective in the treatment of PMS and other conditions, further evaluation of this patient is needed before starting medications.

Vignette 3 Question 2

Answer D: The etiology of PMS is largely unknown and is likely due to a combination of physiological, psychological, and other causes. No single treatment is known, and dozens have been suggested, some of which work for some women but not in all. Reviews of PMS treatment studies have identified a few agents that appear to significantly decrease symptoms associated with PMS. Studies have shown that the use of SSRIs such as Prozac, Paxil, Celexa, and Zoloft are effective for treating both the physical as well as mood symptoms associated with PMS. Prozac is FDA approved for this use.

Older studies do not show OCPs to be effective in treating PMS symptoms. However, newer formulations using the progestin drospirenone (a spironolactone with antimineralocorticoid and antiandrogenic activity) and a 4-day rather than 7-day pill-free interval has been shown to be effective in the treatment of PMS.

Several studies have shown that the use of vitamin supplements including high-dose calcium, vitamin D, vitamin E, vitamin B_6, and magnesium are effective in the treatment of PMS. In small studies, exercise and relaxation techniques have been shown to decrease PMS symptoms.

Vignette 3 Question 3

Answer E: If following 2 months of treatment with vitamin supplementation the patient does not see improvement of symptoms, additional time with this treatment plan is unlikely to work. Similarly, abandoning treatment would not help when the patient continues to complain of significant symptoms. In the past, progesterone was commonly used for the treatment of PMS. However, studies show that they are no more effective than placebo. They are no longer used in the management of PMS. Considering another therapeutic approach with a SSRI is an option; however, there is an additional clue in the patient's presentation at this visit. Review of the symptom calendar reveals that she is having symptoms throughout the cycle and no longer appears to have complete resolution of symptoms following onset of a period. In light of this new information, it is appropriate to revisit the initial diagnosis and consider an underlying mood disorder such as depression. While medications in the SSRI category are very effective in the treatment of mood disorders, to treat mood disorders, they must be given on a daily basis and not limited to the luteal phase as is often done in the treatment of PMS.

Vignette 4 Question 1

Answer B: A common cause of amenorrhea in young women is hypothalamic hypogonadism, which is seen most frequently in athletes who engage in vigorous daily exercise as well as in women with eating disorders including anorexia and bulimia. Inquiring about her daily exercise and diet is the most correct answer in this situation.

Although it is important to obtain a thorough history of all medications including type and dose of oral contraceptives in this patient, any of the OCPs can induce "postpill amenorrhea," which can last for up to 6 months following discontinuation.

Family history, as well, is an important part of any new-patient evaluation. Amenorrhea is not strictly known to be a heritable condition. Some causes of amenorrhea, such as PCOS, can be seen to run in families. Knowing that there are other women in this patient's family that are affected by amenorrhea would not alter the course of this patient's evaluation.

Obtaining a detailed sexual history including use of hormonal and barrier contraceptives, the frequency of intercourse, number or partners, their gender as well as the timing of most recent exposure is an important part of all gynecologic evaluations. In a woman with oligo/amenorrhea and who is sexually active, a pregnancy test is always indicated regardless of the timing of her most recent intercourse as bleeding patterns can be unreliable in determining if a given woman is pregnant.

Vignette 4 Question 2

Answer A: In this patient, you are suspicious for anovulation due to her history of amenorrhea following discontinuation of her oral contraceptives. The most common etiologies for anovulation include PCOS, pregnancy, hypo- or hyperthyroidism, and hyperprolactinemia. 17-OH progesterone, DHEAS, and testosterone are typically used to look for causes of hirsutism. In this case, she is not hirsute and these tests would not be indicated at this point.

Because she has a history of regular spontaneous menses prior to the initiation of oral contraceptives, she is unlikely to have a structural or congenital defect (absence of a uterus or ovaries, imperforate hymen, or vaginal septum). An ultrasound can be used in supporting a diagnosis of PCOS by identifying multiple immature ovarian follicles ("string of pearls"); however, it is not sufficient nor is it required to diagnose the condition. An ultrasound might be used later in the evaluation of this patient but is not an appropriate initial test. Similarly, with a history of prior normal menses, and no intervening pregnancy, trauma, surgery or infection, it would be unusual to have a diagnosis of intrauterine adhesions.

Vignette 4 Question 3

Answer D: In women with PCOS, chronic anovulation often results in oligomenorrhea or amenorrhea, with occasional, irregular episodes of bleeding that can be heavy and prolonged. Prolonged stimulation of the endometrium by estrogen without regular exposure to progesterone (at ovulation) can lead to endometrial hyperplasia as well as endometrial cancer. The choice of a treatment modality depends upon a woman's current desire for contraception. If hoping to become pregnant, we prescribe medication to induce ovulation such as clomiphene citrate or Glucophage. In addition to these medications, general counseling about weight loss is important, as a reduction in BMI alone can lead to a resumption of normal ovulation and regular menses. Weight loss has also been shown to improve insulin resistance, hirsutism, and hyperlipidemia.

In women who desire contraception, options include combination OCPs, as well as progestin-only methods such as the Mirena IUD, progestin-only pills, Implanon, or Depo-Provera. Exposure to progesterone in a cyclic or continuous fashion will protect the endometrium from developing hyperplasia. Caution should be taken with the use of Depo-Provera and possibly Implanon because these agents have been associated with weight gain (in women with a predisposition to gain weight) and may not be the best choice in the overall treatment of obese women with PCOS. Another option in women who do not need contraception, but are not trying to become pregnant is the use of intermittent progestins administered for 12 to 14 days per month to induce regular bleeding and protect the endometrium from hyperplasia and cancer.

Chapter

23 Hirsutism and Virilism

Adults have two types of hair: vellus and terminal. Vellus hair is nonpigmented and soft, and covers the entire body. Terminal hair is, on the other hand, pigmented and thick, and covers the scalp, axilla, and pubic area. Androgens are responsible for the conversion of vellus to terminal hair at puberty, resulting in pubic and axillary hair. An abnormal increase in terminal hair is due to androgen excess or increased 5α-reductase activity; this enzyme converts testosterone to the more potent dihydrotestosterone (DHT). DHT is believed to be the main stimulant of terminal hair development.

Hirsutism refers to the increase in terminal hair on the face, chest, back, lower abdomen, and inner thighs in a woman. Often, the pubic hair is characterized by the development of a male escutcheon, which is diamond shaped as opposed to the triangular female escutcheon. **Virilization** refers to the development of male features, such as deepening of the voice, frontal balding, increased muscle mass, clitoromegaly, breast atrophy, and male body habitus.

The evaluation of hirsutism and virilism in the female patient is complex and requires the understanding of pituitary, adrenal, and ovarian function with detailed attention to the pathways of glucocorticoid, mineralocorticoid, androgen, and estrogen synthesis.

NORMAL ANDROGEN SYNTHESIS

The adrenal gland is divided into two components: the adrenal cortex, which is responsible for glucocorticoid, mineralocorticoid, and androgen synthesis, and the adrenal medulla, which is involved in catecholamine synthesis. The adrenal cortex is composed of three layers. An outer **zona glomerulosa** layer produces aldosterone and is regulated primarily by the renin–angiotensin system. Because this zone lacks 17α-hydroxylase, cortisol and androgens are not synthesized. In contrast, the inner layers, the **zona fasciculata** and the **zona reticularis**, produce both cortisol and androgens but not aldosterone because they lack the enzyme **aldosterone synthase**. These two inner zones are highly regulated by adrenocorticotropic hormone (ACTH).

ACTH regulates the conversion of cholesterol to pregnenolone by hydroxylation and side-chain cleavage. Pregnenolone is then converted to progesterone and eventually to aldosterone or cortisol or shunted over to the production of sex steroids (Fig. 23-1).

In the adrenal glands, androgens are synthesized from the precursor 17α-hydroxypregnenolone, which is converted to **dehydroepiandrosterone** (DHEA) and its sulfate (DHEAS), androstenedione, and finally to testosterone. DHEA and DHEAS are the most common adrenal androgens, whereas only small amounts of the others are secreted.

In the ovaries, the theca cells are stimulated by luteinizing hormone (LH) to produce androstenedione and testosterone. Both androstenedione and testosterone are then aromatized to estrone and estradiol, respectively, by the granulosa cells in response to follicle-stimulating hormone (FSH). Elevations in the ratio of LH to FSH may therefore lead to elevated levels of androgens.

PATHOLOGIC PRODUCTION OF ANDROGENS

Elevation of androgens can be due primarily to adrenal or ovarian disorders. Because synthesis of steroid hormones in the adrenal cortex is stimulated by ACTH at a nondifferentiated step, elevated ACTH levels increase all the steroid hormones, including the androgens. If enzymatic defects are present, the precursor proximal to the defect accumulates and is shunted to another pathway. Thus, enzymatic blockade of either cortisol or aldosterone synthesis can lead to increased androgen production. Because DHEAS is derived almost entirely from the adrenal glands, its elevation is used as a marker for adrenal androgen production.

In the ovary, any increase in LH or in the LH:FSH ratio appears to lead to excess androgen production. Further, tumors of both the adrenal gland and the ovary can lead to excess androgens. Regardless of the source, elevated androgens lead to hirsutism and possibly virilism.

ADRENAL DISORDERS

The adrenal disorders leading to virilization in a woman are divided into two categories: nonneoplastic and neoplastic etiologies. Androgen-producing adrenal tumors may be either adenomas or carcinomas. Adrenal adenomas typically cause glucocorticoid excess and virilizing symptoms are rare. Carcinomas, on the other hand, can be more rapidly progressive and lead to marked elevations in glucocorticoid, mineralocorticoid, and androgen steroids.

CUSHING SYNDROME

Cushing syndrome is characterized by excess production of cortisol. Because the intermediates in production are androgens, there will be a concomitant hyperandrogenic state. Cushing syndrome may be caused by pituitary adenoma, ectopic sources of ACTH, and tumors of the adrenal gland. The most common cause of Cushing syndrome (other than exogenous glucocorticoid intake) is **Cushing's disease, which refers to a** pituitary adenoma that hypersecretes ACTH. Paraneoplastic syndromes, such as nonpituitary ACTH-secreting tumors, may also lead to increased ACTH levels. Adrenal gland tumors usually result in decreased levels of ACTH secondary to the negative feedback from the increased levels of adrenal steroid hormones. All three of these situations lead to the glucocorticoid excess characteristic of Cushing syndrome, as well as hirsutism, acne, and menstrual irregularities related to adrenal androgen production.

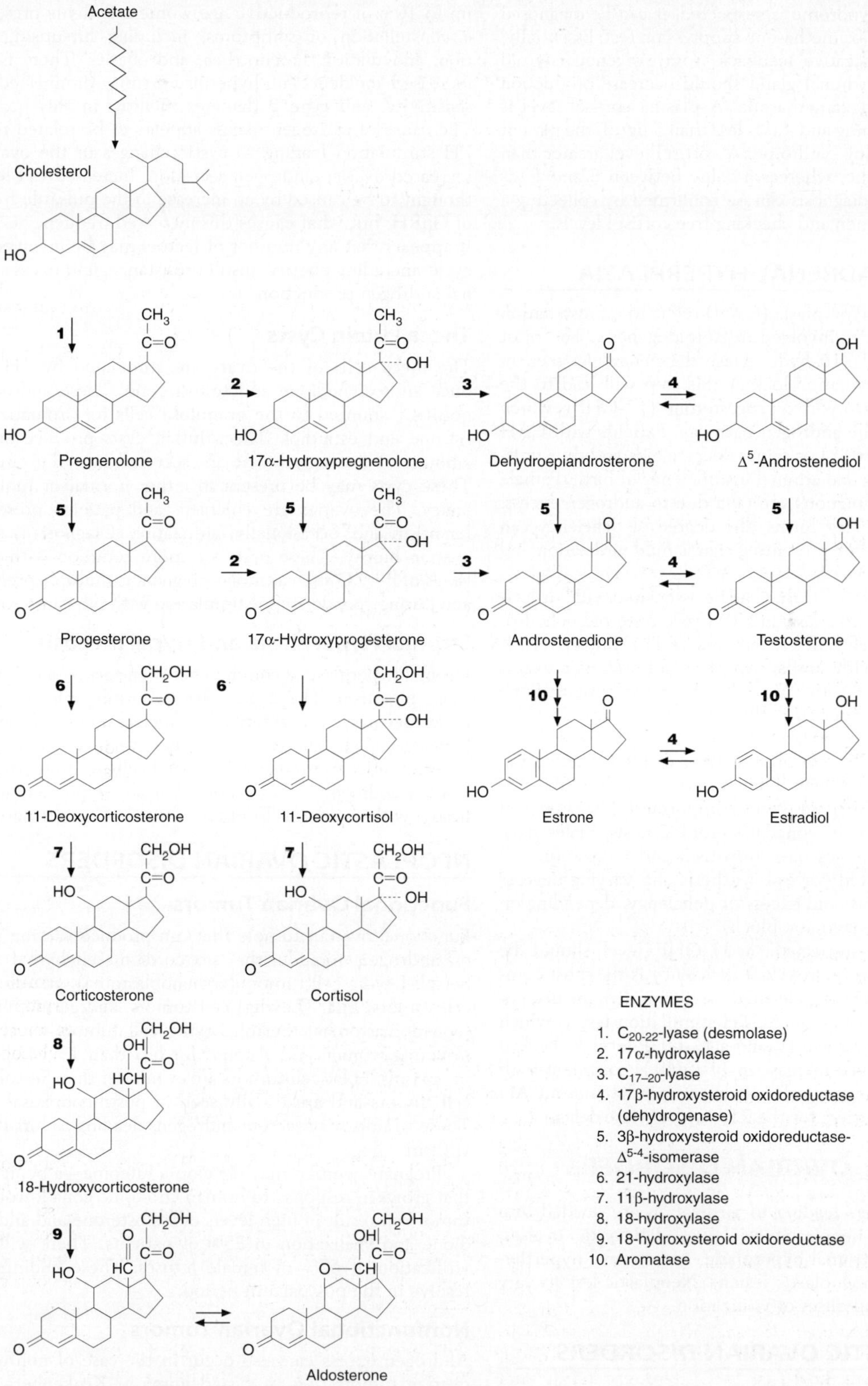

Figure 23-1 • Biosynthesis of androgens, estrogens, and corticosteroids.
(Reproduced with permission from Mishell DR, Davajan V, Lobo RA. *Infertility, Contraception, and Reproductive Endocrinology*, 3rd ed. Cambridge, MA: Blackwell Science; 1991.)

When Cushing syndrome is suspected, it can be diagnosed with the overnight dexamethasone suppression test. Essentially, if there is normal negative feedback from exogenous steroid hormone, then the adrenal gland should decrease production in response to the dexamethasone. A plasma cortisol level is drawn the next morning and if it is less than 5 μg/dL the patient does not have Cushing syndrome. A cortisol level greater than 10 μg/dL is diagnostic, whereas a value between 5 and 10 is indeterminate. The diagnosis can be confirmed by collecting a 24-hour urine specimen and checking free cortisol levels.

CONGENITAL ADRENAL HYPERPLASIA

Congenital adrenal hyperplasia (CAH) refers to a constellation of enzyme deficiencies involved in steroidogenesis. The most common disorder is 21α-hydroxylase deficiency. As seen in Figure 23-1, an enzymatic block at this step will lead to the accumulation of 17α-hydroxyprogesterone (17-OHP), which is then shunted to the androgen pathway. Patients with CAH do not synthesize cortisol or mineralocorticoids and thus present with salt wasting and adrenal insufficiency at birth. Female infants will have ambiguous genitalia due to androgen excess. In milder or adult-onset forms, the degree of deficiency can vary, and often the only presenting sign is mild virilization and menstrual irregularities.

The other types of CAH that can be associated with virilization include 11β-hydroxylase and 3β-hydroxysteroid dehydrogenase (3β-HSD) deficiencies. Patients with 11β-hydroxylase deficiency present with similar symptoms of androgen excess as accumulated precursors are shunted to androstenedione and testosterone production pathways. Patients with 3β-HSD deficiency actually accumulate DHEA because they are unable to convert pregnenolone to progesterone or DHEA down the androgen synthesis pathway. DHEA and its sulfate, DHEAS, both have mild androgenic effects. Importantly, because this defect is also present in gonadal steroidogenesis, males have feminization and females have hirsutism and virilization. All patients have impaired cortisol synthesis and varying degrees of either mineralocorticoid excess or deficiency, depending on the location of the enzymatic block.

When CAH is suspected, a 17-OHP level should be checked because 21α-hydroxylase deficiency is the most common etiology. If 17-OHP is elevated (>200 ng/dL), the diagnosis can be confirmed with an ACTH stimulation test in which Cortrosyn (ACTH) is given IV and a 17-OHP level is checked after 1 hour. A marked increase in 17-OHP is consistent with CAH, with lower elevated values being seen in late-onset CAH and heterozygote carriers for the 21α-hydroxylase deficiency.

FUNCTIONAL OVARIAN DISORDERS

The ovarian disorders leading to virilization are divided into nonneoplastic and neoplastic etiologies. Polycystic ovaries, theca lutein cysts, stromal hyperplasia, and stromal hyperthecosis all involve nonneoplastic lesions. Neoplastic lesions vary and often cause rapid onset of virilization.

NONNEOPLASTIC OVARIAN DISORDERS

Polycystic Ovarian Syndrome

Polycystic ovarian syndrome (PCOS), previously known as the Stein-Leventhal syndrome, is a common disorder affecting up to 10% of reproductive age women. Patients present with a constellation of symptoms, including hirsutism, virilization, anovulation, amenorrhea, and obesity. There is also an increased incidence of hyperinsulinemia, diminished insulin sensitivity, and type 2 diabetes mellitus in this population. The cause of androgen excess appears to be related to excess LH stimulation leading to cystic changes in the ovaries and increased ovarian androgen secretion. Increased LH levels are thought to be caused by an increase in the pulsatile frequency of GnRH, but what causes this increased frequency is unclear. It appears that any number of factors may be involved in this cycle, including obesity, insulin resistance, and excessive adrenal androgen production.

Theca Lutein Cysts

The **theca cells** of the ovary are stimulated by LH to produce androstenedione and testosterone. These androgens are normally shunted to the **granulosa cells** for aromatization to estrone and estradiol. Theca lutein cysts produce an excess amount of androgens that are secreted into the circulation. These cysts may be present in either normal or molar pregnancy. The ovaries are enlarged, and patients present with hirsutism and, occasionally, virilization. Diagnosis is made by ovarian biopsy. These cysts are more common with elevated levels of β-hCG such as molar pregnancy, multiple pregnancies, and during gonadotropin stimulation with infertility treatment.

Stromal Hyperplasia and Hyperthecosis

Stromal hyperplasia is common between ages 50 and 70 and can cause hirsutism. The ovaries are uniformly enlarged. **Stromal hyperthecosis** is characterized by foci of utilization within the hyperplastic stroma. It is more likely than simple hyperplasia to result in virilization as the utilized cells continue to produce ovarian androgens. The ovaries typically appear enlarged and fleshy, with the more florid cases seen in younger patients.

NEOPLASTIC OVARIAN DISORDERS

Functional Ovarian Tumors

Functional ovarian tumors that can produce varying amounts of androgen include the sex-cord mesenchymal tumors, Sertoli-Leydig cell tumors (arrhenoblastoma), granulosa-theca cell tumors, hilar (Leydig) cell tumors, and germ cell tumors (gonadoblastomas). Sertoli-Leydig cell tumors usually occur in young women and account for less than 1% of all ovarian neoplasms. Hilar cell tumors are even rarer than Sertoli-Leydig cell tumors and are usually seen in postmenopausal women. These tumors may secrete androgens, leading to hirsutism and virilism.

Pregnant women may develop a luteoma—a benign tumor that grows in response to human chorionic gonadotropin. This tumor can result in high levels of testosterone and androstenedione and virilization in 25% of patients. There will also be virilization of 65% of female fetuses. These findings should resolve in the postpartum period.

Nonfunctional Ovarian Tumors

Androgen excess can also occur in the case of nonfunctional ovarian tumors (e.g., a cystadenoma or Krukenberg tumor). Although these tumors do not secrete androgens themselves, they do stimulate proliferation in the adjacent ovarian stroma, which in turn may lead to increased androgen production.

DRUGS AND EXOGENOUS HORMONES

A variety of drugs can affect the circulating levels of sex hormone binding globulin (SHBG). SHBG is one of the major proteins that bind circulating testosterone, leaving a small proportion of free testosterone to interact at the cellular level. Androgens and corticosteroids decrease SHBG, leaving a greater percentage of free testosterone circulating. Patients who use anabolic steroids often present with hirsutism and virilization. In addition, drugs such as minoxidil, phenytoin, diazoxide, and cyclosporin will cause hirsutism without using androgenic pathways.

IDIOPATHIC HIRSUTISM

Hirsutism is considered idiopathic in the absence of adrenal or ovarian pathology, an exogenous source of androgens, or use of the above-listed drugs. Patients may actually have occult androgen production, but many will have normal circulating androgen levels. There may be an increase in peripheral androgen production due to elevated 5α-reductase activity at the level of the skin and hair follicles.

Clinical Manifestations

A detailed history including time of onset, progression, and symptoms of virilization/hirsutism should be obtained, as well as a pubertal, menstrual, and reproductive history. Because various medications can affect androgen levels by affecting SHBG or intrinsic androgenic activity, a detailed drug history should be obtained. A family history is also important in order to look for genetic disorders such as CAH.

Physical Examination

On physical examination, the hair pattern should be noted, with attention to facial, chest, back, abdominal, and inner thigh hair, as well as the presence of frontal balding. The body habitus and presence or absence of female contours should be described. Breast examination may reveal atrophic changes, and a careful pelvic examination should include inspection of the escutcheon (pattern of pubic hair), clitoris (for clitoromegaly), and palpation for ovarian masses. Cushingoid features should be ruled out and inspection for acanthosis nigricans (velvety, thickened hyperpigmentation) in the axilla and nape of the neck should be performed because this dermatologic finding is often associated with polycystic ovary syndrome.

Diagnostic Evaluation

Laboratory evaluation should include free testosterone, 17-OHP, and DHEA-S, the latter of which is normally exclusive to the adrenal gland. An elevation in free testosterone confirms androgen excess and a concomitant elevation in DHEAS suggests an adrenal source. An elevated 17-OHP is suggestive of CAH. If an adrenal source is suspected, an abdominal CT should be performed to rule out an adrenal tumor, as well as further tests to diagnose Cushing syndrome or CAH.

If the DHEA-S is normal or minimally elevated, an ovarian source should be considered and a pelvic ultrasound or CT should be performed to rule out an ovarian neoplasm. An elevation in the LH:FSH ratio greater than 3 is suggestive of PCOS. However, most obstetrician-gynecologists do not diagnose PCOS with the LH:FSH ratio any longer. Rather, polycystic ovary syndrome is a diagnosis of exclusion when two out of the three Rotterdam criteria are met: secondary amenorrhea/oligomenorrhea, evidence of hyperandrogenism, or evidence of polycystic ovaries as assessed by ultrasound.

Rapid onset of virilization and testosterone levels >200 ng/dL may indicate an ovarian neoplasm. At times the source of androgen excess is not readily evident and further diagnostic tests such as abdominal MRI and selective venous sampling need to be done for localization. In the hirsute woman with normal free testosterone, an assay for 5α-reductase activity is performed to determine whether increased peripheral enzymatic activity is responsible for the development of hirsutism.

Treatment

Adrenal nonneoplastic androgen suppression can be achieved with glucocorticoid administration, such as prednisone 5 mg qhs. Finasteride inhibits the 5α-reductase enzyme, thus diminishing peripheral conversion of testosterone to DHT. Antiandrogens such as spironolactone have been helpful as well, but are temporizing at best. In the case of ovarian or adrenal tumors, the underlying disorder should be treated. Often surgical intervention is required.

In general, ovarian nonneoplastic androgen production can be suppressed with oral contraceptives that will suppress LH and FSH as well as increase SHBG. Progesterone therapy alone may help patients with contraindications to estrogen use. Progesterone decreases levels of LH and thus androgen production; further, the catabolism of testosterone is increased, resulting in decreased levels. Gonadotropin-releasing hormone (GnRH) agonists can also be used to suppress LH and FSH. However, this leads to a hypoestrogenic state and requires concomitant estrogen replacement.

Patients using exogenous androgens or other drugs leading to increased androgens or hair growth should be advised to discontinue use. For patients with idiopathic hirsutism or contraindications to hormonal use, waxing, depilatories, and electrolysis will often provide cosmetic improvement.

KEY POINTS

- Hirsutism is excess hair growth with a male pattern on the face, back, chest, abdomen, and inner thighs, usually in response to excess androgens.
- Virilism is a constellation of symptoms including hirsutism, deepening of the voice, frontal balding, clitoromegaly, and increased musculature.
- Primary causes of hirsutism and virilization include PCOS, ovarian tumors, adrenal tumors, CAH, and Cushing syndrome.
- Diagnosis is made by history and physical, serum assays for testosterone, DHEAS, and 17-OHP, and imaging studies.
- Management involves primary treatment for the underlying cause; hormonal therapy with OCPs, GnRH, or progestins; and cosmetic treatment of hirsutism.

C Clinical Vignettes

Vignette 1

A 16-year-old female presents to your office with her mother, who is concerned that she is pregnant. Over the past 3 months, the patient and her mother have noticed a swelling in her lower abdomen. The patient notes a sensation of fullness, and occasional left lower pelvic pain. The patient reports that she does have a male partner, but they have not yet been sexually intimate. She reports irregular menses over the past 6 months, but thought it was secondary to stress. She has noted increased hair over her chin and breasts, and her acne seems to have worsened and spread onto her chest and back, whereas it used to be only on her face. Her mother attributes this to "normal puberty stuff." She is otherwise healthy, with no other known medical problems or prior surgeries. She is normotensive, and vital signs are normal. On physical examination, you notice a few dark colored hairs over her upper lip, and several beneath her chin. Her breast development is normal. Pelvic examination reveals a prominent, enlarged clitoris and bimanual examination reveals a 17-cm, mobile, smooth left adnexal mass. An in-office urine pregnancy test is negative.

1. What set of laboratory tests would you first perform to aid in your diagnosis?
   a. Serum testosterone and DHEA-S
   b. TSH, free T4
   c. 24-hour urine collection for metanephrines
   d. Plasma aldosterone and renin
2. Your laboratory tests confirm your suspicions, and you perform a pelvic ultrasound, which reveals a $15 \times 16 \times 17$ cm^3 solid left ovarian mass. Which of the following is the most likely diagnosis?
   a. Polycystic ovary syndrome
   b. Sertoli-Leydig cell tumor
   c. Luteoma of pregnancy
   d. Cushing syndrome
3. You opt to proceed with excision of her left adnexal mass. What procedure do you recommend?
   a. Total abdominal hysterectomy, bilateral salpingo-oophorectomy and staging procedure
   b. Total abdominal hysterectomy, bilateral salpingo-oophorectomy with intraoperative frozen section followed by staging
   c. Laparotomy, left ovarian cystectomy and possible oophorectomy with intraoperative frozen section
   d. Neoadjuvant chemotherapy
4. Another patient presents for her 18-week anatomy ultrasound. She is a 19-year-old African American G1P0 who has had an uncomplicated pregnancy. On your ultrasound, you find normal fetal anatomy in a female appearing fetus. However, you do note bilateral 6 cm masses that appear homogenous. You suspect bilateral ovarian luteomas and perform serum testing of the mother, which reveals elevated testosterone and androstenedione. A subsequent examination of the patient reveals evidence of hirsutism. The patient shrugs and states, "I thought that was normal in pregnancy." What obstetric and perinatal complication is her fetus at risk for?
   a. Pre-eclampsia
   b. Abruption
   c. Virilization of the fetus
   d. Preterm premature rupture of membranes (PPROM)

Vignette 2

A 31-year-old obese woman presents to your office for an infertility consultation. She and her husband have been attempting pregnancy for the preceding 18 months. She states that her menses are irregular, occurring every 25 to 47 days, and sometimes she skips menses altogether. They are sometimes heavy, other times light with just brown spotting. She notes that her menses have always been this way, ever since menarche at age 12. She denies any history of sexually transmitted infections and her husband has proven paternity with a previous wife. She notes that she has never been pregnant. On further questioning, she admits to plucking and shaving excessive hair from her chin, around her navel, and on her lateral thigh. She also admits to bothersome acne and extreme difficulty with weight loss. Physical examination reveals obesity with BMI 31, normal breast development, and presence of excessive hair as described by the patient. Pelvic examination reveals normal external genitalia and unremarkable bimanual examination.

1. What additional information do you need to make your diagnosis?
   a. Day 3 serum FSH and estradiol
   b. Pelvic ultrasound
   c. Serum testosterone, DHEA-S, and prolactin
   d. None of the above
2. What test might you perform to determine whether this patient is ovulatory in any given month?
   a. Urinary ovulation predictor kits
   b. Day 3 progesterone
   c. Day 28 progesterone
   d. Luteal phase endometrial biopsy

3. The patient is grateful to have a syndrome to explain her symptoms; however, she is anxious to hear what you may offer to her in terms of fertility treatment—getting pregnant is all she can really think about now. In addition to starting a prenatal vitamin with folic acid, you recommend:
   a. Attempted weight loss with a sensible diet and regular vigorous exercise
   b. Insulin therapy
   c. Clomiphene citrate ovulation induction
   d. In vitro fertilization
   e. a and c
   f. a, b, and c
   g. a, b, and d

4. Your patient goes on to successfully conceive a pregnancy and delivers a healthy baby boy. During her 6-week postpartum visit, you discuss birth control options. Which of the following contraceptive choices will improve her symptoms of hirsutism and acne?
   a. Condoms
   b. Depo-Provera
   c. Levonorgestrel intrauterine device
   d. Combined estrogen and progestin contraceptive pill

5. Two years later, your patient returns to your clinic for her annual examination. She is now 35 years old and mentions to you that she decided to use condoms for the past few years because she did not like the oral birth control pills you suggested. She admits to very heavy menstrual flow over the past year (lasting 8 days and filling 10 pads on 5 of the 8 days), and her menses continue to be irregular. She has not lost much of her "baby weight" after her delivery and currently has a BMI of 36. She is unsure if she desires more children in the future. You again discuss birth control and suggest the placement of a levonorgestrel IUD, which the patient accepts. What further testing or evaluation would you recommend for her at this time?
   a. Glucose tolerance test, fasting lipid screening test
   b. Thyroid function testing and complete blood count
   c. Endometrial biopsy and pelvic ultrasound
   d. a and b
   e. a, b, and c

Vignette 3

A patient presents to your office for a return OB visit. She is a 25-year-old G5P2204 at 20 weeks 5 days by first trimester ultrasound. She presented with symptoms of excessive weight gain, acne, abdominal and upper extremity striae, migraine headache, fatigue and muscle weakness. So far she has gained 60 lb this pregnancy without significant dietary changes. She complains of facial swelling, bruising, and "stretch marks." She reports excessive hair growth since the onset of this pregnancy and states that she has "furry cheeks, breasts, and arms." The hair is notably darker and of greater quantity than normal for her. This hair growth is also associated with significant worsening of her acne. Regarding her stretch marks—she states that in prior pregnancies, they were a whitish color, while these are purple and extremely pruritic. Migraine headaches are not new for her but worsened during this pregnancy to nearly daily episodes, whereas prior to pregnancy she had a migraine one to two times weekly. She is otherwise a healthy female with no prior history of medical illness (including history of hypertension or diabetes). Regarding her gynecologic history, she reports normal, monthly menses since menarche at age 13. On physical examination, she was noted to have an elevated systolic blood pressure of 140/90, and is tachycardic in the 110 to 120s. Fetal heart tones are 144 bpm. Physical examination confirms the above reported hirsutism, acne, bruising, and abdominal striae. Additionally, she has increased fat deposition on her posterior neck. She has a fundal height of 19 cm, and there are no pelvic masses on sterile vaginal examination.

1. You suspect Cushing syndrome. What is the first step in your workup?
   a. 24-hour urinary free cortisol excretion
   b. Late night salivary cortisol level
   c. Dexamethasone suppression test
   d. a, b, and c
   e. Plasma ACTH concentration
   f. Abdominal ultrasound

2. An ultrasound is performed and reveals an enlarged right adrenal mass, measuring 5.7 × 5.6 × 4.4 cm with well-defined margins. The radiologist tells you that the characteristics of the mass do not appear consistent with a pheochromocytoma; however, because of your patient's additional complaints of worsening headaches, and additionally her hypertension and tachycardia, you are concerned about this rare possibility. To rule out pheochromocytoma, you order the following tests:
   a. 24-hour urine protein collection
   b. Plasma metanephrines
   c. 24-hour urine metanephrines and catecholamines
   d. Complete metabolic panel

3. Another patient with a known diagnosis of Cushing syndrome secondary to chronic glucocorticoid treatment to prevent flares of her rheumatoid arthritis presents to your clinic requesting treatment for her hirsutism. She is a 32-year-old G1P1001 and had a healthy term pregnancy 3 years ago. She has already tried depilatory lotions and plucking with only mild improvement. Which therapeutic option might you offer her initially?
   a. Shaving, plucking, waxing
   b. Oral contraceptive pills
   c. Spironolactone
   d. GnRH agonists

Vignette 4

A 19-year-old female presents to your clinic with her mother for evaluation regarding possible vaginoplasty. She has classic "salt wasting" congenital adrenal hyperplasia and has been moderately controlled with her pediatric endocrinologist. She is controlled on fludrocortisone and prednisone daily. When she was 18 months old, she underwent a U-flap vaginoplasty and clitoroplasty for ambiguous genitalia, which is now stenotic because of lack of use. She reports oligomenorrhea with menses approximately every 4 months. She does have some anxiety, for which she has seen a counselor every 2 weeks regarding anxiety as well as her sexuality. She reports that at this point in her life, she has had relationships with both men and women, and is equally attracted to both. However, she and her mother feel that her lack of a normal vagina inhibits her ability to be fully intimate with a male, therefore inhibiting her from fully exploring her sexuality. On physical examination, the patient is well appearing, with normal breast development. She has a muscular build and is noted to have multiple bruises on her body. Pelvic examination is notable for a prominent clitoris. A normal appearing anus is noted. Between the clitoris and rectum there is a single small opening which is a urogenital sinus, allowing efflux of both menstrual flow and urine. No additional vaginal opening is present. Rectal examination confirms the presence of a uterus.

1. Which protein is deficient in a patient with classic "salt wasting" congenital adrenal hyperplasia?
   a. 21-hydroxylase
   b. 11β-hydroxylase

c. 3β-hydroxysteroid dehydrogenase
d. Aromatase
e. None of the above

2. Your physical examination and a bedside ultrasound confirm the presence of a uterus and ovaries. The presence of a normal appearing uterus and tubes is surprising, given this patient's clitoromegaly and absent lower vagina. However, this is embryologically explained by the fact that females with congenital adrenal hyperplasia have:
   a. Testicles and concomitant development of the uterus and tubes
   b. Ovaries and the lack of testicular derived Mullerian-inhibiting substance
   c. Absent Sertoli cells
   d. Absent 5α-reductase enzyme, which prevents synthesis of DHT

3. What is the most likely reason this patient is having oligomenorrhea?
   a. Oligo-ovulation secondary to polycystic ovary syndrome
   b. Premature ovarian failure
   c. Exercise-induced hypothalamic hypogonadotropic hypogonadism
   d. Inadequate glucocorticoid therapy, leading to relative hyperandrogenemia

4. You decide to proceed with surgical intervention and trial of vaginoplasty. What serious complication is she at risk for during the procedure?
   a. Intractable hemorrhage
   b. Sudden cardiac death
   c. Adrenal crisis
   d. Cerebrovascular accident
   e. Disseminated intravascular coagulopathy (DIC)

A Answers

Vignette 1 Question 1

Answer A: Although each of these tests may be helpful, the first set of testing you should consider is a serum testosterone and DHEA-S, both of which are measurements of serum androgen. If testosterone is elevated, this confirms androgen excess. A DHEA-S level assists with determining if the source of the androgens is adrenal in origin.

Thyroid testing is not helpful in this setting given that the patient has signs and symptoms of virilization rather than hypothyroidism or hyperthyroidism. Because the patient does not display evidence of hypercortisolism, the 24-hour urine collection and plasma aldosterone and renin are not likely to be helpful.

Vignette 1 Question 2

Answer B: The presence of an adnexal mass on examination and the absence of pregnancy make a Sertoli-Leydig cell tumor, although rare, the most likely diagnosis. These are sex-cord stromal tumors of the ovary, which may be benign or malignant. These tumors commonly secrete androgens and building blocks of androgens (testosterone, androstenedione, and 17-hydroxyprogesterone), which lead to the virilizing features seen clinically (in this case, hirsutism, acne, and clitoromegaly). Definitive diagnosis is made histologically after surgical excision of the mass.

Polycystic ovary syndrome does not typically present with an abdominal mass; the polycystic ovaries are typically multiple, small peripheral cysts instead. Luteoma may cause similar symptoms, but this would be the case in a patient with a current or recent pregnancy, neither of which fits this clinical scenario. Cushing syndrome would cause hirsutism and virilization, but typically also presents with evidence of hypercortisolism.

Vignette 1 Question 3

Answer C: Given this patient's young age, a fertility sparing procedure is ideal if possible. Knowing that Sertoli-Leydig cell tumors can be benign or malignant, you correctly elect to have a frozen section performed at the time of your procedure. Because the mass approaches 17 cm, laparoscopic removal is not possible in this case, and she needs an open procedure. You counsel your patient that the best procedure for her would be a laparotomy with left ovarian cystectomy and possible oophorectomy.

Although you should discuss with your patient before going to the operating room the possibility of finding a malignancy, in which case proceeding with hysterectomy and full staging is necessary, your goal will be to preserve her fertility. The most likely scenario is that she will have a benign neoplasm, and oophorectomy alone will be required. There is no role for neoadjuvant chemotherapy in this case.

Vignette 1 Question 4

Answer C: This patient has bilateral luteomas of pregnancy that are ovarian masses and are thought to be caused by elevated circulating levels of β-hCG. They are typically asymptomatic other than mild symptoms of maternal virilism in some but not all cases. Serum studies typically show elevated levels of circulating androgens. This fetus is at risk of virilization in utero. Typically the masses regress postpartum without need for intervention.

Pre-eclampsia, abruption, and PPROM are not known to be associated with ovarian luteomas of pregnancy.

Vignette 2 Question 1

Answer D: Multiple systems of diagnostic criteria for polycystic ovary syndrome (PCOS) have been proposed, but the most commonly used are the Rotterdam criteria, which were established in 2003. These maintain that the diagnosis of PCOS is made on the basis of meeting two out of the following three criteria: oligo/anovulation, clinical or laboratory evidence of hyperandrogenism, and polycystic ovaries on ultrasound. For the patient in this scenario, she already meets the criteria for oligo-ovulation (irregular and skipped menses) and clinical evidence of hyperandrogenism (acne, hirsutism).

Thus the addition of a pelvic ultrasound, testosterone, DHEA-S and prolactin are unnecessary to make the diagnosis. However, the knowledge of the values from these tests may rule out additional disorders and are often checked as well. Day 3 FSH and estradiol may be helpful in determining the underlying quality of her remaining oocytes in terms of her fertility, but are not necessary in making the diagnosis of PCOS.

Vignette 2 Question 2

Answer A: Because this patient's menstrual cycles have been irregular, predicting ovulatory cycles is more difficult than a patient with regular cycles. The use of daily urinary ovulation predictor kits starting at cycle day 11 or 12 can aid in predicting ovulation and timing intercourse for conception. Ovulation predictor kits detect the luteinizing hormone (LH) surge, which occurs approximately 24 to 36 hours prior to ovulation. They can unfortunately be falsely positive in patients with PCOS, however, because of elevated baseline circulating levels of LH.

Measurement of progesterone in the luteal phase may indicate that ovulation has occurred (although it will not help with predicting ovulation in order to time intercourse). In a woman with normal 28-day cycles, it is typically measured on cycle day 21, when you would expect elevated levels secondary to progesterone production by the corpus luteum after ovulation. Neither a Day 3 nor a Day 28 progesterone would be helpful. In the case of a woman with irregular menses, it is also difficult to determine the accuracy of a progesterone level, and therefore this test may be less useful in this particular case. In years past, an endometrial biopsy used to be performed to evaluate for evidence of decidualization of the endometrium as evidence of progesterone effect. This is no longer a standard procedure in the workup of anovulation as there are other, less painful, methods to determine ovulation.

Vignette 2 Question 3

Answer E: The first step in attempting to achieve pregnancy is to attempt weight loss through diet and exercise, and consider the addition of ovulation induction with clomiphene citrate (Clomid). Many women will start to ovulate spontaneously with as little as 10% weight reduction. Clomid is an anti-estrogen that increases the probability that ovulation occurs by removing the negative feedback of circulating estrogen to the brain, thereby increasing circulating levels of FSH seen by the ovary. Administration usually starts with the lowest dose, 50 mg daily starting on cycle day 3 or 5, continuing for 5 days of therapy. Patients should be counseled regarding increased risk of multiple pregnancy (secondary to multiple oocyte released in one cycle) as well as risk of ovarian hyperstimulation.

Although patients with PCOS have increased risk of diabetes, initiating insulin therapy without a diagnosis of diabetes is contraindicated. Although this patient may eventually require ovulation induction with other medications or injectable gonadotropins, in vitro fertilization is not yet indicated.

Vignette 2 Question 4

Answer D: Combined OCPs are the first-line therapy for helping to decrease circulating androgens, and may prevent progressive hirsutism and acne. This is achieved by increasing the levels of SHBG concentrations, in turn decreasing circulating free androgen levels and their stimulatory effect on hair follicles.

Condoms have no effect on SHBG and therefore would not prevent worsening or reduce current levels of circulating androgens. Depo-Provera and the levonorgestrel IUD work well to decrease heavy bleeding and for contraception, but will not be of help in reducing symptoms of hyperandrogenism.

Vignette 2 Question 5

Answer E: Provided that this patient presented today for her annual examination, and your knowledge that she meets the criteria for polycystic ovary syndrome, you astutely test her for diabetes and hyperlipidemia since you know that she is at increased risk for both of these diseases as well as cardiovascular disease. Because of her heavy menstrual flow, you opt to screen her for hypothyroidism and evaluate for the possibility of anemia. Finally, because you know she is at increased risk for endometrial hyperplasia and carcinoma from chronic anovulation and elevated levels of circulating estrogens, you recommend a pelvic ultrasound and an endometrial biopsy.

Vignette 3 Question 1

Answer D: The first step in the evaluation of this patient is to determine whether she truly meets the criteria for Cushing's syndrome, and the next is to determine the etiology. Current recommendations are to start with at least two of the three "first line" tests, which include a 24-hour urinary free cortisol test, late night salivary cortisol measurement, and a dexamethasone suppression test (DST). The urinary and salivary cortisol measurements should be obtained at least twice, and the diagnosis of Cushing's syndrome is confirmed when there are two abnormal tests. Because of the low specificity for these tests, if any of them come back equivocal, additional testing should be performed prior to confirming the diagnosis.

Plasma ACTH testing is used to determine the cause of Cushing's syndrome after the diagnosis is made. A low ACTH indicates the syndrome is caused by ACTH independent disease (for example an adrenal adenoma), whereas an elevated value is indicative of pituitary or ectopic secretion of ACTH. An abdominal ultrasound may be useful in evaluating for the presence of an adrenal adenoma, but a CT scan is more sensitive and more commonly used. In this particular case, an ultrasound may be used first given increased risks of radiation to the fetus with a CT scan compared with an abdominal ultrasound.

Vignette 3 Question 2

Answer C: The collection of a 24-hour urine sample and testing for metanephrines and catecholamines is felt to be the first-line test for evaluating for pheochromocytoma, followed closely by plasma metanephrines. Plasma metanephrines have high sensitivity for pheochromocytoma, but poor specificity.

A 24-hour urine protein collection and complete metabolic panel may enlighten you to other metabolic or renal derangements, but will not aid in diagnosis of a pheochromocytoma.

Your patient undergoes a CT scan, which is concerning for an adrenal adenoma and given that she is at 20 weeks' gestation, she is taken to the operating room for a unilateral adrenalectomy which is uncomplicated. She goes on to have an uncomplicated pregnancy and delivers her infant at term.

Vignette 3 Question 3

Answer B: The patient is presenting to your office already having tried some depilatory strategies, so your first option for treatment would be an oral contraceptive pill. The oral contraceptive pill will reduce circulating levels of androgens by stimulating production of SHBG and in turn decreasing circulating levels of androgens. This method should be tried for at least 6 months before trying another method. Your patient should be counseled that while the pill should improve symptoms of acne and prevent additional hair growth, it will not reduce the already present hirsutism. Waxing, plucking and shaving may decrease her current unwanted hair, and the pill may reduce new hair growth.

Spironolactone (as well as other anti-androgen medications) acts as an androgen receptor antagonist. It is best used in conjunction with combined oral contraceptives after a trial of oral contraceptives alone has failed. GnRH agonists (such as leuprolide) essentially cause a state of menopause, effectively decreasing serum androgen levels as well as serum estrogens. They are very effective in treating hirsutism, but should not be used as a first-line agent given their side-effect profile.

Vignette 4 Question 1

Answer A: Classic "salt wasting" CAH is caused by a deficiency in 21-hydroxylase, leading to elevated levels of 17-hydroxyprogesterone. Female infants present with ambiguous genitalia, as in the above patient, as well as adrenal insufficiency. All infants in the United States are screened at birth by measuring levels of 17-hydroxyprogesterone in the blood. The absence of 21-hydroxylase causes decreased cortisol synthesis and therefore increased stimulation of the adrenals by ACTH. This in turn leads to increased androgen production, leading to virilization of females.

There are other, more mild forms of congenital adrenal hyperplasia, in which the enzymes 11β-hydroxylase and 3β-hydroxysteroid dehydrogenase are absent. Aromatase deficiency can lead to virilization of a female fetus, but is not related to the congenital adrenal hyperplasia spectrum.

Vignette 4 Question 2

Answer B: Female patients with congenital adrenal hyperplasia are chromosomally 46,XX, and develop ovaries. The internal genitalia in both males and females initially develop by means of wolffian and müllerian ducts in both sexes. In males, the presence of testicles and Sertoli cells within them initiates secretion of müllerian-inhibiting substance (MIS), which causes regression of the müllerian ducts (which would have otherwise fused to form the uterus, tubes, and upper vagina). Because this patient is genetically 46,XX, she will by default (and by the absence of MIS) develop a uterus.

The case in which a patient appears to have testicular tissue with a present uterus and tubes may be gonadal dysgenesis or testicular regression (in which testicular function is inadequate or absent). Absent Sertoli cells would lead to absent MIS as well, causing a persistent müllerian system. Additionally, mutations in the gene for MIS may lead to persistence of the müllerian ducts with externally male appearing genitalia. The lack of DHT would lead to abnormal development of external genitalia in a male.

Vignette 4 Question 3

Answer D: The most likely cause of her oligomenorrhea is inadequate control of her congenital adrenal hyperplasia, leading to elevated levels of circulating androgens, leading to anovulation.

Premature ovarian failure is unlikely in this setting, as the more likely explanation is her CAH. Although exercise-induced amenorrhea is possible, she does not give a history of excessive vigorous exercise, and again, the more likely explanation is her CAH. PCOS is a diagnosis of exclusion; therefore it is not the correct answer, given that the patient already carries a diagnosis of CAH.

Vignette 4 Question 4

Answer C: This patient is at risk for adrenal crisis. Because of her underlying adrenal insufficiency, she is unable to mount a response to the stress of surgery. Signs and symptoms of adrenal crisis include hypotension, hyponatremia, hypoglycemia, and shock. She will need "stress dose steroids," which for her age would require 100 mg hydrocortisone IV once followed by a taper over the following several days, in addition to her regular doses of fludrocortisone and prednisone.

Hemorrhage and DIC are unlikely if pre-operative coagulation studies are normal and she has been well controlled in terms of her medications, as long as no additional surgical complications present. Surgical risk for sudden cardiac death and cerebrovascular accidents are not increased above her baseline risk with CAH.

Chapter 24

Contraception and Sterilization

Approximately 90% of women of childbearing age use some form of contraception. Despite this, nearly 50% of pregnancies in the United States are unintentional. Of these, 43% result in live births, 13% in miscarriages, and 44% end in elective abortion. In weighing the risks and benefits of contraception methods, couples must keep in mind that no contraceptive or sterilization method is 100% effective. Table 24-1 outlines relative failure rates or the number of women likely to become pregnant within the first year of using a particular method. **Theoretical efficacy rate** refers to the efficacy of contraception when used exactly as instructed. **Actual efficacy rate** refers to efficacy when used in real life, assuming variations in the consistency of usage.

NATURAL METHODS

The methods of contraception described in this section—periodic abstinence, coitus interruptus, and lactational amenorrhea—are **physiology-based methods** that use neither chemical nor mechanical barriers to contraception. Many couples, for religious, philosophical, or medical reasons, prefer these methods to other forms of contraception. However, these are the **least effective** methods of contraception and should not be used if pregnancy prevention is a high priority.

PERIODIC ABSTINENCE

Method of Action

Periodic abstinence (the rhythm or calendar method) is a physiologic form of contraception that emphasizes **fertility awareness and abstinence** shortly before and after the estimated ovulation period. This method requires instruction on the physiology of menstruation and conception and on methods of determining ovulation. It also requires the woman to have regular, predictable menstrual cycles. **Ovulation assessment methods** may include the use of ovulation prediction kits, basal body temperature measurements (Fig. 24-1), menstrual cycle tracking, cervical mucus evaluation, and/or documentation of any premenstrual or ovulatory symptoms.

Effectiveness

The average effectiveness of periodic abstinence is relatively low (55% to 80%) compared to other forms of pregnancy prevention.

Advantages/Disadvantages

Periodic abstinence uses neither chemical nor mechanical barriers to conception and is therefore the method of choice for many couples for philosophical, medical, and/or religious reasons. However, this method requires a highly motivated couple willing to learn reproductive physiology, predict ovulation, and abstain from intercourse. Periodic abstinence is relatively unreliable compared to the more traditional methods of contraception. This low reliability may require prolonged periods of abstinence and **regular menstrual cycles**, making it less desirable for some couples.

COITUS INTERRUPTUS

Method of Action

Coitus interruptus, or withdrawal of the penis from the vagina before ejaculation, is one of the oldest methods of contraception. With this method, the majority of semen is deposited outside of the female reproductive tract with the intent of preventing fertilization.

Effectiveness

The failure rate for coitus interruptus is quite high (27%) compared to other forms of contraception. Failure can be attributed to the deposition of semen (pre-ejaculate) into the vagina before orgasm, or the deposition of semen near the introitus after intracrural intercourse.

Advantages/Disadvantages

The primary disadvantage of coitus interruptus is its **high failure rate**. Other disadvantages include the need for sufficient self-control to withdraw the penis before ejaculation.

LACTATIONAL AMENORRHEA

Method of Action

Continuation of nursing has long been a widespread method of contraception for many couples. After delivery, the restoration of ovulation is delayed because of a nursing-induced hypothalamic **suppression of ovulation**. Specifically, there is a **prolactin-induced** inhibition of pulsatile gonadotrophin-releasing hormone (GnRH) from the hypothalamus resulting in suppression of ovulation.

Effectiveness

The duration of ovulatory suppression during nursing is highly variable. In fact, 50% of lactating mothers will begin to ovulate between 6 and 12 months after delivery, even while breastfeeding. Importantly, return of **ovulation occurs before the return of menstruation**. As a result, 15% to 55% of mothers using lactation for contraception subsequently become pregnant.

The effectiveness of lactational amenorrhea as a method of contraception can be enhanced by following certain principles. First, breastfeeding should be the only form of nutrition for the infant. Second, this method of contraception should be used

TABLE 24-1 Failure Rates for Various Contraceptive Methods During the First Year of Use in the United States

	Percent of Women Who Become Pregnant	
Method	**Theoretical Failure Rate (%)**	**Actual Failure Rate (%)**
No method	85.0	85.0
Periodic abstinence		
Calendar	9.0	25.0
Ovulation method	3.0	25.0
Symptothermal	2.0	25.0
Postovulation	1.0	25.0
Withdrawal	4.0	27.0
Lactational amenorrhea	2.0	15.0–55.0
Condom		
Male condom	2.0	15.0
Female condom	5.0	21.0
Diaphragm with spermicide	6.0	16.0
Cervical cap with spermicide		
Parous women	26.0	32.0
Nulliparous women	9.0	16.0
Spermicide alone	18.0	29.0
Intrauterine devices		
Copper-T IUD (ParaGard)	0.6	0.8
Levonorgestrel IUS (Mirena)	0.1	0.1
Combination estrogen and progesterone		
Combination pill	0.1	3.0
Transdermal patch (Ortho Evra)	0.3	0.8
Vaginal ring (NuvaRing)	0.3	0.8
Progesterone-only methods		
Progestin-only pill (POPs)	0.5	8.0
Depo-Provera	0.3	0.3
Subdermal implant (Implanon/Nexplanon)	0.4	0.4
Surgical sterilization		
Female sterilization	0.5	0.5
Male sterilization	0.1	0.15

only as long as the woman is experiencing amenorrhea and, even then, it should only be used for a **maximum of 6 months** after delivery. Following these guidelines, lactational amenorrhea as a method of contraception can have a much lower failure rate. In practice, however, most mothers are not able to meet these stringent requirements.

Advantages/Disadvantages

Lactational amenorrhea has no effect on nursing and has no monetary cost. However, while the theoretical failure rates are reasonable, the failure rates for actual practice are so high as to make this an unacceptable and unreliable sole means of contraception.

BARRIER METHODS AND SPERMICIDES

These contraceptive methods work by preventing sperm from entering the endometrial cavity, fallopian tubes, and peritoneal cavity. Figure 24-2 shows the various barrier method contraceptives and spermicides.

MALE CONDOMS

Method of Action

Condoms are latex sheaths placed over the erect penis before ejaculation. They prevent the ejaculate from being released into the reproductive tract of the woman.

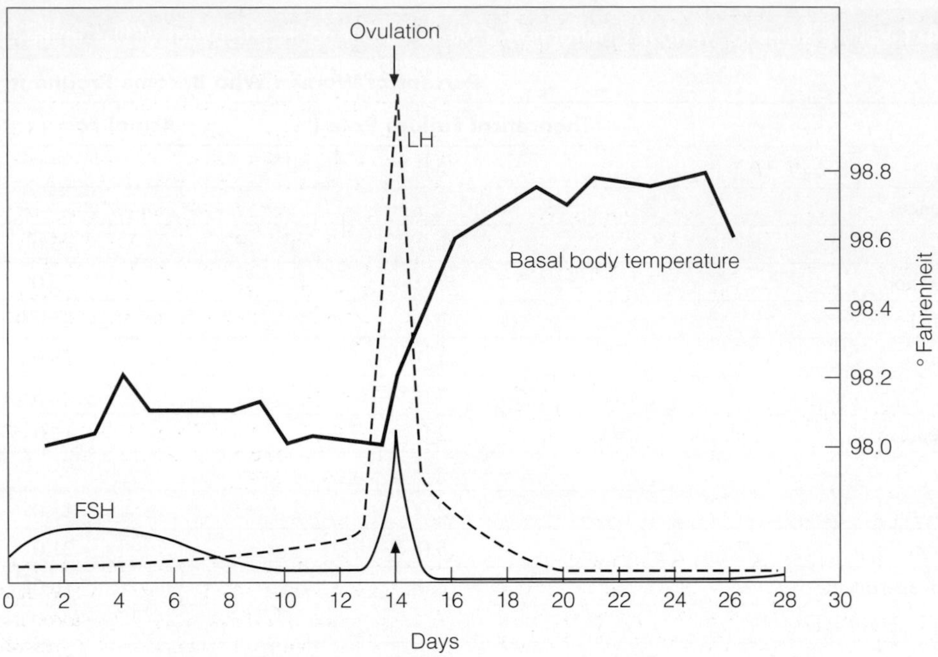

Figure 24-1 • The relationship between ovulation and basal body temperature. LH, luteinizing hormone; FSH, follicle-stimulating hormone.

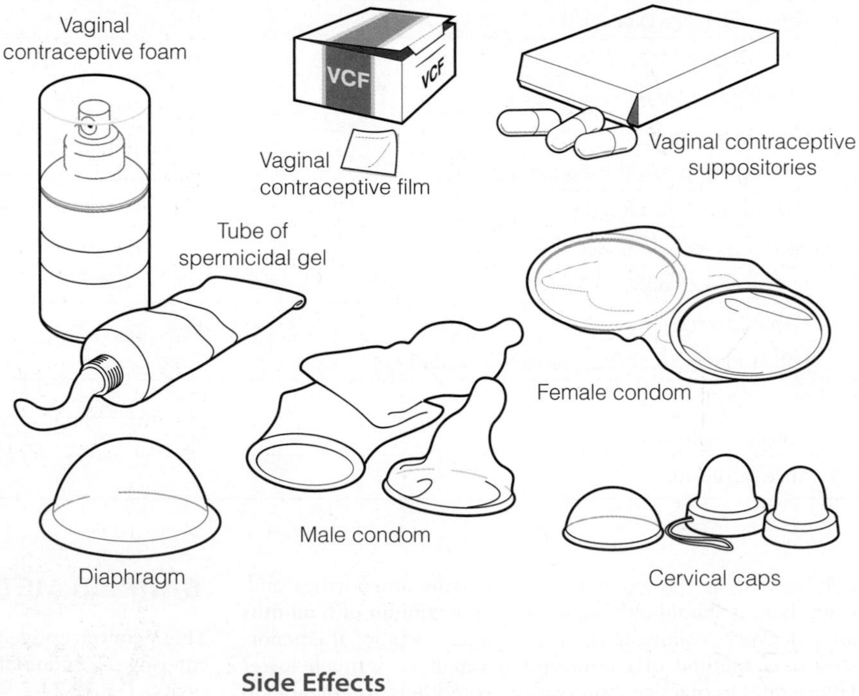

Figure 24-2 • Barrier methods and spermicides.

Effectiveness

When properly used, the condom can be 98% effective in preventing conception. The actual efficacy rate in the population is **85% to 90%**. To maximize effectiveness and decrease the risk of condom breakage, it is important to leave a well at the tip of the condom to collect the ejaculate and to avoid leakage of semen as the penis is withdrawn. Efficacy is also increased by use of spermicide-containing condoms or by using a spermicide along with condoms.

Side Effects

Some individuals may experience a hypersensitivity to the latex, lubricant, or spermicide in condoms.

Advantages/Disadvantages

Condoms are widely available for a moderate cost and carry the added benefit of preventing the transmission of many **sexually transmitted infections** (STIs). Condoms are the only method of contraception that offers protection against human immunodeficiency virus (HIV). Drawbacks of the condom include coital interruption and possible decreased sensation or hypersensitivity.

FEMALE CONDOMS

Method of Action

The female condom (FC; formerly the Reality Vaginal Pouch) is a pouch made of polyurethane that has a flexible ring at each end. One ring fits into the depth of the vagina, and the other stays outside the vagina near the introitus (Fig. 24-3).

Effectiveness

Initial studies show that the failure rate of the female condom is 20% to 25%, somewhat higher than that of the male condom. However, these were short-term studies and may not reflect the failure rate with long-term usage.

Advantages/Disadvantages

Female condoms protect against many STIs while also placing the control of contraception with the female partner. Major drawbacks include cost and overall bulkiness. The acceptability rating is somewhat higher for the male partner (75% to 80%) than for the female partner (65% to 70%).

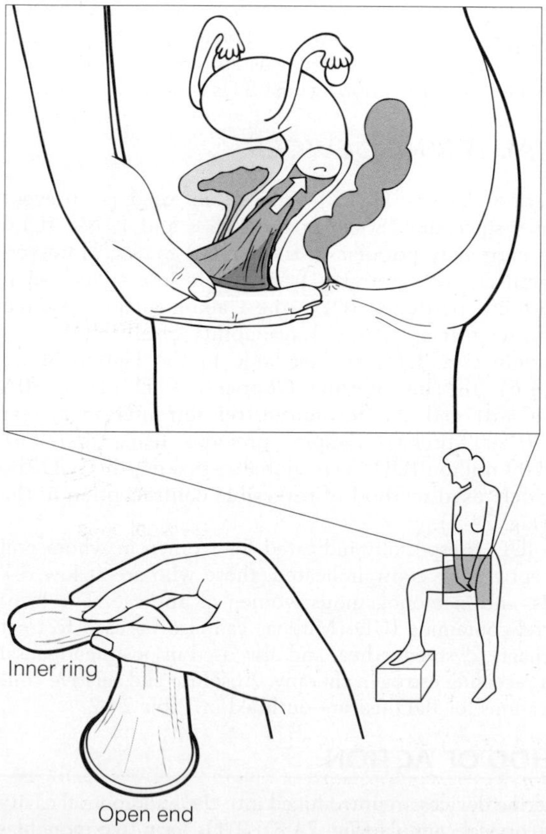

Figure 24-3 • Placement of the female condom.

DIAPHRAGM

Method of Action

The vaginal diaphragm is a dome-shaped latex rubber sheet stretched over a thin coiled rim. Spermicidal jelly is placed on the rim and on either side of the diaphragm, and it is placed into the vagina so that it covers the cervix (Fig. 24-4). The diaphragm and spermicide should be placed in the vagina before intercourse and left in place for **6 to 8 hours** after intercourse. If further intercourse is to take place within 6 to 8 hours after the first episode of intercourse, additional spermicide should be placed in the vagina without removing the diaphragm.

Effectiveness

The theoretical effectiveness of the diaphragm approaches 94%. The actual effectiveness rate of the diaphragm with spermicide is 80% to 85%.

Side Effects

Possible side effects include bladder irritation, which can lead to urinary tract infections (UTIs). If the diaphragm is left in place too long, colonization by *Staphylococcus aureus* may lead to the development of **toxic shock syndrome** (TSS). Some women also experience a hypersensitivity to the rubber, latex, or spermicide.

Advantages/Disadvantages

The diaphragm must be fitted and prescribed by a clinician, making its initial cost significantly higher than over-the-counter methods of contraception. The diaphragm should be replaced every 2 years or when the patient gains or loses more than 20% of her body weight. It should also be checked after each pregnancy. Women who are not comfortable with inserting the diaphragm, or who cannot be properly fitted due to pelvic relaxation defects are poor candidates for the diaphragm, as are women who are at high risk of HIV.

CERVICAL CAP

Method of Action

The cervical cap (FemCap, Lea's Shield) is a small, soft, silicone cap that fits directly over the cervix (Fig. 24-5). It is held in place by suction and acts as a barrier to sperm. The cap must be **fitted by a clinician** and must be used with a **spermicidal jelly**. Because of the variability in cervix size, proper fit and usage of

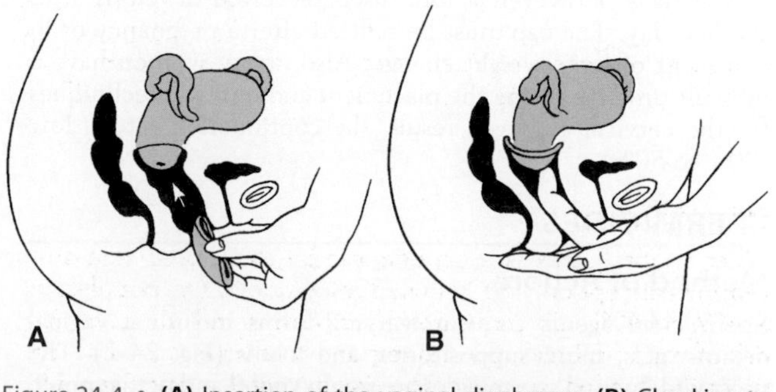

Figure 24-4 • **(A)** Insertion of the vaginal diaphragm. **(B)** Checking to ensure the diaphragm covers the cervix.
(From Beckmann C, Ling F. *Obstetrics & Gynecology*, 5th ed. Philadelphia, PA: Lippincott Williams & Wilkins; 2006.)

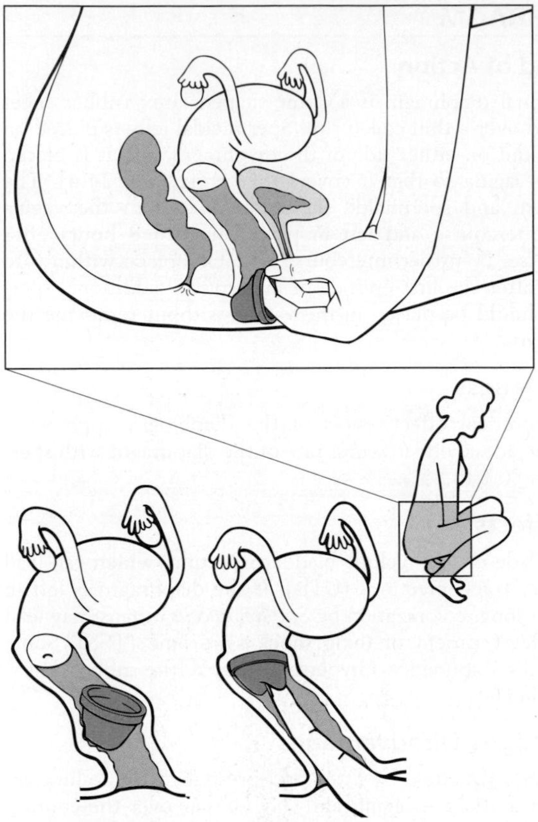

Figure 24-5 • Insertion of the cervical cap.

the cap are essential to its effectiveness. Although it is widely used in Britain and Europe, the cervical cap is not widely available in the United States.

Effectiveness

The actual efficacy rate of the cervical cap is 68% to 84% (16% to 32% failure rate), depending on the woman's parity. There is an increased risk of failure in parous women. **Dislodgment** is the most common cause of failure.

Advantages/Disadvantages

One advantage of the cervical cap is that it can be inserted up to 6 hours prior to intercourse and can be left in place for 1 to 2 days. However, a foul discharge often develops after the first day. The cap must be refitted after a pregnancy or in the event of large weight change. Also, many women have a difficult time mastering the placement and removal techniques for the cervical cap; as a result, the continuation rate is low (30% to 50%).

SPERMICIDES

Method of Action

Spermicidal agents come in varying forms including vaginal creams, gels, films, suppositories, and foams (Fig. 24-2). The most widely used spermicides are **nonoxynol-9** and **octoxynol-9**. Other agents such as menfegol and benzalkonium chloride are used around the world but are not available in the United States. Nonoxynol-9 and octoxynol-9 both disrupt the cell membranes of the spermatozoa and also act as a mechanical barrier to the cervical canal. In general, spermicides should be placed in the vagina at least 30 minutes before intercourse to allow for dispersion throughout the vagina. Spermicides may be used alone but are far more effective when used in conjunction with condoms, cervical caps, diaphragms, or other contraceptive methods.

Effectiveness

When properly and consistently used with condoms, spermicides can have an effectiveness rate as high as 95%. However, in actual usage, the efficacy of spermicides when used alone is only 70% to 75%. This effectiveness is further reduced by failure to wait long enough for the spermicide to disperse in the vagina prior to intercourse.

Side Effects

Spermicides can irritate the vaginal mucosa and external male and female genitalia.

Advantages/Disadvantages

Spermicidal agents are widely available in a variety of forms and are relatively inexpensive. Some formulations can also be messy to use.

In addition to providing contraception, it was initially thought that spermicides might provide some protection against STIs. However, it now appears that these agents **do not** confer any protection against STIs. They may, in fact, make the user **more susceptible to STIs** including HIV by causing vaginal irritation. For this reason, spermicides should not be used by women with HIV or at high risk of contracting HIV. This is of special significance in developing nations where contraception and STI prevention are paramount. For the general public, it is strongly recommended that **consistent condom use** be employed whenever protection against STIs is desired.

INTRAUTERINE DEVICES

Intrauterine devices (IUDs) have been used to prevent pregnancy since the 1800s. In the 1960s and 1970s, IUDs became extremely popular in the United States. However, legal ramifications stemming from pelvic infections associated with one particular IUD—the Dalkon shield—resulted in consumer fear and limited availability of all IUDs. Currently, only two IUDs are available in the United States (Fig. 24-6): the **intrauterine Copper-T IUD** (TCu-380A or ParaGard) and the **levonorgestrel intrauterine system** (LNG-20 or Mirena). Despite previous fears, there are nearly 100 million IUD users globally, making the IUD the **most widely used method of reversible contraception in the world** (Fig. 24-7).

The IUD is especially indicated for women in whom oral contraceptives are contraindicated, those who are at low risk for STIs, and in monogamous women of any age. The levonorgestrel-containing IUD (Mirena) can also be used to treat menorrhagia, dysmenorrhea, and also used in postmenopausal women receiving estrogen therapy. Absolute and relative contraindications for IUD use are outlined in Table 24-2.

METHOD OF ACTION

Intrauterine devices are introduced into the endometrial cavity using a cervical cannula (Fig. 24-8). IUDs have two monofilament strings that extend through the cervix where they can

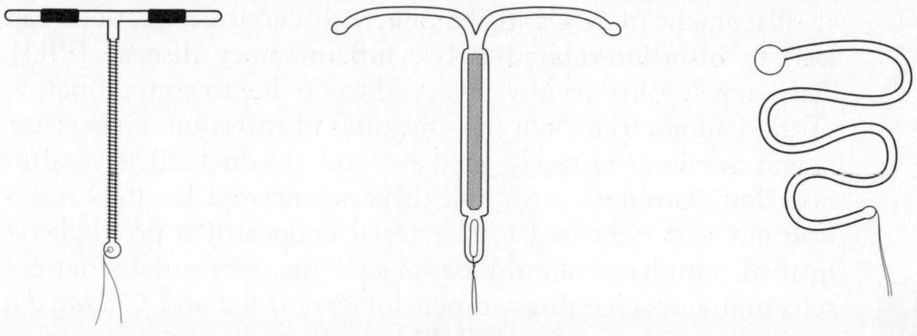

Figure 24-6 • Intrauterine devices (IUD). **(A)** ParaGard Copper T (TCu-380A). **(B)** Mirena (Levonorgestrel IUS). **(C)** Lippes loop (used throughout the world but not available in the United States).
(From Speroff L, Fritz M. *Clinical Gynecologic Endocrinology and Infertility*, 7th ed. Philadelphia, PA: Lippincott Williams & Wilkins; 2005.)

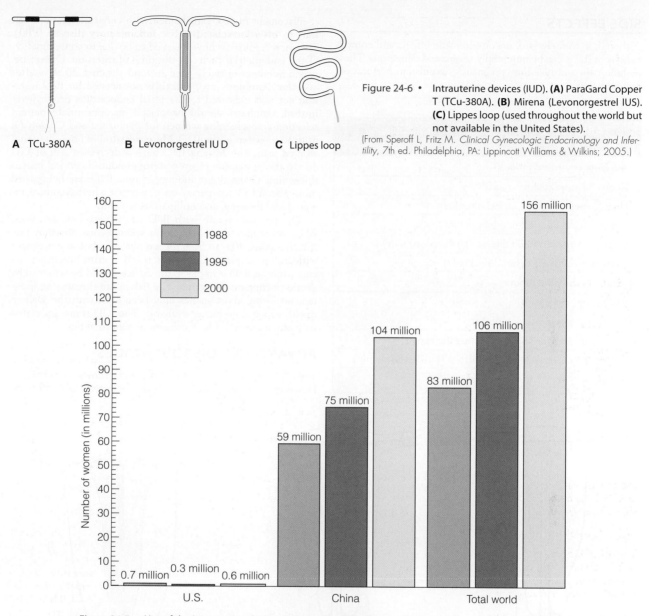

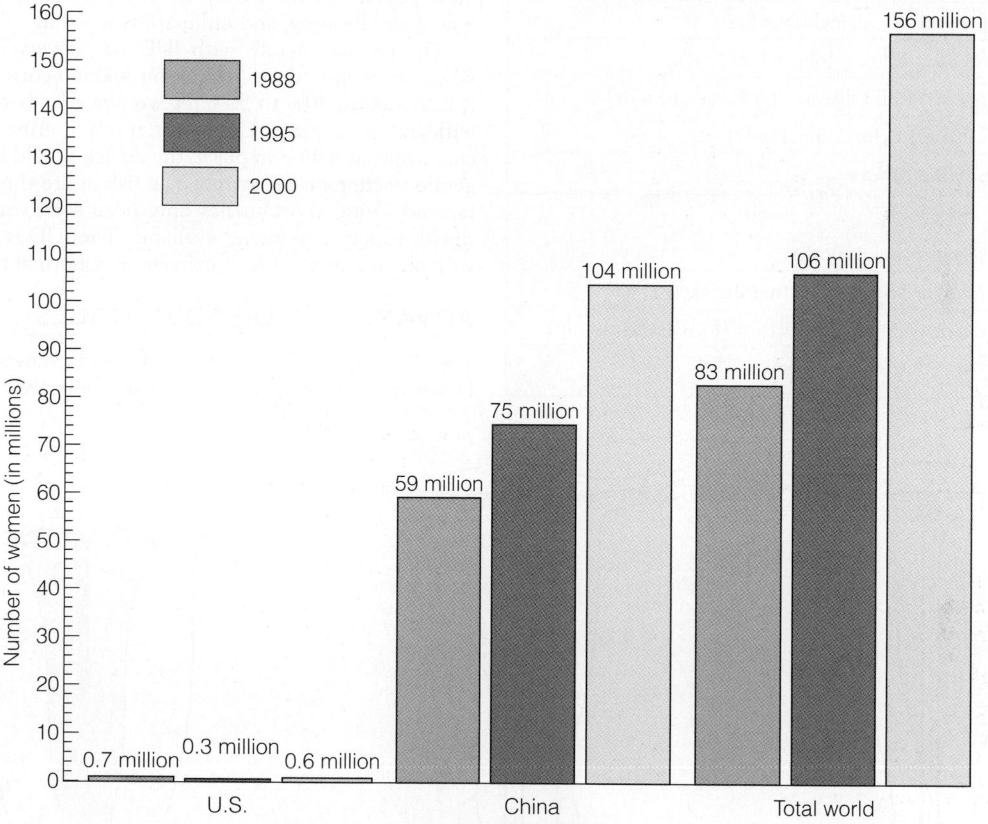

Figure 24-7 • Use of the intrauterine devices (IUD) in the United States, China, and the rest of the world.

be checked to detect expulsion or migration (Fig. 24-8). The strings also facilitate removal of the device by the clinician.

The mechanism of action for IUDs is not completely understood, but they are known to act mainly by killing sperm (spermicidal) and **preventing fertilization**. Specifically, the primary method of action is to elicit a **sterile inflammatory response** resulting in sperm being engulfed, immobilized, and destroyed by inflammatory cells. The IUD is also thought to **reduce tubal motility** that in turn inhibits sperm and blastocyst transport. IUDs do not affect ovulation, nor do they act as abortifacients. Their presumed mechanisms of action are augmented by the addition of levonorgestrel in the Mirena IUD and copper in the ParaGard IUD. Progesterone in the Mirena **thickens the cervical mucus** and **atrophies the endometrium** to prevent implantation. Copper in the ParaGard is thought to hamper sperm motility and capitation so sperm rarely reach the fallopian tube and are unable to fertilize the ovum.

EFFECTIVENESS

The efficacy for IUDs rivals that of permanent sterilization with prolonged use. The failure rate is 0.8% for the ParaGard and 0.2% for the Mirena IUD within the first year of use. The cumulative 10-year failure rate for the ParaGard is approximately 1.9% and the cumulative 5-year failure rate for the Mirena is 0.7%. Some sources state that the failure rate in the first year is closer to 3%, partially due to unrecognized expulsions.

SIDE EFFECTS

Although extremely safe, uncommon side effects and complications of IUDs can be potentially severe and dangerous. These include pain and bleeding, pregnancy, expulsion, perforation, and infection.

TABLE 24-2 Contraindications for Intrauterine Device (IUD) Use

Absolute contraindications
Known or suspected pregnancy
Undiagnosed abnormal vaginal bleeding
Acute cervical, uterine, or salpingeal infection
Copper allergy or Wilson disease (for ParaGard only)
Current breast cancer (for Mirena only)
Relative contraindications
Prior ectopic pregnancy
History of STIs in past 3 months
Uterine anomaly or fibroid distorting the cavity
Current menorrhagia or dysmenorrhea (for ParaGard only)

STI, sexually transmitted infection.

Placement of IUDs in women with cervical infections can lead to **insertion-related pelvic inflammatory disease** (PID). This increased risk is now believed to be due to contamination of the endometrial cavity at the time of insertion. Otherwise, pelvic infection is rarely seen beyond the first 20 days after insertion. Antibiotic prophylaxis is not needed for IUD insertion nor is it indicated for bacterial endocarditis prophylaxis. Instead, emphasis should be placed on appropriate patient selection and screening women for gonorrhea and *Chlamydia* prior to insertion of the IUD. Moreover, studies now show that women using the Mirena IUD have a decreased risk of PID due to the protection of progesterone-induced cervical mucus thickening. Given these findings, Mirena IUDs are being used more liberally in younger women, women who have not completed childbearing, and nulliparous women.

The pregnancy rate with IUD use is very low; however, when pregnancy does occur, the **spontaneous abortion** rate is increased to 40% to 50% for women who become pregnant with an IUD in place. Given this, if intrauterine pregnancy occurs while an IUD is in place, the device should be removed by **gentle traction on the string**. The risk of life-threatening spontaneous septic abortion has only been seen with the Dalkon shield, which is no longer available. The IUD is not associated with any increased risk of congenital abnormalities.

ADVANTAGES/DISADVANTAGES

The IUD must be prescribed, inserted, and removed by a clinician. However, once in place, it is highly effective, cost-effective,

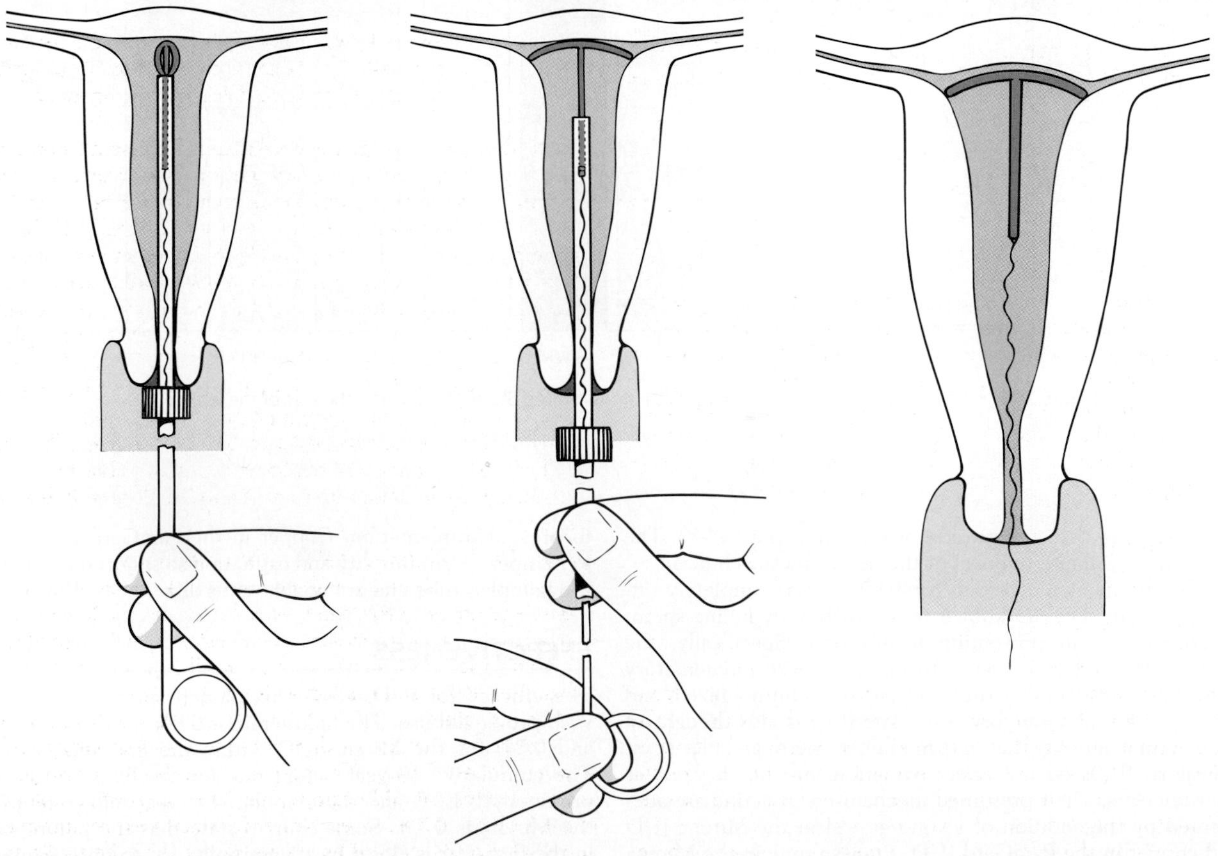

Figure 24-8 • Placement of a ParaGard intrauterine devices (IUD).

long-lasting, and rapidly reversible. The user is encouraged to do a monthly string check to ensure the device has not been expelled. This improves coital spontaneity and decreases fear of pregnancy. In the United States, the **ParaGard IUD has been approved for use for 10 years** but has been shown to maintain its effectiveness for 12 years. The **Mirena IUD has been approved for use for 5 years** but is effective for at least 7 years. One IUD can be removed and another one can be inserted on the same visit. Also, an IUD may be inserted **immediately after induced or spontaneous first trimester abortions** without increased risk of infection or perforation. ParaGard is also approved for emergency contraception when placed within 72 hours of unprotected intercourse or contraceptive failure. The ParaGard IUD can be inserted immediately postpartum (within 10 minutes of placental delivery) with an increased risk of expulsion but no increased risk of infection or perforation. Both the Mirena and ParaGard IUDs can be used safely at **6 weeks postpartum** and are safe in breastfeeding women.

In general, because IUDs are so effective at preventing pregnancy, the risk of **ectopic pregnancy is reduced** in IUD users compared to that of noncontraceptive users. In the rare event that a woman does become pregnant with an IUD in place, however, **the risk of ectopic pregnancy may be as high as 30% to 50%** of those patients. Although controversial, the IUD is an acceptable form of contraception for women with a **prior history of ectopic pregnancy**.

The Mirena IUD has been found to **decrease menorrhagia** (90% less blood loss) and **dysmenorrhea**. It is also as effective as oral progestins in treating endometriosis, endometrial hyperplasia, and cancer. It also protects the user from PID. As a result, this decreases the number of surgeries needed for pain and bleeding (hysterectomies, D&Cs, endometrial ablations). About 20% of women will experience amenorrhea while using a Mirena IUD for 1 year and 60% will experience amenorrhea after using the Mirena for 5 years.

HORMONAL CONTRACEPTIVE METHODS

Hormonal contraceptives are the most commonly used reversible means of preventing pregnancy in the United States and consist of combined (estrogen and progesterone) and progesterone-only methods. Currently, combined hormonal methods are available in oral, transdermal, and vaginal forms, whereas progesterone-only methods are available in oral, injectable, implantable, and intrauterine forms. At this time, there are several hormonal contraceptives in various stages of the FDA approval process in the United States, including new formulations for oral use, new subdermal implants and vaginal delivery systems, self-injectables, and male hormonal methods.

COMBINED ESTROGEN AND PROGESTIN METHODS

Oral Contraceptive Pills

Method of Action

Oral contraceptive pills (OCPs) are composed of progesterone alone or a combination of progesterone and estrogen. (The progesterone-alone pill is described later in the progesterone-only section.) Over 150 million women worldwide—including one-third of sexually active women in the United States—use oral contraceptives.

Oral contraceptives place the body in a **pseudo-pregnancy** state by interfering with the pulsatile release of

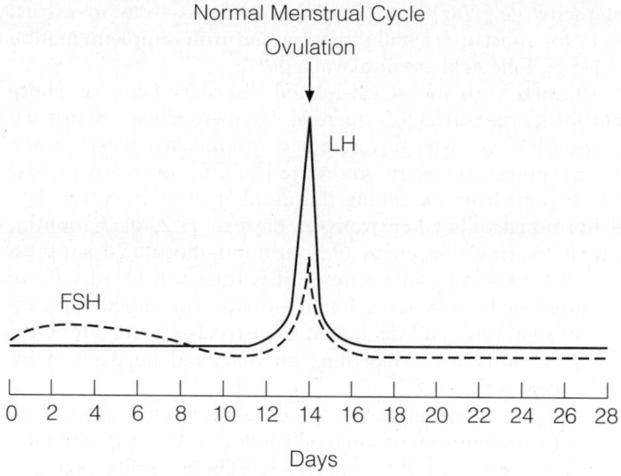

Figure 24-9 • Serum levels of FSH and LH during a normal menstrual cycle. FSH, follicle-stimulating hormone; LH, luteinizing hormone.

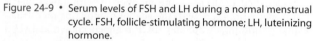

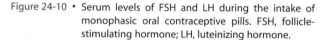

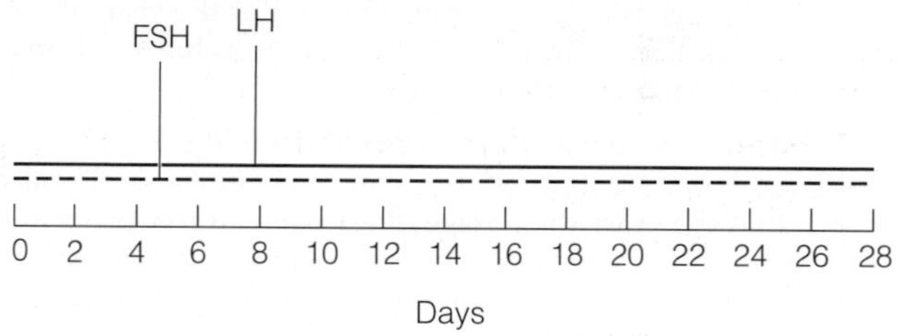

Figure 24-10 • Serum levels of FSH and LH during the intake of monophasic oral contraceptive pills. FSH, follicle-stimulating hormone; LH, luteinizing hormone.

follicle-stimulating hormone (FSH) and luteinizing hormone (LH) from the anterior pituitary. This pseudo-pregnancy state **suppresses ovulation** and prevents pregnancy from occurring. Figure 24-9 illustrates the serum levels of FSH and LH during the normal menstrual cycle, and Figure 24-10 shows FSH and LH levels during a cycle on the combination pill. Because the FSH and LH surges do not occur, follicle growth, recruitment, and ovulation do not occur. The bleeding that takes place during the hormone-free interval is actually a bleed due to the withdrawal of hormone rather than a menstrual period induced by endogenous hormone fluctuation.

Secondary mechanisms of action for OCPs include thickening the **cervical mucus** to render it less penetrable by sperm and changing the **endometrium** to make it unsuitable for implantation.

Monophasic (Fixed-Dose) Combination Pills

Monophasic combination pills contain a **fixed dose of estrogen and a fixed dose of progestin in each tablet**. Nearly 30 combinations of estrogen and progestins are available in the United States. In general, the selection of a particular pill depends on the individual side effects and risk factors for each patient.

The combination pill containing both estrogen and progestin is taken for the first 21 days out of a 28-day monthly cycle. During the last 7 days of the cycle, a placebo pill or no pill is taken. Bleeding should begin within 3 to 5 days of completion of the 21 days of hormones. Newer formulations are now available that give **24 days of hormone** (rather than the traditional 21 days) and a 4-day hormone-free interval. The so-called 24/4 regimens (i.e., Yaz) result in a shorter 3- to 4-day menstrual cycle for most users. Pills that contain **iron supplementation** and even **folic acid** are also available.

Women with menstrual-related disorders (such as endometriosis, menorrhagia, anemia, dysmenorrhea, menstrual irregularity, menstrual migraines, premenstrual syndrome [PMS], polycystic ovary syndrome [PCOS], or ovarian cysts) may benefit from extending the number of consecutive days of hormonal pills taken from 21 days to 1, 2, or 3 months, thus increasing the length of continuous hormonal suppression and decreasing the number of withdrawal bleeds. These **extended or long-cycle regimens** provide continued suppression of ovulation and decreased menstrual-related symptoms (such as pain, heavy bleeding, anemia, and headaches) for their users.

Seasonale, **Seasonique,** and their generic equivalents contains **84 consecutive hormonal pills** followed by 7 placebo pills, or 7 low-estrogen pills, respectively. These dosing regimens were designed to decrease the number of withdrawal bleeds to four per year, again, with the goal of minimizing menstrual-related symptoms. A **365-day OCP regimen** known as Lybrel was approved by the FDA. **Lybrel** provides a combination estrogen and progestin pill each day, 365 days of the year. There is more breakthrough bleeding in this regimen, but no formal monthly or quarterly withdrawal bleed.

Multiphasic (Dose Varying) Combination Pills

Multiphasic oral contraceptives differ from monophasic pills only in that they **vary the dosage of estrogen and/or progestin** in the active hormone pills in an effort to mimic the menstrual cycle. The advantage of the multiphasic dosing is that it may provide a lower level of estrogen and progestin overall, but is still highly effective at preventing pregnancy.

Effectiveness

OCPs are remarkably effective in preventing pregnancy. In fact, the theoretical failure rate for the first year of use is less than 1%. However, the failure rate with **actual real-life usage** is closer to **8%**. Nausea, breakthrough bleeding, and the necessity of taking the pill every day are often cited as reasons for discontinuing the pill.

Several medications are thought to interact with oral contraceptives resulting in reduced effectiveness of the pill. Despite common belief, the only antibiotic which lowers the effective of OCPs is Rifampin. Conversely, oral contraceptives can also reduce the efficacy of many medications (Table 24-3).

TABLE 24-3 Interactions of Oral Contraceptives with Other Medications

Medications That Reduce the Efficacy of Oral Contraceptives	Medications Whose Efficacies Are Changed by Oral Contraceptives
Barbiturates	Chlordiazepoxide (Librium)
Carbamazepine (Tegretol)	Diazepam (Valium)
Griseofulvin	Hypoglycemics
Phenytoin (Dilantin)	Methyldopa
Rifampin	Phenothiazides
St. John's wort	Theophylline
Topiramate (Topamax)	Tricyclic antidepressants

TABLE 24-4 Complications Associated with Oral Contraceptives

Cardiovascular[a]
Deep Vein Thrombosis (DVT)
Pulmonary Embolus (PE)
Cerebrovascular Accident (CVA)
Myocardial Infarction (MI)
Hypertension
Other
Cholelithiasis
Cholecystitis
Benign liver adenomas (rare)
Cervical adenocarcinoma (rare)
Retinal thrombosis (rare)

[a]These complications occur mainly in smokers.
[b]Most MIs and CVAs occur in users of high-dose estrogen products.
DVT, deep vein thrombosis; PE, pulmonary embolism; CVA, cerebrovascular accident; MI, myocardial infarction.

Side Effects

Table 24-4 lists some of the cardiovascular, neoplastic, and biliary complications associated with oral contraceptive use.

Oral contraceptives with estrogen doses greater than 50 mg can increase coagulability, leading to higher rates of myocardial infarction, stroke, thromboembolism, and pulmonary embolism, particularly in women who smoke. Even at lower doses of estrogen (35 mcg or less), women over 35 years who smoke more than one pack of cigarettes per day are still at increased risk of **heart attack**, **stroke**, **deep vein thrombosis (DVT), and pulmonary embolism (PE)** if they use OCPs. The progestins in oral contraceptives have been found to raise low-density lipoproteins while lowering high-density lipoproteins in pill users smoking more than one pack per day. For these reasons, oral contraceptives are **contraindicated in women over age 35 years who smoke 15 or more cigarettes a day**. The advent of new progestins and lower estrogen doses has led to pill formulations that are essentially neutral in terms of cardiovascular effect. However, combination oral contraceptive use is still contraindicated in women over age 35 years who smoke. These women often benefit from progesterone-only IUDs or permanent female or male sterilization.

Neoplastic complications of oral contraceptive use are rare. The effect of long-term oral contraceptive use on breast cancer has been studied extensively over the past decade with no conclusive findings. There is, however, an **increased incidence of gall bladder disease and benign hepatic tumors** associated with oral contraceptive use.

Table 24-5 outlines both the absolute and relative contraindications to oral contraceptive use.

Advantages/Disadvantages

The major advantages of OCPs include their **extremely high efficacy** rates and the **noncontraceptive health benefits** primarily attributable to an overall decreased rate of pregnancy, menstrual flow, dysmenorrhea, and ovulation. These benefits

TABLE 24-5 Contraindications to Combination Estrogen–Progesterone Contraceptives

Absolute Contraindications	**Relative Contraindications**
Thromboembolism	Uterine fibroids
Pulmonary embolism	Lactation
Coronary artery disease	Diabetes mellitus
Cerebrovascular accident	Sickle-cell disease or sickle C disease
Smokers over the age of 35 y	Hepatic disease
Breast/endometrial cancer	Hypertension
Unexplained vaginal bleeding	Lupus (SLE)
Abnormal liver function	Age 40+ and high risk for vascular disease
Known or suspected pregnancy	Migraine headaches
Severe hypercholesterolemia	Seizure disorders
Severe hypertriglyceridemia	Elective surgery

TABLE 24-6 Noncontraceptive Health Benefits of Oral Contraceptives

Decrease risk of serious diseases
Ovarian cancer
Endometrial cancer
Ectopic pregnancy (combination pills only)
Severe anemia
Pelvic inflammatory disease
Salpingitis
Improve quality-of-life problems
Iron deficiency anemia
Dysmenorrhea
Functional ovarian cysts
Benign breast disease
Osteoporosis (increased bone density)
Rheumatoid arthritis
Treat/manage many disorders
Dysfunctional uterine bleeding
Control of bleeding in bleeding disorders and anovulation
Dysmenorrhea
Endometriosis
Acne/hirsutism
Premenstrual syndrome

include a reduced incidence of ovarian cancer, endometrial cancer, ectopic pregnancy, PID, and benign breast disease (Table 24-6). By taking OCPs, nearly 50,000 women avoid hospitalizations; of these, 10,000 avoid hospitalization for life-threatening illnesses.

Disadvantages include cardiovascular complications, increased gallbladder disease, increased incidence of benign hepatic tumors, and the need to take a medication every day. Because they contain estrogen, combination OCPs are not suitable for many women. Many women also complain of nausea, headaches, breakthrough bleeding, and weight gain associated with OCP use. Most of these symptoms are generally mild and transient.

Transdermal Estrogen and Progestin Hormonal Contraception—Ortho Evra

Mechanism of Action

The contraceptive patch (Fig. 24-11) with the brand name **Ortho Evra** releases progestin and **ethinyl estradiol. The patch releases 150 mg per day of the progestin, norelgestromin, and 20 mg per day of ethinyl estradiol**. The overall average estrogen concentration is higher in Ortho Evra users compared to women taking standard OCPs. Therefore, these patients should be made aware of the **increased risk of thromboembolism**, specifically **DVT and PE** in Ortho Evra users compared to women taking standard OCPs. There does not appear to be an increased risk of heart attack and stroke in these patients.

Women apply one patch each week for 3 weeks followed by 1 week patch-free period during which they will have a withdrawal bleed. This hormone-free period can be skipped to allow for continuous 3-month dosing. Again, just like combined OCPs, the primary mechanism of action is suppression of ovulation by decreasing endogenous FSH and LH levels (Figs. 24-9 and 24-10).

Effectiveness

The patch has been shown to have a 1% pregnancy rate in actual use—similar to other combination hormonal methods.

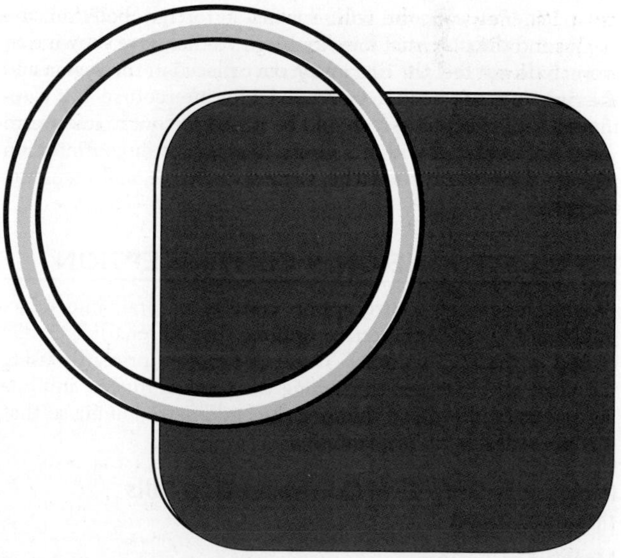

Figure 24-11 • Vaginal contraceptive ring (NuvaRing) and transdermal contraceptive patch (Ortho Evra). Both contain a combination of estrogen and progesterone, which are released over a period of 1 week and 3 weeks, respectively.

(From Speroff L, Fritz M. *Clinical Gynecologic Endocrinology and Infertility*, 7th ed. Philadelphia, PA: Lippincott Williams & Wilkins; 2005.)

Ortho Evra has been found to have a **decreased effectiveness in markedly overweight women (>198 lb or 90 kg)**.

Advantages/Disadvantages

The same primary side effects and noncontraceptive health benefits of OCPs apply to the patch as well. The patch can cause skin irritation in some users. The patch has the added benefit of being self-administered only once a week.

Vaginal Estrogen and Progestin Hormonal Contraception—NuvaRing

Method of Action

The hormone-releasing vaginal ring (Fig. 24-11) with the brand name of **NuvaRing** releases a daily dose of 15 mcg of ethinyl estradiol and 120 mcg of etonogestrel (the active form of desogestrel). The ring is **placed in the vagina for 3 weeks** (it is likely effective for 4 weeks), and is removed for 1 week to allow for a withdrawal bleed. Again, this hormone-free period can be skipped to allow for continuous dosing, typically for 3 months.

Effectiveness

Clinical studies are ongoing, but the vaginal ring is **highly effective** (1% to 2% failure rate in actual use), similar to other forms of combined hormonal contraception.

Advantages/Disadvantages

Because one size of vaginal ring fits all women, the vaginal ring need does not need to be fitted by a clinician. Women place the ring in the vagina themselves for 3 continuous weeks and then remove it for 1 week. Because the ring is left in place continuously, it provides a low, steady release of hormone with lower total hormone exposure compared to other combination hormone methods. And while douching with the NuvaRing in place is discouraged, the use of antifungal agents and spermicides is permitted.

The disadvantages of the vaginal ring include a woman's (or partner's) concern with having a foreign body in the vagina and the potential for expulsion. Studies have shown that women do not feel the ring inside once placed in the vagina and **the ring does not need to be removed for intercourse**. If it is removed for intercourse, it should be rinsed in cool to lukewarm water and replaced within 3 hours. Reasons for discontinuation include discomfort, headache, vaginal discharge, and recurrent vaginitis.

PROGESTERONE-ONLY CONTRACEPTION

Progesterone-only contraception consists of oral, injectable, implantable, and intrauterine options (the Mirena IUS is discussed in the IUD section). These all function primarily using the same mechanisms: thickening the cervical mucus, inhibiting sperm motility, and thinning the endometrial lining so that it is not suitable for implantation.

Progestin-Only Oral Contraception Pills (The Minipill)

Method of Action

Progestin-only pills (POPs; Micronor, Nor-QD) deliver a **small daily dose of progestin** (0.35 mg norethindrone) without any estrogen. POPs have lower progestin doses than combination pills, thus the nickname *minipills*. POPs also differ from traditional pills in that **they are taken every day of the cycle** with no hormone-free days. POPs are believed to **thicken the cervical mucus** making it less permeable to sperm. This effect, however, decreases after 22 hours so the minipill must be **taken at the same time each day**. Other mechanisms of action include endometrial atrophy and ovulation suppression (50% of cycles).

Effectiveness

POPs are generally **not as effective** as combination hormone regimens, with failure rates estimated at greater than 8%. This failure rate increases if punctual dosing is not achieved.

Side Effects

Side effects of the progesterone-only OCP include irregular ovulatory cycles, breakthrough bleeding, increased formation of follicular cysts, and acne. POPs can also cause breast tenderness and irritability.

Advantages/Disadvantages

Because they contain no estrogen, POPs are ideal for nursing mothers and **women for whom estrogens are contraindicated,** including women over 35 years who smoke and women with hypertension, coronary artery disease, collagen vascular disorder (CVD), lupus, migraines, and those with a personal history of thromboembolism. In addition to their contraceptive benefits, POPs can be used to treat abnormal uterine bleeding in high risk medical populations whose bleeding has been adequately evaluated (i.e., anovulatory bleeding and endometrial hyperplasia in poor surgical candidates).

The disadvantages **include irregular menses** ranging from amenorrhea to irregular spotting. Also, POPs must be taken at the same time each day. A delay of more than 3 hours is akin to a missed pill.

Injectable Progesterone-Only Contraception—Depo-Provera

Method of Action

Although it was only approved for contraceptive use in the United States in 1992, Depo-Provera (**medroxyprogesterone acetate; DMPA**) has been used in other countries since the mid-1960s. Depo-Provera (150 mg/1 mL, intramuscular "IM") is injected intramuscularly every 3 months in a vehicle that allows the slow release of progestin over a 3-month period. A **newer low-dose DMPA** (104 mg/0.65 mL, subcutaneous "SC") is also available although not widely used yet. This formulation carries the benefit of lower progestin levels but the same efficacy rates. Depo-Provera acts by suppressing ovulation, thickening the cervical mucus, making the endometrium unsuitable for implantation, and reducing tubal motility. After an injection, ovulation does not occur for 14 weeks; therefore, patients have a 2-week grace period in their every 12-week dosing.

Effectiveness

With a first-year theoretical failure rate of only 0.3%, Depo-Provera is one of the most effective contraceptive methods available. Typical use failure rates are estimated at 3%, mostly attributed to patients failing to return at scheduled times for follow-up injections.

Side Effects

The primary side effects experienced by Depo-Provera users include **irregular menstrual bleeding**, depression, weight gain, hair loss, and headache. Over 70% of patients experience spotting and irregular menses during the first year of use. Irregular bleeding is the primary reason for discontinuing

TABLE 24-7 The Effects of Depo-Provera Use on Bone Mineralization

Bone density is decreased in women using Depo-Provera, due to the decrease in ovarian estradiol production
The decrease in bone density is most rapid in the first year of use
The decrease in bone density increases with length of use
The decrease in bone density is reversible and occurs over 6 mo to 2 y
There is no role for the use of bone density screening (DEXA) in DMPA users
There is no role for the use of bisphosphonates, estrogens, and SERMS in DMPA users
Women on Depo-Provera should be encouraged to take calcium and vitamin D, stop smoking, and do regular weight-bearing exercises.
DMPA, Depo medroxyprogesterone acetate; SERMs, selective estrogen receptor modulator.

Depo-Provera. It is anticipated that **50% of DMPA users will have amenorrhea after 1 year** of use and 80% after 5 years of DMPA use. However, the possibility of amenorrhea makes Depo-Provera a good option for women with bleeding disorders, women on anticoagulation, women in the military, and women who are mentally or physically disabled.

Women using DMPA for more than 2 years may experience a **reversible decrease in bone mineralization** similar to that seen in lactating women, due to the decrease in ovarian estradiol production. The effect of Depo-Provera use on bone mineralization is summarized in Table 24-7. Thus, calcium, vitamin D, weight-bearing exercises, and smoking cessation should be encouraged in all women using Depo-Provera. A recent randomized controlled trial demonstrated the SC and IM forms to be similar in their effects on bone mineral density.

Advantages/Disadvantages

The primary advantages of Depo-Provera are that it is **highly effective**, acts independent of intercourse, and requires infrequent injections (**every 3 months**). Like other progestins, Depo-Provera **reduces the risk of endometrial cancer and PID** and also the amount of menstrual bleeding. It is also useful in the treatment of menorrhagia, dysmenorrhea, endometriosis, menstrual-related anemia, and endometrial hyperplasia. DMPA is especially useful in women who desire effective contraception, but may have **concomitant medical conditions** that prevent the use of estrogen-containing contraceptives, such as women with migraines with auras, seizure disorders, lupus, sickle cell disease, hypertension, coronary artery disease, and smokers.

Irregular bleeding to DMPA use, weight gain, and mood changes are the major disadvantages. Although not contraindicated, Depo-Provera should be used with caution in patients with a history of depression, mood disorders, PMS, and premenstrual dysphoric disorder (PMDD). Similarly, Depo-Provera use is not contraindicated in obese women, but weight monitoring should be employed when using the medicine in women who may be at an increased risk for weight gain.

After discontinuation of Depo-Provera injections, some women may experience a significant **delay in the return of regular ovulation** (range of 6 to 18 months; average of 10 months). This is independent of the number of injections but may be directly related to the weight of the patient. Within 18 months, however, fertility rates return to normal levels.

Implantable Progesterone-Only Contraception—Nexplanon

Method of Action

Nexplanon (the newest generation of the Implanon device) is a **single-rod, subdermal progestin implant** that provides **3 years** of uninterrupted contraceptive coverage. The progestin used in Nexplanon is **etonogestrel**, the same progestin as used in the NuvaRing. The device is 4 cm × 2 mm, contains 68 mg of etonogestrel, and provides a slow release of hormone over 3 years. It is radiopaque and the size of a matchstick . It has a redesigned applicator that facilitates placement in the subdermal skin of the inner side of a woman's upper arm. When appropriate timing of placement is utilized, Nexplanon is effective 24 hours after placement and has quick return to fertility once the device is removed by a clinician. Similar to other contraceptives, it acts by suppressing ovulation, altering the endometrium, and increasing cervical mucous viscosity.

Jadelle is a two-rod implantable subdermal device also approved by the FDA. It uses **levonorgestrel** to provide 5 years of contraceptive coverage. At this time, Jadelle has not yet been marketed in the United States but has been used in many other countries.

Effectiveness

Nexplanon is one of the **most highly effective reversible** contraceptive methods, with only a 0.5% failure rate.

Side Effects

Irregular and unpredictable light bleeding is the major side effect of Nexplanon. In the majority of cases (75%), the bleeding is lighter than a normal menstrual bleed and requires only a panty liner or less for protection. However, irregular bleeding was the reason for approximately 15% of discontinuations, followed by headaches (approximately 12%).

Advantages/Disadvantages

The major advantage of Nexplanon is that it is implantable and provides three uninterrupted years of contraceptive coverage. There is **no maintenance** associated with the device and thus **no interruption of sexual spontaneity**.

The disadvantages include the need for a provider to insert and remove the device and the **unpredictable bleeding profile**.

EMERGENCY CONTRACEPTION

Emergency contraception (EC) is a **safe and effective** means of **preventing pregnancy** after unprotected intercourse or in the case of contraceptive failure (condom break, diaphragm dislodgment, IUD expulsion, missed pill, and late Depo-Provera injection). It is used only if a woman is not already pregnant from a previous act of intercourse. The use of emergency contraceptive pills (ECPs) is not indicated in women with a known or suspected pregnancy. However, there is **no known evidence of harm** to the patient, her pregnancy, or to the fetus if ECPs are unintentionally taken during pregnancy. EC can also be used safely in women in whom continual estrogen might otherwise be contraindicated, such as women with a history of DVT, PE, myocardial infarction (MI), stroke, or migraines with auras.

Emergency contraception works by preventing pregnancy, not by disrupting an implanted pregnancy. In fact, ECP is thought to account for a 40% **decline in therapeutic abortions** in the past 10 years while also **decreasing the number of teen pregnancies**. It is available in three forms: ECPs (also called the *postcoital* or the *morning-after pill*), an emergently inserted Copper T IUD (ParaGard), or a selective progesterone receptor modulator (ulipristal acetate or Ella). Although **mifepristone** (RU 486) has been approved in the United States for the termination of pregnancy up to 49 days of gestation, its use has not been approved for EC. In the United States, EC does not require an examination by a provider, although a pregnancy test should be performed before placing a Copper IUD or giving ulipristal (Ella). The ECPs may be obtained over-the-counter **without a prescription** by men and women 17 years or older.

EMERGENCY CONTRACEPTIVE PILLS

Methods of Action

ECPs use high doses of both estrogen and progestins or progesterone alone (Plan B One Step, Next Choice) to prevent pregnancy after unprotected intercourse has taken place. Several differing regimens exist including those using high doses of regularly prescribed OCPs and some using prepackaged regimens. For those using ECPs, **levonorgestrel methods are preferred** over estrogen–progesterone regimens since levonorgestrel is more effective and has fewer side effects.

The most common prepackaged formulation is **Plan B (progestin only)**. This regimen can be taken as a single 1.5 mg of Levonorgestrel (Plan B One Step) or as two 0.75 mg doses taken 12 hours apart (Next Choice). Studies show that Plan B is equally effective if taken in a single dose with minimal increased side effects. Regardless of the regimen, **the first dose must be taken within 72 hours of unprotected vaginal intercourse.** There is some additional efficacy if initiated within 120 hours, although not as high as within the first 72 hours. An antiemetic is often prescribed at the same time to prevent nausea (more common in estrogen-containing regimens).

The **mechanism of action** for ECPs depends on the point during the cycle when the pills are taken. Emergency contraception is used to prevent pregnancy by inhibiting ovulation, interfering with fertilization and tubal transport, preventing implantation, or causing regression of the corpus luteum.

Effectiveness

When taken within 72 hours of intercourse, ECPs have a failure rate of 0.2% to 3%. The sooner an ECP is taken after unprotected intercourse, the more effective it is. The risk of pregnancy is reduced by 75% to 90% in women who have had unprotected intercourse during the second or third week of their menstrual cycles, when they are most likely ovulating. Of all the oral EC regimens, the progesterone-only formulations (Plan B) are the most effective and have fewer side effects. Thus, **Plan B One Step should be used as a first choice** when it is available, rather than using a combination method.

Side Effects

The primary side effects of EC include **nausea (50%)**, **vomiting (20%)**, headaches, dizziness, and breast tenderness. Most of these symptoms are thought to be secondary to the high doses of estrogen in the combined regimens. The side effects of the progesterone-only formulations are less severe than symptoms experienced with estrogen and progesterone-containing methods.

While there are relative and absolute contraindications for use of oral contraceptives in women with certain medical conditions (history of stroke, heart attack, DVT, and PE), these contraindications do not apply to women using emergency contraceptives. However, repeated use of ECP is not recommended in this high-risk group.

Advantages/Disadvantages

ECPs are extremely effective in preventing pregnancy and are safe for the user. In 2006, the FDA approved over-the-counter dispensing of Plan B emergency contraception without a prescription for men and women aged 17 years and older.

The major disadvantages include the short window of time when they can be used (within 72 to 120 hours of intercourse). Additionally, these cannot be used as long-term contraception.

EMERGENCY IUD INSERTION

Method of Action

The Copper T IUD (Fig. 24-6A) can be inserted in the uterine cavity within 120 hours (or 5 days) of unprotected intercourse as a form of emergency contraception. The IUD functions primarily by eliciting a **sterile inflammatory response** within the uterus, making the environment unsuitable for fertilization.

Effectiveness

Emergency Copper T IUD insertion reduces the risk of pregnancy by 99.8%; therefore, only 1 in 1,000 become pregnant after emergency IUD insertion, **making it the most effective form of emergency contraception**.

Side Effects

The side effects are the same as those discussed in the IUD section. Copper T is not an acceptable form of emergency contraception in women who are not candidates for IUDs, including those with multiple sexual partners, suspected active cervical or uterine infections, and victims of rape.

Advantages/Disadvantages

Emergency Copper T IUD insertion is extremely effective, even more effective than the oral regimens. It differs from ECPs in that it **can be continued for long-term contraception (10 years)**, whereas the ECPs have a one-time-only use. Disadvantages of IUD are that it must be placed by a provider, it has a higher one-time cost than oral regimens, and its potential for rare complications such as infection and perforation (described in the IUD section above). The ParaGard IUD is also associated with heavier menses and dysmenorrhea.

EMERGENCY PROGESTERONE RECEPTOR MODULATORS

Method of Action

The newest form of ECP received FDA approval in August of 2010. Ulipristal (*Ella, EllaOne*) is a derivative of 19-norprogesterone, and acts as a selective progesterone receptor modulator (SPRM) with agonist/antagonist effects at progesterone receptor sites. Its primary mechanism of action is to **delay ovulation** (follicular rupture) and inhibit implantation into the endometrial lining. It is available worldwide and is administered in a single dose of 30 mg within 120 hours (5 days) after unprotected coital event. Small trials suggest that ulipristal is more effective than progestin-only regimens in preventing pregnancy when used between the 72- and 120-hour postcoital time period.

A closely related drug to ulipristal is **mifepristone (RU 486)**. Its mechanism of action is similar to ulipristal. Currently, mifepristone is not available in the United States for prevention of pregnancy, although trials have shown 99% to 100% efficacy (similar to or better than that of current ECPs). The actual dosing has not yet been determined for this indication, and its current use in the United States is limited to medical termination of pregnancy.

Effectiveness

The pregnancy rate when prescribed within the 120-hour window is about 2%.

Side Effects

The most common side effects are similar to ECPs and include self-limited headache, bleeding, nausea, and abdominal pain.

Advantages/Disadvantages

Ulipristal is contraindicated in women who are breastfeeding or currently pregnant, given its antiprogestin effects and potential to terminate an existing pregnancy. A **pregnancy test** is required before the administration of ulipristal. Advantages of its use include one-time dosing and relatively mild side effects.

One disadvantage is that it is available by **prescription only**. Its use is also controversial given its potential use as an abortifactant (although not approved for this indication). This is, in contrast to progestin-only or combined estrogen/progestin ECPs, because they do not terminate an existing pregnancy nor cause teratogenic effects. For these reasons, ulipristal is not as widely prescribed when compared with other ECPs.

SURGICAL STERILIZATION

The rate of surgical sterilization as a method of contraception has increased dramatically over the past three decades. Approximately 30% of reproductive-age couples in the United States and Great Britain choose female sterilization for contraceptive purposes. A similar number of men seek vasectomies each year. The rate of sterilization is higher in women who are **married, divorced, over age 30, or African–American.**

Before performing any sterilization procedure, careful counseling should be provided and informed consent obtained. The patient should understand the **permanent and largely irreversible nature** of the procedure, operative risks, chance of failure, and possible side effects. Sterilization is ideal in stable monogamous relationships where (no additional) children are desired. It is also indicated in women in whom pregnancy would be life-threatening such as those with major cardiac issues.

TUBAL STERILIZATION

Method of Action

Tubal sterilization prevents pregnancy by surgically occluding both fallopian tubes to prevent the ovum and sperm from uniting. Tubal ligation can be performed in the immediate postpartum period (**postpartum sterilization** [PPS]), or outside the postpartum period via a laparoscopic approach (**laparoscopic tubal ligation** [LTL]) or via **hysteroscopic tubal occlusion** (*Essure*).

Tubal ligation can be performed immediately postpartum (**postpartum sterilization** [PPS]) through a small subumbilical incision using epidural or spinal anesthesia. The most commonly used method, the *modified* Pomeroy tubal ligation (aka Parkland), is illustrated in Figure 24-12. Laparoscopically, there are a number of methods by which tubal occlusion can be accomplished including bipolar cautery (Fig. 24-13), Silastic banding with Falope rings (Fig. 24-14), or clipping with Hulka clips or Filshie clips (Fig. 24-15).

Modern techniques have evolved to incorporate sterilization procedures in both operating room and outpatient (in-office) practices that involve **nonincisional hysteroscopic approaches.** The **Essure** was introduced in the United States in 2002. In this method, flexible form-fitting microinserts are introduced into the interstitial (uterine) portions of the fallopian tubes. An outer **spring coil** molds to the shape of the fallopian tube to anchor the microinsert. **Over about 12 weeks, sterilization is accomplished** as in-growth of tissue around the coils results in tissue barrier occlusion in the fallopian tubes.

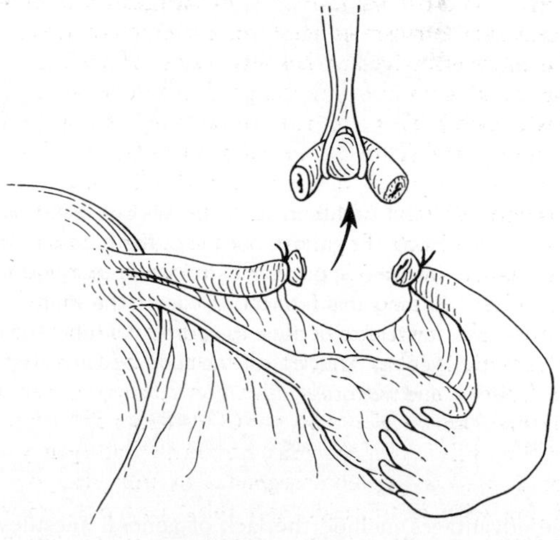

Figure 24-12 • The Parkland (modified Pomeroy) method of postpartum tubal ligation. A 2- to 3-cm segment of the tube is doubly ligated and the intervening segment is removed. This technique is typically performed during the immediate postpartum period through a small subumbilical incision.
(From Rock J, Jones H. *TeLinde's Operative Gynecology*, 10th ed. Philadelphia, PA: Lippincott Williams & Wilkins; 2008.)

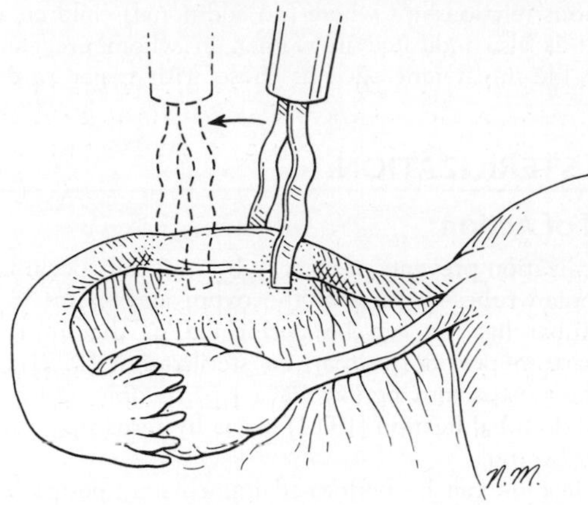

Figure 24-13 • Tubal occlusion with the bipolar cautery. A 3-cm portion of the isthmic tube is desiccated with bipolar forceps.
(From Rock J, Jones H. *TeLinde's Operative Gynecology*, 10th ed. Philadelphia, PA: Lippincott Williams & Wilkins; 2008.)

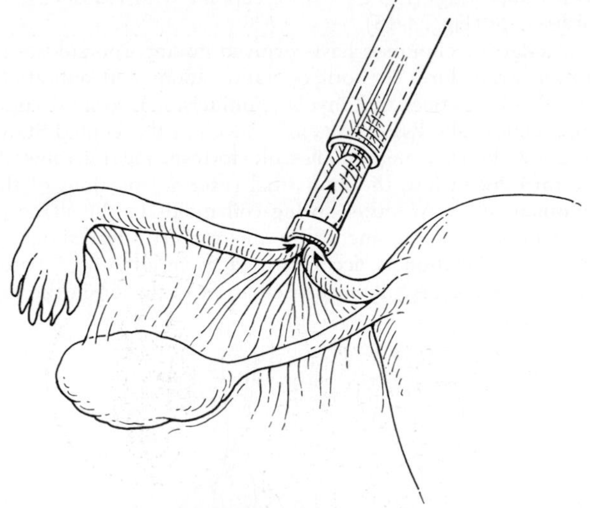

Figure 24-14 • Tubal occlusion with the silicone band (Falope ring). The isthmic portion of the tube is retracted into the applicator barrel using grasping tongs. During this retraction process the ring is rolled forward to occlude the portion of tube. The intervening "knuckle" of the tube becomes ischemic and necroses.
(From Rock J, Jones H. *TeLinde's Operative Gynecology*, 10th ed. Philadelphia, PA: Lippincott Williams & Wilkins; 2008.)

The advantages include the lack of general anesthesia and the lack of a surgical incision. As a result, when hysteroscopic tubal sterilization/occlusion can be performed, very little recuperative time is needed and it provides a **safer, more effective** means of permanent birth control. The Essure procedure can often be performed in the **office setting**, making it a preferable option to surgical sterilization for all women, including obese women, women with prior abdominal surgeries, or those at risk from anesthesia use.

Because the tubal blockage is accomplished over time, a **backup method of birth control** is recommended for 3 months after the procedure until such time that a **hysterosalpingogram** (HSG) can confirm coil location and complete tubal occlusion. Some patients are reassured by this confirmatory test, whereas others are burdened by the additional step to achieving permanent sterilization. Prior to the procedure, patients should understand that tubal occlusion by this method is essentially **irreversible**.

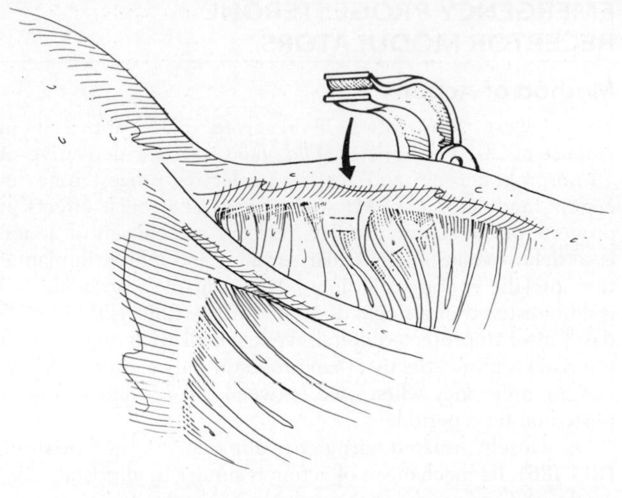

Figure 24-15 • Tubal occlusion with the Filshie clip. The clip is applied to the mid-isthmic portion of the tube about 2 cm from the cornua. The lower jaw of the clip should be visible through the mesosalpinx to ensure inclusion of the entire circumference of the tube.
(From Rock J, Jones H. *TeLinde's Operative Gynecology*, 10th ed. Philadelphia, PA: Lippincott Williams & Wilkins; 2008.)

Effectiveness

Tubal ligation has a failure rate of 0.3% but varies by method, patient age, and surgeon's experience. The **highest success** rates are achieved with **postpartum sterilization and Essure tubal occlusion**. When the laparoscopic approach is undertaken, the Falope ring has been found to be most effective in women under age 28 years. Electrocautery and Falope rings are equally effective in women over age 28. More recently, titanium Filshie clips have been used for tubal ligation, but long-term efficacy rates are not yet available. **Essure** offers the lowest rates of all of these methods when tubal occlusion is achieved (2.6/1,000 pregnancy rate over 5 years, aside from unipolar sterilization, which is no longer used).

Side Effects

There are no side effects associated with tubal sterilization. Some women report pain and menstrual disturbances. This phenomenon was once described as **posttubal ligation syndrome** but has largely been discounted by the literature. In most of these women, symptoms are due to **discontinuation of hormone-containing contraceptives**. As a result, patients may experience heavier baseline menses and dysmenorrhea. In rare circumstances, malplacement of *Essure* coils has contributed to significant pain requiring subsequent surgical removal.

Advantage/Disadvantages

Tubal ligation offers the advantage of permanent effective contraception without continual expense, effort, or motivation. The **mortality rate** of bilateral tubal ligation is 4 in 100,000 women. The major risks are those associated with surgery including the risk of infection, hemorrhage, conversion to laparotomy, viscus injury, vascular damage, and anesthesia complications.

Tubal ligation results in a **very low risk of pregnancy**. However, when pregnancy does occur, there is an **increased risk of ectopic pregnancy** (1 in 15,000). However, nearly 1,000 maternal lives are saved due to sterilization during the period from the time of sterilization to the end of the woman's reproductive life. The rates of ectopic pregnancy after Essure is decreased compared to tubal ligation. Patients may also benefit from a **reduction in the risk of ovarian cancer**. The reason for this is unclear but it is speculated that tubal ligation may limit the migration of carcinogens from the lower genital tract into the peritoneal cavity.

Of women who undergo permanent sterilization, **regret is highest in women who were under 30** years when the procedure was performed. However, it is estimated that less than 2% of women seek reversal of tubal sterilization. The success of reversal varies from 41% to 84% depending on the method used (Table 24-8). The success rate of reanastomosis is highest when clips are used since they destroy a much smaller segment of the tube. When pregnancy is desired after tubal ligation, in vitro fertilization (IVF) offers a greater likelihood of pregnancy than tubal microplasty. However, when multiple future pregnancies are desired, tubuloplasty may be a more economical alternative than multiple IVF cycles.

VASECTOMY

Method of Action

Vasectomy is a simple and safe option for permanent sterilization involving **ligation of the vas deferens**. This procedure may be performed in a provider's office under local anesthesia through a small incision in the upper outer aspect of each scrotum (Fig. 24-16). In 1985, the **no-scalpel vasectomy** technique was introduced. With this procedure both vas are ligated through a single small midline incision that reduces the already low rate of complications associated with vasectomy. Unlike female tubal ligations, **vasectomy is not immediately effective**. Because sperm can remain viable in the proximal collecting system after vasectomy, patients should use **another form of contraception** until azoospermia is confirmed by semen analysis, usually in 6 to 8 weeks.

Effectiveness

The failure rate for vasectomy in actual practice is 0.15%. In fact, with the exception of Essure, vasectomy is **safer, simpler, and more effective than female sterilization**. When pregnancies occur after vasectomy, many are due to having intercourse too soon after vasectomy rather propr to azoospermia than from recanalization of the vas deferens.

Side Effects

Complications after vasectomy are rare and usually involve slight bleeding, skin infection, and reactions to the sutures or local anesthesia. Fifty percent of patients form **antisperm antibodies** after the procedure. However, there are no long-term side effects of vasectomy.

Advantages/Disadvantages

Vasectomy is a permanent, highly effective form of contraception with few, if any, side effects. Vasectomy is generally safer and less expensive than tubal ligation and can be performed as an outpatient under local anesthesia. Vasectomy offers permanent sterilization. The success rate of vasal reanastomosis is 60% to 70%. Pregnancy rates after vasectomy reversal range from 18% to 60%.

TABLE 24-8 Success Rates of Tubal Occlusion Reversal, by Method

Method of Tubal Sterilization	Success Rates for Reversal (%)
Clips	84
Bands	72
Pomeroy	50
Electrocauterization	41

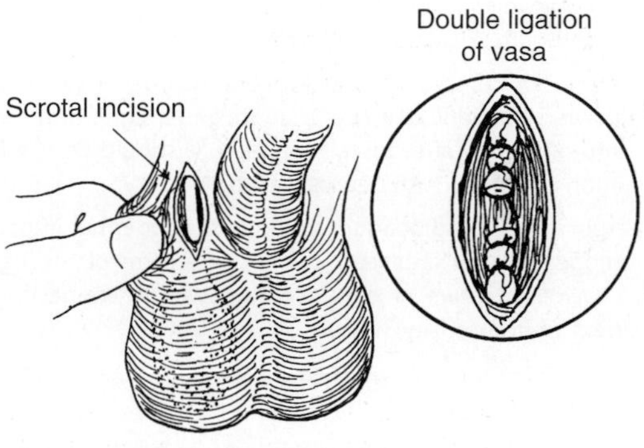

Figure 24-16 • Sterilization by vasectomy. Typically performed in an office setting under local anesthesia.
(From Beckmann C, Ling F. *Obstetrics & Gynecology*, 5th ed. Philadelphia, PA: Lippincott Williams & Wilkins; 2006.)

KEY POINTS

- Natural family planning methods and coitus interruptus are the least effective methods of contraception and should not be used if pregnancy prevention is a high priority.
- Lactational amenorrhea provides a prolactin-induced suppression of GnRH and subsequent suppression of ovulation. It should only be used for a maximum of 6 months after delivery in an amenorrheic woman and breastfeeding should be the only source of nutrition for the infant.
- Condoms, diaphragms, and cervical caps act as mechanical barriers between sperm and egg. Their efficacy rate is 75% to 85% with practical use.
- Male and female condoms carry the added benefit of prophylaxis against STIs.
- Efficacy of spermicides is 70% to 80%, but variability in user technique can significantly lower efficacy. Spermicides DO NOT

protect against STIs and may, in fact, make the vaginal mucosa more susceptible to infections such as HIV.

- IUDs provide long-term, highly effective, and cost-effective contraception. There are currently two IUDs in the US market: ParaGard (copper-containing; 10 years of use) and Mirena (progestin-containing; 5 years of use).
- The primary mechanism of action for IUDs is a sterile spermicidal inflammatory response. Other mechanisms include inhibition of implantation and alteration in tubal motility. Potentially serious side effects include insertion-related PID, uterine perforation, and spontaneous abortion.
- Hormonal contraceptives have extremely low failure rates when used appropriately and are available in oral, injectable, transdermal, implantable, vaginal, and intrauterine forms.
- Combined hormonal contraception methods (OCPs, Ortho Evra, and NuvaRing) prevent pregnancy by suppressing ovulation, altering cervical mucus, and causing atrophic changes in the endometrium.
- Serious complications from combined hormonal contraception use occur mainly in smokers over age 35, including pulmonary embolism, stroke, DVT, and heart attack.
- Benefits of combined hormonal contraception include protection from ovarian and endometrial cancer, anemia, PID, osteoporosis, dysmenorrhea, acne, hirsutism, and benign breast disease.
- Progesterone-only contraception (progestin-only OCPs, Depo-Provera, Nexplanon, and the Mirena IUD) use progestins to suppress ovulation, thicken the cervical mucus, and make the endometrium unsuitable for implantation.
- Primary side effects of Depo-Provera include irregular bleeding, reversible bone demineralization, and a significant delay in return of fertility after discontinuation. It should be used with caution in women with depression and obesity.
- Nexplanon is a radiopaque, single-rod, subdermal implant of etonogestrel that is placed in the upper arm of the patient. It provides 3 years of contraception without impacting the patient's bone density, weight, or mood.
- ECPs contain high doses of estrogen and progestin or progesterone alone and must be taken within 72 hours of intercourse to prevent pregnancy. These pills act to suppress ovulation and to prevent fertilization and implantation. They do not cause abortions.
- A newer form of emergency contraception, ulipristal, is available that blocks progesterone receptor sites. This method is not yet widely used and is controversial due to its ability to affect an existing pregnancy if present. It has a higher effectiveness rate than ECPs.
- When available, a single dose of progesterone-only ECP (Plan B) should be used preferentially, given its increased effectiveness and lower rate of side effects.
- Emergency IUD insertion (Copper T only) must be performed within 120 hours of unprotected intercourse; it can then be used as long-term contraception.
- Both vasectomy and tubal occlusion are highly effective forms of permanent sterilization. Vasectomies are safer, simpler, and more easily reversed than female sterilization.
- Patients requesting sterilization should be counseled of the permanent and largely irreversible nature of the procedures. The risk of regret is highest among women under age 30 regardless of their parity.
- The most effective tubal ligations are those done immediately postpartum or those utilizing the Essure tubal occlusion system.
- When interval laparoscopic approach is undertaken, Falope rings have the highest efficacy in women less than 28 years. Electrocautery and Falope rings have equal efficacy in women 28 years and older.
- Essure offers a hysteroscopic approach to tubal ligation and the safest and most effective means of permanent birth control. It does not require a surgical incision or general anesthesia but it does require use of a backup method for 3 months and an HSG to confirm complete tubal occlusion.
- Reversal rates for tubal occlusion vary from 41% to 84% depending on the method used for sterilization. These procedures are costly and are associated with a higher rate of ectopic pregnancy.

C

Clinical Vignettes

Vignette 1

An 18-year-old G0 F presents to your office for contraceptive counseling. She has never used any method of contraception before and is engaged in a monogamous sexual relationship. Gynecologic history is significant for regular, heavy menstrual cycles using up to eight pads per day, lasting up to 7 days at a time, with severe pain (dysmenorrhea). She smokes one-half pack of cigarettes per day and tells you that her mother and aunt both have Factor V Leiden disease, but that she has never been tested herself or had a thromboembolic event. She will attend college soon and has no plans for a pregnancy in the near future. She indicates her desire for the "most reliable" method of contraception that you can offer.

1. Which of the following methods of contraception has the least efficacy?
   a. Ortho Evra patch
   b. Combined oral contraceptive pills
   c. Mirena IUD
   d. Condoms with spermicide
   e. Coitus interruptus
2. Physical examination in the office reveals a blood pressure of 140/85 mm Hg, pulse of 80, and BMI of 40. Abdomen is soft, nontender, and genitourinary exam is unremarkable with no cervical inflammation. Which of the following would be the best choice of contraception for this patient?
   a. Ortho Evra patch
   b. Combined oral contraceptive pills (COCs)
   c. Mirena (Levonorgestrel) IUD
   d. Condoms with spermicide
   e. Coitus interruptus
3. Of course, during your discussion at this visit, you could encourage smoking cessation and recommend weight loss to help improve her overall health. You and the patient have decided to proceed with IUD placement. Prior to placement, it is important to perform which of the following tests?
   a. FSH level
   b. Prolactin level
   c. Urine pregnancy test
   d. Gonorrhea/Chlamydia testing
   e. Both c and d

Vignette 2

A 37-year-old female G5P5 has come to your office to discuss long-term contraception. A thorough history and office examination reveal a healthy, thin female, in no acute distress. She reports seasonal allergies and has undergone one cesarean section in the past as well as four spontaneous vaginal deliveries, and no additional surgeries. She has never had an STI, and is a nonsmoker. Her Pap smears and HPV screens have all been normal and are up to date. She asks you to explain which methods will be effective for a long period of time, as she has trouble remembering to take a pill daily with five small children at home.

1. You inform her that many methods can be considered "long term," except which of the following?
   a. 1.5 mg Levonorgestrel pill
   b. Etonogestrel rod (Nexplanon)
   c. Copper IUD (ParaGard)
   d. Levonorgestrel IUD (Mirena)
   e. Tubal Ligation/Occlusion
2. She chooses to consider the options presented above, and returns 3 weeks later after discussing the methods with her husband. They have decided to undergo permanent sterilization. She is nervous about "going to sleep" under anesthesia as she's had severe nausea from this in the past, and doesn't want any additional abdominal scars. Which one of the following methods can be performed in the office with local anesthesia and oral pain medication, avoiding the need for general anesthesia?
   a. Falope rings
   b. Filshie clips
   c. Pomeroy method (postpartum tubal)
   d. Essure (microinsert coils)
   e. Bipolar cautery
3. Once you've performed the chosen procedure (above) in the office, you instruct her that she will need a follow-up test in 3 months to confirm that the coils are in the correct location and that tubal occlusion has been achieved. Which of the following tests is used to confirm complete tubal occlusion?
   a. Ultrasound
   b. Flat/upright abdominal X-ray
   c. Hysterosalpingogram (HSG)
   d. CT scan of Pelvis without contrast
   e. MRI of Pelvis with contrast

Vignette 3

A 40-year-old F G3P3 comes to your office to discuss contraception. She has been married for 15 years, and smokes one pack of cigarettes per day. She was diagnosed with systemic lupus erythematosus (SLE)at the age of 20, and has only been hospitalized once for an acute exacerbation of joint swelling and fatigue. Her BMI is 24, and she has light to normal menstrual flow. She has no plans for a future pregnancy, but is not ready to commit to permanent sterilization.

1. You inform her that all of the following are absolute contraindications to combined oral contraceptive pill use, except:
   a. History of or current thromboembolism
   b. Coronary artery disease
   c. Tobacco use of greater than or equal to 15 cigarettes/day over the age of 35 years
   d. Diabetes mellitus
   e. Abnormal liver function

2. Which of the following would *not* be a reasonable method of contraception for this patient?
   a. Ortho Evra patch
   b. Depo-Provera
   c. ParaGard IUD
   d. Mirena IUD
   e. Progestin-only oral pill

3. The patient decides to continue using condoms and spermicide. She is aware of the 95% effectiveness when spermicide is used. Several months later, she calls your office 36 hours after having unprotected intercourse and is very concerned about becoming pregnant. You prescribe her Plan B, and tell her it is most effective if taken within 72 hours of the event. What is the most common side effect of Plan B?
   a. Heavy vaginal bleeding
   b. Fever
   c. Diarrhea
   d. Dizziness
   e. Nausea/vomiting

Vignette 4

A 23-year-old G0 F comes to your office to discuss an effective method of contraception. Her only medical condition is endometriosis—diagnosed by laparoscopy 3 years ago. She was placed on oral contraceptives shortly after her laparoscopy and fulguration of endometriosis. Unfortunately after her surgery, she lost her health insurance, wasn't able to refill the medication, and hasn't resumed care until now. She has been sexually active with the same partner for 3 years, and has monthly menses with moderate flow. She has never had an STI, and is not planning to become pregnant in the near future.

1. You tell her that the mechanism of action of oral contraceptives includes:
   a. Thickening of cervical mucous
   b. Making the endometrial environment unsuitable for implantation
   c. Interfering with pulsatile FSH/LH surges
   d. Suppressing ovulation and follicular recruitment
   e. All of the above

2. She reports severe dysmenorrhea that begins 1 week prior to each menstrual cycle, and is resolved 1 to 2 days after bleeding begins. This pain is only partially relieved with nonsteroidal anti-inflammatory drugs (NSAIDs), and she would like to know what can be done to help with this. To reduce dysmenorrhea caused by endometriosis, you instruct her to take combined oral contraceptive pills in the following manner:
   a. Continuous dosing—take active pills only for 3 months, then take 1 week of placebo to have withdrawal bleed
   b. Take two active pills each day, can take up to three pills per day if pain becomes severe
   c. Tapered dosing—take four pills for 4 days, then three pills for 3 days, and so on until the pack is complete, then resume from the beginning
   d. Take one pill every other day
   e. Change to a progesterone-only "mini pill" and take one each day

3. You have prescribed the appropriate combined oral contraceptive pill regimen to the patient described in the prior question. You now see a 30-year-old G1P0010 F who presents to your office with the diagnosis of menstrual migraines without aura, and otherwise negative workup and medical history. She desires COCs, and you prescribe the same method of use as you did to the previous patient. Taking COCs in this manner can be used as treatment for patients with all of these conditions, **except** which of the following?
   a. PMS
   b. PCOS
   c. Endometrial hyperplasia
   d. Ovarian cysts
   e. Menstrual migraines without aura

A Answers

Vignette 1 Question 1
Answer E: Coitus interruptus has a significantly high failure rate—up to 27%. Ortho Evra patch has a 1% pregnancy rate with recommended use, which is comparable to that of combined oral contraceptive pills. However, actual use of oral contraceptive pills has a failure rate of 8%. Condoms are 85% to 90% efficacious, and up to 95% effective with addition of spermicide.

Vignette 1 Question 2
Answer C: This is a progesterone-only, low maintenance delivery of contraception, also approved for the treatment of heavy menstrual bleeding. We have established the patient's family history of thromboembolic disorder, as well as obesity (BMI: 40), hypertensive, and a smoker; therefore it is prudent to avoid an estrogen-containing method in this patient because of the increased risk of cardiovascular disease, specifically thromboembolic event. Ortho Evra patch and COCs both contain estrogen. Condoms with spermicide would be a good alternative; however, the patient has requested the "most reliable method"—Mirena IUD has a failure rate of 0.8%, whereas condoms with spermicide have approximately 5% failure rate. Mirena IUD could also offer the added benefit of reduced menstrual flow and treatment of dysmenorrhea. Coitus interruptus is not a reliable method of contraception given its high rate of failure.

Vignette 1 Question 3
Answer E: Urine pregnancy and Gonorrhea/Chlamydia testing should be performed prior to IUD insertion in this patient. Absolute contraindications to IUD insertion include: known or suspected pregnancy, undiagnosed abnormal vaginal bleeding, acute cervical/uterine/ or salpingeal infection, Copper allergy or Wilson's disease (for ParaGard only), or current breast cancer (for Mirena only). STI testing is indicated in any "high risk" population (defined as age <25 years or multiple sexual partners). FSH and prolactin level tests are not necessary for this patient, as these are traditionally used in workup of abnormal bleeding and have no bearing on this patient's situation. One additional test that we would recommend to her is Factor V Leiden genetic testing, given her family history.

Vignette 2 Question 1
Answer A: Levonorgestrel pill (Plan B) is a progestin-only method used for emergency contraception. It is available over-the-counter to those aged 17 years and older, and is very effective (up to 97% success rate), when taken within 72 hours of unprotected intercourse. This method is not intended for repeated or long-term use. The Etonogestrel rod (Nexplanon), Copper IUD (ParaGard), and Levonorgestrel IUD (Mirena) are all considered "Long-Acting Reversible Contraception" methods (LARCs). Nexplanon can be used up to 3 years, Mirena up to 5 years, and ParaGard up to 10 years. Tubal ligation and tubal occlusion are permanent forms of birth control are permanent forms of birth control and patients are counseled that this method is not intended to be reversed.

Vignette 2 Question 2
Answer D: The Essure method was approved by the FDA in 2002 and is widely available in the United States today. It consists of micro insert coils containing flexible metal, and induces a mild fibrotic reaction in the tubal lumen resulting in occlusion. Advantages of this method include the ability to perform the procedure in office, thus avoiding the need for general anesthesia. It is performed transcervically, which confers less risk to adjacent organs, therefore avoiding the need for abdominal entry (laparoscopy). Falope rings, Filshie clips, and bipolar cautery are also commonly used methods; however, they require laparoscopic entry into the abdominal peritoneum. The Pomeroy method is commonly performed at the time of cesarean section, or through a small sub-umbilical incision when immediately following a vaginal delivery. During the immediate postpartum period the uterus remains enlarged and sits just beneath the umbilicus, making the fallopian tubes accessible through this small incision.

Vignette 2 Question 3
Answer C: HSG is an X-ray (fluoroscopy) of the pelvis during which radiopaque contrast medium is placed via a catheter through the cervix and injected into the endometrial cavity. The course of the contrast is observed, and the tubes are confirmed to be completely occluded if there is no dye spill through the tubes into the peritoneal cavity. This test is also used during an infertility workup to evaluate tubal patency or uterine cavity shape.

Current studies are assessing the ability of ultrasonography to evaluate tubal occlusion following the Essure procedure; however, this method can only demonstrate coil placement, not tubal patency and is not recommended for confirmation of tubal closure at this time in the United States. The micro coils are radiopaque, and can be seen on a flat/upright X-ray film; however, this does not tell us about their effectiveness, only location. A CT scan and MRI are not recommended to evaluate success of tubal occlusion. MRI for other diagnostic purposes is safe with Essure coils in place.

It is important that the patients have a reliable method of contraception during the 3 months after placement of the microinserts until a confirmatory test has been performed to verify correct coil location and demonstrate bilateral tubal occlusion.

Vignette 3 Question 1

Answer D: Diabetes mellitus is a relative contraindication to administering COCs. It is not recommended for use in patients with longstanding or uncontrolled diabetes, especially those with vascular complications (renal and ophthalmologic involvement). A history of venous thromboembolic event (VTE) is an absolute contraindication, as well as any coronary artery disease, or tobacco use (≥15 cigarettes/day) over the age of 35 years. Other absolute contraindications include: history of cerebrovascular accident, breast or endometrial cancer, suspected or current pregnancy, and severe hypercholesterolemia or hypertriglyceridemia. SLE is a relative contraindication; COCs should be used cautiously in this population and avoided when possible.

Vignette 3 Question 2

Answer A: The Ortho Evra patch is a combination contraception patch, and contains both estrogen and progesterone (ethinyl estradiol and norelgestromin). A patch is placed on the skin for 3 weeks, then removed for 1 week at which time a withdrawal bleed should occur. It carries the same risks as oral contraceptives, and should not be given to women who are smokers over the age of 35 years, as well as the other absolute contraindications listed in Vignette 3 Question 1. Its primary action is suppression of ovulation by decreasing endogenous FSH and LH levels. It should also not be given in women over 198 lb (or 90 kg). Depo-Provera, Mirena IUD, and Progestin-only pills are all non-estrogen containing methods of contraception. There is a negligible risk of thromboembolism with these methods, and they are often used for those patients who are not candidates for estrogen use. The ParaGard IUD is a Copper-T device, and is effective in limiting sperm and tubal motility and also creates a "sterile inflammatory environment" within the uterus. It should not be used in women with a history of menorrhagia or unexplained abnormal bleeding. Given her low BMI and no history of depression, Depo-Provera use would also be reasonable.

Vignette 3 Question 3

Answer E: Nausea is present in approximately 50% and vomiting in 20% of patients who take Plan B. These are slightly less severe in those taking Plan B (progestin-only, single dose) versus prior combination methods (Yuzpe method) containing estrogen. Often providers prescribe antiemetics at the same time as emergency contraception. Headaches, dizziness, and breast tenderness are also side effects, however, not the most common. There are no significant reports of fever or diarrhea when using emergency contraception. The patient should expect her menses to come a couple of days earlier than expected after using ECPs. The Copper IUD is also a method of emergency contraception when used up to 5 days after unprotected intercourse.

Vignette 4 Question 1

Answer E: Oral contraceptives have multiple mechanisms of action. Their primary effect is to suppress the mid-cycle surge by interfering with the pulsatile release of FSH and LH from the anterior pituitary, thus preventing follicular maturation and ovulation. The progesterone component works by thickening the cervical mucus, impairing tubal motility, and making the endometrium less suitable for implantation.

Vignette 4 Question 2

Answer A: Of the dosing regimens shown, the most effective would be the continuous method. Women with endometriosis, PMS, PCOS, ovarian cysts, or menstrual migraines may benefit from extending the number of consecutive days of hormonal pills (up to 1, 2, or 3 months), and decreasing the number of withdrawal bleeds. These extended or long-cycle regimens provide continued suppression of ovulation—reducing the circulating estrogen levels and decreasing the menstrual-related symptoms (i.e., pain, heavy bleeding, anemia, cysts, and/or headaches).

Taking more than one active pill per day for extended periods of time is contraindicated and can lead to thromboembolic events such as DVT and PEs. This method of dosing is used for very short periods of time in selected circumstances such as for emergency contraception and abnormal uterine bleeding. The tapering method is generally reserved for management of extremely heavy and prolonged bleeding. Again, it is used for a short period of time and only in specific circumstances; not as a routine dosing method. Taking one pill every other day increases the risk of both an endometriosis flare and pregnancy.

Progestins may be effectively used in the treatment of endometriosis.The low dose (0.35 mg) of the progesterone-only contraceptive pills (POPs) are less effective at suppressing ovulation and maintaining low levels of estrogen compared with combination OCPs. However, other progesterone-only methods are effective at treating endometriosis including oral medroxyprogesterone acetate (Provera), depot medroxyprogesterone acetate (Depo-Provera), norethindrone acetate (2.5 to 10 mg), and the levonorgestrel-containing IUD (Mirena).

Vignette 4 Question 3

Answer C: Endometrial hyperplasia is abnormal overgrowth of the endometrial cells, which can ultimately develop into endometrial cancer if left untreated. Most commonly, this is a result of excess estrogen effect with inadequate progesterone balance, and is often seen in women with obesity and oligomenorrhea—such as those with PCOS or anovulatory cycles. The treatment for this would be progesterone or surgical treatment, but not COCs, as these contain estrogen. Women with PMS, PCOS, ovarian cysts, or menstrual migraines without auras may benefit from extending the number of consecutive days of hormonal pills (up to 1, 2, or 3 months), and decreasing the number of withdrawal bleeds. These extended or long-cycle regimens provide continued suppression of ovulation—reducing the number of new cysts formed and decreasing menstrual-related symptoms (i.e., pain, heavy bleeding, anemia, and headaches).

Chapter 25 Elective Termination of Pregnancy

In the United States, nearly 50% of all pregnancies are unintended and 40% of these end in elective abortion. Excluding miscarriages, 22% of all pregnancies are electively terminated. As such, the availability of safe and effective means of elective pregnancy termination is an important component of family planning and an integral part of obstetrics and gynecologic care. Of the over **1.2 million abortions** performed annually in the United States, approximately 50% are performed on women in their 20s and 18% are performed on teenagers (<19 years of age). Abortion is a common procedure in the United States, with 3 in 10 women having the procedure done by the age of 45 years. Over 60% of women undergoing abortions have one or more children and 80% are unmarried. Caucasian women account for 36% of procedures; Black women for 30%; and Hispanic women for 25%. The most common reasons women give for choosing to have an abortion include financial burden, familial obligations, interference with work or school, and desire to avoid single parenting.

The abortion procedures used legally in the United States are both **safe and effective**. Since the legalization of abortion in 1973, the risk of death from abortion has declined by 85%. The most recent maternal mortality rate for induced abortion in the United States is **0.1 per 100,000**. This is in comparison to a maternal mortality of 7.7 per 100,000 for completed pregnancy and delivery. The major causes of abortion mortality are complications of hemorrhage and infection, followed by thromboembolism and anesthetic complications. In general, maternal morbidity is lowest if abortion is performed before 8 weeks' gestation (Fig. 25-1). Less than 0.3% of abortions performed in the first trimester result in complications that require hospitalization.

There are several surgical and medical procedures by which pregnancy termination can be achieved (Fig. 25-2). Evacuation of the uterus is an important technique in the field of obstetrics and gynecology. Not only is it used for elective termination of pregnancy, but it is also an integral part of managing spontaneous abortion, missed abortion, intrauterine fetal demise, retained products of conception, and gestational trophoblastic neoplasia. Approximately 88% of induced abortions are performed in the first trimester of pregnancy (75% prior to 9 weeks), utilizing a surgical evacuation of the uterus (D&C).

The options for first trimester abortion include suction curettage, manual vacuum aspiration, and nonsurgical "medical" abortion using either mifepristone or methotrexate. Second trimester options include surgical evacuation of the uterus and medical induction of labor. In general, the technique used for termination is determined by the duration of the pregnancy, provider experience, and patient preference. Table 25-1 outlines the various options available during the first and second trimesters. Nearly 95% of all induced abortions are performed before 16 weeks' gestation, 4% are performed between 16 and 20 weeks' gestation, and less than 1.5% is performed after 21 weeks' gestation. Laws vary from state to state, but generally, terminations are performed up until the fetus has reached viability at about 24 weeks' gestation. After week 24, abortions are generally only performed when necessary for the preservation of maternal life. Though second trimester abortions are rare, access to providers is often reported as a barrier that pushes women into having procedures beyond the first trimester. In 2000, 87% of counties in the United States had no access to an abortion provider.

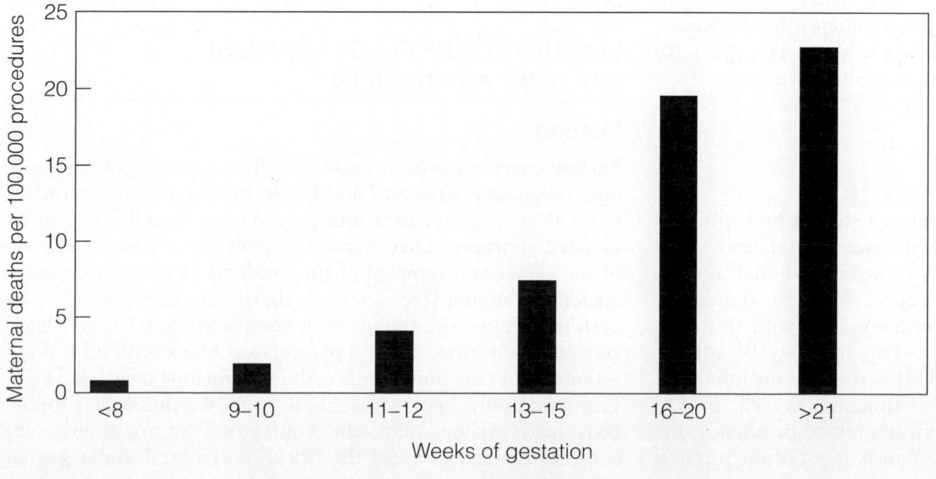

Figure 25-1 • The effect of gestational age on maternal mortality for legal abortions.

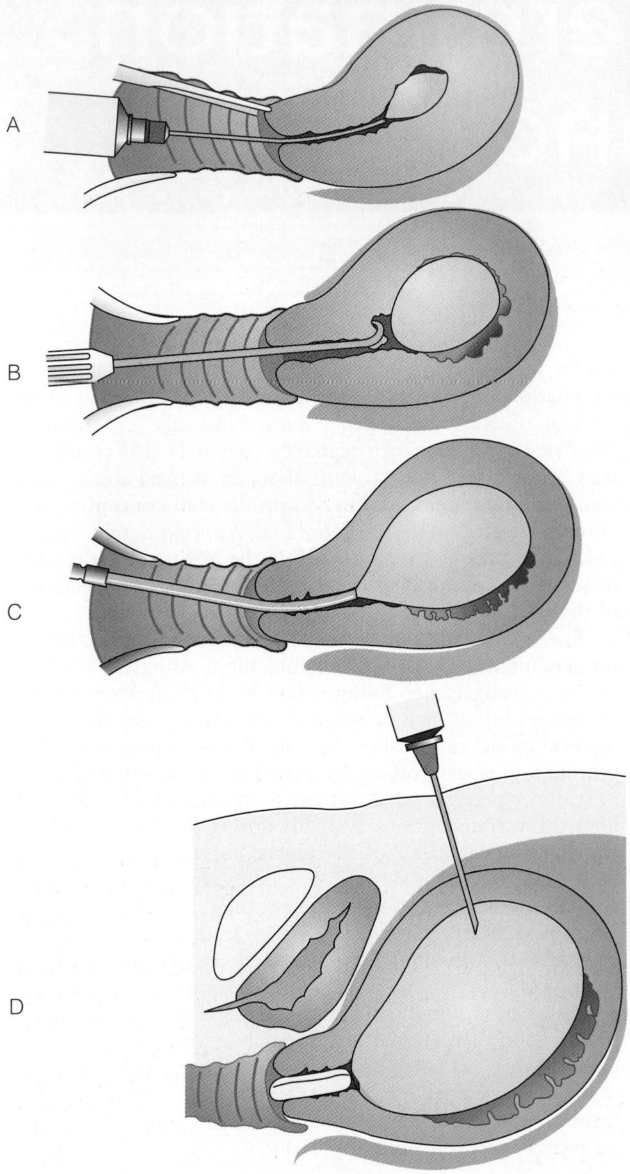

Figure 25-2 • Various techniques used for termination of pregnancy. **(A)** Manual extraction. **(B)** Sharp curettage (D&C). **(C)** Suction dilation and curettage (D&C) or evacuation (D&E). **(D)** Induction of labor by intra-amniotic instillation.
(From Pillitteri A. *Maternal and Child Nursing*, 4th ed. Philadelphia, PA: Lippincott Williams & Wilkins; 2003.)

Prior to termination, **gestational age should be confirmed** by last menstrual period, bimanual examination, and ultrasound evaluation. All Rh–negative women should **receive RhoGAM** at the time of procedure. Women should be counseled on reliable forms of **contraception** with initiation of chosen method, if appropriate. Patients may be offered **sexually transmitted infections (STI) screening for infections** such as gonorrhea and chlamydia at this time as well. Two to four weeks after completion of termination of pregnancy, the routine follow-up should include an assessment of the physical and emotional status of the patient. Clinical, laboratory, or imaging studies should be used as needed to confirm completion of the abortion, and any complications should be treated. This may also be an opportune time to obtain **cervical cytology** if the Pap smear is not up-to-date and to provide indicated immunizations (Rubella, varicella, Tetanus, Diptheria, Pertussis (TDap)), and the influenza vaccine.

TABLE 25-1 Termination of Pregnancy Options, by Gestational Age

First trimester terminations
Suction curettage (D&C)
Manual vacuum aspiration
Nonsurgical medical abortion[a]
Mifepristone plus misoprostol
Methotrexate plus misoprostol
Second trimester terminations
Surgical evacuation of the uterus (D&E)
Medical induction of labor
High-dose oxytocin
Intra-amniotic installation agents
Prostaglandins

[a]Only used up to 63 days from the last menstrual period (LMP).

FIRST TRIMESTER OPTIONS

The majority of all abortions are performed **before 12 weeks' gestation**. Suction curettage (D&C), manual vacuum aspiration, and nonsurgical medical abortions are all methods of inducing abortion in the first trimester. Most first trimester terminations in the United States are achieved using the suction curettage (D&C) procedure. However, an increasing number of terminations (25%) are being accomplished by nonsurgical abortions ever since FDA approval (September 2000) of the use of mifepristone (RU 486) for pregnancy termination in the United States. The maternal mortality for suction curettage is 0.1 in 100,000 patients. In general, the risk of complications after suction curettage is small and directly proportional to the gestational age.

SUCTION CURETTAGE/MANUAL VACUUM ASPIRATION

Method

Suction curettage is both a safe and effective means of terminating a pregnancy between 7 and 13 weeks of gestation. According to CDC surveillance data, this procedure is used for 87% of all induced abortions. D&C typically involves mechanical dilation of the cervix and removal of the products of conception using a **suction cannula** (Fig. 25-3). A **sharp curettage** may then be performed to ensure the uterus is completely evacuated. This is generally performed using a **paracervical block** with a local anesthetic often in conjunction with IV conscious sedation STET. Less commonly, general anesthesia is used. **Antibiotic prophylaxis** (doxycycline, ofloxacin, ceftriaxone, or metronidazole) is recommended to avoid the risk of postabortal upper genital

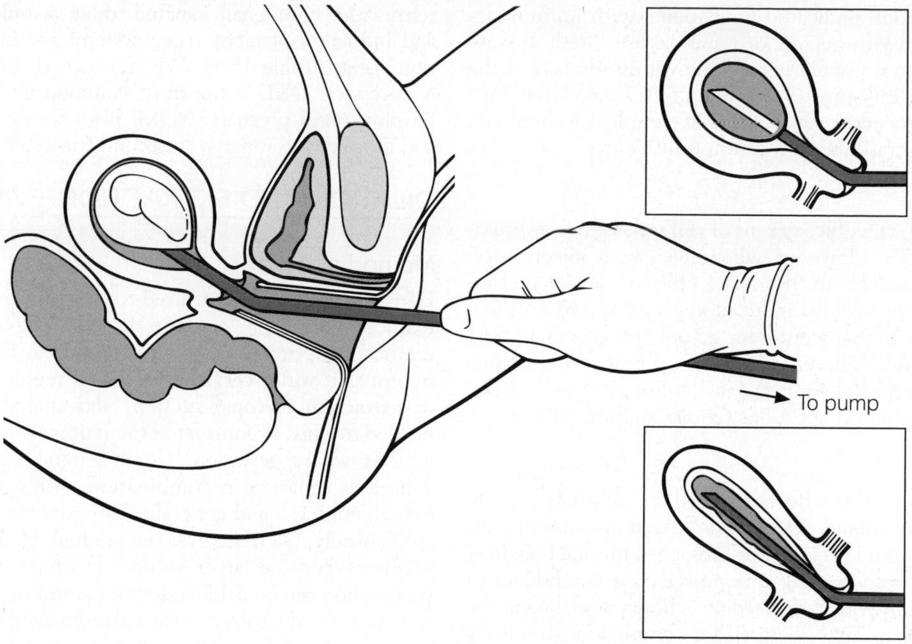

Figure 25-3 • Suction curettage of uterine cavity for termination of pregnancy.

tract infection. Maternal complications are rare with suction curettage and the maternal mortality rate is 0.1 per 100,000.

For early pregnancies up to 10 weeks of gestation, **manual vacuum aspiration** can be performed. This technique involves insertion of a 4- to 12-mm cannula into the cervical os. The uterine contents are then manually extracted using a 50- or 60-mL self-locking vacuum syringe instead of a suction machine. Evacuation is achieved by a gentle in and out motion while also rotating the unit to ensure clearance of all products of conception. Sharp curettage is not performed in this procedure.

Effectiveness

When performed by a trained physician, the success rate for suction curettage is 98% to 99%. After any type of suction curettage procedure, the products of conception (POCs) should be examined to ensure completion. If the gestational age is less than 6 weeks, verification of POCs on pathology report is very important as the embryo is so small at <6 weeks, the D&C procedure may fail to evacuate it from the uterus. In these early pregnancies, an effort should also be made to identify villi after the procedure by floating the evacuated tissue in saline. If no villi are identified, or the patient has persistent vaginal bleeding, then serial β-hCG levels should be taken to rule out ectopic pregnancy, gestational trophoblastic disease, or an ongoing pregnancy.

Complications

First trimester termination using suction curettage (D&C) is the **safest of all surgical termination methods**. Complications of suction curettage are rare and include infection (1% to 5%), excessive bleeding (2%), uterine perforation (1%), and incomplete abortion (1%). Limited data suggest that women who have three or more cervical dilation procedures (for termination, hysteroscopy, D&Cs, etc.) may be at higher risk for cervical insufficiency and uterine scarring (Asherman's syndrome). The maternal mortality rate for D&C is 0.1 per 100,000.

NONSURGICAL ABORTION

Mifepristone (RU 486)

The FDA approved mifepristone for use in termination of pregnancies in the United States in September 2000. Since that time, medication abortion has become increasingly utilized and now accounts for 25% of terminations prior to 9 weeks of gestation. Mifepristone (RU 486) is a **synthetic progesterone receptor antagonist** that binds to progesterone receptors in the uterus, thus blocking the stimulatory effects of progesterone on endometrial growth. Mifepristone thereby disrupts the pregnancy by making the endometrial lining unsuitable to sustain the pregnancy. This leads to detachment of the embryo. Mifepristone can be used up to **63 days from the last menstrual period** (LMP). Although it can be used alone, the success rate of completed pregnancy is greatly improved when used in combination with a **prostaglandin analog** such as misoprostol. This is considered the gold standard for medical termination of pregnancy. The typical protocol used for termination involves a single oral dose (200 to 600 mg) of RU 486 followed by a buccal (400 to 800 mcg) or vaginal (800 mcg) dose of misoprostol (Cytotec) 24 to 48 hours later. Of note, the FDA has only approved the 400-mcg oral dose of misoprostol for medical termination. Approximately 2 weeks after the procedure, the success of completion is typically confirmed with ultrasound or a serum β-hCG level.

Methotrexate

Methotrexate is a chemotherapeutic agent and **dihydrofolate reductase inhibitor** that works by interfering with DNA synthesis, thereby **preventing placental villi proliferation**. Because methotrexate has been approved for use for a variety of medical conditions including ectopic pregnancy, it has been used by clinicians on an off-label basis as an abortifacient. Like mifepristone, methotrexate is also used with a prostaglandin analog.

Methotrexate is contraindicated for patients with immunodeficiency and those with hepatic or renal disease. Methotrexate is administered intramuscularly or orally **within 49 days of the LMP**, followed by misoprostol (Cytotec) 6 to 7 days later. Two weeks after the procedure, the success of completion should be confirmed with ultrasound or a serum β-hCG level.

Effectiveness

When used alone, the efficacy rate of mifepristone is approximately 65% to 85%. However, when given with misoprostol, the **success rate is 92% to 98%**. The efficacy rate of methotrexate with misoprostol for induced abortion is 94% to 96%. Methotrexate is also therapeutic for ectopic pregnancy in 90% to 95% of the cases. The efficacy rates of both mifepristone and methotrexate decline for pregnancies greater than 7 weeks' gestation. Failed medical abortions require suction D&C.

Side Effects

The most common side effects of medical abortion are **abdominal pain and cramps**. Other side effects include nausea, vomiting, diarrhea, and excessive or prolonged **uterine bleeding**. The majority of women using misoprostal as a component of medical termination will start bleeding 2 hours after taking the prostaglandin analog. Time required for completion is typically 24 to 48 hours. Vaginal bleeding averages 10 to 17 days. The rate of endometritis for medical abortion is lower than that after surgical abortion.

Advantages/Disadvantages

Nonsurgical abortion offers the advantages of being a **highly effective noninvasive** means of termination that can be achieved on an **outpatient basis**. However, in a nonsurgical abortion, a miscarriage is induced and the woman must go through the experience of miscarriage, which generally involves substantial uterine cramping and bleeding. Medication abortion typically requires two visits to a health provider: one to obtain the medication, and then a 2-week follow-up visit. The contraindications of nonsurgical abortion are shown in Table 25-2.

SECOND TRIMESTER OPTIONS

Second trimester terminations are performed between weeks 13 and 24 weeks of gestation. **Congenital fetal abnormalities** are the primary reason for second trimester abortions. Other indications include severe hyperemesis, previable preterm premature rupture of membranes (PPROM), life-threatening maternal conditions, and undesired pregnancy. Options for second trimester termination of pregnancy include **dilation and evacuation** (D&E) and **induction of labor** using systemic or intrauterine installation agents (Table 25-1). When a second trimester termination is necessary, **D&E is the most common and safest** method of termination of pregnancy. D&E has a lower maternal mortality and morbidity compared to second trimester induction of labor.

TABLE 25-2 Contraindications of Medication Abortion

Pregnancy >63 days from LMP
Pregnancy with an intrauterine device in place
Obstruction of the cervical canal
Ectopic pregnancy
Gestational trophoblastic disease
Chronic systemic steroid use
Bleeding disorder, chronic adrenal failure
Allergy to mifepristone or misoprostol
Inability to sign the consent agreement because of lack of competence

DILATION AND EXTRACTION/EVACUATION

Method of Action

D&E is the general term used to describe cervical dilation and extraction of uterine contents after 14 weeks of gestation. This method of termination is very similar to first trimester D&C except that **wider cervical dilation** is required. A combination of **extraction forceps**, suction, and sharp curettage may be needed to assist in complete evacuation of the uterus, especially after 16 weeks' gestation. This is generally performed using **IV conscious sedation** in combination with a paracervical block. Spinal, epidural, and general anesthesias are only rarely used.

Typically, D&E involves the gradual dilation of the cervix to accommodate the larger volume of uterine contents. Cervical preparation can be achieved with careful manual dilation, multiple osmotic dilators, or prostaglandin agents. Osmotic dilators are generally preferred given that manual dilation for second trimester terminations may result in increased cervical lacerations and hemorrhage, and prostaglandin agents such as misoprostol can take some time to provide sufficient cervical dilatation.

Osmotic dilators can be synthetic (Lamicel, Dilapan) or natural (seaweed-based laminaria). These dilators are placed into the cervix the day before the procedure and gradually dilate and soften the cervix as they absorb the cervical moisture (Fig. 25-4). These osmotic dilators slowly expand over 12 to 18 hours to dilate the cervix prior to D&E. Once dilated, a large **suction cannula** (12 to 14 mm) can be introduced into the uterus to extract the fetal tissue and placenta. At more advanced gestational ages greater than 16 weeks, **forceps** designed to extract uterine contents are often needed in addition

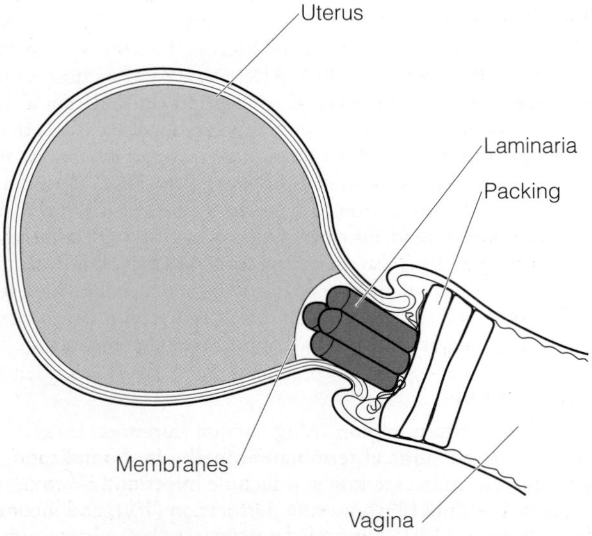

Figure 25-4 • Osmotic dilation of the cervix. Multiple laminaria are placed inside the cervix through both the internal and external os. They slowly expand by absorbing moisture from the vagina, thereby dilating the cervix.

to suction curettage to remove fetal parts. Upon completion of the procedure, the clinician should verify extraction of the major fetal parts. **Ultrasound** can be used to guide the extraction and to rule out retained products of conception.

Effectiveness

When performed by a highly experienced clinician, the success rate for second trimester extraction procedures is 98% to 99%.

Side Effects

Complications from D&E are uncommon but may include **cervical laceration, hemorrhage, uterine perforation, infection, and retained tissues**. These can be lessened by visual inspection of the fetal parts to ensure complete evacuation of the products of conception. For pregnancies at 16 weeks' gestational age and less, D&E has been found to be safer than induction of labor. The maternal mortality rate for D&E is 4 in 100,000.

Advantages/Disadvantages

As a method of second trimester abortion, D&E offers the advantage of being performed on an **outpatient basis,** without the need to undergo induction of labor and delivery. Also, there is no risk of delivering a live-born fetus with extraction procedures. Complications from D&E occur at lower rates than those for intra-amniotic instillation or intravaginal prostaglandin abortions. Some patients may feel the **decreased amount of time** for this procedure is advantageous over an induction of labor; however, other patients may feel that the **delivery of a nonintact fetus** is unacceptable. Perceptions of advantages and disadvantages of these procedures depend greatly on patient preference.

INDUCTION OF LABOR

Method of Action

Termination of a second trimester pregnancy can also be achieved with induction of labor. In the past, installation of intrauterine abortifacient agents such as hypertonic saline, prostaglandin F2α, or hyperosmolar urea was a common method of inducing labor for second trimester terminations. These methods have largely been abandoned for safer methods (D&E or induction of labor). Termination through induction of labor is typically done using **cervical ripening agents**, amniotomy, and **high-dose IV oxytocin infusion**. Vaginal or oral prostaglandins (prostaglandin E2, misoprostol) can be used to ripen the cervix and augment labor in second trimester termination. Prostaglandins usually result in higher rates of fever and gastrointestinal side effects. **Feticidal agents** (intraamniotic saline or digoxin and intracardiac potassium chloride) can be used in conjunction with prostaglandins to circumvent the possibility of live birth.

Effectiveness

Depending on the regimen used, the success rate for second trimester abortions using induction of labor is **80% to 100%.**

Side Effects

General complications of induction of labor for termination of pregnancy include retained placenta, uterine rupture, hemorrhage, and infection (Table 25-3). Oral and vaginal prostaglandins have a higher incidence of **live births** and significant gastrointestinal side effects (**nausea, vomiting, diarrhea**), whereas instillation agents have a higher rate of retained placenta (13% to 46%). The maternal mortality rate for second trimester induction of labor is **8 in 100,000,** similar to that of term delivery (7.7 in 100,000).

TABLE 25-3 Complications Associated with Second Trimester Abortion by Induction of Labor

Complications	Side Effects
Retained placenta	Nausea
Incomplete abortion	Vomiting
Hemorrhage	Diarrhea
Infection	Fever
Cervical laceration	Chills

Advantages/Disadvantages

Induction of labor is a **longer process** than D&E. It requires an **inpatient admission** and can potentially become a **multiday process**. However, induction of labor allows for the potential delivery of an **intact fetus**. This may be emotionally important for some patients and also facilitates a more comprehensive **postmortem evaluation** of the fetus, particularly when fetal anomalies are involved and fetopsy is requested.

KEY POINTS

- First trimester abortion options include suction curettage, manual vacuum aspiration, and medication abortion up until week 9.
- Ninety percent of all abortions in the United States are achieved using suction curettage.
- Suction curettage can be performed anytime during the first trimester but is most effective between 7 and 13 weeks' gestation.
- Complications are rare but can include infection, bleeding, and perforation of the uterus.
- Mifepristone (RU 486) is an abortifacient that blocks progesterone stimulation of the endometrial lining, thus causing detachment of the embryo.
- Methotrexate is a chemotherapeutic agent that blocks dihydrofolate inhibitor that interrupts placental proliferation.
- Both mifepristone and methotrexate are used in combination with a prostaglandin (often misoprostal) and have high efficacy rates (92% to 98%) for medical termination when used within 63 days of the LMP.
- During the second trimester, abortion may be achieved via D&E or induction of labor. D&E has lower maternal mortality and morbidity compared to induction of labor for second trimester abortions.
- D&E is similar to suction curettage (D&C) but requires wider cervical dilation and the use of special forceps and curets to assist with the extraction of the larger volume of fetal parts.
- Complications of D&E include cervical laceration, hemorrhage, infection, uterine perforation, and retained tissue.
- Induction of labor techniques most commonly include cervical ripening with a prostaglandin, and amniotomy along with induction of labor with high-dose oxytocin.
- Complications from induction of labor include retained placenta, hemorrhage, infection, and cervical laceration.
- Maternal morbidity is 4 in 100,000 for D&E and 8 in 100,000 for induction of labor compared to 7.7 in 100,000 for term pregnancy and delivery.

C Clinical Vignettes

Vignette 1

A 36-year-old G3P2002 female presents to a family planning clinic for termination of pregnancy. She states that her last menstrual period was 7 weeks ago. She has no significant past medical history and has had two previous full-term vaginal deliveries. She currently smokes over a half a pack of cigarettes a day and has mild hypertension that is well controlled. Ultrasound confirms a single intrauterine pregnancy of 7 weeks gestation. She reports that she is recently divorced and has a new sexual partner. She is not using any kind of contraception.

1. What is the MOST important test for this patient to undergo prior to her procedure?
   a. Basic metabolic panel
   b. Pulmonary function testing
   c. Rh status
   d. Hematocrit
   e. Gonorrhea and chlamydia screening
2. At 7 weeks gestational age, what methods of termination can be offered to this patient?
   a. Medication abortion
   b. D&C with suction curettage
   c. Manual vacuum aspiration
   d. D&E
   e. a, b, c
3. The patient chooses a medication abortion. She is given mifepristone (RU-486) in the office and counseled to self-administer buccal misoprostol (Cytotec) 24 to 48 hours later. What follow-up is most appropriate for this patient?
   a. No follow-up is needed
   b. She is counseled on signs of complications and instructed to call for an appointment if needed
   c. She is scheduled for 2 weeks to confirm completion of termination via ultrasound or β-hCG
   d. She is scheduled to return weekly for serum β-hCG monitoring until the levels turn negative
   e. She is counseled to return to clinic after her next period
4. The patient is interested in contraception. Which type of contraception would NOT be recommended for her?
   a. Intramuscular medroxyprogesterone
   b. Levonorgestrel intrauterine device (IUD)
   c. Copper-T IUD
   d. Combined oral contraceptive pills
   e. Condoms

Vignette 2

A 19-year-old woman presents to your general practice gynecology office with complaints of irregular menses. She states that she has not had a period for 2 months. Prior to this, her menses have been regular. She complains of nausea and vomiting as well as breast tenderness. She has no significant past medical history. On physical examination, she seems well-appearing, and bimanual examination revealed a slightly enlarged uterus.

1. What is the most helpful test to order at this point?
   a. Complete blood count (CBC)
   b. Urine pregnancy test
   c. Serum β-hCG level
   d. Basic metabolic panel
   e. Rapid plasma reagin
2. The patient's pregnancy test is positive. What is the most appropriate way to convey these results?
   a. Congratulate her on becoming a new mother
   b. Have your medical technician inform her the results so you can continue to see other patients
   c. Tell her that her pregnancy test is positive and ask her how she feels about that
   d. Hand her brochures on pregnancy and tell her you are available to answer any questions
   e. There is no way that is most appropriate
3. You sit down across from the patient and tell her that her pregnancy test is positive. She is visibly upset. You ask her what her thoughts are regarding this pregnancy and she states that she is not ready to become a parent. What is the most appropriate next step?
   a. Tell her you do not believe in abortion and that she would be making a mistake to terminate the pregnancy
   b. Present her with her options, which include carrying the pregnancy to term with parenting, adoption, and induced abortion
   c. Give her the number to a local family planning clinic
   d. Tell her you have a nurse who is interested in adoption
   e. Relate a story about your cousin who went through a similar experience
4. After considering all of her options, she chooses to terminate the pregnancy. You refer her to a local family planning clinic. What additional tests could you offer her at this time?
   a. HIV testing
   b. Complete blood count

c. Gonorrhea and chlamydia
d. Rh status
e. All of the above

Vignette 3

A 24-year-old G2P1001 female is diagnosed with fetal anencephaly, a lethal anomaly, at her first prenatal visit at 16 weeks. She is otherwise healthy. She had a previous term vaginal delivery without complications. She wishes to terminate this pregnancy.

1. Which termination method has the lowest maternal mortality rate at this gestational age?
   a. D&E
   b. Labor induction
   c. Medication abortion
   d. Manual vacuum aspiration
   e. D&C

2. The patient is counseled on the risks and benefits of both D&E and labor induction. She opts for D&E. Which is NOT used for cervical dilation prior to the procedure?
   a. Osmotic dilators
   b. Laminaria
   c. Misoprostol
   d. High dose IV oxytocin
   e. Foley balloon catheter

3. On the day of the procedure, she would like to talk to you about pain management. What method of pain control do you recommend?
   a. General anesthesia
   b. Spinal anesthesia
   c. IV conscious sedation combined with paracervical block
   d. Paracervical block alone
   e. Oral nonsteroidal anti-inflammatory drugs (NSAIDs) only

4. Postoperatively she does well and there are no intraoperative complications. Two weeks later she calls your nurse and says that she is passing large clots and having increased abdominal cramping. What is in your differential diagnosis?
   a. Uterine perforation
   b. Retained products of conception (POC)
   c. Continuing pregnancy
   d. Postabortal endometritis
   e. b and d

Vignette 4

A 30-year-old G2 P0010 female presents to a family planning clinic for termination of her current pregnancy. She has a remote history of pelvic inflammatory disease. She has had one previous spontaneous miscarriage and no other pregnancies. She states that her last menstrual period was 4½ weeks ago. She complains of left lower quadrant pain and she has had vaginal spotting over the past few days.

1. What next steps would be appropriate in her evaluation?
   a. Physical examination
   b. Urine pregnancy test
   c. Rh status
   d. Transvaginal ultrasound
   e. All of the above

2. On physical examination, she has mild left lower quadrant tenderness and her uterus is approximately 5- to 6- weeks in size. She has no rebound, rigidity, or guarding. Urine pregnancy test is positive. She is Rh-positive. Transvaginal ultrasound shows no gestational sac in the uterus and no adnexal masses. What do you recommend next?
   a. You counsel her that she probably has an early intrauterine pregnancy that is too small to be detected on ultrasound and that she should have a medication abortion if she desires
   b. You recommend that she have a suction D&C the same day
   c. You recommend that she have serial serum β-hCG levels starting the same day
   d. You tell her that she has an ectopic pregnancy and needs emergency surgery
   e. You schedule her to come back the next day for repeat ultrasound

3. The patient's serum β-hCG level is 600 mIU/mL. You counsel her on warning signs such as severe abdominal pain and heavy vaginal bleeding for which she should call or go to the emergency room. She returns to the clinic in 72 hours for repeat serum testing and the level is 1,000. You schedule her to come back to the clinic in 72 hours for repeat serum testing and transvaginal ultrasound. She has an appropriate rise in her pregnancy hormone levels and transvaginal ultrasound now detects an intrauterine pregnancy at approximately 5½ weeks gestation. She still desires pregnancy termination. What are her options?
   a. D&C with suction
   b. Manual vacuum aspiration
   c. Medication abortion
   d. D&E
   e. a, b, and c

A Answers

Vignette 1 Question 1

Answer C: It is important to determine Rh status prior to an induced abortion. Regardless of the method of termination that is chosen, all Rh-negative women should be given RhoGAM to prevent isoimmunization, which could occur if an Rh-negative woman is exposed to Rh-positive fetal blood cells. Without RhoGAM, this exposure would cause an Rh-negative woman to form antibodies to the Rh factor. Any future pregnancies with a fetus with Rh factor would be at risk for attack by those maternal antibodies. By giving RhoGAM, future pregnancies are protected from the complications of isoimmunization. There is no need to perform a basic metabolic panel or pulmonary function testing. Hematocrit and STI screening is often obtained prior to an induced abortion but these are not mandated.

Vignette 1 Question 2

Answer E: At this gestational age, the patient is eligible for medication abortion, D&C, or manual vacuum aspiration. D&C with suction curettage is what is most commonly done at this gestational age. Medication abortion can be administered up to 63 days of gestation. At clinics that offer options of surgical and medication abortion, she would be counseled on risks and benefits of both options to enable her to make the decision that is the best for her. Manual vacuum aspiration is a type of suction curettage that may be performed up to 10 weeks of gestation. D&E is a procedure that is used for second trimester procedures greater than 14 weeks of gestation.

Vignette 1 Question 3

Answer C: Most providers prefer to have the patient return in 2 weeks to ensure completion of the abortion. Since 92% to 98% of medication abortions are successful, there will be a small percentage of women who need additional intervention to complete the procedure. It is important to identify those women in a timely fashion, so the answers A and E would not be the best choice. Though it is important to counsel a woman on the signs of complications, a 2-week follow-up appointment would be more appropriate. The correct answer would be D in the absence of an intrauterine pregnancy when ectopic pregnancy is suspected.

Vignette 1 Question 4

Answer D: Estrogen-containing contraceptives are contraindicated in this patient because she has HTN, is over 35, and smokes >15 cig/day. Any of the other options would be reasonable but either the Levonorgestrel or Copper IUD would provide the most effective contraception.

Vignette 2 Question 1

Answer B: This patient presents with symptoms of early pregnancy. The most helpful test at this point would be to get a urine pregnancy test, as this would facilitate the most rapid diagnosis; hence the answer is B. Answer C, serum pregnancy test would also help establish the diagnosis but it is more expensive and would take more time to get the results. Answers A and E are included in standard prenatal labs, but these would not be the most helpful tests at this time prior to the establishment of the diagnosis. Unless her nausea and vomiting is severe, a basic metabolic panel (D) is not warranted.

Vignette 2 Question 2

Answer C: C is the correct answer because the most appropriate and patient-centered way to deliver these results is directly by the clinician and in a nonjudgmental fashion. Answer A is incorrect because it assumes that the pregnancy is desired. Answer B is incorrect because it has another staff member tell her the results. Answer D is incorrect because the results are not given in a straightforward or sensitive manner. Answer E is incorrect because there is an appropriate way to give patient sensitive results.

Vignette 2 Question 3

Answer B: The correct answer is B. Providing options counseling is important because it presents the patient with all of her options without making assumptions on which decision is the best for her. Answer A imposes personal beliefs on to the patient and is judgmental. Answer C assumes that she has already made a decision. Answer D is inappropriate and unethical as it potentially takes advantage of the patient who is in a vulnerable position. Answer E is incorrect because it does not focus on the patient and her needs, but instead makes the situation about someone else.

Vignette 2 Question 4

Answer E: Though several of these tests would be offered to her prior to her procedure, you could order them prior to her visit and send the results. Offering STI screening such as HIV and gonorrhea/chlamydia testing is appropriate as she has had unprotected intercourse and is at risk. CBC would be appropriate as it would be helpful to know if she was anemic prior to any procedure that will induce bleeding. Rh status is important to protect future pregnancies from isoimmunization if she is Rh-negative.

Vignette 3 Question 1

Answer A: The maternal mortality rate for D&E at this gestational age is approximately 4 per 100,000 as compared to 8 per 100,000 for labor induction. Therefore, A is the correct answer. Answer C is incorrect because medication abortions cannot be offered past 63 days gestation. Manual vacuum aspiration, answer D, is offered up to 10 weeks gestation. D&C is generally done up to 14 weeks gestation.

Vignette 3 Question 2
Answer D: D is the correct answer. IV oxytocin is used for labor induction as it stimulates uterine contractions. It is not an agent for cervical ripening. Osmotic dilators, laminaria, misoprostol, and Foley balloon catheters have all been used for cervical ripening to assist with dilation prior to second trimester D&E. Osmotic dilators and prostaglandins such as misoprostol (Cytotec) are most typically used.

Vignette 3 Question 3
Answer C: For most women having second trimester procedures at 16 weeks of gestation, IV conscious sedation combined with a paracervical block would be the most acceptable option. General anesthesia is typically not required in this setting and introduces more risk for the patient. Spinal anesthesia could be offered in the right setting but most women do not require such an intervention. Paracervical block alone may not be adequate. NSAIDs, though an appropriate component of postoperative pain control, would not be adequate in isolation.

Vignette 3 Question 4
Answer E: Uterine perforation would most likely be diagnosed at the time of the procedure and would be unlikely to cause delayed symptoms 2 weeks out from the procedure. Continuing pregnancy is unlikely, as the tissue should have been examined during the procedure. Retained products of conception are a possibility as a small piece of placental tissue can cause delayed bleeding such as this. Intraoperative use of ultrasound assists in decreasing the risk of retained POC's. Postabortal endometritis can cause uterine bleeding and cramping and should be in the differential diagnosis.

Vignette 4 Question 1
Answer E: All of the listed answers would add useful clinical information. A physical examination would give the clinician an indication of the nature of the left lower quadrant pain as well as an estimate of uterine size. A urine pregnancy test could confirm pregnancy. Rh status is not only important because she is seeking termination but would be important to know because she is having vaginal bleeding in the context of pregnancy. Women who are having threatened miscarriages are given RhoGAM if they are Rh-negative. Transvaginal ultrasound is important to determine location and estimated gestational age of the pregnancy.

Vignette 4 Question 2
Answer C: At this point, this patient has a pregnancy of unknown location. The differential diagnosis includes early intrauterine pregnancy, nonviable intrauterine pregnancy, or ectopic pregnancy. Answer C is correct because serial measurement of the pregnancy hormone level can assist in determining the location of the pregnancy. Early intrauterine pregnancies will cause at least a rise of 50% over 48 to 72 hours in serum β-hCG. Hormone levels that decline or plateau are a concern for nonviable pregnancy or ectopic pregnancy. Medication abortion is not appropriate if there is no evidence of an intrauterine pregnancy; so A would be incorrect. Answer B would also not be correct for the same reason. Although it is possible that she has an ectopic pregnancy (D), it is not possible to diagnose this from the available data. It would be appropriate to counsel her on warning signs for ectopic pregnancy and miscarriage. Answer E is not correct because a day is not an appropriate interval to detect changes on an ultrasound. The earliest duration for repeating the ultrasound would be in 1 week.

Vignette 4 Question 3
Answer E: At 5½ weeks gestational age, either medication abortion or manual vacuum aspiration is appropriate. Suction D&C is also an option but is more likely to miss the pregnancy at gestations of less than 7 weeks. D&E procedures are not necessary on early first trimester pregnancies.

Chapter 26 Infertility and Assisted Reproductive Technologies

INTRODUCTION

Infertility is a complex medical disorder that requires the **evaluation and treatment of a couple** rather than an individual. **Infertility** is defined as the failure of a couple to conceive after 12 months of unprotected sexual intercourse. If the female partner is 35 year of age or older, evaluation should be initiated after 6 months of unprotected intercourse. In the United States, 1.2 million women (2% of couples with reproductive aged women) sought medical help in 2002 to become pregnant and 10% of women had received infertility services during their lifetime.

Fecundability, or the ability to achieve pregnancy in one menstrual cycle, is a more accurate measurement to evaluate fertility potential. The **fecundity rate** in a normal couple who has had unprotected intercourse is approximately **20% to 25% for the first 3 months**, followed by 15% during the next 9 months. This means that 80% to 90% of couples are able to spontaneously conceive within 12 months (Table 26-1). The fecundity rate of the cohort decreases over time and with increasing maternal age. For the remaining 10% to 20% of couples who are incapable of conceiving on their own within that time frame, the factors contributing to infertility vary widely.

Of those couples who undergo evaluation for infertility, approximately 45% to 55% is attributed to **female factors** and 35% attributed to **male factors** (Fig. 26-1). After evaluation, 10% of couples will have **no identifiable cause** for their infertility. In as many as 10% to 20% of infertility cases, **both male and female factors** are detected (Table 26-2). Once the cause of infertility is identified, therapy is aimed at correcting reversible conditions or overcoming irreversible conditions. The overview of infertility evaluation is shown in Figure 26-2.

Since its inception in 1981 in the United States, assisted reproductive technology (ART) has become the most technical and expensive therapeutic intervention to help infertile couples. ARTs involve all therapies in which both sperm and/or oocytes are handled in vitro for the purpose of increasing the rate of conception. In 2009, 146,244 ART cycles were conducted in the United States, resulting in 45,870 live births (deliveries of one or more living infants) and 60,190 infants. Currently, more than 1% of all births in the United States result from ART procedures (largely in vitro fertilization [IVF]).

FEMALE FACTOR INFERTILITY

The World Health Organization (WHO) task force on Diagnosis and Treatment of Infertility performed a study of 8,500 infertile couples and found that the most common identifiable female factors were **ovulatory disorders** (32%), **fallopian tube abnormalities** including pelvic adhesions (34%), and **endometriosis** (15%). Other factors that cause infertility include uterine and cervical factors, luteal phase defect, and genetic disorders (Table 26-3 and Fig. 26-3).

OVULATORY DISORDERS

Disruption in the hypothalamic-pituitary-gonadal axis (HPGA) (Fig. 20-1) can result in menstrual disorders and infertility through impairment of folliculogenesis, ovulation, and endometrial maturation (Table 26-4). The WHO has classified ovulatory disorders into four groups: WHO group 1, hypogonadotropic hypogonadal anovulation (hypothalamic amenorrhea); WHO group 2, normogonadotropic normoestrogenic anovulation (polycystic ovarian syndrome [PCOS]); WHO group 3, hypergonadotropic hypoestrogenic anovulation (premature ovarian failure, advanced maternal age); and WHO group 4, hyperprolactinemic anovulation. The most common ovulatory disorders that lead to infertility are **PCOS and advanced maternal age**.

Oocyte aging is an important factor affecting female fertility. During fetal life, the ovary contains the greatest number of germ cells, approximately 6 to 7 million in mid-gestation. The germ cell population then begins an **exponential decline** through gene-mediated apoptosis, numbering 1 to 2 million at birth and 300,000 at the onset of puberty (Fig. 26-4). The number of viable follicles continues to decline throughout the reproductive years and the rate of loss **accelerates after the mid-30s**. At the time of menopause, the ovary contains fewer than 1,000 follicles. Other factors that result in decreased ovarian reserve and primary ovarian insufficiency (commonly known as premature ovarian failure) include tobacco smoking, viruses, radiation and chemotherapy, and autoimmune and genetic disorders.

The age-related decrease in fecundability is due to both the **decline of quantity and quality of the oocytes**. It is generally accepted that oocyte age is the single most important factor affecting the probability of success with ART. The live birth rates for nulliparous women undergoing ART using fresh non-donor eggs exponentially decline after 35 year of age.

TABLE 26-1 Average Conception Rates for All Couples

Percentage of Couples	Length of Time Before Conception
20	Conceive within 1 month
60	Conceive within 6 months
75	Conceive within 9 months
80	Conceive within 12 months
90	Conceive within 18 months

However, if donor eggs are utilized, the live birth rate is determined by the age of the donor (Fig. 26-5). The age-related decrease in fertility may be due to the corresponding increase in the rate of aneuploidy.

PCOS is the most common cause of oligo-ovulation and anovulation among all women and those presenting with infertility (Chapters 21 and 23). The diagnostic criteria of this syndrome have been avidly debated ever since it was first described by Stein and Leventhal in 1935. In general, most clinicians use the minimal criteria set forth by the National Institutes of Health (NIH). These criteria to diagnose PCOS are menstrual irregularity due to **oligo-ovulation or anovulation**, clinical or biochemical evidence of **hyperandrogenism** (hirsutism, acne, male pattern balding, or elevated serum androgen concentrations), and exclusion of other causes of hyperandrogenism and menstrual irregularity.

The prevalence of reproductive-age women with PCOS based on the NIH 1990 criteria is **6.5% to 8%**. Risk factors include obesity, insulin resistance, diabetes, infertility, premature adrenarche, and a positive family history of PCOS among first-degree relatives.

Currently, PCOS is thought to be a complex disorder with a **multifactorial etiology** where multiple genetic variants and environmental factors interact, resulting in the development of this disorder. Suspected genetic variants include genes that are responsible for the regulation of gonadotropin, androgen, or insulin secretion and action (Fig. 26-6). These genetic polymorphisms interplay with diet and obesity. The end result is **hyperinsulinemia,** which contributes to **hyperandrogenism** by stimulating androgen biosynthesis in the ovary and decreasing the circulating level of sex hormone–binding globulin. Hyperandrogenism then leads to disruption of the hypothalamic-pituitary-gonadal axis (HPGA) manifest by infrequent or absent menses due to **chronic anovulation**.

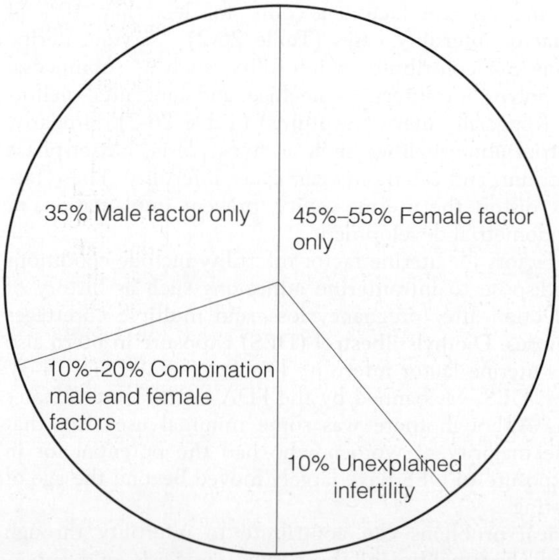

Figure 26-1 • Contribution of male and female factors to infertility.

TABLE 26-2 Contribution of Various Male and Female Factors to the Incidence of Infertility

Etiology	Incidence (%)
Male factor	35
Hypothalamic pituitary disease	2
Testiclar Disease	35
Post-testicular defects in sperm transport	15
Idiopathic	45
Female factor	45–55
Ovulatory factors	32
Peritoneal/tubal factors	34
Endometriosis	15
Uterine and cervical factors	10
Combined male and female factors	10–20
Unexplained infertility	10

TUBAL FACTORS

Tubal disease and pelvic adhesions (Color Plate 12) result in infertility by preventing the transport of the oocyte and sperm through the fallopian tube (Fig. 26-7). The primary cause of tubal factor infertility is **pelvic inflammatory disease (PID; Chapter 17)**. In countries where infection by gonorrhea and *Chlamydia* is increasing and treatment is limited, tubal factor infertility is on the rise. Other conditions that can interfere with normal tubal transport include severe **endometriosis**, history of **ectopic pregnancy**, and pelvic adhesions from **previous surgery** or **non-gynecologic infection** such as appendicitis or diverticulitis.

ENDOMETRIOSIS

Although the true prevalence of endometriosis is unknown, it is believed that approximately **15% of infertile women** have endometriosis. Endometriosis is the presence of endometrial cells outside the uterine cavity (Chapter 15). It can invade local tissues and cause severe **inflammation and adhesions** (Color Plate 12).

Although the presence of endometriosis has been associated with an increased risk of infertility, the exact mechanism is not understood. Endometriosis can interfere with tubal mobility, cause tubal obstruction, or result in tubal or ovarian adhesions that contribute to infertility by holding the fallopian tube away from the ovary, obstructing the tube, or by trapping the released oocyte. However, infertility has also been

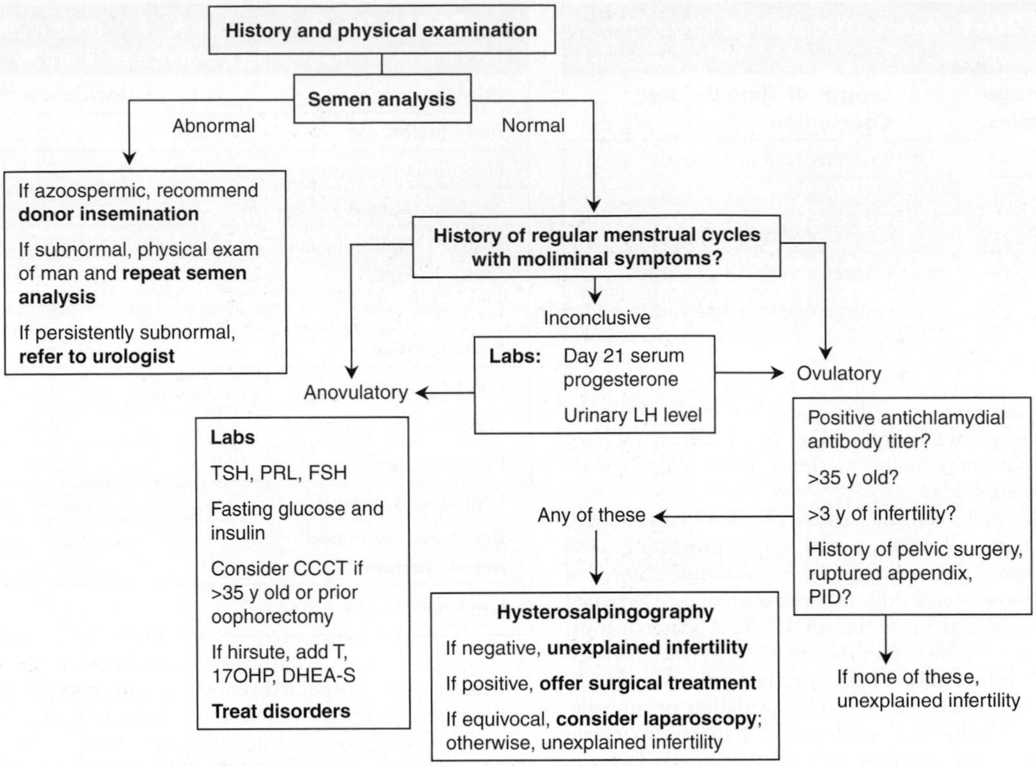

Figure 26-2 • Algorithm for evaluation and treatment of the infertile couple. LH, luteinizing hormone; TSH, thyroid stimulating hormone; PRL, prolactin; FSH, follicle stimulating hormone; CCCT, clomiphene citrate challenge test; DHEA-S, dehydroepiandrosterone sulfate; PID, pelvic inflammatory disease.
(From Curtis M. *Glass' Office Gynecology*, 6th ed. Philadelphia, PA: Lippincott Williams & Wilkins; 2005.)

TABLE 26-3 Causes of Female Factor Infertility

Ovarian
Polycystic ovarian syndrome
Advanced maternal age
Premature ovarian failure
Hypothalamic amenorrhea
Hyperprolactinemia
Tubal factors
Pelvic inflammatory disease/salpingitis
Tubal ligation
Endometriosis
Pelvic adhesions
Uterine factors
Congenital malformations
Submucosal fibroids
Uterine polyps
Intrauterine synechiae (Asherman's syndrome)
Cervical factors
Müllerian duct abnormalities
Cervical stenosis
Cervicitis or chronic inflammation

diagnosed in women with minimal endometriosis and minimal to no adhesive disease. It is thought that endometriosis may stimulate the production of **inflammatory mediators,** which impair ovulation, fertilization, and/or implantation.

UTERINE AND CERVICAL FACTORS

Uterine and cervical factors account for less than **10% of female factor infertility** cases (Table 26-2). Varying **uterine conditions** can contribute to infertility, such as submucosal fibroids, polyps, intrauterine synechiae, and congenital malformations (especially uterine septums) (Table 26-3). Similarly, **endometrial abnormalities** such as hyperplasia, out-of-phase endometrium, and carcinoma can cause infertility. These factors may distort the uterine cavity, prevent implantation, or affect endometrial development.

Risk factors for uterine factor infertility include conditions that predispose to **intrauterine adhesions** such as history of PID, infection after pregnancy loss, and multiple curettages of the uterus. **Diethylstilbestrol (DES) exposure in utero** also increases uterine factor infertility (Table 26-3 and Fig. 14-3). However, DES was banned by the FDA in the United States in 1971. Although there was some minimal use after that date, the majority of women who had the potential for in utero exposure to DES have largely moved beyond the age of childbearing.

Cervical problems can contribute to infertility through structural abnormalities of the cervix, cervicitis, and abnormal cervical mucous production. **Cervical stenosis** may be iatrogenic and may result from cervical scarring after loop

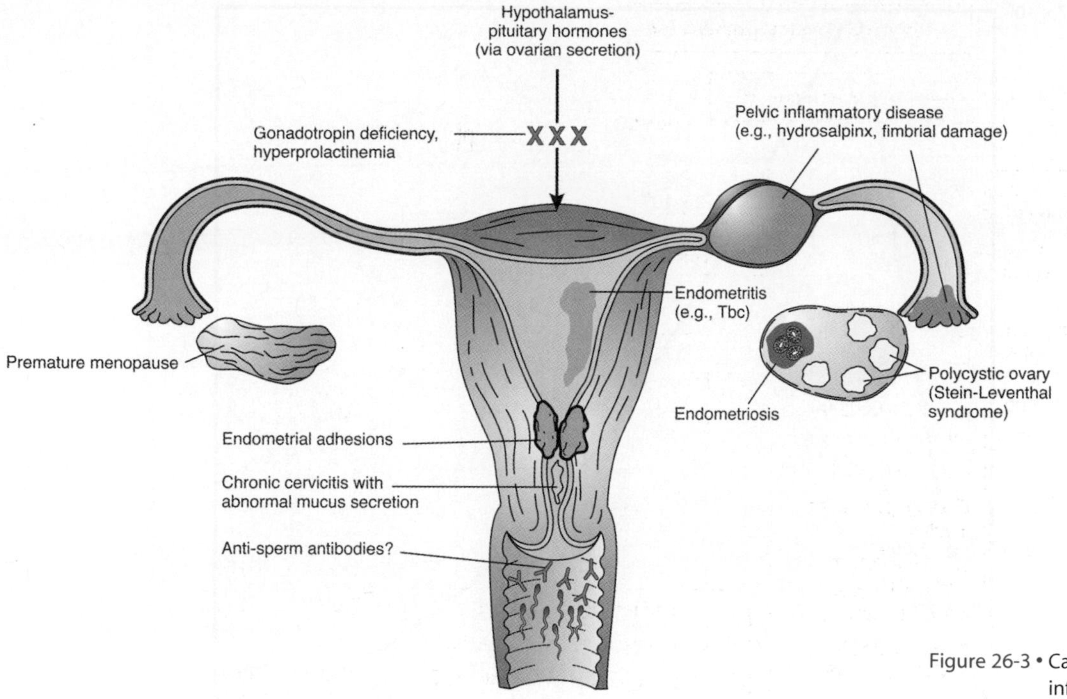

Figure 26-3 • Causes of female factor infertility.

electrocautery excisional procedure (LEEP) conization, mechanical dilations (e.g., cervical dilation for miscarriage, termination of pregnancy, or hysteroscopy), and from extensive laser or cauterization of the cervix. These procedures may result in stenosis as well as destruction of the endocervical epithelium, leading to **inadequate mucous production**. Normal midcycle cervical mucus facilitates the transport of sperm into the endometrial cavity. Disruptions in normal mucus production can thereby lead to difficulty in conceiving.

TABLE 26-4 Causes of Ovulatory Factor Infertility

Central
Pituitary insufficiency (trauma, tumor, congenital)
Hypothalamic insufficiency
Hyperprolactinemia (drug, tumor, empty sella)
Luteal phase defects
Peripheral defects
Gonadal dysgenesis
Premature ovarian failure
Ovarian tumor
Ovarian resistance
Metabolic disease
Polycystic ovarian syndrome (chronic hyperandrogenemic anovulation)
Thyroid disease
Liver disease
Obesity
Androgen excess (adrenal, neoplastic)

OTHER FACTORS

Luteal phase defect is a controversial and poorly understood disorder. The defect may possibly begin with disruption of the HPGA (Fig. 20-1), resulting in inadequate production of progesterone by the corpus luteum and subsequent delay in endometrial maturation. This results in impaired implantation following fertilization.

In couples in which no other cause of infertility can be determined, infertility may be due to **genetic abnormalities** (trisomies, mosaics, translocations, etc.). The most common aneuploidy associated with female infertility is 45X (Turner syndrome).

Clinical Manifestations

History

The evaluation should begin with a thorough **medical history** including a **menstrual history** (Fig. 26-2). The physician should guide the interview systematically while looking for symptoms related to ovarian, tubal, uterine, and cervical factors, which can lead to infertility.

Patients with **ovulatory dysfunction** may report amenorrhea, oligomenorrhea, or menorrhagia. Additional questioning should elicit symptoms related to PCOS, thyroid dysfunction, hyperprolactinemia, and ovarian failure. Patients with PCOS may report hirsutism, irregular menses, and/or weight changes. A detailed social history might reveal reasons for centrally mediated ovulatory dysfunction including eating disorders, extreme exercise, or unusual stress.

Women with **endometriosis** often give a history of cyclic pelvic pain, dysmenorrhea, and/or dyspareunia. Pelvic adhesions may be asymptomatic or may be associated with varying degrees of pelvic pain, especially with movement or lifting.

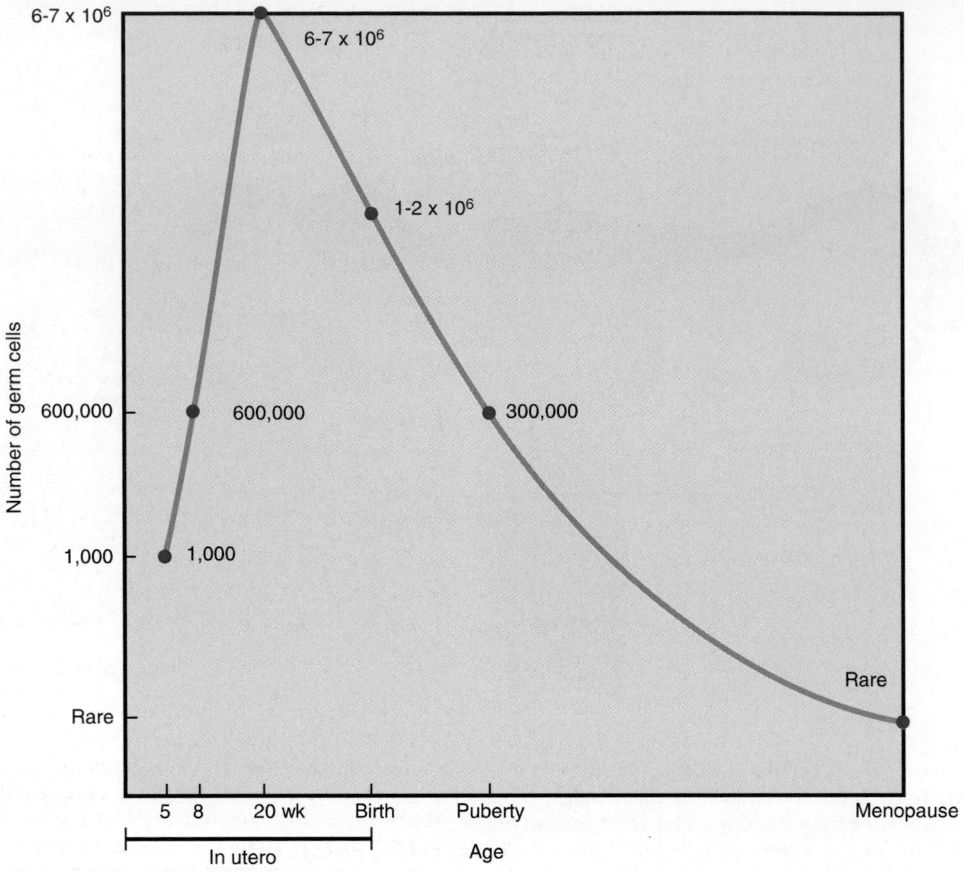

Figure 26-4 • The number of oocytes in the ovary before and after birth and through menopause.
(From Berek JS. *Berek & Novak's Gynecology*, 14th ed. Philadelphia, PA: Lippincott Williams & Wilkins; 2006.)

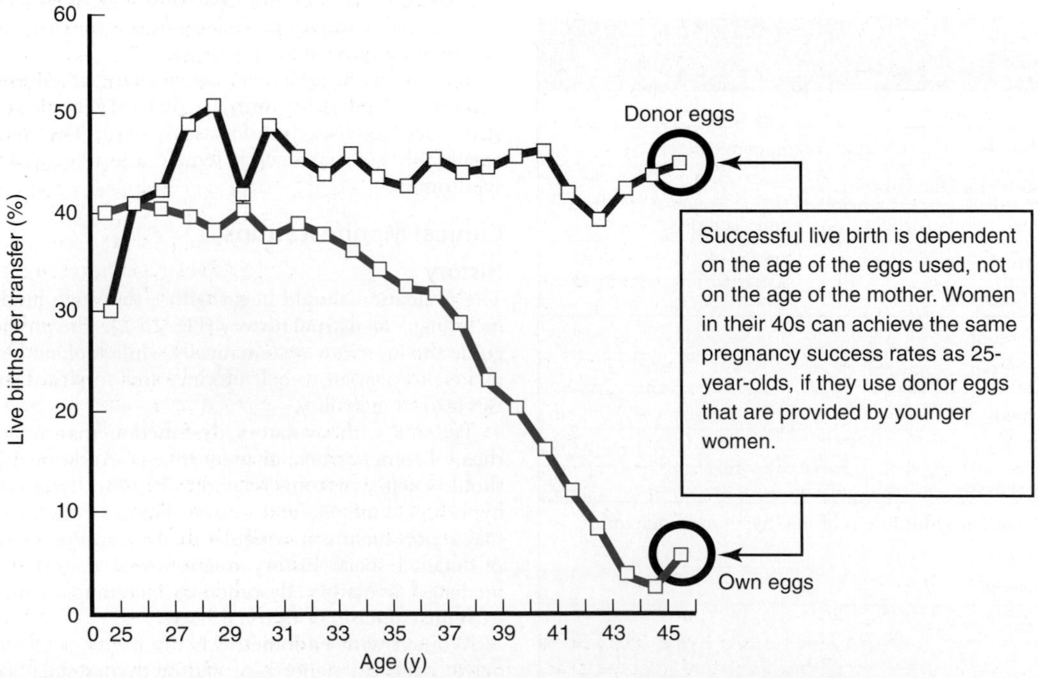

Figure 26-5 • Live births per embryo transfer comparing use of a patient's own versus donor oocytes.
(From Berek JS. *Berek & Novak's Gynecology*, 14th ed. Philadelphia, PA: Lippincott Williams & Wilkins; 2006.)

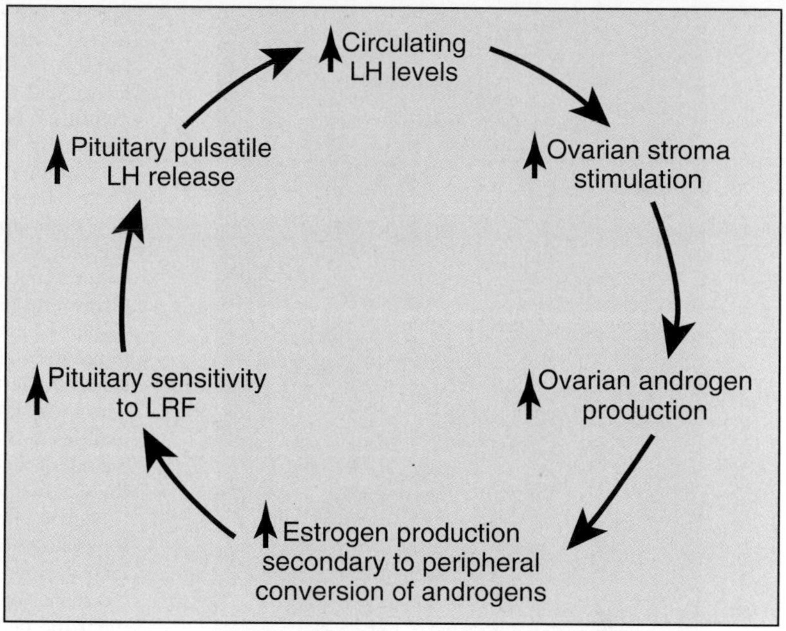

Figure 26-6 • A proposed mechanism for polycystic ovarian syndrome. LH, luteinizing hormone; LRH, luteinizing releasing hormone.
(From Beckmann C, Ling F. *Obstetrics & Gynecology*, 5th ed. Philadelphia, PA: Lippincott Williams & Wilkins; 2006.)

The clinical presentation of **uterine factor** infertility varies with the etiology. For many of these factors, infertility may be the only symptom. Among the most common causes, endometritis may present with pelvic pain and fever; and submucosal fibroids and polyps may present with abnormal uterine bleeding. Uterine anomalies such as uterine septum may present with a history of recurrent pregnancy loss. **Cervical factor** infertility may present with a history of prior cryotherapy, conization, and/or cervical dilations.

Physical Examination

A physical examination should be performed to look for signs that may point toward a disorder associated with infertility. Careful evaluation may uncover **signs of PCOS** such as acne, hirsutism, acanthosis nigricans (Color Plate 13), skin tags, and central obesity (BMI > 27). Similar care should be taken while evaluating for **thyroid dysfunction** (goiter, changes in hair/nails, and tachycardia). The examination should also look for breast development as a sign of past estrogen secretion.

When performing a **pelvic examination**, primary ovarian insufficiency might present with signs of estrogen deficiency such as vaginal atrophy. Visualization of the cervix may demonstrate **cervical stenosis**, signs of infection, or malformations. The findings associated with **endometriosis** or pelvic adhesions include a fixed or retroverted uterus, uterosacral nodularity, or tender fixed adnexa. With **pelvic adhesions**, the pain can sometimes be reproduced on abdominal or pelvic exam. Uterine size should be evaluated and the physician should look for **leiomyoma** and any signs of current or prior pelvic infection. Endometriomas and other **ovarian pathology** may be palpated during the pelvic exam.

Diagnostic Evaluation

The primary tests for the evaluation of ovulatory factor infertility involve looking for **evidence of ovulation** by tracking the menstrual cycle, measuring the basal body temperature (Fig. 24-1), monitoring the cervical mucus, and measuring the **mid-luteal progesterone** (days 21 to 23). Over-the-counter ovulation prediction kits have made predicting the presence and timing of ovulation much easier and have largely replaced daily basal body temperature monitoring.

As it is common for women to delay childbearing, an assessment of ovarian reserve has become an important topic in fertility. This can also be especially useful in women over 30 year of age, those with prior ovarian surgery or only one ovary, those with a history of prior chemotherapy or radiation exposure, and in women who have had a poor response to ovulation induction (OI).

Traditionally, a **clomiphene citrate challenge test** (CCCT) can be used to assess for decreased ovarian reserve—the oocyte-related decline in fertility. The test involves administration of 100 mg of clomiphene citrate (Clomid) on days 5 through 9 of the menstrual cycle. The follicle-stimulating hormone (FSH) level is measured on days 3 and 10. Even small elevations in FSH levels correlate with decreased fecundity. However, the CCCT has largely been replaced by the use of basal FSH/estradiol testing, the antral follicle count (AFC), and the anti-Mullërian hormone (AMH) assay.

Measurement of a **Day 3 FSH level** is based on the notion that women with good ovarian reserve will make enough ovarian hormone early in the menstrual cycle to provide inhibition of FSH, thus keeping it at a low level. Comparatively, women with poor ovarian reserve will have insufficient ovarian hormone production early in the cycle. This insufficiency results in a reflexive increase in FSH level. In general, a Day 3 FSH value less than 10 mIU/mL is indicative of adequate ovarian reserve; 10 to 15 mIU/mL of borderline ovarian reserve, and greater than 20 mIU/mL is indicative of poor ovarian reserve. The greatest value is the correlation between abnormally high levels (>20 mIU/mL) and an inability to conceive using the patient's own eggs. In these cases, the use of donor oocytes will likely be needed.

Measurement of the Day 3 estradiol level may also be used to assess ovarian reserve by looking for elevated basal rates of estradiol. This may be indicative of premature follicle recruitment that can occur in women with poor ovarian reserve. Thus, a higher Day 3 estradiol level (>80 pg/mL) is suggestive

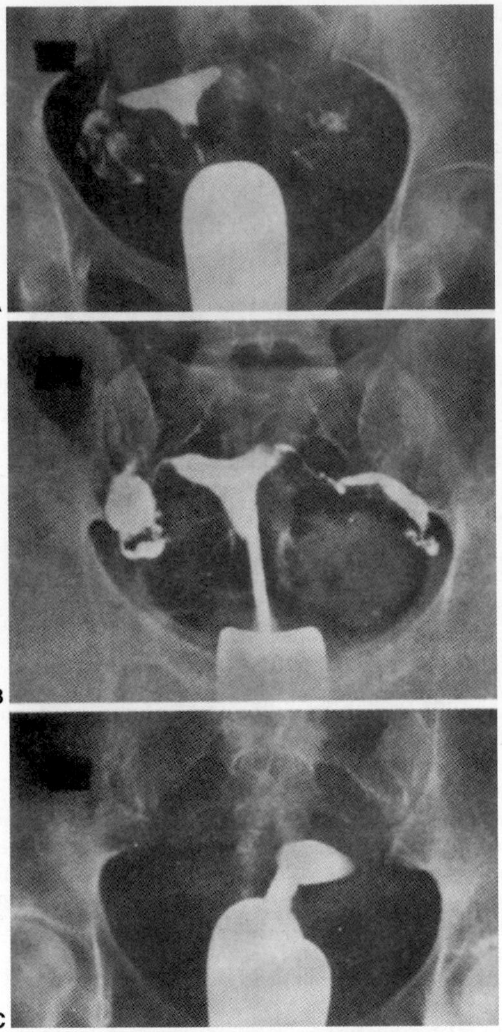

Figure 26-7 • Hysterosalpingograms showing **(A)** normal uterine cavity and patent tubes, **(B)** bilateral hydrosalpinx, and **(C)** bilateral tubal occlusion.
(From Beckmann C, Ling F. *Obstetrics & Gynecology*, 5th ed. Philadelphia, PA: Lippincott Williams & Wilkins; 2006.)

of diminished reserve, whereas a lower level (<80 pg/mL) is suggestive of adequate ovarian capacity.

Measurement of the **antral follicle count (AFC)** can also be used to assess ovarian reserve. This ultrasound test measures the number of antral follicles (2 to 10 mm in diameter) present between Days 2 and 4 of the menstrual cycle. In general, the presence of 4 to 10 antral follicles is a sign of good ovarian reserve, whereas lower follicle numbers suggest poor reserve. Most recently, measurement of **anti-Mullerian hormone (AMH)** has been used in predicting ovarian reserve. It is based on measurement of AMH from the primordial follicle pool. When the pool is robust, a high level of AMH is detected. As women age and the pool declines, a lower amount is found. A level of AMH greater than 0.5 ng/mL is considered adequate ovarian reserve, whereas levels less than 0.15 ng/mL are suggestive of a reduced follicle pool and decreased pregnancy rates.

Endocrine evaluation may include measurements of FSH, luteinizing hormone (LH), prolactin, thyroid function tests (TFTs), and thyroid antibodies. If Cushing's syndrome is suspected, serum testosterone, dehydroepiandrosterone sulfate (DHEA-S), 17-hydroxyprogesterone, 24-hour urine cortisol levels, and an overnight dexamethasone suppression test are helpful. When intracranial lesions are suspected, **MRI or CT imaging** of the head should be done.

Endometriosis or pelvic adhesions may be strongly suspected based on the patient's history, but direct visualization with **laparoscopy or laparotomy** is necessary to confirm the diagnosis. Ovarian endometriomas (cystic collections of endometrial cells on the ovaries) can be diagnosed on **pelvic ultrasound** (Fig. 15-2).

Tubal patency can be demonstrated with a **hysterosalpingogram** (HSG) performed during the follicular phase, or tubal lavage (chromopertubation) performed during laparoscopy. An HSG can also aid in the search for **structural abnormalities** in the endometrial cavity. This involves installation of a contrast dye transcervically to evaluate for filling defects in the cavity and to test for **tubal patency** (Fig. 26-7).

Pelvic ultrasound is one of the primary investagative tools for evaluating the female reproductive tract for structural defects such as fibroids, polyps, adenomyosis, ovarian cysts, and congenial anomalies. A **saline sonohysterogram** can complement the pelvic ultrasound by allowing better visualization of the uterine cavity. This is accomplished by transcervical infusion of saline into the cavity while ultrasound examination of the uterus is being performed.

Hysteroscopy in the office or in the operating room may be used to directly visualize the endocervical canal and endometrial cavity. **MRI** can also be useful in better delineation of adenomyosis and uterine anomalies.

A **Pap smear** and **cervical cultures** for gonorrhea and *Chlamydia* should be performed in all women undergoing an infertility evaluation since cervicitis and cervical dysplasia are often asymptomatic. Other evaluative testing including the postcoital test, endometrial biopsy, basal body temperature measurements, karyotyping, and mycoplasma cultures have **not** been found to have any value in the evaluation of infertility and are no longer routinely used.

Treatment

The **underlying etiology** of infertility should be **identified and corrected**. For uncorrectable cases, ovulation induction (OI) with fertility drugs, **intrauterine insemination** (IUI) with sperm, or **in vitro fertilization** (IVF) can be used.

Regular ovulation can be restored in 90% of infertility cases that are due to endocrine factors by treating the underlying disorder. The most common etiology of ovulatory infertility is **PCOS**. For these patients, weight loss, metformin, and OI with Clomid or letrozole (Femara) have been effective in establishing ovulation and producing viable pregnancies. In PCOS patients, even small amounts of weight loss (5% of initial weight) can result in lowered fasting insulin levels, testosterone, and androstenedione and in restoration of spontaneous ovulation.

Metformin (Glucophage) is an oral biguanide typically used for the treatment of non-insulin–dependent diabetes mellitus. This insulin sensitizer results in inhibition of gluconeogenesis and **increased peripheral glucose uptake**. PCOS patients using metformin experience a decrease in fasting insulin levels and testosterone levels. These improvements can help promote the reestablishment of **spontaneous ovulation** in PCOS patients.

If spontaneous ovulation cannot be established, ovulation-inducing medications can be utilized to stimulate ovulation

TABLE 26-5 Medications Used in the Treatment of Infertility and in Assisted Reproductive Technologies

Commercial Name	Generic Name	Mechanism
Clomid Serophene	Clomiphene citrate	Anti-estrogen, stimulates follicular development for ovulation induction
Glucophage	Metformin	Insulin sensitizer, decreases insulin, testosterone, BMI; promotes ovulation
Novarel Pregnyl Profasi	Human chorionic gonadotropin	Similar structure to LH, triggers ovulation after gonadotropin follicle stimulation
Lutrepulse Factrel	Pulsatile GnRH/ gonadorelin	GnRH agonist, stimulates release of FSH/LH from pituitary
Femara	Letrozole	Aromatase inhibitor, reduces androgen conversion to estrogen, stimulates follicular development for ovulatory induction

BMI, body mass index; GnRH, gonadotropin releasing hormone; FSH, follicle stimulating hormone; LH, luteinizing hormone.

(Table 26-5). Of these medications the most frequently used are **Clomid and letrozole** (Femara). If these treatments are unsuccessful, OI and pregnancy can be attempted with a combination of Clomid, letrozole, or human gonadotropins with IUI or IVF.

For patients with **hypothalamic-pituitary failure** (WHO Group 1), ovulation can usually be achieved with pulsatile gonadotropin-releasing hormone (GnRH) therapy or human gonadotropins (Table 26-5). Of note, there is **no treatment** for WHO Group 3 patients with **primary ovarian insufficiency/ failure** because these patients lack viable oocytes. Patients with this diagnosis should be offered the options of egg donation, gestational surrogacy, or adoption.

Symptomatic relief of **endometriosis** can be achieved medically or surgically. However, **there is no role for medical management in the treatment of infertility caused by endometriosis**. Medical treatments such as Danazol, Lupron, oral medroxyprogesterone (Provera), or continuous oral contraceptives can temporarily relieve symptoms but do not increase fertility rates.

For patients with endometriosis, fertility rates can be improved by surgical ligation of periadnexal adhesions during laparoscopy or laparotomy with excision, coagulation, vaporization, or **fulguration of endometrial implants**. Pregnancy rates after surgical treatment depend on the extent of the disease, but increased fertility through spontaneous conception and in vitro fertilization (IVP) has been demonstrated after surgical treatment of mild, moderate, and severe endometriosis.

Microsurgical **tuboplasty with tubal reanastomosis** or neosalpingostomy has proven to be effective for treating tubal occlusion due to prior infection or from prior tubal ligation. However, because it is more effective, most couples undergo **IVF rather than attempt tuboplasty**. The advantage of tuboplasty is that it allows for more than one future pregnancy without the cost and difficulty of multiple IVF cycles. When tubal occlusion, tubal damage, or hydrosalpinx result from prior salpingitis, reproductive endocrinologists will often remove the damaged tube and opt for **IVF** to treat the resulting infertility.

Operative hysteroscopy is used to treat **uterine factors** such as uterine synechiae, septae, polyps, or submucosal fibroids. Following surgical ligation of synechiae or septae, estrogen therapy or intrauterine devices are often used to **prevent recurrence** of adhesions. Fertility is restored in 50% of these cases. Most surgeons reserve myomectomy for treatment after recurrent pregnancy loss or when symptomatic fibroids have been identified.

Treatment of cervical factor infertility varies with the cause. Cervical stenosis can often be treated with **surgical or mechanical dilation** of the endocervical canal. Both cervical stenosis and abnormal cervical mucus can be treated by **bypassing the cervix with intrauterine insemination** (Fig. 26-8). IUI appears to be the most effective treatment for cervical factor infertility. In cases that are refractory to other treatments, patients should be offered IVF.

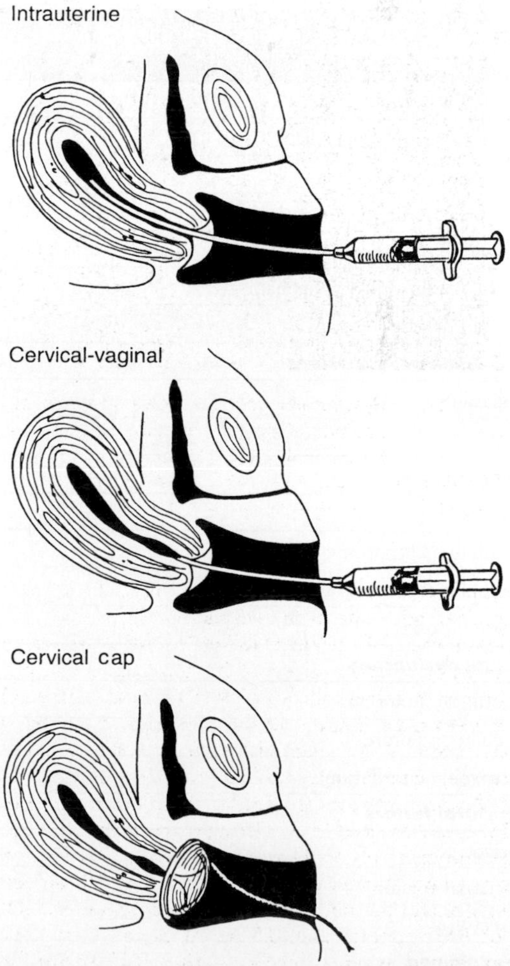

Figure 26-8 • Techniques of artificial insemination.
(From Beckmann C, Ling F. *Obstetrics & Gynecology*, 5th ed. Philadelphia, PA: Lippincott Williams & Wilkins; 2006.)

MALE FACTOR INFERTILITY

PATHOGENESIS

There are multiple causes of male factor infertility (Table 26-6) including endocrine disorders, anatomic defects, problems with abnormal sperm production and motility, as well as sexual dysfunction.

EPIDEMIOLOGY

Thirty-five percent of infertility is due to **purely male factors** (Fig. 26-1). Of couples undergoing infertility evaluation, 10% to 20% are affected by a combination of male and female factors.

RISK FACTORS

Men with **occupational or environmental exposure** to chemicals, radiation, or excessive heat are at increased risk for infertility, as are those with a history of varicocele, mumps, hernia repair, pituitary tumor, anabolic steroid use, testicular injury, and impotence. **Certain medications** have also been found to depress semen quantity and quality, cause erectile dysfunction, or result in ejaculation failure (Table 26-7).

TABLE 26-6 Common Etiologies of Male Factor Infertility

Abnormal semen
Cryptorchidism (congenital)
Mumps orchitis
Antisperm antibodies
Endocrine disorders
Hypogonadotropic hypogonadism
Thyroid disease
Environmental exposures
Radiation
Heat
Chemicals
Genetic
Klinefelter's syndrome
Immobile cilia syndrome
Cystic fibrosis
Sexual dysfunction
Erectile dysfunction
Ejaculation failure
Retrograde ejaculation
Structural factors
Varicocele
Testicular torsion
Vasectomy
Unexplained
No identifiable cause
Idiopathic abnormal semen

TABLE 26-7 Drugs That Decrease Semen Quality and Quantity

Medications		**Exogenous Exposures**
Cimetidine	Metoclopramide	Anabolic steroids
Sulfasalazine	Chemotherapeutic agents	Marijuana
Spironolactone	Beta blockers	Alcohol abuse
Antidepressants	Nitrofurans	Heroin/cocaine abuse

CLINICAL MANIFESTATIONS

History

The physician should ask about previous pregnancies fathered by the patient, environmental exposures, medications, and any history of sexually transmitted infections (STIs), mumps orchitis, hernia repair, and surgery or trauma to the genitals.

Physical Examination

The physical examination should include identification of the urethral meatus, measurement of testicular size, and a search for signs of varicocele, cogenital absence of the vas, and hernias. Testosterone deficiency may be evidenced by increased body fat, decreased muscle mass, loss of pubic, axillary and facial hair, decreased oiliness of the skin, and fine facial wrinkles.

DIAGNOSTIC EVALUATION

A **semen analysis** is the primary investigative tool for male factor infertility. The semen sample is analyzed for sperm count, volume, motility, morphology, pH, and white blood cell count (Table 26-8). In the case of an abnormal semen analysis, an endocrine evaluation should include TFTs, prolactin, LH, and FSH (to assess for parenchymal damage to testes and hypogonadism).

The **postcoital test** is rarely performed but can be used to examine the interaction between the sperm and the cervical mucus. An abnormal postcoital test, sperm agglutination, and reduced sperm motility are suspicious for the presence of **antisperm antibodies**. Several tests are presently available to detect such antibodies.

TREATMENT

In general, the probability of conception can be enhanced by **improvements in coital practice**. This includes having intercourse every other day near ovulation. Men should avoid the

TABLE 26-8 Semen Analysis Normal Parameters

Volume	>2.0 mL
pH	7.2–7.8
Concentration	>20 million/mL
Morphology	>30% normal forms
Motility	>50% with forward progression
WBC	<1 million/mL

use of tight underwear, saunas and hot tubs, and unnecessary environmental exposures such as radiation, excess heat, and certain medications (Table 26-7).

Treatment of male factor infertility **depends upon the etiology**. Hypothalamic-pituitary failure can be treated with injections of human menopausal gonadotropins (hMGs), and varicoceles can be repaired by ligation.

Assisted reproductive technologies (ARTs) can be used to overcome an abnormal semen analysis, when treating the underlying disorder is not effective. Low semen volume, low sperm density, and low sperm motility are most often treated by **washed sperm for IUI** (Fig. 26-8).

Intracytoplasmic sperm injection(ICSI) is another option for patients with low sperm density or impaired motility and has revolutionized the treatment of male factor infertility (Fig. 26-9). This method involves retrieving sperm from the male, preparing it, individually injecting a single sperm directly into an egg, and then placing the fertilized egg into the uterus cavity (IVF). The sperm can be retrieved from the male by ejaculation, or by direct aspiration from the testis (testicular sperm extraction [TSE]) or epididymis either microscopically (microsurgical epididymal sperm aspiration [MESA]) or percutaneously (PESA).

In refractory cases of male factor infertility, artificial insemination with **donor sperm is highly effective**.

UNEXPLAINED INFERTILITY

Among those couples who complete an initial assessment, **10% find no cause for their infertility** (Fig. 26-1). When the initial infertility evaluation reveals no cause, the problem often involves abnormalities in sperm transport, the presence of antisperm antibodies, or problems with penetration and fertilization of the egg. When problems in sperm transport, motility, or functional capacity are identified, **IVF and ICSI** may be used for treatment. If this fails, the use of **donor sperm** may result in pregnancy.

When no cause for infertility is identified after in-depth testing, studies show that most therapies have **no higher success rates than no treatment at all**. Although some patients with unexplained infertility may undergo three to six cycles of gonadotropin stimulation with IUI followed by IVF cycles, many opt for no treatment. The eventual pregnancy rate for couples with unexplained infertility who receive no treatment approaches **60% over 3 to 5 year**. Other options include use of donor sperm, surrogacy, adoption, or acceptance of childlessness.

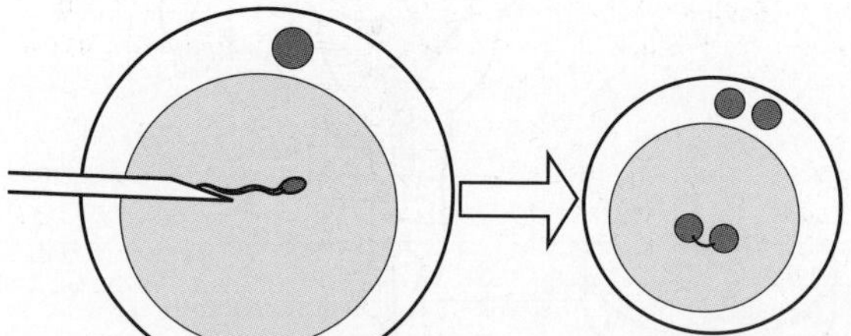

Figure 26-9 • Intracytoplasmic sperm injection (ICSI). A spermatid or spermatozoon is collected by ejaculation or aspiration from the epididymus or testis. One sperm is injected directly into each harvested egg. The embryos are then transferred back into the uterine cavity via IVF.

ASSISTED REPRODUCTIVE TECHNOLOGIES

Since their inception, the treatment of infertility with ARTs has progressed rapidly and now includes not only fertility drugs that stimulate multiple follicular development but also technologies that combine **OI** agents with **IUI, IVF, or ICSI**. Oocytes may also be obtained via natural, nonstimulated cycles, but the number of eggs per cycle is increased by OI.

OVULATION INDUCTION

Clomiphene citrate (Clomid) is a **selective estrogen receptor modulator** (SERM) that **competitively binds to estrogen receptors** in the hypothalamus. In doing so, it blocks the negative feedback effect of endogenous estrogen. This results in increased pulsatile GnRH frequency. Subsequently, **FSH and LH production is increased,** leading to follicular growth and ovulation (Table 26-5). Clomid is generally administered orally to women with absent or infrequent ovulation, starting on day 3 or 5 of the follicular phase of the menstrual cycle for approximately 5 days. Ovulation generally occurs 5 to 12 days after the last day of clomid.

Letrozole is an **aromatase inhibitor** that **decreases the conversion of androgens** (testosterone and androsteindione)**into estrogens** (estradiol and estrone) (Table 26-5). Lower estrogen levels reduce the negative feedback effect on the hypothalamus and pituitary which leads to an increase of FSH and follicular development. It's use for OI is off-label in the United States.

Absent or infrequent ovulation is the major indication for Clomid and letrozole use in women with PCOS or mild hypothalamic amenorrhea. Specific causes of anovulation should be ruled out first, and patients should have normal thyroid stimulating hormone (TSH), FSH, and prolactin levels. Although Clomid is used as a first-line therapy in couples with unexplained infertility, it has no use in patients with primary ovarian insufficiency (POI; formerly known as premature ovarian failure).

The other major category of OI agents is **human menopausal gonadotropins** (hMGs). These are best used when the pituitary gland fails to secrete sufficient FSH and LH to stimulate follicular maturation and ovulation, and when Clomid is also incapable of stimulating ovulation. Patients with mild to severe hypothalamic dysfunction fall into this category and often require hMGs for OI.

The hMGs (Table 26-5) often come in combined preparations of FSH and LH or of FSH alone. They are administered via intramuscular injection during the follicular phase of the menstrual cycle. The patient's response to OI should be **monitored closely** through **serial estrogen levels and pelvic ultrasounds** to measure the number of follicles, size of follicles, and the total estrogen production level.

Each means of **OI** can potentially produce multiple follicular development. Once ovulation occurs, **fertilization** may be attempted by intercourse or IUI. Conversely, after OI, **oocyte retrieval** may be accomplished with **transvaginal aspiration** (Fig. 26-10). The oocytes are then fertilized via **ICSI** (Fig. 26-9) or **in vitro fertilization** is allowed to occur (Fig. 26-11). Selected **embryos are then transferred** into the uterus under ultrasound guidance. Progesterone is often used to promote **endometrial receptivity** beginning after embryo transfer and lasting through the first trimester. Any remaining embryos are saved using **cryopreservation** techniques for future cycles, embryo donation, or research.

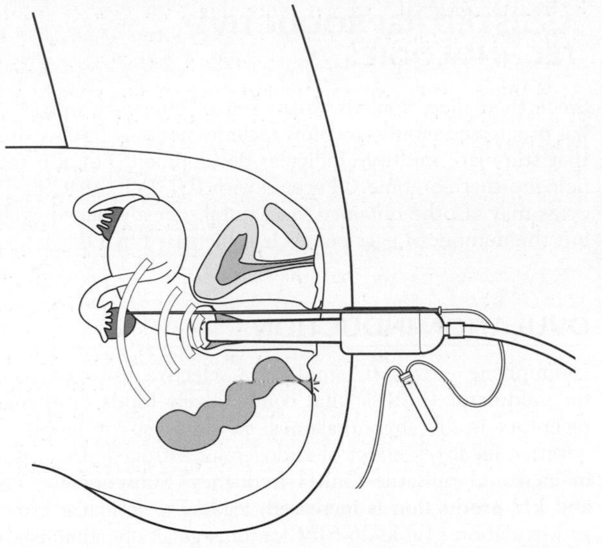

Figure 26-10 • Transvaginal ultrasound-guided needle aspiration of oocytes. Following ovulation induction, multiple eggs are removed from the ovaries by placing a vaginal probe into the vagina. A fine needle is guided toward the ovary while the physician visualizes the follicles on ultrasound. Fluid around the follicles is then collected through a needle connected to a test tube.

Effectiveness

Clomiphene citrate is successful in **inducing ovulation in 80% of correctly selected patients** and **36% become pregnant**. If pregnancy does not occur after three to six cycles of Clomid, more aggressive therapies are needed. Gonadotropins have an **80% to 90% ovulation success rate** and a **10% to 40% pregnancy success rate** per cycle depending on the diagnosis (recall fecundity is only 20% to 25% in the general population). Gonadotropins carry a much higher risk of **ovarian hyperstimulation** (1% to 3%) and **multiple gestation pregnancy** (20%).

Side Effects and Complications

The potential side effects of Clomid are related to its **antiestrogen effects**: hot flashes, abdominal distension and bloating, emotional lability, depression, and visual changes. These side effects are mostly mild and disappear after discontinuation of the medication. Although there is some controversy about the risk of **teratogenesis** with aromatase inhibitors, care should be taken to rule out pregnancy prior to induction of ovulation for this off-label indication.

Multiple gestation pregnancy is a major side effect of OI and ARTs. Multiple gestation pregnancies occur in 8% of Clomid-induced pregnancies and in 20% of pregnancies from gonadotropins.

The other major complication of OI with gonadotropins is ovarian **hyperstimulation syndrome** (OHSS). This is a potentially life-threatening condition caused by overstimulation of the ovaries occurring in 1% to 3% of patients undergoing OI. This completely iatrogenic disorder can range from ovarian enlargement and minimal symptoms to significant ovarian enlargement, torsion, or rupture. This may be complicated by ascites, pleural effusions, hemoconcentration, hypercoagulability, electrolyte disturbances, renal failure, and even death.

The risk of both multiple gestations and OHSS can be mediated by careful monitoring of estradiol production and follicle growth during ovulation induction, and by limiting the number of embryos placed during IVF.

ADVANCED REPRODUCTIVE TECHNOLOGIES (IVF, ICSI, PGD)

Method of Action

ARTs have advanced the treatment of infertility by allowing physicians to successfully **bypass the normal mechanisms of gamete transportation and fertilization**. In conjunction with OI, multiple oocytes may be harvested from the ovary using ultrasound (Fig. 26-10).

During IVF, the oocytes are allowed to mature briefly in vitro before washed sperm are added. **Fertilization** is verified 14 to 18 hours later by the presence of two pronuclei. In the case of IVF, the conceptuses are then **placed into the uterus** through the cervix using a catheter (Fig. 26-11), making IVF a relatively noninvasive procedure.

ICSI has revolutionized the treatment of male factor infertility by allowing a single spermatid or **sperm to be directly injected into the cytoplasm of a harvested oocyte** (Fig. 26-9). The resulting embryos can then be placed back into the uterus for implantation.

Preimplantation genetic diagnosis (PGD) refers to the evaluation of the embryo for genetic abnormalities prior to transfer during an IVF cycle. PGD involves removing one or two cells from a six- to eight-cell embryo, and then screening

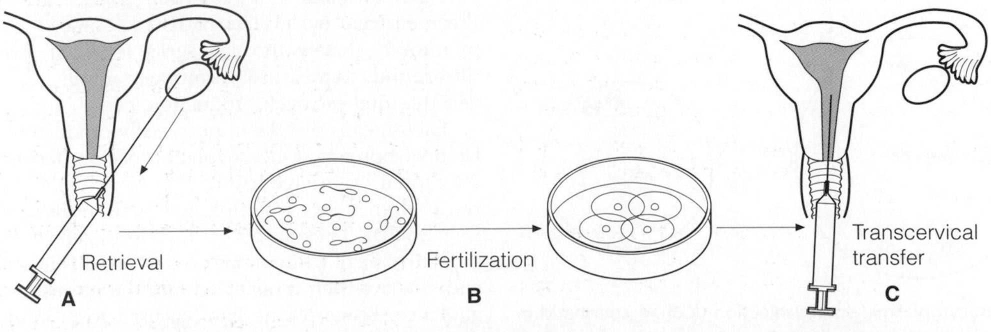

Figure 26-11 • In vitro fertilization (IVF). **(A)** After ovulation induction, oocytes are harvested transvaginally. **(B)** The egg and sperm are placed together in the laboratory and fertilization takes place. **(C)** The fertilized embryos are transferred into the uterine cavity through the cervix.

for common **chromosomal abnormalities** or **genetic mutations** such as sickle cell anemia, Tay-Sachs disease, cystic fibrosis, Down syndrome, hemophilia A, and fragile X syndrome. This technique is usually performed when a patient has a known inherited genetic disease, is a carrier of a chromosomal translocation that has resulted in recurrent miscarriages, has an affected child, or is of advanced maternal age (increased risk of aneuploidy). PGD is used in approximately 5% of ART cycles nationwide.

Effectiveness

The success rate of these advanced reproductive technologies varies from center to center. On average, with IVF, **delivery** is achieved in **34%** of oocyte retrievals **using fresh nondonor embryos** and **55% of transfers using fresh donor embryos**. Success rates are dependent on maternal age, diagnosis, the number and quality of oocytes, sperm, and embryos. The most favorable rates are seen among **women under age 35**, those **without hydrosalpinges**, and women with **adequate ovarian reserve**. Again, keep in mind that the normal fecundity rate in a couple with no fertility factors is approximately 20% to 25% per month.

Multiple gestation pregnancies are a major complication of ART. The Society for Assisted Reproductive Technologies reports that in 2009 the rate of multiple gestations at delivery was **31% for IVF** (29% twins, 3% triplets and higher-order multiples). This compares with a multiple-infant birth rate of slightly more than 3% in the general US population. The rate of multiple gestations is important because these pregnancies are at greater risk for **maternal complications** (preeclampsia, gestational diabetes, placenta previa, premature delivery, and postpartum hemorrhage) and **fetal complications** (intrauterine growth restriction [IUGR], respiratory distress syndrome, intraventricular hemorrhage, neonatal sepsis, low birth weight, and death). Guidelines have been established regarding the number of embryos to transfer in various clinical scenarios with the intent of minimizing the risk for multiple gestation.

KEY POINTS

- Female factor infertility is purely responsible for 45% to 55% of all infertility cases. These can be divided into ovulatory, tubal, uterine, and cervical factors.
- Female factor infertility may be due to ovulatory factors that interrupt the hypothalamic-pituitary-ovarian axis such as polycystic ovarian syndrome, primary ovarian insufficiency, hyperprolactinemia, and thyroid diseases. The most common causes of ovulatory factor infertility are PCOS and advanced maternal age.
- Ovulatory factors are diagnosed by confirming ovulation through menstrual history, ovulation detection kits, midluteal progesterone level, along with endocrine evaluation (TSH, prolactin, FSH, and LH) and assessment of ovarian reserve (Day 3 FSH and estradiol levels, AMH levels, and AFC).
- Ovulatory factors are best addressed by treating the cause of the ovulatory dysfunction. PCOS-related infertility can be treated with weight loss, metformin, and OI with Clomid or letrozole. When refractory to treatment, OI with human gonadotropins can be used along with along with IUI or IVF.
- The most common causes of tubal factor infertility are endometriosis and pelvic adhesions. These factors are diagnosed by history and laparoscopy or laparotomy, and treated surgically to improve fertility rates. Tubal occlusion may be repaired with microsurgical tuboplasty, but most couples opt for IVF.
- Female infertility may be due to uterine factors such as uterine synechiae, polyps, submucosal fibroids, congenital malformations, or endometritis. Uterine factors are diagnosed by pelvic ultrasound, HSG, saline sonohysterogram, hysteroscopy, and laparoscopy.
- Uterine factors are treated according to the cause of the infertility. Synechiae, fibroids, and polyps can be resected; endometritis is treated with antibiotics.
- Female infertility may also be due to cervical factors such as cervical stenosis from surgical or mechanical dilation. These factors are diagnosed on physical exam and treated with surgical or mechanical dilation of the endocervical canal or IUI to bypass the cervix.
- Male factor infertility is purely responsible for 35% of all infertility cases.
- It may be idiopathic or due to improper coital practices, sexual dysfunction, endocrine disorders, or abnormalities in spermatogenesis, sperm volume, density, or mobility.
- Male factor infertility is diagnosed by semen analysis and endocrine evaluation if indicated. The treatment of male factor infertility depends on the causal agent and includes improved coital practices, repair of anatomic defects, ICSI, and the use of donor sperm.
- Ten percent of couples find no explanation for infertility after their initial assessment. When this occurs, further assessment may be done to search for problems with sperm transport, ability to penetrate and fertilize the egg, and antisperm antibodies. IVF/ICSI can be used to treat these patients.
- Most therapies for unexplained infertility have not been shown to have higher success rates than no treatment. Couples with unexplained infertility who choose no treatment will conceive up to 60% of the time over 3 to 5 year.
- Clomiphene citrate is an antiestrogen that binds to estrogen receptors in the hypothalamus to cause increased FSH and LH production, thereby promoting follicular maturation and ovulation. Letrozole is an aromatase inhibitor that decreases the conversion of androgens into estrogens, thereby lowering estrogen levels and increasing FSH and follicular development. Its use for OI is off-label in the United States.
- Clomiphene citrate is best used for OI in women with chronic anovulation or mild hypothalamic insufficiency after specific causes of hypothalamic dysfunction have been ruled out.
- Human menopausal gonadotropins are forms of FSH, or combinations of FSH and LH that directly stimulate follicular maturation in patients for whom Clomid has failed, or those with hypothalamic or pituitary failure or unexplained infertility.
- The primary complications of fertility drugs include ovarian hyperstimulation and multiple gestation pregnancy.
- IVF and ICSI may be used to bypass the normal mechanisms of gamete transport and fertilization with deliveries in about 30% of cases.

C Clinical Vignettes

Vignette 1

A young couple comes in with a chief complaint of infertility. The patient is a 30-year-old G0 who has not undergone any evaluation. Her husband is a 33-year-old who has had a semen analysis, which was reported as normal. He has never fathered a child. The couple reports having unprotected intercourse for the past 14 months. On further history, the patient reports that her periods have been quiet irregular over the last year and that she has not had period in the last 3 months. She also reports hot flashes, vaginal dryness, and decreased libido.

1. The most likely diagnosis for this patient based on her history is
   a. Polycystic ovarian syndrome
   b. Primary ovarian insufficiency/Premature ovarian failure
   c. Endometriosis
   d. Kallmann syndrome
   e. Spontaneous pregnancy
2. To confirm your suspicion you decide to do some lab tests. All of the following would be appropriate test of ovarian reserve, except:
   a. Anti-Mullërian Hormone (AMH)
   b. Day 3 FSH
   c. Day 3 estrodiol level
   d. Progesterone
   e. Clomid Citrate Challenge Test (CCCT)
3. The FSH on the patient comes back at 40 and the estrogen comes back at less than 20 pg/mL. You repeat the labs in 2 weeks and the findings are similar. You have the patient and her husband come back to clinic and gently give them the diagnosis. They have many questions of what this means in terms of their ability to achieve a pregnancy. You let them know that their best chances of achieving a pregnancy are with
   a. Gonadotropins/IUI therapy
   b. IVF with the patient's own eggs
   c. IVF with donor eggs
   d. There is no way for this patient to carry a pregnancy given the diagnosis
   e. OI with aromatase inhibitors

Vignette 2

A 27-year-old patient and her husband present to you with primary infertility. The patient reports regular periods every 28 to 30 days. The patient has no significant medical history and does not take any medications other than prenatal vitamins. Her husband is also in good health, is 30 year of age, and has two children from a previous marriage. When you asked the patient how long they have been trying to achieve a pregnancy, they tell you 6 months.

1. Your instructions to the couple are the following:
   a. They will likely need IVF to achieve a pregnancy
   b. They will likely need Clomid/IUI cycles
   c. Continue trying appropriately-timed intercourse for 6 more months and if no pregnancy is achieved, come back to see you
   d. Consider donor egg
   e. Consider adoption
2. The couple comes back to you after appropriately timed intercourse, not having achieved a pregnancy. At this time you embark on a workup that includes a semen analysis, an HSG, and an endocrine evaluation including FSH, E2, TSH, prolactin levels, and ovarian reserve testing. All of the tests come back normal. Your next recommendation.
   a. Have 6 more months of timed intercourse and if no pregnancy is achieved, come back to see you
   b. Clomiphene citrate with IUI
   c. IVF
   d. Donor egg
   e. Human gonadotropin (hMG)
3. Ovulation was induced successfully in this patient with 6 cycles of Clomid, three of which included IUI. However, after six cycles of Clomid, a pregnancy had not been achieved. How would you proceed?
   a. Have six more cycles of Clomid
   b. Aromatase inhibitors
   c. Donor egg
   d. ICSI
   e. Ovulation induction with human gonadotropins (hMG) followed by IVF

A Answers

Vignette 1 Question 1

Answer B: While the patient's irregular periods and oligomenorrhea are consistent with PCOS, her symptoms of hot flashes, vaginal dryness, and decreased libido are not. The finding of endometriosis is not typically associated with any type of amenorrhea or oligomenorrhea, or any of the other symptoms described. While Kallmann syndrome is associated with amenorrhea, it is primary amenorrhea rather than secondary amenorrhea. This patient reports a lifelong history of regular menses except for the past year. Similarly, although pregnancy could explain the lack of menses for the past 3 months, pregnancy is not associated with hot flashes, vaginal dryness, or decreased libido. The most likely diagnosis for this is patient is answer B—primary ovarian insufficiency. Primary ovarian insufficiency, formerly called premature ovarian failure, is associated with the premature marked decrease in the oocyte pool prior to the age of 40. These women, although young, present with classic menopausal symptoms associated with low estrogen levels including hot flashes, night sweats, decreased libido, and vaginal dryness.

Vignette 1 Question 2

Answer D: There are several available tests for the assessment of ovarian reserve. Traditionally, the CCCT was used to assess ovarian reserve. This involves administration of 100 mg of Clomid on days 5 to 9 of the cycle. The FSH level is then measured at days 3 and 10. The CCCT is still a valid test but has largely been replaced by direct measurement of AMH, Day 3 FSH, and Day 3 estradiol. Measurement of a Day 3 FSH level is based on the notion that women with good ovarian reserve will make enough ovarian hormones early in the menstrual cycle to provide inhibition of FSH, thus keeping it at a low level. In general, a Day 3 FSH value greater than 20 mIU/mL is indicative of poor ovarian reserve. Measurement of the Day 3 estradiol level assesses ovarian reserve by looking for elevated basal rates of estradiol caused by premature follicle recruitment in women with poor ovarian reserve. Thus, a higher Day 3 estradiol level measurement of AMH reflects the size of primordial follicle pool. (>80 pg/mL) is suggestive of diminished reserve. As women age and the pool declines, a lower amount of AMH is found. A level of less than 0.15 ng/mL is suggestive of a reduced follicle pool and is associated with decreased pregnancy rates. Days 21 to 23 progesterone levels are used to assess ovulation for a given cycle, not ovarian reserve.

Vignette 1 Question 3

Answer C: The diagnosis of primary ovarian insufficiency is associated with elevated gonadotropins in response to a markedly decreased ovarian reserve. Giving exogenous gonadotropins or aromatase inhibitors in this case would be of no benefit to this patient because they would not result in maturation of oocytes, given the patient's depleted store. Similarly, having the patient undergo IVF with her own eggs would be of no benefit because the patient's store of eggs has been exhausted. Having the patient undergo IVF using an egg donor is plausible and gives her the most likely chance of a successful pregnancy. In this situation an egg donor would undergo ovarian stimulation and egg retrieval, and the donated eggs would be combined with the patient's husband's sperm and the resulting embryos would be transferred into the patient. D is not the correct answer because while the patient's store of eggs is depleted, primary ovarian insufficiency is not typically associated with any uterine malformation, and thus these patients are typically able to carry a pregnancy to term without complications.

Vignette 2 Question 1

Answer C: The definition of infertility is the inability to conceive after 12 months of unprotected intercourse. Eighty percent to 90% of couples will conceive spontaneously within 12 months of unprotected intercourse. In couples where the woman is under the age of 35 year, infertility evaluation should begin only after the couple has tried on their own for at least 12 months. If the woman is over the age of 35 year, or if there is a history irregular menses, or risk factors for infertility such as endometriosis, or history of PID or uterine anomalies, evaluation might begin after 6 months of unprotected intercourse.

Vignette 2 Question 2

Answer B: At this point the couple has had 12 months of unprotected appropriately timed intercourse, and hence testing and intervention would be the next course of action; so another 6 months of timed intercourse would not be recommended. First-line treatment for infertility of unknown cause is clomiphene citrate (Clomid) with or without intrauterine insemination (IUI). Clomid is one of the oldest and safest infertility drugs that are used. It is associated with a low (4% to 8%) risk of twins and very low risk of triplets or higher order multiples (<1%). Eighty percent of appropriately selected patients will ovulate using Clomid and 40% will become pregnant. Higher pregnancy rates are seen when Clomid is combined with IUI.

Vignette 2 Question 3

Answer D: As the patient successfully ovulated on Clomid and completed six cycles of Clomid, additional cycles are not indicated. Patients who ultimately conceive on Clomid usually do so in the earlier cycles. Moreover, the association between OI and ovarian cancer was primarily seen among women who completed high numbers of Clomid cycles. Donor egg would not be indicated at this time given that the patient is less than 35 year and has adequate ovarian reserve. Similarly, with a normal semen analysis, ISCI would not be indicated. The next step for this couple would be ovulation induction with gonadotropins followed by IVF.

Chapter 27 Neoplastic Disease of the Vulva and Vagina

Benign lesions of the vulva and vagina are discussed in Chapter 13. This chapter discusses preinvasive neoplasia and invasive cancers of the vulva and vagina, respectively (Table 27-1). It is important to distinguish between benign disease and neoplastic disease so that appropriate treatment and follow-up can be offered to patients.

PREINVASIVE NEOPLASTIC DISEASE OF THE VULVA

Preinvasive neoplastic disease of the vulva is divided into two categories: squamous (**vulvar intraepithelial neoplasia; VIN**) and nonsquamous intraepithelial neoplasias (**Paget disease, melanoma in situ**). Histologically, vulvar intraepithelial neoplasia, Paget disease, and melanoma of the vulva can all be quite similar. Therefore, immunohistochemical staining is often used to assist in the diagnosis of vulvar lesions.

VULVAR INTRAEPITHELIAL NEOPLASIA

Pathogenesis

Just as the incidence of cervical dysplasia has been rising in younger women, so has the incidence of VIN. VIN is defined as **cellular atypia contained within the epithelium**. It is characterized by a loss of epithelial cell maturation, cellular crowding, nuclear hyperchromatosis, and abnormal mitosis. The lesions are designated as VIN I (mild dysplasia), II (moderate dysplasia), or III (severe dysplasia), based upon the depth of epithelial involvement. In 2004, the classification for VIN was revised. What was formerly VIN I is now classified as koilocytic atypia, and VIN 2 and 3 are categorized as VIN and subdivided into two distinct clinicopathologic subtypes: Usual VIN and Differentiated VIN (Table 27-2). The newer terminology has not been widely implemented, and therefore for the purposes of this chapter, we will be using the older terminology. Twenty percent of patients with VIN will have a **coexistent invasive carcinoma**, which has penetrated the basement membrane.

The concomitant rise in VIN and cervical intraepithelial neoplasia (CIN) is not surprising because both cervical and vulvar neoplastic diseases are correlated with **human papillomavirus (HPV) infection**; 80% to 90% of VIN lesions will have DNA fragments from HPV, and 60% of women with VIN have cervical neoplasia as well. Additional risk factors for VIN include **cigarette smoking** and an **immunocompromised state.**

This disease has **two distinct forms**, which differ by the age of the patient. Younger premenopausal women are more likely to have more aggressive multifocal lesions (Fig. 27-1) that rapidly become invasive and are associated with HPV 75% to 100% of the time. Older postmenopausal women have another form that is more likely to involve focal lesions that are slow to become invasive and are not typically associated with HPV.

Epidemiology

In the past, VIN was thought of as a disorder primarily affecting postmenopausal women. However, in the past few decades, the incidence of VIN has nearly doubled. Today, the majority of cases occur in **premenopausal women (75%)** and the median age is 40 years. Interestingly, despite the increased incidence in VIN, the incidence of vulvar cancer has stayed relatively stable over the same period of time. Risk factors for VIN include infection with **HPV** types 16 and 18, **cigarette smoking**, immunodeficiency, and **immunosuppression**. The incidence of HPV-associated VIN decreases as age increases. There is no racial predisposition to VIN.

Diagnosis

As many as 50% of patients with VIN are **asymptomatic**. This highlights the need for a **thorough inspection** of the vulva for masses, ulcerations, and color changes at the annual examination. When symptoms are present, the most common are **vulvar pruritus** or vulvar irritation. Patients may also experience a **palpable abnormality, perineal or perianal burning, or dysuria**. Often, these women would have been examined several times and diagnosed with candidiasis, but experience no relief of symptoms with antifungal treatments or topical steroids. Any time a pruritic area of the vulva does not respond to topical antifungal creams—particularly in the postmenopausal woman—further evaluation with **vulvar biopsy should be undertaken** (Fig. 13-6).

On **physical examination,** there may be a variety of lesions that are discrete and often multifocal. Lesions may appear white, red, or pigmented and may be raised or flat. When the patient is symptomatic and there are no obvious lesions, **colposcopic-directed vulvar biopsy** may be performed. Extensive colposcopy of the entire vulvar region often reveals multiple suspicious lesions that can be biopsied to make a pathologic diagnosis (Fig. 27-1). VIN appears as distinct acetowhite lesions with or without punctations. Associated vascular abnormalities are more commonly associated with invasive disease.

Treatment

Treatment depends on the degree of the disease. Unlike CIN, VIN encompasses a mixed group of lesions with varying potential for **progression to invasive vulvar cancer**. Although spontaneous regression can be seen in women under 40 years, the risk of progression of untreated disease may be as high as **100% for women over the age of 40**. The options for treatment include wide local excision, laser vaporization, and superficial skinning vulvectomy with and without split-thickness skin grafting.

TABLE 27-1 Classification of Neoplastic Diseases of the Vulva and Vagina

	Vulvar Disease	Vaginal Disease
Premalignant	VIN	VAIN
Malignant	Squamous cell (85%)	Squamous cell (90%)
		Adenocarcinomas (6%)

VIN, vulvar intraepithelial neoplasia; VAIN, vaginal intraepithelial neoplasia.

If all of the biopsies taken reveal VIN without any evidence of invasion, then **wide local excision** can be used for distinct, unifocal disease. The goal is to have a **disease-free margin of at least 5 to 10 mm**. When multifocal disease is diagnosed, a simple vulvectomy or skinning vulvectomy may be used. **Split-thickness skin grafts** are often used to replace the excised lesions. More recently, **laser vaporization** has been used to eradicate multifocal lesions; this results in less scar tissue and decreased healing time, but it provides no pathologic specimen and should therefore only be used when previous biopsies show no invasive disease.

In younger patients, conservative treatment with topical **5-fluorouracil** (5-FU) and imiquimod (Aldara) has been attempted to preserve vulvar anatomy. Effectiveness varies from 40% to 75%. These therapies require thorough evaluation to rule out invasive disease prior to use.

Follow-Up

These therapies can be curative for VIN; however, studies have reported recurrence rates from 18% to 55%. Recurrence is more common with multifocal lesions, moderate and severe dysplasia, and in patients with positive margins. Patients should have follow-up colposcopy of the entire genital tract every 6 months for 2 years and then annually. There is not a recommended timeline for follow-up; however, close follow-up is recommended secondary to the high likelihood of recurrence.

PAGET DISEASE OF THE VULVA

Extramammary Paget disease (EMPD) is an uncommon apocrine gland neoplasia most often affecting the anogenital areas of both women and men. It typically presents between the ages of 50 and 80 years in Caucasian women. EMPD is commonly an intraepithelial disease that tends to recur locally with minimal propensity to invade. Only about 20% of patients with Paget disease will have **coexistent adenocarcinoma** underlying the outward changes. When this occurs, metastasis is common. When adenocarcinoma is not present, Paget disease can be treated locally without concern for metastases.

TABLE 27-2 Classification of Squamous Intraepithelial Lesions of the Vulva (ISSVD, 2004)

Older Terminology	Current Terminology
VIN 1	Reactive changes/HPV effect/ Condyloma
VIN 2	VIN, usual type[a]
VIN 3	VIN, usual type[a]
Differentiated VIN	VIN, differentiated type

[a]Encompasses VIN, warty type; VIN, basaloid type; and VIN, mixed type, warty, and basaloid.
VIN, vulvar intraepithelial neoplasia.

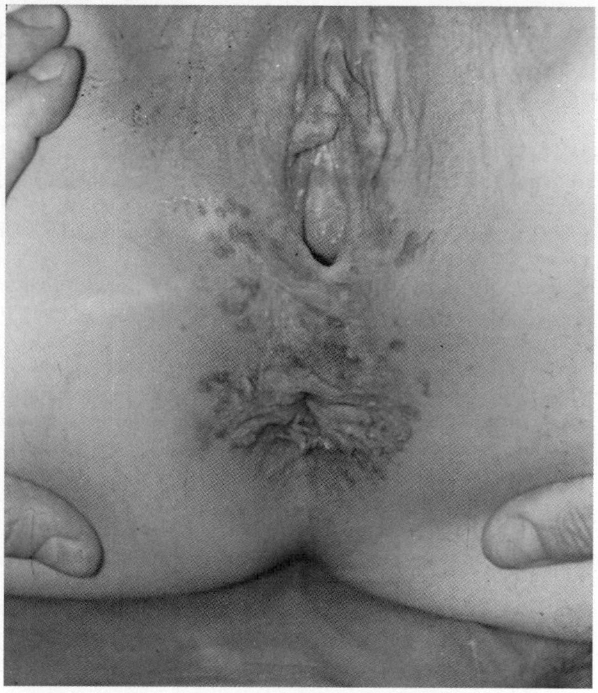

Figure 27-1 • Severe vulvar intraepithelial neoplasia (VIN III). (From Rock J, Jones H. *TeLinde's Operative Gynecology*, 10th ed. Philadelphia, PA: Lippincott Williams & Wilkins; 2008.)

Diagnosis

The lesions of Paget disease are consistent with **chronic inflammatory changes**—hyperemic, sharply demarcated, and thickened with areas of excoriation and induration. Commonly, there is a long standing **pruritus** that accompanies **velvety red lesions** of the skin that eventually become eczematous and scar into **white plaques**. These lesions may be focal on the labia, perineum, or perianal region or may encompass the entire region. The disease is most common in **patients over age 60 years**, but the symptoms of **vulvar pruritus and vulvodynia** can precede the diagnosis by years. Absolute diagnosis is made only with vulvar biopsy (Fig. 13-6).

Treatment

In the absence of invasion, EMPD is generally treated with **wide local excision** of the circumscribed lesion. Because microscopic Paget disease often extends beyond the obvious gross lesions, wide margins should be taken, and excised segments checked in pathology for clean margins. It is also important to rule out underlying adenocarcinoma during pathologic evaluation. Finally, even with clean margins, Paget disease has a **high recurrence rate** and may require multiple local excisions. Without nodal metastases, the disease is commonly cured with local excision; however, the disease is **almost invariably fatal if it spreads to lymph nodes**.

CANCER OF THE VULVA

Pathogenesis

Cancers of the vulva may arise from the skin, glandular tissue, subcutaneous tissue, or the mucosa of the lower vagina. The most common type of vulvar cancer is **squamous cell carcinoma** (SCC), which makes up 87% of the cases. The other types of vulvar cancers include malignant melanoma (6%), Bartholin's adenocarcinoma (4%), basal cell carcinoma (<2%), and soft tissue sarcomas (<1%). Although lesions can appear anywhere on the vulva, most are on the **labia majora**. These lesions range in appearance from cauliflower-like masses to hard indurated ulcers (Fig. 27-2). The spread of disease is primarily via the **lymphatics** to the superficial inguinal lymph nodes, with a smaller degree of spread via **direct extension** to vagina, urethra, and anus. In patients without metastases to the inguinal nodes, it is rare for the disease to spread to the intra-abdominal pelvic nodes.

Epidemiology

Vulvar cancer accounts for only **5% of gynecologic malignancies**, with over 3,800 new cases diagnosed and 800 deaths reported in the United States each year. Although the rate of noninvasive neoplasia of the vulva has increased dramatically over time, the rate of vulvar carcinoma has **remained relatively stable**. This is thought to be due to the disproportionate increase in VIN in younger women. These women are more likely to undergo early detection and treatment, resulting in cancer prevention.

Risk factors for vulvar cancer include menopausal status, cigarette smoking, VIN, CIN, HPV, immunosuppression, and history of cervical cancer. The average age of diagnosis is 65 years. Young women are more likely to have associated HPV infections and VIN.

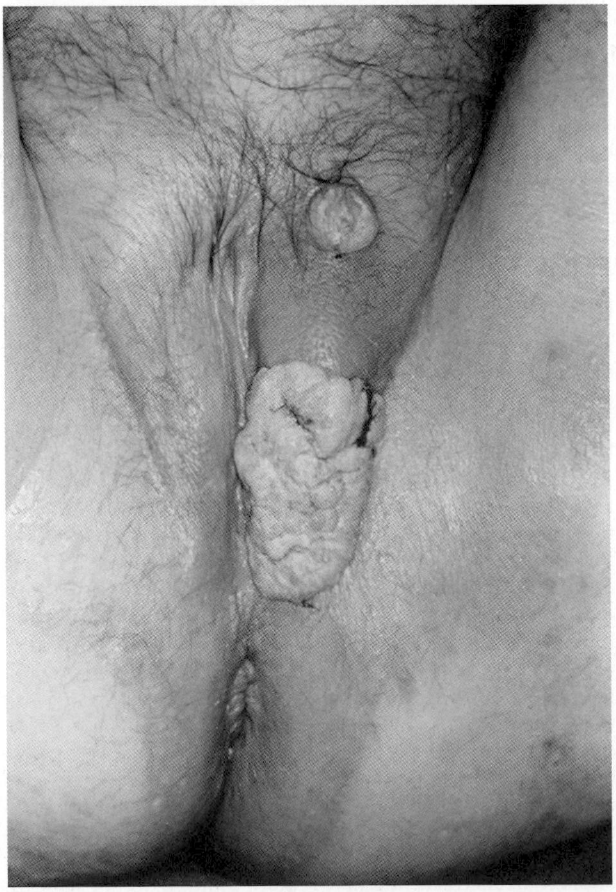

Figure 27-2 • Multifocal carcinoma of the vulva.
(From Rock J, Jones H. *TeLinde's Operative Gynecology*, 10th ed. Philadelphia, PA: Lippincott Williams & Wilkins; 2008.)

Diagnosis

Annual examination of the vulva by a healthcare provider is an important component in the diagnosis of vulvar cancer. Patients with vulvar cancer often present with long histories of **vulvar pruritus, pain, and bleeding**. Focal lesions tend to be merely inflamed and erythematous in early cancers and heaped up or ulcerated in later stages. They may also present with a **vulvar mass** that may be fleshy, nodular, or warty (Fig. 27-2).

The most common location is the labia majora. Ninety percent of lesions are **unifocal**. Final diagnosis is made by pathologic examination of a biopsy specimen, which should be taken even if the patient is asymptomatic. Twenty percent of patients will have a **secondary neoplasia** (usually cervical). The presence of bleeding, discharge, or a clear mass is strongly suggestive of invasive carcinoma.

Staging

Vulvar carcinoma is **surgically staged** using the International Federation of Gynecology and Obstetrics (FIGO) staging criteria based on tumor size, level of invasion, nodal involvement, and distant metastases (Table 27-3). Staging is the most important prognostic factor for vulvar cancer. The most common surgical approach is **radical local excision** with **inguino-femoral lymph node dissection**. Patients with superficial (<1 mm invasion) and unilateral disease can forego unilateral lymph node dissection. Patients with deeper disease (>1 mm invasion), bilateral disease, or disease which crosses the midline may require ipsilateral bilateral lymph node dissection depending on the location of the lesion.

Given its method of spread, **inguinal lymph node dissection** is required to definitely stage vulvar cancer. Staging may be approximated by a thorough examination for palpable lymph nodes, although 25% of those with positive nodes will have no palpable nodes on physical examination. The use of **sentinel node biopsy,**as a means of preventing some of the complications associated with complete inguinal node dissection, is under investigation. Metastasis to the intra-abdominal pelvic lymph nodes is very unlikely if the inguinal nodes are disease-free.

Treatment

Prior to definitive treatment, women with vulvar cancer should undergo a **complete pelvic examination** including palpation of the inguinal nodes, collection of cervical cytology, and colposcopy of the cervical vagina, vulva, and perianal areas.

For a primary occurrence of invasive squamous cell carcinoma of the vulva, **wide radical local excision** with **inguinal lymph node dissection** is the treatment of choice. Stage I disease rarely has positive contralateral lymph nodes, and thus **ipsilateral lymphadenectomy** is sufficient. Most stage II diseases can be treated with **modified radical vulvectomy** and separate inguinal incisions for resection of lymph nodes. Stage III and stage IV diseases may require **radical vulvectomy,**

TABLE 27-3 FIGO Staging of Vulvar Cancer

Carcinoma of the Vulva	
Ia	Tumor confined to the vulva or perineum, ≤2 cm in size with stromal invasion ≤1 mm, negative nodes
Ib	Tumor confined to the vulva or perineum, >2 cm in size or with stromal invasion >1 mm, negative nodes
II	Tumor of any size with adjacent spread (one-third lower urethra, one-third lower vagina, anus), negative nodes
IIIa	Tumor of any size with positive inguinofemoral lymph nodes
	(i) One lymph node metastasis ≥5 mm
	(ii) One to two lymph node metastasis(es) of <5 mm
IIIb	(i) Two or more lymph nodes metastases ≥5 mm
	(ii) Three or more lymph nodes metastases <5 mm
IIIc	Positive node(s) with extracapsular spread
IVa	(i) Tumor invades other regional structures (two-third upper urethra, two-third upper vagina), bladder mucosa, rectal mucosa, or fixed to pelvic bone
	(ii) Fixed or ulcerated inguinofemoral lymph nodes
IVb	Any distant metastasis including pelvic lymph nodes

FIGO, International Federation of Gynecology and Obstetrics.

bilateral inguino-femoral lymph node dissection (Fig. 27-3), and **pelvic exenteration**. Preoperative radiation therapy and chemoradiation have been used to avoid the morbidity and mortality associated with pelvic exenteration.

If lymphadenectomy reveals metastatic disease, **pelvic radiation** is used as adjunct therapy. In patients for whom extensive surgery is contraindicated, the procedure may be confined to vulvectomy. In these patients, preoperative radiation therapy with and without chemotherapy has been used to reduce tumor burden. For recurrence, secondary excision or chemoradiation therapy can be used. Recurrences are usually near the primary site.

Melanoma of the vulva occurs predominantly in postmenopausal Caucasians. It can be treated similarly to SCC, except that **lymphadenectomy is rarely performed**. Depth of invasion is the key prognostic factor. **Once the melanoma has metastasized, the mortality rate is near 100%**. Basal cell carcinoma can be treated with wide local excision. These lesions rarely metastasize to the lymph nodes; thus, lymphadenectomy is not required.

Prognosis

The 5-year survival rate for all patients after surgical treatment of invasive SCC is approximately 75%. The **most important prognostic factor is the number of positive inguinal lymph nodes**. In patients with metastases to local lymph nodes, 5-year survival rates are 90% to 95% for one positive lymph node, 50% to 80% for two positive lymph nodes, and less than 15% for three or more positive lymph nodes.

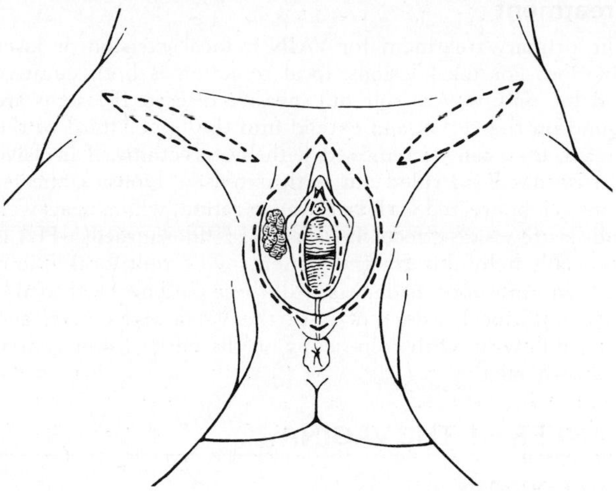

Figure 27-3 • Incision for radical vulvectomy with separate incisions for bilateral inguinofemoral lymph node dissection.
(From Rock J, Jones H. *TeLinde's Operative Gynecology*, 10th ed. Philadelphia, PA: Lippincott Williams & Wilkins; 2008.)

PREINVASIVE DISEASE OF THE VAGINA

Pathogenesis

Vaginal intraepithelial neoplasia (VAIN) is a **premalignant lesion** similar to that of the vulva and cervix. However, VAIN is much less common than either VIN or CIN. By definition, the squamous cell atypia seen in VAIN is limited to the epithelium. Lesions are designated as VAIN I, II, or III based upon the amount of epithelium with cellular changes. VAIN I and II encompass the lower one-third and two-thirds of the epithelium, respectively. **VAIN III** involves greater than two-thirds of the epithelium as well as full thickness abnormalities (**carcinoma in situ**). VAIN occurs most commonly as **multifocal lesions** in the **vaginal apex**. VAIN is associated with CIN, cervical cancer, condyloma, and history of **infection with HPV**.

Epidemiology

The peak incidence occurs in patients in their mid- to late 40s. At least 50% to 90% of patients with VAIN will have **coexistent or prior neoplasia,** or cancer of the vulva or cervix.

Diagnosis

Patients with VAIN are **almost always asymptomatic**; however, some patients can present with vaginal discharge or postcoital spotting. Many patients are diagnosed due to an abnormality on **Pap smear**. In particular, suspicion of vaginal neoplasia should be raised in patients with **persistently abnormal Pap smears but no cervical neoplasia** detected on colposcopy or cervical biopsy. Patients who have undergone hysterectomy for a history of high grade CIN should continue to have annual Pap smears to screen for VAIN until three consecutive negative Pap tests have been obtained.

VAIN can be diagnosed with a thorough colposcopy of the cervix (if present) and upper vagina using both acetic acid and Lugol's solution. The identified lesions **should then be biopsied** to give a final pathologic diagnosis and rule out invasive disease.

Treatment

The primary treatment for VAIN is **local excision or laser ablation**. For focal lesions, local resection is both curative and the only way to rule out invasive disease. If lesions are found on the cervix and extend into the upper third of the vagina, they can be removed with hysterectomy. If invasive disease has been ruled out with extensive biopsies, the lesions can be treated with **laser vaporization,** which heals well and has few side effects. Intravaginal **5-fluorouracil**(5-FU) is especially helpful in treating patients with multifocal lesions and immunosuppression. Many of these patients tend to also have multifocal lesions of both the vulva and cervix, and close follow-up with colposcopy on the entire lower genital tract is needed.

CANCER OF THE VAGINA

Pathogenesis

Vaginal cancer is extremely rare and comprises only 1% to 2% of malignant neoplasms of the female genital tract. The most common histologic type of vaginal cancer is squamous cell carcinoma (SCC) (85%); adenocarcinoma (6%), sarcomas, and melanomas are found in a much smaller percentage of patients. In the 1970s, **clear cell adenocarcinoma** was found to be associated with in utero exposure of **diethylstilbestrol** (DES).

SCC may appear ulcerated, nodular, or exophytic and usually involves the **posterior wall and upper one-third** of the vagina. Spread may occur via **lymphatic** drainage to the inguinal nodes and deep pelvic nodes or via **direct extension** to the bladder or rectum. Late in the disease process, **hematogenous spread** to liver, lungs, and bone is possible.

Epidemiology

Primary vaginal cancers make up only **1% to 4% of all gynecologic cancers**. In fact, secondary carcinoma of the vagina is more common than primary disease. The mean age for diagnoses of squamous cell cancer of the vagina is 60 years. The cause of SCC of the vagina is **unknown**. Similar to vulvar and cervical cancers, vaginal cancers can be associated with HPV infection. However, because the vaginal mucosa is not undergoing constant metaplasia like cervical epithelium, the vagina is much less susceptible to the oncogenic effects of the virus.

Women who were exposed in utero to DES have a propensity to develop **clear cell adenocarcinoma** of the vagina. Even then, the incidence in DES-exposed women is only 0.1%. These cancers are typically found in DES exposed women under age 20 years. They can present as polypoid masses palpated on the anterior aspect of the vagina.

Diagnosis

Many patients (20%) with vaginal cancer are asymptomatic. The most common presenting symptoms are **pruritis, postmenopausal vaginal bleeding, postcoital spotting, and/or watery, blood-tinged discharge**. With more advanced disease, urinary (dysuria, hematuria, frequency) and gastrointestinal (constipation, melena) symptoms may be reported as well. As in VAIN, vaginal cancer may be diagnosed during Pap smear screening and follow-up colposcopy and biopsy. The differential diagnosis for vaginal cancer includes Gartner duct cyst, endometrial implants, and cancer of the urethra, bladder, or rectum.

Staging and Treatment

Invasive SCC of the vagina is often complicated by involvement with local structures such as the rectum or bladder (Table 27-4). Given this, patients diagnosed with vaginal cancer should undergo preoperative chest imaging, cystoscopy, proctosigmoidoscopy, and intravenous pyelogram (IVP) to assess for disease spread. At the time of presentation, 26% of vaginal cancer patients have stage I disease, 37% have stage II, 24% have stage III, and 13% have stage IV disease.

Small stage I lesions (<2 cm) in the upper third of the vagina are amenable to **surgical resection** (radical hysterectomy, upper vaginectomy, and bilateral pelvic lymph node dissection). Lesions greater than 2 cm, those in the lower two-thirds of the vagina, and stage III and IV lesions are treated with external and internal **radiation therapy** alone (see Table 27-4). Comprehensive treatment should also include addressing the **psychosexual ramifications** of treatment.

Adenocarcinoma of the vagina is treated similarly to SCC. However, a clear-cut therapy for clear cell carcinoma has not been established. These lesions are often treated similarly with resection of earlier staged lesions, and radiation for stage III and IV lesions and those involving the lower vagina.

Prognosis

The 5-year survival rate for SCC of the vagina is highly dependent on the clinical stage and tumor size at the time of diagnosis. The overall survival rate for primary vaginal cancer has improved over time and is now about 45% to 55%.

TABLE 27-4 FIGO Staging for Carcinoma of the Vagina

Stage	Clinical/Pathologic Findings
Stage I	The carcinoma is limited to the vaginal wall
Stage II	The carcinoma has involved the subvaginal tissue but has not extended to the pelvic wall
Stage III	The carcinoma has extended to the pelvic wall
Stage IV	The carcinoma has extended beyond the true pelvis or has clinically involved the mucosa of the bladder or rectum; bullous edema as such does not permit a case to be allotted to stage IV
Stage IVa	Spread of the growth to adjacent organs and/or direct extension beyond the true pelvis
Stage IVb	Spread to distant organs

KEY POINTS

- VIN is a premalignant disease confined to the vulvar epithelium. Histologic grades include VIN I, II, and III.
- VIN is often asymptomatic but can present with vulvar pruritus and vulvar irritation that are unresponsive to treatment with antifungals or steroids.
- Risk factors for VIN include HPV 16 and 18, cigarette smoking, immunodeficiency, and immunosuppression.
- VIN lesions are quite varied and vulvar biopsy is required for diagnosis and to rule out invasive disease.
- Treatments include wide local excision, simple or skinning vulvectomy, or laser vaporization of tissue with close colposcopic follow-up.
- Extra Mammary Paget disease (EMPD) is another preinvasive intraepithelial neoplasia of the vulva; it is rare but is associated with adenocarcinoma 20% of the time.
- EMPD lesions are often velvety red in appearance and can eventually scar into white plaques. Diagnosis is made only by biopsy.
- Treatment for EMPD is with wide local excision; there is a high recurrence rate and close follow-up is important.
- Vulvar carcinoma is surgically staged; it makes up <5% of all gynecologic cancers. Risk factors include HPV, HIV, and history of cervical cancer.
- Patients with vulvar cancer often present with vulvar itching, pain, and bleeding, and the diagnosis is made by vulvar biopsy.
- The most common histologic type of vulvar cancer is SCC (90%).
- Most treatments include radical local excision (stage I) or radical vulvectomy (stages II, III, IV), and regional lymphadenectomy; pelvic exenteration or preoperative chemoradiation may also be used for advanced disease.
- Five-year survival rates for vulvar cancer are excellent for two or fewer positive nodes, but drops to 15% for three or more positive nodes.
- VAIN lesions are often asymptomatic but may present with vaginal discharge or postcoital spotting. They can also be picked up on cervical cytology.
- VAIN is much less common than CIN or VIN. Most lesions are multifocal and located in the vaginal apex. Diagnosis is made by colposcopically directed biopsy.
- At least 50% to 90% of patients with VAIN have a coexistent intraepithelial lesion or invasive lesion of the cervix or vulva.
- Local excision, laser vaporization, and topical 5-FU are common therapies for VAIN.
- Patients require close follow-up with colposcopy to rule out recurrence.
- Vaginal cancer is often asymptomatic, but can present with vaginal pruritis, discharge, or bleeding.
- Diagnosis is made by colposcopic-assisted vaginal biopsy. Prior to treatment, patients should undergo chest imaging, cystoscopy, proctosigmoidoscopy, and IVP to assess for the extent disease.
- Small stage I malignancies of the upper vagina can be treated with surgical excision; all other lesions are treated with internal and external radiation therapy for an overall 5-year survival rate between 45% and 55%.

C Clinical Vignettes

Vignette 1

A 38-year-old obese white female presents to your office with complaints of "something is not right down there. It feels like worms crawling all over." While obtaining her health history you learn that she underwent a total vaginal hysterectomy 5 years ago for a history of high grade cervical dysplasia and heavy menses. She says she was told that she no longer needed gynecologic care. She denies any post-menopausal bleeding but complains of vulvar itching and discomfort. She has smoked one pack of cigarettes per day for the past 15 years. On pelvic examination, you note a rash under her pannus and bilaterally in her groin folds, consistent with *Candida*. Her vulva is notable for erythema, hyperpigmentation of the labia, and small fissures. The patient declines speculum examination stating that it would be too uncomfortable.

1. What test(s) are you likely to perform at this visit?
   a. KOH wet prep of the vulva
   b. Colposcopy of the vulva with acetic acid
   c. Biopsy of the hyperpigmented lesion
   d. Referral to gynecologic oncologist
   e. Both a and c
2. A microscopic evaluation reveals yeast buds and hyphae. It is negative for WBCs. You discuss with the patient that you would like to treat her Candida and would like her to return to see you in 1 week to discuss the biopsy result. Biopsy returns as VIN III. Your recommendation for treatment of her VIN III includes:
   a. Radical vulvectomy
   b. High-dose steroid ointment
   c. Observation
   d. Wide local excision
   e. chemordilation
3. The patient questions how she got this since she has not been sexually active in over 7 years. You explain that she has many risk factors for the development and persistence of VIN. Which of the following is **not** a risk factor?
   a. Smoking
   b. History of CIN
   c. Obesity
   d. HPV infection
   e. Immunosuppression

Vignette 2

Your next patient is a 28-year-old African–American female with a history significant for a renal transplant 3 years ago. She presents to the clinic for a colposcopy for further evaluation of an HGSIL Pap smear. On colposcopic examination there were no lesions seen or identified on her cervix. She returns 6 months later for another repeat Pap test, which remains HGSIL. On colposcopic examination her results are satisfactory, and she continues to have no colposcopic changes on her cervix.

1. There are no cervical lesions to biopsy. Your next recommendation is:
   a. Perform endocervical curettage
   b. Colposcopic examination of the entire vagina
   c. Molecular testing for HPV types
   d. All of the above
   e. Both a and b
2. You have performed an ECC and examination of the vagina. In the posterior vaginal fornix you note a single acetowhite lesion with punctation. Your next recommendation is to:
   a. Biopsy
   b. 5-FU
   c. LEEP conization of the cervix
   d. Wide local excision
   e. Laser vaporization
3. The pathology report returns as VAIN III, now what is your recommendation?
   a. Imiquimod
   b. 5-FU
   c. Local excision
   d. Intravaginal clindamycin
   e. Intralesional steroid injection

Vignette 3

A 75-year-old female living in a nursing home is referred to you for a velvety red vulvar lesion with associated white plaques. The lesion has been slowly expanding in size and causing burning and itching over the past 5 years. She has been treated with various topical agents without relief, although she does get some relief from the itching and pain from the use of a steroid cream.

1. Which conditions are in your differential diagnosis?
   a. Contact dermatitis
   b. Eczema
   c. Invasive vulvar cancer
   d. Paget's disease
   e. All of the above

2. Her biopsy returns and shows Paget's disease of the vulva. You recommend further evaluation because she is at increased risk for:
   a. Melanoma
   b. SCC of the vulva
   c. Crohn's disease
   d. Adenocarcinoma
   e. Ulcerative colitis

3. Treatment recommendations would include:
   a. Laser vaporization
   b. Wide local excision
   c. Radical vulvectomy
   d. Pelvic exenteration
   e Chemoradiation

Vignette 4

A 54-year-old female presents to the clinic with a complaint of vulvar pain for 2 years. On examination you note a 1.5-cm lesion on her vulva. She does not have palpable inguinal adenopathy and the remainder of her examination is unremarkable.

1. What is her stage?
   a. Stage I
   b. Stage II
   c. Inadequate information for staging
   d. Stage III
   e Stage IV

2. Patient goes to the OR for a wide radical local excision with lymph node dissection, with final pathology showing a 1.5-cm lesion with depth of invasion of 1.2 mm. There are no nodal metastases. She is staged as
   a. Stage Ia
   b. Stage Ib
   c. Stage IIIc
   d. Stage 0
   e Stage IV

3. What is the most important prognostic factor?
   a. Size of lesion
   b. Depth of invasion
   c. Number of positive lymph nodes
   d. High risk HPV status
   e. Smoking history

A Answers

Vignette 1 Question 1

Answer E: A wet prep obtained from the vulva and groin will confirm the diagnosis of cutaneous Candida. It is also important to inspect the vulva and to biopsy the lesions for definitive diagnosis.

Colposcopy of the vulva would not be inappropriate; however, she has already commented to her provider that she has significant discomfort and application of acetic acid would likely cause significant burning and pain. If indicated, the colposcopy may be better done at a follow-up visit once the biopsy results are available.

A referral to a gynecologic oncologist at this time would be inappropriate unless you are suspecting a cancer or have a biopsy-proven diagnosis.

Vignette 1 Question 2

Answer D: A radical vulvectomy is not an appropriate treatment for preinvasive disease of the vulva. A high-dose steroid ointment would not treat the VIN III or yeast. Observation of VIN III is not recommended. While spontaneous regression of VIN can be seen in women under 40 years, the risk of progression of untreated disease may be as high as 100% in women over 40 years. Surgical therapy with wide local incision is the recommended treatment for VIN III.

Vignette 1 Question 3

Answer C: Although obesity has multiple comorbidities associated with it, it is not in itself considered to be a risk factor for VIN.

The patient has been a heavy smoker for many years. Smoking is a known risk factor for the development and persistence of VIN. She has a documented history of CIN. Both cervical and vulvar neoplastic diseases are correlated with HPV infection. Nearly 90% of all VIN lesions are HPV positive. Immunosuppression is also a major risk factor for VIN.

Vignette 2 Question 1

Answer E: Her Pap test continues to remain with a high grade abnormality and there are no abnormalities on her cervix. An endocervical curettage (ECC) would be a helpful diagnostic tool to ensure that there are no abnormalities in the canal that you are unable to visualize. A Pap test does often pick up abnormalities in the vagina as well as cervix. Molecular testing for HPV would not be beneficial or cost effective because the result would not change our management of the current results.

Vignette 2 Question 2

Answer A: Biopsy is the appropriate choice at this time to obtain a histologic diagnosis. 5-FU is not a good choice because we do not have a diagnosis yet. Wide local excision would give a histologic diagnosis; however, there is more morbidity associated with it and the finding may not require such an extensive surgery. Laser vaporization would not be a good choice again because there is no diagnosis. Moreover, based on laser criteria there needs to be reasonable certainty that there is no microinvasive or invasive cancer.

Vignette 2 Question 3

Answer C: The primary treatment for VAIN is local excision or laser ablation. For focal lesions, local excision can be both curative and the only way to rule out invasive disease. Imiquimod and intravaginal clindamycin treatments are currently not approved for VAIN III. 5-FU is helpful in treating patients that have multifocal disease or are immunosuppressed.

Vignette 3 Question 1

Answer E: Because of its eczematoid appearance, it is not unusual for Paget's disease to be misdiagnosed as eczema or contact dermatitis.

Vignette 3 Question 2

Answer D: Studies have shown that around 20% of patients with Paget's disease have a coexistent adenocarcinoma underlying the outward changes.

Vignette 3 Question 3

Answer B: Current recommended first-line therapy is a wide local excision. Laser vaporization will not provide a tissue sample to rule out other pathologies. A radical vulvectomy and pelvic exenteration are not indicated for the treatment of preinvasive disease.

Vignette 4 Question 1

Answer C: Vulvar cancer is surgically staged and the information provided is inadequate to properly stage her cancer.

Vignette 4 Question 2

Answer B: Tumor confined to the vulva or perineum, greater than 2 cm in size or with stromal invasion greater than 1 mm, negative nodes. Stage Ia = Tumor confined to the vulva or perineum, less than or equal to 2 cm in size with stromal invasion less than or equal to 1 mm, negative nodes. Stage IIIc = Positive node(s) with extracapsular spread. With the new updated FIGO staging guidelines from 2009, there is no longer a stage 0, which was previously carcinoma in situ.

Vignette 4 Question 3

Answer C: Vulvar carcinoma is **surgically staged** using the FIGO staging criteria based on tumor size, depth of invasion, nodal involvement, and distant metastases (Table 27-2). Staging is the most important prognostic factor for vulvar cancer.

Chapter 28 Cervical Neoplasia and Cervical Cancer

Prior to the 20th century, cervical cancer was the most common cancer in women and the most common cause of cancer death in women in the United States. Since the advent of the **Papanicolaou (Pap) smear**, which gained widespread acceptance in the 1950s and 1960s, it has been easier to detect and treat premalignant changes before they develop into cancer (Fig. 28-1). As a result of public health initiatives involving population-based screening, detection, and treatment, cervical cancer has dropped to the 11th leading cause of death from cancer in women in the United States, accounting for about 4,000 deaths per year.

Further advances in detection and screening have resulted from identification of the **human papillomavirus (HPV) as the causal agent** in the vast majority of cervical intraepithelial neoplasias (CIN) and cervical cancers. By allowing us to pick up premalignant changes of the cervix, the combination of **Pap smear screening** and **HPV testing** reduces a woman's risk of dying of cervical cancer by 90%. Fortunately, vaccines have been developed that protect against HPV infection and reduce the risk of cervical cancer by 70%.

Because developing countries often lack available screening, vaccination, and treatment modalities, cervical cancer continues to be the second most common cancer in women worldwide and is the **number one cancer killer of women in the developing world**.

CERVICAL INTRAEPITHELIAL NEOPLASIA

PATHOGENESIS

CIN (formerly cervical dysplasia) refers to **premalignant changes in the cervical epithelium** that have the potential to progress to cervical cancer. The histologic features most commonly associated with cervical dysplasia include cellular immaturity, cellular disorganization, nuclear abnormalities, and increased mitotic activity. The severity of CIN is determined by the **portion of epithelium showing disordered growth and development**. The changes start at the basal layer of the epithelium and can expand to encompass the entire epithelium (Fig. 28-2).

The nomenclature for cervical neoplasia divides the epithelial thickness into thirds to express the degree of abnormality (Table 28-1). In CIN I (formerly mild dysplasia), the changes are restricted to the lower one-third of the epithelium. In CIN II (formerly moderate dysplasia), two-thirds of the epithelium is involved. And, in CIN III (formerly severe dysplasia), more than two-thirds of the epithelium shows abnormal changes. The atypical cells in CIN III can expand the full thickness of the epithelium (formally CIS or carcinoma in situ).

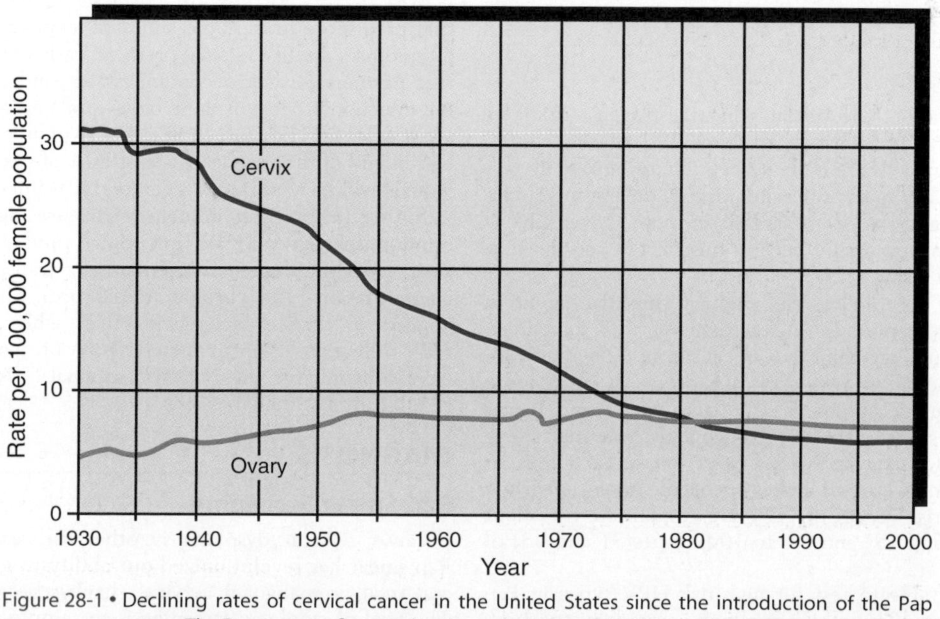

Figure 28-1 • Declining rates of cervical cancer in the United States since the introduction of the Pap smear. The Pap test was first used in the early 1930s and 1940s and became more commonly used in the 1950s.

(From Beckmann CRB, Ling FW, Laube DW, et al. *Obstetrics and Gynecology*, 4th ed. Baltimore, MD: Lippincott Williams & Wilkins; 2002.)

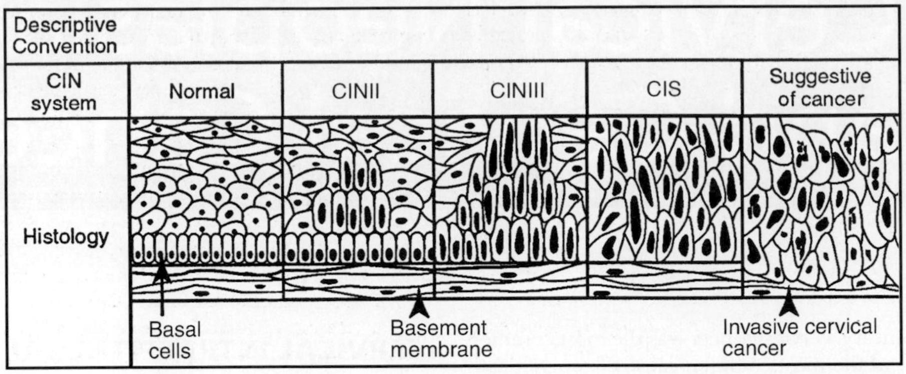

Figure 28-2 • Histologic classification of cervical intraepithelial neoplasia (CIN). The degree of CIN is determined by the portion of epithelium showing disordered growth and development. Changes are restricted to the lower one-third of the epithelium in CIN I. The lower two-thirds of the epithelium is involved in CIN II, and more than two-thirds of the epithelium shows abnormal changes in CIN III. If the entire epithelium is abnormal, this represents CIS, but is still within the CIN III category. In invasive cervical cancer, the abnormalities invade through the basement membrane into the cervical stroma.
(From Beckmann CRB, Ling FW, Laube DW, et al. *Obstetrics and Gynecology*, 4th ed. Baltimore, MD: Lippincott Williams & Wilkins; 2002.)

TABLE 28-1 Classification of Cervical Intraepithelial Neoplasia (CIN)
CIN I: Cellular dysplasia confined to the basal third of the epithelium (formerly mild dysplasia)
CIN I: Cellular dysplasia confined to the basal third of the epithelium (formerly mild dysplasia)
CIN III: Cellular dysplasia encompassing more than two-thirds of the epithelial thickness (formerly severe dysplasia), including full-thickness lesions (formerly carcinoma in situ or CIS)

During menarche, the production of estrogen stimulates metaplasia in the transformation zone (TZ) of the cervix. These metaplastic cells are more susceptible to oncogenic factors; therefore, CIN **most commonly occurs during menarche and after pregnancy** when metaplasia is most active. CIN is thought to begin as a single focus in the TZ but can develop into a **multifocal lesion**.

HPV is now accepted as the **primary causative agent in CIN and cervical cancer**. DNA fragments of HPV have been found incorporated into the DNA of cells from 80% of all CIN lesions and 90% of all invasive cervical cancers. There are more than 100 different serotypes of HPV. Serotypes 6 and 11 are among the types with the **lowest oncogenic potential**. They are responsible for causing 90% of **condylomas**. Serotypes 16 and 18 and 31 and 41 are of higher oncogenic potential. These so-called "high risk" types of HPV are responsible for about 70% (types 16 and 18) and 5% to 10% (types 31 and 45) of cervical cancers.

We are now able to test for high-risk HPV types in Pap smear specimens. This testing allows providers to more accurately predict which precancerous lesions have the potential to progress to cancer if left untreated and which will most likely spontaneously regress. Moreover, HPV vaccines are now available (e.g., Gardasil and Cervarix) that prevent HPV infections and reduce the risk of cervical cancer by 70%. Gardasil immunizes against types 6, 11, 16, and 18. Cervarix immunizes against types 16, 18, 31, and 45. Both are given as three injections over 6 months to males and females age 9-26.

EPIDEMIOLOGY

CIN is most commonly diagnosed in **women in their 20s**; CIS is diagnosed most commonly in women of age 25 to 35 years; and invasive cancer is typically diagnosed after the age of 40.

Risk factors for cervical dysplasia include characteristics that predispose to multiple and early **exposure to HPV** (early intercourse, multiple sexual partners, early childbearing, "high-risk" partners, low socioeconomic status, and sexually transmitted infections). Most of these behavioral and sexual risk factors are **proxies for HPV** infection rather than independent risk factors in and of themselves. At least **80% of sexually active individuals** will have acquired a genital HPV infection by age 50.

Other factors that influence CIN are **cigarette smoking, immunodeficiency** (HIV infection), **and immunosuppression** (systemic lupus erythematosus, transplant recipients, chemotherapy, and chronic steroid use). Cigarette smoking appears to have a synergistic effect when combined with HPV infection. Approximately 10% of women with CIN have concomitant vulvar (VIN), vaginal (VAIN), or perianal (PAIN) intraepithelial lesions.

DIAGNOSIS

Pap Smear Screening

Because cervical dysplasia is otherwise **asymptomatic**, the Pap smear has revolutionized our ability to identify, monitor, and treat premalignant cervical changes before cancer arises. The goal of cytologic screening is to sample the TZ, the area where transformation from squamous epithelium to columnar endocervical epithelium takes place and where dysplasia and cancer arise.

The Pap smear involves scraping endocervical and ectocervical cells from the external os of the cervix with a spatula to sample cells from the **TZ** (Fig. 28-3A). Because the squamocolumnar junction (SCJ) may be in the endocervical canal, it is important to also sample the **endocervical canal** with a cytobrush. The sample is then placed directly on a glass slide (conventional Pap smear) or into a liquid-based medium that is then used to make a slide. The prepared slides are then examined by a cytopathologist with or without aid of an automated cytology (Fig. 28-3B).

Liquid-based Pap tests, such as ThinPrep and SurePath, have proven to be more sensitive than conventional glass slide Pap smears because the cells do not clump on top of each other in the liquid-based medium and there is **less debris** on the resulting slide. Additionally, fewer cells are required to make an adequate liquid-based specimen than with a conventional glass slide Pap smear. As a result, with liquid-based cytology tests, more **intraepithelial lesions are identified,** and fewer Pap smears are considered nondiagnostic secondary to "insufficient material."

In 2012, the American Cancer Society (ACS) guidelines for cervical dysplasia and cancer were updated after a systemic review of the evidence and contributions from the American Society of Colposcopy (ASCCP), the American Society for Clinical Pathology, among other major professional organizations. The findings are supported by the American College of Obstetrics and Gynecology (ACOG). The new guidelines recommend that all women should begin cervical cancer screening at age 21 regardless of risk factors, including age of onset of sexual activity. Women aged 21 to 29 should have Pap testing every 3 years. The preferred option for women aged 30 and above is to screen with both a Pap test and an HPV test, and if both are negative, to re-screen no sooner than every 5 years. Co testing with a Pap and an HPV test is 95% to 100% sensitive for CIN III. If HPV testing is unavailable, screening with pap smear alone every 3 years is acceptable for women 30 and over.

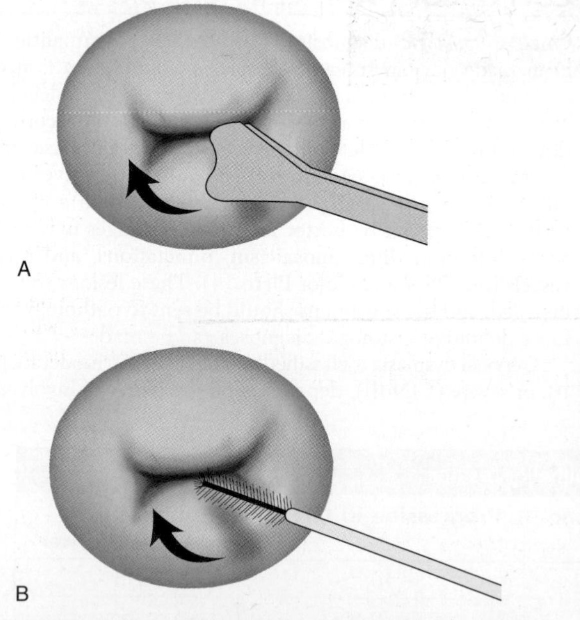

Figure 28-3 • Performing a Pap. **(A)** Spatula. **(B)** Endocervical brush. (From Bickley LS, Szilagyi P. *Bates' Guide to Physical Examination and History Taking*, 8th ed. Philadelphia, PA: Lippincott Williams & Wilkins; 2003.)

It is reasonable for **women over age 65 to 70 to stop cervical cancer screening** if they have had three or more normal Pap tests in a row have not had CIN 2/3 or higher in the past 20 years, or if a woman has had a **total hysterectomy** (removal of both the uterine corpus and cervix) for benign indications (such as bleeding or fibroids) and she does not have a history of CIN 2/3 or higher, she may stop pap screening at the time of her hysterectomy. Women with a **history of CIN II or III** who undergo hysterectomy may safely discontinue Pap smear screening after three consecutive negative screening tests (either the three most recent Pap smears prior to the hysterectomy or three consecutive screening examinations subsequent to the hysterectomy).

Importantly, women who have undergone a **supracervical hysterectomy** and have an intact cervix still need to continue routine Pap smear screening appropriate for their age. Most organizations recommend **continued cytologic screening after hysterectomy** for women with a history of invasive cervical cancer and other GYN malignancies. Women with risk factors such as in utero diethylstilbestrol (DES) exposure, HIV infection, or **immunosuppression** due to organ transplant, chemotherapy, or chronic steroid use should also continue annual vaginal screening.

Abnormal Pap Smear Management

Pap smear reports may show findings consistent with normal cellular material, inflammatory changes, infection, dysplasia, or cancer. Nearly 3.5 million American women have abnormal Pap smear findings each year; this represents approximately 5% to 7% of Pap smears performed. Table 28-2 shows the major **classes of epithelial abnormalities** as they are reported using the 2001 Bethesda classification system.

Cytological abnormalities occur because actively replicating **HPV produces characteristic cellular changes**, such as nuclear enlargement, multinucleation, hyperchromasia, and perinuclear cytoplasmic clearing (halos), which are detected during cytopathologic evaluation. These cytological features are used to categorize the abnormal Pap smear. Resolution of active HPV infection is associated with regression of these abnormalities.

The cellular changes ascribed to the atypical squamous cells (ASC) category may represent benign inflammatory response to infection or trauma but may also herald a preinvasive neoplastic lesion. In fact, it is estimated that **10% to 15% of ASC Pap smears harbor severe dysplasia** histology that should be treated. To better differentiate Pap smears with more benign appearing features from those which are more concerning, for dysplasia the ASC category has been divided into two groups: **ASC-US** (atypical squamous cells of unknown significance) and **ASC-H** (atypical squamous cells—cannot rule out high-grade lesion). Patients in the ASC-H category should be evaluated

TABLE 28-2 Major Classes of Epithelial Cell Abnormalities Found on Pap Smears

ASC-US: Atypical squamous cells of undetermined significance
ASC-H: Atypical squamous cells cannot exclude high-grade squamous intraepithelial lesion
LSIL: Low-grade squamous intraepithelial lesion
HSIL: High-grade squamous intraepithelial lesion
SCC: Squamous cell carcinoma
AGC: Atypical glandular cells

with colposcopy. **Patients with ASC-US should undergo HPV testing to determine whether colposcopy is indicated or not.**

Patients who receive an ASC-H, low-grade squamous intraepithelial lesion (LSIL), or high-grade squamous intraepithelial lesion (HSIL) Pap smear result should **proceed directly to colposcopy** (Table 28-3). Because of the potential for both cervical and endometrial **adenocarcinoma**, patients with a Pap smear reading of **atypical glandular cells** (AGC) should undergo **colposcopy**, high-risk HPV testing, and endocervical sampling. Moreover, when AGCs are identified, patients aged 35 and older and those younger than 35 with risk factors for endometrial hyperplasia or endometrial cancer should also have an **endometrial biopsy** (Table 28-3).

TABLE 28-3 Management of Abnormal Pap Smear Results in Adult Women[a]

NILM pap, High-risk HPV positive	Repeat both pap and HPV in 1 year OR screen for HPV 16 and 18. If either is positive then immediate colposcopy
ASC-US, High-risk HPV negative	Continue routine pap smear screening
ASC-US, High-risk HPV positive	Colposcopy and cervical biopsies if indicated
ASC-H	Colposcopy and cervical biopsies if indicated
LSIL	Colposcopy and cervical biopsies if indicated
HSIL	Colposcopy and cervical biopsies if indicated
SCC	Colposcopy , HPV screen, and cervical biopsies, potential cold-knife conization (CKC)
AGC	Colposcopy and cervical biopsies, endometrial biopsy*

*In women aged 35 or older and in women with risk factors for endometrial hyperplasia and endometrial cancer.

HPV Testing

With the advent of **HPV DNA testing**, it is now recommended that women with an ASC-US result be tested immediately for the presence of high-risk HPV subtypes. This process is known as **reflex HPV testing**. "Reflex" testing can be achieved using either the residual liquid from the liquid-based Pap test or a separate sample collected at the time of the initial Pap for HPV testing. The HPV results are added to the initial Pap smear interpretation. This eliminates the need for the patient to return for repeat testing, and it allows the clinician to predict a patient's risk for a high-grade lesion with more accuracy and to better direct the plan of care.

If the woman with an ASC-US Pap test is **positive for a high-risk HPV type, she should be evaluated with colposcopy** (Table 28-3), where directed biopsies can be performed if indicated. However, if the patient with an ASC-US Pap **test is negative for a high-risk HPV type**, she can continue with routine screening appropriate for her age (pap every 3 years from age 21-29 and pap plus HPV every 5 years for ≥ 30 year old). For women aged 30 or older who are screened with a pap and a high risk HPV, a normal pap and positive high-risk HPV screen should be followed by repeating both the pap and HPV screen in 12 months. If either result is subsequently abnormal, colposcopy should be performed. Conversely, in facilities where specific HPV typing is available, a patient ≥ 30 with a normal pap and positive screen for high-risk HPV can be sub-typed for HPV 16 and 18. If positive for either, colposcopy should be performed. If negative for both, the pap had HPV screens should be repeated in one year and managed with colposcopy if either is abnormal.

Not all providers are using HPV testing in their management of ASC-US Pap smears; some providers repeat the cytology in 6 months and then refer to colposcopy if the repeat Pap smear results are ASC or higher. Likewise, **no high-risk HPV testing is recommended for ASC-H, LSIL, and HSIL**, because nearly all of these lesions will be positive for high-risk HPV types.

Fortunately, many epithelial abnormalities found on Pap smears will **regress to normal** over 6 months to 2 years. Some of the abnormalities will **persist at their current level,** and the remainder will **progress to more serious lesions** or cervical cancer (Table 28-4). ASC and LSIL lesions usually represent a transient infection with HPV, so the majority will regress spontaneously over time. However, HSIL lesions are more likely to be associated with persistent infection and progression to cancer. Therefore, patients who receive an ASC-H, LSIL, or HSIL Pap smear result should **proceed directly to colposcopy** (Table 28-3).

COLPOSCOPY AND CERVICAL BIOPSY

Once a *cytologic* diagnosis of epithelial abnormalities has been made on Pap smear, a *histologic* examination is needed to make the diagnosis of cervical dysplasia or cancer. This histologic evaluation can be achieved during **colposcopy with directed biopsies** to determine the severity of dysplasia and to identify any invasive carcinoma. The colposcope gives a magnified view of the cervix and, when stained with acetic acid, cervical lesions can be better identified. Changes may include **acetowhite epithelium, mosaicism, punctations, and atypical vessels** (Fig. 28-4 and Color Plate 14). These lesions should be biopsied, and the specimens should be sent to pathology where more definitive histologic diagnoses can be made.

Cervical dysplasia is classified as mild (CIN I), moderate (CIN II), or severe (CIN III), depending on the depth of involvement

TABLE 28-4 Natural History of Cervical Intraepithelial Lesions

CIN Level	Regress Spontaneously (%)	Persist at Same Level	Progression to CIN III	Progress to Invasive Cancer
CIN I	60	30	10	<1
CIN II	40	35	20	5
CIN III	30	50	N/A	12–22

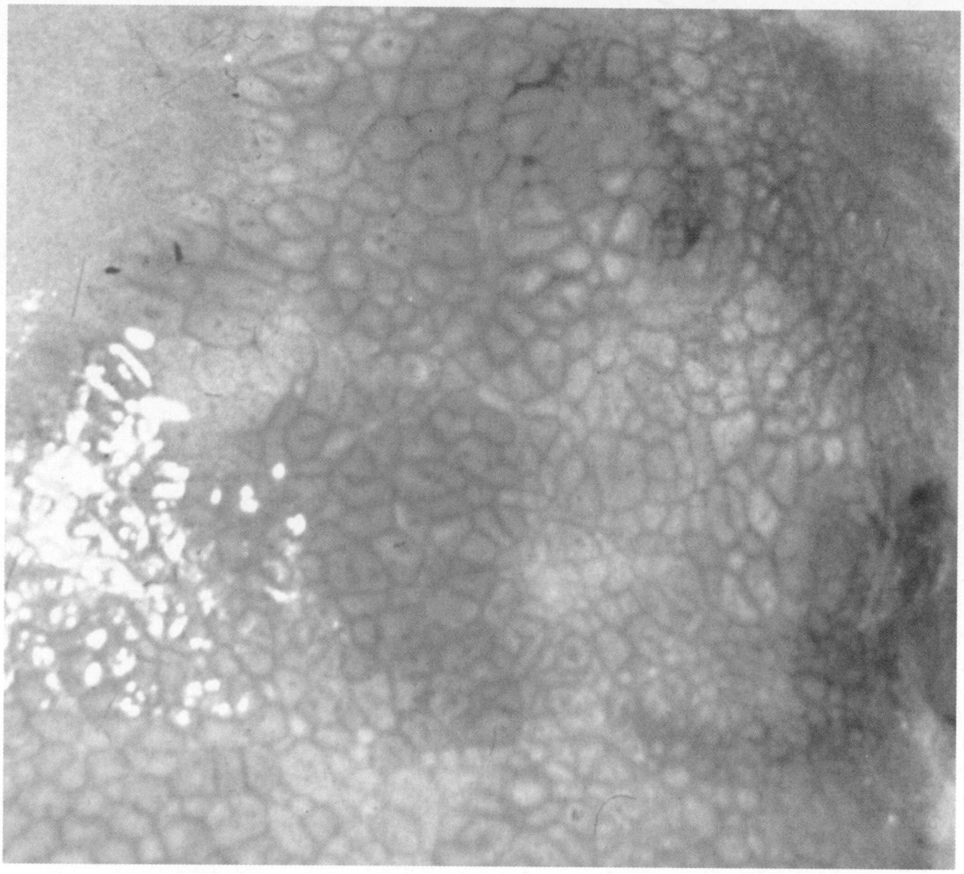

Figure 28-4 • Colposcopic view of the cervix. Abnormalities shown include acetowhite epithelium, punctations, and mosaic patterns.
(From Rubin E, Farber JL. *Pathology*, 3rd ed. Philadelphia, PA: Lippincott Williams & Wilkins; 1999.)

TABLE 28-5 Management of Cervical Intraepithelial Neoplasia by Level

CIN I	Repeat Pap smear every 6 mo × 1 y; or high-risk HPV screen in 1 y; if persistent × 2 y then offer LEEP procedure
CIN II	LEEP procedure; or repeat pap and colpo every 6 mo for 2 y for young women
CIN III	LEEP procedure

of the epithelium on cervical biopsy (Fig. 28-2). The treatment plan is then determined by the level of cervical dysplasia. In general, **CIN I** lesions can be followed with **repeat cytology** (every 6 months × 2) or **repeat HPV testing** (in 1 year). Because of their potential to progress to cervical cancer, **CIN II** and **CIN III** are typically treated with **surgical excision** (Table 28-5).

Treatment of Cervical Dysplasia

When the diagnosis of CIN is made on cervical biopsy, several treatments may ensue. **CIN I** is commonly followed with **repeat Pap smears** (every 6 months for 12 months) or **HPV testing** in 1 year. If either the repeat Pap smears are abnormal or if the testing for high-risk HPV is positive, the patient should have a **repeat colposcopy and biopsy** if indicated. If the repeat Pap smears are all within normal limits or if the patient is found to be HPV negative, the patient can return to routine cervical screening appropriate for her age (pap every 3 years from age 21-29 and pap and HPV every 5 years ≥ 30 yo).

Women with **CIN I that persists** for more than 2 years or with CIN II may be treated with cryotherapy or surgical excision. An alternative to treatment in young women with **CIN II** is observation with colposcopy and Pap testing every 6 months for 24 months. Women with CIN III are treated with surgical excision. Historically, a **cold-knife conization** (CKC) was performed, which removes a wedge-shaped portion of the cervical stroma and endocervical canal (Fig. 28-5). This is no longer the standard of care for CIN. The **loop electrosurgical excision procedure** (LEEP) **or large-loop excision of the transformation zone** (Lletz) is now more commonly performed to treat CIN II and CIN III. LEEP, loop, and Lletz all refer to the same procedure that involves removing a cone-shaped piece of cervical portio (conization), typically with a cauterized fine-wire loop or with a laser (Fig. 28-6). The LEEP can be performed as an office procedure under local anesthesia and is quicker and has less blood loss than the CKC.

Table 28-6 describes the suggested means of surgical excision of CIN based on characteristics of the lesion or patient. For small lesions confined to the ectocervix, an **in-office LEEP** is the most common means of excision, although cryotherapy

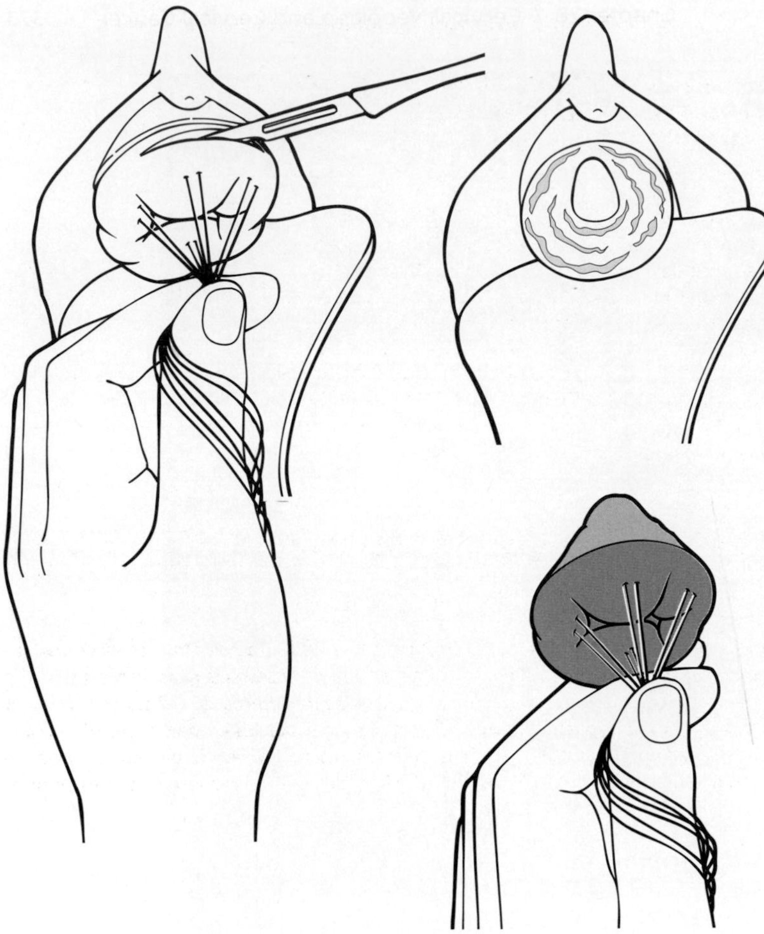

Figure 28-5 • Cold-knife cone of the cervix.

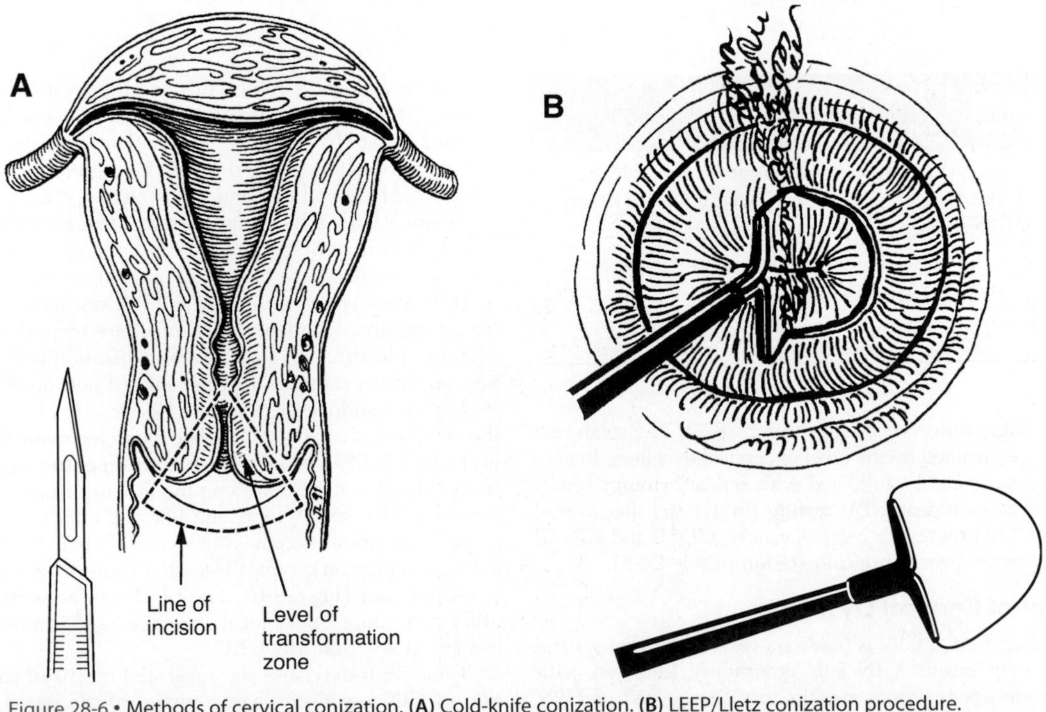

Figure 28-6 • Methods of cervical conization. (A) Cold-knife conization. (B) LEEP/Lletz conization procedure.
(From Beckmann CRB, Ling FW, Laube DW, et al. *Obstetrics and Gynecology*, 4th ed. Baltimore, MD: Lippincott Williams & Wilkins; 2002.)

or laser therapy may be used. Lesions involving the endocervix are usually treated with **CKC or a two-stage LEEP** to allow more of the endocervix to be removed. In the two-stage LEEP procedure, the first LEEP is performed to remove the ectocervix and a second smaller, deeper LEEP is then done to remove a portion of the endocervical canal. This is also known as a "top hat" because the resulting defect in the cervix resembles the shape of a top hat. Lesions that are large, multifocal, or those involving the vagina are often treated with **laser conization.** This allows for more precise removal of only abnormal tissue and removal of less normal cervix.

In general, cervical excision procedures remove cervical tissue without causing extensive damage to the stroma of the cervix, although scarring of the endocervical canal may still ensue. Infrequent complications include **cervical stenosis, cervical insufficiency, infection, or bleeding**. The persistence rate is about 4% for CIN II and CIN III and the recurrence rate is 10% and 15%, respectively. Therefore, after surgical conization, patients should be followed every 6 months with a repeat Pap smear or repeat Pap smear and colposcopy for 1 year. If the results all remain normal, the patient can return to routine screening **for at least 20 years.** Alternatively, after a cervical conization with unsatisfactory colposcopy, the patient can be followed with HPV testing every 6 months for 1 year after the procedure. If not high risk, the patient can return to routine screening **for at least 20 years.** In either scenario, any abnormal cytology or the presence of high-risk HPV should result in repeat colposcopic examination and cervical biopsies if indicated.

TABLE 28-6 Various Surgical Excision Options Based on Characteristics of the Lesion or Patient

Characteristics	Suggested Procedure
Confined to ectocervix	LEEP[a]
Endocervix involved	2-stage LEEP or CKC
Large lesion	Laser conization
Upper vagina involved	Laser conization

[a]Cryotherapy is acceptable if lesion is small, limited to CIN I or CIN II, and there is no endocervical involvement.

CERVICAL CANCER

PATHOPHYSIOLOGY

Squamous cell carcinoma (SCC) accounts for 80% of all cervical cancers. The route of metastasis is most often by direct extension (Fig. 28-7). **Adenocarcinoma** accounts for most of the remaining 20% of cervical cancers. One type of adenocarcinoma is clear cell carcinoma, which is correlated with in utero **DES exposure**. Very rarely is a sarcoma or lymphoma of the cervix found.

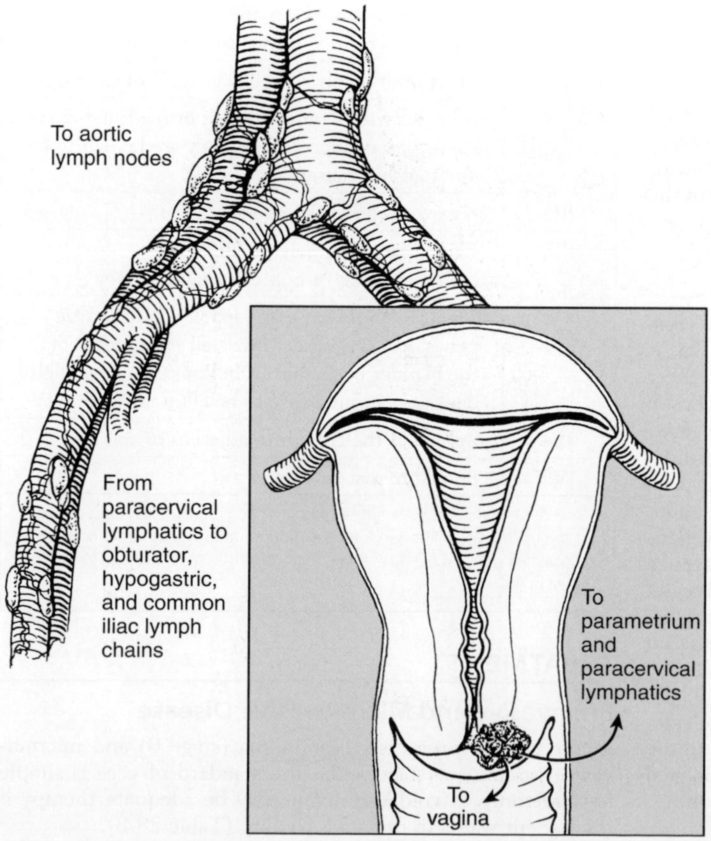

Figure 28-7 • Spread patterns of cervical carcinoma.

EPIDEMIOLOGY

There are approximately 11,000 cases of invasive cervical cancer diagnosed annually in the United States, leading to an estimated 3,600 deaths. Routine Pap smear screening combined with HPV typing decreases a woman's risk of cervical cancer by 90%.

The median age of diagnosis of cervical cancer is 52, and the average is 45. Risk factors for cervical cancer and dysplasia include **high-risk HPV serotypes** (16, 18, 31, and 45), cigarette smoking, high number of sexual partners, early age at onset of sexual activity, and **immunosuppression**. Additionally, patients with poorly controlled HIV (high viral loads and low CD4 counts) have an increased progression, persistence, and recurrence of disease. In fact, cervical cancer was classified an **AIDS-defining illness**.

CLINICAL MANIFESTATIONS

Even though the Pap smear has been proved to be an excellent screening method for cervical dysplasia, some patients who still do not get routine Pap smears occasionally present with advanced stages of cervical cancer. Early disease is **usually asymptomatic**. When symptoms are present, the most common is **postcoital bleeding**. Other signs and symptoms that accompany cervical cancer include any abnormal vaginal bleeding, watery discharge, pelvic pain or pressure, and rectal or urinary tract symptoms. On speculum examination, a friable, bleeding cervical lesion or mass may be seen with possible invasion into the upper vagina. On bimanual examination, a mass within the cervix may be palpated as well as invasive lesions into the upper vagina, cul-de-sac, or adnexa.

DIAGNOSIS

Pap smears are not sufficient to diagnose cancer. Cervical cancer can be diagnosed only with a tissue biopsy. If an abnormal Pap smear is found, a colposcopy and cervical biopsies should be obtained. If a visible lesion is found, it should also be **biopsied**. If the physical examination is abnormal, ultrasound or computed tomography (CT) may be performed to confirm the findings and define the extent of disease.

CLINICAL STAGING

Cervical cancer is the only gynecologic cancer that is **still clinically staged** (Table 28-7) rather than surgically staged. This is due in large part to the fact that it is the leading cause of cancer death in women in developing nations, where many diagnostic tools are not readily available. Clinical staging involves evaluating the patient for **invasion into adjacent structures** and metastatic involvement (Figs. 28-7 and 28-8). Acceptable diagnostic tools for staging of cervical cancer include examination under anesthesia, chest X-ray, cystoscopy, proctoscopy, intravenous pyelography (IVP), and barium enema. Magnetic resonance imaging and CT may be used to define the extent of the disease, but **cannot be used to determine the stage of the disease**. Likewise, once the stage has been assigned, it **does not change based on intraoperative findings** or progression of disease.

Stage I is confined to the cervix (Table 28-7 and Fig. 28-7). Stage II extends beyond the cervix but not to the pelvic sidewalls or the lower third of the vagina. Stage III extends to the pelvic sidewalls or lower third of the vagina. Stage IV is defined as extension beyond the pelvis, invasion into local structures, including the bladder or rectum, or distant metastases.

TABLE 28-7 FIGO Staging for Carcinoma of the Cervix Uteri

Stage	Clinical/Pathologic Findings
0	CIS, intraepithelial carcinoma
I	The carcinoma is strictly confined to the cervix (extension to the corpus should be disregarded)
Ia	Invasive cancer identified only microscopically. All gross lesions—even with superficial invasion—are stage Ib cancers. Invasion is limited to measured stromal invasion with maximum depth of 5.0 mm and no wider than 7.0 mm[a]
Ia-1	Measured invasion of stroma no greater than 3.0 mm in depth and no wider than 7.0 mm
Ia-2	Measured invasion of stroma greater than 3.0 mm and no greater than 5.0 mm and no wider than 7.0 mm
Ib	Clinical lesions confined to the cervix or preclinical lesions greater than stage Ia
Ib-1	Clinical lesions no greater than 4.0 cm in size
Ib-2	Clinical lesions greater than 4.0 cm in size
II	The carcinoma extends beyond the cervix but has not extended to the pelvic wall. The carcinoma involves the vagina but not as far as the lower third
IIa	No obvious parametrial involvement
IIb	Obvious parametrial involvement
III	The carcinoma has extended to the pelvic wall. On rectal examination, there is no cancer-free space between the tumor and the pelvic wall
	The tumor involves the lower third of the vagina
	All cases with hydronephrosis or nonfunctioning kidney are included unless they are known to be due to other causes
IIIa	No extension to the pelvic wall
IIIb	Extension to the pelvic wall and/or hydronephrosis or nonfunctioning kidney
IV	The carcinoma has extended beyond the true pelvis or has clinically involved the mucosa of the bladder or rectum. A bullous edema as such does not permit a case to be allotted to stage IV
IVa	Spread of the growth to adjacent organs
IVb	Spread to distant organs

[a]The depth of invasion should be no more than 5 mm taken from the base of the epithelium, either surface or glandular, from which it originates. Vascular space involvement, either venous or lymphatic, should not alter the staging.

TREATMENT

Preinvasive and Microinvasive Disease

In the case of preinvasive carcinoma (stage 0) and microinvasive carcinoma (stage Ia-1), the standard of care is **simple hysterectomy**. A **cold-knife cone** may be adequate therapy if the patient wants to maintain fertility (Table 28-8).

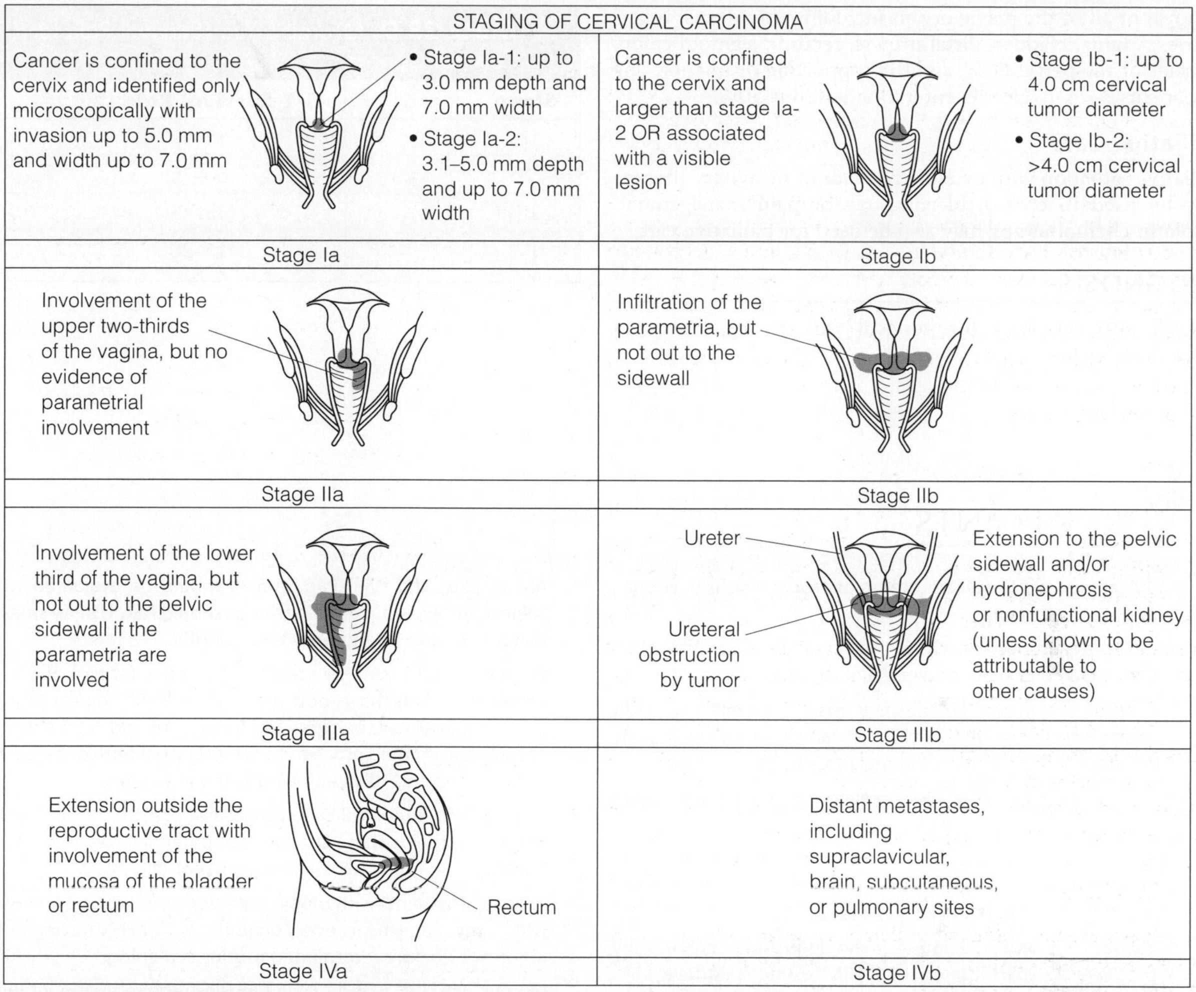

STAGING OF CERVICAL CARCINOMA
Cancer is confined to the cervix and identified only microscopically with invasion up to 5.0 mm and width up to 7.0 mm
• Stage Ia-1: up to 3.0 mm depth and 7.0 mm width
• Stage Ia-2: 3.1–5.0 mm depth and up to 7.0 mm width
Stage Ia
Cancer is confined to the cervix and larger than stage Ia-2 OR associated with a visible lesion
• Stage Ib-1: up to 4.0 cm cervical tumor diameter
• Stage Ib-2: >4.0 cm cervical tumor diameter
Stage Ib
Involvement of the upper two-thirds of the vagina, but no evidence of parametrial involvement
Stage IIa
Infiltration of the parametria, but not out to the sidewall
Stage IIb
Involvement of the lower third of the vagina, but not out to the pelvic sidewall if the parametria are involved
Stage IIIa
Ureter
Ureteral obstruction by tumor
Extension to the pelvic sidewall and/or hydronephrosis or nonfunctional kidney (unless known to be attributable to other causes)
Stage IIIb
Extension outside the reproductive tract with involvement of the mucosa of the bladder or rectum
Rectum
Stage IVa
Distant metastases, including supraclavicular, brain, subcutaneous, or pulmonary sites
Stage IVb

Figure 28-8 • **Staging of cervical carcinoma.**

TABLE 28-8 Treatment of Cervical Cancer by Stage of Disease Invasion

Level	Stage	Treatment
Preinvasive disease	0-Ia to 1	CKC or simple hysterectomy
Early disease	Ia-2 to IIa	Radical hysterectomy or radiation
Advanced disease	IIb to IV	Chemoradiation[a]

[a]External beam radiation, cisplatin-based chemotherapy, and intracavitary radiation.

Early Disease

Early disease (stages Ia-2 to IIa) may be treated with either **radiation therapy or radical hysterectomy** (with bilateral pelvic lymph node dissection) (Table 28-8). In addition to removing the uterus, a radical hysterectomy also removes the parametria, upper vaginal cuff, uterosacral/cardinal ligament complex, and local vascular and lymphatic supplies. For early disease, both radical hysterectomy and radiation therapy have **similar recurrence and survival rates**. The choice of treatment depends on the patient's age, ability to tolerate surgery, and proximity to radiation facilities. Young patients who are otherwise healthy are often treated with surgery to maintain ovarian function that would be diminished or terminated by radiation therapy.

Advanced Disease

For more advanced lesions (stages IIb to IV) that have spread to the pelvic sidewall or beyond (Fig. 28-8), the treatment is **chemoradiation therapy**. Both external beam radiation and intracavitary radiation are used in combination with **cisplatin-based chemotherapy**. The goals of chemoradiation are to eradicate local disease and prevent metastatic disease. This combined treatment regimen has led to significantly prolonged disease-free survival when compared with radiation therapy alone.

Recurrent Disease

When cervical cancer recurs in a patient initially treated with surgery alone, radiation can be used to treat the recurrence. When the cancer recurs in a patient already treated with radiation, surgical treatment with **pelvic exenteration** can be used if the recurrence is centrally located. Exenteration involves removal of all of the pelvic organs including the uterus, tubes, ovaries, vagina, bladder, distal ureters, rectum, sigmoid colon, muscles of the pelvic floor, and the supporting ligaments. The 5-year survival rate after exenteration is about 50%.

Palliative Care

Palliative **radiation** with external beam or intracavitary therapy may be used to control bleeding or for pain management. Cisplatin **chemotherapy** may also be used for palliative care.

PROGNOSIS

Overall survival rates for cervical cancer are shown in Table 28-9.

TABLE 28-9 Overall 5-Year Survival Rate for Cervical Cancer

Stage	5-Y Survival Rate (%)
I	85–90
II	60–75
III	35–45
IV	15–20

KEY POINTS

- Cervical cancer is the leading cause of cancer deaths in women in developing nations.
- HPV is the causative agent in CIN and cervical cancer. HPV types 16, 18, 31, and 45 are considered high-risk types.
- HPV testing can be used in the diagnosis and surveillance of CIN and cervical cancer. HPV vaccination can protect against some HPV infections, thereby preventing 70% of cervical cancer.
- Regular Pap and high-risk HPV testing can reduce a woman's risk of cervical cancer by 90%.
- Regular pap testing should begin at age 21 regardless of the onset of sexual activity. Pap smears should then be repeated every 3 years through age 29.
- Screening in women 30 and over should include Pap and HPV typing every 5 years (preferred). If HPV testing is not available, Pap every 3 years is acceptable.
- For women with no history of CIN 2/3 or higher, Pap smear screening can be stopped after age 65.
- Women with a history of CIN 2/3 or higher, should continue to have routine screening for at least 20 years after CIN 2/3. They can stop routine surveillance at that time or at age 65, whichever comes last.
- Women who have a complete hysterectomy for benign indications and who have no history of CIN 2/3 or higher can stop routine Pap screening at the time of hysterectomy.
- Women who have a history notable for CIN 2/3 who undergo a complete hysterectomy should continue to have routine vaginal Pap smear surveillance at least 20 years after the CIN 2/3 diagnosis. They can stop routine surveillance at that time or at age 65, whichever comes last.
- Pap smears are classified as negative for intraepithelial lesions and malignancy, atypical squamous cells (ASC-US and ASC-H), LSIL, HSIL, or SCC.
- ASC-H, LSIL, and HSIL Pap smears should be evaluated with colposcopy and directed biopsies as should ASC-US Pap smears that are positive for high-risk types of HPV.
- Women with normal Pap screen but positive for high-risk HPV screen can either have both the Pap and HPV repeated in 1 year, or, if available, be subtyped for HPV 16 and 18. If either is present, they should proceed to colposcopy. If both or negative, both the Pap and HPV can be repeated in 1 year.
- CIN I reflects abnormalities in the basal one-third of epithelial cells of the cervix. These changes can potentially lead to cancer, but a high number (70%) will regress spontaneously.
- In general, patients with biopsies showing CIN I can be followed with repeat Pap smears every 6 months × 2 or HPV testing in 12 months × 1 before returning to routine screening.
- Women with CIN II and CIN III biopsies require treatment with surgical excision, typically with loop/LEEP/Lletz. Young women with CIN II may be observed with Pap and colposcopy every 6 months for up to 24 months.
- Complications of cervical conization include bleeding and infection and, much less likely, cervical stenosis or cervical insufficiency.
- Preinvasive (stage 0) and microinvasive disease (stage Ia-1) can be treated with cone biopsy or simple hysterectomy. Stage Ia-2 should be treated with radical hysterectomy.
- Early disease stages Ia-2 to IIa are equally responsive to radical hysterectomy or radiation therapy.
- More advanced lesions stage IIb or greater are treated with internal and external radiation, usually in combination with cisplatin chemotherapy.
- Radiation and/or chemotherapy may be used for palliative care.
- Five-year survival rates for cervical cancer vary from 85% to 90% for stage I disease, and 15% to 20% for stage IV disease.

C Clinical Vignettes

Vignette 1

A 24-year-old G1P1 female comes to the office for colposcopy due to LSIL pap 1 month prior. Her pap was normal 3 years ago. She began sexual activity at age 16 and has had five partners. She has had Chlamydia and vulvar warts in the past, both of which have been treated and resolved. She is a smoker of approximately 15 cigarettes per day since she was 15. She uses Depo Provera for contraception. Her mother died last year of cervical cancer at age 44.

1. What are her risk factors for CIN?
   a. Age 16 at onset of sexual activity
   b. Five sex partners
   c. Her history of STDs
   d. Smoking 15 cigarettes a day
   e. All of the above

2. You perform colposcopy and see a condylomatous acetowhite lesion on her cervix with punctation. The biopsy of the lesion confirms CIN I consistent with HPV changes. What do you recommend for management?
   a. Imiquimod (Aldara)
   b. LEEP procedure
   c. HPV test in 1 year
   d. Repeat pap in 6 months then return to routine screening
   e. Repeat pap in 12 months then return to routine screening

3. She returns in 1 year, and her HPV test is positive. She returns for colposcopy, and on examination you see a dense acetowhite area on the anterior cervix in the TZ. You can easily see the entire SCJ. Biopsy of this lesion returns CIN II. What is your recommendation?
   a. Repeat Pap test in 1 year
   b. Repeat Pap test and colposcopy in 6 months
   c. Repeat pap and colposcopy in 6 months
   d. Cold knife cone procedure
   e. Simple hysterectomy

Vignette 2

A 30-year-old G0 comes in for her annual examination and tells you that she plans to become pregnant sometime in the next year. She had a LEEP procedure 5 years ago at another facility for moderate dysplasia. You verify her Pap tests have all been negative since the LEEP, but her last pap was 2 years ago.

1. What is the recommended cervical cancer screening for this patient?
   a. Pap testing every 6 months
   b. Pap testing and colposcopy every 6 months
   c. Pap testing every 3 years
   d. Pap testing and high-risk HPV testing every 5 years
   e. She has been treated with the LEEP, so she no longer needs pap smears

2. Her Pap test returns HSIL and she is high-risk HPV positive. You have her return for colposcopy. After the application of acetic acid, you see a large, dense, white area with mosaic vessels encompassing the entire anterior cervix and extending into the endocervical canal. You obtain a biopsy of this area and perform an endocervical curettage. The pathology report for both biopsies is CIN III. What treatment do you recommend?
   a. LEEP in office
   b. Cryotherapy
   c. Cold-knife cone or two-stage LEEP in OR
   d. Simple hysterectomy
   e. Radical hysterectomy

3. What are the complications of surgical excisional procedures of the cervix?
   a. Cervical stenosis, cervical insufficiency, infection, bleeding
   b. Cervical stenosis, infertility, infection, bleeding
   c. Cervical insufficiency, increased vaginal discharge, infection, bleeding
   d. Vaginitis and bleeding
   e. There are no known complications

Vignette 3

1. She relates that her mother sent her for a Pap smear. How do you respond?
   a. Since she is sexually active, you perform a Pap smear and offer an STI screen
   b. Since she is sexually active, you perform a Pap smear and low-risk HPV screen
   c. Since she is sexually active, you perform a Pap smear and high-risk HPV screen
   d. You inform her that she doesn't need a Pap smear until age 21
   e. You inform her that she doesn't need a Pap smear until age 30

2. She has seen a lot of information about abnormal Pap smears and cervical cancer in school and in the community, and she wants to know how she can decrease her own risk. You tell her
   a. Cervical cancer doesn't usually affect women before age 40 so she doesn't have anything to worry about

b. You recommend she start and complete the Gardasil vaccine series
c. You inform her that the Gardasil vaccine won't work for her because she's already sexually active
d. You inform her that that she is too old for HPV vaccination and should have had it at age 11 or 12
e. You inform her there are no interventions that will decrease her risk

3. She wants to know more about HPV immunization. You tell her
a. It will lower her risk of cervical dysplasia
b. It will lower her risk of cervical cancer
c. It will lower her risk of genital warts
d. It will lower her risk of other cancers
e. All of the above

4. She returns a year later for routine GYN care. She has completed the Gardasil immunization series. She wants to know how the vaccine will change her recommended Pap smear screening.
a. No. She will still need a Pap every year.
b. No. She will still need a Pap every 3 years.
c. Yes. She can now space out her Paps to every 3 years.
d. Yes. She can now increase her screening interval to a Pap every 5 years.
e. Yes. She can increase her interval screening to a Pap and HPV every 5 years.

Vignette 4

A 62-year-old woman presents to the office complaining of watery vaginal discharge and bleeding for the past 2 months. She has not had a Pap test in 14 years. She states she had a mildly abnormal pap in her 30s, but that was treated with cryotherapy. She states she went through menopause at age 50 and has never been on hormone replacement therapy. She does admit to smoking one-half pack a day for 40 years. Her husband is deceased, and she has not been sexually active in 10 years. Her examination reveals a cervical necrotic mass approximately 5 cm in size. Rectovaginal examination is suspicious for left parametrial involvement. There is no evidence of adnexal masses, but examination of the uterus and adnexa is limited by the patient's body habitus.

You suspect this may be cervical cancer. You obtain a Pap smear and take a biopsy of her cervical abnormality. The Pap test returns with a reading of SCC, and the biopsy confirms this diagnosis. She also received a cystoscopy for hematuria with positive urine cytology. The biopsy also shows SCC. You order a CT scan, which shows a cervical mass measuring 7.7 × 5.0 cm as well as an avid left internal iliac lymph node consistent with locally metastatic disease.

1. What is the International Federation of Gynecology and Obstetrics (FIGO) stage for her cancer?
a. Stage I
b. Stage II
c. Stage III
d. Stage IV

2. What do you recommend for the next step treatment of her cervical cancer?
a. Cold-knife cone
b. Simple hysterectomy
c. Radiation and chemotherapy
d. Chemotherapy alone
e. Palliative care

3. She is treated with chemoradiation and 3 years later has a recurrence. You proceed with pelvic exenteration for her recurrent cancer. What is her 5-year survival rate after pelvic exenteration?
a. 5%
b. 10%
c. 25%
d. 50%
e. 90%

A Answers

Vignette 1 Question 1
Answer E: Risk factors for cervical dysplasia include characteristics that predispose patients to multiple and early exposure to HPV (early intercourse, multiple sex partners, early childbearing, "high-risk" partners, low socioeconomic status, sexually transmitted infections, cigarette smoking, immunodeficiency, and multiparity). Most of these behavioral and sexual risk factors are associated with HPV infection rather than independent risk factors in and of themselves.

Vignette 1 Question 2
Answer C: Women with CIN I have high rates of regression to normal. LSIL lesions usually represent a transient infection with HPV, so the majority will regress spontaneously over time. Imiquimod is a treatment for perineal condyloma, but is not indicated for vaginal or cervical HPV. LEEP procedure should be used for persistent CIN II or for CIN III in a woman her age. CIN 1 can be followed with HPV screening in 1 year or pap alone at 6 **and** 12 months.

Vignette 1 Question 3
Answer D: For young women with CIN II, it is acceptable to offer observation with colposcopy and Pap testing every 6 months for 24 months. Squamous intraepithelial lesions have a very high rate of spontaneous regression. Repeat Pap testing only is not a recommended follow-up for CIN II in any age group. Treatment with cold knife cone is an acceptable option, but due to her age and the likelihood of future childbearing, observation is an appropriate plan.

Vignette 2 Question 1
Answer D: Pap testing and high-risk HPV testing every 5 years is routine screening for women aged 30 and above. She does have history of a prior abnormal pap and LEEP, but with normal screening for the year following the LEEP, she can return to routine screening. Screening recommendations for women aged 21 to 29 is to have Pap testing every 3 years. A colposcopy is not indicated unless she has another abnormal Pap test.

Vignette 2 Question 2
Answer C: A result of CIN III needs to be excised and due to the size of the area and the extension into the endocervical canal, an OR procedure is recommended. Cryotherapy is acceptable for small lesions confined to the ectocervix when LEEP is not available. LEEP in the office is appropriate for focal lesions confined to the ectocervix. Hysterectomy is not indicated because she does not have cervical cancer.

Vignette 2 Question 3
Answer A: Complications of cervical excision procedures are cervical stenosis, cervical insufficiency, infection, and bleeding. These risks are infrequent. Infertility has not been found to be affected by cervical excision.

Vignette 3 Question 1
Answer D: The current recommendation for screening for cervical dysplasia and cancer should begin at age 21 regardless of the onset of sexual activity. The appropriate screening for women from age 21 to 29 is to have a Pap smear every 3 years. Routine HPV screening is not indicated in this population. There is no role for low-risk HPV screening in the detection or management of cervical dysplasia and cancer.

Vignette 3 Question 2
Answer B: This patient is at the appropriate age to receive HPV immunization. There are two current HPV vaccines available in the United States, Gardasil and Cervarix. These are recommended for girls aged 11 to 12 (but may be given as early age 9) up through women aged 26. Smoking cessation would also decrease her risk of cervical dysplasia and cancer.

Vignette 3 Question 3
Answer E: Gardasil protects against the two most common HPV subtypes responsible for genital warts (6 and 11) and for cervical dysplasia and cancer (16 and 18). It also lowers the risk of vaginal and vulvar dysplasia as well as some cancers of the head and neck. It is given in a series of three injections over 6 months.

Vignette 3 Question 4
Answer B: The current recommendation for screening for cervical dysplasia and cancer for women aged 21 through 29 is for Pap smear screening every 3 years. HPV vaccination does not change the screening guidelines.

Vignette 4 Question 1
Answer D: Cervical cancer is *clinically staged* as opposed to surgically staged. The FIGO staging system is largely based on physical examination. This clinical staging process can include physical examination, examination under anesthesia, cervical biopsy and/or conization, chest X-ray, hysteroscopy, cystoscopy, proctoscopy, and IVP and/or barium enema, if indicated. Other imaging studies, laboratory tests, and surgical procedures are often used to assess for lymph node involvement and metastases. However, these results *do not* alter the FIGO stage.

Stage I disease is confined to the cervix. Stage II involves the upper two-thirds of the vagina and/or involvement of the parametria. Stage III involves the lower vagina, extension to the pelvic side wall, and/or hydronephrosis from ureteral obstruction by the tumor. Stage IV involves extension outside the reproductive tract including involvement of the bladder mucosa and distant metastases.

This patient has a large lesion with likely parametrial involvement. The CT information is not used for FIGO staging, but the cystoscopy showing bladder involvement is. This would place her at stage IV, given involvement of the mucosa of the bladder.

Vignette 4 Question 2

Answer C: For stages I and II of cervical cancer, radial hysterectomy and radiation have similar survival rates. The choice of treatment depends on the patients' age, ability to tolerate surgery, and proximity to radiation facilities. Young patients are often treated with surgery to maintain ovarian function that would be diminished or eliminated by radiation.

More advanced stage III or stage IV disease requires chemoradiation in order to treat local disease and prevent metastatic disease. This typically involves the use of both external beam radiation and intracavitary radiation (brachytherapy) in concert with cisplatin-based chemotherapy.

Vignette 4 Question 3

Answer D: When cervical cancer recurs in a patient initially treated with surgery alone, radiation can be used to treat the recurrence. When the cancer recurs in a patient who has already been treated with radiation, surgical treatment with pelvic exenteration can be used if the recurrence is centrally located (vaginal apex or pelvis without pelvic sidewall involvement) and there is no metastatic disease. Exenteration involves removal of the pelvic organs, including the uterus, tubes, ovaries, vagina, bladder, rectum, sigmoid colon, and muscle and support structures of the pelvic wall. The 5-year survival rate after pelvic exenteration for recurrent cervical cancer is about 50%.

Chapter

29 Endometrial Cancer

Endometrial carcinoma is the fourth most common cancer in American women, exceeded only by cancer of the breast, bowel, and lung. Over 43,000 women are diagnosed with this disease each year in the United States alone, accounting for 6% of all cancers in women. Although endometrial cancer is the **most** commonly encountered gynecologic malignancy in the United States, it is associated with a favorable survival profile because the majority of disease is diagnosed early. In fact, 72% of women are diagnosed with stage I disease, thus rendering the surgical staging itself as curative treatment. Fortunately, **early symptoms and accurate diagnosis modalities** contribute to the fact that despite being the most common GYN cancer, endometrial cancer is only the third most common cause of gynecologic cancer deaths (behind ovarian and cervical cancer). It accounts for 7,900 deaths each year in the United States.

Factors such as obesity, chronic anovulation, nulliparity, late menopause, unopposed estrogen use (i.e., without progesterone), hypertension, and diabetes mellitus lead to an increased risk of both endometrial hyperplasia (see Table 14-6) and endometrial cancer.

PATHOGENESIS

There are **two distinct pathogenic etiologies** of endometrial cancer. The most common type, type I (80%), occurs in **women** with a history of chronic estrogen exposure unopposed by progestin. These are referred to as **estrogen-dependent neoplasms**. These tumors usually start as atypical endometrial hyperplasia and progress to carcinomas. The tumors tend to be well differentiated (endometrioid type) with lower grade nuclei and usually have a more **favorable prognosis**.

Type II (20%) endometrial cancer is believed to be an **estrogen-*in*dependent** neoplasm that is *not* related to unopposed estrogen stimulation or endometrial hyperplasia. These tumors often occur within a background of atrophic endometrium or polyps. These cancers often have high-grade nuclear atypia with **serous or clear cell histology**. Many are associated with a mutation in the **p53 tumor supression gene.**

Grossly, endometrial cancer itself may appear as a single mass within the endometrium, or it may be spread diffusely throughout the endometrium. **Depth of myometrial invasion** is an important component in the staging and prognosis of endometrial cancer. The prognosis is dramatically worsened when the cancer has invaded more than one-half of the thickness of the myometrium.

Endometrial carcinoma has four primary routes of spread. The most common route is **direct extension** of the tumor downward to the cervix or outward through the myometrium and serosa. When there is significant myometrial penetration, cells may spread through the **lymphatic system** to the pelvic and para-aortic lymph nodes. Exfoliated cells may also be shed **transtubally** through the fallopian tubes to the ovaries, parietal peritoneum, and omentum. **Hematogenous** spread occurs less frequently, but can result in metastasis to the liver, lungs, and/or bone.

The most common type of endometrial cancer is **endometrioid adenocarcinoma** (75% to 80%). Other nonendometrioid tumor types include mucinous carcinomas (5%), clear cell carcinomas (5%), papillary serous carcinomas (4%), and squamous carcinomas (1%). These types are less common but also tend to be more aggressive. Invasive adenocarcinoma usually results from **proliferation of the glandular cells** of the endometrium in a back-to-back fashion without intervening stroma.

Histologic grade is the most important prognostic factor for endometrial carcinoma (Table 29-1). Poorly differentiated tumors have a higher grade and a higher percentage of solid (nonglandular) growth. High-grade tumors have a much poorer prognosis due to the likelihood of spread outside of the uterus. The **histologic type** of carcinoma also affects prognosis. Other prognostic factors are shown in Table 29-2.

TABLE 29-1 Prognostic Factors for Endometrial Cancer: Histologic Grade—Degree of Differentiation

Grade	Percentage Solid Growth	Differentiation
Grade 1 (G1)	5% or less of the tumor shows a solid growth pattern	Highly differentiated
Grade 2 (G2)	6%–50% of the tumor shows a solid growth pattern	Moderately differentiated
Grade 3 (G3)	More than 50% of the tumor shows a solid growth pattern	Poorly differentiated

TABLE 29-2 Major Independent Prognostic Factors for Endometrial Cancer

Age
Depth of myometrial invasion
Histologic grade
Histologic type
Surgical stage
Peritoneal cytology
Tumor size
Lymphovascular invasion
Pelvic lymph node metastasis

TABLE 29-4 Risk Factors for Endometrial Cancer

Risk Factor	Relative Risk
Nulliparity	2–4
Late menopause	2–4
Chronic anovulation (PCOS)	3
Diabetes mellitus	2–8
Tamoxifen use	3–8
Obesity	
21–50 lb overweight	2–4
>50 lb overweight	10
Unopposed estrogen therapy	2–10

EPIDEMIOLOGY

Endometrial cancer occurs in both premenopausal (25%) and postmenopausal (75%) women. Five percent to 10% of those with premenopausal diagnoses are less than 40 years of age. The **average age of diagnosis is 61**; the largest affected group is between age 50 and 59. Most tumors are caught early when they are of low grade and low stage (Table 29-3); therefore, the overall prognosis for the disease is good and overall mortality rates are declining. Eighty percent of women have type I endometrial cancer, while 20% have the more aggressive type II cancers.

RISK FACTORS

Several risk factors have been identified for type I endometrial cancer. These include a history of **unopposed estrogen exposure**, obesity, nulliparity, late menopause, chronic anovulation, and tamoxifen use (Table 29-4). Other risk factors include diabetes mellitus; hypertension; cancer of the breast, ovary, or colon; and a family history of endometrial cancer.

Excess exogenous estrogen exposure can result from unopposed use of **estrogen replacement therapy** (ERT) in the absence of progesterone in a woman with a uterus. Studies show that 20% to 50% of women who are given ERT without progesterone will develop endometrial hyperplasia within 1 year. Similarly, **tamoxifen**, a selective estrogen receptor modulator (SERM), can also act as a source of exogenous estrogen. It is typically used in women with estrogen–progesterone receptor positive breast cancer (see Chapter 32) to competitively inhibit estrogen at the estrogen receptor. Therefore, it works to block stimulation of breast tissue in women with estrogen–progesterone receptor positive breast cancer. However, in endometrial tissue, tamoxifen acts as a **partial agonist/weak estrogen** to stimulate endometrial proliferation.

Endometrial cancer can also be caused by prolonged exposure to **excess endogenous estrogen** without concomitant progesterone exposure. This mechanism of action is demonstrated in **obese women**. These women have higher endogenous estrogen levels due to **peripheral conversion of androgens to estrone and estradiol** in the adipocytes. These women also have lower sex hormone binding globulin levels. Many are anovulatory as well.

Women with chronic anovulation and/or polycystic ovary syndrome **(PCOS)** typically have more central obesity and therefore have more peripheral conversion of androgens to estrone and estradiol. Additionally, these patients have a **relative lack of progesterone** in the luteal phase due to their **anovulatory cycles**. This mechanism of action may also explain the higher rates of endometrial cancer in **nulliparous women**. These women are thought to be at higher risk of infertility and subfertility secondary to **anovulatory cycles**. The increased risk of endometrial cancer with **early menarche** and **late menopause** is presumably due to prolonged endogenous estrogen stimulation.

Diabetes (type II > type I) and hypertension also increases a patient's risk of endometrial cancer. This is partially attributed to the comorbid risk of **obesity and chronic anovulation** in this patient population. Even when controlling for these factors, diabetes and hypertension are still independent risk factors for endometrial cancer. It is hypothesized that the presence of hyperinsulinemia, insulin resistance, and insulin-like growth factors may lead to **abnormal endometrial proliferation** in these patients.

There is an increased risk of endometrial cancer in women who have at least one **first-degree relative** (mother, sister, or daughter) with uterine cancer. Women with a known **family history of Lynch II syndrome** have an increased risk of endometrial cancer as well. Lynch II syndrome is also known as hereditary nonpolyposis colorectal cancer (HNPCC) and is associated with a genetic predisposition to breast, ovarian, colon, and endometrial cancers. Specific **germline gene mutations** are responsible for the cancers in the majority of these women with Lynch II syndrome. Patients with a **personal history of breast cancer** also have an increased risk of endometrial cancer. This is attributed to the presence of similar risk factors (**obesity, nulliparity, and high-fat diet**) in both cancers. It is unclear whether the presence of *BRCA1* (the breast cancer susceptibility gene) plays a role in the development of endometrial cancer.

Endometrial hyperplasia is another risk factor for endometrial cancer. The degree of risk of malignant transformation of endometrial hyperplasia to endometrial cancer depends on the type of hyperplasia (see Table 14-5). Its mildest form, simple hyperplasia *without* atypia, poses a 1% risk of endometrial cancer, whereas its most severe form, complex hyperplasia *with*

TABLE 29-3 Stage at Which Endometrial Cancer Is Diagnosed

Stage I	72%
Stage II	12%
Stage III	13%
Stage IV	3%

atypia, poses a 29% risk of developing endometrial cancer if left untreated. Furthermore, women with atypical endometrial hyperplasia may have a coexistent endometrial cancer as often as 17% to 52% of the time.

Despite these known risk factors for type I endometrial cancer, there are **no effective screening mechanisms** for endometrial carcinoma. Neither annual Pap smears nor endometrial biopsies have been shown to offer cost-effective screening in asymptomatic patients.

Conversely, protective factors include those that **decrease lifetime estrogen exposure** including combination oral contraceptive pills (OCPs), progestin-containing contraceptives, and combination estrogen and progesterone hormone replacement (HRT). These patients have a lower rate of endometrial cancer compared with nonusers. The protection conferred on a woman who takes combination OCPs lasts for 15 years after discontinuation. Other **protective factors** include high parity, pregnancy, physical activity (decreased obesity, favorable immune function, and endogenous hormone levels), and smoking (causes increased hepatic metabolism of estrogen). Women can also lower their risk of endometrial cancer by **avoiding obesity, hypertension, and diabetes**, and by eating a **healthy diet and exercising**. Women who exercise regularly have one-half the risk of endometrial cancer as those who do not exercise.

Unfortunately, there are **no identifiable risk factors** for women who may be at risk for type II endometrial cancer.

CLINICAL MANIFESTATIONS

HISTORY

Ninety percent of women with endometrial cancer have either **postmenopausal bleeding** or some form of **abnormal vaginal bleeding** (menorrhagia, postcoital spotting, or intermenstrual bleeding). Ten percent of women may also present with a nonbloody vaginal discharge. As a result of these early symptoms, most endometrial cancers are diagnosed at an early stage (Table 29-3). **Pelvic pain**, **pelvic mass**, and **weight loss** are seen in women who present with more advanced disease.

PHYSICAL EXAMINATION

The physical examination may reveal obesity, acanthosis nigricans, hypertension, or stigmata of diabetes. The clinician should look for signs of metastatic disease, including pleural effusion, ascites, hepatosplenomegaly, general lymphadenopathy, and abdominal masses.

Women with endometrial carcinoma typically have a **normal pelvic examination**. In more advanced stages of the disease, the cervical os may be patulous, and the cervix may be firm and expanded. The uterus may be of normal size or enlarged. The adnexae should be carefully examined for evidence of extrauterine metastasis and/or coexistent ovarian carcinoma.

DIFFERENTIAL DIAGNOSIS

Most women with endometrial cancer present with a complaint of **abnormal uterine bleeding**. This may include menorrhagia, metrorrhagia, menometrorrhagia, postcoital spotting, or even oligomenorrhea. The differential diagnosis for premenopausal bleeding includes uterine fibroids, endometrial polyps, adenomyosis, endometrial hyperplasia, ovarian cysts, and thyroid dysfunction (see Fig. 22-1).

The differential diagnosis for **postmenopausal bleeding** is shown in Table 29-5. Note that endometrial cancer is responsible for up to 20% of postmenopausal hyperplasia and/or bleeding. However, the older the patient and the higher the number of years since menopause, the higher the probability of malignancy. The amount of bleeding does not correlate with risk of malignancy.

TABLE 29-5 Differential Diagnosis of Postmenopausal Bleeding

Cause of Bleeding	Frequency (%)
Endometrial atrophy	60–80
Exogenous estrogens/HRT	15–25
Endometrial cancer	10–15
Endometrial or cervical polyps	2–12
Endometrial hyperplasia	5–10
Miscellaneous	10

DIAGNOSTIC EVALUATION

Although dilation and curettage (D&C) was once the gold standard for the evaluation of irregular bleeding, office endometrial biopsy (EMB) has an accuracy of 90% to 98% without the need for anesthesia and operative time. In postmenopausal women, **transvaginal ultrasound** can be helpful in triaging suspicious lesions from the most common source of postmenopausal bleeding-atrophy. An endometrial thickness of 4 mm or less is indicative of low risk for malignancy. These women do not require EMB unless their bleeding is persistent/recurrent or they are at high risk for malignancy. Premenopausal women are subject to a high degree of variability in the thickness of the endometrial lining. **Therefore, persistent abnormal bleeding**, even in the setting of normal imaging **warrants a tissue diagnosis** for women ≥ 45 and those at risk for malignancy regardless of age.

If an adequate EMB cannot be performed due to patient discomfort, cervical stenosis, or insufficient tissue sample, **D&C** (± hysteroscopy) should be done to sample the endometrium. A D&C should also be done if there are suspicious findings (atypical hyperplasia or necrosis) on EMB or if the patient continues to have symptoms after a negative EMB.

In addition to endometrial sampling, the initial workup for a woman with abnormal vaginal bleeding should also include a thyroid stimulating hormone **(TSH)**, a **prolactin level** (if oligomenorrheic), and possibly a follicle stimulating hormone **(FSH)** and estradiol level (to distinguish whether the patient is menopausal). A complete blood count **(CBC)** should be obtained to rule out anemia preoperatively if bleeding is heavy or prolonged. Similarly, a **CA-125 level** is often drawn preoperatively. Very high CA-125 levels are suggestive of spread beyond the uterus. These levels can also be followed postoperatively to assess the effectiveness of treatment.

An up-to-date **Pap smear** should also be obtained in women with abnormal bleeding although only 30% to 40% of patients with endometrial cancer will have an abnormal Pap smear. When the Pap cytology shows **endometrial cells** in a woman greater than or equal to 40 years, an EMB should be considered to rule out endometrial cancer. These cytology reports are particularly concerning when **atypical endometrial cells** are found.

A **pelvic ultrasound** should also be performed to look for fibroids, adenomyosis, polyps, and endometrial hyperplasia.

Postmenopausal women with an endometrial stripe less than or equal to 4 mm are unlikely to have endometrial hyperplasia or cancer. However, even if the endometrial stripe and the remainder of the pelvic ultrasound appear normal, the physician is still obliged to **obtain an endometrial sampling** via EMB or D&C **if the bleeding is persistent**. Likewise, even if another potential source for bleeding is identified, the endometrium must still be sampled. If bone pain is present, a chest radiograph, CT, or bone scan can be performed.

More than 50% of women at risk for **Lynch II syndrome (or HNPCC)** will develop endometrial and/or ovarian cancer before developing colon cancer. Given this, these women who carry Lynch II syndrome-associated mutations or who have a family member known to carry such a mutation should undergo yearly EMB beginning at age 35.

TREATMENT

Although endometrial cancer was once clinically staged, in 1988, the International Federation of Gynecology and Obstetrics (FIGO) changed to a **surgical staging system** that more accurately reflects the true degree of disease progression. This system relies on **pathologic confirmation** of the extent of spread of the disease (Table 29-6).

STAGE I AND STAGE II DISEASE

In general, treatment for endometrial carcinoma includes systematic surgical staging, including **total abdominal hysterectomy and bilateral salpingo-oophorectomy** (TAH-BSO), pelvic washings, pelvic and para-aortic lymph node resection, and complete resection of visible tumor for all stages of the disease (Table 29-7). Exceptions to complete surgical staging are young women with grade I endometrioid carcinoma who desire future fertility or women with a high-mortality risk related to surgery. When practical and feasible, referral to a gynecologic oncologist is recommended in order to facilitate the most appropriate treatment modality.

Patients with greater than 50% myometrial invasion have a poorer prognosis even if they have stage I or stage II disease confined to the uterus. These patients and those with other poor prognostic factors such as large tumor mass (>2 cm or filling the cavity), grade 3 tumor type (more than 50% of the tumor is solid), papillary serous or clear cell histologic types, or enlarged lymph nodes, may also require **radiation therapy** even if the disease is confined to the uterus.

TABLE 29-6 FIGO Surgical Staging of Endometrial Carcinoma

Stages	Extent of Disease
Stage I	
Ia	Limited to the endometrium no myometrial invasion or invasion
Ib	Invasion limited to less than one-half of myometrium
Ic	Invasion is greater than one-half of the myometrium
Stage II	
IIa	Spread to the endocervical glands only
IIb	Invasion of cervical stroma
Stage III	
IIIa	Tumor invades serosa and/or positive peritoneal cytology
IIIb	Vaginal or parametrial metastases
IIIc	Metastases to pelvic and/or para-aortic lymph nodes
IIIc1	Positive pelvic nodes
IIIc2	Positive para-aortic nodes
Stage IV	
IVa	Tumor invasion of bladder and/or bowel mucosa
IVb	Distant metastases including intra-abdominal and/or inguinal lymph nodes

STAGE III AND STAGE IV DISEASE

When the malignancy has spread to the uterine serosa or beyond it (stage III and IV disease), patients will also require **pelvic radiation** therapy in addition to their surgical treatment.

ADVANCED AND RECURRENT DISEASE

Chemotherapy may be used in advanced or recurrent disease, but the best regimen and duration of use have yet to be determined.

PROGNOSIS

Because most endometrial cancers are stage I at diagnosis and endometrioid subtype, the **overall 5-year survival rate is quite good—65%**. Survival rates for the various stages of endometrial cancer are 87% for stage I, 76% for stage II, 59% for stage III, and 18% for stage IV. The presence of certain high-risk features (Table 29-8) confers a higher risk of recurrence and lower survival rates.

TABLE 29-7 Treatment Recommendations for Endometrial Cancer by Stage

Stage I	TAH-BSO, pelvic and para-aortic LN sampling; if high risk[a], then radiation
Stage II	TAH-BSO, pelvic and para-aortic LN sampling; if high risk, then radiation
Stage III	TAH-BSO, pelvic and para-aortic LN sampling, radiation
Stage IV	TAH-BSO, pelvic and para-aortic LN sampling, radiation
Recurrence, pelvic	High-dose progestins, ± chemotherapy
Recurrence, vaginal	Vaginal radiation

[a]Grade 3 lesions, grade 2 lesion greater than 2 cm, lower uterine segment involvement, cervical involvement, poor histologic differentiation, papillary serous or clear cell histology, greater than one-third myometrial penetration.

TABLE 29-8 High-Risk Features for Endometrial Cancer

>50% Myometrial invasion
Papillary serous or clear cell tumors
Grade 3 tumors (>50% solid growth)
Large tumor (>2 cm or filling cavity)
Spread beyond the uterine fundus (stages III and IV)
Lymphovascular involvement

FOLLOW-UP

Follow-up should include physical examination (with speculum and rectovaginal exam) every 3 months for 3 years, followed by twice yearly examinations for the subsequent 2 years. If without evidence for recurrent disease, the patient can likely be followed annually.

Recurrence is influenced by the original treatment received, as well as the patient's previous history of metastasis and the presence of high-risk features (Table 29-8). The risk of recurrence is greatest within the first 3 years after treatment. About 50% of all recurrences are local, 30% are distant, and 20% are combined. Treatment options for recurrent disease are radiotherapy (if not previously radiated), **chemotherapy,** or **high-dose progestin therapy** (Table 29-7). These therapies, typically megestrol (Megace) or medroxyprogesterone (Provera), have been used with a 30% response rate and minimal side effects.

The use of **ERT** in patients treated for endometrial carcinoma has been controversial. A few preliminary studies suggest that ERT may not affect the rate of recurrence of endometrial cancer. However, at this time, it is usually reserved for those patients whose cancer was well differentiated and minimally invasive. Even then, it is initiated no sooner than 6 to 12 months after treatment. As with traditional use of hormone replacement, use of ERT should be initiated only for severe symptoms and should be given at the lowest effective dose, for the shortest possible duration.

KEY POINTS

- Endometrial cancer is the most common gynecologic cancer but has the best survival rates because it is associated with early symptoms and easy and accurate diagnostic modalities. It is thus diagnosed and treated early.
- Endometrial cancers are classified as type I (80%) or type II (20%). Type I endometrial cancers can be caused by prolonged exposure to exogenous or endogenous estrogen in the absence of progesterone. Endometrial hyperplasia is the typical precursor to type I disease.
- Type II endometrial cancers are *not* estrogen-dependent neoplasms. They are not generally associated with endometrial hyperplasia. They tend to be more aggressive and have a poorer prognosis than type I cancers.
- The most common type of endometrial cancer (80%) is endometrioid adenocarcinoma. Other types have poorer prognosis, including papillary serous and clear cell carcinomas.
- Endometrioid cancer is diagnosed at a median age of 61 with 25% of patients being diagnosed premenopausally and 75% postmenopausally.
- The major risk factors for type I endometrial cancer include unopposed estrogen exposure, endometrial hyperplasia, obesity, chronic anovulation, nulliparity, and late menopause. Hypertension and diabetes are also important risk factors.
- The most common presenting symptom is abnormal uterine bleeding.
- EMB is the standard of care for diagnosing endometrial cancer.
- Currently, there are no cost-effective screening tools for endometrial cancer; however, because of abnormal bleeding, most women are diagnosed early with 75% of lesions being at stage I at the time of diagnosis.
- Endometrial cancer is surgically staged. Treatment may involve TAHBSO with pelvic and para-aortic lymphadenectomy for low-risk, low-stage disease (stages I and II).
- In addition to TAHBSO, pelvic and para-aortic lymph node dissection and pelvic radiation is used to treat women with stage III or IV disease and those with high-risk features (including papillary serous or clear cell types, grade 3 differentiation, large tumor size, lymphovascular invasion, or enlarged lymph nodes).
- Advanced or recurrent disease can be treated with chemotherapy or high-dose progestin therapy.
- Overall 5-year survival rate is 65% with 85% to 100% of recurrences occurring in the first 3 years after treatment.

C Clinical Vignettes

Vignette 1

A 63-year-old G4 P4 woman presents to your office with a chief complaint of vaginal spotting. She reports an isolated episode 1 week prior to presentation that consisted of scant vaginal bleeding. She denies any associated symptoms including pelvic pain, pressure, or early satiety. She also denies any family history of gynecologic malignancy. Her past medical history is significant for morbid obesity, hypertension, and inflammatory bowel disease.

1. What is the most likely diagnosis?
   a. Atrophic endometrium
   b. Endometrial cancer
   c. Endometrial polyp
   d. Ovarian cancer
   e. Adenomyosis
2. After obtaining a thorough history and performing a physical examination (including a pelvic exam), what is the next best step in evaluation?
   a. CA 125
   b. MRI
   c. Cervical cytology
   d. Transvaginal ultrasound and possible EMB
   e. Mammography
3. What is the patient's most significant risk factor for endometrial cancer?
   a. Multiparity
   b. History of prior tobacco use
   c. Remote history of oral contraceptive use
   d. Inflammatory bowel disease
   e. Morbid obesity
4. Upon further questioning, the patient's family history is significant for breast and colon cancer. You are considering a referral to genetic counseling for further evaluation. What familial syndrome (gene mutation) is associated with these malignancies?
   a. BRCA
   b. HER 2 NEU
   c. Lynch II syndrome (hereditary nonpolyposis colorectal cancer)
   d. Cowden syndrome
   e. Peutz–Jeghers syndrome

Vignette 2

A 30-year-old nulligravid patient presenting for her annual examination reports a family history positive for breast and ovarian cancer. Upon further discussion, she notes that her mother developed breast cancer at age 39 and her grandmother passed away from ovarian cancer. After having recently watched an episode about hereditary cancers on her favorite medical talk show, she is wondering if she is a candidate for genetic testing.

1. Which of the following should be recommended?
   a. No testing recommended at this time
   b. Schedule an appointment with a genetic counselor
   c. Order a BRCA test yourself
   d. Recommend a risk-reducing bilateral salpingo-oophorectomy
   e. Recommend surveillance with mammograms every 6 months
2. The patient does accept the referral but is hesitant to pursue the appointment secondary to concerns about losing her health insurance if she tests positive for a genetic predisposition. How do you counsel her?
   a. Reassure her that her results can be kept out of her medical record if she pays cash
   b. Tell her that it is a risk that she must be willing to take
   c. Reassure her that current legislation protects against genetic discrimination
   d. Recommend that a different family member undergoes testing instead
   e. Recommend testing in another country
3. The patient undergoes genetic counseling and tests positive for a BRCA mutation. She is most concerned with her risk for ovarian cancer. After considering the limitations of surveillance for ovarian cancer, she is eager to pursue risk-reducing surgery and declines any fertility sparing measures. Which procedure do you offer the patient?
   a. Bilateral oophorectomy only
   b. Exploratory laparotomy, hysterectomy, and bilateral oophorectomy
   c. Laparoscopic ovarian biopsies, with removal of any cysts
   d. Bilateral salpingo-oophorectomy only
   e. Exploratory laparoscopy, pelvic washings, and bilateral salpingo-oophorectomy

Vignette 3

Your patient is a postmenopausal woman who was recently diagnosed with ductal carcinoma in situ (DCIS) of the breast. Her oncologist has initiated treatment with tamoxifen, and she presents to your office for an annual visit. Her oncologist counseled her to report any postmenopausal bleeding immediately, and she makes an inquiry about the significance of this.

1. In this patient, use of tamoxifen is associated with an increased risk of which of the following?
   a. Endometrial hyperplasia
   b. Invasive carcinoma
   c. Uterine sarcoma
   d. Endometrial polyps
   e. All of the above

2. After receiving the above information, the patient asks whether she warrants any special testing or treatment. She is otherwise asymptomatic. Which do you recommend?
   a. Routine care with pelvic examination, no additional measures unless bleeding develops
   b. Annual transvaginal ultrasound
   c. Annual EMB
   d. Defer to the recommendation of the prescribing oncologist
   e. Serial CA-125 levels

Vignette 4

A 37-year-old patient reports lifelong oligmenorrhea with limited previous evaluation. Her last menstrual period was 10 months ago. She does bring images and report of a recent outside ultrasound that is negative for any anatomic pathology. Her physical examination is significant for obesity (BMI 43) and moderate facial hirsutism, but no other signs of hyperandrogenism. She does not have any other significant comorbidities.

1. What is the most likely diagnosis?
   a. Congenital adrenal hyperplasia
   b. Androgen producing tumor
   c. Conn syndrome
   d. Polycystic ovary syndrome
   e. Anabolic steroid administration

2. In addition to serum testing, what is your next step in the evaluation of this patient?
   a. EMB
   b. Pelvic MRI
   c. Pelvic angiogram
   d. ACTH stimulation test
   e. Transabdominal ultrasound

A Answers

Vignette 1 Question 1
Answer A: Although any vaginal bleeding in a postmenopausal woman warrants a thorough evaluation to rule out endometrial carcinoma, up to 80% of patients will be diagnosed with a benign condition—most commonly endometrial atrophy. The differential diagnosis also includes exogenous estrogens, endometrial or cervical polyps, endometrial hyperplasia, fibroids, ovarian cysts, and endometrial and cervical cancer.

Vignette 1 Question 2
Answer D: Office EMB has an accuracy of 90% to 98% in the detection of endometrial carcinoma. Another option includes transvaginal sonography to assess the thickness of the endometrial lining. An endometrial thickness of 4 mm or less in a postmenopausal woman is indicative of low risk for malignancy. If the endometrial stripe is more than 4 mm or if the patient continues to experience postmenopausal vaginal bleeding, consideration should be given to an EMB or a hysteroscopy, D&C for direct visualization and sampling of the endometrial cavity. Lastly, laboratory studies (TSH, FSH, CBC, prolactin level, cervical cytology, and CA-125) are commonly included in the evaluation of abnormal bleeding, but in the patient described above, pelvic ultrasound with possible EMB are the next best steps.

Vignette 1 Question 3
Answer E: Multiparity, tobacco use, and hormonal contraceptive use are all considered protective factors that decrease the lifetime risk of endometrial cancer. Obesity does confer an increased risk for the development of endometrial cancer, with a relative risk of 10 for those patients who are more than 50 lb overweight. Exogenous unopposed estrogen exposure, nulliparity, late menopause, chronic anovulation (PCOS), hypertension, and diabetes mellitus are also risk factors for endometrial cancer.

Vignette 1 Question 4
Answer C: More than 50% of women who are identified as "at risk" for Lynch syndrome will develop a gynecologic malignancy (ovarian or endometrial) before they develop colorectal cancer. For known carriers of this mutation, annual EMB is recommended, starting at age 35. Ovarian cancer screening with transvaginal ultrasound and CA 125 are recommended at age 30 to 35, or 5 to 10 years earlier than the earliest age of the first diagnosis of these cancers in the family (whichever is earlier). Discussion of prophylactic hysterectomy and salpingo-oophorectomy at around age 35 or at the end of childbearing is appropriate. These patients are not candidates for ovarian preservation if they undergo hysterectomy. Patients who carry the BRCA 1 or 2 germline mutations have an increased risk of breast and ovarian cancer. Patients with Cowden syndrome are at risk for multiple noncancerous hamartomas of the mouth, nose, and intestines. They are also at increased risk for some cancers, including breast, thyroid and endometrial malignancies. Peutz–Jeghers syndrome (PJS) is a hereditary polyposis syndrome notable for benign hamartomatous polyps in the gastrointestinal tract and brown macules on the lips and oral mucosa. Patients with PJS are also at increased risk for certain cancers, including lungs, breast, uterus, and ovaries.

Vignette 2 Question 1
Answer B: Although all patients should be evaluated with a thorough family history, a hereditary cancer risk assessment is best performed by an expert in cancer genetics. These providers have received special training in risk assessment, education, and counseling—and may or may not include genetic testing. Genetic testing may raise several psychological and familial issues, therefore thorough discussion is merited before obtaining the patient's consent. In general, patients with a first-degree relative (mother, sister, or daughter) with breast cancer, mammograms start 5 to 10 years before the age at which the earliest diagnosis was made. This patient would start at age 29—10 years prior to her mom's diagnosis at 39.

Vignette 2 Question 2
Answer C: The Federal Genetic Information Nondiscrimination Act of 2008 protects individuals against health and employment discrimination based on genetic testing. In addition, many state laws protect against the same. However, these laws do *not* apply to other forms of insurance such as life insurance or disability insurance.

Vignette 2 Question 3
Answer E: For risk reducing procedures, either open or laparoscopic procedures can be performed, although laparoscopy may be preferred secondary to morbidity. For either approach, a thorough inspection of all peritoneal surfaces is warranted, along with pelvic washings. Any abnormal areas should be biopsied or resected. Because carriers of the BRCA mutation are at an increased risk for fallopian tube carcinoma, all ovarian and fallopian tissue should be resected.

Vignette 3 Question 1
Answer E: Postmenopausal women taking tamoxifen are at an increased risk for endometrial proliferation, hyperplasia, polyp formation, invasive endometrial carcinoma, and uterine sarcoma. The risk

of developing endometrial cancer is related to dose and duration of tamoxifen use and is greatest in women over 50. A large multicenter study confirmed that the risk of developing endometrial cancer among tamoxifen users was approximately 1.6 per 1,000 person years. But because the use of tamoxifen significantly increased the 5-year survival of patients with breast cancer, the authors concluded that the small risk of developing endometrial cancer is outweighed by the significant survival benefit provided by the drug.

Vignette 3 Question 2
Answer A: Postmenopausal patients on tamoxifen should be vigilant for symptoms of endometrial hyperplasia or cancer; *any* vaginal bleeding, spotting, bloody discharge, or staining should be reported and warrants further evaluation. Routine sonographic evaluation in asymptomatic women has not proven effective, as tamoxifen is known to induce subepithelial stromal hypertrophy (which may not be clinically significant). Similarly, studies have not supported the use of routine EMB for asymptomatic women.

Vignette 4 Question 1
Answer D: In reproductive age women, up to 10% may have hyperandrogenic chronic anovulation (i.e., polycystic ovary syndrome). The clinical hallmarks of this entity are noncyclic menstrual bleeding, hirsutism, and obesity. Adult women with menstrual irregularities should undergo an evaluation that includes TSH, FSH, and prolactin levels. In women with rapid virilization, a tumor can be ruled out by obtaining a pelvic ultrasound and checking levels of testosterone and DHEA-S, and 17-OH progesterone.

Vignette 4 Question 2
Answer A: Although the overall risk of endometrial cancer is very low in women under 45 years, those at high risk for endometrial hyperplasia and cancer who are <45 and present with abnormal uterine bleeding require evaluation. In younger patients with chronic unopposed estrogen exposure, prolonged amenorrhea or other risk factors for uterine carcinoma, endometrial assessment should be performed regardless of age. In this case, the patient is <45 but is at high risk for hyperplasia with a prolonged period of amenorrhea. She should undergo laboratory evaluation ultrasound and endometrial biopsy.

Chapter

30 Ovarian and Fallopian Tube Tumors

TUMORS OF THE OVARIES

There are many types of benign and malignant tumors of the ovaries (Table 30-1), each possessing its own characteristics. Fortunately, 80% of ovarian tumors are benign. In the United States, ovarian cancer is the **second most common cancer of the female genital tract** (Fig. 30-1). Moreover, it is the fifth most common cause of cancer death and the most common cause of gynecologic cancer death. Fallopian tube carcinoma is extremely rare, but the incidence is likely underestimated.

Although ovarian carcinoma accounts for 25% of all gynecologic malignancies (21,990 new cases per year), it is responsible for over **50% of deaths from cancer of the female genital tract** (15,460 deaths per year). This high mortality is due in part to the **lack of effective screening tools** for early diagnosis and presentation at late stages of disease when tumors have spread throughout the peritoneal cavity and the chance for cure is low. Because the overall **5-year survival rate** for women with ovarian carcinoma is only **25% to 45%**, a high degree of suspicion and prompt diagnosis and intervention are critical.

PATHOGENESIS

Tumors of the ovaries are associated with one of the three distinct components of the ovary: the surface **epithelium**, the ovarian **germ cells,** or the ovarian **stroma** (Fig. 30-2). Over 65% of all ovarian tumors and **90% of all ovarian cancers are epithelial tumors** on the ovary capsule. About 5% to 10% of ovarian cancer is metastatic from other primary tumors in the body, usually from the gastrointestinal tract, known as **Krukenberg tumors**, or the breast and endometrium.

Ovarian cancer is spread primarily by **direct exfoliation** of malignant cells from the ovaries. As a result, the sites of metastases often follow the broad circulatory path of the peritoneal fluid. **Lymphatic spread** can also occur, most commonly to the retroperitoneal pelvic and para-aortic lymph nodes (Fig. 28-7). **Hematogenous spread** is responsible for more rare and distant metastases to the lung and brain. In advanced disease, intraperitoneal tumor spread leads to accumulation of ascites in the abdomen and encasement of the bowel with tumor. This results in intermittent bowel obstruction known as a **carcinomatous ileus**. In many cases, this progression results in malnutrition, slow starvation, cachexia, and death.

Although the cause of ovarian carcinoma is unclear, it is believed to result from **malignant transformation of ovarian tissue** after prolonged periods of **chronic uninterrupted ovulation**. Ovulation disrupts the epithelium of the ovary and activates the cellular repair mechanism. When ovulation occurs for long periods without interruption, this mechanism is believed to provide the opportunity for somatic **gene deletions** and **mutations** during the cellular repair process. An emerging theory is that serous ovarian cancers originate in the distal fallopian tube.

About 10% to 15% of women with ovarian cancer have a **familial cancer syndrome**. Patients with mutations in the **BRCA1** gene have an 85% chance of developing breast cancer and a 30% to 50% chance of developing ovarian cancer. A smaller proportion of patients with **BRCA2** gene mutations (25%) also have an increased risk of ovarian cancer. Patients with **Lynch II syndrome** (hereditary nonpolyposis colorectal cancer syndrome [HNPCC]) have a high rate of familial breast, ovarian, colon, and endometrial cancer. High dietary fat and agents such as talc and asbestos have also been proposed as possible etiologic agents in the pathogenesis of ovarian carcinoma.

EPIDEMIOLOGY

An average woman has a **1 in 70 chance of developing ovarian carcinoma** over her lifetime and a 1 in 95 chance of dying from invasive ovarian cancer. The median age of diagnosis is 61 years with two-thirds of women with ovarian cancer being over the age of 55 at the time of diagnosis. Hereditary ovarian cancers typically occur in women who are, on average, 10 years younger than those with nonhereditary ovarian cancer, whereas nonepithelial ovarian cancers are more common in girls and young women. There is a slightly increased frequency in Caucasian women compared to the incidence in Hispanic, Asian, and African American women.

RISK FACTORS

Table 30-2 highlights the major risk factors and protective factors for ovarian cancer. Women with a **familial ovarian cancer syndrome** (BRCA1, BRCA2, or Lynch II syndrome/HNPCC) have the highest risk of ovarian cancer (30% to 50%). Women with a **family history** of ovarian cancer have the next highest risk (5% to 15%). Women with a mother, sister, or daughter with ovarian cancer are at increased risk of developing the disease. The younger the relative is at the time of diagnosis, the higher the risk to first-degree relatives. Similarly, women with a personal history of **breast cancer** have a twofold increase in the incidence of ovarian cancer.

Because the mechanism of ovarian cancer is thought to be linked to mutations occurring during ovulation, women with a history of long periods of **uninterrupted ovulation** (early menarche, infertility, nulliparity, delayed childbearing, late-onset menopause) are at increased risk of ovarian cancer. For the same reason, **increasing age** is another major risk factor for ovarian cancer. Fifty percent of all women diagnosed with ovarian cancer are 63 years of age or older. Other proposed

TABLE 30-1 Benign and Malignant Ovarian Tumors

Epithelial tumors	Serous tumors
	Serous cystadenoma
	Borderline serous tumor
	Serous cystadenocarcinoma
	Adenofibroma and cystadenofibroma
	Mucinous tumors
	Mucinous cystadenoma
	Borderline mucinous tumor
	Mucinous cystadenocarcinoma
	Endometrioid carcinoma
	Clear cell adenocarcinoma
	Brenner tumor
	Undifferentiated carcinoma
Germ cell tumors	Teratoma
	Benign (mature, adult)
	Cystic teratoma (dermoid cyst)
	Solid teratoma
	Malignant (immature)
	Monodermal or specialized (e.g., carcinoid, struma ovarii) Dysgerminoma
	Endodermal sinus tumor
	Choriocarcinoma
	Embryonal carcinoma
	Polyembryoma
	Mixed germ cell tumors
Sex cord–stromal tumors	Granulosa–theca cell tumors
	Granulosa cell tumor
	Thecoma
	Fibroma
	Sertoli–Leydig cell tumor (androblastoma)
	Gonadoblastoma
Unclassified	Ex. lipoid-cell tumors and sarcomas
Metastatic tumors	Ex. from GI tract, female genital tract, or breast

Reproduced with permission from Robbins S, Cotran R, Kumar V. *Robbins' Pathologic Basis of Disease.* Philadelphia, PA: WB Saunders; 1991:1158.

risk factors include the use of talcum powder on the perineum and obesity (BMI > 30).

PROTECTIVE FACTORS

Many of the factors found to be protective from ovarian cancer (Table 30-2) are also linked to the **incessant ovulation** hypotheses. This speculates that ovulation suppression results in less disruption of the ovarian epithelium and less need for activation of the cellular repair mechanism. Thus, there are fewer opportunities for gene deletions and mutations. **Oral contraceptives** (OCPs) have been found to have a protective effect against ovarian cancer by suppressing ovulation. Use of OCPs for greater than 5 years can reduce the risk of ovarian cancer by 50%. Similarly, **breastfeeding**, **multiparity**, and **chronic anovulation** have also been found to be protective agents that act by interrupting or suppressing ovulation. **Tubal ligation** and **hysterectomy** have been associated with a 67% and 30% reduction in ovarian cancer, respectively, even in patients with a familial cancer syndrome. This may be due to impairment of ovarian blood supply by these procedures and/or decreased migration of carcinogens from the lower genital tract up to the ovaries.

CLINICAL MANIFESTATIONS

History

Patients with ovarian cancer are most often **asymptomatic** or have **vague, nonspecific complaints** until the disease has progressed to the advanced stages. Some patients may present with **vague lower abdominal pain**, abdominal distension, bloating, and **early satiety** (Table 30-3). As the tumors progress, other symptoms may develop, including gastrointestinal complaints (nausea, anorexia, indigestion), urinary frequency, dysuria, and pelvic pressure. Ascites may develop in later stages and cause shortness of breath secondary to pleural effusion. Ventral hernia may also be seen owing to increased intra-abdominal pressure.

Physical Examination

There is no evidence to suggest that routine pelvic examination improves the early diagnosis of ovarian cancer. As the disease progresses, the primary findings on examination are a **solid, fixed, irregular pelvic mass** (Table 30-4) that may extend into the upper abdomen and **ascites** (Color Plate 15). Ovarian cancer metastasis to the umbilicus is known as **Sister Mary Joseph nodule**. When a mass is located on examination, there is an increased likelihood of cancer in postmenopausal women (30% to 60%) compared to premenopausal women (5% to 15%).

DIAGNOSTIC EVALUATION

Pelvic ultrasound is the primary diagnostic tool for investigating an adnexal mass. These sonographic traits help to distinguish between benign and malignant tumors (Table 30-5). Other studies, including **computed tomography** (CT) and **magnetic resonance imaging** of the pelvis and abdomen, can assist in diagnosis and in delineation of the spread of disease. Because malignant cells can spread via direct exfoliation, paracentesis and cyst aspiration should be avoided. Once the diagnosis is made, studies are undertaken to look for **metastatic disease** and to distinguish between primary and secondary ovarian cancer. **Barium enema and intravenous pyelography** are helpful in looking for gastrointestinal (GI) and genital urinary sources of disease.

Depending on the type of tumor, ovarian malignancies can be monitored using the **serum tumor markers** CA-125,

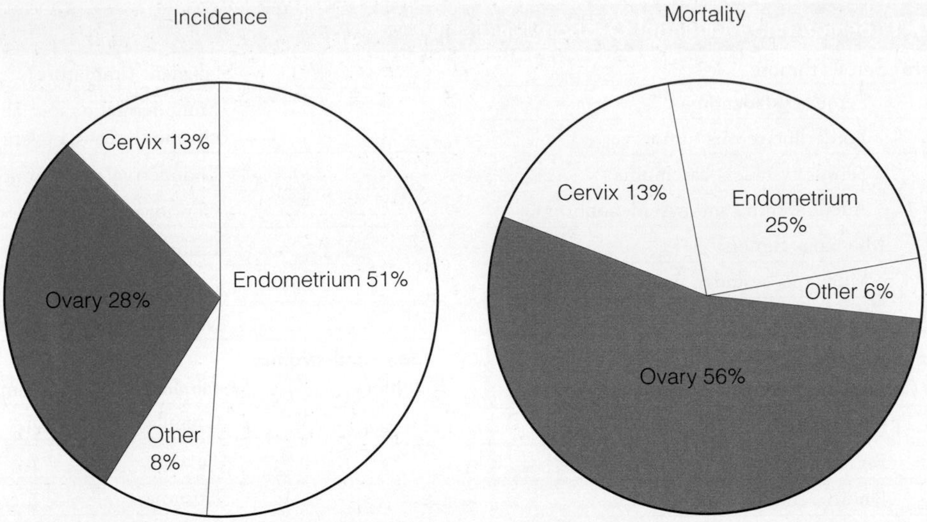

Figure 30-1 • Relationships of ovarian cancer to other gynecologic cancer for incidence and mortality; United States, 1996.
(Modified from Parker SL, Tong T, Bolden S, et al. Cancer statistics. *CA Cancer J Clin.* 1996;46:5–27.)

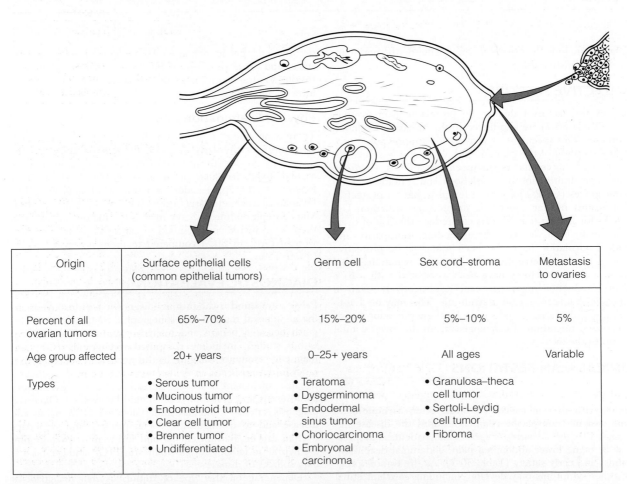

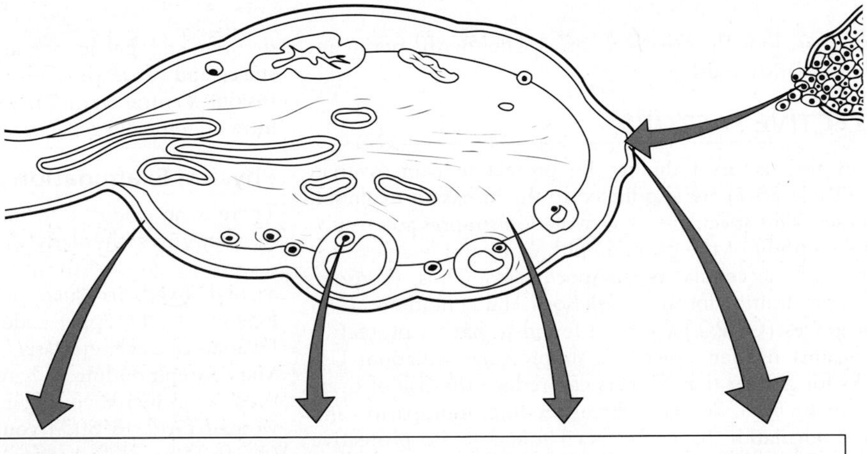

Origin	Surface epithelial cells (common epithelial tumors)	Germ cell	Sex cord–stroma	Metastasis to ovaries
Percent of all ovarian tumors	65%–70%	15%–20%	5%–10%	5%
Age group affected	20+ years	0–25+ years	All ages	Variable
Types	• Serous tumor • Mucinous tumor • Endometrioid tumor • Clear cell tumor • Brenner tumor • Undifferentiated	• Teratoma • Dysgerminoma • Endodermal sinus tumor • Choriocarcinoma • Embryonal carcinoma	• Granulosa–theca cell tumor • Sertoli-Leydig cell tumor • Fibroma	

Figure 30-2 • Classification of various ovarian neoplasms (benign, borderline, and malignant).

TABLE 30-2 Risk Factors and Protective Factors for Ovarian Cancer

Risk factors	
	Familial ovarian cancer syndrome
	Family history of breast and/or ovarian cancer
	Personal history of breast cancer
	Increasing age
	Early menarche (<12 y)
	Infertility
	Nulliparity
	Late-onset menopause (>50 y)
	Obesity (BMI > 30)
Protective factors	
	Use of OCPs (5+ y)
	Multiparity
	Breastfeeding
	Tubal ligation
	Hysterectomy

TABLE 30-3 Symptoms of Ovarian Cancer

Initial symptoms
Bloating
Early satiety
Dyspepsia
Abdominal pain
Pelvic pain
Later symptoms
Back pain
Urinary frequency/urgency
Constipation
Fatigue
Dyspareunia
Menstrual changes

a-fetoprotein (AFP), lactate dehydrogenase (LDH), and human chorionic gonadotropins (hCG).

SURGICAL STAGING

Ovarian carcinoma is **surgically staged** (Table 30-6). Primary staging includes total abdominal hysterectomy, bilateral salpingo-oophorectomy (**TAHBSO**), **omentectomy, peritoneal washings,** Pap smear of the diaphragm, and **sampling the pelvic and para-aortic lymph nodes**. Because there are no reliable screening tools for ovarian cancer and few early symptoms, nearly 75% of patients present with stage III or IV. Subsequently, the 5-year survival is low overall (25% to 45%) and decreases with increasing age. The different types of ovarian cancers are discussed below.

TABLE 30-4 Evaluation of Pelvic and Abdominal Masses Found on Physical Examination

	Benign	**Malignant**
Mobility	Mobile	Fixed
Consistency	Cystic	Solid
Tumor surface	Smooth	Irregular
Bilateral or unilateral	Unilateral	Bilateral

TABLE 30-5 Ultrasound Findings in Patients with a Pelvic Mass

	Benign	**Malignant**
Size	<8 cm	>8 cm
Consistency	Cystic	Solid or cystic and solid
Solid components	Not present	Nodular, papillary
Septations	Not present or singular	Multilocular, thick (>2 mm)
Doppler flow	Not present	Present in solid component
Bilateral or unilateral	Unilateral	Bilateral
Associated features	Calcification, especially Teeth	Ascites, peritoneal masses, lymphadenopathy

EPITHELIAL TUMORS

PATHOGENESIS

Epithelial cell tumors of the ovaries are derived from malignant transformation of the **epithelium cells** of the surface of the ovary. These cells come from the primitive mesoderm and are capable of undergoing metaplasia. The six primary types of epithelial tumors are serous, mucinous, endometrioid, clear cell, Brenner, and undifferentiated (Fig. 30-2). The neoplasms in this group range in malignant potential from benign to borderline (tumors of **low malignant potential**) to frankly malignant. **Serous cystadenocarcinomas** are the most common malignant epithelial cell tumors.

Malignant epithelial tumors extend from the surface capsule of the ovary to seed the peritoneal cavity. In more than 75% of patients, tumors have spread beyond the ovary at the time of diagnosis; thus the prognosis is very poor.

EPIDEMIOLOGY

Epithelial tumors tend to occur in patients who are in their 50s with a peak incidence from 56 to 60 years of age. **Epithelial cell cancers account for 65% of all ovarian tumors** and more than **90% of ovarian cancers. Serous tumors** (serous cystadenocarcinomas) are the most common type of epithelial ovarian cancer. These tumors are large, cystic, and bilateral 65% of the time.

TABLE 30-6 Staging of Ovarian Carcinoma

Stage I: Growth limited to the ovaries
Ia—one ovary involved
Ib—both ovaries involved
Ic—Ia or Ib and ovarian surface tumor, ruptured capsule, malignant ascites, or peritoneal cytology positive for malignant cells
Stage II: Disease extension from the ovary to the pelvis
IIa—extension to the uterus or fallopian tube
IIb—extension to other pelvic tissues
IIc—IIa or IIb and ovarian surface tumor, ruptured capsule, malignant ascites, or peritoneal cytology positive for malignant cells
Stage III: Disease extension to the abdominal cavity
IIIa—abdominal peritoneal surfaces with microscopic metastases
IIIb—tumor metastases >2 cm in size
IIIc—tumor metastases >2 cm in size or metastatic disease in the pelvic, para-aortic, or inguinal lymph nodes
Stage IV: Distant metastatic disease
Malignant pleural effusion
Pulmonary parenchymal metastases
Liver or splenic parenchymal metastases (not surface implants)
Metastases to the supraclavicular lymph nodes or skin

TABLE 30-7 Gynecologic and Nongynecologic Conditions Associated with Elevated CA-125 Levels

Gynecologic cancers
Epithelial ovarian cancer
Fallopian tube cancer
Endometrial cancer
Endocervical cancer
Nongynecologic cancers
Pancreatic cancer
Lung cancer
Breast cancer
Colon cancer
Benign gynecologic conditions
Normal and ectopic pregnancy
Endometriosis
Fibroids
Pelvic inflammatory disease
Benign nongynecologic conditions
Pancreatitis
Cirrhosis
Peritonitis
Recent laparotomy

CLINICAL MANIFESTATIONS

The serum tumor marker **CA-125** is elevated in 80% of epithelial cell cancers. Because CA-125 levels correlate with the progression and regression of these tumors, it has been useful in **tracking the effect of treatment and recurrence** of epithelial ovarian carcinoma. Its value as a screening tool for the detection of ovarian cancer has not yet been established. One reason for this is the high number of benign and malignant gynecologic and nongynecologic conditions associated with an elevated CA-125 level (Table 30-7).

TREATMENT

Surgery is the mainstay of treatment for epithelial cell tumors, including TAHBSO, omentectomy, cytoreduction or "debulking," and bilateral pelvic and para-aortic lymph node sampling. The goal of debulking is to leave behind no visible tumors or tumor nodules no greater than 1 cm. When this is achieved, the patient is said to have undergone optimal debulking. When optimal debulking is not achieved, there is a greater chance of recurrent or persistent disease.

After surgery, epithelial ovarian cancer is treated with combination chemotherapy, most commonly intravenous **carboplatin and paclitaxel** (Taxol) or docetaxel (Taxotere). Patients who have had optimal debulking are offered **intraperitoneal cisplatin and paclitaxel chemotherapy** along with intravenous chemotherapy, which increases overall survival, but also has more side effects than traditional intravenous chemotherapy.

The tumor marker **CA-125** and **CAT scan imaging** are most commonly used to evaluate the success of treatment and to diagnose recurrent disease. Unfortunately, tumors **frequently recur** despite aggressive treatment. Recurrent or persistent cancer is treated with chemotherapy. Recurrent ascites is treated with paracentesis.

The overall **5-year survival rate is 20%** for patients with epithelial ovarian cancer (80% to 95% for stage I, 40% to 70% for stage II, 30% for stage III, and <10% for stage IV disease).

GERM CELL TUMORS

PATHOGENESIS

Germ cell ovarian tumors arise from primordial germ cells of the ovary and may be benign (95%) or malignant (5%). These undifferentiated, totipotent germ cells are capable of differentiating into any of the three germ cell layers: yolk sac, placenta, and fetus. This accounts for the various subtypes of germ cell tumors (Fig. 30-3).

The most common type of germ cell tumor is the **benign cystic mature teratoma**, also known as **dermoid cysts**. Dermoids are cystic masses containing mature adult tissue such as skin, hair, and teeth mixed in sebaceous material, giving them a very characteristic appearance (Color Plate 16). Cystectomy is recommended for definitive diagnosis and to rule out malignancy.

The most common malignant germ cell tumors are **dysgerminomas (50%)**, **immature teratomas (20%)**, and endodermal

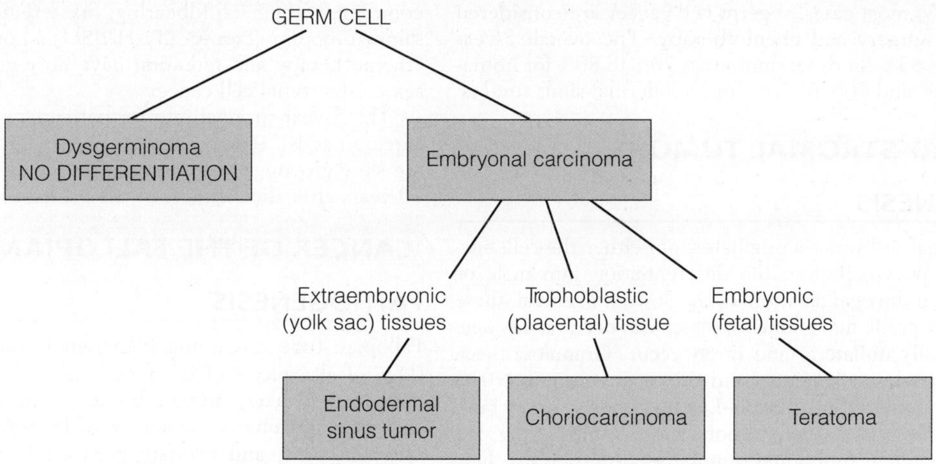

Figure 30-3 • Histogenesis of tumors of germ cell origin. Because they are totipotent, germ cells may remain undifferentiated, or they may develop into any of the three germ layers: yolk sac or placental or fetal tissue.

sinus (yolk sac) tumors (20%). Embryonal carcinoma (composed of undifferentiated cells), nongestational choriocarcinoma (composed of placental tissue), and mixed germ cell tumors are much less common.

Many germ cell tumors produce **serum tumor markers** that can be useful in the diagnosis of a pelvic mass and in assessing a patient's response to therapy (Table 30-8). Although there is wide variation in the type of serum tumor markers, in general, dysgerminomas produce LDH, endodermal sinus (yolk sac) tumors produce AFP, and choriocarcinomas produce hCG. The undifferentiated embryonal carcinomas that give rise to the more differentiated germ cell tumors produce both AFP and hCG.

In contrast to epithelial tumors, most germ cell tumors **grow rapidly**, are **limited to one ovary**, and are at **stage I** at the time of diagnosis. The prognosis for germ cell tumors is therefore far better than that for epithelial tumors. In most cases, **these tumors are considered curable.**

EPIDEMIOLOGY

Germ cell tumors account for 20% to 25% of all ovarian tumors but make up less than 5% of ovarian cancers. Although **95% are benign**, the remaining 5% of germ cell tumors are malignant and found primarily in children and in young women. This makes germ cell tumors the **most common ovarian malignancy in women less than 20 years of age**. Malignant germ cell tumors are three times more common in **black and Asian women** compared to Caucasian women.

TABLE 30-8 Primary Serum Tumor Marker for Germ Cell Cancers

Tumor Type	Primary Tumor Marker
Dysgerminoma	LDH
Immature teratoma	N/A
Endodermal sinus (yolk sac) tumor	AFP
Embryonal carcinoma	AFP and hCG
Choriocarcinoma	hCG

CLINICAL MANIFESTATIONS

Unlike the slow-growing epithelial ovarian cancers, germ cell tumors **grow rapidly** and thus cause symptoms leading to earlier diagnosis. Most commonly, distension of the ovarian capsule from rapid growth, **hemorrhage, and necrosis** results in acute **pelvic pain**. Patients may also complain of **pressure symptoms** on the bladder or rectum or pain from **torsion or rupture** of the tumor. Eighty-five percent of women will have abdominal pain and a pelvic mass at the time of presentation.

TREATMENT

Women with benign germ cell tumors such as mature teratomas (dermoid cysts) are diagnosed and cured by removing the part of the ovary containing the tumor (ovarian cystectomy) or by removing the entire ovary (oophorectomy).

Because most germ cell cancers are diagnosed in the early stage and are **rarely bilateral**, surgery is typically limited to **unilateral salpingo-oophorectomy** if fertility is desired. However, complete surgical staging should still be performed. If childbearing is complete or if the cancer is bilateral, total abdominal hysterectomy and bilateral salpingo-oophorectomy (TAH/BSO) is required along with surgical staging.

With the exception of stage Ia dysgerminomas and immature teratomas, all germ cell malignancies require **multiagent chemotherapy** after surgery. The most common regimen is bleomycin, etoposide, and cisplatin (Platinol) (BEP). In patients who have elevated **serum tumor markers** prior to treatment, these markers can be used to judge the effectiveness of therapy between chemotherapy cycles.

In the past, **radiation therapy** was used as the primary treatment for **dysgerminomas**, which are exquisitely sensitive to radiation. However, current combination chemotherapy regimens have proven to be as good as or better than radiation therapy. Chemotherapy is also more protective of future fertility when only one ovary is removed.

Fortunately, most cases of germ cell cancer are **considered curable** with surgery and chemotherapy. The overall 5-year survival rate is 85% for dysgerminomas, 70% to 80% for immature teratomas, and 60% to 70% for endodermal sinus tumors.

SEX CORD-STROMAL TUMORS

PATHOGENESIS

Ovarian stromal cell tumors originate from either the cells surrounding the oocyte (before the differentiation into male or female) or from the ovarian stroma (Fig. 30-2). In general, these tumors are **low-grade malignancies,** which can **occur at any age**. They are **usually unilateral** and **rarely recur**. Granulosa-theca cells are low-grade malignancies and the most common (70%) type of tumor in this group. Sertoli–Leydig tumors are very rare.

Both granulosa-theca cell tumors and Sertoli–Leydig cell tumors are known as **functional tumors** because they are characterized by **hormone production**. Ovarian stroma can develop into an ovary or a testis. As a result, ovarian **granulosa-theca cell tumors** resemble fetal ovaries and produce large amounts of estrogens. Microscopically, the granulosa cells have grooved "coffee-bean" nuclei, and the cells are arranged in small clusters around a central cavity. These histologic configurations are known as **Call–Exner bodies**, which are pathognomonic for granulosa cell tumors. Conversely, ovarian **Sertoli–Leydig cell tumors** resemble fetal testes and produce testosterone and other androgens.

The third type of stromal cell tumor, the **ovarian fibroma**, is derived from mature fibroblasts and, unlike the other sex cord-stromal tumors, is not a functioning tumor. Occasionally, fibromas are associated with ascites. The triad of an ovarian **tumor, ascites, and right hydrothorax** is known as **Meigs syndrome.**

EPIDEMIOLOGY

Sex cord-stromal ovarian tumors can affect women of any age but occur most commonly in women between ages **40 and 70**. The mean age at diagnosis is 50. Because of estrogen stimulation, 25% to 50% of women with granulosa cell tumors will have **endometrial hyperplasia** and 5% will have concurrent **endometrial cancer**. Most Sertoli–Leydig tumors occur in women under 40.

CLINICAL MANIFESTATIONS

Granulosa-theca cell tumors often produce **estradiol and inhibin A/B**. The estrogen stimulation can cause feminization, precocious puberty, menstrual irregularities, secondary amenorrhea, or postmenopausal bleeding. This estrogen stimulation can lead to endometrial hyperplasia and/or endometrial cancer; therefore, **endometrial sampling** is very important in this setting. Sertoli–Leydig cell tumors produce **androgens** (testosterone, androstenedione) that can cause **virilizing effects** in 75% of patients, including breast atrophy, hirsutism, deepened voice, acne, clitoromegaly, and receding hairline. Patients may also have oligomenorrhea or amenorrhea.

TREATMENT

Because most sex cord-stromal tumors are low-grade lesions, unilateral, and do not often recur, the usual treatment is **unilateral salpingo-oophorectomy**. In women who have completed their childbearing, hysterectomy and bilateral salpingo-oophorectomy (TAH/BSO) should be performed. Chemotherapy and radiation have no regular role in treating sex cord-stromal cell cancers.

The 5-year survival rate for patients with sex cord-stromal carcinomas is 70% to 90%. However, granulosa cell tumors are slow growing, and late recurrences can be detected 15 to 20 years after the removal of the primary lesion.

CANCER OF THE FALLOPIAN TUBES

PATHOGENESIS

Fallopian tube carcinoma is **extremely rare**, comprising only 0.5% of all cancers of the female genital tract. However, the incidence is likely underestimated. An emerging theory is the fallopian tube is the source of high-grade serous ovarian, fallopian tube, and primary peritoneal cancers. The disease progression of these tumors is **similar to that of ovarian cancer**, including wide **peritoneal spread** and **ascites** accumulation. However, the exact etiology of fallopian cancer is unknown. Most fallopian tube cancers are **adenocarcinomas** arising from the mucosa of the tube. The tube is often hugely dilated, and the lumen is filled with papillary growth of solid tumor. The fimbriated end is closed in 50% of cases. Fallopian cancer is bilateral in 10% of cases and is **often the result of metastasis** from other primary tumors. Sarcomas and mixed tumors are less common.

EPIDEMIOLOGY

Primary fallopian tube carcinoma is very rare. These tumors can occur at any age (18 to 80), but the mean age at diagnosis is 55 to 60. Like epithelial ovarian cancers, fallopian tube cancers occur **more frequently in Caucasian women** as compared to African American women. Risk factors include **familial cancer syndromes** (BRCA1 and BRCA2), **nulliparity**, and **infertility**.

CLINICAL MANIFESTATIONS

Fallopian tube cancer is typically **asymptomatic** and is usually diagnosed during pelvic surgery for other indications. The classic triad of **profuse watery discharge, pelvic pain,** and **pelvic mass** is known as Latzko's triad. Although the triad is seen in only 15% of cases, it is considered pathognomonic for fallopian tube carcinoma. The same is true for **hydrops tubae profluens** (intermittent hydrosalpinx), the phenomenon of spontaneous or pressure-induced discharge of watery or blood-tinged vaginal discharge resulting in shrinkage of the adnexal mass. Patients may also report low back pain.

DIAGNOSIS

The diagnosis of fallopian tube cancer is almost never made preoperatively. **Ultrasound** may reveal a complex adnexal mass or ascites. The **CA-125** is often elevated in these patients and **cervical cytology** may rarely show malignant cells with subsequent negative cervical and endometrial biopsy.

TREATMENT

Fallopian tube cancers are **surgically staged**. One-third of patients are stage I at the time of diagnosis, one-third are stage II, and one-third are stage III or IV. The treatment of fallopian tube cancer is the same as that of epithelial ovarian cancer, including TAHBSO, omentectomy, cytoreduction, peritoneal cytologic studies, and retroperitoneal lymph node sampling. After surgery, adjunctive chemotherapy is given including intravenous chemotherapy with **carboplatin and paclitaxel (Taxol) or** with intrperitoneal and intravenous chemotherapy for optimally debulked advanced stage cancers. CA-125 levels and CT imaging can be used to monitor the effectiveness of treatment.

The prognosis for fallopian tube cancer is reported to be slightly better than that of epithelial ovarian cancer. The overall 5-year survival rate is 45% (71% for stage I, 48% for stage II, 25% for stage III, and 17% for stage IV disease).

KEY POINTS

- Epithelial tumors of the ovary account for 90% of ovarian cancers.
- Most patients diagnosed with epithelial tumors of the ovary are diagnosed at stage III or higher.
- When symptoms are present, they might include low abdominal pain, bloating, early satiety, pelvic mass, and ascites. Pelvic ultrasound and abdominal-pelvic CT often reveal a fixed, solid, nodular mass.
- Epithelial ovarian cancers are staged surgically and treated with surgery (TAHBSO, omentectomy, pelvic and para-aortic lymph node sampling, and cytoreduction) followed by Taxol and carboplatin chemotherapy.
- The tumor marker CA-125 can be used to evaluate the success of treatment and look for recurrence of disease but is not appropriate to use as a screening tool for ovarian cancer.
- The 5-year survival rate for epithelial ovarian cancer is less than 20%.
- Germ cell tumors arise from totipotential germ cells capable of differentiating into yolk sac, placental or fetal tissues; 95% are benign and 5% are malignant.
- The most common germ cell tumor is the benign mature cystic teratoma (dermoid cyst). The most common malignant germ cell tumors are dysgerminomas (50%) and immature teratomas (20%).
- Germ cell tumors occur primarily in women under age 20, grow rapidly, are usually unilateral, and are diagnosed at early stages. They often produce serum tumor markers (LDH, AFP, and/or hCG) that can be used in the diagnosis of a pelvic mass and to assess response to therapy.
- Most germ cell tumors are treated by removal of the affected ovary, staging, and combination chemotherapy with BEP with good 5-year survival rates (60% to 85%), depending on the type of tumor.
- Sex cord-stromal germ cell tumors are derived from the cells surrounding the oocyte that produce steroid hormones or from the ovarian stroma.
- Sex cord-stromal tumors are slow-growing tumors with low malignant potential and are often found only incidentally, usually in women between 40 and 70 years old. Sertoli–Leydig cell tumors are rare and occur most often in women under age 40.
- Granulosa cell tumors are the most common type (70%) of sex cord-stromal tumor. They secrete inhibin and estradiol, resulting in feminization and potentially endometrial hyperplasia and/or cancer. Microscopic Call–Exner bodies are pathognomonic for granulosa cell tumors.
- Sertoli–Leydig cell tumors are rare. They secrete androgens causing virilization in patients.
- Ovarian fibromas are derived from mature fibroblasts. These are nonfunctioning tumors. Meigs syndrome consists of the triad of ovarian tumor, ascites, and right hydrothorax.
- The sex cord-stromal tumors are treated surgically, usually with unilateral salpingo-oophorectomy in younger women or TAHBSO in women who have completed their childbearing.
- Sertoli–Leydig cell tumors do not frequently recur, but granulosa cell tumors often have late recurrences 15 to 20 years later.
- Fallopian tube cancers are rare malignancies that can occur at any age. They behave very similar to epithelial ovarian cancers.
- These are usually adenocarcinomas arising from the mucosa or metastases from other primary tumors. Fallopian tube cancers are usually asymptomatic and are rarely diagnosed preoperatively.
- The classic triad of pain, profuse watery discharge (hydrops tubae profluens), and pelvic mass is considered pathognomonic for fallopian tube carcinoma but only occurs in 15% of patients.
- Fallopian tube cancers are treated similar to epithelial ovarian cancers with TAHBSO, omentectomy, cytoreduction, and pelvic lymph node sampling followed by combination chemotherapy.
- The overall 5-year survival rate is 45%.

C Clinical Vignettes

Vignette 1

1. A 17-year-old Asian teen presents to the ED with left lower quadrant (LLQ) pain. Her pregnancy test, UA, and cervical cultures are all negative. She denies sexual activity. On pelvic ultrasound, she is found to have a unilateral complex ovarian mass. What is the most likely diagnosis?
   a. Serous cystadenocarcinoma
   b. Dysgerminoma
   c. Granulosa-theca cell tumor
   d. Mature teratoma
   e. Any of the above

2. What tumor marker is associated with this type of tumor?
   a. hCG
   b. AFP
   c. Ca-125
   d. LDH
   e. All of the above

3. Expected treatment would likely include which of the following?
   a. Unilateral salpingo-oophorectomy plus surgical staging
   b. Bilateral salpingo-oophorectomy plus surgical staging
   c. Total abdominal hysterectomy and bilateral salpingo-oophorectomy with surgical staging
   d. Chemotherapy only
   e. Radiation only

Vignette 2

1. A 56-year-old G3 P2 presents with postmenopausal bleeding. Transvaginal ultrasound reveals a 12-mm endometrial stripe and an 8-cm complex left adnexal mass. An endometrial biopsy reveals endometrial hyperplasia. What characteristics of the mass make it concerning for malignancy?
   a. Fixed, nonmobile location
   b. Internal septations
   c. Surface excrescences
   d. Papillary and nodular solid components
   e. All of the above

2. What is the most likely diagnosis in this patient?
   a. Mucinous cystadenocarcinoma
   b. Benign teratomas
   c. Granulosa-theca cell tumor
   d. Endometrioma
   e. Choriocarcinoma

3. During her preoperative evaluation, she undergoes an abdominal-pelvic CT and chest X-ray for imaging. She is found to have ascites and a right hydrothorax. This combination of adnexal mass, ascites, and hydrothorax is known as:
   a. Latzko's triad
   b. Hydrops tubae profluens
   c. Syndrome X
   d. Meigs syndrome
   e. Metabolic syndrome

Vignette 3

1. A 63-year-old G0 presents to you with a complaint of LLQ pain, intermittent nausea, abdominal pressure, and bloating. Her history is notable for mild obesity, right breast cancer, and hypertension. She and her husband desired children but were never able to conceive. Her family history is notable for premenopausal breast cancer in her mother and maternal aunt. She had a pelvic ultrasound showing a normal appearing uterus with a 7-cm left ovarian mass containing internal septations and papillary excrescences. She has moderate ascites and her Ca-125 was 719. Which of the following is associated with an increased risk of ovarian cancer?
   a. Personal history of breast cancer
   b. Multiparity
   c. Breastfeeding
   d. Tubal ligation
   e. Hysterectomy

2. She underwent TAH, BSO, collection of pelvic washings, omentectomy, cytoreduction or "debulking," and bilateral pelvic and para-aortic lymph node sampling. The mass had spread beyond the ovary to the omentum, peritoneum, and bowel. She was found to have ascites, and pelvic washings were positive. There did not appear to be any liver or lymph node involvement. What stage of ovarian cancer does she have?
   a. Stage I
   b. Stage II
   c. Stage III
   d. Stage IV
   e. None of the above

3. Postoperative chemotherapy is most likely to include which regimen?
   a. Cisplatin
   b. Carboplatin and Taxol
   c. Cisplatin and Taxol

d. Methotrexate
e. Methotrexate and actinomycin-D

Vignette 4

A 64-year-old G2 P2 presents for her annual examination. She complains of abdominal bloating and has noted some difficulty zipping her pants despite a recent unplanned 10-lb weight loss. She has also noticed copious watery vaginal discharge, often preceded by a sharp pain in her LLQ.

1. This complex of symptoms is suspicious for what condition?
   a. Epithelial ovarian cancer
   b. Germ cell
   c. Dysgerminoma
   d. Fallopian tube cancer
   e. Endometrial cancer
2. Which of the following is *not* true regarding this patient's cancer?
   a. It is extremely rare
   b. It often results as a metastasis from another site
   c. It is bilateral 90% of the time
   d. It spreads along the circulatory path of the peritoneal fluid
   e. It is associated with an elevated Ca-125 and ascites, but rarely with abnormal cervical cytology
3. Fallopian tube cancer behaves most like what other GYN cancer?
   a. Vulvar
   b. Vaginal
   c. Cervical
   d. Endometrial
   e. Ovarian

A Answers

Vignette 1 Question 1
Answer B: In a young patient, immature teratomas and dysgerminomas are most common. This patient likely has a dysgerminoma. Eighty-five percent of patients with dysgerminomas present similar to this with abdominal pain and a pelvic mass. These occur most commonly in children and young girls. They are more common in Black and Asian females. They tend to be rapid growing and present with pelvic pain, pressure, and rupture. Serous cystadenocarcinoma is an epithelial ovarian cancer—which make up 80% of all ovarian cancers. These occur most commonly in the sixth decade and tend to be bilateral.

Vignette 1 Question 2
Answer D: Many ovarian tumors produce serum tumor markers that aid in the diagnosis and clinical monitoring of treatment. Dysgerminomas most commonly produce LDH. hCG secretion is common in embryonal sinus tumors and choriocarcinomas. Ca-125 can be found in ovarian neoplasms that are derived from the epithelium of the ovary. The Ca-125 tumor marker can also be seen in any number of benign and malignant gynecologic and nongynecologic conditions such as pancreatic cancer, lung cancer, breast cancer, endometriosis, pregnancy, fibroids, PID, pancreatitis, cirrhosis, and peritonitis.

Vignette 1 Question 3
Answer A: Because most germ cell tumors are diagnosed in the early stages and are rarely bilateral, most can be treated with unilateral salpingo-oophorectomy. However, complete surgical staging should be done. If childbearing is complete, or if the cancer is bilateral, total abdominal hysterectomy and bilateral salpingo-oophorectomy should be done along with surgical staging. Dysgerminomas are very sensitive to radiation therapy and chemotherapy. Either can be used after surgical treatment in all but stage Ia patients.

Vignette 2 Question 1
Answer E: Some characteristic findings on pelvic examination and imaging are concerning for malignancy. On examination, a fixed, solid, irregular, bilateral tumor is more likely to be malignant than a mobile, cystic, smooth, unilateral tumor. Similarly, on imaging, masses that are above 8 cm with solid components, internal septations, surface nodules, or excrescences are more concerning for a malignant process. Associated features such as ascites, peritoneal masses, and lymphadenopathy are more suggestive of a malignant process.

Vignette 2 Question 2
Answer C: Although many of these options are possible, the presentation of the endometrial hyperplasia along with the ovarian mass is more characteristic of a granulosa-theca cell tumor. These sex cord-stromal tumors resemble cells of the fetal ovaries and thus produce high amounts of estrogens. They are often unilateral, low-grade and functional tumors. This endogenous unopposed estrogen production results in stimulation of the endometrium, a thickened endometrial stripe on pelvic ultrasound, and bleeding in this postmenopausal patient. Microscopically, the nuclei of the granulosa cell tumors are grooved and "coffee-bean" shaped, and the cells are arranged in microclusters known as Call–Exner bodies. These are pathognomonic for granulosa cell tumors. Mucinous adenocarcinomas tend to be quite large and may be associated with mucinous tumors of the appendix as well. Benign cystic mature teratomas (dermoid tumors) are the most common type of germ cell tumor. Dermoids and endometriomas both have very characteristic appearances. Dermoids can contain tissue from skin, hair, teeth, bone, and sebaceous material. Endometriomas have a ground glass appearance.

Vignette 2 Question 3
Answer D: Meigs syndrome is the presentation of ascites and hydrothorax along with an ovarian fibromas or other pelvic tumor. Latzko's triad is associated with the classic triad of profuse watery discharge (hydrops tubae profluens), pelvic pain, and pelvic mass seen in association with fallopian tube cancers. Hydrops tubae profluens (or intermittent hydrosalpinx) is the phenomenon of spontaneous or pressure-induced release of watery or blood-tinged vaginal discharge resulting in shrinkage of a pelvic mass. This is likewise associated with fallopian tube cancers.

Syndrome X is also known as metabolic syndrome and insulin-resistance syndrome. This syndrome is characterized by hypertension, obesity, insulin resistance or NIDDM along with hypertriglyceridemia, increased peripheral vascular disease, and elevated catecholamine levels.

Vignette 3 Question 1
Answer A: Risk factors for ovarian cancer include familial ovarian cancer syndromes (Lynch II/hereditary nonpolyposis colon cancer, BRAC1 and 2), family history of breast and/or ovarian cancer, personal history of breast cancer, increasing age, early menarche and late menopause, infertility, nulliparity, and obesity (BMI $>$ 30). Most of these characteristics are associated with prolonged or increased ovulation. Conversely, many of the protective factors for ovarian cancer include those which decrease the lifetime number of ovulations such as multiparity, breastfeeding, and greater than 5 years of OCP use. Other protective factors include hysterectomy and tubal ligation.

Vignette 3 Question 2
Answer C: Ovarian cancer is surgically staged with TAH, BSO, collection of pelvic washings, omentectomy, cytoreduction or "debulking," and bilateral pelvic and para-aortic lymph node sampling. Stage I

ovarian cancer is confined to the ovary or ovaries. Stage II describes disease extending to the pelvis (uterus, fallopian tubes, and peritoneal washings). Stage III disease includes spread to the abdomen, and stage IV includes distant metastases including positive pleural effusion and disease of the liver.

Vignette 3 Question 3

Answer B: The most common chemotherapeutic regime following treatment for epithelial ovarian cancer is carboplatin and Taxol. The same is used to treat fallopian tube carcinoma. Methotrexate has many therapeutic indications, including treatment of ectopic pregnancy and rheumatoid arthritis. Methotrexate or actinomycin-D may be used to treat persistent/invasive molar pregnancies.

Vignette 4 Question 1

Answer D: Symptoms most characteristic of fallopian tube cancer are watery vaginal discharge and intermittent hydrosalpinx. Latzko's triad is the classic triad of profuse watery discharge, pelvic pain, and pelvic mass seen in association with fallopian tube cancers. Hydrops tubae profluens (AKA intermittent hydrosalpinx) is the phenomenon of spontaneous or pressure-induced discharge of watery or blood-tinged vaginal discharge resulting in shrinkage of a pelvic mass. Both are characteristic of fallopian tube cancers. Epithelial ovarian cancer could present with abdominal pain, bloating, and increasing abdominal girth in the setting of a pelvic mass. However, the watery vaginal discharge and intermittent hydrosalpinx are more commonly associated with fallopian tube cancer. Dysgerminomas occur most commonly in girls and young women and in Asian and African American women. Eighty percent of patients with endometrial cancer present with abnormal uterine bleeding and would not necessarily have a pelvic mass.

Vignette 4 Question 2

Answer C: Fallopian tube adenocarcimonas are extremely rare tumors. Primary disease is rarely picked up preoperatively and most are discovered incidentally, and many result from metastasis from other tumors of the ovaries, endometrium, GI tract, or breast. They are associated with both ascites and elevated Ca-125 levels. They are most often unilateral and are only bilateral 10% of the time.

Vignette 4 Question 3

Answer E: Primary fallopian tube cancer is very rare. Like epithelial ovarian cancers, the mean age is 55 to 60, it is more common in Caucasian women, and its risk factors include familial cancer syndromes, nulliparity, and infertility. The treatment for both fallopian tube and epithelial ovarian cancers include TAH, BSO, omentectomy, debulking, pelvic and para-aortic lymph node sampling. Likewise, postsurgical chemotherapeutic regime includes carboplatin and Taxol. The prognosis for fallopian tube cancer is slightly better than that of epithelial ovarian cancer.

Chapter 31 Gestational Trophoblastic Disease

Gestational trophoblastic disease (GTD) is a diverse group of interrelated diseases resulting in the **abnormal proliferation of trophoblastic (placental) tissue**. It can be grouped into four major classifications (Table 31-1): molar pregnancies (80%), persistent/invasive moles (10% to 15%), choriocarcinoma (2% to 5%), and very rare placental site trophoblastic tumors (PSTTs). These tumors are unique in that the maternal tumor results from **abnormal fetal tissue** rather than maternal tissue. These neoplasms also share the ability to **produce human chorionic gonadotropin** (hCG), which serves both as a tumor marker for diagnosing the disease and as a tool for measuring the effects of treatment. GTD is also **extremely sensitive to chemotherapy** and is therefore the most curable gynecologic malignancy and one of the few that may allow for the **preservation of fertility**.

BENIGN GESTATIONAL TROPHOBLASTIC DISEASE

Benign GTD consists of molar pregnancies, also known as **hydatidiform moles**. Complete and partial moles account for 80% of all GTD. Ninety percent of molar pregnancies are classified as **classic** or **complete moles** and are the result of molar degeneration but have no associated fetus. Ten percent of molar pregnancies are classified as **partial or incomplete moles** and are the result of molar degeneration in association with an abnormal fetus. The characteristics of complete and partial molar pregnancies are compared in Table 31-2.

EPIDEMIOLOGY

The incidence of molar pregnancy is about **1 in 1,000 pregnancies** among white women in the United States. There is a decreased rate of GTD in black women in the United States. The worldwide incidence of molar pregnancy **varies from region to region**. Low and intermediate rates are seen in North America and Europe, whereas Latin America and Asia have moderate to high rates. The global rate is **highest among Asian women**, particularly in Japan, where molar pregnancies occur in 1 in 500 pregnancies.

RISK FACTORS

Extremes in age and **prior history of GTD** are two of the major risk factors for molar pregnancy. There is a slight increase in women under 20 and a significant increase in women over 35 years of age. Women over 35 also have an increased risk of malignant disease. Similarly, women with a **history of GTD** are at increased risk to have subsequent pregnancies affected by GTD. The baseline risk of GTD in a woman with no previous history of the disease is 0.1%. That risk increased to 1% in women with one prior molar pregnancy and can be as high as 16% to 28% in a woman with two prior molar pregnancies.

Over 70% of women with GTD have never given birth, making **nulliparity** another important risk factor. Conversely, the rate of GTD seems to decrease with increasing parity. Higher incidences have also been found in geographic areas where the **diet is low in beta-carotene, folic acid, and animal fat**. Other possible associated factors include **smoking, infertility, spontaneous abortion, blood group A**, and a history of oral contraceptive pill **(OCP) use**.

COMPLETE MOLAR PREGNANCIES

PATHOGENESIS

Although the cause of molar pregnancy is unknown, it is believed that most **complete moles** result from the fertilization of an enucleate ovum or **empty egg**, one whose nucleus is missing or nonfunctional, by **one normal sperm** which then replicates itself (Fig. 31-1). All of the resultant chromosomes are therefore **paternally derived**. The most common chromosomal pattern for complete moles is **46,XX**. Rarely, a complete mole may be formed by the fertilization of an empty egg by two normal sperm. In this case as well, all chromosomes are parentally derived.

The placental abnormality in a complete mole is characterized by noninvasive **trophoblastic proliferation** associated with diffuse swelling of the chorionic villi. This **hydropic degeneration** gives the complete mole the appearance of grape-like vesicles filling the uterus in the **absence of fetus** villi (Fig. 31-2).

In complete molar pregnancy, there is abnormal proliferation of the syncytiotrophoblasts that produce hCG. This is responsible for the extremely **high hCG levels** (>100,000 mIU/mL) that can be associated with complete moles. These high hCG levels explain many of the signs and symptoms associated with complete moles. Recall that hCG has both an alpha and a beta subunit. Although the beta subunit is unique to hCG, the **alpha subunit is also found in luteinizing hormone (LH), follicle-stimulating hormone (FSH), and thyroid-stimulating hormone (TSH)**. Therefore, high hCG levels associated with complete moles can act as a homolog to LH and FSH, resulting in stimulation of **large theca lutein cysts** (>6 cm). hCG can similarly act as a homolog to TSH, resulting in **hyperthyroidism** in patients with complete moles. The high hCG levels can also cause **hyperemesis gravidarum** and early **preeclampsia** in these patients as well.

Although most molar pregnancies are benign, complete moles have a **higher malignant potential** than do partial moles (Table 31-2).

TABLE 31-1 Classification of GTD

Benign GTD (80%)	
Complete mole (classic mole)	
Partial mole (incomplete mole)	
Malignant GTD (20%)	
Persistent/invasive mole	
Choriocarcinoma	
Placental site trophoblastic tumors	

TABLE 31-2 Comparison of Characteristics of Complete and Partial Molar Pregnancies

Features	Complete (Classic) Mole (90%)	Partial (Incomplete) Mole (10%)
Genetics		
Most common karyotype	46,XX	69,XXY
Chromosomal origin	All paternally derived	Extra paternal set
Pathology		
Coexistent fetus	Absent	Present
Fetal red blood cells	Absent	Present
Chorionic villi	Hydropic (swollen)	Few hydropic
Trophoblasts	Severe hyperplasia	Minimal/no hyperplasia
Clinical presentation		
Associated embryo	None	Present
Symptoms/signs	Abnormal vaginal bleeding	Missed abortion
Classic symptoms[a]	Common	Rare
Uterine size	50% large for dates	Size equals dates
Theca lutein cysts	Present in 25%	Rare
hCG levels	High (>100,000)	Slightly elevated
Malignant potential		
Nonmetastatic disease	15%–25%	2%–4%
Metastatic disease	4%	0%
Follow-up		
Weeks to normal hCG	14 wk	8 wk

[a]Hyperemesis gravidarum, early preeclampsia, hyperthyroidism, anemia, excessive uterine enlargement.

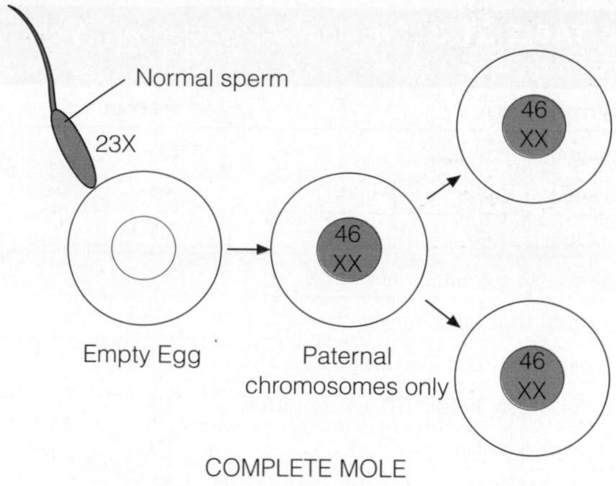

Figure 31-1 • A complete mole arises from the fertilization of an empty enucleate egg by a normal sperm. The sperm duplicates its own chromosomes, resulting in a 46,XX diploid karyotype; all of the chromosomes are, therefore, of paternal origin. (From Beckmann C, Ling F. *Obstetrics & Gynecology*. 5th ed. Philadelphia, PA: Lippincott Williams & Wilkins; 2006.)

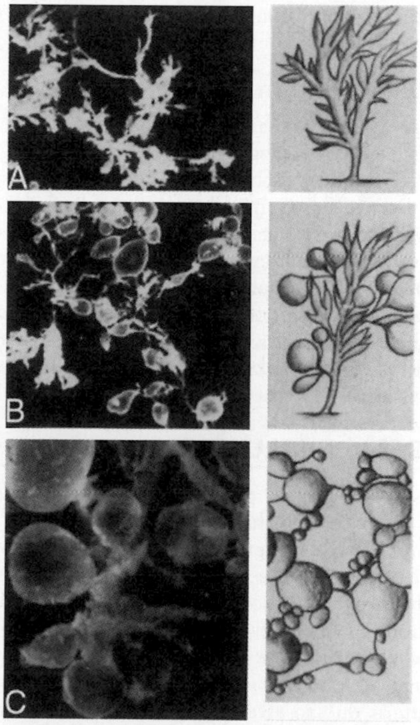

Figure 31-2 • Gross morphology of villi. **(A)** Normal chorionic villi. **(B)** Partial mole with normal villi admixed with swollen ones (case of triploidy, 69,XXY). **(C)** Complete mole with swollen, vesicular villi.

CLINICAL PRESENTATION

History

The most common presenting symptom of molar pregnancy is **irregular or heavy vaginal bleeding** during early pregnancy (97%). The bleeding is due to separation of the tumor from the underlying decidua, resulting in disruption of the maternal vessels. Table 31-3 lists other conditions associated with complete molar pregnancy, in descending order of frequency. Many of these symptoms can be attributed to the **high hCG levels,** including severe nausea and vomiting (from **hyperemesis gravidarum**); irritability, dizziness, and photophobia (from **preeclampsia**); or nervousness, anorexia, and tremors (from **hyperthyroidism** although subclinical hyperthyroidism is more

TABLE 31-3 Symptoms Associated with Molar Pregnancy

Symptoms	Percent
Vaginal bleeding	90–97
Passage of molar vesicles	80
Anemia	50
Uterine size greater than dates	30–50
Bilateral theca lutein cysts	25
Hyperemesis gravidarum	10–25
Preeclampsia before 20 wk gestation	10–15
Hyperthyroidism	10
Trophoblastic pulmonary embolic	2

common than overt hyperthyroidism). In fact, in the absence of chronic hypertension, preeclampsia occurring prior to 20 weeks' gestation is pathognomonic for molar pregnancy. Fortunately, because of earlier diagnosis and treatment of molar pregnancy, these conditions are seen less often than they were historically.

Physical Examination

In complete molar pregnancy, the physical examination may show sequelae of **preeclampsia** (hypertension) or **hyperthyroidism** (tachycardia, tachypnea). The abdominal examination in molar pregnancy may be remarkable for the **absence of fetal heart sounds** because there is no associated fetus in complete molar pregnancy. The **uterine size is greater** than the anticipated "gestational age" due to the presence of tumor, hemorrhage, and clot in the uterus. The pelvic examination may reveal the expulsion of **grape-like molar clusters** into the vagina or blood in the cervical os. Occasionally, the provider may palpate large bilateral **theca lutein cysts** (Fig. 31-3).

DIAGNOSTIC EVALUATION

In the presence of a molar pregnancy, quantitative serum **hCG levels can be extremely high** (>100,000 mIU/mL), relative to values for normal pregnancy. The hCG level reflects the amount of tumor volume and can be used for diagnosis and risk stratification and assessment of treatment effectiveness. Confirmation of GTD is usually made using **pelvic ultrasound**. In the case of a complete mole, no fetus or amniotic fluid is present. Instead, the intrauterine tissue appears as a **"snowstorm" pattern** due to swelling of chorionic villi (Fig. 31-3). The scan may also reveal **bilateral theca lutein cysts (15% of cases)**, which appear as large (>6 cm) multilocular cysts on both ovaries. The definitive diagnosis of molar pregnancy is made on **pathologic examination of the intrauterine tissue** once the uterus is evacuated.

DIFFERENTIAL DIAGNOSIS

The differential diagnosis for GTD includes conditions that can result in abnormally high hCG levels, vaginal bleeding in pregnancy, and/or enlarged placentas such as multiple gestation pregnancy, erythroblastosis fetalis, intrauterine infection, uterine fibroids, threatened abortion, ectopic pregnancy, or normal intrauterine pregnancy.

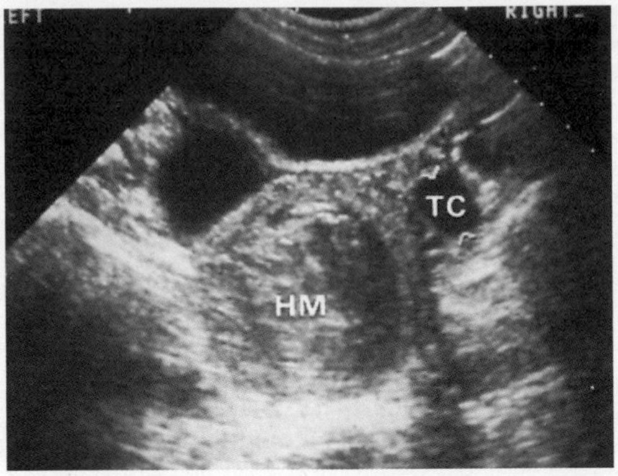

Figure 31-3 • Ultrasound scan of a complete molar pregnancy demonstrating the classic "snow storm" appearance. Large theca lutein cysts can sometimes be seen on the ovary (not pictured here).

TREATMENT

The treatment for molar pregnancy, regardless of the duration of pregnancy, is **immediate removal of the uterine contents** with suction curettage (D&C). Prior to evacuation of the uterus, laboratory examination should include a baseline hCG level, a complete blood count (CBC), coagulation studies, along with renal, thyroid, and liver function tests. Maternal blood type and antibody screen should also be obtained to determine **Rh(D) status** and to prepare for the possibility of heavy vaginal bleeding during the procedure. A chest X-ray (CXR) is no longer routinely necessary. If a patient is demonstrating signs of preeclampsia, **antihypertensives** may be used to decrease risk of maternal stroke. Similarly, patients with sequelae of hCG-induced hyperthyroidism benefit from the use of **beta blockers** such as propranolol to avoid precipitation of **thyroid storm** by the anesthesia and the surgical procedure.

Prior to the procedure, **cross-matched blood** should be made available in case of heavy bleeding and **intravenous (IV) access** should be optimized. **General anesthesia** is typically used, given the risk of hemorrhage and complications such as thyroid storm and **trophoblastic embolization**. Dilation and suction curettage **(D&C)** is the definitive treatment for most patients with complete molar pregnancy. After the uterine contents have been removed, **IV oxytocin** can be administered to stimulate uterine contraction and minimize blood loss. Even though no fetal tissue is present, Rh immunoglobulin **(RhoGAM)** should be given to all Rh-negative women. Patients with **theca lutein cysts** should be managed expectantly. In general, the cysts will spontaneoulsy involute as the hCG levels decrease following the procedure.

If the patient with a molar pregnancy has completed childbearing, **hysterectomy** is an alternate therapy. Although this will eliminate the risk of local invasion, hysterectomy does not prevent metastasis of the disease.

FOLLOW-UP

The prognosis for molar pregnancy is excellent, with **95% to 100% cure rates** after suction curettage. Persistent disease will develop in 15% to 25% of patients with complete moles and in 4% of patients with partial moles. For this reason, close follow-up is essential even after hysterectomy.

After evacuation of a molar pregnancy, **serial hCG titers** should be monitored to ensure complete resolution of the disease. For this monitoring, a radioimmunoassay specific for GTD should be used, and the same lab should be used for each measurement. Levels should be measured within 48 hours of uterine evacuation and then **weekly until negative for 3 consecutive weeks**. The levels should then be followed monthly for 6 months. Figure 31-4 demonstrates the normal regression of hCG titers after molar evacuation. The average time to normalization of levels is **14 weeks** for a complete mole compared to 2 to 4 weeks following a normal pregnancy, miscarriage, or termination. A **plateau or rise** in hCG levels during monitoring or the presence of **hCG greater than 6 months after the D&C** is indicative of persistent/invasive disease.

To ensure resolution of the disease, hCG monitoring is critical. Therefore, it is essential to **prevent pregnancy** during the follow-up period. OCPs are typically used, given their low failure rate and low risk of irregular bleeding.

Patients who are cured of the disease can have normal pregnancies after treatment with no increase in the rate of spontaneous abortion, complications, or congenital malformations. However, all subsequent pregnancies should be closely monitored with **early ultrasound** and **hCG levels** to exclude recurrent disease. Following delivery, an **hCG level** should be checked at the 6-week postpartum visit. It is no longer necessary to send the placenta for pathologic examination, but any tissue obtained from a miscarriage or termination should be evaluated for molar tissue. The risk of developing **recurrent GTD** is approximately **1% to 2% after one molar pregnancy** (compared to 0.1% in the general population), but as high as 16% to 28% after two molar pregnancies. This holds true even after hysterectomy.

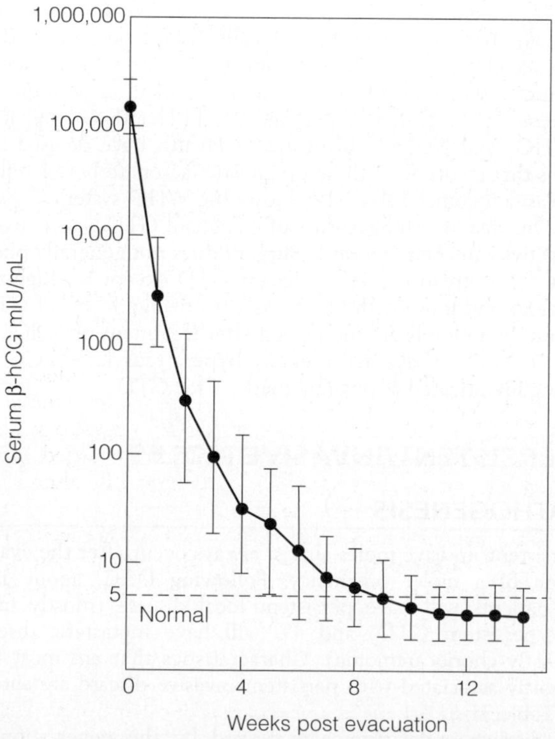

Figure 31-4 • Normal regression of β-hCG levels after molar evacuation of the uterus. The average time to normalization of levels is 8 to 14 weeks.

PARTIAL MOLAR PREGNANCY

PATHOGENESIS

A **partial or incomplete mole** is formed when a normal ovum is fertilized by two sperm simultaneously (Fig. 31-5). This results in a **triploid karyotype** with 69 chromosomes, of which two sets are paternally derived. The most common karyotype is **69,XXY** (80%). The placental abnormality in a partial mole is characterized by focal hydropic villi and trophoblastic hyperplasia primarily of the cytotrophoblast. As cytotrophoblasts do not produce hCG, hCG levels in partial molar pregnancies are **normal or only slightly elevated** compared to the extreme elevations seen in complete moles.

Partial moles are the only histologic type of GTD associated with the **presence of a fetus**. In fact, amniotic fluid and a fetal heart rate may also be present. The karyotype of the fetus may be normal diploid or triploid. These fetuses often have **multiple anomalies** such as syndactyly and hydrocephalus and are often **growth restricted**. Most fetuses associated with partial moles survive only several weeks **in utero** before being spontaneously aborted in the late first or early second trimester. As a result, partial moles are often misdiagnosed as spontaneous or missed abortions. Partial moles are almost always benign and have a much **lower malignancy potential** than complete moles.

CLINICAL PRESENTATION

History

Partial molar pregnancy often presents with **delayed menses** and **a pregnancy diagnosis**. The hCG levels are **normal or only slightly elevated**. As a result, patients with partial moles may have similar but **much less severe symptoms** than those with complete molar pregnancy. Ninety percent of patients with partial moles present with **vaginal bleeding** from miscarriage or incomplete abortion in late first trimester or early second trimester. Consequently, partial moles may be **diagnosed somewhat later** than complete molar pregnancies. Diagnosis is often made on pathologic examination of the products of conception.

PHYSICAL EXAMINATION

In partial molar pregnancy, the physical examination is **typically normal**. Given the relatively normal hCG levels, hyperemesis, hyperthyroidism, and preeclampsia are rarely seen in women with partial moles. Fetal heart sounds may be present because there is a **coexistent fetus**. These pregnancies are often complicated by intrauterine growth restriction (IUGR), so the abdominal examination may be notable for **size less than dates**.

DIAGNOSTIC EVALUATION

Unlike complete molar pregnancy, quantitative serum **hCG levels** are likely to be relatively normal in partial molar pregnancies. **Pelvic ultrasound** may reveal a fetus with cardiac activity, congenital malformations, and/or IUGR. **Amniotic fluid** is usually present but **reduced,** and these patients generally do not have theca lutein cysts seen in complete molar pregnancy. The intrauterine tissue may contain anechoic spaces juxtaposed against chorionic villi giving the tissue a **Swiss-cheese appearance**. The definitive diagnosis of molar

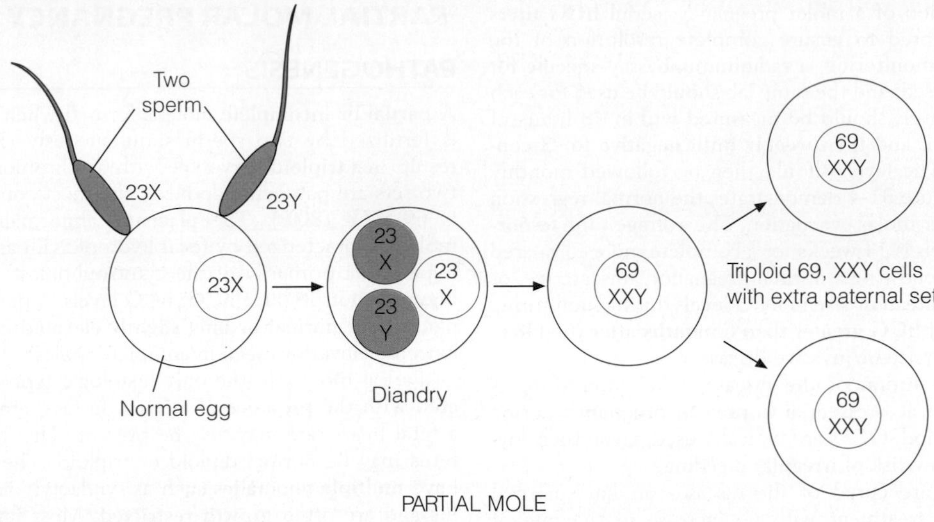

Figure 31-5 • An incomplete mole arises from the simultaneous fertilization of a normal ovum by two sperm (diandry). The resulting triploid karyotype is most commonly 69,XXY.

pregnancy is made on **pathologic examination of the intrauterine tissue** once the uterus is evacuated.

TREATMENT

Treatment is immediate removal of the uterine contents via **suction curettage (D&C)** as described in the complete molar pregnancy treatment section. Less than 4% of patients with partial moles will develop persistent malignant disease (Table 31-2).

FOLLOW-UP

Meticulous follow-up with **serial hCG levels**, as described in the previous section on complete molar pregnancy, is critical to the treatment of this disease. The average time to normalization of levels is **8 weeks** for a partial mole compared to 2 to 4 weeks following a normal pregnancy, miscarriage, or termination and 14 weeks for a complete mole. **Reliable contraception** is also important to prevent pregnancy and allow accurate hCG measurement and monitoring.

MALIGNANT GESTATIONAL TROPHOBLASTIC DISEASE

OVERVIEW

Molar pregnancies (complete and partial) are typically benign and make up 80% of all GTD; however, 20% of patients with GTD are diagnosed with a malignant form of the disease so named because of their potential **for local invasion and metastasis**. Malignant GTD is divided into three histologic types (Table 31-1): **persistent/invasive moles (75%), choriocarcinoma (25%), and PSTT (extremely rare)**. In 50% of cases, malignant GTD occurs **months to years after a molar pregnancy**. Another 25% occur after an antecedent normal pregnancy and 25% occur after a miscarriage, ectopic pregnancy, or abortion. Malignant GTD that occurs after a molar pregnancy is most commonly persistent/invasive GTD, and malignant GTD that occurs after a nonmolar pregnancy is most commonly choriocarcinoma.

For the purpose of treatment and prognosis, malignant GTD (persistent/invasive moles, choriocarcinoma, PSTT) can be classified as **nonmetastatic** if the disease is confined to the uterus or **metastatic** if the disease has progressed beyond the uterus (Fig. 31-6). Metastatic disease can further be classified as **good prognosis or poor prognosis,** depending on factors such as length of time since antecedent pregnancy, hCG level, presence of brain or liver metastases, type of antecedent pregnancy, and the result of prior chemotherapy trials (Fig. 31-6).

The staging for GTD is shown in Table 31-4. This system has not been found to be clinically useful because it does not account for important prognostic factors such as degree of metastasis, type of antecedent pregnancy, or duration of disease. In the United States, the World Health Organization (WHO) and National Institutes of Health have devised systems that incorporate these prognostic factors to better reflect disease outcome. Table 31-5 shows the WHO system.

One distinguishing feature of malignant GTD is its **extreme sensitivity to chemotherapy. Surgery does not generally play a role** in the treatment of malignant GTD except for high-risk patients and those with PSTT. As with benign forms of GTD, **serum hCG levels** are monitored after treatment of malignant GTD. Newer assays that measure hyperglycosylated hCG are being investigated as possible markers for GTD.

PERSISTENT/INVASIVE MOLES

PATHOGENESIS

Persistent/invasive moles almost always occur after the evacuation of a molar pregnancy. Following D&C, about 15% of patients will have persistent local disease (mostly invasive/persistent GTD) and 4% will have metastatic disease (mostly choriocarcinoma). Characteristics that are most frequently associated with persistent/invasive disease are shown in Table 31-6.

Invasive moles are characterized by the penetration of large, swollen **(hydropic) villi and trophoblasts** into the myometrium. This proliferation can sometimes extend through the myometrium to the peritoneal cavity to invade the uterine

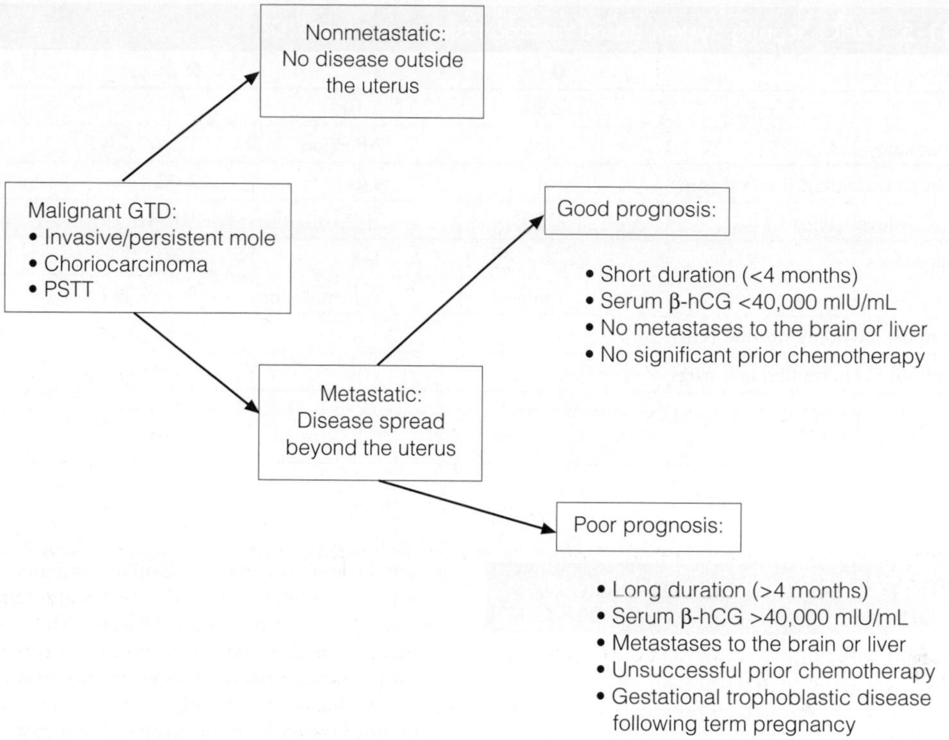

Figure 31-6 • Classification of malignant GTD Anatomic spread as well as clinical presentation impacts the prognosis of malignant disease.

TABLE 31-4 Staging of Gestational Trophoblastic Tumors

Stage	Extent of Disease[a]
I	Confined to the uterus
II	Metastases to the pelvis or vagina
III	Metastases to the lung
IV	Distant metastases

[a]Metastasis sites in order of frequency are lung, vagina, pelvis, brain, and liver.

vasculature. In rare cases, persistent/invasive GTD can cause uterine rupture, hemoperitoneum, and severe anemia. Despite this, invasive moles **rarely metastasize** and are capable of **spontaneous regression**.

EPIDEMIOLOGY

Invasive moles have an overall incidence of 1 in 15,000 pregnancies.

CLINICAL PRESENTATION

History

Most patients with persistent/invasive moles are identified as a result of **plateauing or rising hCG** after treatment for a molar pregnancy and are usually asymptomatic at the time of diagnosis. The most common symptom is **abnormal uterine bleeding.**

Physical Examination

The physical examination in patients with invasive moles is similar to that for molar pregnancy. Women with persistent/invasive GTD are more likely to have hCG levels above 100,000 mIU/mL, excessive uterine size for dates, and prominent theca lutein cysts.

DIAGNOSTIC EVALUATION

As with benign forms of GTD, **hCG levels and pelvic ultrasound are the cornerstones of diagnosis**. **Pelvic ultrasound** may reveal one or more **intrauterine masses** with possible invasion of the myometrium. Doppler examination typically shows **high vascular flow**. A repeat suction curettage (D&C) can be considered in patients with plateauing hCG and without evidence of metastatic foci.

TREATMENT

Persistent/invasive moles are typically **nonmetastatic** and respond well to **single-agent chemotherapy,** typically **methotrexate or actinomycin-D**. When metastases are present, low-risk patients are treated with **single-agent chemotherapy,** and high-risk patients are treated with **multiagent chemotherapy**.

FOLLOW-UP

As with other forms of GTD, careful follow-up with **serial hCG levels** as described is critical to demonstrating resolution of the disease (Fig. 31-4). Likewise, **reliable contraception** is critical in order to maintain accurate measurement of hCG levels and verify resolution of the disease.

TABLE 31-5 WHO Scoring System Based on Prognostic Factor for GTD[a]

Risk Factors	0	1	2	4
Age (y)	≤39	≥40		
Antecedent pregnancy	Mole	Abortion	Term	
Pregnancy event to treatment interval (mo)	<4	4–6	7–12	>12
Pretreatment hCG level (IU/mL)	$<10^3$	10^3–10^4	10^4–10^5	$>10^5$
Number of metastases		1–4	4–8	>8
Site metastases	Lung	Spleen, kidney	Bowel, liver	Brain
Largest tumor mass, including uterine (cm)			3–5	>5
Prior number of failed chemotherapy drugs			Single drug	Two +

[a]The total score for a patient is obtained by adding the individual scores for each prognostic factor. Total score: less than 4 = low risk; 5 to 7 = mid-level risk; greater than or equal to 8 = high risk.

TABLE 31-6 Risk Factors for Persistent/Invasive Moles

hCG >100,000 mIU/mL
Uterine size >14–16 wk
Large theca lutein cysts
Coexistent viable fetus

CHORIOCARCINOMA

PATHOGENESIS

Choriocarcinoma is a **malignant necrotizing tumor** that can arise weeks to years after any type of pregnancy. Although 50% of patients who develop choriocarcinoma have had a **preceding complete molar pregnancy**, 25% develop the disease after a normal-term pregnancy and 25% after miscarriage, abortion, or ectopic pregnancy.

Choriocarcinoma is a **pure epithelial tumor**. The characteristic histologic pattern of choriocarcinoma includes **sheets of anaplastic cytotrophoblasts and syncytiotrophoblasts in the absence of chorionic villi**. Choriocarcinoma invades the uterine wall and uterine vasculature, causing destruction of uterine tissue, necrosis, and potentially severe hemorrhage. These tumors are often metastatic and usually **spread hematogenously** to the lungs, vagina, pelvis, brain, liver, intestines, and kidneys. These lesions tend to be very vascular and bleed easily.

EPIDEMIOLOGY

Choriocarcinoma is very rare in the United States, where its incidence is only 1 in 20,000 to 40,000 pregnancies, but is more common in women of Asian or African ethnicity.

CLINICAL PRESENTATION

History

Patients with choriocarcinoma often present with **late postpartum bleeding** (beyond 6 to 8 weeks postpartum), but can also present with **irregular uterine bleeding** years after an antecedent pregnancy. Unlike patients with persistent/invasive moles, patients with choriocarcinoma often present with symptoms of **metastatic disease**. Metastases to the **lungs** may cause cough, dyspnea, respiratory distress, or hemoptysis. Central nervous system **(CNS) lesions** may cause headaches, dizziness, blackouts, or other symptoms common to space-occupying lesions. Hepatic, urologic, and gastrointestinal symptoms are often signs of metastatic disease. Vaginal metastases may cause **vaginal bleeding**.

PHYSICAL EXAMINATION

Patients with choriocarcinoma often have **signs of metastatic disease**, including uterine enlargement, vaginal masses, bilateral theca lutein cysts, and neurologic signs from CNS involvement.

DIAGNOSTIC EVALUATION

The primary workup for choriocarcinoma includes measurement of quantitative **hCG levels** and assessment for metastasis to the lungs, liver, kidneys, spleen, and brain. This entails **laboratory tests** including a CBC, coagulation studies, along with renal and hepatic function tests. **Pelvic ultrasound** may reveal a uterine mass with hemorrhage and necrosis. These tumors are typically **highly vascular** as demonstrated by Doppler analysis. Other imaging studies might include a **CXR** or **chest CT** to look for lung metastases as well as an **abdominal/pelvic CT or MRI** to look for metastatic disease if indicated. If vaginal or lung metastases are present, **a CT or MRI of the brain** should also be obtained.

DIFFERENTIAL DIAGNOSIS

Choriocarcinoma has been found to metastasize to virtually every tissue in the body. It is known as **"the great imitator"** because its signs and symptoms are similar to those of many disease entities. Also, given that choriocarcinoma can occur from weeks to years after any type of gestation and is relatively rare, the **diagnosis is often delayed** when the disease occurs outside the context of a prior molar pregnancy.

TREATMENT

Classification and treatment of choriocarcinoma mirror those of persistent/invasive GTD (Fig. 31-6). Nonmetastatic and good-prognosis metastatic diseases are treated with **single-agent**

chemotherapy. Poor-prognosis metastatic choriocarcinoma is treated with **multiagent chemotherapy**. The cure rate for good prognosis disease is 95% to 100%, and the cure rate for poor prognosis disease is 50% to 70%.

FOLLOW-UP

As with all other forms of GTD, choriocarcinoma requires close monitoring of **hCG levels** in conjunction with **reliable contraception**.

PLACENTAL SITE TROPHOBLASTIC TUMORS

PATHOGENESIS

PSTTs are extremely rare tumors that arise from the **placental implantation site**. In this form of malignant GTD, intermediate cytotrophoblasts from the placental site infiltrate the myometrium and then invade the blood vessels. Histologically, these tumors are characterized by the **absence of villi** and the proliferation of intermediate trophoblasts and excessive production of **human placental lactogen (hPL;** as opposed to proliferation of syncytiotrophoblasts and cytotrophoblasts seen in other forms of GTD).

CLINICAL PRESENTATION

Persistent **irregular vaginal bleeding** is the most common symptom of PSTT and may occur weeks to years after an antecedent pregnancy. Physical examination may reveal an **enlarged uterus**.

DIAGNOSTIC EVALUATION

Unlike other forms of GTD, these tumors produce **chronic low levels of hCG** because these tumors lack proliferation of syncytiotrophoblasts (the placental layer responsible for hCG production). Serum **hPL** may be used as a diagnostic tool. The **pelvic ultrasound** may show a uterine mass, but there is typically less hemorrhage than seen in choriocarcinomas. Both cystic and solid components may be present. Like other forms of malignant GTD, the tumor can invade the uterine wall and surrounding tissues.

TREATMENT

PSTTs are also generally **not sensitive to chemotherapy** but, fortunately, they rarely metastasize beyond the uterus. Therefore, **hysterectomy is the treatment of choice** for PSTT. Multiagent chemotherapy is given 1 week after surgery to prevent recurrent disease.

KEY POINTS

- GTD is a group of related diseases resulting from abnormal proliferation of trophoblastic (placental) tissue.
- Eighty percent of GTD is benign disease (complete and partial moles) and 20% is malignant disease (persistent/invasive moles, choriocarcinoma, and PSTTs).
- Of benign GTD, 90% are complete moles. Complete moles result from the fertilization of an empty ovum by one sperm that then duplicates. The most common karyotype is 46,XX—all chromosomes are paternally derived.
- There is no associated fetus in complete molar pregnancy, and patients usually present with irregular vaginal bleeding, an enlarged uterus, or passage of vesicles.
- Complete molar pregnancy can have very high hCG levels (>100,000 mIU/mL), resulting in classic symptoms of hyperemesis gravidarum, preeclampsia before 20 weeks' gestation, hyperthyroidism, and/or large bilateral theca lutein cysts.
- Complete molar pregnancy is diagnosed by hCG levels and pelvic ultrasound showing a "snowstorm" pattern and is treated with immediate suction D&C to empty the uterus. Oxytocin is often given to avoid hemorrhage.
- Complete molar pregnancy requires close follow-up with weekly, then monthly, hCG levels for 6 months. Concurrent reliable contraception is imperative during this time.
- Complete molar pregnancy results in persistent malignant disease in 15% of cases and has a risk of recurrence of 1% after one molar pregnancy and 16% to 28% after two molar pregnancies.
- Partial moles account for 10% of molar pregnancies and result from the simultaneous fertilization of a normal ovum by two sperm. The most common karyotype is 69,XXY.
- Partial moles have a coexistent abnormal fetus and usually present with vaginal bleeding from spontaneous or incomplete abortion.
- Partial moles are diagnosed by hCG levels and pelvic ultrasound and treated with D&C. Persistent malignant disease develops in only 4% of cases. Follow-up is similar to complete moles with serial hCG levels and reliable contraception.
- Persistent/invasive moles make up 75% of malignant GTD. They are usually diagnosed by detecting plateauing or rising hCG levels after molar evacuation.
- These moles have an overall incidence of 1 in 15,000 normal pregnancies. They are generally confined to the uterus and respond well to single-agent chemotherapy (95% to 100% cure rate).
- Choriocarcinoma is a rare form of GTD with an overall incidence of 1 in 20,000 to 40,000 pregnancies in the United States. It is a malignant, necrotizing tumor that can occur weeks to years after any type of gestation.
- Patients can present with signs and symptoms of metastases to the lungs, vagina, liver, brain, or kidneys. Choriocarcinoma is diagnosed by pelvic ultrasound, hCG levels, and a thorough workup for metastatic disease.
- Choriocarcinoma is treated with single- or multiagent chemotherapy, depending on the presence of disease outside the uterus and on the disease prognosis category.
- PSTTs are extremely rare tumors that arise from the placental implantation site. They are characterized by the absence of villi and the proliferation of cytotrophoblasts. This results in chronic low levels of hCG (<100 mIU/mL) and elevated levels of hPL.
- PSTTs spread by invasion into the myometrium and blood vessels. Patients most commonly present with vaginal bleeding and persistently low levels of hCG (<100 mIU/mL).
- PSTTs are treated by hysterectomy followed by multiagent chemotherapy to prevent recurrences.

C Clinical Vignettes

Vignette 1

A 27-year-old woman presents to your office with a positive home pregnancy test and a 3-day history of vaginal bleeding. She is concerned that she may be having a miscarriage. On examination, the uterine fundus is at the level of the umbilicus. By her last period, she should be around 8 weeks gestation. On pelvic examination, there is a moderate amount of blood and vesicle-like tissue in the vaginal vault, and the cervix is closed. The lab then calls you to say that her serum β-hCG result is greater than 1,000,000 mIU/mL.

1. Which of the following is the best next step in this patient's evaluation?
   a. Complete pelvic ultrasound
   b. Determination of Rh status
   c. Surgical intervention (suction curettage)
   d. Methotrexate administration
   e. Schedule a follow-up visit in 2 to 4 weeks to recheck a β-hCG level

2. The patient undergoes an uncomplicated suction D&C. The pathology report is available the next day and is consistent with a complete molar gestation. What is the best next step in the care of this patient's condition.
   a. Repeat pelvic imaging
   b. Radiation therapy
   c. Chemotherapy
   d. Surveillance of serum β-hCG
   e. No further follow-up is required

3. During post-operative surveillance, you meet with her in your office about 3 months after the index visit. Which of the following interventions is most important to emphasize during her follow-up period?
   a. No further pregnancies are recommended
   b. Await pregnancy attempt for 2 years
   c. Reliable contraception during surveillance
   d. Prophylactic antibiotic use during surveillance
   e. Prophylactic chemotherapy to decrease the risk of persistent and recurrent disease

Vignette 2

A 42-year-old G4 P3 woman presents to your emergency department with a 6-month history of irregular bleeding and a new onset of coughing up blood. Her history reveals three term vaginal deliveries, her last being approximately 6 months ago. That delivery was uncomplicated. On physical examination, vital signs are stable, her uterus is approximately 10 to 12 weeks size, and there is a moderate amount of blood in the vaginal vault. CXR shows a new single nodule in the left lower lobe suspicious for a metastatic lesion from unknown location.

1. Which of the following laboratory tests will most likely assist in her diagnosis?
   a. CA 125
   b. Serum β-hCG
   c. CBC
   d. Prothrombin time
   e. Fibrinogen

2. The quantitative serum β-hCG is 108,000 mIU/mL. Which of the following is the most likely diagnosis?
   a. Incomplete molar pregnancy
   b. Complete molar pregnancy
   c. Persistent molar pregnancy
   d. Choriocarcinoma
   e. Placental site trophoblastic tumor

3. The pelvic ultrasound reveals bilateral multicystic ovarian masses along with an enlarged uterus. What is the most likely diagnosis and most appropriate management of this finding?
   a. Metastatic lesions/surgical intervention
   b. Primary epithelial ovarian carcinoma/surgical intervention
   c. Theca lutein cysts/percutaneous drainage
   d. Metastatic lesions/chemotherapy
   e. Theca lutein cysts/conservative surveillance

4. You refer the patient to a gynecologic oncologist for evaluation and management of choriocarcinoma. What is the most likely intervention to be recommended?
   a. Total abdominal hysterectomy
   b. Serum β-hCG surveillance
   c. Chemotherapy
   d. Whole pelvis radiation
   e. Pulmonary wedge resection

Vignette 3

A 17-year-old G1 P0 patient presents to your office with vaginal bleeding at approximately 10 weeks' gestation by her last menstrual period. Her examination is benign with a 10-week-sized uterus, a closed cervical os, and a small amount of blood within the vaginal vault. You order a complete pelvic ultrasound that shows an intrauterine gestational with a fetus measuring approximately 8 weeks' gestation. A yolk sac is identified. Doppler sonography is unable to demonstrate any fetal heart beat. The placenta demonstrates marked thickening and increased echogenicity with suggestion of small cystic spaces within the placenta. A serum β-hCG is 282,000 mIU/mL.

1. What is the most likely diagnosis?
   a. Missed abortion
   b. Inevitable abortion
   c. Incomplete abortion
   d. Complete molar pregnancy
   e. Incomplete molar pregnancy

2. You decide to perform a suction D&C. When giving informed consent, you discuss the risk most commonly encountered in this operation. Which of the following is the most common risk associated with suction D&C?
   a. Infection
   b. Uterine perforation
   c. Uterine bleeding
   d. Damage to the bladder
   e. Need for future surgery

3. After pathology returns, you discuss the findings with your patient in follow-up at your office. Which of the following is most accurate when discussing risk of persistent gestational trophoblastic disease?
   a. Less than 1%
   b. 2% to 5%
   c. 6% to 10%
   d. 11% to 15%
   e. Greater than 20%

Vignette 4

A 44-year-old woman presents to your emergency department with profuse vaginal bleeding. Her medical history is unremarkable. She has had two term vaginal deliveries, her last being 10 years ago. An initial workup shows a solid intrauterine mass and a serum β-hCG level of 220 mIU/mL. You decide to proceed with endometrial sampling, which is uncomplicated. Final surgical pathological diagnosis is consistent with PSTT.

1. Which of the following elevated serum markers is most associated with PSTT?
   a. Prolactin
   b. Serum β-hCG
   c. Human placental lactogen
   d. CA-125
   e. Inhibin-A

2. Which of the following is typically the primary treatment of choice for PSTT?
   a. Directed external beam radiation therapy
   b. Systemic chemotherapy
   c. Hysteroscopy, D&C
   d. Hysterectomy
   e. Serum β-hCG surveillance

3. In the preoperative workup of your patient, a CXR shows bilateral solid masses within the middle lung lobes. According to the FIGO stratification which stage of the disease does she have?
   a. I
   b. II
   c. III
   d. IV

A Answers

Vignette 1 Question 1

Answer A: This patient's vignette is most consistent with GTD, which is a proliferative disorder of trophoblastic placental tissue. The initial workup should include a pelvic ultrasound to determine the exact etiology of the patient's examination and laboratory findings. Rh status would be included in this patient's workup after a diagnosis had been established. Suction curettage is the treatment of choice for GTD and allows for an exact diagnosis to be made but should not be entertained until the sonographic diagnosis has been confirmed. Methotrexate is not generally a treatment of choice in the early diagnosis of GTD. It can be used as adjuvant therapy if malignant GTD is discovered. Conservative management is never an option in patients with suspicion for GTD as the therapy of choice is surgical intervention.

Vignette 1 Question 2

Answer D: Persistent GTD after evacuation of a complete molar gestation can occur in approximately 20% to 30% of patients (compared to a <5% risk in partial incomplete molar gestation). Risks factors for persistence typically include hCG level over 100,000 mIU/mL, the presence of large (>6 cm in diameter) theca lutein cysts, and significant uterine enlargement (all of which are consistent with larger amounts of trophoblastic tissue). Serum β-hCG surveillance, usually lasting approximately 6 months, proves reliable in confirming that all proliferative trophoblastic cells have disappeared. Conservative management without hCG surveillance is not appropriate in this patient. Chemotherapy would be entertained if persistent GTD were confirmed. However, during the initial surveillance period, it is reasonable to allow the serum β-hCG to decrease spontaneously. Repeat imaging of the pelvis is not indicated at this time.

Vignette 1 Question 3

Answer C: Reliable contraception is paramount during surveillance of serum β-hCG after a molar gestation. This will decrease confusion with the possibility of a new pregnancy during the interval period. Typically, the most common method used is combination oral contraception. Medroxyprogesterone acetate injection is an appropriate alternative. Implants are typically avoided given the high rate of irregular bleeding with these devices. Pregnancy should be avoided during the 6-month surveillance period; however, after persistent GTD has been ruled out, attempt at pregnancy is reasonable. Prophylactic antibiotics and/or prophylactic chemotherapy are not warranted in these cases.

Vignette 2 Question 1

Answer B: This patient's clinical history and physical examination are most consistent with metastatic GTD. A quantitative serum β-hCG is the most important initial diagnostic test that will confirm the presence of proliferative trophoblastic tissues. CA-125 is a very nonspecific lab test that is unlikely to assist given this patient's clinical history. Although CBC, prothrombin time, and fibrinogen level are reasonable to order, they will not lead to a diagnosis in this patient.

Vignette 2 Question 2

Answer D: The malignant forms of GTD include persistent/invasive gestational trophoblastic neoplasia (after complete or incomplete molar pregnancy), choriocarcinoma, and PSTT. The most likely diagnosis in this patient is metastatic choriocarcinoma. This is a rare condition occurring most commonly after evacuation of a complete molar gestation (50%), and less commonly after term pregnancies (25%) and spontaneous abortions or ectopic pregnancies (25%). When malignant GTD is encountered after a *nonmolar* pregnancy, the diagnosis is almost always choriocarcinoma and rarely placental site trophoblastic tumor. Choriocarcinoma is an aggressive tumor and most commonly presenting with abnormal uterine bleeding. The most common site of metastasis is the lung (80%). Other sites include the vagina (30%), liver and brain (10%). Complete and incomplete molar pregnancies are potentially malignant. If there is evidence of metastasis, malignant GTD is the diagnosis. Invasive or persistent molar pregnancy usually occurs after evacuation of a molar gestation and rarely metastasizes. PSTT is exceedingly rare, associated with a persistent *low* β-hCG levels, and is typically confined to the uterus.

Vignette 2 Question 3

Answer E: Theca lutein cysts result from overstimulation of ovarian parenchyma from high levels of serum hCG. The typical appearance is multiseptated cysts, commonly occurring bilaterally. Conservative management of these cysts is recommended, as they resolve once the hCG has been eliminated. Ovarian metastasis from choriocarcinoma is not common. Epithelial ovarian carcinoma is unlikely in this particular patient.

Vignette 2 Question 4

Answer C: Malignant GTD is extremely sensitive to chemotherapy and is therefore the mainstay of treatment in these patients. Single or multiagent therapies are used, guided by the presence or absence of certain prognostic factors. The International Federation of Gynecology and Obstetrics (FIGO) established a four-tiered staging system based mostly on the location of metastatic lesions. Other risk factors for recurrence include serum β-hCG greater than 100,000 mIU/mL and greater than 6 months from the index pregnancy. Surgical intervention and radiation therapy are typically reserved for tumor that is resistant to initial chemotherapy and/or cerebral tumor involvement, respectively.

Vignette 3 Question 1

Answer E: The combination of findings including an intrauterine fetus, marked thickening and cystic formation within the placenta, and a significantly increased serum β-hCG is highly suggestive of an incomplete (partial) molar pregnancy. Partial molar pregnancies are triploid karyotpyes, compared to diploid in complete molar pregnancies. Typically, these pregnancies present and are often confused with missed and/or incomplete abortions. Diagnostic accuracy using pelvic ultrasound is the gold standard in the evaluation of this patient.

Vignette 3 Question 2

Answer C: Vaginal bleeding is commonly encountered during these cases mostly because of the high vascularity of the pregnancy and the abnormal placental tissue. Uterotonics (oxytocin, methylergonivine, misoprostol) are frequently used in these cases to help prevent and minimize excessive bleeding. Other choices are associated risks but are less common.

Vignette 3 Question 3

Answer B: Incomplete (partial) molar gestation is associated with approximately a 2% to 5% risk of persistent disease (compared to approximately 20% risk of persistence with a complete molar pregnancy). The importance of serial β-hCG surveillance is paramount in the management of these patients postoperatively. If levels plateau during surveillance or begin rising, further workup for persistent disease should be initiated.

Vignette 4 Question 1

Answer C: PSTT is a slowly growing malignant tumor that arises from placental cytotrophoblasts. These cells produce low amounts of β-hCG and high amounts of hPL. This can be used in the diagnosis of PSTT. These tumors have persistently low levels of serum β-hCG. The remaining choices are not typically used in this condition.

Vignette 4 Question 2

Answer D: Definitive hysterectomy is typically the treatment of choice for patients with PSTT. This is in contrast to all other forms of malignant GTD, which typically involves treatment of primary disease with systemic chemotherapy.

Vignette 4 Question 3

Answer C: Stage I is defined as persistently elevated serum β-hCG levels with tumor confined to the uterus. Stage II is defined by the presence of tumor outside the uterus, but limited to the vagina and/or pelvis. Stage III is defined as pulmonary metastasis with or without uterine, vaginal, or pelvic tumor metastasis. Stage IV includes all other metastatic lesions most commonly including the brain, liver, kidneys, and the gastrointestinal tract.

Chapter

32 Benign Breast Disease and Breast Cancer

Breast cancer is the most common malignancy in women in the United States (except for skin cancers), representing approximately 30% of female cancers and 230,000 **new diagnoses** each year in the United States. It is also the second most common cause of **cancer deaths** in women (after lung cancer deaths), accounting for some 40,000 deaths per year. A woman has a **one in eight chance (12%)** of developing invasive breast cancer over her lifetime. Yet, despite its incidence, the cause of breast cancer remains unknown.

In addition to breast cancer, as many as 50% of women will have benign breast lesions over their lifetime. Therefore, understanding the range of benign and malignant breast lesions and their symptoms is enormously important. Obstetrician-gynecologists, primary care providers, and surgeons perform evaluations of breast pain, nipple discharge, and breast masses and also screen for breast cancer. The anatomy and physiology of the breast as well as how to diagnose and treat these lesions should be understood by all physicians involved in the care of women.

ANATOMY

Breast parenchyma is divided into segments containing **mammary glands** that consist of 20 to 40 lobules drained by **lactiferous ducts** that open individually into the nipple (Fig. 32-1). Fibrous bands spanning between two fascia layers—called **Cooper suspensory ligaments**—support the breast. The breast is divided into four quadrants for ease of description: upper outer quadrant (UOQ), lower outer quadrant, upper inner quadrant (UIQ), and lower inner quadrant (LIQ).

The **major blood supply** to the breast is from the **internal mammary** and **lateral thoracic arteries** (Fig. 32-2). The medial and central aspects are supplied by the anterior perforators of the internal mammary artery, and the UOQ is supplied by the lateral thoracic.

The **axillary lymph nodes** drain up to 97% of the ipsilateral breast, and secondarily drain the supraclavicular and jugular nodes. These nodes are subdivided into three levels for the purposes of specifying disease progression. The **internal mammary nodes** are responsible for 3% of drainage, mainly of the UIQ and LIQ. The interpectoral nodes (Rotter nodes) lie between the pectoralis major and pectoralis minor muscles.

The **innervation** of the breast requires careful attention during surgical dissection. Nerves at risk of injury include the **intercostobrachial nerve** that transverses the axilla to supply sensation to the upper medial arm; the **long thoracic nerve** (of Bell) of C5, C6, and C7 that innervates the serratus anterior muscle, injury of which can lead to the "winged" scapula; the **thoracodorsal nerve** that innervates the latissimus dorsi muscle; and the lateral pectoral nerve that innervates the pectoralis major and minor muscles.

PHYSIOLOGY

Breast development is classified into **Tanner stages 1 to 5** (see Chapter 20 and Fig. 20-3). The breast responds to cyclic hormones, as well as to changes during pregnancy and menopause. **Estrogen** promotes ductal development and fat deposition. **Progesterones** promote the lobular-alveolar (stromal) development that makes lactation possible. **Prolactin** is involved in milk production, whereas **oxytocin** from the posterior pituitary causes milk letdown. In **postmenopausal women**, the hypoestrogenic state is associated with **tissue atrophy**, loss of stroma, and replacement of atrophied lobules with fatty tissue.

EVALUATION OF THE BREAST

ROUTINE EVALUATION—WOMEN AT AVERAGE RISK

There are three major components of breast cancer screening of **women at average risk**. These include the clinical breast examination, the breast self-examination, and screening mammography. Guidelines for breast cancer screening vary between leading medical organizaions such as the American Cancer Society (ACS) and the American College of Obstetricians and Gynecologists.

Most of these organizations support routine **clinician breast evaluation** every 1 to 3 years for all women above age 20. After age 40, clinical breast evaluation should be done annually. Physical examination involves careful **inspection of the skin** for contour or color changes, dimpling, and retractions with the patient in upright and supine positions. This is followed by **palpation** of the axilla for lymphadenopathy and the breast for masses, nipple discharge, or pain.

Most of the leading medical organizations consider **breast self-examination** for women aged 20 and over to now be optional. For those that do support breast self-examination, emphasis has moved from the monthly breast self-examination toward general **"breast self-awareness."** The latter encourages women to become familiar with their breasts and to report any changes from baseline. Breast self-awareness should be reviewed at each annual gynecology visit.

In addition to the clinical breast examination and patient self-examinations, the third part of routine breast care for the patient at average risk is **screening mammography** (Fig. 32-3). Although there has been some controversy over frequency of mammograms between ages 40 and 50, current mammography screening guidelines by the ACS include a mammogram every year starting at age 40 and continuing for as long as a woman is in good health. There is no agreed upon consensus of an **upper age limit** at which mammogram screening can be stopped.

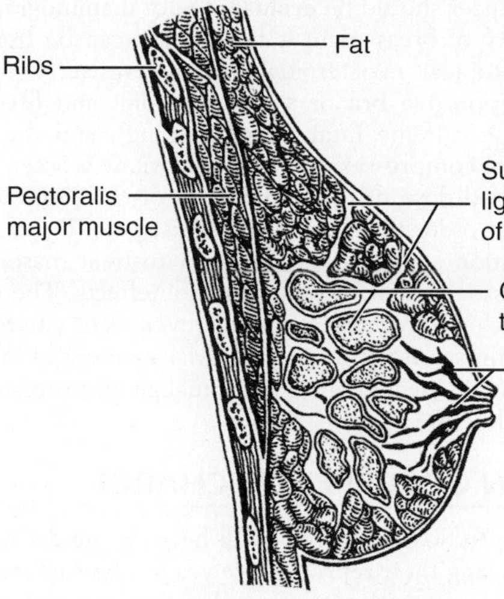

Figure 32-1 • Clinical anatomy of the female breast and chest wall.
(From Beckmann C, Ling F. *Obstetrics & Gynecology*. 5th ed. Philadelphia, PA: Lippincott Williams & Wilkins; 2006.)

ROUTINE EVALUATION—WOMEN AT HIGH RISK

Women at **highest risk of** breast cancer are those who have a known **BRCA1 or BRCA2** gene mutation, a first-degree relative (mother, sister, or daughter) with either mutation, and those deemed to be at high risk based on a validated risk assessment tool (e.g., Gail or Claus model). Other women at high risk of breast cancer include those who underwent radiation to the chest between the ages of 10 and 30, or who have a hereditary syndrome associated with multiple cancer diagnoses (e.g., Li–Fraumeni, Lynch II syndrome). Women at **moderate risk** are those deemed to be at moderate risk based on a validated screening tool, those with a personal history of breast cancer or its precursor lesions, or those who have particularly dense breast tissue on mammogram.

Screening recommendations for these women vary, but typically include teaching of breast self-awareness, clinical breast examination every 6 to 12 months, and annual mammogrphy starting at age 25 or 5 to 10 years before the age of the youngest cancer diagnosis in the family. Women at highest risk for breast cancer might also have interval breast **MRIs** along with the annual screening mammogram. Women at moderate risk can consider adding MRI screening to their annual mammography.

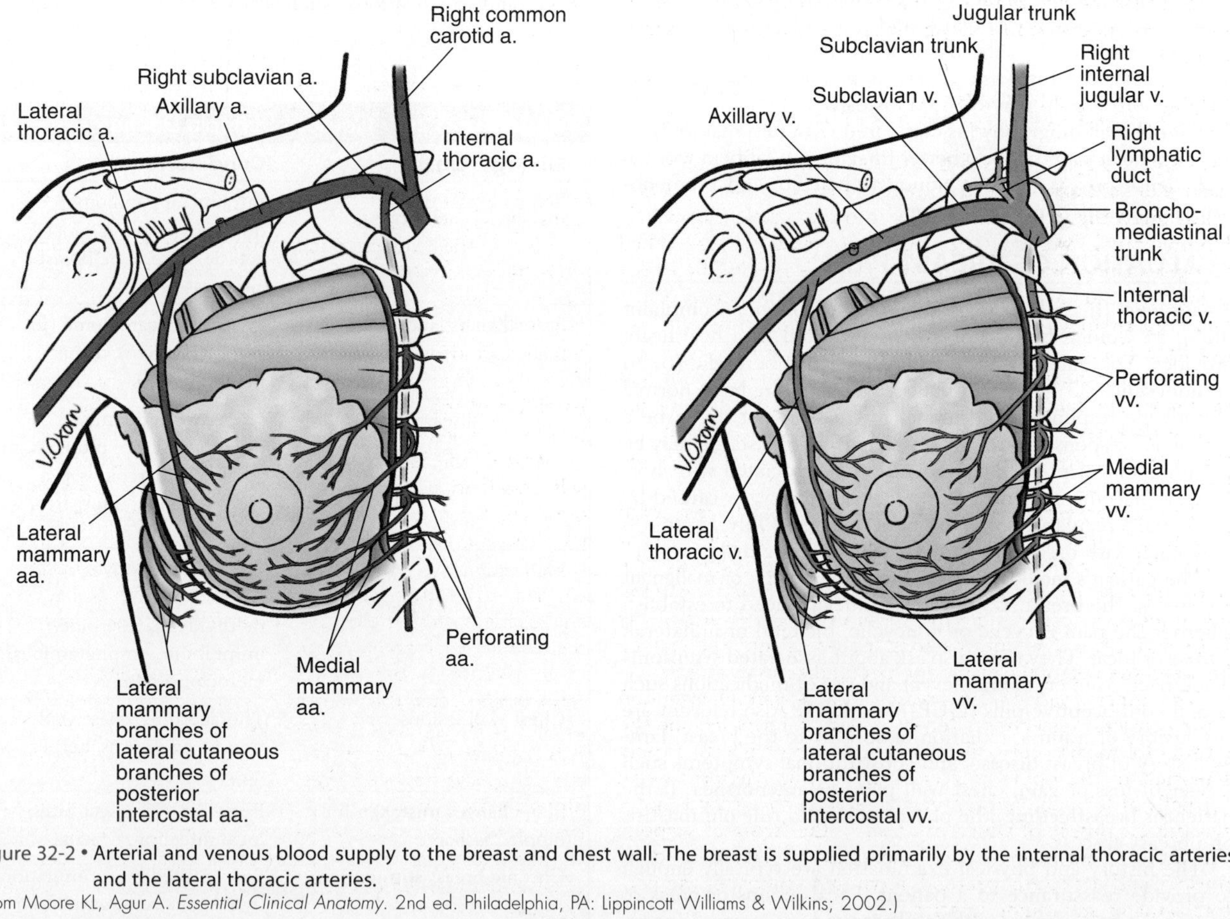

Figure 32-2 • Arterial and venous blood supply to the breast and chest wall. The breast is supplied primarily by the internal thoracic arteries and the lateral thoracic arteries.
(From Moore KL, Agur A. *Essential Clinical Anatomy*. 2nd ed. Philadelphia, PA: Lippincott Williams & Wilkins; 2002.)

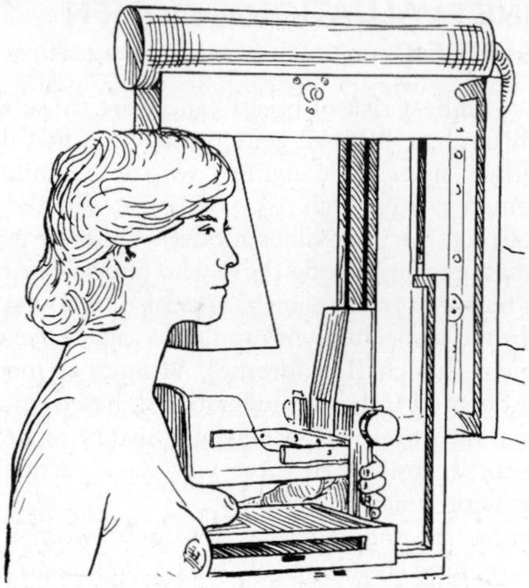

Figure 32-3 • Mammogram.

Other Tools

Ultrasonography has been established as a useful addition to mammography. It can be helpful in the evaluation of uncertain mammographic findings, in women younger than 40, in women with dense breast tissue, and as a tool to guide a needle for breast biopsies. It is also useful in distinguishing a cyst from a solid mass. If a high-risk patient is unable to undergo MRI imaging, ultrasound may be used instead.

Digital mammography (as compared with film mammography) has been found to be a better imaging modality in women with dense breasts, women younger than 50, and premenopausal or perimenopausal women.

EVALUATION OF BREAST PAIN

Breast pain (mastalgia, mastodynia) is a **common complaint** (65%) in women but is not always reported to a healthcare provider. The pain is typically **mild** and may be **cyclic** (67%) or **noncyclic** (33%) in nature. Breast pain can be a normal physiologic response to hormonal fluctuations, or it can be a pathologic response to trauma or malignancy. Mastalgia may be a component of premenstrual syndrome, associated with hormone replacement therapy (HRT) or pregnancy, or caused by menstrual irregularities or fibrocystic change. Only 1% to 7% of women with breast pain will have underlying malignancy.

The patient's **medical history**, including benign or malignant diseases of the breast, is relevant. Clinicians need to establish whether the pain is cyclic or noncyclic, bilateral or unilateral, diffuse or focal. They must also ask about **associated symptoms** (back/neck pain, erythema, fever) and use of medications such as oral contraceptive pills (OCPs) and HRT. Also relevant are any history of trauma, radiation or surgery to the breast, family history of breast disease, and constitutional symptoms such as weight loss or gain, chest wall pain, or amenorrhea. If the patient is **breastfeeding**, the physician should rule out mastitis or a breast abscess.

The history and physical examination are typically enough to provide **reassurance** to a patient. Focal lesions or areas of trauma can be evaluated with an **ultrasound** in women. Women at high risk of cancer should be evaluated with **mammography**. The vast majority of breast pain is benign and can be treated with oral and topical nonsteroidal anti-inflammatory drugs **(NSAIDs)**, a **supportive bra** or sports bra, diet and lifestyle changes (decrease caffeine intake and smoking), and the use of warm and cool **compresses** and massage. Many women will require a decreased dose or discontinuation of oral contraceptions and HRT in order to relieve their breast pain. Danazol is the only medication approved by the FDA to treat mastalgia. However, it is associated with signficant side effects. The data have been inconclusive regarding the effectiveness of vitamin E and evening primrose oil on breast pain. Management of breast pain associated with specific benign and malignant processes is further discussed below.

EVALUATION OF NIPPLE DISCHARGE

As many as 50% to 80% of women will have nipple discharge at some point during their reproductive years. The vast majority of nipple discharge is due to normal physiology or benign processes, and only 5% is associated with underlying malignancy (Table 32-1). The **most concerning** discharge is spontaneous, **bloody** or serosanguineous, **unilateral**, **persistent**, from a **single duct** and **associated with a mass**. Bilateral, nonbloody, multiductal secretion is usually benign regardless of color.

The most common cause of **bloody nipple discharge** is an **intraductal papilloma,** although invasive papillary cancer can also present in this manner. **Galactorrhea** is associated with pregnancy, pituitary adenomas, hypothyroidism, stress, and medications such as OCPs, antihypertensives,

TABLE 32-1 Causes of Nipple Discharge

Etiology Class	Conditions
Benign breast disease	Intraductal papilloma, ductal hyperplasia, duct ectasia, fibrocystic breast changes
Premalignant and malignant breast disease	Intraductal carcinoma (in situ or invasive), diffuse papillomatosis
Systemic disease	Hyperprolactinemia, hypothyroidism, pituitary adenomas, sarcoidosis, chronic renal failure, liver cirrhosis
Medications	Oral contraceptives, phenothiazines, methyldopa, reserpine, imipramine, amphetamines, metoclopramide
Chest wall lesions	Thoracotomy, chest wall trauma and burns, herpes zoster
Skin changes mistaken for nipple discharge	Paget disease, insect bites, local infection, eczema
Chronic breast stimulation	Poorly fitted bra, stimulation by partner, self-stimulation

and psychotropic drugs. **Serous discharge** is associated with normal menses, OCPs, fibrocystic change, or early pregnancy. **Yellow-tinged discharge** is associated with fibrocystic change or galactocele. **Green, sticky discharge** is associated with duct ectasia. **Purulent discharge** indicates superficial or central breast abscess.

When a patient presents with nipple discharge, it is important to delineate the nature of the discharge: its **color, bilaterality**, the number of **duct openings** involved, and whether it occurs **spontaneously** or with manual expression. The physical examination should look for **skin changes**, associated **masses** or lymphadenopathy. An attempt should be made to elicit secretion by applying pressure to the base of the areola. Bloody or serosanguineous discharge should be tested on a **guaiac card** and sent for **cytologic evaluation**. Routine culture is not indicated. Women with associated amenorrhea, menstrual irregularities, headaches, or visual disturbances should have **prolactin and thyroid levels** drawn. Women with associated masses should have **ultrasound and/or mammography** evaluation, depending on their age (generally ultrasound <30 and mammogram ≥30).

Most nipple discharge is benign and does not require treatment. When indicated, treatment should be individualized to the specific cause of the discharge.

EVALUATION OF BREAST MASSES

If a patient is found to have a **breast mass** on the clinician's examination or her own self-examination, a thorough history and examination are crucial. Importantly, up to **10% to 15% of new breast cancers are not seen or detected via mammography**; therefore, a suspicious mass should never be dismissed just because the mammogram is negative. The most common causes of breast masses are **fibroadenomas and breast cysts**.

When evaluating a breast mass, it is important to ascertain the manner in which it was discovered, associated tenderness or trauma, and the relationship of changes to the menstrual cycle. Likewise, its location, size, shape, consistency, and mobility should be noted, as well as any overlying skin changes. Worrisome lumps are dominant, discrete, and dense. **Malignant masses are classically single, firm, nontender, and immobile with irregular borders**. Lymph nodes are worrisome if larger than 1 cm, fixed, irregular, firm, or multiple.

Abnormal breast masses should also be **evaluated radiographically**. For **women younger than 30 years, ultrasound** is the preferred initial method of imaging. Ultrasound is also useful in distinguishing **solid versus cystic** masses in women of any age. For **women aged 30 or older, mammography** is used to further evaluate suspicious masses. To standardize mammogram reporting, a collaborative scoring system was devised and published by the American College of Radiology. It is known as the **Breast Imaging Reporting and Database System** (BI-RADS). This system (Table 32-2) categorizes mammographic findings to translate the radiologist's opinion of the absence or likelihood of breast cancer. Findings that are most suggestive of malignancy include a spiculated mass; architectural distortion with retraction; asymmetric localized fibrosis; microcalcifications with linear, branched patterns; increased vascularity; or altered subareolar duct pattern (Fig. 32-4).

Any concerning palpable mass or abnormality seen on radiologic imaging should be evaluated with mammography (if not previously performed) and biopsied to obtain a **pathologic diagnosis** (Table 32-3). The goal of tissue biopsy is to obtain an adequate sample for diagnosis using the least invasive sampling possible. If a palpable cystic mass is found on examination and confirmed on ultrasound, it can be drained and sampled for diagnosis using **needle aspiration** (Fig. 32-5). This treats the cyst and also provides fluid for cytology if indicated by turbid or bloody aspirate. The **cyst should be excised** if the fluid is bloody, a mass persists after fluid is removed, the cyst is persistent after two aspirations, or if the fluid reaccumulates within 2 weeks.

When a **palpable solid mass** is found on examination and confirmed with ultrasound or mammography, a tissue sample should be obtained for diagnosis. In women less than 30 years old, **fine-needle aspiration** (FNA) can be used to sample solid masses (Fig. 32-6). This technique involves an experienced cytopathologist making multiple passes through the mass from different angles while aspirating the syringe on a 20G to 22G needle. Diagnostic accuracy approaches 80% to 90%. An **excisional biopsy** is performed if the FNA does not obtain fluid or tissue. Excisional biopsy is also performed if cytology or histology is nondiagnostic. In women aged 30 years or older with a palpable solid mass, a **core-needle biopsy** is recommended.

When a **nonpalpable lesion** is found by mammography, excisional biopsy can also be performed under **needle or wire guidance**. The goal should be to excise the abnormal tissue along with a 1-cm rim of normal tissue to qualify for lumpectomy, thus avoiding the need for repeat surgery if the mass is malignant.

TABLE 32-2 Breast Imaging Reporting and Database System (BI-RADS) for Characterization of Mammogram Findings

Cat	Assessment Category	Recommended Action	Risk of Malignancy
0	Incomplete	Additional imaging needed	N/A
1	Negative	Routine follow-up	0%
2	Benign finding(s)	Routine follow-up	0%
3	Probably benign	Short-interval (6 mo) follow-up	≤2%
4	Suspicious of malignancy	Core-needle biopsy ASAP	2%–95%
5	Highly suspicious of malignancy	Core-needle biopsy ASAP	≥95%
6	Known, biopsy-proven malignancy	Definitive treatment ongoing	100%

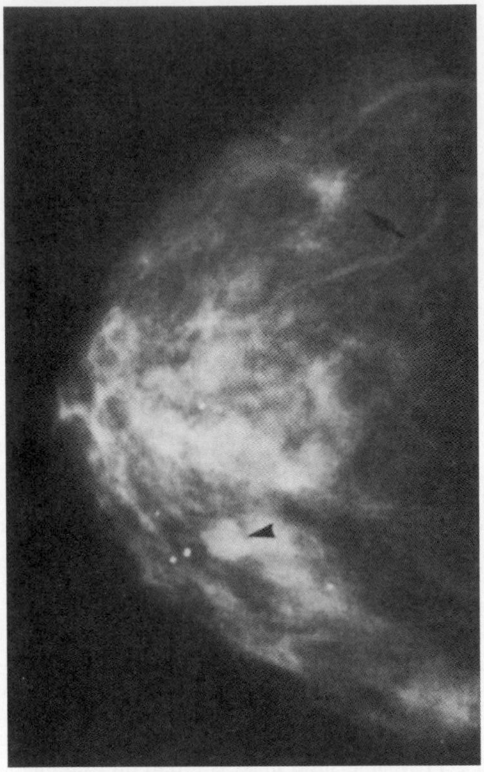

Figure 32-4 • A cephalocaudal mammogram film contrasting a small speculated mass carcinoma (*arrow*) versus a well-marginated fibroadenoma (*arrowhead*).
(From Beckmann C, Ling F. *Obstetrics & Gynecology*. 5th ed. Philadelphia, PA: Lippincott Williams & Wilkins; 2006.)

TABLE 32-3 Evaluation of Abnormal Breast Masses and Abnormal Mammogram Findings

Abnormal Findings		Appropriate Evaluation
Palpable cystic lesion	→	Needle drainage
Recurrent cyst, bloody fluid	→	Excision
Solid, palpable mass (<30 y)	→	FNA
Nondiagnostic FNA of solid mass	→	Excisional biopsy
Solid, palpable mass (≥30 y)	→	Core-needle biopsy
Nondiagnostic core-needle biopsy	→	Excisional biopsy
Nonpalpable abnormal mammogram finding	→	Wire-guided excision

BENIGN BREAST DISEASE

Benign breast symptoms and findings are common and occur in approximately 50% of women, with a higher incidence in younger women. The decision to biopsy any abnormal breast findings for definitive diagnosis is influenced by the patient's risk factors for malignant disease. Two-thirds of tumors in reproductive-age women are benign, whereas half of palpable masses in perimenopausal women and the majority of lesions in postmenopausal women are malignant.

FIBROCYSTIC BREAST CHANGES

Pathophysiology

Fibrocystic change of the breast includes a spectrum of clinical findings due to **exaggerated stromal response** to hormones and growth factors. It typically presents as **painful breast masses** that are **often multiple and usually bilateral**. There can be rapid fluctuation in the size of the masses. The associated breast changes can include cystic change, nodularity, stromal proliferation, and epithelial hyperplasia. In the absence of atypical hyperplasia, **fibrocystic change is not associated with increased cancer risk**.

Epidemiology

Peak incidence is between ages 30 and 40, but changes can persist throughout a woman's entire life. The changes are rare in postmenopausal women.

Diagnosis

Patients with fibrocystic changes present with breast swelling, pain, and tenderness. Fibrocystic disease may have more focal symptomatic areas, involve both breasts, and vary throughout the menstrual cycle. The pain is commonly worse as the mass size increases during the **premenstrual part of the cycle**. Evaluation with mammogram, ultrasound, and/or biopsy should be performed for suspicious lesions (dominant mass that does not fluctuate in size).

Treatment

The pain of fibrocystic breast changes can be ameliorated with **reduction of caffeine, tea, and chocolate** although the role of caffeine reduction is controversial. **Avoiding trauma and wearing a support bra** may also help decrease the pain associated with fibrocystic change. Although the data have been inconsistent, other recognized treatments include **evening primrose oil, vitamins E and B_6, danazol, progestins, bromocriptine, and tamoxifen** (not approved for this indication).

FIBROADENOMA

Pathogenesis

Breast fibroadenomas are benign tumors with glandular and stromal components (Fig. 32-4). Most masses are 1 to 5 cm in diameter at the time of detection. Lesions larger than 5 cm are termed *giant fibroadenomas*. In these cases, cystosarcoma phyllodes should be ruled out. Fibroadenomas are **usually solitary** but can be multiple. These are bilaterally up to 25% of the time. The etiology is unknown but is likely related to the hormonal milieu.

Epidemiology

Fibroadenomas are the most common benign tumors of the breast. They usually occur in women aged 15 to 35. They are more common than breast cysts in women younger than 25 years. They very rarely occur and often regress after menopause.

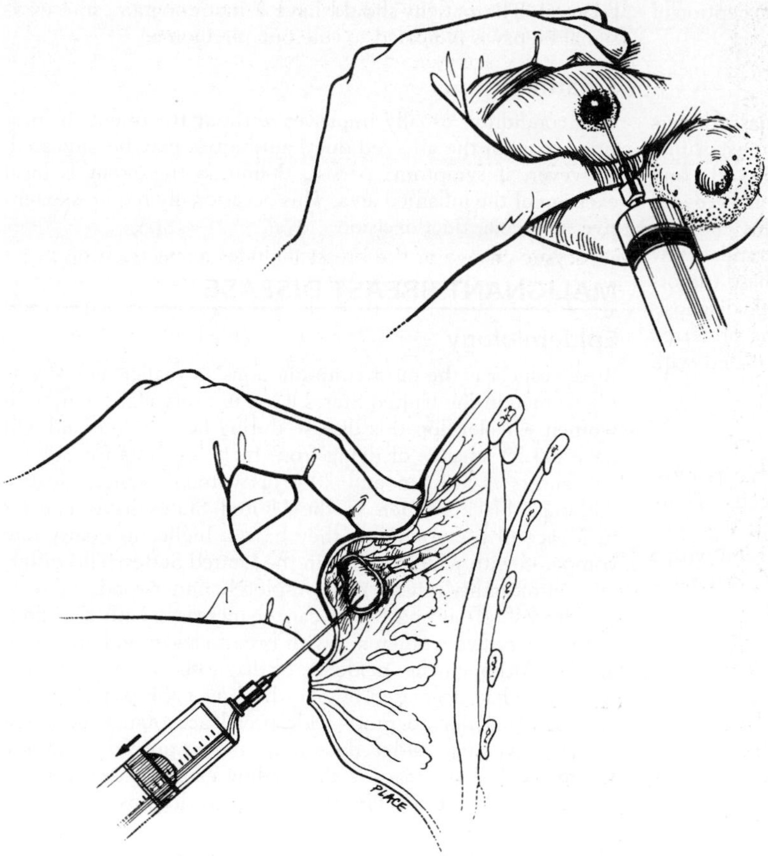

Figure 32-5 • Needle aspiration of a breast cyst.
(From LifeART image copyright © 2006 Lippincott Williams & Wilkins. All rights reserved.)

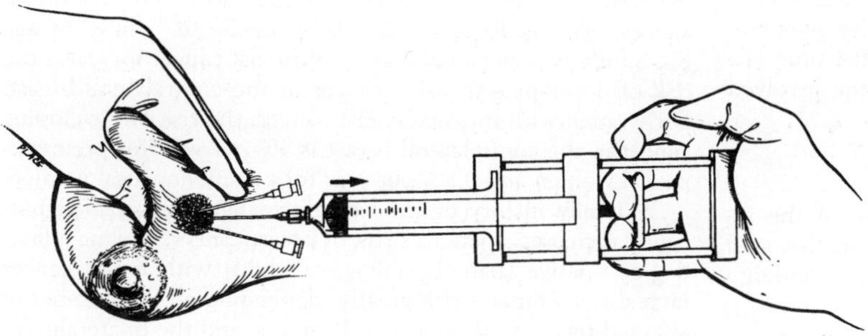

Figure 32-6 • Fine-needle aspiration of a solid breast mass.
(From Beckmann C, Ling F. *Obstetrics & Gynecology*. 5th ed. Philadelphia, PA: Lippincott Williams & Wilkins; 2006.)

Diagnosis

Fibroadenomas are often palpated on physical examination as round, well-circumscribed, mobile, firm lesions that are **rubbery and nontender**. The patient may report changes in the lesion during the menstrual cycle, pregnancy, and with OCP use. Classic fibroadenoma in a woman less than 30 years old may be the only solid breast mass that does not require tissue diagnosis.

Treatment

A young patient (<30 years old) with classic presentation of a simple fibroadenoma with no adjacent proliferative damage and no family history of breast cancer can be **followed clinically if stable**. Otherwise, FNA for cytology is highly sensitive for detecting cancer or phyllodes tumors. If simple fibroadenoma is confirmed by biopsy, **and is asymptomatic it can be left in place or treated with cryoablation**. If the fibroadenoma is large or worrisome, excisional biopsy is recommended to remove the tumor and establish pathologic diagnosis.

CYSTOSARCOMA PHYLLODES

Pathogenesis

Phyllodes tumors are a **rare variant of fibroadenoma** and involve epithelial and stromal proliferation.

Epidemiology

These tumors are diagnosed most commonly in premenopausal women, although they can occur at any age. There have been no etiologic or predisposing factors identified, with the exception of Li–Fraumeni syndrome.

Diagnosis

This lesion appears as a **large, bulky, mobile mass that is painless**. The overlying skin is warm, erythematous, shiny, and engorged. The mass is **large** (4 to 7 cm), smooth, and well circumscribed and is characterized by **rapid growth**. Most lesions are benign; however, some physicians consider cystosarcoma phyllodes a **low-grade malignancy,** and a few tumors do develop true sarcomatous potential. These tumors are worrisome for aggressive malignancies; pathologic diagnosis must therefore be made. **Core-needle biopsy** is the preferred method for diagnosis, but should be strongly correlated with clinical suspicion.

Treatment

The clinical course of these tumors is unpredictable as most appear benign, but **10% do contain malignant cells**. There is also a high rate of local recurrence after simple excision. Recommended therapy is therefore **wide local excision** with a 1-cm margin for small tumors and simple mastectomy for large lesions not amenable to wide local excision.

INTRADUCTAL PAPILLOMA

Pathogenesis

Intraductal papilloma is a benign solitary lesion that involves the **epithelial lining of lactiferous ducts**. It is the most common cause of **bloody nipple discharge** in the absence of a concurrent mass.

Diagnosis

Intraductal papilloma usually appears with bloody nipple discharge in premenopausal women. The serosanguineous discharge is **sent for cytology** to rule out invasive papillary carcinoma, which has similar symptoms 25% of the time. To identify the papilloma, the physician can open the involved duct to visualize the tumor.

Treatment

Definitive diagnosis and treatment is by **excision of the involved ducts** after localization by physical examination and core-needle biopsy. Intraductal papillomas rarely undergo malignant transformation.

MAMMARY DUCT ECTASIA (PLASMA CELL MASTITIS)

Pathogenesis

This subacute inflammation and fibrosis of the ductal system causes dilated mammary ducts. There are infiltration of plasma cells and significant periductal inflammation.

Epidemiology

This lesion most commonly occurs **at or after menopause**, but is also a cause of breast mass in adolescents.

Diagnosis

Patients present with **nipple discharge**, noncyclic **breast pain**, **nipple retraction**, or subareolar masses. The discharge is multicolored, sticky, originating from multiple ducts, and **often bilateral**. The patient should have a mammogram, and excisional biopsy is indicated to rule out carcinoma.

Treatment

This condiditon usually improves without treatment. If mastitis occurs in the affected duct, antibiotics may be indicated. However, if symptoms persist, definitive treatment is **local excision** of the inflamed area. This occasionally requires extensive subareolar duct excision.

MALIGNANT BREAST DISEASE

Epidemiology

Breast cancer is the most common nonskin malignancy affecting women in the United States. One in every eight American women will develop this disease during her lifetime and will have a 3.5% chance of dying from it. It accounts for 30% of all cancers in women and 20% of women's cancer deaths. Although black women in the United States have a lower incidence of breast cancer, they have a higher mortality rate compared with white women in the United States. This difference in mortality rates is not completely understood.

The risk of getting breast cancer increases with age. Four out of every five women are with breast cancer and are above age 50. Although the incidence of diagnosis is increasing, the death rate had decreased by one-third over the past 25 years. This is likely due to more widespread acceptance of breast cancer screening, earlier detection, and improved therapies. Currently, breast cancer is the leading cause of death in US women aged 40 to 59. The average age of diagnosis is 61.

Risk Factors

Numerous risk factors are associated with breast cancer (Table 32-4). One major risk factor is **increasing age**. For example, an American woman's annual risk of invasive breast cancer increases from 1 in 2,000 by age 30 to "1 in 8" by age 80. Similarly, **a personal history of breast cancer** increases the risk of developing invasive cancer in the contralateral breast. For women with invasive breast cancer, the risk of developing cancer in the contralateral breast is 1% per year for premenopausal women and 0.5% per year for postmenopausal women.

A **family history** of gynecologic malignancies also significantly increases a patient's risk of breast cancer. Having a first-degree relative (parent, sibling, or child) with breast cancer increases a woman's risk greatly, depending on the number of affected relatives, their age at diagnosis, and the bilaterality of their disease. Having one affected first-degree family member increases the patient's risk by nearly two times and having two first-degree family members increases a patient's risk by nearly three times. These risks are even further amplified if the family member was premenopausal at the time of diagnosis.

A strong family history is suspicious for a **genetic predisposition**. Although **10% of women with breast cancer have a family history** of the disease, inherited genetic mutations are still rare. Six familial syndromes have been identified with an increased risk of breast cancer. The best known of these are the BRCA1 and BRCA2 genes associated with **bilateral premenopausal breast cancer** and breast cancer associated with ovarian cancer.

Exposure to **ionizing radiation** of the chest at a young age (such as used in the treatment of Hodgkin lymphoma) and alcohol abuse can significantly increase the risk of breast cancer. Diagnosis of atypical **ductal or lobular hyperplasia** on

TABLE 32-4 Breast Cancer Risk Factors

Risk Factors	Category at Risk	Comparison Category	Relative Risk
Alcohol intake	Two drinks per day	Nondrinker	1.2
Body mass index	80th percentile, age 55 or greater	20th percentile	1.2
HRT with estrogen and progesterone	Current user for at least 5 y	Never used	1.3
Radiation exposure	Repeated fluoroscopy	No exposure	1.6
	Radiation therapy for Hodgkin's disease	No exposure	5.2
Early menarche	Younger than 12 y	Older than 15 y	1.3
Late menopause	Older than 55 y	Younger than 45	1.2–1.5
Age at first childbirth	Nulliparous or first child after 30	First child before 20	1.7–1.9
Current age	65 or older	<65	5.8
Past history of breast cancer	Invasive breast carcinoma	No history of invasive breast carcinoma	6.8
Other histologic findings	LCIS	No abnormality detected	16.4
	DCIS	No abnormality detected	17.3
Breast biopsy	Hyperplasia without atypia[a]	No hyperplasia	1.9
	Hyperplasia with atypia	No hyperplasia	5.3
	Hyperplasia with atypia and positive family history	No hyperplasia, negative family history	11
Cytology (FNA, nipple aspiration fluid)	Proliferation without atypia[a]	No abnormality detected	2.5
	Proliferation with atypia	No abnormality detected	4.9–5
	Proliferation with atypia and positive family history	No abnormality detected	18.1
Family history	First-degree relative 50 y or older with postmenopausal breast cancer	No first- or second-degree relative with breast cancer	1.8
	First-degree relative with premenopausal breast cancer	No first- or second-degree relative with breast cancer	3.3
	Second-degree relative with breast cancer	No first- or second-degree relative with breast cancer	1.5
	Two first-degree relatives with breast cancer	No first- or second-degree relative with breast cancer.	3.6
Germline mutation	Heterozygous for BRCA1, age <40	Not heterozygous for BRCA1, age <40	200[b]
	Heterozygous for BRCA1, age 60–69	Not heterozygous for BRCA1, age 60–69	15[b]

[a]There is controversy over whether pathologic hyperplasia detected in breast biopsy samples is directly equivalent to cytologic hyperplasia detected in samples obtained through FNA or nipple aspiration.
[b]Begg has suggested that these relative risks are subject to ascertainment bias and may overestimate the true risk associated with germline mutations in BRCA genes.

biopsy increases risk by a factor of 5. The presence of ductal or lobular carcinoma in situ (LCIS) or noninvasive carcinomas also increases cancer risk.

Between 0.5% and 4.0% of breast cancer is diagnosed surrounding **pregnancy or lactation**. Compared to nonpregnant women with breast cancer at similar stage and age, **survival rates seem equivalent** for pregnant or lactating women with breast cancer. Younger age at menarche, nulliparity, later date of first live birth, and later age at menopause have all been linked with increased risk of breast cancer. This is thought to be due to cumulative **lifetime estrogen exposure**.

The question of whether or not **postmenopausal HRT** changes the risk of breast cancer has been hotly debated. It is now generally believed that patients who use combination HRT for more than 5 years are at a slightly **increased risk** of developing invasive breast cancer. This risk has not been seen in women using estrogen-only hormone therapy (ERT). **Past and current** OCP use has not been shown to **increase the risk** of breast cancer, nor has the use of caffeine, breast implants, electric blankets, or hair dyes.

Prevention

Early pregnancy, prolonged lactation, chemical or surgical sterilization, exercise, abstinence from alcohol, and a low-fat diet may help prevent breast cancer. The studies linking phytoestrogens to a reduction of breast cancer risk have been inconclusive. These are naturally occurring plant substances similar to estradiol and are composed mainly of isoflavones such as those found in soybeans—a major component of tofu. Similarly, no protective effect has been proven with the use of aspirin and other NSAIDs.

Tamoxifen, a selective estrogen receptor modulator (SERM), is effective in suppressing the development of breast cancer. By binding to the estrogen receptor (ER), tamoxifen **competitively inhibits estrogen binding** and thereby blocking stimulation of breast cancer cells. Tamoxifen is currently used as adjuvant therapy in patients with early stage, surgically treated, ER-positive breast cancer and has been shown to decrease the rate of recurrent breast cancer by 40% and breast cancer mortality by 35%.

Diagnosis

The trifecta of routine breast care is **breast self-awareness**, the annual **clinician breast examination**, and annual **mammography** for women aged 40 and over or those who are at high risk for breast cancer. Thirty percent to 50% of breast cancers are diagnosed as a result of an abnormality detected via mammography.

Patients may present clinically with **breast masses**, **skin change**, **nipple discharge**, or symptoms of metastatic disease. **Skin dimpling** can occur due to tethering of Cooper ligaments from the mass underneath. The skin can appear erythematous and warm, with **nipple retraction** or inversion. Tissue edema or a **peau d'orange appearance** may occur due to dermal lymphatic invasion and blockage. The superficial epidermis of the nipple may appear eczematous or ulcerated, as in Paget disease.

Bloody discharge needs to be evaluated to rule out invasive papillary carcinoma although the most common cause is benign intraductal papilloma. Palpable masses are often detected by the patient or the partner on self-examination and are usually nontender, irregular, firm, and immobile. **Fifty percent of tumors occur in the UOQ** (Fig. 32-7). These tumors can be multifocal, multicentric, or bilateral. Mammography is the best tool to detect early lesions, reducing mortality by 32% to 50%. Recent studies have shown that mammography is less effective in women with dense breast tissue—for example, in African American women. Furthermore, up to **20% of new breast cancers are not detectable on mammography,** so any suspicious lesion should be biopsied if clinically indicated, even if the mammogram is negative.

A nonpalpable suspicious lesion found on mammogram requires **localized needle biopsy** or **stereotactic FNA** for pathologic diagnosis.

The evaluation for metastatic disease with a thorough history, physical, and imaging is also an important part of breast disease management. Breast cancer tends to metastasize to the **bone, liver, lung, pleura, brain,** and **lymph nodes**. Patients may present with constitutional symptoms of weight loss, anorexia, night sweats, and fatigue. They may also have dyspnea, cough, and/or bone pain.

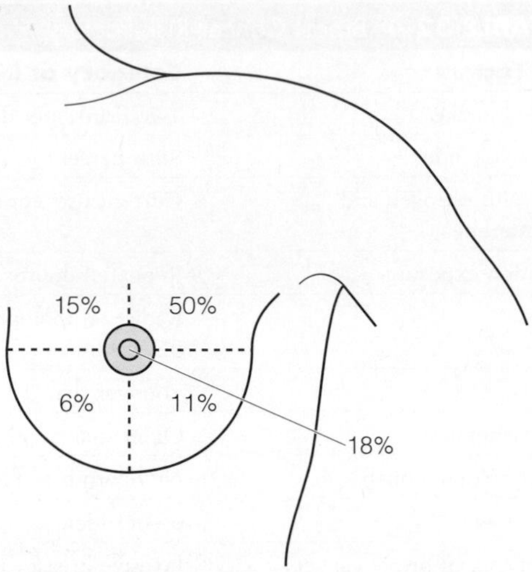

Figure 32-7 • Most common locations of malignant lesions.

NONINVASIVE DISEASE

Lobular Carcinoma in Situ

Pathogenesis

LCIS is the proliferation of **malignant epithelial cells** contained within breast lobules with no invasion of the stroma (Fig. 32-8). It is usually multicentric and is bilateral 50% to 90% of the time. It is considered by some to be a premalignant lesion that is, itself, not a true cancer. However, most agree that the importance of LCIS is as **an indicator for subsequent risk of invasive breast cancer** (25% to 30% within 15 years) in the ipsilateral or contralateral breast or in both breasts.

Epidemiology

The average age at diagnosis is the mid-40s. Patients are typically premenopausal.

Diagnosis

LCIS is usually diagnosed incidentally on biopsy for another finding as it **is not palpable** and **not seen on mammograms**.

Treatment

Because its significance is controversial, there is debate regarding optimal treatment. Currently, there are three options: **observation without further therapy**, prophylactic chemoprevention with **SERMs** such as tamoxifen or raloxifene, or bilateral mastectomy. SERMs may reduce the risk of subsequent cancer by 50%. Before deciding on treatment, invasive cancer or ductal carcinoma in situ (DCIS) must be ruled out. Subsequent cancers may be intraductal, invasive ductal, or lobular carcinoma and may be in the ipsilateral or contralateral breast.

Ductal Carcinoma in Situ

Pathogenesis

DCIS—also called intraductal carcinoma—involves proliferation of **malignant epithelial cells** in mammary ducts without spread to the breast stroma (Fig. 32-8). It is more common than LCIS, and, if left untreated, has a **higher potential to progress to invasive carcinoma** than does LCIS.

Epidemiology

Average age at diagnosis is mid-50s.

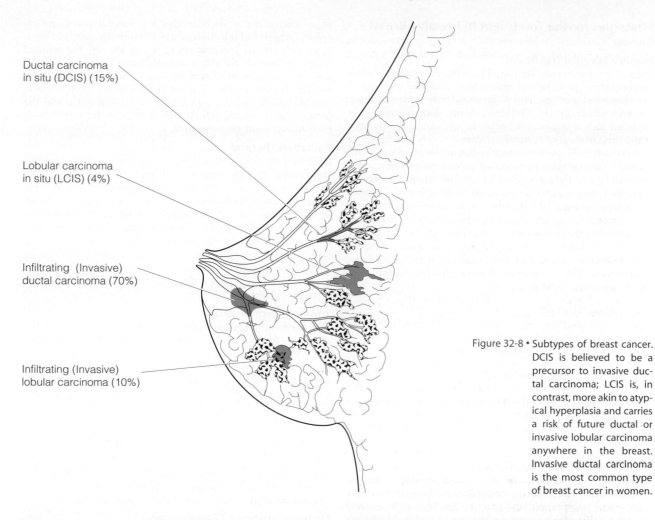

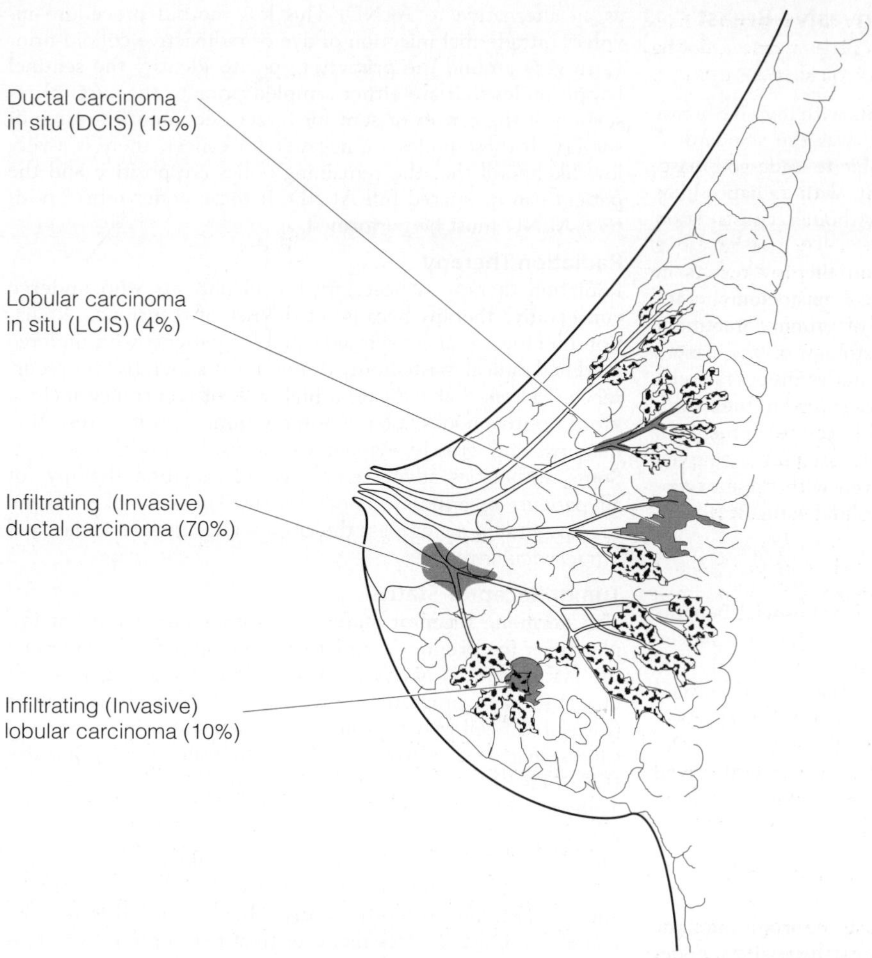

Figure 32-8 • Subtypes of breast cancer. DCIS is believed to be a precursor to invasive ductal carcinoma; LCIS is, in contrast, more akin to atypical hyperplasia and carries a risk of future ductal or invasive lobular carcinoma anywhere in the breast. Invasive ductal carcinoma is the most common type of breast cancer in women.

Diagnosis

Ninety percent of DCIS is detected by **screening mammography** revealing **clustered microcalcifications**. Ten percent present with a **palpable mass**. Diagnosis can be established by needle localization biopsy or excisional biopsy of a palpable lesion. Thirty-five percent of lesions are multicentric; bilateral disease is rare.

Treatment

Current treatment involves conservative surgical **excision of all microcalcifications with wide margins**. Simple **mastectomy** is occasionally necessary for extensive lesions, but is considered overly aggressive for the treatment of all women with DCIS. If resection margins are inadequate (<10 mm), **radiation therapy** may be used to reduce the risk of local recurrence but has no impact on survival. The risk of subsequent invasive ductal carcinoma or local recurrence of intraductal carcinoma is approximately 5% per year. Of recurrent disease, 50% will be DCIS; the other 50% will be invasive carcinoma.

INVASIVE BREAST CANCERS

Infiltrating Ductal Carcinoma

This is the **most common breast malignancy**, accounting **for 76% of all invasive breast cancers**. The tumor arises from the ductal epithelium and infiltrates the supporting stroma (Fig. 32-8). Less common but more favorable subtypes include medullary carcinoma, colloid carcinoma, tubular carcinoma, and papillary carcinoma.

Invasive Lobular Carcinoma

Lobular carcinoma arises from the lobular epithelium and infiltrates the breast stroma (Fig. 32-8). It accounts for 8% of all invasive breast cancers and tends to be bilateral.

Paget Disease of the Nipple

Paget disease accounts for 1% to 3% of all breast malignancies. It is often concomitant with DCIS or invasive carcinoma in the subareolar area. The malignant cells enter the **epidermis of the nipple**, causing the classic eczematous changes of the nipple. Examination reveals crusting, scaling, erosion, discharge, and possibly a breast mass.

Inflammatory Breast Carcinoma

This is an **extremely aggressive** malignancy, accounting for 0.5% to 2% of all breast cancers in the United States. It is a poorly differentiated tumor characterized by **dermal lymphatic invasion**. Symptoms include edema, erythema, warmth, and diffuse induration of the skin described as **peau d'orange**. It is usually accompanied by axillary lymphadenopathy and has distant metastases on presentation 17% to 36% of the time.

Strategies for the Treatment of Invasive Breast Cancer

Primary Surgical Treatment

Surgical resection is required in all patients with invasive breast cancer. In the past, radical mastectomy was the standard of care; however, most patients today are able to undergo breast-conserving therapy (BCT) (lumpectomy with radiation), or modified radical mastectomy with or without reconstruction at the time of surgery or at a later date.

BCT with **lumpectomy and radiation therapy results in identical survival rates as modified radical mastectomy** in appropriately selected patients. The type of primary treatment depends largely upon the **size and histology** of the cancer and on the presence of **palpable lymph nodes** preoperatively. Large tumors (>5 cm) and those that have spread to the lymph nodes tend to recur more often, so BCT is not recommended. Patients with large tumors benefit from mastectomy coupled with postoperative radiation therapy. Even with these exceptions, **60% to 75% of women will be candidates for BCT** with lumpectomy and radiation.

Breast Reconstruction

Breast reconstruction carries significant **psychosocial benefits** for women with breast cancer. Reconstruction can be achieved with **implants or with autogenous tissue** (Fig. 32-9). The need for reconstruction is determined by the type of primary surgery. BCT does not typically require reconstruction unless a large mass is removed from a small breast. Also, reconstruction can be performed **at the time of initial surgery or deferred** until later without any adverse oncologic impact. In either case, the reconstructive surgeon should be consulted before the initial surgery.

Axillary Lymph Node Evaluation

As **axillary node status** is one of the **most important outcome predictors** of breast cancer, evaluation of the axillary nodes must always take place. In the past, this has been accomplished using full **axillary lymph node dissection** (ALND). ALND has been proven to increase survival, decrease recurrence, and provide valuable prognostic information. However, it can also result in arm morbidity, including arm edema, seroma formation, loss of sensation, and shoulder dysfunction. As a result, many centers now utilize **sentinel lymph node biopsy** (SLNB) as an alternative to ALND. This less morbid procedure involves intradermal injection of dye or radioactive colloid prior to surgery around the primary tumor to identify the sentinel lymph nodes that are either sampled prior to the surgical resection of the cancer or sent for frozen section at the time of surgery. If these nodes are negative for cancer, there is a very low likelihood that the remaining nodes are positive and the patient can be spared full ALND. If these nodes return positive, ALND must be performed.

Radiation Therapy

Radiation therapy is necessary for **all patients who undergo conservative therapy** because of the risk of recurrence. Radiation therapy has also been indicated for patients who undergo modified radical mastectomy if they are at a high risk for recurrence. Factors that indicate a **high risk of recurrence** include ≥four positive nodes, a large primary tumor, positive resection margins, and grossly evident extracapsular nodal resection. Some authorities advocate the use of radiation therapy for all patients regardless of node status. The field of radiation therapy should encompass the chest wall, supraclavicular, and infraclavicular regions.

Tumor Receptor Status

The **hormone receptor status** of a tumor has significant implications for **prognosis and treatment** options. To ascertain the status, special assays are run to look for estrogen receptors (ERs) and progesterone receptors (PR), S-phase analysis (measure of cell growth), and HER2/neu status in the excised tumor. In general, **estrogen and progesterone receptor positive** (ER+, PR+) tumors are well differentiated and exhibit a less aggressive clinical behavior, including lower recurrence rate and lower capacity to proliferate. Estrogen and progesterone-positive status therefore carries a **more favorable prognosis** than negative hormone receptor status. In addition to estrogen and progesterone receptor status, **HER2/neu status** has become an important assessment for treatment options. Overexpression of HER2/neu indicates more **aggressive tumors**.

Systemic Adjuvant Chemotherapy

Systemic adjuvant therapy with hormonal therapy, chemotherapy, or both may also be indicated based on lymph node status, tumor size, tumor grade, menopausal status, and tumor receptor status (ER, PR, HER2). Adjuvant chemotherapy results in significantly **decreased risk of recurrence** and **decreased morbidity**.

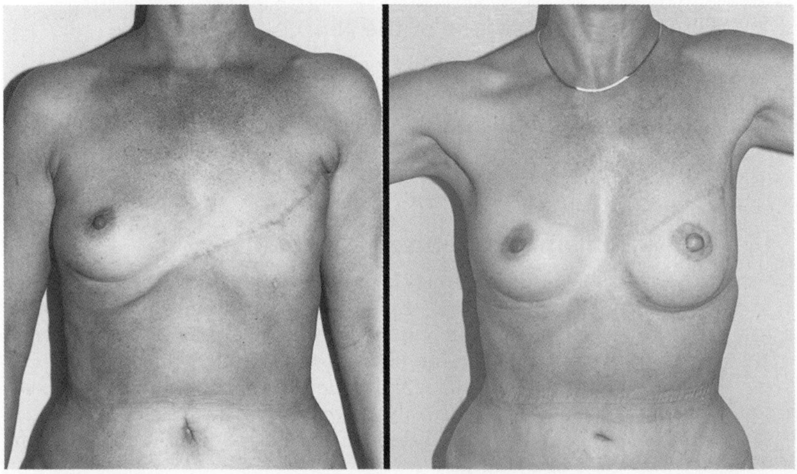

Figure 32-9 • Postmastectomy breast reconstruction. (From Georgiade NG, Reifkohl R, Levine LS. *Georgiade Plastic, Maxillofacial and Reconstructive Surgery.* 3rd ed. Baltimore, MD: Lippincott Williams & Wilkins; 1997.)

Women with **positive lymph node status** are twice as likely to metastasize to other parts of the body, and chemotherapy is indicated. Women with **negative lymph node status but at higher risk** (tumor size >1 cm, high tumor grade) should also undergo chemotherapy with the goal of controlling micrometastases. Various chemotherapy regimens are currently in use. A typical regimen might include a combination of cyclophosphamide (C), methotrexate (M), and 5-fluorouracil (F).

Systemic Adjuvant Hormone Therapy

Systemic hormonal therapy with or without chemotherapy is also utilized for patients with receptor positive cancers (ER+, PR+) regardless of the patient's age or menopausal status. **Tamoxifen** is available for women with positive ER and/or PR status. This antiestrogen works by competitively binding ERs, thus inhibiting the effect of estrogen on breast tissue. Tamoxifen stops estrogen from stimulating the growth of the cancer cells. It is generally used for 5 years after the primary surgical treatment. It is currently the first-line postsurgical treatment for premenopausal breast cancer patients and second-line therapy after **aromatase inhibitors** for postmenopausal patients. **Fulvestrant** is a new ER antagonist that has no agonist effects. It has been approved by the FDA for use in postmenopausal women with hormone-receptor positive breast cancer. It also has positive treatment effects on HER2-positive breast cancer.

Aromatase inhibitors such as letrozole, anstrozole, and exemstane are now available for postmenopausal women with receptor-positive cancers. These newer agents have **antiestrogenic properties** and have been shown to have a longer disease-free survival when compared with tamoxifen.

HER2/neu status is another prognostic factor for more aggressive tumors. Monoclonal antibodies such as trastuzumab are used for adjuvant treatment. Trastuzumab works by binding to the HER2/neu receptor and preventing proliferation.

Treatment of Metastatic or Recurrent Disease

ER negative patients with metastatic or recurrent disease are best treated with combination chemotherapy that may include doxorubicin (Adriamycin [A]) and vincristine (V), in addition to CMF. There is a 75% response to chemotherapy, but this is only temporary (6 to 8 months) with the average additional survival being 1.5 to 2 years from the time of recurrence.

ER positive patients with metastatic or recurrent disease benefit most from hormonal therapy rather than chemotherapy. Premenopausal women may be treated with oophorectomy or gonadotropin-releasing hormone (GnRH) antagonists, whereas postmenopausal women are treated with tamoxifen or aromatase inhibitors.

The choice to continue or reenter treatment should balance the impact on survival with the effects on quality of life.

Prognosis

The most reliable predictor for survival is the **stage of breast cancer** at the time of diagnosis (Table 32-5). Staging is determined by the size of the primary tumor and the absence or

TABLE 32-5 TNM Staging of Breast Cancer

Cancer Stages	Primary Tumor Size	Lymph Node Involvement	Distant Metastases
0	T_{is}	N_0	M_0
I	T_1	N_0	M_0
IIa	T_0	N_1	M_0
	T_1	N_1	M_0
	T_2	N_0	M_0
IIb	T_2	N_1	M_0
	T_3	N_0	M_0
IIIa	T_0	N_2	M_0
	T_1	N_2	M_0
	T_2	N_2	M_0
	T_3	N_1	M_0
	T_3	N_2	M_0
IIIb	T_4	Any N	M_0
	Any T	N_3	M_0
IV	Any T	Any N	M_1
Key: TNM Classification			
T	Primary tumor		
T_x	Primary tumor unassessable		
T_0	No evidence of primary tumor		
T_{is}	Carcinoma in situ; intraductal carcinoma, LCIS, or Paget disease of the nipple with no tumor		
T_1	Tumor ≤2 cm in largest dimension		

Key: TNM Classification	
T_{1c}	Tumor <2 cm but >1 cm
T_2	Tumor ≤ 5 cm but >2 cm in greatest dimension
T_3	Tumor >5 cm in greatest dimension
T_4	Tumor any size extending to chest wall or skin
N	Regional lymph nodes
N_x	Regional lymph nodes cannot be assessed
N_0	No regional lymph node metastases
N_1	Metastasis to mobile ipsilateral axillary lymph node (s)
N_2	Metastasis to the ipsilateral axillary lymph node, fixed and/or internal mammary nodes
N_3	Metastasis to ipsilateral intraclavicular and/or supraclavicular lymph node (s)
M	Distant metastasis
M_x	Presence of distant metastasis cannot be assessed
M_0	No clinical or radiographic evidence of distant metastasis
M_1	Distant metastasis, determined by clinical or radiographic means

Adapted from American Joint Committee on Cancer. *Manual for Staging of Cancer*, 7th edition (2010).

presence of regional lymph node involvement and/or distant metastases. Other prognostic indicators include lymph node status, hormone receptor status, tumor size, nuclear grade, histologic type, proliferative rate, and oncogene expression. The current overall 5-year survival rate for stage 0 breast cancer has increased to 93%. The 5-year disease-free survival rate is 88% for stage I, 74% to 81% for stage II, 41% to 67% for stage III, and 15% for stage IV disease. **Positive estrogen and progesterone receptor status carries a more favorable prognosis as does negative lymph node status.**

Follow-Up

Follow-up after breast cancer treatment should include **a physical examination** every 3 to 6 months for 3 years, every 6 to 12 months for years 4 and 5, and annually thereafter. In women who receive breast-conserving surgery, the first **follow-up mammogram** is usually performed 6 months after completion of lumpectomy and radiation treatment and annually after that. Women who had a mastectomy should continue to have **yearly mammograms** on the remaining breast.

Routine CBC, blood chemistries, tumor markers, chest X-ray, CT, and bone scans are not recommended for routine breast cancer follow-up or for asymptomatic patients. These tests have been replaced with **clinical monitoring for metastatic disease** (dry cough, exertional dyspnea, bone and body pains, pleuritic chest pain, etc.). Women taking **tamoxifen** should be followed for irregular bleeding given the possibility of increased endometrial cancer with tamoxifen use. Endometrial biopsy should be performed for abnormal uterine bleeding.

Hormone Use after Breast Cancer Treatment

Some premenopausal patients may wish to become pregnant after breast cancer treatment. Traditionally, this has been discouraged for fear that pregnancy-related estrogens may stimulate dormant cancer cells. Studies now suggest that **there is no difference in survival rates in women who become pregnant after breast cancer treatment**. For women who wish to avoid fertility after cancer treatment, there has been **no adverse effect shown with the use of oral contraceptives** containing estrogen.

The use of postmenopausal HRT in breast cancer survivors has been widely debated. Several well-constructed, long-term studies such as the Women's Health Initiative have identified an increased risk of breast cancer in women utilizing combination hormone therapy (HRT). For this reason, **HRT use is not recommended in women with a personal history of breast cancer.**

KEY POINTS

- Breast cancer is the most common noncutaneous neoplasm in women, with a lifetime risk of 1 in 8 women in the United States.
- Clinical breast examination every 1 to 3 years is recommended for all women over age 20. Greater emphasis is placed on overall breast self-awareness.
- Current routine mammogram recommendations include a mammogram every 1 to 2 years from age 40 to age 50, and yearly after age 50. No upper age limit has been identified.
- Women with a strong family history of breast cancer should begin screening mammograms 5 years earlier than the age of diagnosis of the youngest family member with breast cancer; 10 years earlier in the case of premenopausal breast cancer.
- Evaluation of breast masses includes careful physical examination, evaluation with mammography and ultrasound of any abnormal findings, and biopsy of suspicious findings to rule out malignancy.
- Benign breast symptoms and findings are common and occur in approximately 50% of women, with a higher incidence in younger women.
- Two-thirds of tumors in reproductive-age women are benign, whereas half of palpable masses in perimenopausal women and the majority of lesions in postmenopausal women are malignant.
- The most common benign breast conditions are breast cysts and fibroadenomas.
- Patients with fibrocystic change often have cyclic breast pain and masses due to an exaggerated stromal response to hormones and growth factors. Reduction in caffeine, tea, and chocolate, and treatment with progestins, danazol, and tamoxifen, have been found to help symptoms.
- Fibroadenomas are benign rubbery breast tumors that are usually solitary. They can be followed with expectant management. When large, they should be biopsied to rule out cystosarcoma phyllodes.
- Benign intraductal papilloma is the most common cause of bloody nipple discharge.
- Numerous risk factors have been identified for breast cancer (increasing age, family history, high-fat diet, ionizing radiation, late childbearing, atypical hyperplasia; prolonged HRT use); however, most patients have no known risk factors.
- Only 5% to 10% of breast cancer is related to genetic predisposition.
- DCIS (15%) is a preinvasive disease and is treated with lumpectomy and radiation therapy. LCIS (4%) is treated with observation and possible use of tamoxifen to prevent subsequent invasive breast cancer.
- Invasive breast disease—including infiltrating ductal carcinoma (76%) and infiltrating lobular carcinoma (8%)—is treated with lumpectomy and radiation or with modified mastectomy with equal risk of recurrence and survival in properly selected patients.
- Breast reconstruction can be an important part of recovering from breast cancer. It can be done during the primary surgery or delayed until later.
- All women with invasive breast disease should have ipsilateral lymph node evaluation with ALND or sentinel node dissection. The resected tumors should also be checked for hormone receptor status.
- The standard adjuvant treatment for women with positive lymph nodes is combination chemotherapy.
- All hormone receptor positive patients should receive hormone therapy aimed at suppressing estrogen, and thereby suppressing stimulation of cancer cells. This is most commonly achieved with tamoxifen (an estrogen agonist/antagonist) or aromatase inhibitors (e.g., letrozole, anastrazole), which have antiestrogen activity.
- Follow-up for patients with invasive breast cancer includes annual bilateral mammography in women who underwent lumpetomy and radiation and annual mammography of the contralateral breast in women who underwent mastectomy.
- Frequent physical examination to evaluate for recurrent metastatic disease is also indicated. Other routine blood and imaging studies are not indicated in the asymptomatic patient.
- The use of HRT and ERT should be avoided in breast cancer survivors.

C Clinical Vignettes

Vignette 1

A 38-year-old female G0 presents to your office for her annual gynecologic examination. She has just moved to your area, and this is the first time you have seen her. During her history, she reports regular, monthly menses with moderate flow. Her mother was diagnosed with breast cancer at age 48, and her paternal aunt was diagnosed with breast cancer at age 67. She has no other family history for cancer. Her previous gynecologist diagnosed her with fibrocystic breast change, and this worries her. She notices pain in both breasts often, and she has a clear discharge from both nipples around the time of her menses. Her breast examination shows Tanner stage 5 breasts that are symmetric and without palpable mass or abnormal skin changes. Upon palpation of the nipples of both breasts, a clear discharge is noted.

1. Which element of her history and examination is most associated with an increased risk of breast cancer over the general population?
   a. Mother with breast cancer at age 48
   b. Paternal aunt with breast cancer at age 67
   c. History of fibrocystic breast change
   d. Breast pain
   e. Nipple discharge
2. Which element of her history and examination is most associated with a low risk of breast cancer?
   a. Age
   b. Gravidity and parity
   c. Regular menses
   d. Normal breast examination
   e. Paternal aunt with breast cancer at age 67
3. What is the most appropriate evaluation of the nipple discharge?
   a. Express the discharge and send for culture
   b. Express the discharge, perform guaiac, and sent for cytology
   c. Breast ultrasound
   d. Breast mammography
   e. Expectant management

Vignette 2

A 42-year-old female G4P3 presents to your office with complaint of a palpable breast mass that she noticed while performing her breast self-examination. After taking her history, you perform a clinical breast examination which reveals a solitary, 3-cm, mobile, nonpainful, rubbery mass.

1. On the basis of her clinical examination, what is most likely her diagnosis?
   a. Fibrocystic breast change
   b. Fibroadenoma
   c. Cystosarcoma phyllodes
   d. Intraductal papilloma
   e. Invasive breast cancer
2. She undergoes the recommended diagnostic tests for a palpable breast mass in her age group. You are surprised that on biopsy the pathologist finds epithelial and stromal proliferation consistent with a fibroadenoma, but with few scattered malignant cells. She later reports that this mass has grown in size quickly. Her diagnosis is now most consistent with:
   a. Fibrocystic breast change
   b. Fibroadenoma
   c. Cystosarcoma phyllodes
   d. Intraductal papilloma
   e. Invasive breast
3. She returns to your office to discuss the treatment plan. The most appropriate management of her diagnosis is:
   a. Expectant management with serial imaging
   b. Lumpectomy with radiation
   c. Wide local excision with 1-cm margins
   d. Modified radical mastectomy
   e. Bilateral modified radical mastectomy

Vignette 3

A 35-year-old G0 woman presents to your office with complaints of bloody nipple discharge. She is most distraught. Her mother was diagnosed with breast cancer at age 45. When asked about breast self-examination, she denies feeling a mass at home but states she is also not very consistent in examining herself. You perform a guaiac test and cytology of nipple discharge and breast examination.

1. The most likely diagnosis associated with her nipple discharge is:
   a. Fibrocystic breast change
   b. Fibroadenoma
   c. Cystosarcoma phyllodes
   d. Intraductal papilloma
   e. Invasive papillary carcinoma
2. The cytology shows malignant cells, and you can palpate a breast mass just lateral to the nipple. She is sent for diagnostic imaging.

On mammogram, a spiculated mass is identified. Now her most likely diagnosis is:

a. Fibrocystic breast change
b. Fibroadenoma
c. Cystosarcoma phyllodes
d. Intraductal papilloma
e. Invasive papillary carcinoma

3. You refer her to a specialist for treatment. She is very worried because she would still someday like to have a child. What is the most appropriate counseling for this patient?

a. Breast cancer patients should never become pregnant in the future due to the increased risk of recurrence with a pregnancy (regardless of type of tumor)
b. There is no difference in survival among premenopausal patients who become pregnant after treatment and those who do not
c. If her tumor is ER positive only, she is at increased risk of recurrence if she becomes pregnant
d. If her tumor is PR positive only, she is at increased risk of recurrence if she becomes pregnant
e. If her tumor is estrogen *and* progesterone receptor positive, she is at increased risk of recurrence if she becomes pregnant

Vignette 4

A 59-year-old female G4P4 presents to her OB/GYN for her annual examination. She goes for her routine screening mammogram. The radiologist gives her a score of BI-RADS 4 (suspicious of malignancy). She then undergoes stereotactic FNA for biopsy. The result is infiltrating ductal carcinoma. The tumor is ER+, PR+, and HER2/neu neg. The tumor is less than 4 cm in size. You cannot palpate any lymphadnopathy on examination.

1. The most appropriate treatment plan for her is:

a. Bilateral radical masectomy with full ALND followed by radiation therapy
b. Wide local excision with periodic surveillance with breast examination and annual mammogram
c. Modified radical mastectomy with ALND, followed by trastuzumab
d. BCT with lumpectomy and SLNB, followed by tamoxifen for 5 years
e. BCT with lumpectomy, SLNB, and breast reconstruction, followed by radiation and letrozole

2. During surgery, the tumor was found to be 4 cm in size, with negative sentinel node biopsy and negative margins after excision. After she undergoes her treatment, she wants to discuss her prognosis with you. The most appropriate counseling regarding her prognosis is:

a. The current overall 5-year survival rate is 94%; however, the most reliable predictor of survival is the stage of breast cancer at the time of diagnosis
b. Her tumor's estrogen and progesterone receptor status (both positive) is a marker of poor prognosis and decreased survival
c. Her tumor's HER2/neu receptor status (negative) is a marker of poor prognosis and decreased survival
d. Tumor size is not a predictor of prognosis
e. Because she received radiation anyway, her lymph node status is not a predictor of survival

3. She has completed her treatment and is curious how to follow up with her doctor. She does not want to miss a recurrence. The most appropriate recommendations for follow-up are:

a. Physical examination every year with annual mammogram
b. Physical examination every month for 12 months, mammogram every 3 months for 1 year, then annually thereafter for both
c. Physical examination every 6 months with annual mammogram and tumor markers
d. Physical examination every 3 to 6 months for 3 years, then every 6 to 12 months for years 4 and 5, with annual mammogram (beginning 6 months after radiation)
e. Physical examination every year with CBC, chest X-ray, and tumor markers, and annual mammogram

A Answers

Vignette 1 Question 1
Answer A: The risk for breast cancer with a first-degree relative (mother, sister, or daughter) diagnosed before menopause is 1.8–8.8 to 1 (depending on unilaterality or bilaterality of the disease). This risk with having a second-degree relative diagnosed with breast cancer is 1.5 to 1. Fibrocystic change is not associated with an increased risk of breast cancer. Only 1% to 6% of women with breast pain will have an underlying malignancy. Only 5% of patients presenting with nipple discharge will have a malignancy, and this is more likely with unilateral or bloody discharge.

Vignette 1 Question 2
Answer A: The average age of breast cancer diagnosis is 61 years, and four out of every five women with breast cancer are over age 50; thus, this patient's young age is her most protective quality. Nulliparity is associated with a 3:1 risk of breast cancer compared to parous women. Regular menses are theoretically protective due to a constant monthly control of estrogen exposure, but are not as protective as young age. A normal breast examination is a reassuring clinical sign, but 30% to 50% of breast abnormalities are diagnosed by mammography because a lesion is not palpable. Having a second-degree relative with breast cancer is a risk factor and is not protective against breast cancer.

Vignette 1 Question 3
Answer E: With a normal exam and bilateral clear nipple discharge with expression only expectant management and reassurance are appropriate. Bloody nipple discharge should be evaluated by testing with a guaiac card and sent for cytology. This helps rule out a bloody component. The most common cause of bloody nipple discharge is benign intraductal papilloma. The differential includes potential underlying malignancy. Culture, especially without a foul odor or sign of infection, is not necessary in this case. Ultrasound, mammography, and biopsy are reserved for the evaluation of breast masses.

Vignette 2 Question 1
Answer B: A solitary, mobile, nonpainful, rubbery mass is most likely a fibroadenoma. Fibrocystic breast change is typically multiple, painful, bilateral, and fluctuates throughout the menstrual cycle. Cystosarcoma phyllodes is a rare variant of fibroadenoma that is usually associated with overlying skin changes. Intraductal papilloma usually presents as bloody nipple discharge in the absence of a mass. Invasive breast cancer is not usually mobile and rubbery, but is a firm, fixed mass.

Vignette 2 Question 2
Answer C: Cystosarcoma phyllodes is a rare variant of fibroadenoma that grows quickly and is considered a low-grade malignancy due to a small proportion of malignant cells found on biopsy. Fibrocystic breast change and fibroadenoma are not associated with malignant cells. Intraductal papilloma does not present as a mass. Invasive breast cancer would be constituted almost completely of malignant cells.

Vignette 2 Question 3
Answer C: The most appropriate treatment of cystosarcoma phyllodes is wide local excision with 1-cm margins or simple mastectomy. Because it is considered a low-grade malignancy, expectant management is contraindicated. One-centimeter margins are necessary due to the high rate of local recurrence after simple excision. Lumpectomy with radiation and modified radical mastectomy are reserved for treatment of invasive breast cancers.

Vignette 3 Question 1
Answer D: Intraductal papilloma is the most common cause of bloody nipple discharge. The second most common cause is invasive (papillary) breast cancer. Fibrocystic breast change, fibroadenoma, and cystosarcoma phyllodes typically present as painful and nonpainful breast masses.

Vignette 3 Question 2
Answer E: Invasive papillary carcinoma is the second most common cause of bloody nipple discharge, and it is a malignancy (unlike intraductal papilloma). Fibrocystic breast change and fibroadenoma are not malignant. Cystosarcoma phyllodes is not associated with bloody nipple discharge.

Vignette 3 Question 3
Answer B: Studies have shown that there is no difference in survival rates in women who become pregnant after successful breast cancer treatment, regardless of tumor type or receptor status. However, it is generally recommended that pregnancy be delayed until 2 to 3 years after completion of treatment, not because of any influence of the pregnancy on the malignancy, but rather to defer childbearing until after the period of greatest risk of recurrence.

Vignette 4 Question 1
Answer E: Tumors less than 5 cm in size and with no palpable lymph nodes are candidates for BCT. SLNB or full axillary lymph node biopsy may be considered; however, full axillary lymph node biopsy results in greater morbidity, and many patients can be thoroughly evaluated with sentinel nodes alone. Radiation therapy is necessary for all patients who undergo conservative therapy. Breast reconstruction should be considered when a large mass is removed from the breast as it carries significant psychosocial benefits. Estrogen/

progesterone-receptor positive tumors should be treated with an antiestrogen agent or aromatase inhibitor following surgical resection. Postmenopausal women (like this patient) with ER+ and PR+ tumors should be first treated with an aromatase inhibitor, like letrozole with hormone receptor positive cancers. Tamoxifen is the first-line hormone therapy for *premenopausal* women. Trastuzumab is a monoclonal antibody for adjuvant treatment in tumors that are HER2/neu positive.

Vignette 4 Question 2

Answer A: Currently, the overall 5-year survival rate is 94%, and the most reliable predictor of survival is the stage of breast cancer at the time of diagnosis. Positive estrogen and progesterone receptor status are favorable prognostic signs. Negative HER2/neu is also a favorable prognostic sign, as HER2/neu positive tumors are more aggressive. Other prognostic indicators are lymph node status, tumor size, nuclear grade, histologic type, proliferative rate, and oncogene expression.

Vignette 4 Question 3

Answer D: Follow-up after breast cancer treatment should include a physical examination every 3 to 6 months for 3 years, every 6 to 12 months for years 4 and 5, and annually thereafter. In women who receive breast-conserving surgery, the first follow-up mammogram is usually performed 6 months after completion of radiation treatment. Unless otherwise indicated, breast cancer patients should have annual mammograms. Women with BCT should have bilateral mammograms and women who are status post masectomy should have unilateral mammograms of the contralateral breast. Routine CBC, blood chemistries, tumor markers, chest X-ray, CT, and bone scans are not recommended for routine breast cancer follow-up. They should only be used in symptomatic patients in whom metastasis is suspected.

Questions

1. A 38-year-old woman presents to your emergency department with complaints of irregular vaginal bleeding for the past 1 year. Upon evaluation of her surgical history, she tells you she had a procedure outside of the country for an "abnormal pregnancy" about 1 year ago. She has had no follow-up since then. On review of systems, she tells you she has been coughing up blood for the past 1 week. Physical examination reveals old blood in the vaginal vault. Your lab data are significant for a serum β-hCG of 112,000 mIU/mL. The most likely diagnosis is:
   a. Complete molar pregnancy
   b. Metastatic persistent GTD
   c. Placental site trophoblastic tumor
   d. Dysfunctional uterine bleeding
   e. Partial molar pregnancy

2. A 37-year-old woman presents to your office with a 3-month history of intermenstrual bleeding and intermittent pelvic pain. She is sexually active and reports one new sexual partner in the last year. She uses condoms for contraception. A pelvic ultrasound is found to be normal. Subsequently, an endometrial biopsy is performed. The biopsy specimen shows leukocytic infiltrate with plasma cells. Which of the following is the most appropriate course of action?
   a. Doxycycline 100 mg orally twice daily for 14 days
   b. Insertion of a levonorgestrel intrauterine system (LNG-IUS)
   c. Hysteroscopy
   d. Total abdominal hysterectomy
   e. Cefoxitin 2 g IV every 6 hours

3. A 24-year-old G2P0010 presents for an initial prenatal visit. Gestational age by known LMP is 15 weeks. This is a desired pregnancy and she shares that she believes she had a miscarriage 6 months ago while traveling abroad. Medical history is complicated by migraine headaches. Bedside ultrasound demonstrates intrauterine pregnancy with fetal heartbeat of 154. You order a prenatal lab panel and Quad screening test for the patient. The prenatal panel reveals the patient is Rh-negative and antibody positive. You order a titer level on your patient and offer her partner testing. The father of the baby is Rh-positive, making the fetus at risk for fetal hydrops. What is the lowest titer level that you would begin with to be concerned about development of fetal hydrops and start serial amniocentesis to check for RBC hemolysis?
   a. 1:4
   b. 1:8
   c. 1:16
   d. 1:64
   e. 1:256

4. A 25-year-old woman presents to your office requesting a mammogram immediately. She just found out that her paternal grandmother has breast cancer at age 75, and she is very concerned. She wants to make sure that she also doesn't have breast cancer. What is your most appropriate recommendation for her?
   a. Immediate mammogram
   b. Immediate breast MRI
   c. Reassurance and counseling about risk factors, breast self-examination overall breast awareness, and annual clinical breast examination
   d. Monthly breast self-examination with annual breast ultrasound, beginning now
   e. Reassurance and counseling about risk factors with follow-up at age 40 for first mammogram

5. Maternal serum screening screens for all of the following conditions, except:
   a. Down syndrome
   b. Trisomy 18
   c. Fragile X syndrome
   d. Abdominal wall defects
   e. Neural tube defects

6. A 36-year-old G4P4004 woman comes to you for contraceptive advice. She had an IUD placed last year; however, it was noted to be perforated so it was removed. She does not want any additional intrauterine or vaginal inserts, and asks if she is a candidate for the birth control pill. Her medical history is significant for a single venous thromboembolism during her last pregnancy, and Type II diabetes mellitus. She has a remote history of tension headaches but none in the past year. She is a nonsmoker, and otherwise has had only uncomplicated vaginal deliveries and no surgeries. Which of the following is an absolute contraindication to starting combined oral contraceptive pills in this patient?
   a. Age greater than 35 years
   b. History of venous thromboembolism
   c. Diabetes mellitus
   d. History of tension headaches
   e. History of uterine perforation

7. A common complication of both epidural and spinal anesthesia includes:
   a. Maternal hypotension
   b. Maternal hyperventilation

c. Fetal tachycardia
d. Tetanic uterine contractions
e. Chorioamnionitis

8. Which of the following is not a sign of active labor?
a. Bloody show
b. Palpable contractions
c. Nausea and vomiting
d. Fever and chills
e. Maternal pain

9. A 36-year-old G3P1103 at 10 weeks 3 days presents to establish prenatal care. In addition to advanced maternal age, her antenatal issues include chronic hypertension and type 2 diabetes mellitus. She currently smokes approximately one pack of cigarettes per day. Additionally, she reports that her last pregnancy was induced at 35 weeks for severe preeclampsia. Risk factors for the development of preeclampsia include all of the following, except:
a. Smoking
b. Diabetes mellitus
c. History of preeclampsia in a prior pregnancy
d. Advanced maternal age
e. Chronic hypertension

10. A 17-year-old woman presents to your office with her mother with no menses for 2 months. A pregnancy test is positive, and ultrasound confirms an intrauterine pregnancy at 8 weeks' gestation. She and her mother request information regarding termination of pregnancy. How many first trimester abortions have complications that require hospitalization?
a. 0.3%
b. 3%
c. 13%
d. 30%

11. A 25-year-old G1P0 at 31 weeks' gestation presents with blood pressures in the 160 to 170/110 to 120 ranges and a severe headache that does not decrease with acetaminophen treatment. On laboratory testing, her platelets are 72,000; AST is 226; and Creatinine is 1.4. Your plan is:
a. Betamethasone and expectant management
b. Hydralazine and expectant management
c. Magnesium sulfate and expectant management
d. Immediate delivery
e. Magnesium sulfate, hydralazine, betamethasone, and immediate delivery

12. A 34-year-old G4P1112 presents at 40 weeks 3 days to labor and delivery with onset of painful contractions 3 hours ago. She denies leaking fluid or vaginal bleeding. Her obstetric history is significant for a prior vaginal delivery at 41 weeks after induction for oligohydramnios. Her second pregnancy was complicated by a placental abruption at 35 weeks after a motor vehicle accident and required emergent delivery by cesarean section. This pregnancy has been complicated by low back pain, secondary to her history of MVA. She has chosen a trial of labor after cesarean. Cervical examination on arrival is 4 cm dilation, 80% effaced, and −1 station. Contractions are regular every 3 minutes. The contractions are more painful 2 hours later and she requests an epidural. Cervical examination at that time is 5 cm dilated, 100% effaced, and zero station. She receives an epidural with good pain relief. You are called to her room 1 hour later as she suddenly developed worsening abdominal pain. The nurse reports that the fetus has had a few deep variable decelerations to the 70s that are new. You lift the sheet to perform a cervical examination and notice bright red blood at the introitus and on the sheets. Cervical examination is still 5 cm dilated, 100% effaced, but is now −3 station. There is a moderate amount of vaginal bleeding now. The fetus is now having a prolonged deceleration. You get the patient's consent for an emergent cesarean section. What do you expect to find at time of fetal delivery?
a. Placental abruption
b. Vasa previa
c. Uterine rupture
d. Fetal nuchal cord
e. No abnormality noted

13. A 24-year-old G1P0 at 28 weeks 5 days' gestation presents to routine prenatal care with complaint of increased discharge today. She first noticed it after going to the bathroom. When she stood up she felt as if a little urine continued to leak out. Throughout the afternoon, she has continued to feel like water is leaking from the vagina. There is no vaginal bleeding or abdominal pain. The discharge is clear and odorless. Her pregnancy has been otherwise uncomplicated. Which of the following is the first step in evaluating this patient?
a. Amnio dye test/tampon test
b. Ultrasound to check for Amniotic Fluid Index (AFI)
c. Sterile speculum examination
d. AmniSure test
e. Amniocentesis to rule out chorioamnionitis

14. Your next patient is a 34-year-old who was diagnosed with endometriosis 10 years earlier. She and her husband have been unable to conceive after 1.5 years of unprotected intercourse. Which of the following is most likely to improve their chance of conceiving?
a. NSAIDs
b. OCPs for 6 months to suppress endometrial implants
c. Oral medroxyprogesterone acetate
d. Depot Lupron
e. Surgery for lysis of adhesions and fulguration of endometriosis

15. Which of the following is most likely to improve pregnancy outcomes in a patient with PPROM?
a. Tocolysis for 48 hours with nifedipine
b. Administration of betamethasone
c. Hospital observation and bed rest
d. Augmentation of labor

16. A 33-year-old G2P0101 at 34 weeks' gestation is evaluated in fetal ultrasound for fetal size less than dating by fundal height. The fetus has been lagging in growth throughout the pregnancy, but recently the obstetrician did not notice interval growth in the fundal height. Fundal height today measures 31 weeks. She had an ultrasound at 18 weeks, which showed normal anatomy and growth in the 30th percentile. The patient's medical history is complicated by a history of oxycodone abuse, and she is currently taking methadone in pregnancy. She has had negative urine drug screening at each prenatal visit. She delivered her first child vaginally at 36 weeks secondary to PPROM. You are covering for her provider today and are looking at the ultrasound report, which shows that her fetus is small with head and abdominal circumferences at the 5th percentile and femur length less than the 10th percentile. There are abnormal findings with the placenta. Which of the following placental conditions do not increase a fetus's risk of IUGR?
a. Chronic placental abruption
b. Placenta previa
c. Thrombosis
d. Chorioamnionitis
e. Marginal cord insertion

17. A 26-year-old G1P0 at 33 weeks 3 days presents for routine prenatal visit. She reports contractions, which have been off and on for the past few weeks but today she notes that they have become regular, occurring every 5 minutes, and uncomfortable. She denies leaking fluid or vaginal bleeding. The baby is very active. Pregnancy is notable for elevated 1-hour glucose tolerance test but a normal 3-hour glucose tolerance test. Upon examination you note that the fundal height measures 37 weeks. You palpate two moderately firm contractions while listening to the fetal heart tones. You decide to send the patient over for evaluation on the labor and delivery ward. Monitoring there reveals contractions every 2 to 3 minutes and category 1 fetal tracing. Cervical examination is notable for a closed cervix, 25% effacement, and −3 station. Bedside ultrasound demonstrates an AFI of 28 cm, fetus in cephalic presentation and posterior placenta. An hour later you recheck the patient's cervix and it is unchanged. She continues to have contractions but they are now every 5 minutes and less painful. Polyhydramnios is not associated with which of the following conditions?

a. Gestational diabetes
b. Congenital anomalies
c. Multiple gestations
d. Potter's syndrome
e. Neural tube defects

18. A 19-year-old G1P0 presents to routine prenatal follow-up visit at 35 weeks' gestation. Her blood pressure is 142/88 mm Hg and a urine dip is negative for protein. She has no headache, no visual symptoms, and no right upper quadrant pain. You send preeclamptic labs (CBC, LFTs, Cr, and LDH), which are all within normal limits. What is her diagnosis and plan?

a. Gestational hypertension—expectant management
b. Preeclampsia—expectant management
c. Rule out preeclampsia—send 24-hour urine protein
d. Gestational hypertension—delivery
e. Preeclampsia—delivery

19. A 23-year-old G_1P_0 Caucasian woman at 12 weeks GA presents for a routine prenatal visit. Her medical history is unremarkable. Her temperature is 37.3°C, blood pressure is 120/84 mm Hg, pulse is 85 per minute, and respirations are 13 per minute. BMI is 24. Her best friend was diagnosed with gestational diabetes, and the patient is concerned she may develop it as well. Gestational diabetes is seen at higher rates in all of the following except?

a. Caucasian race
b. Family history of diabetes
c. Hispanic ethnicity
d. Increasing maternal age
e. Native American race

20. A 36-year-old G_3P_2 woman at 35 weeks' gestation presents for a routine prenatal visit. Her previous two pregnancies 10 and 12 years ago, respectively, resulted in healthy vaginal deliveries. In the past decade, she has gained weight, and her BMI today is 29. She was diagnosed with gestational diabetes a few weeks ago, which is well-controlled with insulin. She asks you about expectations for her delivery management. All of the following would be appropriate steps in her management except?

a. Induce labor at 39 weeks of gestation
b. Offer patient an obstetric ultrasound for estimated fetal weight at 35 weeks
c. Offer patient an elective cesarean birth if EFW is greater than 4,500 g
d. Upon admission, regulate blood glucose levels with insulin and dextrose drips
e. Utilize forceps and vacuum if macrosomia is suspected to assist the mother in delivery

21. A 25-year-old G1 at 9 weeks' gestational age (GA) comes to her initial prenatal visit, and in addition to a series of blood tests, a screening urine culture is obtained. She is asymptomatic and asks why this additional test must be performed. You counsel her that:

a. Even though she is asymptomatic, she is still at risk for STIs and this is one way to screen for those types of infections
b. Asymptomatic bacteriuria if not treated has been associated with higher rates of chorioamnionitis and neonatal sepsis
c. She is at increased risk of having asymptomatic bacteriuria compared to nonpregnant patients
d. Asymptomatic bacteriuria increases her risk of cystitis, pyelonephritis, and preterm birth
e. You are worried that she has pyelonephritis

22. A 34-year-old G3P0020 at 11 weeks GA presents for a follow-up prenatal care visit. You review her screening prenatal labs, which are significant for a positive hepatitis B surface antigen. She remembers being told she had hepatitis as a child, but has never been symptomatic. She asks how this might affect her pregnancy and you counsel her that her pregnancy and delivery will not be managed any differently.

a. She likely has chronic hepatitis B, and there is an increased risk of transmission to the neonate around the time of delivery
b. There is no way to tell if this is an acute or chronic infection, so she will need close monitoring during her pregnancy
c. Chronic hepatitis B has been associated with increased risk of congenital anomalies, and she will need a detailed anatomy ultrasound between 18 and 20 weeks, which includes a fetal echo
d. Reactivation of hepatitis B is more common during pregnancy and places her at risk for hepatic failure

23. Congenital toxoplasmosis infection is associated with what fetal manifestations?

a. Chorioretinitis, intracranial calcifications, and hydrocephalus
b. Deafness, saber shins, mulberry molar, Hutchinson's teeth, and a saddle nose
c. Deafness, cardiac abnormalities, cataracts, and mental retardation
d. Hepatomegaly, splenomegaly, thrombocytopenia, jaundice, cerebral calcifications, and chorioretinitis
e. Disseminated granulomatous lesions with microabscesses, placental lesions, and chorioamnionitis

24. A 23-year-old G2P0101 at 28 weeks GA comes to the office for an urgent visit. She complains of vaginal irritation and increased thin, grey discharge. She denies leakage of fluid, vaginal bleeding, or contractions. The baby is moving well. She is in a monogamous relationship and last had intercourse 2 weeks ago. She has not noticed any dysuria or urinary frequency. She has no history of sexually transmitted infections. You perform a sterile speculum examination, and there is no evidence of ruptured membranes. You collect a sample of discharge and perform a wet mount and KOH, which shows clue cells, a positive whiff test, and no hyphae. The pH of the discharge is less than 5.0. You diagnose her with bacterial vaginosis. If this had gone untreated, how would it have increased her risk during this pregnancy?

a. Increased risk of neonatal blindness
b. Increased risk of neonatal sepsis and admission to the NICU

c. Increased risk of preterm premature rupture of membranes (PPROM)
d. Increased risk of placental abruption
e. Increased risk of congenital malformations

25. While working on labor and delivery, you admit a 32-year-old G4P3003 at 40 2/7 weeks GA in active labor. Her contractions occur every 5 minutes and started 2 hours ago. She denies any leakage of fluid or vaginal bleeding. Her fetal heart tracing is Category 1. During your evaluation, you can find no record of group B *streptococcus* (GBS) testing done at her clinic. You review her obstetrical history and find that she has had three previous vaginal deliveries that were all uncomplicated. What would be an indication to treat her with GBS prophylaxis?

a. Evidence of ruptured membranes
b. Previous history of GBS positive test in prior pregnancy
c. GBS bacteriuria on her initial prenatal urine screening culture
d. If the pregnancy was less than 40 weeks GA
e. Prior infant with *E. Coli* sepsis

26. You are paged to the emergency room to see a patient with an early pregnancy. She is an 18-year-old G1P0 at 8 weeks gestational age (GA) by a self-reported last menstrual period (LMP). She has not previously been seen in clinic for this pregnancy. She states that since the beginning of her pregnancy, she has had progressive nausea and vomiting. She has not been able to keep anything down for the past 24 hours and has vomited seven times in the past day. She denies diarrhea, but had a normal bowel movement yesterday. She feels very weak and lightheaded, especially when standing. She denies any fevers or chills, dysuria, headaches, or other symptoms. She has had no sick contacts. She is tachycardic, but otherwise her vital signs are normal. Her abdominal examination is benign. You get a urinalysis and it shows a specific gravity of greater than 1.030 and moderate ketonuria. There are no urinary nitrates or leukocyte esterase. A complete metabolic panel is significant for mild hypokalemia and hypochloridemia. The CBC is normal. Her serum β-hCG is 150,000. You plan to admit her for IV fluids, antiemetics, and electrolyte replacement. What should be the next step in her care?

a. Order an obstetric ultrasound
b. Place a nasogastric tube for nutritional supplementation
c. Order blood cultures and a chest X-ray to evaluate for an infectious etiology for her symptoms
d. Consult general surgery, given your concern for a small bowel obstruction
e. Place a PICC line and start total parenteral nutrition (TPN)

27. A 32-year-old woman comes to your clinic for preconception counseling. She was diagnosed with epilepsy at age 12 and is currently taking phenytoin and carbamazepine. She has been seizure-free for 1½ years. She and her husband are planning to conceive within the next year. What should you advise to decrease the risks for the upcoming pregnancy?

a. Stop all seizure medications
b. Optimize her seizure regimen to include only one medication
c. Start taking a prenatal vitamin and 400 mcg of folic acid
d. Keep the same dose of both medications and start taking 4 mg of folic acid
e. Recommend she transition off both her current medications and start taking valproic acid for monotherapy

28. A 35-year-old G4P0030 presents to the office for her initial prenatal visit. She is 8 weeks pregnant, dated by her last normal menstrual period. Her obstetric history is significant for an elective termination of pregnancy as a teenager and two losses at 16 weeks' gestation in the past 3 years. With both of her later pregnancy losses, she reports that she presented to the hospital with mild spotting, was found to be 4 to 5 cm dilated, and delivered very shortly thereafter. Genetic analysis of both fetuses was normal. Her medical history is significant for a history of cervical dysplasia leading to a LEEP procedure at age 27. She denies any history of bleeding or clotting disorders. She is in a monogamous relationship, and her current partner is also the father of her two most recent pregnancies. This is a highly desired pregnancy. What recommendation would you give this patient?

a. She and her husband should undergo karyotyping to look for a balanced translocation
b. She should have a hysterosalpingogram after this pregnancy to look for uterine abnormalities
c. She should undergo chorionic villus sampling to evaluate the chromosomes of the fetus
d. She should start progesterone supplementation for presumed luteal phase defect
e. She should have a prophylactic cerclage placed between 12 and 14 weeks for presumed cervical incompetence

29. Which of the following treatments is most appropriate for varicose veins that develop in pregnancy?

a. Diuretics
b. Pressure stockings and lower extremity elevation
c. Low sodium diet and fluid restriction
d. Surgical intervention
e. Antihypertensive medication

30. A 39-year-old G1P0 presents at 12 weeks for fetal nuchal translucency (NT) screening. Her medical history is noncontributory. Her family history is unremarkable. After genetic counseling today, the patient states she desires screening, given her risk of chromosomal disorders associated with advanced maternal age. The patient proceeds with the ultrasound screen, which reveals a thickened NT. What is the most appropriate next step?

a. Repeat the test in 1 week
b. Repeat the test in 2 weeks
c. Offer CVS now
d. Offer amniocentesis now
e. Offer termination of the pregnancy

31. A 34-year-old G2P0010 at 39 weeks GA presents to labor and delivery in active labor. Her pregnancy has been complicated by a bicuspid aorta with moderate aortic stenosis. She has had a recent ECHO that shows a normal ejection fraction of greater than 65%, a gradient across the aorta of 30 mm Hg (moderate 25 to 40 mm Hg), and a valve area of 1.4 cm^2 (moderate 1.0 to 1.5 cm^2). She has had no symptoms of heart failure or arrhythmia during this pregnancy. What is the best management plan to minimize her cardiovascular risks during the intrapartum and postpartum period?

a. Start ampicillin for endocarditis prophylaxis
b. Monitor strict intake and output, place an early epidural and plan for an assisted vaginal delivery with forceps or vacuum once the fetus is +2 station
c. Proceed immediately to cesarean delivery to minimize cardiac stress
d. Admit to the ICU and place a central venous line
e. To maintain cardiac output give lasix to decrease afterload

32. You are called to see a 21-year-old G3P2002 at 28 weeks gestational age who has had limited prenatal care. She has diffuse complaints of abdominal pain, cold sweats, anxiety, and insomnia. Upon review of her history, she tells you that she usually has two to three vodka drinks every day. For the past 3 days, she has not been able to afford to purchase any alcohol. She denies any other significant medical or surgical history. You diagnose her with alcohol withdrawal and admit her to the hospital for treatment. What is the most significant long-term complication of alcohol dependence during pregnancy?

a. Fetal alcohol syndrome
b. Maternal withdrawal
c. Neonatal withdrawal
d. Low fetal birth weight
e. Neonatal admission to the NICU

33. A patient in your clinic is a 22-year-old G2P1001 at 26 weeks GA. Her pregnancy is complicated by tobacco use and she is currently smoking one pack per day (PPD). This is down from two PPD at the start of her pregnancy. You continue to counsel her to quit at each visit. Which of the following are not adverse outcomes of maternal tobacco use during pregnancy?

a. Placental abruption
b. Decreased birth weight
c. Cardiac defects
d. Preterm birth
e. Spontaneous abortion

34. You are assisting in a gynecologic oncology clinic when you see a 57-year-old G3 P3 female patient who is a former nurse. She presents with 6 months of pelvic discomfort, increasing abdominal girth, and early satiety. Physical examination reveals a large abdominopelvic mass. A pelvic ultrasound and CT scan show a 10-cm right ovarian mass, ascites, and studding of the peritoneum. In your discussion with the patient you predict that this most likely represents a malignant ovarian neoplasm. She asks about the primary method of treatment for ovarian carcinoma. You explain that the mainstay of treatment for epithelial ovarian cancer is:

a. Radiation therapy alone
b. Surgery alone
c. Surgery followed by chemotherapy
d. Surgery followed by radiation therapy
e. Chemoradiation alone

35. A 20-year-old African American G_2P_2 is seen in the hospital on postpartum day number 1, after a spontaneous vaginal delivery of a healthy male infant with APGAR score of 8 and 9. Her pregnancy was uncomplicated. Her delivery was complicated only by a second degree perineal laceration that was repaired in standard fashion. Her medical history is significant for having Hepatitis C. She also reports a history of breast augmentation. She received an intramuscular injection of Depo-Provera for postpartum contraception. This morning she appears very tired and although doing well from a physical standpoint, is noted to be bottle-feeding her infant. She acknowledges the benefits of breast-feeding but explains that bottle-feeding has its merits as well. Which of the following describes one of the benefits of bottle-feeding over breast-feeding?

a. She decreases her risk of vertical transmission of Hepatitis C by bottle-feeding
b. She will be unable to breast-feed because of her history of breast augmentation
c. Breast-feeding is contraindicated in women receiving Depo-Provera for contraception
d. Bottle-feeding ensures a more adequate supply of milk to her baby during the first few days of life
e. Breast-feeding may not provide enough Vitamin D for some infants compared with that supplemented in formula

36. A 34-year-old Caucasian G3P2002 presents to labor and delivery at 41 weeks and 1 day for induction of labor for post-dates pregnancy. Her pregnancy was uncomplicated. Her medical history is significant only for mild intermittent asthma; she denied any history of hypertension. Her surgical history is significant for a cesarean section during her last pregnancy for Stage II arrest. Her induction is started with a Foley bulb for cervical ripening, followed by Pitocin, which succeeds in progressing her to Stage II of labor. She delivers a viable male infant in three pushes with APGAR score of 8 and 9. She subsequently delivers a normal-sized, normal-appearing placenta with membranes intact and a centrally inserted three-vessel cord. She has an intact perineum. Her cervix is intact on examination. She is noted to have continued brisk bleeding from her vagina. Her fundus is noted to be above the umbilicus and boggy despite fundal massage. Which of the following medications would be contraindicated in the management of her hemorrhage?

a. 10 mg Intramuscular Pitocin
b. 200 mcg Intramuscular Methylergonovine
c. 800 mcg Rectal Misoprostol
d. 250 mcg Carboprost
e. 20 mg IV Pitocin in 1,000 mL Lactated Ringer's

37. A 27-year-old Caucasian G_1P0_{1001} is seen in the hospital on postpartum day number 2, after a spontaneous vaginal delivery of a healthy female infant with APGAR score of 9 and 9. She reports feeling febrile and has intermittently moderate uterine cramping. She is tolerating a regular diet, breast-feeding without difficulty, voiding spontaneously without discomfort, and having minimal lochia. She has been slow to ambulate, having only recently had her epidural catheter removed. Her pregnancy was complicated solely by her rubella nonimmune status. Her delivery was complicated only by a superficial vaginal laceration that was repaired in standard fashion. Her medical and surgical histories are noncontributory. She is taking an iron supplement and recently received her MMR and TDaP vaccines. Her vitals are significant for a temperature of 38.0°C; her pulse 85, blood pressure 112/72. She is comfortably breathing room air. Her physical examination shows no acute distress, with regular heart rate and rhythm, clear lungs, a soft abdomen with a firm, though mildly tender, uterus, and nontender symmetric lower extremities significant for 2+ pitting edema. Which of the following is the most likely cause of her postpartum fever?

a. Postpartum endometritis
b. Urinary tract infection
c. Deep vein thromboembolism
d. Vaccine reaction
e. Breast fever

38. A 36-year-old Hispanic American now G6P6006 at 41 weeks and 2 days gestation arrives on labor and delivery and precipitously delivers a viable male infant followed by a large gush of fluid. Her infant was notable for an APGAR score of 8 and 9 and weight of 9 lb. She subsequently delivered a normal-sized, normal-appearing placenta with a centrally inserted three-vessel cord over an intact perineum. Her cervix was intact on examination. Her pregnancy was complicated by A1 gestational diabetes, which was suboptimally controlled. Her medical history is significant for a 2 × 3 cm intramural fibroid noted in the anterior wall during routine pregnancy ultrasound. She denied any history of asthma or hypertension. Her surgical history is significant for a cesarean section during her last pregnancy for Stage II arrest. Review of her previous pregnancy ultrasounds is significant for a low-lying placenta without previa. During her medical interview conducted postpartum she is noted to have continued brisk bleeding from her vagina. Which of the following is not a risk factor for her postpartum hemorrhage?

a. Her parity
b. Her fibroid

c. Her baby's weight
d. Her low lying placenta
e. All of the above

39. A 21-year-old G0 presents for her first gynecologic examination. She states that she became sexually active 2 weeks ago for the first time. She has no significant medical history. She has regular menses with some mild dysmenorrhea. During the speculum examination, you observe a small raised 0.5cm lesion 0.5 cm. It is smooth and light-bluish in color with the appearance of a bubble under the epithelial surface and a blood vessel running over the top. What is your diagnosis?
a. Bartholin's gland cyst
b. Cervical dysplasia
c. Nabothian cyst
d. Skene's gland cyst
e. Cervical cancer

40. A 68-year-old woman presents with vulvar pruritus since the previous year that has been increasing over the last few months. She has tried antifungal medications, which seem to help, but the symptoms keep recurring. She went through menopause at age 49 and has not been sexually active for 10 years. She does not use any douching products and is not taking any antibiotics. On physical examination, you note thin white epithelium of the labia minora with red oval-shaped erosions, varying in size from 0.5 to 1.5 cm. How would you proceed?
a. Culture the vagina and treat with high-dose antifungal
b. Wide local excision of the lesions
c. Cryotherapy to eradicate the lesions
d. Punch biopsy of the vulvar lesions
e. Treat with moderate-high potency topical steroids

41. A 40-year-old woman with regular menstruation returns for assessment of vulvar pruritus. She has had itchy vulvar skin for over a year; the symptoms vary in severity over time. She has been treated with oral and topical antifungal creams. She has adhered to vulvar skin care guidance. She had a prior vulvar biopsy that described squamous cell hyperplasia without evidence of a fungal infection. She has been applying a moderate-potency topical steroid since her last visit with you; she says it helps for a while and then her symptoms recur and she has to use it again. On examination, you note thickened epithelium of the inner labia majora and labia minora, with several small red erosions suggestive of excoriation. What do you recommend?
a. Punch biopsy of vulvar skin
b. Topical clobetasol ointment
c. Laser vaporization of affected area
d. Prolonged course of antifungals
e. Topical estrogen cream

42. A 13-year-old girl presents with severe lower abdominal pain of 24 hours' duration. She states that the pain is sharp and constant and that she has had similar pain for several days, approximately every month over the past 4 months. She has no vomiting or diarrhea with the pain, but she is constipated frequently, having a bowel movement about every 3 to 4 days. She feels that her jeans are getting tighter around the waist, although she remains active, playing soccer daily. She has never had a menstrual period and denies ever being sexually active. She has normal vital signs, normal stature, Tanner 3 breast development, and has Tanner stage 3 pubic hair. Abdominal examination reveals a firm and tender midline mass that is inferior to the umbilicus. The patient refuses a pelvic examination, but agrees to a visualization of the vulva; when parting the labia minora, a tense bulging membrane can be seen. Of the following, the most likely diagnosis is
a. Megacolon
b. 45 XO, Turner's syndrome
c. Hematocolpos
d. Endometriosis
e. Ovarian cyst

43. A 22-year-old G2P1001 at 39 weeks 2 days presents with history of contractions every 3 minutes for the past 2 hours. Her prior pregnancy was induced at 41 weeks and 3 days. Her first stage of labor lasted 9 hours and during her second stage of labor she pushed for 2 hours, resulting in delivery of a male infant weighing 3,800 g. She denies rupture of membranes, vaginal bleeding, or decreased fetal movement. Her initial cervical examination is 2 cm dilation, 50% effacement, and −2 station. Per the records, her cervical examination in the clinic last week was 2 cm, 25% effaced, and −2 station. You decide to have her ambulate and repeat her cervical examination in 2 hours to assess if she is in labor. Two hours later you evaluate the patient and see that she is painfully contracting and requesting epidural placement. Your cervical examination reveals 4 cm dilation, 100% effacement, and −1 station. You admit the patient to labor and delivery for expectant management and she receives an epidural for pain control. Which of the following findings will cause you to recommend a cesarean delivery at this time?
a. Fetus in right occiput posterior (ROP) presentation
b. Maternal hypotension
c. Development of vaginal bleeding with change in hematocrit from 33 to 32
d. Repetitive fetal decelerations to 80 beats per minute with absent variability

44. A healthy 28-year-old G1 P0 comes to you for established prenatal care. She has always had regular menstrual cycles, but she was not in the habit of tracking them. This pregnancy was desired but unplanned. An early ultrasound for dating shows that the embryo is in the left horn of a bicornuate uterus. This diagnosis is new to her and she is concerned about the implications for her pregnancy. You explain that the most common pregnancy-related risk associated with a bicornuate uterus is
a. Infertility
b. Antepartum bleeding
c. Recurrent first trimester miscarriage
d. Cervical insufficiency
e. Preterm labor and delivery

45. A 32-year-old G0 comes in for consultation for an enlarged fibroid uterus. She and her husband are planning their first attempt at conception in the next month or two but she wants to have her fibroids treated before she becomes pregnant. A review of her outside medical records reveals a recent transvaginal ultrasound showing a 7-cm uterus with a 2- and 1-cm intramural fibroid. There are no signs of adenomyosis and the endometrial stripe and ovaries are all normal. She has a history of mild dysmenorrhea but no history of menorrhagia, menometrorrhagia, postcoital spotting, or intermenstrual bleeding. Her examination at your visit is unremarkable. What treatment options would you recommend to her for management of her uterine fibroids?
a. Intrauterine device (IUD)
b. Endometrial ablation
c. Hysteroscopic resection
d. Uterine artery embolization
e. Expectant management

46. A 48-year-old G3 P3 patient comes to see you for a complaint of heavier, longer menses. She is healthy with no major medical problems and a BMI of 27. Her only medication is a daily multivitamin. She has always had regular menstrual periods until recently. She is also experiencing increased pain with her menstrual cycles. Her last pap and high risk HPV screen were negative less than a year ago. She denies any postcoital spotting but has had a few episodes of intermenstrual bleeding. A transvaginal ultrasound reveals a normal myometrium with an endometrial stripe of 22 mm. An endometrial biopsy reveals proliferative endometrium without evidence of glandular crowding or cytologic atypia. What is the most likely diagnosis?

a. Fibroids
b. Thyroid disease
c. Perimenopause
d. Endometrial polyp
e. Endometrial hyperplasia

47. A new female patient presents to your office on referral from her primary care physician. She is 62 years old, G2P2, postmenopausal for more than 10 years, and has occasional right lower quadrant discomfort. Ultrasound from their office showed a 4-cm complex ovarian mass with cystic and solid components, two internal nodules, septations, and increased Doppler flow. A thorough history is taken. On your physical examination you do not observe any abnormalities, and you discover that she has undergone a hysterectomy as there is no cervix or uterus palpable. You explain to the patient your assessment and plan. Which of the following is the next best step in the management of this patient?

a. Surgical evaluation
b. Repeat ultrasound in 3 months
c. Colonoscopy
d. Pregnancy test
e. CT scan of abdomen

48. A 24-year-old G0 Caucasian woman presents to your office with the complaint of worsening dysmenorrhea over the last 6 months. She was recently married and reports stopping her oral contraceptives, which she started as a teenager for dysmenorrhea. She also complains of deep dyspareunia. On further questioning she reports that her mother has a history of endometriosis. You suspect that your patient also may have endometriosis. Which of the following conditions should you counsel her about as potential results of endometriosis?

a. Pelvic inflammatory disease
b. Abnormal uterine bleeding
c. Hirsutism
d. Infertility
e. b and d

49. A 28-year-old G0 woman presents to your office with complaints of a palpable breast mass discovered by her husband. You perform a clinical breast examination and can palpate the mass as well. She is sent for diagnostic imaging. A solid mass is confirmed by imaging and a tissue sample needs to be obtained for diagnosis. The most appropriate method to obtain tissue in this patient would be:

a. Fine-needle aspiration (FNA)
b. Excisional biopsy
c. Core-needle biopsy
d. Needle or wire-guided excision
e. Lumpectomy

50. A 27-year-old G1P0010 presents to the clinic for a postoperative visit. Two weeks earlier, she underwent a laparoscopic left salpingostomy for an ectopic pregnancy. A review of her medical history reveals a history of infection with chlamydia 2 years ago. Both she and her partner received a single dose course of antibiotics. They have been mutually monogamous since that time. She denies any abnormal pap smears. On physical examination, she is afebrile with stable vital signs. Her abdomen is nontender and she has three well-healed surgical incisions from the laparoscopic port sites. This was a desired pregnancy and she and her partner hope she becomes pregnant again in the future. What counseling should you give her regarding her future risk?

a. Her history of chlamydia makes it unlikely that she will ever conceive normally and she should consider in vitro fertilization
b. Her risk of a subsequent ectopic pregnancy is 10%
c. Her risk of a subsequent ectopic pregnancy is 25%
d. She should avoid using an IUD for contraception as it increases her risk of ectopic pregnancy
e. She should receive a single dose of methotrexate to ensure that all of the pregnancy tissue has been evacuated

51. A 32-year-old G3P1021 woman returns to your clinic for a follow-up visit. She has a history of endometriosis proven by biopsy at the time of laparoscopy. She has been using a combination oral contraceptive in a continuous fashion to manage her cyclic pelvic pain. She has been experiencing some nausea and breast tenderness and would like to know what other medical options she has to treat her symptoms. You explain to her that there are several options, and they include all except which of the following?

a. Nonsteroidal anti-inflammatory drugs (NSAIDs)
b. Oral progestins
c. Selective serotonin reuptake inhibitors (SSRI)
d. Gonadotropin-releasing hormone (GnRH) agonists
e. Levonorgestrel-releasing intrauterine system

52. A 43-year-old G3 P3 presents to your clinic for an annual examination. She is a longtime patient of yours and reports that a friend of hers recently had a hysterectomy. When the pathology report returned, adenomyosis was noted. Your patient is concerned and wonders if she may have adenomyosis. Which finding on history or examination would *not* be suggestive of the diagnosis of adenomyosis?

a. Metrorrhagia
b. Menorrhagia
c. Secondary dysmenorrhea
d. An enlarged globular uterus
e. A boggy, tender uterus

53. A 45-year-old G2P2 returns for follow-up after endometrial biopsy for heavy menstrual bleeding that has developed over the last 6 months. Her biopsy revealed normal secretory endometrium. You suspect that she most likely has adenomyosis. She is not familiar with this condition and would like for you to explain it to her. Which of the following most accurately describes the condition?

a. The presence of endometrial cells outside the endometrium with the hallmark of cyclic pelvic pain
b. An extension of endometrial tissue into the uterine myometrium leading to menorrhagia and dysmenorrhea
c. Local proliferations of smooth muscle cells within the uterus, often surrounded by a pseudocapsule
d. A cystic collection of endometrial cells on the ovary
e. Inflammation or irritation of the lining of the uterus (endometrium), typically caused by infection

54. A 32-year-old woman comes to the gynecologist with 1 week history of vulvar ulcers. She first noticed two red "bumps," which subsequently opened up and are now extremely painful. She is sexually active and reports three new sexual partners in the last month. She reports a remote history of gonorrhea, which was treated. On pelvic examination, there are two 1.5-cm ulcers on the left labia minora. The ulcer bases are erythematous and the borders are irregular but well demarcated. There is tender inguinal lymph node enlargement on the left side. Bacterial and viral cultures from the ulcer base are negative. Venereal Disease Research Laboratory (VDRL) and HSV testing are negative. What is the best initial treatment for this patient?

a. Benzathine penicillin G 2.4 million units IM once
b. Ceftriaxone 250 mg IM once
c. Doxycycline 100 mg orally twice daily for 14 days
e. Erythromycin 500 mg orally four times daily for 21 days
e. Acyclovir 200 mg five times daily for 7 days

55. A 25-year-old nulligravid woman comes to the gynecologist for sexually transmitted infection screening. She has been sexually active since age 16 and reports eight new partners in the last year. She is currently asymptomatic. Testing results include hepatitis B surface antigen negative, rapid plasma reagin (RPR) positive, HIV antibody negative, and nucleic acid amplification test (NAAT) for *Chlamydia* and gonorrhea negative. What is the next best step in the management of this patient?

a. Venereal Disease Research Laboratory (VDRL) testing
b. Treatment with benzathine penicillin G 2.4 million units IM once
c. Fluorescent treponemal antibody absorption (FTA-ABS) testing
d. Serial rapid plasma reagin (RPR) titers
e. Treatment with benzathine penicillin G 2.4 million units IM weekly for three doses

56. A 25-year-old G1P1 woman presents to urgent care with a 4-day history of suprapubic pain, increased urinary frequency, burning with urination, and increased vaginal discharge. She reports a history of similar symptoms 1 month ago when she was treated empirically for a urinary tract infection. All of the following are appropriate in the management except?

a. Administer trimethoprim-sulfamethoxazole PO twice daily for 3 days
b. Send urine specimen for urinalysis
c. Send urine specimen for urine culture
d. Perform microscopy of the vaginal discharge
e. Perform nucleic acid amplification test (NAAT) for *Chlamydia* and gonorrhea

57. A 27-year-old woman presents to her gynecologist for evaluation of new vulvar lesions. She first noticed several "bumps" on her outer labia 3 weeks ago. She is otherwise without any associated symptoms. On pelvic examination there are six flesh-colored, nontender, 1- to 3-mm verrucous papules. Which of the following is the most likely cause of the patient's vulvar lesions?

a. Human papillomavirus (HPV) serotype 16
b. Herpes simplex virus (HSV) type 1
c. Pox virus
d. Human papillomavirus (HPV) serotype 6
e. *Haemophilus ducreyi*

58. A 37-year-old G2P1 presents at 12 weeks for prenatal diagnosis. She does not currently have any medical issues and takes no medications. After genetic counseling, the patient states she wishes to proceed with a chorionic villus sampling (CVS). She undergoes CVS, which reveals normal chromosomes. What further prenatal testing do you offer?

a. Maternal serum alpha fetoprotein
b. Amniocentesis
c. Repeat CVS
d. Fetal echocardiography
e. Cordocentesis

59. A 17-year-old nulligravid woman presents to the emergency department with a 2-week history of abdominal pain. The pain started in her lower abdomen, but has become progressively generalized to include her upper abdomen, especially on her right side. The pain is worse with deep breathing, coughing, and movement. She reports intermittent nausea and vomiting for the past day. Six months ago, she was treated for *N. gonorrhoeae* and *T. vaginalis* infection. She uses a contraceptive implant (Implanon) and reports five new sexual partners in the last year. Her temperature is 38.3°C (100.9°F), pulse is 94 per minute, respirations are 20 per minute, and blood pressure is 118/70 mm Hg. Abdominal examination shows diffuse tenderness, especially in the right upper quadrant. On pelvic examination, there is foul smelling frothy discharge. There is tenderness with manipulation of the cervix and uterus. There is no adnexal fullness or tenderness. What is the most likely diagnosis?

a. Tubo-ovarian abscess
b. Disseminated gonorrhea
c. HELLP syndrome
d. Fitzhugh-Curtis syndrome
e. Secondary syphilis

60. A 22-year-old woman comes to the emergency department with acute onset of fever, myalgias, abdominal pain, vomiting, and diarrhea. She is sexually active in a monogamous relationship and uses an oral contraceptive pill. Her menses began 3 days prior to onset and she reports using super tampons. Her temperature is 39.5°C (103.1°F), pulse is 124 per minute, respirations are 26 per minute, and blood pressure is 80/50 mm Hg. On examination there is a diffuse, red, macular rash. Her abdomen is tender, slightly distended with guarding. All of the following are included in the diagnostic criteria except?

a. Positive blood culture
b. Fever greater than 38.9°C
c. Hypotension
d. Multisystem involvement
e. Diffuse erythematous macular rash

61. A 42-year-old G4P4 woman presents to the gynecologist for an annual examination. She was recently diagnosed with HIV and is receiving treatment with highly active antiretroviral therapy. Her most recent viral load was 12,000 copies/mL and CD4 count 940 cells/mm^3. She is otherwise healthy. She is not currently in a sexual relationship. She denies any history of CIN 2 or CIN 3 and she has had three consecutive negative cervical cytology screening tests. How often should cervical cancer screening be performed?

a. Pap smear every 6 months
b. Pap smear annually
c. Pap smear twice in the first year after diagnosis of HIV and annually thereafter if both are normal
d. Colposcopy every 6 months
e. Pap smear every 3 years

62. A 67-year-old patient presents with a chief complaint consistent with pelvic organ prolapse. This is subsequently confirmed by your physical examination. All of the following risk factors may have contributed to this pathologic process except?

a. Genetic predisposition
b. Chronic constipation with a lifelong history of straining
c. Postmenopausal status
d. Chronic obstructive pulmonary disease
e. Sexual inactivity

63. You are consulted on an 89-year-old inpatient in a nursing facility. Your patient has complete eversion of the vagina. What is another term for this?
a. Cystocele
b. Procidentia
c. Rectocele
d. Urethrocele
e. Enterocele

64. A 45-year-old presents for evaluation because her primary care physician has diagnosed her with pelvic organ prolapse while performing annual care. She denies any pelvic pressure, bulge, or difficulty with urination. Her only medical comorbidity is obesity. For asymptomatic grade 1 pelvic organ prolapse, what do you recommend?
a. Conservative management with pelvic floor muscle exercises and weight loss
b. Colpocleisis obliterative procedure
c. Gellhorn pessary
d. Round ligament suspension
e. Hysterectomy

65. A postmenopausal woman with symptomatic vaginal vault prolapse elects to proceed with surgical correction of the descensus. You determine that she is an appropriate candidate for an uterosacral ligament suspension. After completion of the surgery, successful anatomic restoration is noted. Before you conclude the surgery, what additional procedure is indicated?
a. Hysteroscopy
b. Defecography
c. Cystoscopy
d. Episiotomy
e. Anterior colporrhaphy

66. A 62-year-old G2 P2 presents to the urogynecology clinic with complaints of urinary incontinence. She has urinary urgency and can't make it to the bathroom before leaking a large amount of urine. She gets up two to three times per night to urinate. A urinalysis and urine culture done 1 week ago at her PCP's office are both negative. What is the most likely diagnosis and appropriate treatment option for this type of urinary incontinence?
a. Stress incontinence, mid-urethral sling
b. Urgency incontinence, oxybutynin (anticholinergic medication)
c. Overflow incontinence, oxybutynin (anticholinergic medication)
d. Urinary fistula, surgical repair
e. Functional incontinence, bladder suspension

67. A 42-year-old G2 P2 complains of urinary leakage when exercising. She recently began jogging for exercise in an effort to lose weight. She does wear a pad when she jogs and reports that it is approximately 75% soaked when she finishes her run. She denies loss of urine at any other time. Urinalysis and urine cultures were negative. Her BMI is 32. Which of the following would you recommend as part of the initial treatment plan for this patient?
a. Mid-urethral sling
b. Detrol LA (anticholinergic medication)
c. Tibial nerve stimulation
d. Pelvic floor muscle exercises
e. Vaginal hysterectomy

68. Urinary incontinence, the involuntary loss of urine is . . .
a. Rare, affecting fewer than 3% of women in the United States in 2010
b. Common, and expected to affect more than 28 million women by 2050
c. Not considered a significant cost burden, since it affects so few women
d. Rarely seen in nursing home residents
e. Almost always due to stress incontinence

69. Labor is divided into stages and phases. These delineations are used to communicate where patients are in the progress of labor. In particular, the first stage of labor:
a. Begins at the time of full cervical dilation
b. Has a latent phase that ends with dilation exactly at 6 cm
c. Has an active phase that begins with repetitive contractions
d. Has an active phase wherein at least 1.0 cm per hour of dilation is expected in the nulliparous patient
e. Has a latent phase with a rapid rate of cervical change

70. Micturition is voluntary and occurs with relaxation of the urethra and sustained contraction of the bladder until emptying is complete. Sustained contraction of the detrusor muscle of the bladder requires parasympathetic stimulation. Parasympathetic control of the detrusor is supplied by which of the following nerves?
a. Hypogastric nerve
b. Pudendal nerve
c. Peroneal nerve
d. Pelvic nerve
e. Sciatic nerve

71. A long-term patient of yours brings her 14-year-old daughter in to see you for concern over irregular menses. The daughter started menstruating at age 13. Her cycles are irregular in that they may come monthly but she often skips a month. The daughter is of normal weight without any hirsutism, abnormal acne, or acanthosis. Her breast development and height are appropriate for her age. She is a high school soccer player and practices twice a week. She also does yoga and light weight lifting two to three times a week. They want your opinion about how to proceed. How do you counsel them?
a. You recommend checking FSH, LH, estradiol, and progesterone levels to look for etiology of her menstrual irregularity
b. You recommend a pelvic ultrasound to look for a structural abnormality and verify normal anatomy
c. You recommend a hysteroscopy to better evaluate the endometrial cavity and lining
d. You advise expectant management for now with completion of menstrual calendar over the upcoming year
e. You refer her to a reproductive endocrinologist or pediatric gynecologist as this issue is beyond the scope of your practice

72. A 52-year-old G3 P3 comes in to see you for management of her hot flashes and night sweats. She stopped having menses 1.5 years ago and still has her ovaries and uterus in situ. She has been suffering with recurrent hot flashes and night sweats, which interfere with her quality of life. She had hoped to avoid taking hormones but her symptoms have not improved over the past 1.5 years and she is now ready for treatment. In counseling her about treatment options for her hot flashes and night sweats, which of the following would *not* be an appropriate option?
a. Oral estrogen and progesterone
b. Topical estrogen and progesterone patch
c. Low dose vaginal estrogen cream
d. A selective serotonin reuptake inhibitor (SSRI) such as paroxetine (Paxil) or fluoxetine (Prozac)
e. Topical clonidine (Catapres) patch

73. Your next patient is here with her husband to inquire about attempting pregnancy. She is a 28-year-old G0 P0 pulmonary fellow with regular 28 to 30 days' menstrual cycles without menorrhagia or dysmenorrhea. Her last pap was done 6 months ago and was normal. Both she and her husband are healthy and have no major medical problems. They do not have any children. She is up-to-date on her immunizations and has had a recent flu shot. She has started a prenatal vitamin and takes no other medications. She confesses that she's forgotten a lot about the menstrual cycle since medical school, but is excited to learn when their most fertile time of the month would be. Which of the following is true about ovulation and fertilization?

a. Fertilization occurs in the uterine cavity
b. Fertilization of the ovum must occur within 72 hours of ovulation or else it degenerates
c. Ovulation is triggered by the production of estrogen, which triggers an LH spike from the anterior pituitary
d. She will be most fertile during the luteal phase of her cycle and they should increase sexual activity during this time
e. It's impossible to predict the most fertile time period for a given patient

74. A 28-year-old G1P0 woman presents at 10 weeks' gestation for her initial prenatal visit. In addition to the routine prenatal screening tests, she wishes to obtain screening for aneuploidy. The prenatal diagnostic screening modality for Down syndrome that will give the highest sensitivity is:

a. Nuchal translucency at 11 weeks
b. Combined screening (nuchal translucency + PAPPA and free β-hCG) at 12 weeks
c. Maternal serum triple screen (MSAFP + estriol + β-hCG) at 17 weeks
d. Second trimester ultrasound
e. Sequential screening with combined screening in first trimester and quad screening in the second

75. You are consulted to see a 16-year-old G0 who presented to the emergency department with primary amenorrhea and cyclic abdominal pain. She notes that her symptoms have been worsening over the past 6 months, such that she most recently had to miss school secondary to abdominal pain and now she presents to the emergency room. You are consulted because an ultrasound revealed a normal appearing uterus with a 4-cm cystic heterogeneous mass in the vagina below the cervix, and bilateral adnexal masses with low level echoes. You perform a physical examination, which reveals normal breast development and normal distribution of pubic hair. She has a tender, but non-acute abdomen, and her vital signs are normal. Pelvic examination reveals a normal appearing hymenal ring, with no visible cervix. Instead, you visualize a bulging, bluish purple pouch at the apex of the vagina. What is the most likely diagnosis?

a. Uterine didelphys
b. Uterine agenesis
c. Transverse vaginal septum
d. Imperforate hymen
e. Uterine septum

76. A 32-year-old G0 presents to your office with absent menses for 1 year. She notes that her menses had become closer together over the previous 2 years, and she attributed this to increased stress in her life. She is otherwise healthy, with no prior surgeries, and actually is hoping to get pregnant soon. She and her husband got married a little over a year ago and have been having unprotected intercourse for the past 3 months. She has been increasingly alarmed as she has been reading online about fertility because of her absent menstrual cycles. She does endorse some vague symptoms of "temperature deregulation." You perform a physical examination, which is normal. You perform a series of tests, including a TSH (normal), β-hCG (negative), prolactin (normal), a complete blood count (normal), FSH (elevated), and Estradiol (low). What is the next step in your diagnosis?

a. Serum LH to determine if she is ovulating
b. Serum progesterone on Day 21 to determine if she is ovulating
c. Karyotype
d. Pelvic ultrasound and MRI to evaluate for Müllerian anomalies
e. Nothing, you have enough information to determine your diagnosis

77. A 33-year-old G3P2012 woman presents to your office with a complaint of absent menses for the past 6 months. She has a history of tubal ligation, and did a urine pregnancy test earlier that morning, which was negative, and further, she states she is not sexually active. She has noted that she has been increasingly fatigued lately, and has noted that her hair has become more brittle and coarse, and she seems to be losing more hair than usual in the shower and on her hairbrush. She attributed many of these symptoms to stress at home related to recent separation with her husband as well as feeling exhausted chasing after her two young children. She denies any other medical problems, and other than the tubal ligation, has had no surgeries. She does note that she breastfed for 6 months after her most recent child without difficulty. She takes only occasional ibuprofen for a headache and a multivitamin. She denies allergies to medication. On physical examination, you note a heart rate of 58, normal blood pressure. Her skin is notably coarse and dry, but otherwise your examination is unremarkable. You perform a series of laboratory studies including a urine pregnancy test, complete blood count, prolactin, FSH and estradiol, and thyroid function testing. All are normal with the exception of her TSH, which is markedly elevated, and T4, which is low. You recommend treatment with T4 replacement. She is hoping to have another pregnancy sometime in the future and wonders about how the medication will affect her pregnancy. You inform her that:

a. She will need less thyroid medication during pregnancy
b. She will be able to stop her thyroid medication in pregnancy
c. Her thyroid medication will not need adjustment because the fetus autoregulates its own thyroid
d. She will need more medication during her pregnancy
e. The dose of her thyroid medication will be tripled upon confirmation of pregnancy and will continue at the same dose throughout gestation

78. A 29-year-old G2P0020 presents to your office with a chief complaint of irregular menses for the past 6 months. She denies any medical problems and has a history of having her wisdom teeth extracted, but otherwise has had a negative surgical history. She is taking a multivitamin only and is using no contraception at the current time (but she denies sexual activity in the past year). Her two prior pregnancies were therapeutic abortions induced with misoprostol. She previously had normal menses, every month, not too heavy or too painful until 6 months ago. Since then she has only had two periods, the first, which seemed normal, and the second, which was light and during which she spotted for 2 weeks. For the past 2 months she has not had any menses. She has no history of STDs, and is up-to-date with her Pap smears, all of which have been normal. On review of systems, she denies symptoms of acne or excessive hair growth, but does admit to a small amount of bilateral nipple discharge, and occasional headaches. Physical examination is performed and reveals normal vital signs, and a wholly normal examination with the exception of confirmation of bilateral clear white nipple discharge. You perform an in-office urine pregnancy test, which is negative. What is the next test or series of tests you might perform?

a. Karyotype
b. Urinary LH predictor kit
c. Pelvic ultrasound and pelvic MRI
d. TSH and PRL
e. FSH and serum estradiol

79. Your 38-year-old G4 P3 calls for a work-in appointment for worsening pain with her menses. She has had regular menses all of her life with a normal amount and length of flow. She occasionally had mild to moderate cramping, which was easily treated with a dose or two of ibuprofen. Her last pap smear was 8 months ago and was within normal limits. Her high risk HPV screen was negative at that time. She has no history of cervical dysplasia and has never had an STI. Six months ago, she underwent an elective repeat cesarean section that was complicated by endomyometritis. Since the birth of her daughter 6 months ago, she had noticed that her periods are progressively more painful. Most months she finds herself curled up in a ball, using a heating pad and missing work during her cycle. She also finds that she is having pain associated with activities such as intercourse, exercise, and lifting the baby. She is now taking ibuprofen "like it's candy" but not getting much relief. She tried a couple of pain killers left over after her husband's knee surgery. This gives her some relief but the pain still recurs. On examination, she has a normal sized uterus, which is nontender, but her pain is exacerbated with movement of her uterus. Her gonorrhea and chlamydia cultures are both negative. You order a pelvic U/S and CT, which both show a normal upper abdomen, uterus, tubes, and ovaries. You maximize her pain regimen but she is still in significant pain with activity and menses. What is the most likely next step?

a. Tell her you've done all you can given her negative workup
b. Start her standing narcotic order
c. Counsel her for a diagnostic laparoscopy for likely lysis of pelvic adhesions
d. Counsel her for a hysterectomy
e. Refer her to the local pain clinic and/or psychiatric evaluation

80. A 34-year-old African American woman and her partner present to their first prenatal visit. She is currently 12 weeks with diamniotic dichorionic twin gestation. Dating is by sure LMP. The patient has a history of chronic hypertension, which has been poorly controlled. She is currently taking labetalol 200 mg t.i.d. and her blood pressure today is 134/80. She quit smoking prior to conception but used to smoke one-half pack per day. Her mother and sister both have diabetes and she has been told she had prediabetes a few years ago, but has not had any follow-up care or testing. You are counseling her that her pregnancy is at risk for a number of complications due to her twin gestation, history of chronic hypertension, and history of insulin resistance. You explain that she is at increased risk for preterm labor, preterm birth, preterm premature rupture of membranes, preeclampsia, need for cesarean section, and IUGR. What is the difference between the terms SGA and IUGR?

a. SGA refers to the fetus, whereas IUGR is specific for neonates
b. IUGR specifically describes growth disorders related only to placental or maternal disease
c. SGA refers to growth disturbance due to chromosomal abnormalities or toxins
d. SGA refers to a neonate in whom cause of small size is uncertain, whereas IUGR describes the fetus and suggests an intrauterine etiology for growth restriction
e. IUGR refers to a neonate in whom the cause of growth disruption is not identified, whereas SGA refers to a fetus and suggests a known cause for growth restriction

81. A 42-year-old G2P2 comes to see you with a complaint of 14 months of "irregular bleeding." She previously had regular monthly menses but over the past 2 years they have become totally unpredictable. Sometimes she will bleed for 2 to 3 weeks off and on and then she may go 2 months without a cycle at all. Her pelvic examination, pap smear, cervical cultures, pregnancy test, TFTs, PRL, and FSH are all within normal limits. She has no hot flashes, night sweats, or vaginal dryness. Her pelvic ultrasound shows a normal uterus and adnexa. Her endometrial biopsy shows proliferative endometrium without hyperplasia or malignancy. How would you define her bleeding pattern?

a. Menorrhagia
b. Polymenorrhea
c. Oligomenorrhea
d. Metrorrhagia
e. Dysfunctional uterine bleeding (DUB)

82. A mother brings in her 17-year-old G0 daughter to see you for heavy painful periods. Her menarche was at age 13 and she has had fairly regular cycles for the past 2 years. However, her bleeding has often been so heavy that she soaks through a tampon and pad every 2 to 3 hours. She routinely bleeds for 7 to 9 days each cycle. She's been chronically anemic with a hematocrit of 31 despite fair compliance with iron supplementation. She also bruises easily with eccymoses that may be 5 cm or greater. She has a history of nosebleeds and recalls how her stuffed bunny rabbit always had dried blood on it from her frequent nose bleeds when she was a child. Her mother also shares that she had a difficult time with persistent bleeding after her tonsillectomy and again after her wisdom teeth extraction earlier this year. How do you proceed?

a. Check a pregnancy test, TFTs, PRL and, if normal, start her on oral contraceptive pills to decrease her menorrhagia
b. Check a pregnancy test, CBC, TFTs, CBC, PT, PTT, von Willebrand's antigen, ristocetin cofactor, and refer to hematology to rule out bleeding disorder
c. Check a pelvic ultrasound to rule out congenital malformation and fibroids. If normal, recommend a Mirena IUD to control her bleeding
d. Recommend a trial of tranexamic acid (Lysteda) to be taken with each menstrual period
e. Get a saline sonohysterogram to evaluate the endometrial cavity and consider endometrial ablation, given her severe level of bleeding

83. Historically, before the development of the standard pregnancy test, it was diagnosed by history and physical examination. Which of the following is not a sign of pregnancy?

a. Chadwick sign
b. Goodell's sign
c. Ladin's sign
d. Development of linea nigra
e. Cullen's sign

84. A 27-year-old G0 presents to your clinic with irregular menses. She reports 4 to 5 menstrual cycles per year for the past year. She also complains of worsening acne, and having to pluck dark hairs from her upper lip, chin, and abdomen. Your physical examination is remarkable only for the hair and acne she described, as well as obesity. You perform a bedside ultrasound that reveals multiple small follicular cysts on her bilateral ovaries. You correctly

diagnose her with polycystic ovary syndrome. In PCOS, patients are likely to have which of the following physiologic changes:
a. Increased levels of FSH
b. Increased frequency of GnRH pulses
c. Low estradiol concentrations
d. Low free testosterone
e. Low inhibin levels

85. An 18-year-old woman presents to the emergency room with abdominal cramping and vaginal bleeding. Her vital signs are temperature 37.3°C, blood pressure 110/70, pulse 82 beats per minute, and respiratory rate 18 breaths per minute. Abdominal examination reveals mild lower abdominal tenderness to palpation without rebound tenderness or guarding. Pelvic examination reveals a mildly enlarged uterus with right adnexal fullness. A urine pregnancy test is positive. You obtain a quantitative β-hCG, complete blood count, type and screen, complete metabolic panel, and pelvic ultrasound. Her β-hCG level is 9,000 mIU/mL. Her complete blood count and complete metabolic panels are normal. Her blood type is A negative, antibody negative. The pelvic ultrasound reveals an ectopic pregnancy and a moderate amount of fluid in the pelvis. What is the next best step in treating this patient?
a. Multidose methotrexate therapy
b. Emergent laparotomy for evacuation of the ectopic pregnancy
c. Laparoscopic evacuation of the ectopic pregnancy
d. Misoprostol therapy
e. Administer RhoGAM

86. You are covering the postpartum ward and are asked to perform an examination of a 1-day-old female infant. The examination is normal with the exception of an enlarged clitoris, and only one opening other than the rectum. What is the most common cause of ambiguous genitalia in females?
a. Polycystic ovary syndrome
b. Müllerian agenesis
c. Transverse vaginal septum
d. Congenital adrenal hyperplasia

87. A 30-year-old patient with polycystic ovary syndrome returns to your clinic for a follow-up visit after starting the oral contraceptive pill to reduce her symptoms of acne and hirsutism. After 6 months of use, she is pleased with the aesthetic improvements to her appearance. She wonders how the birth control pill works to improve her symptoms. You explain that the effects are due to the oral contraceptive causing:
a. Increased 5-alpha reductase activity in the skin
b. Lower sex hormone–binding globulin and therefore lower circulating testosterone
c. Increased sex hormone–binding globulin and therefore higher circulating testosterone
d. Increased sex hormone–binding globulin and therefore lower circulating testosterone
e. Stimulation of LH production leading to lower circulating testosterone

88. A 20-year-old G1P1001 presents to your clinic for her annual examination. She denies any significant past medical history or surgical history. Her pregnancy, which was 1 year prior, was uncomplicated other than gestational diabetes. She has a family history of type 2 diabetes mellitus and hypertension. On physical examination, you note that her BMI is 32, and that she has a gray–brown velvety discoloration on her neck and around her vulva. Her examination is otherwise normal. These findings prompt you to add which test to her health care maintenance testing?
a. Fasting glucose
b. Vulvar biopsy
c. Papanicolaou test
d. Cholesterol screening
e. Mammogram

89. A 27-year-old G1P1001 woman comes to your office 8 months following an uncomplicated vaginal delivery of a healthy male newborn. She and her husband have been trying to conceive a second pregnancy for 3 months, but she has been unsuccessful and is very anxious about this. After a thorough history, you find that she is still breastfeeding her newborn routinely and is not menstruating. Assuming that she has not yet ovulated, what is the likely underlying cause of the findings in this patient?
a. Thyroid hormone suppression of the anterior pituitary
b. Abnormal endometrial regeneration causing failure of implantation
c. Prolactin-induced inhibition of pulsatile GnRH from the hypothalamus
d. Reduced tubal motility secondary to elevated prolactin levels
e. Pathologically decreased sperm count of the male partner

90. A 24-year-old G3P3003 woman presents to your practice requesting the best contraception that you have available. She has undergone three uncomplicated vaginal deliveries and has no underlying chronic medical conditions. She is agreeable to taking a pill daily and states that she is "very responsible." Which of the following, has the highest actual efficacy in preventing pregnancy?
a. Coitus interruptus
b. Combined oral contraceptive pill
c. Diaphragm
d. Progesterone-only pill
e. Intrauterine device

91. A 35-year-old woman has been your patient for at least 5 years. You have recently placed her on a progestin-only birth control pill (POP), given her history of smoking one PPD for nearly 20 years. All of the following are mechanisms of action for progestin-only contraceptive methods except:
a. Suppress ovulation
b. Thicken the cervical mucous
c. Make the endometrium unsuitable for implantation
d. Inhibit sperm motility
e. Cause regression of the corpus luteum

92. A 33-year-old G2P1001 woman at 15 weeks EGA presents to your office for a return visit after a fetal diagnosis of Trisomy 18. She desires pregnancy termination. You discuss that options include labor induction and dilation and evacuation (D&E). She opts for labor induction. Which risk below would you *not* include on the consent form?
a. Infection
b. Bleeding
c. Uterine perforation
d. Possible need for additional procedures
e. Transfusion

93. A 15-year-old adolescent female presents to a family planning clinic for termination of pregnancy. Her father accompanies her. Ultrasound confirms that she has an intrauterine gestation of 6 weeks' gestation. She was recently diagnosed with chlamydia and has completed treatment. Her medical history is significant for Lupus for which she is taking daily prednisone. She desires medication abortion. Which is a contraindication to medication abortion?
a. Age less than 18
b. Gestational age less than 8 weeks
c. Chronic steroid use
d. Recent diagnosis of chlamydia
e. Teen pregnancy

94. A 26-year-old G1 P0 woman had a medication abortion 2 weeks ago at 6 weeks' gestation. She had light bleeding in the first few days and has had no bleeding since then. She presents for her follow-up appointment and ultrasound shows a gestational sac. What is the best next step?

a. Repeat dose of misoprostol
b. Repeat dose of mifepristone
c. Serial ultrasounds
d. Perform D&C
e. Perform D&E

95. Which of the following is *not* a major cause of infertility?

a. PCOS
b. Endometriosis
c. PID and pelvic adhesions
d. Uterine fibroids
e. Advanced maternal age

96. Which of the following are potential causes for male factor infertility?

a. Anabolic steroid use
b. Erectile dysfunction
c. Varicocele
d. a and c
e. All of the above

97. A 20-year-old G1 at 34 weeks 0 day is being induced for severe preeclampsia. She is receiving magnesium sulfate 2 g per hour IV for seizure prophylaxis. In the fourth hour of her labor induction, she experiences a tonic clonic seizure lasting approximately 2 minutes. After ensuring her airway, breathing, and circulation are intact and normal, the next step in treating this patient is:

a. Administer hydralazine 5 mg IV push
b. Deliver the baby immediately via cesarean section
c. Stop the magnesium infusion and convert to phenytoin
d. Rebolus magnesium sulfate 2 g IV
e. Administer furosemide 40 mg IV

98. As part of routine prenatal care, there are a series of tests offered throughout pregnancy. Usually, these tests are delineated by the trimester in which they are offered. Which of the following tests is routinely offered in the second trimester?

a. GBS
b. Hematocrit
c. Amniocentesis
d. Transvaginal ultrasound for dating
e. Fern test

99. Which are potential treatments for unexplained infertility?

a. Ovulation induction with Clomid
b. IVF (in vitro fertilization) with ICSI (intracytoplasmic sperm injection)
c. Expectant management
d. a and b
e. a, b and c

100. A 28-year-old G_2P_1 woman at 30 weeks gestational age presents to the clinic for a routine OB visit. She was diagnosed with gestational diabetes 4 weeks ago and was started on a diabetic diet and exercise regimen. She adhered to the recommendations, measured her glucose levels four times a day, and recorded results for the past week. Her average fasting glucose value is 84 mg/dL and 1-hour postprandial values after all three meals range from 135 to 165 mg/dL. What is the best next step in the management of this patient?

a. Continue diabetic diet plus exercise
b. Start the patient on Lispro and NPH in the morning and Lispro at dinner
c. Start the patient on Lispro in the morning, and Lispro and NPH at dinner
d. Start the patient on Metformin 500 mg PO daily
e. Start the patient on NPH in the morning and NPH at dinner

101. On the basis of the 2004 ISSVD classification of squamous intraepithelial lesions of the vulva, VIN is divided into two categories. Which of the following are the correct categories?

a. HPV effect / differentiated type
b. Reactive changes / condylomatous type
c. Usual type / differentiated type
d. High risk HPV / Low risk HPV
e. Benign / malignant

102. A 24-year-old G_1P_0 patient at 25 weeks GA presents for a routine OB visit. She is sexually active with her boyfriend of 4 years. Her BMI is 29. Physical examination is otherwise unremarkable. She was surprised when you told her she screened positive for diabetes. She is uninsured and prior to this pregnancy, had only utilized Student Health for acute illnesses, but has never been told she had diabetes before. Which of the following is the most likely diagnosis and etiology of her diabetes?

a. Type 2 diabetes mellitus—Autoimmune destruction of β-islet cells
b. Type 1 diabetes mellitus—Elevated progesterone levels
c. Gestational diabetes—Human chorionic somatomammotropin
d. Type 1 diabetes mellitus—Preexisting peripheral insulin resistance
e. Gestational diabetes—Recently acquired HCV infection

103. Based on current knowledge of Paget disease of the vulva, all of the following are true except:

a. It is a disease of elderly women and may present with a concomitant adenocarcinoma elsewhere
b. It may present with an invasive component
c. Recurrences may be treated with CO_2 laser ablation
d. The overall lifetime risk of invasive squamous cell carcinoma is approximately 5%
e. Paget disease can be found in vulva, breast, and bone

104. A 58-year-old G0 with systemic lupus and renal failure presents to clinic with a diagnosis of superficially invasive vulvar cancer based on a biopsy. She was sent to you and underwent a modified radical vulvectomy with ipsilateral lymph node sampling with a diagnosis of invasive, moderately differentiated squamous cell carcinoma, 2.9 cm in greatest dimension, four nodes were negative for invasion. According to FIGO staging, what stage is this patient?

a. Stage Ib
b. Stage II
c. Stage IIb
d. Stage IIIa
e. Stage 0

105. A 23-year-old G0 who has never had a Pap test or pelvic examination comes to the office to start on birth control pills. She tells you her periods are regular but heavy and last 7 days, and she has terrible cramps. She has been sexually active for the past 2 years with three different partners. She uses condoms most of the time. You perform an examination including STI testing and a Pap test and prescribe a trial of oral contraceptive pills. Her STI testing is negative but her Pap test result is "atypical squamous cells of undetermined significance (ASCUS)" and a reflex HPV test is negative. What is your recommendation for this Pap test result?

a. Return for colposcopic exam
b. Repeat the Pap test in 3 months

c. Repeat the Pap test in 3 years
d. Repeat the HPV test in 1 year
e. LEEP conization of the cervix

106. A 38-year-old G2P2002 comes for her annual examination and Pap testing. Her periods are very light and infrequent since she had Mirena placed 3 years ago. She is recently divorced and has a new partner. She tells you her last Pap was normal 3 years ago. Her Pap test result is "negative for intraepithelial lesion or malignancy" (NILM) and the HPV test is positive. What do you recommend?
a. Colposcopy
b. Repeat Pap test and HPV in 1 year
c. Repeat Pap test in 3 months
d. Repeat HPV test only in 1 year
e. LEEP conization of the cervix

107. A 28-year-old G0 had a low-grade squamous intraepithelial lesion (LSIL) Pap result at age 26 followed by colposcopic examination findings of CIN 1. An HPV test at her annual examination last year was positive and colposcopy was again consistent with CIN 1. The HPV test was repeated this year and remains positive. At her colposcopy examination, you see a faintly acetowhite lesion at the squamocolumnar junction (SCJ) and biopsy of the area again returns CIN 1. The examination is satisfactory (the entire SCJ is seen) and the entire lesion is viewed. She is very concerned and would like to know what she should do now. What is *not* one of the recommended options?
a. Repeat Pap every 3 months for 1 year
b. Cryotherapy
c. Excisional procedure (LEEP)
d. Repeat HPV test again in 1 year
e. Pap at 6 and 12 months after colposcopy

108. A 16-year-old G0 is accompanied by her mother who requests you to perform STI testing, check a Pap test, and prescribe birth control pills for her daughter. The patient recently told her mother she had been sexually active for the past 2 years. She tells you she has used condoms most of the time but wants to try pills to help control her painful periods. What is not one of your recommendations for this patient?
a. HPV vaccination
b. Pap testing in 2 years
c. HIV, chlamydia, and gonorrhea testing
d. Wait 5 years to perform Pap testing
e. Pregnancy testing

109. A 73-year-old woman presents with a chief complaint of scant vaginal spotting. After obtaining a thorough history and physical examination, what test would you likely order as your next step in evaluating this patient?
a. FSH
b. Transvaginal ultrasound
c. CA-125
d. Hepatic enzymes
e. Estradiol levels

110. Staging for endometrial cancer generally entails which of the following?
a. Clinical staging with physical examination, pyelogram, chest X-ray, and anoscopy
b. Clinical staging with physical examination, pyelogram, chest X-ray, and cat scan
c. Surgical staging with TAH, BSO, and possible pelvic and para-aortic lymphadenectomy
d. Surgical staging with TAH, BSO, pelvic nodes, pelvic washings, and omentectomy
e. Surgical staging with hysterectomy only

111. Which of the following is *not* a protective factor against the development of endometrial cancer?
a. Parity
b. Smoking
c. Physical activity
d. Oral contraceptive use
e. Tamoxifen use

112. Which of the following is the most commonly diagnosed gynecologic malignancy in the United States?
a. Endometrial
b. Cervical
c. Ovarian
d. Tubal
e. Vulvar

113. A 22-year-old G0 presents for routine examination. She is without complaints. Her LMP was 3 weeks ago and was normal. On pelvic examination, she has a mobile 8-cm mass. Her urine pregnancy test is negative. Pelvic ultrasound shows a right ovarian 6 $\times$ 8 cm cystic mass with a focal solid component and calcifications. What is the next step in the management of this patient?
a. Repeat ultrasound in 6 weeks
b. Exploratory laparotomy, TAH/BSO
c. Right ovarian cystectomy
d. Removal of the right ovary and tube (RSO)
e. Expectant management

114. A 37-year-old G2P2 reports irregular menses, intermittent pelvic pain, and a recent increase in facial and body hair. On physical examination, the patient has acne, facial hair, and a 10-cm left adnexal mass. Pelvic ultrasound confirms a solid lobulated 10-cm mass arising from the left ovary. Which of the following serum concentrations were most likely elevated?
a. Progesterone
b. Estradiol
c. Testosterone
d. AFP
e. Ca-125

115. A 20-year-old woman presents to your emergency department for new onset vaginal bleeding. She is found to be pregnant with a serum β-hCG level of 300,000 mIU/mL. Both her heart rate and blood pressure are elevated. On physical examination, you palpate her uterus to be at the umbilicus, whereas her last menstrual period places her at about 8 weeks' gestation. On ultrasound examination, there is a profound amount of vesicular appearing material without an identifiable fetus. Which of the following is *not* part of the immediate initial management plan?
a. Determination of Rh status
b. Surgical intervention (Suction curettage)
c. Methotrexate administration
d. Evaluation of thyroid status
e. Complete blood count

116. A 25-year-old G1P0 presents to the emergency room with vaginal bleeding. Her last normal menstrual period was 6 weeks earlier. She reports that she is sexually active with male partners and does not use any hormonal or barrier methods for contraception. On arrival, her temperature is 37°C, blood pressure is 115/80, pulse is 75 beats per minute, respiratory rate is 16 breaths per minute, and she has 100% oxygen saturation on room air. A pelvic examination reveals a small amount of dark blood in the vagina. The external cervical os appears 1 to 2 cm dilated. Her uterus is mildly enlarged, anteverted, and nontender. A urine pregnancy test is positive. A pelvic ultrasound is obtained and shows an intrauterine gestational sac with a yolk sac. No fetal pole or cardiac motion is seen. Bilateral adnexa are normal. What is her diagnosis?

a. Incomplete abortion
b. Threatened abortion
c. Ectopic pregnancy
d. Missed abortion
e. Inevitable abortion

117. A 21-year-old woman undergoes hysteroscopy and curettage for persistent irregular uterine bleeding after her term vaginal delivery 8 months ago. Final pathologic findings from the D&C are consistent with choriocarcinoma with invasion into the myometrium. Baseline serum β-hCG is 200,000 mIU/mL. Which of the following is *not* currently indicated?

a. Imaging for distant metastatic lesions
b. Surgical intervention (hysterectomy)
c. Chemotherapy
d. Close surveillance of serum β-hCG
e. Reliable contraception

118. An 18-year-old G1 sees you in your office and tells you she missed her last period and had a positive home urine pregnancy test. You perform your normal first obstetrical examination and obtain basic prenatal labs as well as a first trimester viability ultrasound. The radiologist calls you to discuss the findings, which demonstrate a gestational sac with a fetus measuring approximately 8 weeks' gestation. There is no fetal heartbeat demonstrated. The placenta is markedly thickened and echogenic, more than would be expected in the first trimester. There are multiple areas of small cystic spaces within the placenta as well. The most likely diagnosis and corresponding karyotype is:

a. Complete Mole, 46 XX
b. Incomplete Mole, 46 XY
c. Incomplete Mole, 69 XXY
d. Complete Mole, 69 XXX
e. Incomplete Mole, 69 XYY

119. A 33-year-old G2P2 woman presents to your office with a complaint of nipple discharge. She states it is milky in color, comes from both breasts, and is present even when she doesn't express it. You perform a breast examination, and express milky discharge from both breasts. You diagnose her with galactorrhea. Which condition is *not* associated with galactorrhea?

a. Pregnancy
b. Breast abscess
c. Pituitary adenoma
d. Psychotropic medications
e. Hypothyroidism

120. A 42-year-old G1P1 presents to your office with a complaint of bloody nipple discharge. She undergoes excision of the involved duct for an intraductal papilloma. On pathology, she is also noted to have lobular carcinoma in situ. Which of the following statements about this diagnosis is *not* true?

a. LCIS is considered a premalignant lesion (but not a true cancer itself) because it is an indicator for subsequent risk of breast cancer
b. It is not palpable or seen on mammogram
c. The recommended treatment is observation; however, selective estrogen receptor modulators may reduce the risk of subsequent invasive cancer
d. Subsequent cancers are always on the same side as the LCIS
e. Subsequent cancers may be intraductal, invasive ductal, or lobular carcinoma

121. Which of the following would be most reassuring when assessing a fetal heart tracing?

a. Fetal heart rate of 140 with marked variability
b. Fetal heart rate of 100 with minimal variability
c. Fetal heart rate of 150 with moderate variability
d. Fetal heart rate of 90 with absent variability
e. Fetal heart rate of 190 with moderate variability

122. A 30-year-old G2P1 at 30 weeks' gestation is transported to the emergency department (ED) via ambulance after motor vehicle accident (MVA). The accident involved the patient who was driving her car at approximately 40 miles per hour when she was hit on the driver's side by another car going 30 miles per hour. She was restrained by her seatbelt and her airbag deployed. She was found on the scene of the accident by the paramedics to be awake, alert, oriented despite significant pelvic pain, bruises on her abdomen from the seat belt, and a few minor lacerations. She is afebrile, BP 120/70 mm Hg, HR 120 bpm, arterial oxygen saturation 100%, RR 18 per minute. The OB team arrives in the ED and places the baby on continuous external fetal monitoring. She is noted to have contractions every 2 minutes and the fetal heart rate is approximately 110 bpm with late decelerations noted with every contraction. The paramedics report that they have not noted any vaginal bleeding. On sterile speculum examination, the cervix appears to be closed with no blood noted in the vaginal vault. On bedside ultrasound, there appears to be a normal amniotic fluid index and an anterior placenta low-lying placenta and a small retroplacental fluid collection. What is the most likely cause of the late decelerations on the continuous fetal monitoring?

a. Umbilical cord compression
b. Preterm labor
c. Concealed placental abruption
d. Fetal head compression
e. Placenta previa

123. A 25-year-old Hispanic G2P1 at 36 weeks' gestation by 24 week ultrasound presents to L&D complaining of painful uterine contractions every 2 to 4 minutes for the last hour. She was late to prenatal care and had her first US at 28 weeks' gestation. On her ultrasound at 28 weeks, she was noted to have normal fluid and growth, no anomalies, and an anterior placenta with a posterior velamentous cord insertion. When Doppler was used during the ultrasound, it was noted that there appeared to be fetal vessels coursing across the internal os connecting to the posterior velamentous cord insertion. After her last ultrasound the patient was lost to follow-up until she presented today. The patient denies any leakage of fluid or vaginal bleeding. On SVE, the cervix is noted to be 6 cm/90% effaced/0 station. FHR tracing is reactive with no decels. Which of the following is the most appropriate delivery plan for this patient?

a. Expectant management, vaginal delivery
b. Artificial rupture of membranes with placement of IUPC, vaginal delivery
c. Emergent cesarean section
d. Oxytocin augmentation
e. None of the above

124. In prenatal genetic testing, which of the following is *not* a trait commonly screened for in parents from high-risk populations?

a. Sickle cell disease
b. Cystic fibrosis
c. Thalassemia
d. Prader-Willi
e. Tay-Sachs

125. A 38-year-old African American G1P0 presents to L&D at 34 weeks complaining of painful uterine contractions for the last 2 hours. She denies leakage of fluid, or discharge. She does report vaginal bleeding that started 30 minutes ago. She has no significant PMH but has a past surgical history of a prior abdominal myomectomy in which she had a large anterior fibroid removed. Per the operative report, the endometrial cavity was entered to remove the fibroid. On examination, she is afebrile, vital signs stable. On ultrasound, the fetus is vertex, normal AFI, no evidence of retroplacental clot, posterior placenta. On sterile speculum exam (SSE), she has approximately 100 cc bright blood in the vaginal vault, no pool, no ferning. Nitrazine is positive. Her cervix appears to be approximately 3 cm dilated. On the FHR tracing, the FHTs are 120s with moderate variable decelerations down to the 60s with each contraction; on tocometry she appears to be contracting every 2 to 4 minutes. Which of the following is the most likely etiology of the antepartum hemorrhage in this clinical situation?

a. Preterm premature rupture of membranes
b. Uterine rupture
c. Cervical laceration
d. Placenta previa
e. Vasa previa

126. A 34-year-old Asian woman G4P3003 at 34 weeks' gestation presents to L&D triage complaining of hematuria, dysuria, and occasional contractions for 1 week. She also notes some occasional vaginal spotting over the last 3 days. She denies any leakage of fluid or discharge. She denies back or flank pain but has had some suprapubic discomfort. She had an anatomy ultrasound at 18 weeks where she was noted to have normal fetal anatomy, normal AFI, and an anterior complete placenta previa. She has no significant PMH. She has surgical history of three previous cesarean sections at term. Her first cesarean section was 8 years ago in China for breech at term. Due to her social situation, she has not been able to schedule a repeat ultrasound at 30 weeks, as was recommended at the time of her anatomy ultrasound. She has not had recent intercourse. Which of the following is *not* an appropriate initial test to determine the etiology of this patient's hematuria?

a. Urine analysis
b. Urine culture
c. Sterile speculum examination
d. CT scan of abdomen and pelvis
e. Abdominal ultrasound of uterus

127. A 33-year-old G7P1224 at 34 weeks 1 day's gestation, with a history of prior preterm birth at 35 weeks for diamniotic–dichorionic twins and at 33 weeks with a singleton PPROM, presents with sudden onset vaginal bleeding and abdominal pain. Her medical history is significant for ruptured appendectomy requiring emergency surgery at age 19. Social history is complicated. She lives with her mother and older sister in a two-bedroom apartment with her four children. She does not work outside the home and smokes one-half pack per day of tobacco. She takes methadone for history of heroin use. Current medications include methadone, prenatal vitamin, and iron supplement. Which of the following is not associated with risk of preterm birth?

a. Socioeconomic status
b. PPROM
c. Placental abruption
d. Her age
e. Her BMI of 18

128. Your next patient is a 62-year-old G2 P2 with biopsy proven VIN III who is returning for discussion of results. While counseling her you explain the risk factors for the development of VIN including . . .

a. Immunosuppression
b. Smoking
c. High risk HPV infection
d. Asian ethnicity
e. a, b and c

A Answers

1. b (Chapter 31)
Metastatic persistent GTD most commonly (90%) presents after evacuation of a molar pregnancy. This patient's history is consistent with a suction curettage performed a year ago, probably for molar pregnancy. Most patients with persistent GTD will have localized disease in the uterus (typically due to invasive mole), but rarely, metastasis can occur. Metastatic foci are more associated with choriocarcinoma than invasive molar pregnancy. This patient's symptoms are probably due to pulmonary foci, the most common site for metastasis. The brain, liver, bowel, kidney, and vagina are other potential sites of metastasis.

2. a (Chapter 17)
The histologic finding of plasma cells in the endometrial stroma is indicative of chronic endometritis. Both acute and chronic inflammatory cells are often seen histologically. Chronic endometritis is often asymptomatic but can be linked to infertility. Symptomatic women usually present with abnormal uterine bleeding and lower abdominal pain or cramping. Doxycycline is the treatment of choice.

b. Insertion of an LNG-IUS is not a treatment for chronic endometritis. LNG-IUS may be used to treat women with endometrial hyperplasia. Histologic findings of endometrial hyperplasia include proliferation of endometrial glands and an increased gland-to-stroma ratio. Other non-contraceptive uses of the LNG-IUS include treatment of dysmenorrhea, pelvic pain, and menorrhagia.

c. Hysteroscopy is a minimally invasive surgical approach that can be utilized to view the inside of the endometrial cavity. It is used for the evaluation and treatment of a variety of conditions including abnormal uterine bleeding, polyps, fibroids, Müllerian anomalies, and infertility. In this case, the patient has already undergone a pelvic ultrasound and endometrial biopsy. No further evaluation is needed as a diagnosis of chronic endometritis has already been made.

d. Chronic endometritis is not an indication for hysterectomy.

e. Cefoxitin is commonly used in the treatment of puerperal endomyometritis.

3. c (Chapter 7)
Amniocentesis should be performed when a titer of 1:16 or greater (1:256) is identified. Once Rh sensitization is discovered, titers should be checked every 4 weeks. You would begin fetal testing between 16 and 20 weeks' gestation when the titer reaches 1:16. Testing is performed by serial amniocenteses and the amniotic fluid is analyzed by a spectrophotometer that measures the light absorption (DOD_{450}) by bilirubin, which will accumulate in the amniotic fluid with increasing fetal hemolysis. The results are plotted on the Liley curve (Fig. 7-5), which predicts the severity of disease. Fetal cells can also be analyzed for Rh status. If fetal Rh status is negative, Rh incompatibility is no longer a concern for the pregnancy. Depending on the level of hemolysis, further monitoring with amniocentesis or more invasive procedures such as fetal intrauterine transfusion may be indicated.

Answers a and b describe titer levels that are not concerning. At levels of 1:4 and 1:8, the patient can continue to be monitored but does not require further intervention until the titer reaches 1:16.

Answers d and e. Both these titer levels warrant further testing with amniocentesis but they are not the lowest answer choices available in this scenario.

4. c (Chapter 32)
Many patients' fears over breast cancer can be alleviated by counseling and discussion of risk factors with them. Genetic counseling and breast center referral are available for patients who require additional reassurance. Overall breast awareness is the recommended surveillance for her age group, coupled with clinical breast examination every 1 to 3 years. She may participate in breast self-examinations if she chooses. If a mass is palpated or she turns 40, she is then a candidate for imaging. Women at high risk should include MRI with the screening mammography every year, beginning at age 40. However, she is not in the high-risk category with her history. High-risk groups include women who have a known BRCA1 or BRCA2 gene mutation, have a first-degree relative with either mutation, are at high risk based on an evaluation by a validated risk assessment tool, underwent radiation to the chest between the ages of 10 and 30, or have a hereditary syndrome associated with multiple cancer diagnoses. These women should begin screening at age 30. Ultrasound is used in the evaluation of uncertain mammographic findings, in women under 40, in women with dense breast tissue, as a tool to guide a needle for breast biopsies Ultrasound may also be used in women who are candidates for breast MRI but can't receive one due to gadolidium contrast allergy or other barriers.

5. c (Chapter 3)
Maternal serum screening is both for aneuploidy such as Trisomy 21, 18, or 13 as well as for neural tube defects via the MSAFP. Of note, an elevated MSAFP screens for fetal abdominal wall defects as well. Fragile X syndrome is an X-linked disorder whose etiology is a triplet repeat. Carriers usually have the pre-mutation with 40 to 49 triplet repeats, which then can expand to a full mutation. Because it is X-linked, women are usually only mildly affected, but women with cognitive disabilities related to the Fragile X mutation have been identified. Fragile X is not screened for with maternal serum screening.

6. b (Chapter 24)
A history of venous thromboembolism is an absolute contraindication to using combined oral contraceptives. Other absolute contraindications include history of coronary artery disease, cerebrovascular accident, breast or endometrial cancer, and abnormal liver function. All of the others listed are relative contraindications. Migraine headaches, instead of tension headaches, are a relative contraindication to use, unless a patient has vascular compromise or visual aura where it is generally regarded as absolute.

7. a (Chapter 4)
Maternal hypotension, secondary to decreased systemic vascular resistance, is a complication associated with both epidural and spinal anesthesia, though it is a bit more common with spinal anesthesia. In severe cases it can lead to decreased placental perfusion and fetal heart rate decelerations or even bradycardia. Occasionally, if the anesthetic reaches the innervations of the diaphragm it can cause maternal respiratory depression as opposed to hyperventilation. Increased contraction strength is not associated with either spinal or epidural analgesia, though a decrease in contractions has been seen with both. Finally, chorioamnionitis is not associated with spinal or epidural anesthesia, though increased maternal fever is seen with epidural analgesia, particularly over time.

8. d (Chapter 4)
All of the answer choices are signs of active labor with the exception of fever and chills, which is not normal and could be a sign of infection.

9. a (Chapter 8)
There are a wide range of risk factors for developing preeclampsia, including extremes of maternal age, nulliparity, chronic hypertension, renal disease, diabetes, lupus, African American race, short cohabitation time, history of preeclampsia, molar pregnancy, and so on. However, smoking has been associated with a decreased risk of preeclampsia in several studies.

10. a (Chapter 25)
First trimester abortion is very safe with a complication rate that requires hospitalization of 0.3%. It is important to counsel the patient and her mother on possible risks of the procedure but they can be reassured that the risk of serious complication is very low.

11. e (Chapter 8)
In this setting, there are two indications for immediate delivery. The first is the severe headache that does not resolve with acetaminophen. The second is HELLP syndrome with markedly elevated LFTs and platelets less than 100,000. Although expectant management of severe preeclampsia is the standard of care in most settings, severe symptoms and HELLP are two of the reasons to abandon with expectant management. However, one can still give betamethasone as an induction of labor may take 24 hours and the fetus will get the acute steroid benefits. During the induction, one would control blood pressures in the 140 to 150/80 to 100 ranges to minimize risk from severe blood pressures, but to avoid hypotension as well. Magnesium sulfate would be given for seizure prophylaxis.

12. c (Chapter 6)
This scenario describes a uterine rupture. History of prior cesarean section is a risk factor for uterine rupture. In this case, the patient experienced a sudden change in pain, vaginal bleeding, followed by a change in fetal status, and a change in fetal station with the fetus moving back out of the pelvis. Placental abruption can present with similar findings of vaginal bleeding, abdominal pain, and change in fetal status; however, this scenario is most suggestive of uterine rupture, given the history of prior cesarean section. Vasa previa presents with painless vaginal bleeding and fetal distress, often precipitated by rupture of membranes. Fetal nuchal cord can cause changes in fetal heart rate such as variable decelerations, but generally does not occur until the patient is in the second stage of labor, and is not associated with vaginal bleeding.

13. c (Chapter 6)
Standard evaluation for ruptured membranes includes a sterile speculum examination. Findings of liquid pooling in the vagina, positive nitrazine test, and ferning on microscopy are diagnostic of ruptured membranes. AmniSure, ultrasound, and amnio dye tests are all tests that can be used to diagnose rupture when standard sterile speculum findings are not conclusive. Amniocentesis is helpful if you are concerned about infection, which is suspected based on maternal fever, elevated WBC, or abdominal tenderness.

14. e (Chapter 26)
All of these are methods of treating endometriosis. However, in women who are trying to conceive, medical management has no role in decreasing infertility. It is thought that endometrial implants result in infertility by causing disruption of normal tissue, formation of adhesions and fibrosis, and severe inflammation. The resulting adhesions and inflammation can also result in distortion of the fallopian tubes and other anatomic structures. Surgical resection of endometrial implants has been found to increase the fertility rate in women with mild, moderate, and severe endometriosis.

15. b (Chapter 6)
Betamethasone is the only choice that has been shown to improve pregnancy outcomes. Betamethasone, if given 48 hours prior to delivery, reduces neonatal morbidity. Tocolytics can be used for up to 48 hours to administer corticosteroids for fetal well-being. With prolonged ruptured membranes, hospital observation and bed rest are the standard of care due to the risk of development of chorioamnionitis, cord prolapse, and placental abruption, but they do not have as great a benefit as corticosteroids. Lastly, augmentation of labor would not be recommended until after completion of corticosteroids and at least 32 weeks' gestation unless there was a non-reassuring fetal heart rate tracing or signs of fetal infection.

16. d (Chapter 7)
Chorioamnionitis occurs in approximately 1% to 5% of pregnancies and is generally the result of an ascending infection from organisms normally present in the vaginal flora. Occasionally, it may result from hematogenous dissemination. Young age, low socioeconomic status, nulliparity, prolonged rupture of membranes, and preexisting infection in the genital tract are all risk factors for chorioamnionitis. It is not associated with IUGR.

Answers b, c, d, and e are all placental problems that can result in IUGR. Abnormal placental vascular development or disruptions in the vascular network all can lead to growth disruption in the fetus. Chronic placental abruption reduces the functioning surface of the placenta. Placenta previa is believed to increase the risk for IUGR because the placenta is located in the lower uterine segment, which is felt to a suboptimal location for nutrient exchange. Placental thrombosis or infarction decreases the volume of functioning placenta and thereby decreases the nutrient and oxygen exchange interface between the mother and the fetus. Lastly, marginal cord insertion is associated with IUGR because of its abnormal vascular formation and likely effect on nutrient exchange.

17. d (Chapter 7)
Polyhydramnios is associated with gestational diabetes, congenital anomalies, multiple gestations, and neural tube defects. Polyhydramnios is not found in Potter's syndrome. In fact, Potter's syndrome is characterized by anhydramnios secondary to renal agenesis and therefore decreased production of amniotic fluid.

Answer a. Gestational diabetes is a common cause of mild polyhydramnios presenting later in pregnancy.

Answer b. Congenital anomalies such as esophageal atresia or other intestinal obstructions limit fluid passage uptake in the GI tract and result in polyhydramnios.

Answer d. Twin–twin transfusion syndrome can cause polyhydramnios in the recipient twin. TTTS occurs in monochorionic gestations where vascular connections exist between the veins and the arteries on the surface of the placenta. The donor twin shunts arterial blood to the recipient via arterial–venous connections. The recipient twin therefore sees a larger volume of blood flow and as a result, may develop polyhydramnios.

Answer e. Neural tube defects contribute to polyhydramnios by leaking CSF into the amniotic environment.

18. c (Chapter 8)
This patient has only had one elevated blood pressure, so she doesn't have a diagnosis yet. To make the diagnosis of gestational hypertension, one must have two elevated blood pressures 6 hours apart. A patient with a mildly elevated blood pressure, no symptoms, and normal labs would go home to do the 24-hour urine protein to bring it back for a recheck of BPs and labs. In some institutions, the initial evaluation would occur entirely in the hospital. Even though she has a negative urine dip for protein, a significant proportion of such patients will have significant proteinuria on a 24-hour collection; thus, it is important to do a 24-hour urine collection. Patients with mild gestational hypertension or preeclampsia are usually managed expectantly until 37 weeks and then delivered.

19. a (Chapter 9)
About 1% to 12% of pregnant women will develop gestational diabetes, depending on the population. In the United States, the range is between 5% and 8%. Gestational diabetes is seen at higher rates in women of Hispanic/Latina, Native American, and Asian/Pacific Islander descent. GDM is also seen with increasing maternal age, obesity, presence of family history of diabetes, previous stillborn infant, or birth of a previous infant weighing more than 4,000 g. Initial studies found African American women to have higher rates of GDM compared with Caucasians. However, when controlled for maternal body mass index (BMI) in subsequent studies, little difference in incidence was observed between African Americans and Caucasians.

20. e (Chapter 9)
Forceps and vacuum should generally not be used when macrosomia is suspected due to increased risk of shoulder dystocia, except in the case of true outlet forceps for non-reassuring fetal monitoring.

a. Class A2 gestational diabetics, who by definition are on insulin or a hypoglycemic agent, are generally scheduled to be induced at 39 weeks of gestation.

b. Because of increased risk of macrosomia in A2 GDM patients, they commonly receive an obstetric ultrasound to estimate fetal weight between 34 and 37 weeks of gestation.

c. Patients with an EFW greater than 4,000 g have increased risk of shoulder dystocia. However, elective cesarean delivery is not routinely offered to women until the EFW is greater than 4,500 g.

d. Upon admission to labor and delivery, long-acting hypoglycemics are withheld to closely monitor blood glucose levels. Dextrose and insulin drips are used to maintain blood glucose between 100 and 120 mg/dL. If levels increase above 120 mg/dL, insulin can be increased. If levels drop between 80 and 100 mg/dL, dextrose can be started or increased.

21. d (Chapter 10)
A urine culture is performed at the initial prenatal visit to screen for asymptomatic bacteriuria, defined as greater than 100,000 colony forming units. The rate of asymptomatic bacteriuria during pregnancy is approximately 5% and is the same for nonpregnant women. However, in pregnant women they are at increased risk of progression to cystitis or pyelonephritis, which has significant morbidity. In addition, presence of asymptomatic bacteriuria also increases the risk of preterm birth, and this risk can be decreased with appropriate treatment.

a. You can screen for gonorrhea and chlamydia by performing a DNA probe analysis of an unclean urine sample; however, these STIs are not detected by urine culture.

b. There is no data to support an association between asymptomatic bacteriuria and chorioamnionitis or neonatal sepsis. During pregnancy, screening for group B streptococcus is performed between 35 and 37 weeks, and if a woman is found to be positive, she is treated during labor with penicillin to decrease her risk of chorioamnionitis and neonatal sepsis.

c. Rates of asymptomatic bacteriuria are the same in pregnant and nonpregnant women. Increased bacterial ascent up the urinary system is thought to be caused by progesterone-induced increased smooth muscle relaxation and ureteral dilation. This leads to an increased risk of cystitis and pyelonephritis compared with nonpregnant women.

e. The patient is clinically well and has no symptoms of pyelonephritis (fever, dysuria, or costovertebral angle tenderness).

22. b (Chapter 10)
Chronic hepatitis B is diagnosed by serum studies showing persistent hepatitis B antigen. Pregnancy is generally well-tolerated by these women and the reactivation of the virus or exacerbation of the disease rarely occurs. The placenta acts as a barrier to the hepatitis B virus, and as a result intrauterine infection with the virus is exceptionally rare. This patient's main risk is that of vertical transmission at the time of delivery due to exposure to maternal blood. To decrease this risk, the neonate should be given both the hepatitis B vaccine and hepatitis B antibody (HBIG) at birth. There is no evidence that cesarean delivery decreases vertical transmission and vaginal delivery should be encouraged. Women who have high HBV viral loads may be candidates for treatment with antivirals (lamivudine) to further decrease rates of vertical transmission.

a. We would recommend that this patient be referred to a physician that specializes in chronic liver disease. She may be a candidate for serial liver function tests based on the duration of her disease and viral load.

c. Hepatitis B screening is performed by testing for hepatitis surface antigen. The chronic carrier state for HBV is defined by the persistence of HBsAg and the absence of hepatitis B surface IgG antibody (anti-HBs). Acute infection with hepatitis B is diagnosed by the presence of IgM antibody to the hepatitis B core antigen (IgM anti-HBc), which is then present for approximately 6 months after initial infection.

d. Chronic hepatitis B has not been associated with fetal malformations because the virus does not cross the placenta.

e. See description to answer b.

23. a (Chapter 10)
The classic triad of congenital toxoplasmosis includes chorioretinitis, intracranial calcifications, and hydrocephalus. Severe congenital infection can involve fevers, seizures, chorioretinitis, hydro- or microcephaly, hepatosplenomegaly, and jaundice.

b. Although vertical transmission of syphilis can occur at any time during pregnancy and during any stage of disease, because there must be spirochetemia for vertical transmission to occur, approximately half of prenatal transmission occurs in pregnant women with primary or secondary syphilis. If early congenital syphilis is untreated, manifestations of late congenital syphilis can develop, including eighth nerve deafness, saber shins, mulberry molar, Hutchinson's teeth, and a saddle nose.

c. Rubella infection can be transmitted to the fetus and cause congenital rubella infection, which may lead to congenital rubella syndrome (CRS). The maternal–fetal transmission rate is highest during the first trimester, as are the rates of congenital abnormalities. The congenital abnormalities associated with CRS include deafness, cardiac abnormalities, cataracts, and mental retardation. Specifically, if maternal rubella infection occurs during the period of organogenesis, any fetal organ system may be affected.

d. CMV causes in utero infections in approximately 1% of all newborns. Of these infected infants, approximately 10% will be symptomatic at birth. Infants who are symptomatic can develop cytomegalic inclusion disease manifested by a constellation of findings including hepatomegaly, splenomegaly, thrombocytopenia, jaundice, cerebral calcifications, chorioretinitis, and interstitial pneumonitis. Affected infants have a high mortality rate of up to 30% and may develop mental retardation, sensorineural hearing loss, and neuromuscular disorders. Of the remaining 90% of asymptomatic infants, 15% will go on to develop late disabilities, while 85% will have no sequelae of the infection.

e. Fetal infection with listeria causes disseminated granulomatous lesions with microabscesses, chorioamnionitis, and placental lesions. The overall mortality from listeriosis is about 25% in reported cases.

24. c (Chapter 10)

A large Cochrane review has shown that in women with prior preterm birth, similar to this patient, screening and treatment for bacterial vaginosis may decrease the risk of preterm premature rupture of membranes. There have been some studies to suggest that screening and treatment for bacterial vaginosis may decrease preterm birth, but this finding was not seen in the Cochrane meta-analysis. Screening and treating women who are at average risk for preterm birth has not been shown to decrease rates of preterm birth or PPROM.

a. Untreated gonorrhea at the time of delivery can lead to ophthalmia neonatorum and blindness. In the United States, this is uncommon due to routine screening at the beginning of pregnancy and the application of prophylactic erythromycin eye therapy after delivery.

b. During pregnancy, screening for group B streptococcus is performed between 35 and 37 weeks, and if a woman is found to be positive she is treated during labor with penicillin to decrease her risk of chorioamnionitis and neonatal sepsis.

d. Placental abruption is most commonly due to hypertensive disorders of pregnancy, preterm premature rupture of membranes, trauma, and cocaine or tobacco use, among other etiologies.

e. Bacterial vaginosis has not been shown to increase risk of congenital malformations. Oral metronidazole is the recommended treatment during pregnancy. A meta-analysis found no evidence that the use of oral metronidazole in the first trimester leads to congenital malformations.

25. c (Chapter 10)

Group B *Streptococcus* is a major pathogen in neonatal sepsis, which has severe implications. Although early-onset neonatal sepsis occurs in 2 to 3 per 1,000 live births, the mortality rate with group B *Streptococcal* sepsis ranges from 5% to 50%, depending on gestational age at the time of delivery. To protect infants from group B *Streptococcus* infections, widespread screening programs have been implemented utilizing a rectovaginal culture for group B *Strep* colonization between 35 and 37 weeks. Large prospective studies have demonstrated that these screening programs do decrease the rate of neonatal sepsis from group B *Strep*. Women with positive group B *Strep* cultures are subsequently treated with IV penicillin G in labor. Treatment is also recommended on the basis of risk factors for women with an unknown group B *Strep* status and one of the following risk factors: Gestational age before 37 weeks, rupture of membranes greater than 18 hours, GBS bacteriuria in the current pregnancy, previous infant with invasive GBS disease, or intrapartum fever greater than 100.4°F.

a, b, d, e: See explanation to answer C.

26. a (Chapter 11)

This patient likely has hyperemesis gravidarum based on clinical symptoms of persistent nausea and vomiting with ketonuria and electrolyte disturbances. This occurs with approximately 0.3% to 2% of pregnancies. Once diagnosed, the main goal is to correct any underlying electrolyte disturbances and admit for IV fluids and antiemetics for symptom control. Your next step should be to order an obstetric ultrasound to confirm an intrauterine pregnancy. Hyperemesis gravidarum is more likely to occur with molar pregnancies and your management would be to proceed with dilatation and curettage.

b. The initial goal for treatment of hyperemesis gravidarum is to control symptoms. This often means replacement of IV fluids due to dehydration and IV electrolytes given persistent emesis in addition to IV antiemetics. Most patients will improve with conservative management and begin to tolerate a bland diet. A nasogastric tube is indicated for severe cases that are refractory to all pharmacologic and non-pharmacologic interventions.

c. This patient's clinical presentation is consistent with hyperemesis gravidarum. She is afebrile and has no symptoms concerning for an infectious etiology.

d. This patient has had a recent bowel movement and currently has a benign abdominal examination, which is inconsistent with a diagnosis of small bowel obstruction.

e. Initial treatment for hyperemesis gravidarum is to control symptoms. TPN has significant risk of liver dysfunction, lipid abnormalities and sepsis and should be avoided during pregnancy.

27. b (Chapter 11)

To minimize the risk of congenital malformations, the goal should be to optimize her regimen with a plan to transition to one medication. There is evidence that epileptic women have an increased risk of fetal malformations even without AED use. The data suggest that monotherapy does not increase that baseline risk, and decreasing her regimen to one medication should be the goal to minimize her risk during the upcoming pregnancy. There is evidence that with each additional AED medication there is an increased incidence in fetal malformations.

a. She should be counseled not to stop her seizure medications because this puts her at risk of increased seizure activity. Women who are seizure-free for 2 to 5 years may want to trial being off all therapy because they have an improved chance of remaining seizure-free when off medications.

c. Women with epilepsy have an increased incidence of neural tube defects, even if not on antiepileptic medication. In a randomized controlled trial, supplementation with 4 mg of folic acid significantly reduced that risk. As a result, women with epilepsy should be counseled to take 4 mg of folic acid, not the standard 400 mcg that all women are counseled to take prenatally.

d. Because this patient has been seizure-free for almost 2 years, she has a good chance of weaning down to one medication. Monotherapy has the lowest rates of fetal malformations, and that should be the goal. Simply increasing the folic acid to 4 mg is not sufficient to decrease her risk.

e. The recommendation is to attempt to transition to monotherapy, but valproic acid would not be the medication of choice, given the increased rates of fetal malformations with this medication.

28. e (Chapter 2)
The patient's reported history of two second trimester losses with rapid delivery after mild spotting is suggestive of cervical incompetence. Cervical incompetence accounts for 15% of all second-trimester miscarriages. The patient has also had a prior LEEP, which places her at increased risk for cervical incompetence. She should be offered a prophylactic cerclage, which may have as much as a 90% success rate (e). With both of her prior losses, genetic analysis of fetal tissue was normal. Karyotyping and chorionic villus sampling of the patient and her partner are less appropriate first steps (a, c). Although a hysterosalpingogram may reveal a uterine anomaly, this test cannot be performed during pregnancy and thus will not help your patient during her current pregnancy (b). There is no evidence of a luteal phase defect in this patient (d).

29. b (Chapter 1)
Conservative therapy such as lower extremity elevation and pressure stockings during pregnancy can help to minimize existing varicose veins and prevent new ones from forming. If varicose veins don't improve by 6 months postpartum, surgery can be considered, but it isn't the first line in treatment. The other answer choices are not indicated for the treatment of varicose veins.

30. c (Chapter 3)
Fetal nuchal translucency screening in the first trimester offers an evaluation of risk of trisomy 21, 13, and 18 early in pregnancy between 11 and 14 weeks. One of the benefits of this early test is that information is gained early and if it is a positive screen, it can be followed by a diagnostic test. CVS and amniocentesis can both provide diagnostic testing for chromosomal disorders, but CVS can be done much earlier in pregnancy. Offering CVS testing to this patient is the most appropriate next step. Although one would also offer amniocentesis in several weeks as an alternative, it would not be appropriate at the current gestation. It appears that the pregnancy loss risk may be slightly higher with CVS, so some individuals will choose to wait. Repeating the ultrasound is not an appropriate option if the nuchal region of the fetus was adequately seen. Lastly, termination of the pregnancy without definitive diagnostic testing in a desired pregnancy would not be the most appropriate next step.

31. b (Chapter 11)
This patient has a moderate-risk cardiac lesion, and pregnancy is not contraindicated. If she were to come for preconception counseling, a referral to a cardiologist would have been recommended to discuss valve replacement, as that could decrease her risk of complications during this pregnancy. At the time of her presentation to labor and delivery, the most important plan for management is strict fluid monitoring with a goal to maximize afterload to maintain cardiac output. Strict intake and output will allow for appropriate fluid balance to be maintained. In addition, for most cardiac patients, the stress of labor and delivery is minimized with an early epidural to diminish pain response, and possibly an assisted vaginal delivery (using forceps or vacuum) to diminish the effects from Valsalva.

a. This patient does not have a high-risk cardiac lesion, and therefore it is not recommended that she receive antibiotic prophylaxis against subacute bacterial endocarditis (SBE). The 2007 American Heart Association Guidelines state that routine vaginal delivery and cesarean section are not indications for SBE prophylaxis. SBE prophylaxis may be considered for women with high-risk lesions (mechanical or prosthetic valves, unrepaired cyanotic lesions, etc.) and an infection that could cause bacteremia (chorioamnionitis or pyelonephritis).

c. There have been no clinical benefits shown with cesarean delivery in patients with cardiac lesions. As a result, vaginal delivery is the preferred option to minimize recovery time.

d. Patients with moderate risk cardiac lesions can often be managed on labor and delivery with strict intake and output and close observation. Patients with high-risk lesions or evidence of cardiovascular compromise may be admitted to the ICU for more intensive monitoring.

e. To maintain adequate cardiac output in aortic stenosis, adequate afterload is necessary. Giving lasix would decrease afterload, decrease cardiac output, and may precipitate cardiovascular compromise.

32. a (Chapter 11)
A constellation of abnormalities in the infants born to women who abuse alcohol during pregnancy have been included in the diagnosis of fetal alcohol syndrome (FAS). FAS, which includes growth retardation, CNS effects, and abnormal facies, is estimated to occur in approximately 1 in 2,000 live births. The syndrome has a spectrum of increasing severity in children of women who drink more heavily (two to five drinks/day) during pregnancy. However, there is no safe amount of alcohol in pregnancy that confers no risk. The diagnosis is made by a history of alcohol abuse in the mother combined with the constellation of infant abnormalities. Other teratogenic effects of alcohol include almost every organ system. Cardiac defects are particularly associated with alcohol abuse.

Maternal and neonatal withdrawal, low fetal birth weight and neonatal admission to the NICU are all complications of alcohol dependence in pregnancy; however, these are self-limited.

33. c (Chapter 11)
Tobacco use during pregnancy has not been shown to increase rates of fetal malformations. In contrast, maternal alcohol use in pregnancy has been shown to increase the risk of cardiac defects and fetal alcohol syndrome (growth retardation, abnormal facies, and CNS effects). a, b, d and e: Cigarette smoking in pregnancy has been associated with increased risk of spontaneous abortions, preterm births, abruptio placentae, and decreased birth weight. Further, infants exposed to cigarette smoking in the womb are at an increased risk for sudden infant death syndrome (SIDS) and respiratory illnesses of childhood. A dose-response effect has been noted for many of these outcomes. In the Ontario Perinatal Mortality Study, smokers were divided into less than one pack per day (PPD) and more than one PPD. A 20% increase in the risk of fetal death was found in those pregnancies in which patients smoked less than one PPD and a 35% increase in the more than one PPD group.

34. c (Chapter 30)
The mainstay of treatment for ovarian cancer is surgery with complete surgical staging, including total abdominal hysterectomy, bilateral salpingo–oophorectomy (TAHBSO), collection of peritoneal washings, sampling of pelvic and paraaortic lymph nodes, omentectomy, and cytoreduction of any visible tumor. The patient then undergoes chemotherapy with paclitaxel or docetaxel combined with carboplatin or cisplatin. For advanced stage disease, if the patient has undergone optimal tumor debulking, a combination of intravenous and intraperitoneal chemotherapy is recommended.

35. e (Chapter 12)
Infants who are not exposed to adequate amounts of sun will not generate sufficient quantities of vitamin D if exclusively breast-feeding. Breast milk alone does not provide adequate amounts of vitamin D (25 IU/L). Published case reports of rickets in breast-fed infants in the United States exist. Consequently, in 2008 the American Academy of Pediatrics (AAP) published guidelines for the supplementation of

breast-feeding infants with 400 IU of vitamin D per day, beginning in the first few days of life. At risk breast-feeding infants include those living at high latitudes, in areas of high pollution or cloud cover, or those using sunscreen or with darker skin.

a. Maternal hepatitis C is not a contraindication to breast-feeding. Though the virus is transmissible via the breast milk, the rate of infant infection is the same as that seen among bottle-fed infants owing to baseline risk of infection with vaginal delivery (4%). There is similarly no contraindication to breast-feeding among patients with active hepatitis B so long as their infants receive hepatitis B IgG passive prophylaxis and vaccine active prophylaxis.

b. Breast augmentation is not a contraindication to breast-feeding, although 65% of women who have undergone augmentation mammoplasty have lactation insufficiency. This is most common among patients who undergo a periareolar approach, which is more likely to sever ducts and damage breast tissue. Though some patients with a history of augmentation may initially have a low supply, there is no reason not to try as it can become sufficient if suckling is continued regularly.

c. Depo-Provera is a progesterone-only method that is compatible with breast-feeding. Methods that may affect breast-feeding include combined methods such as pills, rings, and patches.

d. Many young parents are often concerned about their milk supply during the first days of feeding, resorting to bottle-feeding to satiate their infant. However, parents should be reminded of the small volume of the newborn stomach that needs relatively small amounts initially. Continuous attempts at suckling should be encouraged to stimulate lactation and ultimately ensure an adequate supply in the future.

36. d (Chapter 12)

Carboprost is a synthetic prostaglandin analogue of $PGF_{2\alpha}$. As $PGF_{2\alpha}$ is also an inflammatory mediator of bronchial smooth muscle, case reports have been written on the incidence of bronchospasm associated with the use of Carboprost (Hemabate) in asthmatic patients. Given that there are other readily available pharmaceutical options for the treatment of postpartum hemorrhage including oxytocin, misoprostol, and methergine, the general consensus is that Carboprost should be avoided when possible in patients with any history of asthma.

a. Contraindications to oxytocin in the immediate postpartum period are few. Case reports exist of patients exhibiting severe water intoxication, with convulsions and coma, as a function of slow oxytocin infusion over a 24-hour period. Maternal death has been reported. Acute injection of Pitocin is considered a safe option and is sometimes routinely used in Stage III of labor for active, expeditious delivery of the placenta.

b. Methylergonovine is an ergot-alkaloid that functions by stimulating blood vessel constriction and smooth muscle contraction. It is frequently used to both prevent and control postpartum hemorrhage. Given its vessel constricting properties, methylergonovine can raise the blood pressure, making it contraindicated in patients with a history of hypertension or preeclampsia.

c. In this patient's case, misoprostol may have been contraindicated in the management of her labor due to an increased risk of uterine rupture with a history of cesarean section; however, in the postpartum period, misoprostol is a valuable medication for postpartum hemorrhage that can be given per oral, sublingual, buccal, or rectum. Though less acutely effective than injectables, misoprostol is a shelf-stable, inexpensive uterotonic that is gaining in popularity, even for the prevention of hemorrhage during cesarean sections.

e. As per response a, Pitocin is not contraindicated in the treatment of postpartum hemorrhage; however, in a patient who is acutely hemorrhaging, a slow drip of Pitocin may be less effective than any of the above listed methods.

37. d (Chapter 12)

Fever from a vaccine should be a diagnosis of exclusion, which is the case in this particular vignette, given the patient's lack of signs and symptoms. Mild fever is a common side effect of the measles, mumps, and rubella (MMR) vaccine, occurring in one in every six recipients, according to the CDC. Recipients may report temporary pain and stiffness in the joints (one in four). A mild rash can also be seen commonly (1 in 20). Severe problems are very rarely encountered and the vaccine is not contraindicated in breastfeeding.

a. Postpartum endometritis is a bacterial infection of the deciduas that may also extend into the myometrium, in which case it is known as endomyometritis. Classic signs and symptoms include a fever greater than or equal to 38.0°C, uterine tenderness, and sometimes foul-smelling uterine discharge. A boggy uterus is sometimes encountered, which may be accompanied by bleeding. Though this patient has a fever and uterine tenderness, her fundus is firm and the degree of tenderness she reports may be more consistent with that experienced by normal uterine involution postpartum.

b. Though the patient complains of mild pelvic cramps, has fevers, and a history of Foley catheter use that together point toward a possible urinary tract infection, she is voiding comfortably and denies any urgency. Classic symptoms or signs of urinary tract infection would include dysuria, hematuria, and foul-smelling urine. As multiple vaginal examinations, catheterizations during labor, and obstruction from periurethral edema can be associated with urinary tract infections, it should remain part of the differential diagnosis of postpartum fever.

c. Fever and swelling are two of the classic symptoms of deep vein thrombosis, along with pain and erythema of the involved extremity. For patients who are pregnant and have had epidural catheters and sometimes been immobilized for prolonged periods of time, providers should recognize their increased risk of thromboembolism. In this case, however, the patient's swelling is bilateral, which is more likely to be caused by postpartum fluid shifts than bilateral thrombi. Tenderness to palpation of the patient's calf would be more predictive of a thrombus.

e. Fever is common after the start of lactation, which is often associated with engorgement of the breasts. The fever is transient, self-limited, and often resolves with pumping or manual expression of breast milk. For patients not planning on breast-feeding, suppression of lactation can be facilitated with binding. Pain associated with engorgement can be relieved with ice or nonsteroidal anti-inflammatory medications. Breast fever differs from mastitis in its lack of infection as manifested by erythema, induration, and tachycardia.

38. a (Chapter 12)

Several studies have cited grand multiparity, defined as carriage of the fifth baby, as a risk factor for postpartum hemorrhage. Though parity may be associated with age and accumulation of comorbidities that might predispose a patient to postpartum hemorrhage, the effect of parity has been shown to be independent of such confounders. One possible etiology for postpartum hemorrhage in these patients is their association with precipitous deliveries where the uterus contracts so forcefully that it becomes hypotonic postpartum, leading to hemorrhage from the placental bed.

b. Hemorrhage is significantly more likely in women with fibroids as they can distort the uterine architecture and interfere with myometrial contractions necessary for the prevention of atony and postpartum hemorrhage. Hemorrhage risk is greater in cases of larger intramural fibroids located behind the placenta.

c. Her baby's weight, in this case meeting the criteria for macrosomia (birth weight of 4,000 to 4,500 g, 8 lb 13 oz to 9 lb 15 oz), increases her risk of postpartum hemorrhage. The suspected mechanism for increased risk is uterine distension by the baby's size and based upon the description of a large fluid gush, likely polyhydramnios associated with poor control of gestational diabetes. Multiple gestations would also increase the risk of hemorrhage by the same mechanism.

d. The lower uterine segment is comprised of the thinnest layer of myometrium, making it the least contractile. Though this property makes it the ideal region for entry during a cesarean section, its lack of contractility when coincident with a low-lying placenta leads to an inability to adequately constrict a bleeding placental bed, leading to increased risk of postpartum hemorrhage. In patients with a history of cesarean section with incision in the lower uterine segment, placentas are likelier to grow into the wound, also known as accreta, leading to increased risk of retained products and subsequent hemorrhage as well.

39. c (Chapter 13)

The lesion described is a nabothian cyst, a normal variant among menstruating women. They appear as a bubble under the surface of the cervix and are often bluish in color. Cervical dysplasia or cancer would not have this appearance and would not appear within 2 weeks of sexual debut. Bartholin's gland cysts are found in the labia majora. Skene's gland cysts are located near the urethral meatus.

40. d (Chapter 13)

Vulvar pruritus is a common symptom of many benign and malignant diseases of the vulva. When a postmenopausal patient presents with vulvodynia or vulvar pruritus that is refractory to treatment, a punch biopsy should be performed to identify the lesion and guide the choice of treatment. In this patient, where lichen planus or lichen sclerosus are most likely, biopsy should be performed to confirm the diagnosis and rule out any underlying malignancy prior to starting therapy. Surgical therapy is not indicated at this point in the evaluation, since lichen planus or lichen sclerosus can be treated with topical steroids such as clobetasol. Destruction of the lesion(s) with cryotherapy should never be performed without a pathologic diagnosis.

41. b (Chapter 13)

The patient history and findings are pathognomonic of lichen simplex chronicus, with thickened skin. The first course of action would be consistent use of high-potency topical steroid clobetasol. The patient should be advised to continue use even when she begins to have improvement in symptoms. This lesion is not associated with a higher risk of squamous cell cancer and the patient has had a prior biopsy, so repeat biopsy is not necessary. There is no evidence of a current fungal infection. The woman is in her reproductive phase, so estrogen cream would not be indicated. Laser vaporization is not an appropriate intervention for lichen simplex chronicus.

42. c (Chapter 13)

The adolescent described has a clinical history and physical examination compatible with an imperforate hymen, which is the most common obstructive anomaly of the female reproductive tract. An adolescent patient who has an imperforate hymen may be asymptomatic or may have a history of cyclic abdominal pain that may occur for several years before the diagnosis is made. A bluish, bulging hymen may be seen on genital inspection, and a distended vagina (hematocolpos) causes bulging of the imperforate hymen. It may also have a mass effect in the rectal space including elevation of the distended uterus (hematometra), which may be palpated on rectoabdominal or abdominal examination. If the vagina becomes substantially enlarged with accumulated blood, the patient may experience back pain, pain with defecation that can result in constipation, nausea and vomiting, or difficulty in urinating. Treatment is excision of the hymen, under anesthesia, which allows the retained menses to drain and normal menstruation to commence. As this is an isolated anatomic problem, the karyotype should be 46XX. Bladder outlet obstruction occurs rarely, and although it produces a suprapubic mass, it does not cause cyclic abdominal pain. Megacolon also is unlikely and does not cause cyclic pain, although colonic irritation may develop from the pressure produced by the mass. An ovarian cyst typically causes a right- or left-sided (not midline) mass, and endometriosis is an unlikely cause of a palpable mass, although it can cause cyclic and acyclic pain in adolescents.

43. d (Chapter 6)

Cesarean delivery should be considered in any patient with repetitive fetal decelerations not responsive to conservative measures and who is remote from delivery. In the setting of placental abruption, fetal decelerations may indicate worsening of the abruption. Although vaginal bleeding is a clinical sign of placental abruption, concealed bleeding can also exist. Vaginal bleeding and a small change in hematocrit is not a cause for serious concern and recommendation of cesarean delivery unless other mitigating factors are present such as change in maternal or fetal status. If the fetal and maternal statuses are reassuring, serial hematocrits should be checked, two peripheral IVs in place, and active type and screen sent. This patient should be counseled on the change in fetal tolerance of labor and recommendations for cesarean section. Upon transfer to the operating room, the patient should have a repeat cervical examination, as multiparous patients can progress rapidly in labor, and vaginal delivery could then be considered. Fetuses in the ROP position are likely to spontaneously rotate during the birthing process. Therefore, cesarean delivery is not indicated for this reason. Placement of an epidural can cause maternal hypotension, but this usually responds to fluid bolus, repositioning, or vasoactive medications such as ephedrine. If hypotension persists in addition to fetal decelerations, other sources of hypotension should be considered and investigated.

44. e (Chapter 14)

Unlike a uterine septum, a bicornuate uterus is not associated with an increased risk of infertility or recurrent miscarriage. In the case of the uterine septum, the septum is often avascular and thus, an implanted pregnancy is more likely to be aborted due to the lack of vascularized endometrium. Because each horn of the bicornuate uterus is smaller than the normal-sized endometrial cavity, there is less room for fetal growth. The first trimester is largely uneventful in a pregnancy complicated by a bicornuate uterus, so there is not an increased risk of first trimester bleeding. However, as the fetus grows larger in later pregnancy there is less room for growth. As a result, malpresentation, second trimester loss, and preterm labor and preterm delivery are more commonly seen in women with bicornuate (and unicornuate) uteri. Cervical insufficiency (CI), on the other hand, is painless, cervical dilation and effacement often seen in the second trimester. CI is associated with a history of in utero DES exposure and with cervical trauma and multiple instrumentations of the cervix. CI is not more common in women with bicornuate uteri.

45. e (Chapter 14)

This patient does have uterine fibroids but they are small and asymptomatic. At this time, there is no indication for treatment. Endometrial ablation and uterine artery embolization are not indicated for these small fibroids which are in the myometrium (intramural) but not impinging on the endometrium (submucosal). Furthermore, these two procedures are contraindicated in patients who wish to conceive in the future. Likewise, while hysteroscopic resection is an appropriate treatment option for women with submucosal fibroids, it is not indicated here. Resection of submucosal fibroids has been shown to improve pregnancy rates in women with infertility and submucosal fibroid. Intrauterine devices are long-acting reversible contraceptives (LARC) and should not be used in a patient planning a pregnancy in the next month or two. The progesterone-containing IUD (Mirena) is sometimes used to treat dysmenorrhea and menorrhagia associated with intramural fibroids. It is not indicated in this situation.

46. d (Chapter 14)
Changes in the menstrual cycle are very common as women approach the age of menopause. The differential diagnosis includes each of the options. With a normal myometrium, it is very unlikely that she has fibroids as the etiology of her bleeding. Thyroid disorders and perimenopause can each cause a change in the menstrual cycle, but her thickened endometrial stripe is more indicative of a structural source for her bleeding. The normal endometrial bilayer in a premenopausal woman is typically less than 12 mm. At 22 mm, this patient's endometrial lining is significantly enlarged; again concerning for a mass or other structural issue. The endometrial biopsy reveals normal findings. Although hyperplasia is possible, she does not have risk factors for hyperplasia such as obesity, oligomenorrhea, hypertension, diabetes, and PCOS. Furthermore, the lack of glandular crowding and cytologic atypia on endometrial biopsy make this diagnosis much less likely. The most likely diagnosis is an endometrial polyp. In this case, the diagnosis could be confirmed with a saline sonohysterogram and/or hysteroscopy. Polyps are most commonly benign; however, they can have abnormal cells where the stalk attaches to the endometrial wall. Given this, and the fact that the polyp is large and symptomatic, the recommendation would be for surgical removal.

47. a (Chapter 14)
Any ovarian mass or cyst that contains thick septations, nodularity, solid components, abnormal Doppler flow, cyst wall thickening, or presence of ascites is concerning for malignancy. Any cyst greater than 1 cm in a postmenopausal patient requires further evaluation; however, this particular situation adds multiple concerning characteristics that indicate a higher risk for malignancy.

A follow-up ultrasound is incorrect in this scenario, as well as a pregnancy test and colonoscopy. CT scan of the abdomen may be warranted to evaluate for additional intraperitoneal lesions or lymphadenopathy; however, your examination was not concerning for any of these, and surgical evaluation is the next best step.

This patient would need to be consented for bilateral oophorectomy and salpingectomy (removal of fallopian tubes) with removal of cyst, as well as potential for ovarian cancer staging, which includes collection of peritoneal washings, removal of omentum and any visible tumor, and sampling of pelvic and periaortic lymph node.

48. e (Chapter 15)
Some of the common clinical manifestations of endometriosis are cyclic pelvic pain, particularly just prior to menses, dyspareunia, dysmenorrhea, abnormal bleeding, and infertility. An adnexal mass noted on examination is not uncommon for women with endometriomas. Also, women with first degree relatives who have endometriosis are more likely to develop endometriosis themselves.

49. a (Chapter 32)
In women less than 30 years of age, fine-needle aspiration can be used to sample solid masses. Excisional biopsy is only performed if FNA does not obtain enough fluid and/or tissue. Core-needle biopsy is recommended in women greater than 30 years of age with a solid mass. Needle or wire-guided excision is reserved for lesions that are seen on imaging but are not palpable. Lumpectomy is the excision technique that accompanies needle- or wire-guided excision.

50. b (Chapter 2)

b, c. After one prior ectopic pregnancy, the risk of subsequent ectopic pregnancy is 10%. This increases to 25% after more than one prior ectopic pregnancy.

a. Although an increase in sexually transmitted infections is thought to have contributed to the incidence of ectopic pregnancy, we cannot be certain that this patient will be unable to conceive a normal pregnancy. Given the single dose treatment, it is more likely that she had a chlamydia cervicitis and not pelvic inflammatory disease. If there was concern for a history of PID or infertility, the patient might be offered a hysterosalpingogram to evaluate tubal patency.

d. A history of one prior ectopic pregnancy does not preclude the use of an IUD for contraception. In fact, an IUD is the most effective type of reversible contraception and decreases the overall risk of pregnancy significantly. It is true that in the case of a contraceptive failure the rate of ectopic pregnancy is as much as 25% to 50%, but the absolute risk remains exceedingly low.

e. As long as the pathologic report suggests that pregnancy tissue was removed at the time of surgery, there is no indication for additional methotrexate therapy.

51. c (Chapter 15)
NSAIDs, combination oral contraceptives, oral and IM progestins, GnRH agonists, danazol, and the levonorgestrel-releasing intrauterine system are all potentially effective medical treatments for the symptoms of pelvic pain or abnormal bleeding associated with endometriosis. Patients with endometriosis may develop depression or anxiety over the debilitating nature of endometriosis and require an SSRI for that condition. However, SSRIs are not used specifically for the treatment of endometriosis. They have been shown to be effective in the treatment of anxiety, depression, PMS, PMDD, and postmenopausal vasomotor symptoms (hot flashes and night sweats). It is important to note that up to 30% of women with endometriosis are asymptomatic.

52. a (Chapter 15)
Although increasingly heavy or prolonged menstrual bleeding (menorrhagia) is common (50%) in women with adenomyosis, irregular bleeding between menses (metrorrhagia) is not common. Thirty percent of women with adenomyosis have secondary dysmenorrhea. On examination the uterus is often diffusely enlarged up to two to three times the normal size, boggy, and mildly tender.

53. b (Chapter 15)
Choice b is the most accurate description of adenomyosis. In the past it was described as endometriosis interna; however, this nomenclature is not typically used any longer. Choice a most accurately describes endometriosis. Choice c most accurately describes a leiomyoma (fibroid). Choice d most accurately describes an endometrioma. Choice e most accurately describes endometritis.

54. b (Chapter 16)
This patient has chancroid, a sexually transmitted infection caused by *Haemophilus ducreyi*. Since it is often difficult to culture *H. ducreyi*, the diagnosis is usually made clinically after ruling out syphilis and genital herpes. There are many treatment options for chancroid, including ceftriaxone 250 mg IM once, azithromycin 1 g orally once, ciprofloxacin 500 mg orally twice a day for 3 days, or erythromycin 500 mg four times a day for 7 days. Sexual partner(s) should receive treatment as well.

a. Benzathine penicillin G is used to treat primary, secondary, or early latent syphilis. Syphilis is a systemic sexually transmitted infection caused by the spirochete Treponema pallidum. The hallmark lesion of primary syphilis is known as a chancre, which is characterized by a nontender, red, round, firm ulcer approximately 1 cm in size with raised edges. It is usually associated with lymphadenopathy.

c. Doxycycline can be used to treat chlamydial infections and is an alternative treatment for primary, secondary, or early latent syphilis in penicillin-allergic patients.

d. A 21-day regimen of erythromycin is used to treat lymphogranuloma venereum (LGV), which is caused by Chlamydia trachomatis L-serotypes L1, L2, or L3. The primary stage of LGV is characterized by nontender papules or shallow ulcers, which heal quickly and often go unnoticed. Painful inguinal lymphadenopathy typically occurs 2 to 6 weeks after the primary lesion.

e. Acyclovir is used to treat herpes simplex virus (HSV). The first episode of primary genital herpes is often the most severe and described as a painful cluster of small vesicles and ulcers. The lesions are often preceded by systemic flulike symptoms. The diagnosis of HSV should be confirmed with laboratory testing (viral culture, serum HSV antibody testing).

55. c (Chapter 16)
There are two nontreponemal serologic tests for syphilis available: The Venereal Disease Research Laboratory (VDRL) test and the rapid plasma reagin (RPR) test. False–positive nontreponemal tests can occur with various autoimmune conditions, other infections, malignancy, pregnancy, and IV drug use. Therefore, a positive result must be confirmed with specific treponemal antibody studies, such as the fluorescent treponemal antibody absorption (FTA-ABS) test and the *Treponema pallidum* particle agglutination assay (TPPA).

a. The Venereal Disease Research Laboratory (VDRL) test is another nontreponemal serologic test for syphilis. Only a specific treponemal antibody study can confirm the diagnosis of syphilis.

b. The diagnosis of syphilis should be confirmed with a specific treponemal antibody study prior to initiating treatment with penicillin. Benzathine penicillin G 2.4 million units IM once is the treatment of choice for primary, secondary, or early latent syphilis.

d. The treatment of syphilis can be verified by following RPR or VDRL titers at 6, 12, and 24 months. Prior to monitoring titers, the diagnosis of syphilis must be confirmed and treatment initiated.

e. The diagnosis of syphilis should be confirmed with a specific treponemal antibody study prior to initiating treatment with penicillin. Benzathine penicillin G 2.4 million units IM weekly for three doses is the treatment of choice for late latent or latent of unknown duration syphilis.

56. a (Chapter 16)
In otherwise healthy, nonpregnant women with dysuria, urinary frequency, or suprapubic pain in the absence of vaginal discharge, more than 90% will have a urinary tract infection. In those cases, treatment can be initiated without further workup. For patients with recurrent/frequent symptoms or concurrent vaginal discharge, it is not appropriate to initiate treatment for a urinary tract infection until further workup has been completed. This workup should include sending the urine specimen for urinalysis and more importantly, a urine culture. In addition, the vaginal discharge should be evaluated to rule out an underlying sexually transmitted infection.
b, c, d, e: See explanation to a.

57. d (Chapter 16)
The findings are most consistent with genital warts or condyloma acuminate. Approximately 90% of are genital warts caused by HPV serotypes 6 and 11.

a. Cervical cancer is associated with HPV serotypes 16, 18, and 31.

b. The classic findings of HSV genital lesions are painful clusters of small vesicles and ulcers.

c. Molluscum contagiosum is caused by a pox virus. The lesions are typically described as small, 1 to 5 mm, domed papules with an umbilicated center.

e. Haemophilus ducreyi causes chancroid, which is an ulcerated genital lesion. The lesion presents initially as an erythematous papule, which evolves to a pustule and ulcer. The ulcer is painful with an erythematous base and irregular, well-demarcated borders.

58. a (Chapter 3)
The patient's normal karyotype as obtained via CVS is entirely reassuring regarding aneuploidy. However, she still needs a screening test for neural tube defect, so should undergo the maternal serum alpha fetoprotein (MSAFP) screen between 15 and 20 weeks' gestation. She doesn't need to bear the risk of an amniocentesis unless the MSAFP is elevated. Because a second trimester anatomy scan has a high sensitivity for neural tube defects, some clinicians have stopped offering the MSAFP, but in most practices, it is still the standard of care. Fetal echocardiography is to rule out fetal cardiac anomalies in women who are at increased risk for such anomalies (e.g., pregestational diabetes). The CVS does not need to be repeated. A cordocentesis or percutaneous umbilical blood sampling (PUBS) is utilized to obtain fetal cells when getting a karyotype immediately is important or if one needs to know the fetal hematocrit as in Rh-alloimmunization.

59. d (Chapter 17)
Fitzhugh-Curtis syndrome is a perihepatitis from ascending PID infection. It is associated with *Chlamydia* and gonorrhea infections. Fitzhugh-Curtis syndrome should be suspected in women with right upper quadrant pain or pleuritic pain in the context of pelvic inflammatory disease. It can be associated with elevated liver enzymes, but this is less common as the inflammation is usually confined to the liver capsule. Laparoscopy is the gold standard for diagnosis. In practice, the diagnosis is usually made clinically. If laparoscopy is performed, classic "violin-string" adhesions can be seen between the anterior liver capsule and the anterior abdominal wall or diaphragm. Treatment is the same as for PID.

a. Tubo-ovarian abscess (TOA) is an important sequela of pelvic inflammatory disease (PID). It is estimated that 3% to 16% of PID cases will progress to TOA. The diagnosis of TOA is made clinically in the setting of PID and the appreciation of an adnexal or cul-de-sac mass or fullness. In this case, there is no adnexal fullness, making TOA less likely.

b. Disseminated gonococcal infections are characterized by fever and erythematous macular skin lesions that proceed to a tenosynovitis and septic arthritis.

c. HELLP syndrome (Hemolysis, Elevated Liver Enzymes, Low Platelets) is a disease specific to pregnancy.

e. Although secondary syphilis can involve multiple organs (including the liver), the classic presentation includes a maculopapular rash on the palms and soles.

60. a (Chapter 17)
This patient has staphylococcal toxic shock syndrome (TSS). In 1981, the CDC established a case definition, which continues to serve as the criterion for TSS. To meet the case definition for a confirmed case, patients must have a fever greater than 38.9°C, hypotension, diffuse erythematous macular rash, desquamation, and involvement of at least three organ systems. The isolation of *Staphylococcus aureus* is not required for the diagnosis of TSS. In fact, blood cultures are often negative. Although menstrual-related TSS has decreased over time, use of high-absorbency tampons remains a risk factor.
b, c, d, e: See explanation to a.

61. c (Chapter 17)
Owing to the high incidence of cervical cancer in HIV-infected women, more aggressive screening is recommended by the CDC. In this case, a pap smear should be performed at first evaluation and 6 months after. Yearly screening can be performed if both pap smears are normal.

a. Cervical cancer screening should be done every 6 months in HIV-infected women with prior HPV infection, squamous intraepithelial neoplasia, or symptomatic HIV disease.

b. Closer interval cervical cancer screening is recommended at initial evaluation.

d. Routine colposcopy is recommended for HIV-infected women with ASC-US or higher grade cervical cytology abnormality.

e. Women with HIV infections are not eligible to extend the interval between cervical cancer screenings to more than 1 year.

62. e (Chapter 18)
A number of factors have been hypothesized to play a role in the development of pelvic organ prolapse. Genetics, menopausal status and associated lack of estrogen, age, history of pelvic surgery, and connective tissue disorders are risk factors for pathologic pelvic relaxation. Additional factors may be those that contribute to a state of elevated intra-abdominal pressure: Chronic constipation, chronic obstructive pulmonary disease, obesity, and heavy lifting. Although some degree of debate exists regarding the roles of mode of delivery versus pregnancy itself, parity is also considered a risk factor for the development of prolapse. There are no data to indicate whether sexual activity plays any part in the development of prolapse.

63. b (Chapter 18)
Procidentia refers to complete eversion of the vagina, with or without a uterus. Historically, pelvic floor defects were named for the organ presumed to be behind the defect. For example, a rectocele implies herniation of the rectum into the vagina. Because a physical examination cannot definitively identify the organ behind the vaginal wall (rectum versus small bowel, rectocele versus enterocele), the preferred nomenclature is to describe the defect in broader terms, that is, posterior wall defect.

64. a (Chapter 18)
Pelvic organ prolapse is considered a benign entity, and treatment is indicated when the patient specifies bother from the condition. With an asymptomatic patient, expectant or conservative management may be offered. Although there is no strong data to support the role of pelvic floor muscle exercises in preventing progression of prolapse, there is evidence that it may improve coexistent issues such as stress urinary incontinence. Similarly, even modest weight loss has been shown to improve pelvic floor pathology. In a young asymptomatic patient, colpocleisis would likely not be an acceptable or logical option. Round ligament suspensions are not effective for any types of prolapse. A Gellhorn pessary may be used for conservative management in symptomatic women, often in high grade prolapse. A hysterectomy, in and of itself, will not correct the prolapse.

65. c (Chapter 18)
Vaginal suspension procedures are associated with the following advantages: Shorter operative time, faster patient recovery, and overall low complication rates. Although both short- and long-term complication rates for vaginal suspensions are low, *all* prolapse and incontinence procedures carry a risk of injury to the bladder, ureters, or urethra. Intraoperative cystoscopy should be performed to check the integrity of these structures. In particular, ureteral injury rates as high as 11% have been reported with uterosacral ligament suspension. Defecography is sometimes used in the evaluation of posterior vaginal wall defects. Episiotomy can be used to improve access during a vaginal hysterectomy. Anterior colporrhaphy is not indicated with an isolated vault defect, especially if the anatomy has successfully been restored with a vault suspension procedure Hysteroscopy would not be indicated in this setting..

66. b (Chapter 19)
This patient has symptoms consistent with urgency incontinence. An appropriate treatment choice would be oxybutynin, an anticholinergic medication. Stress incontinence presents with leakage of urine on physical exertion (e.g., sporting activities), or on sneezing, laughing, or coughing. Mid-urethral slings such as tension free vaginal slings (TVT) and transobturator slings (TOT) are common surgical options for stress incontinence. Overflow incontinence secondary to urinary retention from an underactive detrusor or bladder outlet obstruction is treated based upon the etiology. Continuous incontinence from a urinary fistula usually requires surgical repair.

67. d (Chapter 19)
This patient's history is consistent with stress incontinence. Initial treatment with lifestyle and behavioral modifications should include weight loss, caffeine restriction, fluid management, bladder training, pelvic floor muscle exercises, and possibly physical therapy. Detrol LA (anticholinergic medication) and tibial nerve stimulation are both used in the treatment of urgency incontinence. A mid-urethral sling is used in the treatment of stress incontinence, but is usually not considered first line therapy; lifestyle and behavioral modifications should be tried first. Vaginal hysterectomy is not indicated in the treatment of urinary incontinence in most circumstances.

68. b (Chapter 19)
The involuntary loss of urine is common, having affected an estimated 18.3 million American women in 2010, with an expected 55% increase to 28.4 million in 2050. Nearly 50% of all women experience occasional urinary incontinence, and 20% of women over age 75 are affected daily. Urinary incontinence is often a major reason for placing individuals in nursing homes, with some 30% of nursing home residents suffering from urinary incontinence. In a large survey study of noninstitutionalized US women, 49.6% reported incontinence symptoms, of which 49.8% reported stress incontinence, 34.3% reported mixed incontinence, and 15.9% reported pure urge incontinence. It is estimated that over $12 billion are spent annually on the treatment of stress incontinence.

69. d (Chapter 4)
The first stage of labor includes a latent phase characterized by slow cervical change classically described to 3- to 4-cm dilation, but may persist up to 6-cm dilation. This is followed by an active phase characterized by more rapid cervical change of at least 1.0 cm per hour of dilation in nulliparous women and 1.2 cm per hour dilation in multiparous women. The first stage ends when the cervix is completely dilated.

70. d (Chapter 19)
Normal voiding is voluntary and occurs through parasympathetic innervations via the pelvic nerve, which originates at levels S2 through S4. Inhibition of the pudendal, a somatic nerve allows relaxation of the external urethral sphincter. Sympathetic control of the bladder is achieved via the hypogastric nerve originating from T10 to L2 of the spinal cord. The sciatic nerve supplies the skin of the leg, the muscles of the back of the thigh, and the leg and foot. The common peroneal nerve is a branch of the sciatic nerve. These two nerves are important to the gynecologist because they can be injured during patient positioning for surgery; they are not involved in micturition.

71. d (Chapter 20)
You advise expectant management for now with completion of menstrual calendar over the upcoming year.

This patient is exhibiting typically developmental changes. She started menstruating at an appropriate age and has been menstruating for 1 year so far. It is very typical for adolescents to have irregular menses for the first 1 to 2 years after menarche. This is reflective of anovulatory cycles. It is very reasonable to follow her cycles with menstrual calendar over the next year. If the irregularity persists, you could then begin looking for other etiologies. A common cause of amenorrhea and delayed menarche in young women is hypothalamic hypogonadism, which is seen most frequently in athletes who engage in vigorous daily exercise (such as gymnasts, ice skaters, and long distance runners) as well as in women with eating disorders including anorexia and bulimia. Irregular menses, particularly oligomenorrhea, can also be seen in teens with polycystic ovarian syndrome. PCOS is often accompanied by signs of androgen access (hirsutism, acne) and insulin resistance (obesity, acanthosis nigricans). None of these are present in this patient.

72. c (Chapter 20)
Vasomotor symptoms such as hot flashes and night sweats should be treated when they are moderate or severe and interfere with the patient's quality of life during the start of menopause. All of the treatment options are appropriate for management of the patient's symptoms except vaginal estrogen cream. Low dose vaginal estrogen cream is an effective treatment for postmenopausal vaginal atrophy. However, vaginal estrogen cream has a localized effect and the systemic levels of estrogen are very low. Thus, systemic vasomotor symptoms are not treated with this medication. Any of the other options would be appropriate for this patient. She still has a uterus in situ so both estrogen and progesterone would be needed. Both oral and transdermal forms would be appropriate. SSRIs and clonidine have both been studied and found to be effective nonhormonal treatments of hot flashes and night sweats. A serotonin and norepinephrine reuptake inhibitors (SNRI) such as venlafaxine (Effexor) is another option.

73. c (Chapter 20)
This patient has a regular menstrual period and should be able to predict her most fertile period for conception. Regardless of cycle length, the fixed portion of the menstrual cycle in an ovulatory patient is the 14 days from ovulation to the start of menses. As the dominant follicle matures during the follicular portion of the menstrual cycle, it produces estrogen and later progesterone that enhances follicular maturation. The increased estrogen level then triggers the release of LH from the anterior pituitary (the LH surge), and this triggers the follicle to rupture and release the mature ovum 36 hours after the surge (ovulation). Fertilization occurs in the fallopian tube, not in the uterine cavity. Fertilization of the ovum must occur within 24 hours of ovulation or else it degenerates. After ovulation, the luteal phase of the cycle begins and fertility drops. Increased sexual activity during the luteal phase would be too late for fertilization. Instead, they should increase sexual activity just before ovulation and at the time of ovulation when fertility is at its peak.

74. e (Chapter 3)
Nuchal translucency screening with or without first trimester serum screening and second trimester maternal serum screening are two accepted strategies for Down syndrome screening among women of low-risk for chromosomal abnormalities. When using the combined first trimester screen using nuchal translucency (NT) plus the serum screens of PAPPA and free β-hCG, 80% sensitivity is reached. The second trimester triple screen has only about 50% sensitivity in women under age 35, but the quad screen which is the triple screen plus inhibin A is approximately 80% as well. Thus, the highest sensitivity would be a test that combines the combined first trimester test with the second trimester quad screen, and such testing achieves a sensitivity above 90%. A Level II ultrasound has only about 50% sensitivity for Down syndrome as well, and routine obstetric ultrasounds are probably even less sensitive.

75. c (Chapter 21)
Because a normal-appearing hymen is visualized upon your examination, you can rule out imperforate hymen and your most likely diagnosis would be a transverse vaginal septum. This is supported by the ultrasound findings, which showed a normal-appearing uterus, with a mass below the cervix: This is hematocolpos from menstrual flow that is unable to egress because of the transverse septum. The bilateral adnexal masses are most likely endometriomas secondary to retrograde menstrual flow.

a. Uterine didelphys is less likely given the normal uterus on ultrasound, although it is true that MRI is more sensitive in detecting abnormalities than ultrasound.

b. Uterine agenesis is incorrect as a uterus is noted on ultrasound.

d. Imperforate hymen is incorrect because you note a normal hymen on physical examination.

e. A uterine septum may additionally be present, although from the case description the most likely cause of her discomfort is a transverse septum preventing egress of menstrual flow.

76. c (Chapter 21)
A karyotype is indicated given that your concern is for premature ovarian failure. You may also consider screening her for Fragile X by checking for mutations in the FMR1 gene.

a, b. Given the absence of menses for the past year, you can assume that she is not ovulating. Therefore, performing a test for LH and/or progesterone would not be clinically useful in determining your diagnosis.

d. An ultrasound and/or an MRI of the pelvis is not indicated in this case. Because she had normal menses in the past, prior to the past year, you can assume that she does not have a Müllerian anomaly causing her secondary amenorrhea.

e. Technically, you have enough information with the tests above to make your diagnosis; however, your workup is incomplete prior to confirming that the patient has a normal karyotype, as the results from the karyotype may give you a different answer (e.g., Turner syndrome).

77. d (Chapter 21)
Patients with hypothyroidism typically need to increase their dose during pregnancy, often to as much as 50% of their prepregnancy dose. Patients with hypothyroidism are followed closely with serial testing of TSH to ensure that they are in a euthyroid range, increasing the dose of T4 replacement as needed.

a, b. It would be highly unusual for a patient to require less thyroid medication during pregnancy, given that normally requirements for T4 are increased.

c. This statement is false. During the first trimester and well into the second trimester until about 20 weeks, the fetus is able to produce only small amounts of thyroid hormone, and is therefore dependent on maternal production.

e. Typically, providers increase the dose of T4 medication by 30% in the first trimester, and follow TSH levels every 6 weeks to adjust as necessary. Tripling the dose of thyroid medication would be inappropriate and may lead to side effects of palpitations, anxiety, and nausea.

78. d (Chapter 21)
The positive review of systems revealing galactorrhea and headaches should increase your suspicion for a prolactinoma. You would test a TSH as well, given that derangements in her thyroid may cause her secondary amenorrhea. Should her prolactin come back elevated

in this case, you may consider repeating it to confirm hyperprolactinemia, and then proceed with an MRI of the head to evaluate for a prolactinoma.

a. While a karyotype may be helpful to rule out Turner's syndrome, this is less likely the cause of her secondary amenorrhea, given her additional symptoms of galactorrhea and headaches.

b. The use of urinary LH testing kits is for the most part aimed at detecting an LH surge for timed intercourse in patients experiencing infertility, rather than as a diagnostic test to determine whether the patient is ovulatory. In this case, the patient's oligomenorrhea indicates that she is also oligoovulatory.

c. Pelvic ultrasound and/or MRI might be useful if she was also experiencing pain or had primary amenorrhea.

e. FSH, in the context of serum estradiol, is a test designed to evaluate ovarian reserve and egg quality, and evaluate for premature ovarian failure. Although they would be included in a general infertility workup, they are not the tests that would lead to the diagnosis in this case.

79. c (Chapter 22)
This patient's secondary dysmenorrhea is most likely due to pelvic adhesions. The etiology is most likely the repeat cesarean delivery complicated by additional adhesions from the endomyometritis. The adhesions may be structurally impacting the uterus and adnexa, resulting in pain with menses. Moreover, adhesions often cause pain with activity as well. The fact that the pain is reproduced with movement of the uterus is further evidence that adhesions may be present. Pelvic adhesions are generally not identifiable on imaging such as ultrasound or CT. Moreover, there's no evidence of other causes of her pain on evaluation such as cervicitis, fibroids, polyps, adenomyosis, and ovarian cysts. If she had endometriosis she would have most likely had a longstanding history of cyclic pelvic pain, and it would have likely been identified during her cesarean sections. Routine narcotic use is inappropriate, as is expectant management, given the level of her pain. Severe dysmenorrhea may be an indication for hysterectomy, but generally, less invasive treatments should be attempted first. Patients with chronic pelvic pain often benefit from pain management consultation and/or psychiatric therapy. This patient's examination and history point to a structural etiology for her pain, which should be evaluated first.

80. d (Chapter 7)
Small for gestational age (SGA) refers to a neonate whose birth weight is less than the 10th percentile. It describes neonates who do not reach their growth potential and in whom there is evidence of fetal growth disruption but where a cause or etiology is not known. The term intrauterine growth restriction (IUGR), describes an intrauterine process of fetal growth restriction due to maternal, uterine, placental, or fetal disorders. All other answer choices are incorrect.

81. e (Chapter 22)
By definition, the diagnosis of DUB is reserved for patients with idiopathic heavy or irregular bleeding with no identifiable causes. The normal menstrual cycle is defined as regularly spaced menses ranging from every 21 to 35 days, lasting 3 to 5 days with an average blood loss of 30 to 50 mL/cycle. She does not have menorrhagia, which is regularly spaced menses that are either prolonged (>7 days) or heavy (>80 mL/cycle). Etiologies often include fibroids, adenomyosis, and endometrial polyps. Polymenorrhea is defined as regularly spaced frequent periods (less than every 21 days). It is most typically caused by anovulatory cycles. Conversely, oligomenorrhea is described as irregular cycles that are greater than 35 days apart. The most frequent cause is chronic anovulation—most commonly due to polycystic ovarian syndrome. Metrorrhagia is intermenstrual bleeding or spotting that occurs between otherwise normal menstrual cycles. Endometrial and cervical polyps can cause this type of bleeding pattern.

82. b (Chapter 22)
Teenagers who present with menorrhagia should be evaluated for a possible underlying bleeding this order. In this patient, the large ecchymoses, history of surgical bleeding, history of epistaxis, and gingival bleeding further support the diagnosis of a likely bleeding disorder. Further examination of her family history would also be helpful. Some initial coagulation studies and referral to hematology for further evaluation is appropriate. A pregnancy test, TFTs, and PRL are also reasonable. However, while she may eventually be started on OCPs, tranexamic acid, or even a Mirena IUD to help treat her menorrhagia, she should first be evaluated for a bleeding disorder. Although heavy, her bleeding is not life-threatening and does not require emergent treatment. An endometrial ablation is much too invasive and extreme and should not be performed on anyone who desires future fertility.

83. e (Chapter 1)
Development of linea nigra from pubis to umbilicus, bluish discoloration of vagina and cervix (Chadwick sign), softening and cyanosis of the cervix (Goodell's sign), and softening of the uterus (Ladin's sign) are all common signs associated with pregnancy. The Cullen sign is pathological and is not associated with pregnancy.

84. b (Chapter 23)
Patients with PCOS have been shown to have increased pulsatile frequency of GnRH, which in turn leads to high levels of LH. These elevated LH levels cause the increased production of androgens, leading to hirsutism, acne, and anovulation.

a. Patients with PCOS typically have normal or low levels of FSH. Patients with decreased ovarian reserve or premature ovarian insufficiency have elevated levels of FSH.

c. Estrogen levels would be normal in PCOS, not decreased.

d. Patients with PCOS have elevated levels of free testosterone.

e. Inhibin is a substance produced by the ovaries that inhibits release of FSH and GnRH from the hypothalamus. It is typically normal or slightly elevated in PCOS patients.

85. c (Chapter 2)

c, b. The patient needs to have surgical evacuation of the pregnancy given the blood in her pelvis, the elevated hCG well above 5,000 mIU/mL. Given that she is hemodynamically stable, it is appropriate to first attempt laparoscopy with conversion to laparotomy only if needed.

a. Multidose methotrexate doses have a higher success rate than single dose therapy (93% vs. 88%); however, both regimens are generally only indicated if the β-hCG is less than 5,000 mIU/mL.

d. Misoprostol is not indicated for the treatment of ectopic pregnancy.

e. Although the patient should have RhoGAM during her hospitalization for Rh-negative status, this is not the next best step.

86. d (Chapter 23)
Congenital adrenal hyperplasia, caused by 21-hydroxylase deficiency, is the most common cause of ambiguous genitalia. Prenatal diagnosis and treatment can prevent the formation of ambiguous genitalia. This infant is at presumed risk for adrenal crisis secondary to inability to produce mineralocorticoids and glucocorticoids, and prophylactic replacement of both compounds is indicated until a definitive diagnosis is made (by measuring the levels of 17-hydroxyprogesterone).

a. Polycystic ovary syndrome does not present in the infant years; rather, it usually presents in adolescence or early 20s. Further, it does not typically cause ambiguous genitalia.

b. Müllerian agenesis leads to abnormalities of the internal, Mullërian system, and would not lead to ambiguous external genitalia.

c. A transverse vaginal septum would not lead to ambiguous genitalia and typically presents around the time of menarche with cyclic abdominal pain and hematocolpos.

87. d (Chapter 23)
Testosterone (both free and bound) is elevated in patients with polycystic ovary syndrome, and the use of oral contraceptive pills to decrease the levels of circulating androgens is effective, especially after 6 to 12 months of treatment. The contraceptive pill suppresses production of ovary-derived androgens by suppressing LH secretion by the pituitary (e). Additionally, they function by increasing circulating levels of sex hormone–binding globulin secondary to the estrogen in the combined OCP. This elevated level leads to lower free androgens (b, c). Finally, the improvements in acne and hirsutism are thought to be secondary to the fact that combined contraceptive pills decrease the activity of 5-alpha reductase in the skin (a).

88. a (Chapter 23)
This patient has multiple risk factors for diabetes mellitus, including her obesity, her family history of diabetes, and her personal history of gestational diabetes. Furthermore, the finding of acanthosis nigricans on her neck and vulva increase your suspicion for insulin resistance and hyperinsulinemia. You correctly suggest a diabetes screening test for her, by way of fasting serum glucose.

b. The velvety brown discoloration around the vulva is acanthosis nigricans and a biopsy is not necessary.

c. This patient is less than 21 years old; a Papanicolaou test is not indicated.

d. Cholesterol screening is a good suggestion; however, at her age and without a family history, it is less pressing an issue than screening for diabetes.

e. A mammogram is not indicated at the age of 20 without a mass or concerning finding, and without family history.

89. c (Chapter 24)
During breastfeeding, prolactin levels are elevated, causing suppression or inhibition of pulsatile GnRH from the hypothalamus. Thyroid hormone abnormalities can also cause menstrual irregularities, and subsequently fertility problems; however, this is not primarily suggested by the case presentation but should remain a consideration. Prolactin is not thought to affect tubal motility, and given her recent pregnancy, it is not likely that her partner's sperm count is a factor.

90. e (Chapter 24)
Intrauterine device failure rates average between 0.7% and 1.9% with adequate placement and nonexpulsion. Failure rates with combined contraceptive pills or progesterone-only pills approach 8% or greater, owing to imperfections in actual use and less-than-ideal adherence. The least effective methods are coitus interruptus and the diaphragm.

91. e (Chapter 24)
Progestin-only pills act to suppress ovulation, thicken cervical mucous, create an unsuitable environment for implantation, and inhibit sperm motility. It does not cause regression of the corpus luteum.

92. c (Chapter 25)
Uterine perforation is a risk of surgical D&E, not of labor induction. However, labor induction of second trimester gestations does include infection, bleeding, uterine rupture, and need for additional procedures including D&C if the placenta does not deliver vaginally.

93. c (Chapter 25)
Concurrent long-term steroid corticosteroid use is a contraindication to medication abortion. These medications may interfere with the immune response and increase the risk of infection. Although a state may require parental consent for ages less than 18, her age itself is not a contraindication for medication abortion. Medical termination can be done up to 49 days' gestation; therefore, her gestational age is appropriate for medication abortion. She has been treated for chlamydia, so this is also not a contraindication.

94. d (Chapter 25)
The presence of a gestational sac indicates an ongoing pregnancy. The best management would be to recommend suction D&C. Repeating a dose of misoprostol is more likely to be effective at evacuating clot from the uterus rather than ending a continuing pregnancy. Serial ultrasounds or repeating mifepristone would not be indicated. D&E is the term used for uterine evacuation in the second trimester.

95. d (Chapter 26)
PCOS and advanced maternal age are two of the major causes of ovulatory factor infertility. Both endometriosis and pelvic inflammatory disease are associated with pelvic adhesions, tubal blockage, and infertility. Fibroids are not a significant cause of infertility. In general, women with uterine fibroids are able to conceive without difficulty. Large fibroids can lead to fetal overdistension of the uterus during pregnancy with subsequent risk for preterm labor and/or delivery. Fibroids can also restrict fetal movement in the uterus and result in a higher rate of fetal malpresentation. If fibroids grow rapidly during pregnancy, they can result in degeneration and pain. Women with infertility who have submucosal fibroids that project into the cavity have increased pregnancy rates when these fibroids are removed or partially resected.

96. e (Chapter 26)
Male factor infertility is responsible for about 35% of infertility cases. The etiologies vary widely but include all of the choices listed. In addition, mumps, antisperm antibodies, and congenital cryptorchidism (undescended testes) can result in an abnormal semen analysis and infertility. Thyroid disease and hypogonadotropic hypogonadism (e.g., from tumors, infection, and Kallmann syndrome) are the primary endocrine abnormalities that result in male factor infertility. Environmental exposures that can result in male factor infertility include radiation, heat, and chemicals. Sexual dysfunction (erectile dysfunction, retrograde ejaculation, and ejaculation failure) and structural factors (varicocele, testicular torsion, and vasectomy) also contribute to causality. Medications such as cimetidine, sulfasalazine, and spironolactone and chemotherapy can all result in impaired male fertility as well.

97. c (Chapter 8)
The seizure prophylaxis of choice for preeclampsia is magnesium sulfate. The assumption is that if a woman seizes while on magnesium sulfate, then the serum level is not high enough. Thus, in this setting, one would rebolus, though not the original 4 or 6 g, but a 2 g rebolus. It is rare that another antiseizure medication such as phenytoin would be used. Hydralazine is used commonly in women with preeclampsia to control severe-range blood pressures, which is not mentioned in this case. It is rare that the fetus requires emergent delivery. Usually, the best approach is to stabilize the mother and follow the fetal heart tracing closely and deliver for fetal indications if necessary. Furosemide generally has little use in the management of severe preeclampsia.

98. c (Chapter 1)
Second trimester tests routinely offered include serum screening for neural tube defects and aneuploidy with the MSAFP and Quad screens, second trimester screening ultrasound for fetal anatomy, and amniocentesis. Hematocrit is offered in the first and third trimesters. GBS is collected late in the third trimester. The fern test is used to determine whether rupture of membranes has occurred, on the basis of a maternal history of leaking fluid. In the first trimester, a transvaginal ultrasound is commonly performed to confirm dating of the pregnancy.

99. e (Chapter 26)

Ten percent of couples who undergo infertility evaluation have no identifiable cause for their infertility. In these patients, ovulation induction with Clomid is the safe, initial approach to management. When problems in sperm transport, motility, or functional capacity are identified ISCI can be utilized. However, it is important that couples realize that most therapies have no higher success rates than no treatment at all. Therefore, expectant management is a very reasonable approach. In this group, 60% will conceive spontaneously in 3 to 5 years.

100. b (Chapter 9)

The target range for fasting blood glucose value is less than 90 mg/dL and 1-hour postprandial values less than 140 mg/dL or 2-hour postprandial values less than 120 mg/dL. If more than 25% to 35% of glucose levels are elevated, medication is indicated. These patients are considered class A_2, or medication-controlled gestational diabetics in the White classification of gestational diabetes. Since her average glucose values were elevated, diet and exercise alone are not sufficient to control her diabetes. True gestational diabetics will commonly have normal fasting glucose values with elevated postprandial values. This is due to the pathophysiology being related to metabolism of large carbohydrate boluses rather than carbohydrate boluses at baseline. Therefore, it is appropriate to treat patients with a short-acting insulin (Lispro) to cover breakfast, and intermediate-acting insulin (NPH) to cover lunch. This combined insulin saves the patient a prelunch injection. Then, a short-acting insulin (Lispro) predinner dose will cover evening postprandial values.

If the blood sugar levels were within target range, continuing to adhere to a diabetic diet and exercise regimen would have been appropriate. Such patients are classified as class A_1, or diet-controlled gestational diabetics in the White classification of gestational diabetes. The patient's fasting levels have been normal. Starting the patient on NPH in the evening would cause her to become hypoglycemic in the mornings. Historically, oral hypoglycemics have not been used in pregnancy due to concerns of placental transfer, and subsequently, fetal hypoglycemia. However, recent studies have indicated that adequate glucose control may be achieved with oral hypoglycemics in some patients without harm to the fetus. Insulin, on the other hand, has been shown to be safe in pregnancies, with no placental transfer. There is debate in the literature and among clinical providers regarding the use of oral hypoglycemics, but in this patient it would be unusual to start metformin.

101. c (Chapter 27)

With the newer classification, the term VIN is subdivided into two categories. Usual VIN correlates with what was formerly known as VIN 2 and VIN 3 or warty, basaloid, and mixed types. It is characterized by full thickness atypia and is associated with HR HPV. Differentiated VIN is not related to high-risk HPV infection. It is associated with inflammatory dermatosis (lichen sclerosis or lichen planus).

102. c (Chapter 9)

This patient has gestational diabetes (GDM). Insulin resistance in pregnancy stems from placental secretion of diabetogenic hormones, which include human chorionic somatomammotropin (placental lactogen), growth hormone, corticotropin-releasing hormone, and progesterone. These hormones increase with the size of the placenta, and thus abnormal carbohydrate metabolism is usually not apparent until the late second or early third trimester. Somatomammotropin is lactogenic, preparing mammary gland growth for lactation, in addition to regulating maternal glucose, fat, and protein so that they are available to the fetus. Many patients with gestational diabetes likely have elevated baseline insulin resistance as well and are at high risk of developing frank Type 2 diabetes mellitus over the ensuing decade.

103. d (Chapter 27)

Around 20% of patients with Paget disease will have a concomitant invasive adenocarcinoma underlying the outward changes. Although the initial treatment recommended for Paget disease is excision, it is acceptable to treat recurrences with ablative modalities. There is not a known risk of invasive squamous cell carcinoma with Paget disease.

104. a (Chapter 27)

According to the most recent FIGO classification system revised in 2009: Tumor confined to the vulva or perineum, greater than 2 cm in size or with stromal invasion greater than 1 mm, negative nodes is stage Ib. Stage II disease is a tumor of any size with adjacent spread (one-third lower urethra, one-third lower vagina, and anus), negative nodes. Stage IIIa disease is tumor of any size with positive inguinofemoral lymph nodes. With the reclassification of the FIGO grading in 2009, stage 0 was dropped.

105. c (Chapter 28)

The ASCUS category includes minor changes due to inflammation or injury, but can also indicate the presence of a more severe abnormality. Reflex HPV testing is recommended to triage the ASCUS Pap results and help to guide providers with the plan of care. If the HPV test is negative, the Pap can be repeated in 1 year. If the HPV test is positive, then a colposcopy is indicated. LEEP conization is reserved for moderate-severe dysplasia (CIN 2 and CIN 3), persistent CIN 1 for greater than 2 years, and for patients with a HGSIL Pap smear and greater than a two step difference in biopsy result.

106. b (Chapter 28)

The cervical cancer screening interval for women aged 30 and over can be increased to 2 to 3 years after three consecutive normal Pap tests have been obtained. It is also recommended that an HPV test be performed and if both are negative, to be rescreened with Pap smear and high-risk HPV every 3 years. Screening more often than every 3 years may identify transient HPV infections and minor cytologic abnormalities that would have resolved on their own if wider screening intervals were given. If the Pap test is negative but the HPV test is positive, both should be repeated in 1 year. At that time if either of the tests is abnormal, then a colposcopy is indicated. LEEP conization is reserved for moderate–severe dysplasia (CIN 2 and CIN 3), persistent CIN 1 for greater than 2 years, and for HGSIL pap smear with greater than two step difference in biopsy result.

107. a (Chapter 28)

CIN 1 that persists for less than 2 years may continue to be followed with or without treatment. If the patient chooses not to treat the lesion, she should continue to have HPV testing in 1 year or Pap testing at 6 and 12 months after the colposcopy. If the patient chooses treatment, either ablative (e.g., cryotherapy) or excisional procedure is acceptable. Excision would be the preferred treatment if the colposcopy is unsatisfactory, the endocervical curettage (ECC) was positive, or if the patient had been previously treated.

108. a (Chapter 28)

Pap screening recommendations are to start testing at age 21 regardless of onset of sexual activity. More than 90% of HPV infections resolve within 3 years in adolescents. There is very little chance that even CIN 2 or 3 will progress to cancer in adolescents. The HPV vaccination is indicated for ages 9 to 26 years, regardless of possible prior exposure to HPV.

109. b (Chapter 29)

The question asks about the evaluation of vaginal bleeding in a postmenopausal woman. The leading etiologies on the differential diagnosis are atrophic endometrium versus endometrial cancer, and the use of ultrasound can help in differentiating between the two. An endometrial thickness of 4 mm or less is indicative of low risk for malignancy. If bleeding is persistent or if the lining appears thickened (>4 mm) or is not adequately visualized, then further tissue evaluation (i.e., endometrial biopsy, hysteroscopy, dilation and curettage) is recommended.

110. c (Chapter 29)
Endometrial cancer is surgically staged with TAH, BSO, pelvic and para-aortic lymphadenectomy when depth of invasion is more than one third of the myometrial thickness. Answer choice (d) describes staging for ovarian cancer and (a) describes clinical staging for cervical cancer. With endometrial cancer, when indicated, it is important to evaluate *both* pelvic and para-aortic lymph nodes because it is possible to have nodal spread to one group while sparing the other. Nodal status does have significant staging and prognostic implications.

111. e (Chapter 29)
All of the answer choices, with the exception of Tamoxifen, are considered protective and lower the lifetime risk of developing endometrial cancer. Tamoxifen is a selective estrogen receptor modulator and as such, contains both agonist and antagonist properties. Tamoxifen does promote endometrial proliferation, hyperplasia, polyp formation, carcinoma, and sarcoma while decreasing the risk of recurrent breast cancer. Any abnormal bleeding with Tamoxifen use warrants further investigation.

112. a (Chapter 29)
Although endometrial cancer is the most commonly encountered gynecologic malignancy in the United States, it is associated with a favorable survival profile as the majority of disease is diagnosed early. In fact, 72% of women are diagnosed with stage I disease, thus rendering the surgical staging itself as curative treatment. Fortunately, early symptoms and accurate diagnosis modalities contribute to the fact that endometrial cancer is only the third most common cause of gynecologic cancer deaths worldwide (behind ovarian and cervical cancer). Endometrial cancer accounts for 7,900 deaths each year in the United States.

113. c (Chapter 30)
The most common type of germ cell tumor is the benign cystic mature teratoma, also known as dermoid cysts. Dermoids are cystic masses containing mature adult tissue such as skin, hair, and teeth mixed in sebaceous material, giving them a very characteristic appearance (Color Plate 16). Cystectomy is recommended for definitive diagnosis and to rule out malignancy.

114. c (Chapter 30)
Both granulosa-theca cell tumors and Sertoli-Leydig cell tumors are known as functional tumors because they are characterized by hormone production. Ovarian Sertoli-Leydig cell tumors resemble fetal testes and produce androgens (testosterone, androstenedione). These elevated hormone levels can cause virilizing effects in 75% of patients including breast atrophy, hirsutism, deepened voice, acne, clitoromegaly, and receding hairline. Patients may also have oligomenorrhea or amenorrhea. Progesterone, estradiol, and AFP are less commonly elevated in Sertoli-Leydig cell tumors. Ca-125 levels can be elevated in a number of benign and malignant processes (such as pancreatitis, diverticulitis, and epithelial ovarian cancer), but it is not generally elevated in Sertoli-Leydig cell tumors.

115. c (Chapter 31)
Molar pregnancies are surgically managed by suction evacuation of the uterine contents. This patient most likely has a complete molar pregnancy that requires surgical intervention. Prior to the operation, Rh(D), thyroid, blood counts, liver, and renal status should be evaluated. Evaluation for theca lutein cysts should also be part of your diagnostic workup prior to proceeding with D&C. Chemotherapy is not part of the initial plan of care in these patients. Only when persistent disease is present should methotrexate be considered.

116. e (Chapter 2)

e. An inevitable abortion is a pregnancy complicated by vaginal bleeding with a dilated cervix such that the pregnancy is likely to pass soon.

a. An incomplete abortion is partial expulsion of POC prior to 20 weeks. This patient has not had any tissue expelled.

b. A threatened abortion does present with vaginal bleeding, but in this type of abortion the patient does not have cervical dilation.

c. This patient has an intrauterine pregnancy, as confirmed by an intrauterine gestational sac and yolk sac.

d. Missed abortion is the death of an embryo with complete retention of all POCs. If the patient does not pass any tissue spontaneously, a missed abortion may develop. However, this is not the best initial diagnosis.

117. b (Chapter 31)
Choriocarcinoma is a pure epithelial tumor (absent chorionic villi) that is highly sensitive to chemotherapy. This patient will require chemotherapy, single or multiagent, depending on the presence of metastasis. Hysterectomy is an option in selected patients; but given her age and likely desire for future fertility, chemotherapy is a better choice in this clinical situation. Contraception is paramount during treatment as is close hCG surveillance.

118. c (Chapter 31)
This patient likely has an incomplete (partial) molar pregnancy based on the ultrasound findings. The workup and treatment is similar to a complete molar pregnancy. Incomplete molar pregnancies are most commonly triploid, 69 XXY (one haploid maternal sets and two haploid paternal sets). These pregnancies have approximately one-fifth the risk for persistent GTD as compared with complete molar pregnancies.

119. b (Chapter 32)
Galactorrhea is a result of pituitary stimulation most commonly by either pregnancy, pituitary adenoma, changes in thyroid function, or psychotropic medications. Breast abscess results in a purulent discharge, erythema, and pain.

120. d (Chapter 32)
LCIS is a premalignant lesion that carries subsequent increased risk of invasive breast cancer—25% to 30% within 15 years. It does not require immediate treatment, but the use of a SERM may reduce the risk of subsequent cancer by 50%. It is usually found incidentally on biopsy for another finding because it is not palpable or seen on mammogram. The subsequent cancer can occur on either side or in both breasts, and may be any of the types mentioned.

121. c (Chapter 4)
When assessing fetal heart tracings, the baseline should be in the normal range (110 to 160 beats per minute) with moderate variability. Although minimal variability is not reassuring, it can also be a sign that the fetus is asleep or inactive. Absent variability is always worrisome. Tachycardia can be a sign of maternal fever, fetal infection, fetal anemia, and even fetal arrhythmia.

122. c (Chapter 5)
The classic presentation of placental abruption is third-trimester vaginal bleeding associated with severe abdominal pain and/or frequent, strong contractions. However, in 20% of placental separations, bleeding is confined within the uterine cavity and is referred to as a concealed hemorrhage. In this case, there is a retroplacental clot noted on ultrasound, which is consistent with a relatively large concealed placenta abruption. This is the most likely cause, particularly in the setting of an MVA with a "seat belt sign" (i.e., bruises from the seat belt) as the sudden stop as well as the direct trauma of the seat belt can cause shearing of the placenta from the uterine wall, causing uteroplacental insufficiency, which is reflected in late decelerations on external fetal monitoring (EFM).

a. The fetal heart rate tracing described is more consistent with uteroplacental insufficiency (recurrent late decelerations) rather than umbilical cord compression. Umbilical cord compression is usually seen on the EFM as recurrent variable decelerations.

b. Although the patient is contracting every 2 minutes, there is no evidence of preterm labor on examination. Additionally, labor itself does not usually cause late decelerations.

d. The fetal heart rate tracing described is more consistent with uteroplacental insufficiency (recurrent late decelerations) rather than fetal head compression. Fetal head compression usually manifests on EFM as early decelerations rather than late. Also, the fetal head must be in the pelvis for compression to occur.

e. Although it is possible to have a placenta abruption in the setting of placenta previa, contractions in the setting of placenta previa do not usually cause late decelerations. Furthermore on ultrasound, there is no evidence of placenta previa. This would need to be confirmed on TV US if it was felt that the placenta was close to the internal os of the cervix.

123. c (Chapter 5)

The most appropriate delivery plan in this case is to proceed with emergent (or at least urgent) cesarean section. Given the ultrasound findings, the patient has a known vasa previa and velamentous cord insertion, so to prevent rupture of the fetal vessels as a result of spontaneous rupture of membranes with labor, it is imperative that the cesarean delivery be done expeditiously.

a. Expectant management with the plan for a vaginal delivery in the setting of a vasa previa is an option but does carry significant risk of rupture of the fetal vessels during labor and with spontaneous rupture of the membranes. The patient should be counseled regarding this risk and that if the fetal vessels rupture, it is a surgical emergency with up to 56% perinatal mortality rate associated. Given the significant risk of perinatal mortality associated with rupture of fetal vessels, most obstetricians proceed with cesarean section in the setting of a known vasa previa.

b. In a patient with a known vasa previa, artificial rupture of membranes is generally considered to be contraindicated as both the amniohook or the actual rupture of the membranes can cause the fragile fetal vessels to rupture, resulting in perinatal morbidity/mortality.

d. Although not absolutely contraindicated in this setting of known vasa previa, just as with expectant management, the patient should be counseled regarding the risk of vaginal delivery before either expectant or active management of labor. Oxytocin is more appropriately started when it is apparent that the patient is not continuing to labor on her own.

e. Emergent cesarean section is the most appropriate course of action.

124. d (Chapter 1)

Of the answer choices listed, only Prader-Willi is not routinely offered for genetic screening in high-risk populations. For the other four traits commonly screened and listed in the question, the traits are recessive. Thus, if both parents are found to be positive carriers, the fetus can be genetically tested through amniocentesis or chorionic villus sampling.

125. b (Chapter 5)

The clinical presentation of uterine rupture is variable. If there is vaginal bleeding, it can range from spotting to passing large clots. In this case, the patient's risk factor for uterine rupture is her prior abdominal myomectomy. It is possible to have a trial of labor after a myomectomy if the endometrial cavity has not been entered during the surgery as the risk of uterine rupture is low; however, this patient had a large fibroid removed that required entry into the endometrial cavity, which increases her risk for uterine rupture significantly. Typically, patients with a history of myomectomy requiring entry into the cavity, prior classical cesarean section, and other major uterine surgery (e.g., corneal wedge resection for ectopic pregnancy) are counseled to avoid labor because they are at high risk for uterine rupture and are usually scheduled for a cesarean section at 36 to 37 weeks, pending fetal lung maturity testing so as to avoid the patient going into labor.

a. There is no evidence of PPROM in this patient. She had a normal AFI, no pool, and no ferning seen on SSE. The nitrazine test was positive most likely secondary to blood in the vaginal vault.

c. There was no evidence of cervical laceration on examination and no factors concerning for this in the patient's history.

d. The patient's placenta was noted to be posterior. There was no mention of the placenta being close to the internal os on ultrasound, so previa is an unlikely source of the antepartum hemorrhage.

e. Vasa previa is a rare cause of antepartum hemorrhage and usually associated with a succenturiate placental lobe or velamentous cord insertion. There was no evidence of vasa previa on ultrasound.

126. d (Chapter 5)

A CT scan of the abdomen and pelvis is not an appropriate initial test in this patient. In particular, you are concerned about the risk of accreta or percreta invading into the bladder. Although CT scan would help determine whether nephrolithiasis is the source of the patient's hematuria, it is more appropriate to start with a less invasive test with less radiation if at all possible. If imaging is going to progress beyond ultrasound, MRI is the modality of choice.

a. Urine analysis would be an appropriate initial test to rule out a urinary tract infection as the source of the patient's hematuria. It would also confirm hematuria and determine whether there are RBC or WBC casts.

b. Urine culture would be an appropriate initial test in conjunction with the urine analysis as urinary tract infections can cause hematuria and suprapubic pain.

c. A sterile speculum examination would be an appropriate initial test to determine whether the patient's bleeding is coming from the cervix, urethra, or both. It would also help determine whether the patient has vaginal bleeding as a result of labor/cervical dilation or cervicitis.

d. Abdominal ultrasound of the uterus would be an appropriate initial test as the patient has a history of three previous cesarean sections, had a complete anterior previa on her anatomy ultrasound at 18 weeks, and has not been reassessed with ultrasound to determine whether the previa has resolved. Additionally, if the placenta previa has not resolved, this patient is at increased risk for a placenta accreta, increta, or percreta. This is particularly concerning for placenta percreta with bladder invasion if she does still have a placenta previa.

127. d (Chapter 6)

While extremes of age have some association with preterm birth, age 33 is not at particularly increased risk. In terms of BMI, studies have shown that underweight individuals are at increased risk of PTB. Low socioeconomic status, PROM, placental abruption, and history of abdominal surgery are risk factors for PTB. Other risk factors include chorioamnionitis, multiple gestations, uterine anomalies such as a bicornuate uterus, previous preterm delivery, and other maternal diseases including preeclampsia and infections.

128. e (Chapter 27)

Risk factors for VIN, usual type, include infection with HPV types 16 and 18, cigarette smoking, immunodeficiency, and immunosuppression. The incidence of VIN, usual type, decreases as age increases and there is no racial predisposition to VIN.

Index

Page numbers followed by *t* refer to tables; page numbers followed by *f* refer to figures.